OPERATIVE ARTHROSCOPY

THIRD EDITION

OPERATIVE ARTHROSCOPY

THIRD EDITION

Editor-in-Chief

JOHN B. McGINTY, MD

Chief Medical Editor, Orthopedics Today
Retired Professor and Chairman,
Department of Orthopaedic Surgery
Medical University of South Carolina
Charleston, South Carolina

Section Editors

STEPHEN S. BURKHART, MD

Clinic Associate Professor
The University of Texas Health Science Center at San Antonio
Director of Medical Education
The Orthopaedic Institute
San Antonio, Texas

ROBERT W. JACKSON, OC, MD, FRCSC

Chief, Department of Orthopaedic Surgery
Baylor University Medical Center;
Clinical Professor, Orthopaedic Surgery
University of Texas Southwestern
Dallas, Texas

DONALD H. JOHNSON, MD, FRCSC

Director, Sports Medicine Clinic
Carleton University;
Associate Professor, Orthopedic Surgery
University of Ottawa,
The Ottawa Hospital
Ottawa, Ontario, Canada

JOHN C. RICHMOND, MD

Professor of Orthopaedic Surgery
Tufts University School of Medicine
Boston, Massachusetts

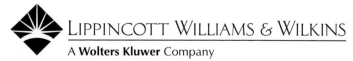

LIPPINCOTT WILLIAMS & WILKINS
A **Wolters Kluwer** Company
Philadelphia · Baltimore · New York · London
Buenos Aires · Hong Kong · Sydney · Tokyo

Acquisitions Editor: *Jim Merritt*
Developmental Editor: *Michelle LaPlante*
Production Editor: *Patrick Carr*
Manufacturing Manager: *Benjamin Rivera*
Cover Designer: *Co.Laborative Design*
Indexer: *Prottsman Indexing*
Compositor: *Maryland Composition*
Printer: *Quebecor-World*

Printed in the United States of America

9 8 7 6 5 4 3 2 1

Library of Congress Cataloging-in-Publication Data

Operative arthroscopy / editor-in-chief, John B. McGinty ; section editors, Stephen S. Burkhart . . . [et al.].—3rd ed.
   p. ; cm.
  Includes bibliographical references and index.
  ISBN 0-7817-3265-4
   1. Joints—Endoscopic surgery. 2. Arthroscopy. I. McGinty, John B., 1930-
  [DNLM: 1. Joints—surgery. 2. Arthroscopy—methods. WE 312 061 2002]
  RD686 .O64 2002
  617.4′72059—dc21   2002141569

CONTENTS

CONTRIBUTING AUTHORS

Gregory M. Alberton, MD, MS
Orthopaedic Surgery
Tri-City Orthopaedic Surgery
Oceanside, California

F. Allegra, MD
Director
Department of Orthopaedics
Guarnieri Clinic
Rome, Italy

Antonello Amelina, MD
Department of Orthopaedic Surgery
Guarnieri Clinic
Rome, Italy

Ned Amendola, MD
Associate Professor
Department of Orthopedics
University of Iowa Hospitals
Iowa City, Iowa

James R. Andrews, MD
American Sports Medicine Institute
Birmingham, Alabama

Wayne K. Augé II, MD
Medical Director
Center for Orthopaedic and Sports Performance
    Research
Northern New Mexico Orthopaedic Center
Department of Orthopaedic Surgery
Los Alamos Medical Center
Espanola-Presbyterian Medical Center
and the United States Department of Health and
    Human Services
Santa Fe, New Mexico

Champ L. Baker, Jr., MD
Staff Physician
Department of Orthopaedic Surgery
Tulane University School of Medicine
New Orleans, Louisiana
The Hughston Clinic
Columbus, Georgia

Wael Barsoun, MD
New England Baptist Hospital
Boston, Massachusetts

Richard A. Berger, MD
Department of Orthopaedic Surgery
Mayo Clinic
Mayo Graduate School of Medicine
Rochester, Minnesota

Louis U. Bigliani, MD
Chief
Columbia Center for Shoulder, Elbow, and Sports Medicine
Department of Orthopaedic Surgery
Chairman
New York Orthopaedic Hospital
Department of Orthopaedic Surgery
New York, New York

Robert C. Bray, MD
Associate Professor
Department of Surgery
University of Calgary
Department of Orthopaedics
Peter Lougheed Centre
Calgary General Hospital
Calgary, Alberta, Canada

Stephen S. Burkhart, MD
Clinical Associate Professor
Department of Orthopaedics
University of Texas Health Science Center at San Antonio
Baylor College of Medicine
Waco, Texas

Robert T. Burks, MD
Professor of Orthopedic Surgery
Department of Orthopedics
University of Utah
Salt Lake City, Utah

Charles A. Bush-Joseph, MD
Associate Professor
Orthopaedic Surgery
Rush Presbyterian St. Luke's Medical Center
Chicago, Illinois

J.W. Thomas Byrd, MD
Assistant Clinical Professor
Department of Orthopaedics and Rehabilitation
Vanderbilt University School of Medicine
Nashville Sports Medicine and Orthopaedic Center
Nashville, Tennessee

E. Lyle Cain, Jr.
American Sports Medicine Institute
Birmingham, Alabama

W. Dilworth Cannon, MD
Professor of Clinical Orthopaedic Surgery
Co-Director of Sports Medicine
Department of Orthopaedic Surgery
University of California, San Francisco

W.G. Carson, Jr., MD
University of South Florida College
Tampa, Florida
The Sports Medicine Clinic of Tampa
Tampa, Florida

K. Casey Chan, MD
Adjunct Professor
Department Of Orthopaedic Surgery
National University Hospital
National University of Singapore
Singapore

James C.Y. Chow, MD
Department of Surgery
Southern Illinois University School of Medicine
Springfield, Illinois

R. Sean Churchill, MD
Department of Orthopaedics and Sports Medicine
University of Washington
Seattle, Washington

Brian Cole, MD
Medical Director
Rush Cartilage Restoration Center
Rush–Presbyterian–St. Luke's Medical Center
Chicago, Illinois

William P. Cooney III, MD
Professor of Orthopaedic Surgery
Department of Orthopaedic Surgery
Mayo Clinic and Mayo Graduate School of Medicine
Rochester, Minnesota

Randall W. Culp, MD
The Philadelphia Hand Center
King of Prussia, Pennsylvania

Jeffrey R. Dugas, MD
American Sports Medicine Institute
Birmingham, Alabama

James C. Esch, MD
Associate Clinical Professor
Department of Orthopaedics
University of California, San Diego, School of Medicine
Tri-City Orthopaedic Surgery
Oceanside, California

Adil N. Esmail, MD
McKay Orthopaedic Research Laboratory
University of Pennsylvania
Philadelphia, Pennsylvania

Nick A. Evans, MD
Southern California Center for Sports Medicine
Long Beach, California

Richard Ferkel, MD
Director of Sports Medicine Fellowship
    and Attending Surgeon
Southern California Orthopedic Institute
Van Nuys, California
Clinical Instructor of Orthopaedic Surgery
University of California, Los Angeles
Los Angeles, California

Larry D. Field, MD
Co-Director
Upper Extremity Service
Mississippi Sports Medicine and Orthopaedic Center
Clinical Instructor
Department of Orthopaedic Surgery
University of Mississippi School of Medicine
Jackson, Mississippi

James M. Fox, MD
Founding Partner/Attending Surgeon
Southern California Orthopedic Institute
Van Nuys, California

Cyril B. Frank, MD
Department of Surgery
The University of Calgary
Calgary, Alberta, Canada

Simon P. Frostick, MA, DM, FRCS
Professor of Orthopaedics
Head of Department of Musculoskeletal Science
University of Liverpool
Honorary Consultant
Trauma and Orthopaedic Directorate
Royal Liverpool University Hospital
Liverpool
United Kingdom

Mehrdad Ganjianpour, MD
Tower Orthopaedics and Sports Medicine Medical
    Group
Los Angeles, California

Ariane Gerber, MD
Harvard Shoulder Service
Massachusetts General Hospital
Boston, Massachusetts

J. Robert Giffin, MD
Assistant Professor
Department of Orthopaedic Surgery
Fowler Kennedy Sport Medicine Clinic
University of Western Ontario
London, Ontario, Canada

Scott D. Gillogly, MD
Director of Sports Medicine
Orthopaedic Residency Program
Atlanta Medical Center
St. Joseph's Hospital of Atlanta
Atlanta, Georgia

James M. Glick, MD
Clinical Professor
Department of Orthopaedic Surgery
University of California
San Francisco, California

Julie Glowacki, PhD
Associate Professor
Orthopaedic Surgery
Harvard Medical School
Director
Skeletal Biology
Orthopedic Surgery
Brigham and Women's Hospital
Boston, Massachusetts

E. Marlowe Goble, MD
Department of Orthopedics
University of Utah
Salt Lake City, Utah

Michael D. Gordon, MD
Department of Orthopaedic Surgery
Rush Presbyterian St. Luke's Medical Center
Chicago, Illinois

Patrick E. Greis, MD
Assistant Professor of Orthopedic Surgery
Department of Orthopedics
University of Utah
Salt Lake City, Utah

Timothy S. Hamby, MD
Atlanta Sports Medicine & Orthopaedic Center
Atlanta, Georgia

Gregory J. Hanker, MD
Hand Surgical Consultant
Southern California Orthopedic Institute
Van Nuys, California
Assistant Clinical Professor
Division of Plastic and Reconstructive Surgery
University of Southern California, Los Angeles
Los Angeles, California

Jo A. Hannafin, MD, PhD
Associate Professor of Orthopaedic Surgery
Weill Medical College of Cornell University
Orthopaedic Director
Womens Sports Medicine Center
Hospital for Special Surgery
New York, New York

Christopher D. Harner, MD
Blue Cross of Western Pennsylvania
Director
Section for Sports Medicine
University of Pittsburgh
Pittsburgh, Pennsylvania

Douglas T. Harryman II, MD
Deceased

Richard J. Hawkins, MD
Steadman Hawkins Clinic
Vail, Colorado

Donald L. Hilton, MD
Department of Neurosurgery
Southwest Texas Methodist Hospital
Neurological Associates of San Antonio
San Antonio, Texas

Robert E. Hunter, MD
Aspen Foundation for Sports Medicine, Education, and
    Research
Aspen, Colorado

Sandra J. Iannotti, MD
Attending Surgeon
Department of Orthopaedics
Saint Catherine of Siena Medical Center
Smithtown, New York

Douglas W. Jackson, MD
Medical Director
Orthopaedic Research Institute
Long Beach Memorial Medical Center
President
Memorial Orthopaedic Group
Long Beach, California

Robert W. Jackson, MD
Department of Orthopaedic Surgery
University of Texas Southwestern Medical Center
Chief
Department of Orthopaedics
Baylor University Medical Center
Dallas, Texas

Donald H. Johnson, MD, FRCSC
Director
Sports Medicine Clinic
Carleton University
Associate Professor
Orthopaedic Surgery
University of Ottawa
The Ottawa Hospital
Ottawa, Ontario
Canada

Christopher K. Jones, MD
Fellow
Mississippi Sports Medicine and Orthopedic Center
Jackson, Mississippi

Ronald P. Karzel, MD
Attending Orthopedic Surgeon
Southern California Orthopedic Institute
Van Nuys, California.

Sumant G. Krishnan, MD
Shoulder Service
W. B. Carrell Memorial Clinic
Dallas, Texas

Jo-Ann Lee, RN
New England Baptist Hospital
Boston, Massachusetts

Richard G. Levine, MD
Department of Orthopaedic Surgery
The Union Memorial Hospital
Baltimore, Maryland

David M. Lichtman, MD
Clinical Professor
Orthopadic Surgery
U.T. Southwestern Medical Society
Dallas, Texas
Chairman/Director
Orthopaedic Surgery
JPS Health Network
Fort Worth, Texas

Ralph T. Lidge, MD
Department of Orthopaedic Surgery
University of Illinois Medical School at Chicago
Chicago, Illinois

Ian K.Y. Lo, MD
Department of Surgery
University of Toronto
Toronto Hospital
Toronto, Ontario, Canada

Frederick A. Matsen III, MD
Department of Orthopaedics and Sports Medicine
University of Washington
Seattle, Washington

Leslie S. Matthews, MD
Chief
Department of Orthopaedic Surgery
The Union Memorial Hospital
Baltimore, Maryland

Augustus D. Mazzocca, MD
University of Connecticut
Department of Orthopaedic Surgery
Farmington, Connecticut

Joseph C. McCarthy, MD
Clinical Professor
Orthopedic Surgery
Tufts University School of Medicine
New England Baptist Hospital
Boston, Massachusetts

John B. McGinty, MD
Professor (*retired*)
Department of Orthopaedic Surgery
Medical University of South Carolina
Charleston, South Carolina

John F. Meyers, MD
Tuckahoe Orthopaedic Associates, Ltd.
Richmond, Virginia
Medical College of Virginia
Richmond, Virginia

Tom Minas, MD
Brigham Orthopedic Associates, Inc.
Boston, Massachusetts

Anthony Miniaci, MD
Department of Surgery
University of Toronto
Toronto Hospital
Toronto, Ontario, Canada

Craig D. Morgan, MD
Department of Orthopaedic Surgery
Thomas Jefferson University
Jeffereson, Pennsylvania
A.I. Dupont Institute
Wilmington, Delaware

Mayo Noerdlinger, MD
Atlantic Orthopaedic Sports Medicine
Portsmouth, New Hampshire

David J. Novak, MD
Fellow
Orthopaedic Sports Medicine
Southern California Orthopaedic Institute
Van Nuys, California

Darrell J. Ogilvie-Harris, MB, ChB, BSc, MSc
Associate Professor, Department of Surgery
Toronto Western Hospital
Toronto, Ontario, Canada

A. Lee Osterman, MD
Hand and Orthopedic Surgery
Philadelphia Hand Center
Division of Hand Surgery
Department of Orthopedic Surgery
Thomas Jefferson University Hospital
Philadelphia, Pennsylvania

Peter M. Parten, MD
Shoulder Fellow
The San Antonio Orthopaedic Group
San Antonio, Texas

Fernando A. Pena Gomez, MD
Departmento Cirugía Ortópedica y Traumatología
Clinica Santa Elena
Madrid
Spain

Marc J. Philippon, MD
Sports Medicine/Hip Disorders
Golf Medicine Program
University of Pittsburgh Medical Center–Center for Sports
    Medicine
Department of Orthopaedic Surgery
University of Pittsburgh School of Medicine
Pittsburgh, Pennsylvania

Gary G. Poehling, MD
Chairman
Department of Orthopaedic Surgery
Wake Forest University Baptist Medical Center
Comprehab Plaza
Orthopaedic Surgery
Wake Forest University Baptist Medical Center
Winston-Salem, North Carolina

Lalit Puri, MD
New England Baptist Hospital
Boston, Massachusetts

Jerome B. Rattner, MD
Department of Surgery
Faculty of Medicine
University of Calgary
Calgary, Alberta, Canada

Robert S. Richards, MD, FRCSC
Associate Professor
Division of Plastic Surgery and Orthopedic Surgery
Department of Surgery
University of Western Ontario
Hand and Upper Limb Centre
St. Joseph's Health Centre
London, Ontario
Canada

John C. Richmond, MD
Professor
Orthopaedic Surgery
Tufts University School of Medicine
Vice-Chairman
Orthopaedic Surgery
New England Medical Center
Boston, Massachusetts

Anthony Romeo, MD
Director
Shoulder Section
Associate Professor
Department of Orthopaedic Surgery
Rush–Presbyterian–St. Luke's Medical Center
Chicago, Illinois

James H. Roth, MD, FRCSC
Professor
Department of Surgery
University of Western Ontario
Director
Hand and Upper Limb Centre
St. Joseph's Health Care, London
London, Ontario
Canada

Neil S. Roth, MD
Assistant Professor
Columbia Center for Shoulder, Elbow, and Sports
    Medicine
Department of Orthopaedic Surgery
Attending Physician
Department of Orthopaedic Surgery
New York Presbyterian Hospital
New York, New York

Thomas G. Sampson, MD
Associate Clinical Professor
Department of Orthopaedic Surgery
University of California, San Francisco
Director of Arthroscopy and Orthopaedics
Healthsouth Surgery Center: Medical Direct
Total Joint Center
Saint Francis Memorial Hospital
San Francisco, California

Felix H. Savoie III, MD
Co-Director
Upper Extremity Service
Mississippi Sports Medicine and Orthopaedic
    Center
Clinical Associate Professor
Department of Orthopaedic Surgery
University of Mississippi School of Medicine
Jackson, Mississippi

Robert C. Schenck, Jr., MD
Professor and Division Chief
Division of Sports Medicine
Department of Orthopaedics and Rehabilitation
University of New Mexico
Health Sciences Center
Department of Orthopaedics
University Hospital
Albuquerque, New Mexico

Walter R. Shelton, MD
Mississippi Sports Medicine and Orthopedic Center
Jackson, Mississippi

John A. Sidles, PhD
Professor
Department of Orthopaedics and Sports Medicine
University of Washington
Seattle, Washington

Neal C. Small, MD
Department of Orthopaedic Surgery
University of Texas Southwestern Medical Center
Associated Arthroscopy Institute
Plano, Texas

Stephen J. Snyder, MD
Southern California Orthopedic Institute
Van Nuys, California.

Louis J. Soslowsky, MD, PhD
Associate Professor
Departments of Orthopaedic Surgery and Bioengineering
Director of Orthopaedic Research
McKay Orthopaedic Research Laboratory
University of Pennsylvania
Philadelphia, Pennsylvania

Maria E. Squire, BS
McKay Orthopaedic Research Laboratory
University of Pennsylvania
Philadelphia, Pennsylvania

James P. Tasto, MD
Clinical Professor
Orthopedic Surgery
University of California, San Diego
Clinical Director
San Diego Medicine & Orthopedic Center
San Diego, California

Gail Thornton, MD
Department of Surgery
University of Toronto
Toronto Hospital
Toronto, Ontario, Canada

Edwin M. Tingstad, MD
Clinical Instructor
Orthopaedics and Sports Medicine
University of Washington
Seattle, Washington
Chief of Surgery
Pullman Memorial Hospital
Pullman, Washington

Todd J. Tucker, MD
Tucson Orthopedic Institute
Tucson, Arizona

Patricia A. Velázques
Center for Orthopaedic and Sports Performance Research
Santa Fe, New Mexico

Jon J.P. Warner, MD
Associate Professor
Orthopaedic Surgery
Harvard Medical School
Massachusetts General Hospital
Brigham and Women's Hospital
Chief
Harvard Shoulder Service
Orthopaedics
Massachusetts General Hospital
Boston, Massachusetts

Stephen C. Weber, MD
Assistant Clinical Professor
University of California, Davis
Davis, California
Sacramento Knee & Sports Medicine Medical
   Corporation
Sacramento, California

Terry L. Whipple, MD
Clinical Associate Professor
Department of Orthopaedic Surgery
Medical College of Virginia
Director
Orthopaedics and Rehabilitation
American Self
Richmond, Virginia

Ethan R. Wiesler, MD
Assistant Professor
Department of Orthopaedic Surgery and Rehabilitation
Wake Forest University School of Medicine
Winston-Salem, North Carolina

W. Howard Wu, MD
Sports Medicine Fellow
New England Medical Center
Tufts University School of Medicine
Boston, Massachusetts

PREFACE

It has been forty years since arthroscopy was reborn in North America. It has had a tremendous effect in decreasing morbidity from musculoskeletal surgery, and has markedly reduced—and in most cases, eliminated—the need for hospitalization. Forty years ago it was not unusual for a patient to be in the hospital for three or four days after a meniscectomy. Anterior cruciate ligament surgery was rarely done. It gradually became apparent, through the work of many innovators, that most intraarticular surgery in the knee could be done without large incisions and damage to surrounding tissues. Over a period of time these approaches and techniques have been expanded to all joints. Arthroscopic surgery has become the most commonly performed musculoskeletal operation. The changes in this exciting branch of orthopaedics continue to accelerate.

The purpose of this third edition of *Operative Arthroscopy* is to again bring together the leaders in this field and have them share their most recent developments. We have attempted to create a new edition of a textbook that has served as a compendium of the various operative procedures available for the orthopaedic surgeon. It is our aim to show surgeons what is available on the cutting edge, but not to necessarily endorse it. It is up to the surgeon to evaluate the procedure in terms of the needs of the patient. This text is intended for surgeons who are experienced arthroscopists and those wishing to learn the necessary skills. The scope of this text is probably beyond medical students, but is certainly of value to orthopaedic residents who are experiencing arthroscopic procedures in their training programs. It must be emphasized that in many of these procedures practice is necessary before performing them on a patient. There are many avenues available to learn these skills, such as cadaver labs, the Orthopaedic Learning Center in Rosemont, Illinois, or even models and simulators. It will not be long before surgery can be practiced in virtual environments.

There is a great deal of work that goes into creating a text of this magnitude. I would like to acknowledge and express my appreciation to the many authors and their staffs, to the hardworking staff of Lippincott Williams & Wilkins, and to the families of all contributors who were deprived of time with their loved ones.

John B. McGinty, MD
Editor-in-Chief

OPERATIVE ARTHROSCOPY

THIRD EDITION

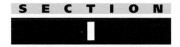

SECTION
I

HISTORY AND DEVELOPMENT

1

HISTORY OF ARTHROSCOPY

ROBERT W. JACKSON

The earliest evidence of humans' insatiable desire to explore the interior of body cavities is documented by references to vaginal specula in the ancient Hebrew literature and by the discovery of proctoscopes in the ruins of Pompeii. The bladder, however, was the most intriguing organ and also provided the major incentive in the development of endoscopic devices. In 1806, Botzini (1773–1809) (1) presented his "Lichtleiter" to the Joseph Academy of Medical Surgery in Vienna, but the concept was not well received. His apparatus consisted of two simple tubes and a candle as a light source. The candlelight was reflected into the bladder of a patient through one of the tubes, and the surgeon looked through the other tube to visualize the contents. In 1853, Désormaux (1815–1882) produced the gazogene endocystoscope. A mixture of turpentine and alcohol was used to provide the fuel for a fire in a small combustion chamber, the light of which was transmitted by mirrors into the bladder through a fairly large tube that was also used for visualization. In 1876, Max Nitze (1848–1906) developed the first modern cystoscope. A platinum loop heated by electricity and encased in a water-cooled goose quill provided the light source within the bladder. In 1880, Edison developed the incandescent lamp, which solved all the previous problems of illumination and proved to be a milestone in the science of endoscopy. Cystoscopy then flourished, and arthroscopy, originally called arthroendoscopy, or the exploration of joint cavities, was a natural evolution.

THE FIRST ARTHROSCOPIST

In April 1912, at the forty-first Congress of the German Society of Surgeons in Berlin, a report was presented dealing with endoscopy of the knee (2). Severin Nordentoft (Fig. 1.1), a relatively unknown Danish surgeon, presented his self-built "trokart-endoscope" to the assembled Congress and described how it could be used not only for cystoscopy, but also for laparoscopy and for endoscopy of the knee joint.

R. W. Jackson: Department of Orthopaedics, Baylor University Medical Center, Dallas, Texas.

His contribution was published in the *Proceedings* of the Society and described an excellent view of the anterior portion of the joint. Nordentoft stated (translated) "you get a view of the bright and smooth synovial membrane and the floating villi and you may easily diagnosis tuberculous degeneration of the synovial membrane and see the difference of a syphilitic inflammation. You can see the back of the patella, and look upwards to the quadriceps bursa, and very often can see the sharp plica marking the boundary of the main joint." He also commented that "although you can see the anterior portions of the meniscus, it is difficult to see the posterior horns which are hidden by the condyles." Difficulty in visualizing the posterior parts of the knee was probably the result of poor illumination and inferior lenses. Nordentoft used the Latin term *arthroscopia genu* to describe his technique.

Severin Nordentoft lived from 1866 to 1922 in Aarhus, Denmark. After a career as a general practitioner and surgeon, he dedicated the last decade of his life to radiotherapy and was not only a pioneer in that area of medicine but also a victim. Without knowing about the dangers of radiation, he received excessive exposure and died of aplastic anemia (3).

DUAL BEGINNINGS

Eastern Pioneers

Professor Kenji Takagi (1888–1963) of Tokyo University (Fig. 1.2) was previously given credit for being the first to apply the principles of endoscopy successfully to a knee joint, a distinction now given to Nordentoft. In 1918, Takagi viewed the interior of a cadaver knee using a cystoscope. The stimulus for his work, as was probably the case with Nordentoft, was the disastrous end result of tuberculosis of the knee, which was rampant at that time and usually resulted in an ankylosed knee. To Japanese citizens, stiff knees represented a serious social as well as physical disability, because they were unable to kneel and squat, both important motions in their society. Professor Takagi hoped to detect tuberculous arthritis early and to provide more

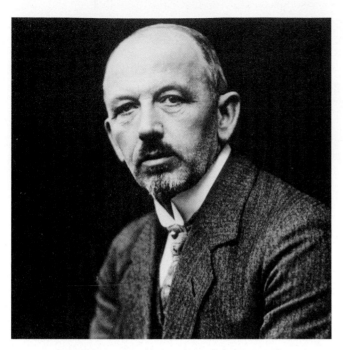

FIGURE 1.1 Severin Nordentoft (1866–1922).

Japanese Orthopaedic Association in Tokyo. He illustrated his report with black-and-white photographs taken through the scope. In 1936, he was successful in obtaining color pictures and a movie film. During this developmental phase, Dr. Saburo Iino worked closely with Takagi in documenting the pathologic features seen within the knee joint and was the first to describe and name the various plicae, or folds of synovium, within the joint.

Unfortunately, from 1939 to 1945, World War II significantly disrupted advances in this area of science. After World War II, Dr. Masaki Watanabe (1921–1994) (Fig. 1.3), a student of Professor Takagi's, continued his work (5). In 1951, the no. 13 arthroscope was developed and was attributed to Dr. Watanabe. In 1958, he released the Watanabe no. 21 arthroscope, which proved to be the first truly successful arthroscope.

The Watanabe no. 21 arthroscope had a magnificent lens with an angle of vision of 102 degrees and a depth of focus from 0.5 mm to infinity. The lenses were produced by a craftsman named Fukuyo, who ground each lens by hand. The incandescent light bulb at the end of the scope was offset and protruded slightly beyond the lens. It provided excellent illumination and was also useful for pushing synovial fronds out of the visual field. However, when the instrument was used by inexperienced arthroscopists, the bulb was also the "Achilles' heel" of the instrument because it was frequently caught on synovial folds within the joint, and this caused it to bend away from the lens and sometimes to break off.

"Cold light" or fiber light was the next major advance and was a feature of the Watanabe no. 22 arthroscope. Smaller-

appropriate and successful treatment (4). In 1919, he used a 7.3-mm cystoscope to explore the knee joint of a patient. The evolution of the technique was slow at first, but over the next few years he developed specific instruments for arthroscopic use and numbered them consecutively. In 1931, the no. 1 Takagi scope was available, and on July 6, 1932, he gave the first report of this instrument to the

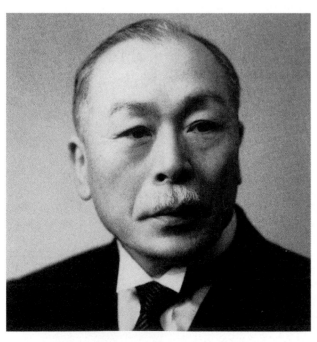

FIGURE 1.2 Professor Kenji Takagi (1888–1963).

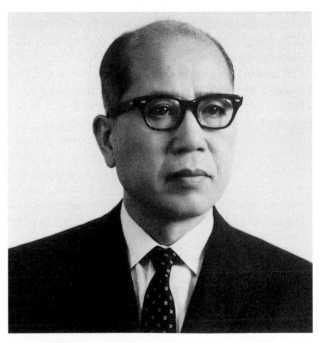

FIGURE 1.3 Dr. Masaki Watanabe (1921–1994).

diameter scopes, such as the no. 24, which measured 2 mm in diameter and consisted of a single fiber of glass, soon followed. With the development of usable instruments, the next major technical advance was the mass production of the instruments.

Recognizing the potential significance of his pioneering efforts, Dr. Watanabe kept immaculate records. His first surgical procedure under arthroscopic control was the removal of a xanthomatous giant cell tumor on March 9, 1955. His first meniscectomy under arthroscopic control was performed on May 4, 1962. His colleagues, Dr. Hiroshi Ikeuchi and Dr. Sakae Takeda, also deserve much credit, because they played a significant role in the early development of the technique of operative arthroscopy.

In 1957, the first edition of Watanabe's *Atlas of Arthroscopy* (6) was published, with Takeda and Ikeuchi as coauthors. This classic atlas was beautifully illustrated by S. Fujihashi. It was revised and republished in 1969 (7), with actual photographs of joint disease.

Western Pioneers

Simultaneous with the development of arthroscopy in the East, Dr. Eugen Bircher (1882–1956) (Fig. 1.4) intro-

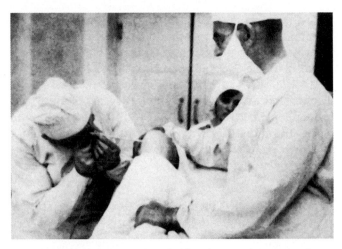

FIGURE 1.5 Dr. Eugen Bircher *(left)* and Dr. Paul Foster performing arthroendoscopy (1922).

duced the Jacobaeus laparoscope into a knee in 1921 and called the technique *arthroendoscopy*. He used gas (carbon monoxide) to distend the joint and wrote about posttraumatic arthritis and the accurate diagnosis of meniscal disease in articles published in 1921 and 1922 (8). One of Bircher's early assistants was identified as Dr. Paul Foster, but little is known about this surgeon (Fig. 1.5). Dr. Bircher's son was a general surgeon in Switzerland and graciously provided information about his father and the early days of arthroscopy.

The first article on arthroscopy in the United States appeared in 1925 (9), when Dr. Phillip Kreuscher (1884–1943) published a plea for the use of arthroscopy in the early recognition and treatment of meniscal lesions. The type of arthroscope he used is not known.

In 1930, Dr. Michael Burman (1901–1975) (Fig. 1.6) of the Hospital for Joint Diseases in New York spent a fellowship year in Berlin studying endoscopic techniques. He returned to the United States and, with a 4-mm diameter arthroscope constructed by Mr. R. Wappler, examined every joint of the body using cadavers. Along with Drs. Mayer, Finkelstein, and Sutro, Burman then published several classic articles (10–13) on this new method of examining joints. His subsequent applications to human patients proved innovative but were met with skepticism by his colleagues. He also had numerous problems with the technology of the time and experienced frequent breakage of his equipment. He did, however, prepare a text for a monograph on arthroscopy, which was never published, and he was the first to experiment with intravital staining to delineate degenerative articular cartilage.

In the German literature, Sommer in 1937 (14) and Vaubel in 1938 (15) reported on their experiences with the technique. Because of the turmoil surrounding World War II and the general dedication of science to military

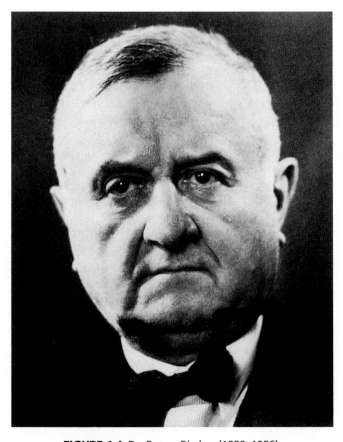

FIGURE 1.4 Dr. Eugen Bircher (1882–1956).

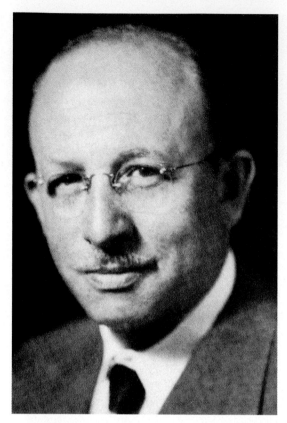

FIGURE 1.6 Dr. Michael Burman (1901–1975).

matters, there were no significant advances in arthroscopy from 1939 to 1945. After World War II, Hurter published an article in the French literature in 1955 (16), and Imbert also published an article in a French journal in 1956 (17).

THE REAWAKENING

In 1964, I went to Tokyo University with the primary purpose of studying tissue culture techniques. On meeting Watanabe and observing arthroscopic procedures (Fig. 1.7), I became convinced that the technique offered a major contribution to the diagnosis and treatment of joint disorders. I returned to the Toronto General Hospital in 1965 and began to practice arthroscopy using the Watanabe no. 21 arthroscope. In 1966, Dr. Isao Abe from Tokyo joined me in Toronto and helped to develop the present technique. In 1967, a short presentation on the subject of arthroscopy was given at the inaugural meeting of the Association of Academic Surgeons held in Toronto, and, in 1968, I gave the first instructional course on the subject, at the annual meeting of the American Academy of Orthopaedic Surgeons. The only other people in the Western world doing any significant amount of arthroscopy at that time were rheuma-

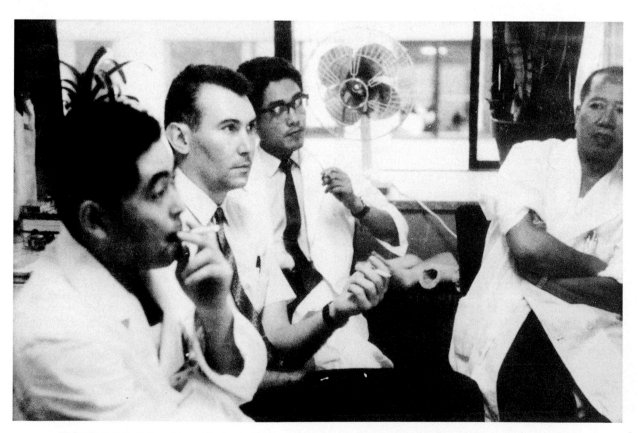

FIGURE 1.7 Drs. Ikeuchi and Jackson discuss cases with Dr. Watanabe at Tokyo Teishin Hospital (1964).

tologists such as Drs. Jason and Dixon in England and Dr. Robles Gil in Mexico.

THE SPREADING AWARENESS

Interest in the technique spread rapidly. Among the early pioneers were Drs. Ward Casscells and Jack McGinty, who visited me in 1967 and began to make their own significant contributions to this field. In 1969, Dr. Richard O'Connor visited Watanabe in Tokyo and soon began to explore new avenues in arthroscopic surgery. Other North American surgeons who played important roles in the development of instruments, techniques, and teaching were Drs. Lanny Johnson, John Joyce III, Ken DeHaven, and Ralph Lidge.

In Europe, Dr. Harold Eikelaar defended his thesis on arthroscopy in 1973 and received the highest degree possible in surgery from the University of Groningen in Holland. Drs. Jan Gillquist and Ejnar Eriksson in Sweden, Dr. Hans Rudolph Henche in Switzerland, and Dr. John Ohnsorge in Germany also played pivotal roles in teaching and developing new techniques of arthroscopy. In 1974, Dr. David Dandy, doing a fellowship year in Toronto, reviewed my experience and coauthored the first English monograph text on the subject of arthroscopy (4).

In 1974, the International Arthroscopy Association (IAA) was founded in Philadelphia, and Professor Watanabe was elected the first chairman. The primary purpose of the IAA was to educate orthopaedic surgeons in the value of the technique and to spread awareness of arthroscopy to all parts of the world. Numerous courses were developed thereafter, under the aegis of both the IAA and various universities. The first major course in arthroscopy was given in 1973 at the University of Pennsylvania under the chairmanship of Dr. John Joyce III (1914–1991). A tremendous boom in arthroscopic teaching occurred over the next 10 years as more and more people became increasingly aware of the potential of this technique. In 1982, the Arthroscopy Association of North America was founded and is now one of the largest such associations in the world.

THE THERAPEUTIC ADVANTAGE

Although Drs. Watanabe and Ikeuchi had performed the first arthroscopic meniscectomy in 1962, the early operative procedures done under arthroscopic control were somewhat limited by the equipment available at that time. Biopsies, removal of loose bodies, and trimming of menisci were all that was possible with the early equipment. However, as special instruments were designed and developed, the therapeutic applications became more apparent. Dr. Richard O'Connor (1933–1980) deserves credit for his pioneering work in this area. Drs. Robert Metcalf (1936–1991), Lanny Johnson, Jim Guhl, George Schonholtz, and Dinesh Patel were early proponents and teachers of operative arthroscopy. Each developed techniques and instruments with the help of various surgical instrument companies. With the increasing ability to perform definitive surgical procedures on pathologic features identified at arthroscopy, the interest and awareness in the technique spread rapidly throughout the world.

THE SOPHISTICATED FUTURE

With the growing number of young, enthusiastic arthroscopists, along with better instrumentation, the basic techniques developed for knee surgery have been applied to shoulders, ankles, hips, and virtually every other joint in the body. Increasing numbers of techniques and surgical procedures are being performed under endoscopic control. Stabilizing and resurfacing procedures are being perfected. New surgical instruments are being developed, such as laser surgery and electrosurgery. The revolution in joint surgery, which began in 1912, has already reached the stage at which arthroscopy must be considered one of the greatest contributions to orthopaedic surgery in the twentieth century, ranking alongside joint arthroplasty.

Where this revolution will end is impossible to predict. The next historian may have the same delightful challenge to outline even greater advances in the field of arthroscopic surgery.

REFERENCES

1. Staff of the National Museum for the History of Science, Leiden, Netherlands. *From lichtleiter to fiber optics.* Catalogue prepared for the 16th Congress of the International Society for Urology, Amsterdam, 1973.
2. Nordentoft S. Ueber Endoskopie geschlossener Kavitäten mittels Trokarendoskops. *Zentralbl Chir* 1912;39:95–97.
3. Kieser CW, Jackson RW. "Severin Nordentoft: The first arthroscopist. *Arthroscopy* 2001;17:532–535.
4. Jackson RW, Dandy DJ. *Arthroscopy of the knee.* London: Grune & Stratton, 1976.
5. Watanabe M. The development and present status of the arthroscope. *J Jpn Med Instr* 1954;25:11.
6. Watanabe M, Takeda S, Ikeuchi H. *Atlas of arthroscopy.* Tokyo: Igaku-Shoin, 1957.
7. Watanabe M, Takeda S, Ikeuchi H. *Atlas of arthroscopy,* 2nd ed. Tokyo: Igaku-Shoin, 1969.
8. Bircher E. Die Arthroendoskopie. *Zentralbl Chir* 1921;48:1460–1461.
9. Kreuscher P. Semilunar cartilage disease: a plea for early recognition by means of the arthroscope and early treatment of this condition. *Ill Med J* 1925;47:290–292.

10. Burman MS. Arthroscopy or direct visualization of joints: an experimental cadaver study. *J Bone Joint Surg* 1931;13:669–695.

11. Burman MS, Finkelstein H, Mayer L. Arthroscopy of the knee joint. *J Bone Joint Surg* 1934;16:255–268.

12. Burman MS, Mayer L. Arthroscopic examination of the knee joint. *Arch Surg* 1936;2:846.

13. Burman MS, Sutro CJ. Arthroscopy by fluorescence: experimental study. *Arch Phys Ther* 1935;16:423.

14. Sommer R. Die Endoskopie des Kniegelenkes. *Zentralbl Chir* 1937;64:1692.

15. Vaubel E. Die Arthroskopie (Endoskopie des Kneigelenkes) eibeitrag zur Diagnostiek der Gelenkkrankheiten. *Z Rheumaforsch* 1938;9:210–213.

16. Hurter E. L'arthroscopie, nouvelle méthode d'exploration du genou. *Rev Chir Orthop* 1955;41:763–766.

17. Imbert R. Arthroscopy of the knee: its technique. *Mars Chir* 1956;8:368.

2

ETHICS

ROBERT W. JACKSON
JOHN B. MCGINTY

Ethics involves moral principles and values, which become the guidelines for practice of individuals or groups of individuals, such as a professional organization. Consequently, each issue of the official publication of the Arthroscopy Association of North America, *Arthroscopy: The Journal of Arthroscopic and Related Surgery,* contains a statement prepared by the association's Committee on Ethics and Standards. This chapter provides a precis of that statement, in addition to some comments on ethical behavior encountered in other aspects of arthroscopic surgery.

CREDENTIALING IN ARTHROSCOPY

When arthroscopic surgical privileges are requested by a physician, a board-certified orthopaedic surgeon or an equivalent specialist with considerable experience in the field of arthroscopic surgery should be involved with the hospital in the decision-making process leading up to the granting of such privileges. Medical (as opposed to surgical) practitioners, who wish to use arthroscopy for diagnostic purposes only (including synovial biopsy), should have an appropriate period of training to learn the pertinent anatomy and the correct techniques and should be competent in the recognition and management of complications.

The recommended training for the practice of arthroscopic surgery includes the completion of an accredited orthopaedic surgery residency or equivalent surgical training with adequate training in arthroscopic surgery. The arthroscopic surgeon should be fully trained in basic surgical principles and techniques to perform "open" procedures safely on any specific part of the body before he or she learns or undertakes arthroscopic or "closed" surgical procedures.

R. W. Jackson: Department of Orthopaedic Surgery, Baylor University Medical Center, Dallas, Texas.

J. B. McGinty: Department of Orthopaedic Surgery, Medical University of South Carolina, Charleston, South Carolina.

The Practice of Arthroscopy

It is strongly emphasized that the arthroscopist do the following:

- Perform an adequate history and physical examination and obtain appropriate laboratory data on the patient or determine that these have already been performed.
- Explain the procedure to the patient including its benefits, possible risks, and complications.
- Exercise due consideration in selecting the correct arthroscopic procedure for a particular condition and be prepared for additional or alternative procedures.
- Prepare an operative report of the procedure that includes the indications for the operation, a description of the operation itself, and a systematic reporting of the findings in each anatomic area.

Continuing Education

It is recommended that the arthroscopist maintain a high level of expertise in arthroscopy through the process of continuing education. To remain informed, the arthroscopist should update his or her knowledge by regular attendance at postgraduate arthroscopic meetings and should continually review the current arthroscopic literature.

New Procedures

As arthroscopic procedures can be very precise, they can also be very difficult. Therefore, adequate training and practice must be undertaken before a surgeon performs a procedure on a patient for therapeutic reasons. There is no excuse today, with modern technology and available learning centers, to fail in performing a procedure or to obtain a harmful result from lack of experience. It is not in the interest of good patient care to look once at a videotape of a complex procedure and then try to do it. In most instances, some hands-on experience is necessary before it is tried on a patient. This ethical decision is the surgeon's, assuming his or her first interest is the welfare of the patient.

Reevaluation of Skills

It is recommended that the performance of an arthroscopic surgeon should be reviewed regularly, and the number of procedures, indications, results, and complications should be made available to appropriate medical staff committees of individual hospitals, which are charged with granting, reviewing, and renewing clinical privileges.

Teaching Arthroscopic Surgery

When a surgeon is presenting a paper or teaching an instructional course on a subject in which he or she has special expertise, it is important that the surgeon make any individual biases known to the audience or students. It is considered unethical to promote an instrument or a procedure in which the educator has a direct financial interest without first making the attendees aware of the situation, so they can place the speaker's remarks in perspective.

Clinical Research

In clinical research in arthroscopy, adequate follow-up is a *sine qua non*. New developments in arthroscopy are frequently accompanied by new instrumentation. The originator of a new procedure often develops new tools to perform the procedure more effectively. Many of these instruments not only are expensive but also provide a royalty to the developer. This is certainly appropriate and ethical, with one caveat. These new instruments and procedures should not be marketed by the industry to the surgical community until adequate trials and follow-up have been performed. It is quite unethical to accept royalties from an unproven procedure. A corollary to this is that new instruments should be developed to perform a procedure with clinical value more efficiently. A procedure should not be developed to market instruments.

Ethics of Industry

Using nonmedical experts in the training of surgeons in the environment of a learning center to teach difficult procedures is ethical and appropriate. Sending a salesperson into the operating room to educate (over the shoulder) in the performance of an actual case is not ethical. The surgeon should carefully plan any actual operative case using arthroscopy before the patient and the surgeon enter the surgical theatre and should not have to rely on instructions during the procedure.

Financial Considerations

In this current economic environment, it is common for insurance companies to manipulate their surgeon providers financially. In spite of that situation, when submitting an account to an insurer or to a patient, the ethical arthroscopist should avoid "unbundling" the work that was done and should not charge for each individual portion of the procedure. A submitted bill should truly reflect the importance of the overall nature of the procedure, and the ancillary procedures performed in the treatment of the patient should *not* be reflected with additional charges.

One must also avoid the tendency to abuse the system by advising arthroscopic procedures on patients without significant clinical evidence to warrant such procedures. In this regard, one of the best quality-assurance measures has been the routine use of closed-circuit television in the performance of a case, so everyone in the operating room is aware of what is going on inside the joint that is being treated.

An issue has arisen involving team physicians. Most team physicians are orthopaedists and are also accomplished arthroscopists. Within the last decade, however, groups of team physicians have bought the "privilege" of caring for professional teams for substantial sums of money. One has to question the ethics of physicians who buy this privilege for the purpose of marketing and advertising. A team should seek the best available care and should pay their consultant physicians for that care—not the other way around.

Avoiding "Overtreatment"

Part of the Hippocratic Oath states: "do no harm." The surgeon should avoid overtreatment, such as dividing every plica that is identified, resecting minor tears of otherwise asymptomatic menisci, and so on. There is also a definite propensity to do harm by doing too much, especially with some of the newer technologic advances. Until modalities such as laser or thermal energy have been fully developed, procedures using such energy sources should be restricted to a few, careful, and scientifically involved practitioners. It is anticipated that many more techniques and energy sources will be developed in the future. It behooves the arthroscopist truly to learn how to perform new techniques and to learn the pros and cons of new modalities before becoming involved with every new procedure.

SUMMARY

These common sense statements add up to what is good and bad and what is essentially our moral duty and obligation to the treatment of patients. Ethical practice is not carved in stone. Ultimately, it is up to the choices made by an individual person in the conduct of his or her professional life. It boils down to the responsibility that a physician has to the patient and the community and, more importantly, to his or her personal integrity.

Operative Arthroscopy, third edition. Edited by John B. McGinty, Stephen S. Burkhart, Robert W. Jackson, Donald H. Johnson, and John C. Richmond.
Lippincott Williams & Wilkins © 2003.

3

OPERATIVE ARTHROSCOPY ENVIRONMENT, ANESTHESIA, AND PATIENT FLOW

NEAL C. SMALL
RALPH T. LIDGE
DONALD H. JOHNSON

The operating room environment is of paramount importance when operative arthroscopy is to be performed. Johnson (1) was the first to make us aware of the need for creating an environment appropriate for arthroscopic surgery. Operative arthroscopy is demanding, and a proper environment is necessary to minimize stress for the surgeon and patient. An efficient system maximizes the environment for arthroscopy. Operating time is minimized, and everyone involved benefits from improved efficiency.

The appropriate environment for operative arthroscopy includes pleasant and efficient operating room personnel. Needless to say, this staff must perform in a professional manner. The surgeon should be allowed to focus on the operative arthroscopy being performed. The staff should minimize the number of distractions that could affect the surgeon's concentration during the procedure.

The purpose of this chapter is to present environmental factors that affect arthroscopic surgery. These factors include choice of facility, anesthesia, operating room layout, operating room staff, and sterilization of instruments.

ANESTHESIA

Today, most arthroscopic procedures are performed on an outpatient basis (2). Excellent references are available for outpatient anesthesia, such as *Anesthesia for Ambulatory Surgery* by Wetchler (3). The choices for anesthesia in the outpatient setting include general anesthesia, regional anes-

thesia, intravenous sedation with monitored anesthesia care (MAC), and local anesthesia.

The advantages of general anesthesia include complete amnesia, a higher level of muscle relaxation, and the ability to use a tourniquet for prolonged periods. Currently, general anesthesia is used in most arthroscopic procedures performed on an outpatient basis. The disadvantages of general anesthesia include the sometimes unpleasant recovery and the potential risks and complications.

Regional anesthesia includes epidural anesthesia, spinal anesthesia, and various nerve blocks. The advantages of regional anesthesia include the somewhat lesser risk of cardiopulmonary complications and the ability for the patient to be responsive during the procedure. For several reasons, regional anesthesia has not become the preferred form of anesthesia for outpatient arthroscopy. Among these reasons are the prolonged time required to establish complete regional anesthesia and the potential risks and complications inherent in the various forms of regional anesthesia.

MAC has become increasingly popular for arthroscopic surgery. This technique basically involves the administration of an intravenous medication rendering the patient into a sedated state. Monitoring is necessary (Table 3.1). Basic monitoring would include a pulse oximeter, blood pressure monitor, and electrocardiographic monitor. Anesthesia records are maintained. MAC is useful for outpatient arthroscopy in the hospital outpatient department, the ambulatory surgery center, and the orthopaedic office. It is usually used in conjunction with local anesthesia. One of the advantages of MAC is that the patient is responsive or can rapidly become responsive. A tourniquet can be used for brief periods even if the sedation is quite minimal. The unpleasant aftereffects of general anesthesia are avoided. The disadvantages of MAC include the need for monitoring and the presence of very little, if any, muscle relaxation.

N. C. **Small:** Department of Orthopaedic Surgery, University of Texas Southwestern Medical Center; Associated Arthroscopy Institute, Plano, Texas.

R. T. **Lidge:** Department of Orthopaedic Surgery, University of Illinois Medical School at Chicago, Chicago, Illinois 60612.

D. H. **Johnson:** Department Orthopaedic Surgery, University of Ottawa, The Ottawa Hospital, Ottawa, Ontario, Canada.

TABLE 3.1 STANDARDS FOR PATIENT MONITORING DURING ANESTHESIA

These standards apply for any administration of anesthesia involving department of anesthesia personnel and are specifically referable to preplanned anesthetics administered in designated anesthetizing locations (specific exclusion: administration of epidural analgesia for labor or pain management). In emergency circumstances in any location, immediate life support measures of whatever appropriate nature come first, with attention turning to the measures described in these standards as soon as possible and practical. These are minimal standards that may be exceeded at any time based on the judgment of anesthesia personnel. These standards encourage high-quality patient care, but observing them cannot guarantee any specific outcome. These standards are subject to revision from time to time, as warranted by the evolution of technology and practice.

Anesthesiologist's or nurse anesthetist's presence in operating room

For all anesthetics initiated by or involving a member of the department of anesthesia, an attending or resident anesthesiologist or nurse anesthetist shall be present in the room throughout the conduct of all general anesthetics, regional anesthetics, and monitored intravenous anesthetics. An exception is made when there is a direct known hazard, such as radiation, to the anesthesiologist or nurse anesthetist, in which case some provision for monitoring the patient must be made.

Blood pressure and heart rate

Every patient receiving general anesthesia, regional anesthesia, or managed intravenous anesthesia shall have arterial blood pressure and heart rate measured at least every 5 minutes, when not clinically impractical.

Electrocardiogram

Every patient shall have the electrocardiogram continuously displayed from the induction or institution of anesthesia until the patient prepares to leave the anesthetizing location, when not clinically impractical.

Continuous monitoring

During every administration of general anesthesia, the anesthetist shall employ methods of continuously monitoring the patient's ventilation and circulation. The methods shall include, for ventilation and circulation each, at least one of the following or the equivalent:

For ventilation: Palpation or observation of the reservoir breathing bag, auscultation of breath sounds, monitoring of respiratory gases such as end-tidal carbon dioxide, or monitoring of expiratory gas flow. Monitoring end-tidal carbon dioxide is an emerging standard and is strongly preferred.

For circulation: Palpation of a pulse, auscultation of heart sounds, monitoring of a tracing of intraarterial pressure, pulse plethyamography/oximetry, or ultrasound peripheral pulse monitoring.

It is recognized that brief interruptions of continuous monitoring may be unavoidable.

Breathing system disconnection monitoring

When ventilation is controlled by an automatic mechanical ventilator, there shall be in continuous use a device capable of detecting disconnection of any component of the breathing system. The device must give an audible signal when its alarm thresholds is exceeded. (It is recognized that in certain rare or unusual circumstances such a device may fail to detect a disconnection.)

Oxygen analyzer

During every administration of general anesthesia using an anesthesia machine, the concentration of oxygen in the patient breathing system will be measured by a functioning oxygen analyzer with a low-concentration-limit alarm in use. This device must conform to the American National Standards Institute No. Z.79.10 standard.

Ability to measure temperature

During every administration of general anesthesia, there shall be readily available a means to measure the patient's temperature.

Rationale: A means of temperature measurement must be available as a potential aid in the diagnosis and treatment of suspected or actual intraoperative hypothermia and malignant hyperthermia. The measurement/monitoring of temperature during every general anesthetic is not specificially mandated because of the potential risks of such monitoring and because of the likelihood of other physical signs giving earlier indication of the development of malignant hyperthermia.

Adapted from Eichhorn JH, Cooper JB, Cullen DJ, et al. Standards for patient monitoring during anesthesia at Harvard Medical School. *JAMA* 1986;256:1019. Copyright 1986 American Medical Association.

TABLE 3.2 SUGGESTED MAXIMUM DOSES OF LOCAL ANESTHETICS FOR A HEALTHY 70-KG ADULT

Local Anesthesia	Plain Solutions (mg)	Solutions Containing Epinephrine (mg)
Lidocaine	300	500
Bupivacaine	175	225

Adapted from Raj PP, Winnie A. *Complications in anesthesiology.* Philadelphia: JB Lippincot, 1985:59, with permission.

Local anesthesia is used for arthroscopic surgery in numerous arthroscopy centers. Local anesthesia has the advantages of being cost-effective and associated with a low risk of adverse effects (Table 3.2). The major disadvantage of local anesthesia is that no muscle relaxation occurs. With posterior medial compartment problems, such as posterior horn tears of the medial meniscus, the amount of distraction available to open the medial compartment is less than with general anesthesia, regional anesthesia, and MAC. Local anesthesia is used frequently in the office setting for diagnostic arthroscopy of the knee and shoulder.

A combination of local anesthesia and MAC has been effective for arthroscopy in the hospital, ambulatory surgery center, and office setting. This combination of anesthetic techniques allows adequate sedation, fair muscle relaxation, and complete anesthesia. For relatively brief knee procedures, a tourniquet can also be used. The combination of MAC and local anesthesia has been the anesthetic regimen of choice for office operative arthroscopy of the knee, shoulder, and ankle.

CHOICE OF FACILITY

Hospital

Arthroscopy in the modern era was introduced to North America by Dr. Robert Jackson in Toronto in 1964 (4). Because arthroscopy was used by orthopaedic surgeons performing knee surgery at that time, it was performed in the hospital operating room. Day surgery and ambulatory surgery centers were not well-known concepts at that time. Many arthroscopists continue to use hospital operating rooms even today. Increasing numbers of larger hospitals have constructed outpatient surgery units, which allow patients the convenience of easy check-in and check-out for same-day surgical procedures.

Although most operative arthroscopy procedures are now performed in either a hospital outpatient surgery unit or a free-standing ambulatory surgery center, some patients prefer a full-service hospital for their surgical procedure. Some patients actually prefer an overnight stay in the hospital for 1 or 2 days. These patients also use the hospital services, including physical therapy, for the early recovery period. Although some third-party payers will not pay for such services on an inpatient basis, certain patients are willing to pay for these services.

Ambulatory Surgery Center

In 1970, anesthesiologists Wallace Reed and John Ford pioneered the first free-standing surgery center (5). Since then, numerous facilities of this type have been constructed and provide a similar type of care to patients across the United States. In 1972, Davis and Detmer proposed that the term *ambulatory surgery* be defined as "surgery of an uncomplicated nature that traditionally has been done on an inpatient basis but that can be done with equal efficiency and safety without hospital admission" (6).

The ambulatory surgery center is a free-standing center. Many such centers have been approved by the Accreditation Association for Ambulatory Health Care (Fig. 3.1). Most centers are endorsed by the Health Insurance Institute and are certified by Medicare. Most ambulatory surgery centers are more cost-effective than a full-service hospital for minor ambulatory surgical procedures. The cost of facility use, equipment, and supplies is usually one-half to one-third the cost for the same surgical procedure performed in a full-service hospital. The average total stay at an ambulatory surgery center is now approximately 4 hours. Patients return home the same day. Thus, ambulatory surgery is frequently referred to as same-day surgery.

The ambulatory surgery center should be fully equipped and safe. Medicare certification is an indication that the center has been designed specifically with patient safety and quality control in mind. Most free-standing ambulatory surgery centers are staffed by anesthesiologists who are experienced in outpatient anesthesia techniques. This approach allows for efficient patient flow and thus reduces costs. Most third-party payers encourage the use of outpatient surgery. For most patients, the out-of-pocket expenditure not covered by the third-party payer is minimized when an ambulatory surgery center is used.

Surgical procedures performed in a free-standing ambulatory surgery center should be approached in a manner similar to surgical procedures performed in a full-service hospital. Preoperatively, the patient should be evaluated by the surgeon and cleared medically for the surgical procedure. The patient should also be instructed regarding the advantages of the ambulatory surgery center and the likely patient flow on the day of the surgical procedure. The surgeon's office should be responsible for making sure that all appropriate medical records are at the ambulatory surgery center on the day of the surgical procedure. A preoperative checklist used by the staff in the surgeon's office is helpful. A standard surgical consent form appropriate for the particular state should be reviewed and signed. The patient should be given appropriate instructions for preoperative eating or drinking.

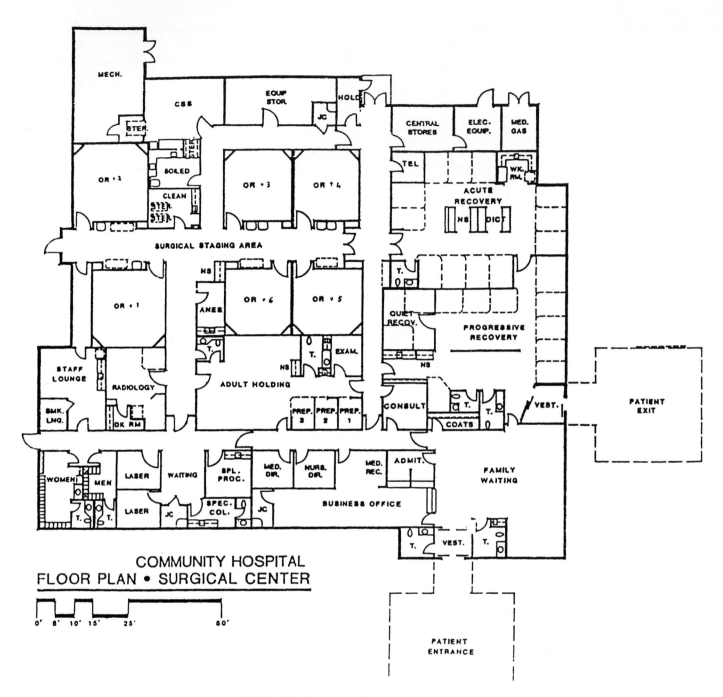

FIGURE 3.1 Floor plan of a typical surgical center.

A complete history and physical examination are performed if general anesthesia is to be used. Appropriate testing, such as a chest radiograph, electrocardiogram, and laboratory work, is performed. It is also appropriate for the patient to be interviewed by the anesthesiologist either in person or over the telephone before the surgical procedure.

After the surgical procedure in an ambulatory surgery center, recovery from general anesthesia requires the use of a postanesthesia recovery room. When regional anesthesia is used, the patient may bypass the postanesthesia recovery room and may go directly to the progressive recovery room before discharge. As a general rule, the patient remains in the acute recovery room after general anesthesia for about 1 hour. When intravenous sedation is used, the patient is observed in the acute recovery room for 1 hour. When regional block anesthesia is used, the patient is kept in the progressive recovery unit until full motion and sensation have been regained.

In many situations, the nurse checks the patient and arranges for discharge from the recovery room when the patient's condition is stabilized. Although physicians may delegate this task to the recovery room nurse or the progressive recovery nurse, the liability still lies with the anesthesiologist and the surgeon. Patients who have received a general anesthetic or intravenous sedation should not be allowed to drive home.

The patient should be informed of the possibility that hospitalization may be necessary after the surgical procedure in the ambulatory surgery center. Arrangements are usually made with a local hospital to accept patients if the need arises.

Written postoperative instructions should be given to the patient when the patient is ready to be discharged. These instructions should be signed by both the nurse and the patient. In most ambulatory surgery centers, the patient receives a phone call from a member of the staff within the first 48 hours after the surgical procedure.

Office Operative Arthroscopy

In recent years, operative arthroscopy has been introduced to the orthopaedic office and clinic (7). Rising health care expenditures have created an awareness among health care providers that cost containment is also a factor in providing optimal care. Procedures can be performed safely in an office environment at a fraction of the cost that is incurred in the hospital or even the ambulatory surgery center (8).

OPERATING ROOM DESIGN

Most hospitals and ambulatory surgery centers have a specific room or several rooms dedicated to arthroscopic surgery. Standards for operating room design, construction, and management have been published by several organizations, including the American College of Surgeons. The American College of Surgeons Committee on Operating Room Environment has, since the 1980s, presented operating room design and safety to surgeons and others. LoCicero and Nichols (9) described environmental health hazards in the operating room. There are three categories to consider:

1. Physical hazards: architecture (room design), lighting and ventilation, electrical hazards (macroshock, microshock, and burns), radiation, and acoustics.
2. Chemical hazards: gaseous (inhalation side effects, explosion) and liquid or solid (contact sensitivity and dermatitis).
3. Biologic hazards: infections transmitted between patient and team or transmitted through the environment.

To minimize physical hazards, appropriate design is important. The design should allow for easy cleaning of the room. Proper illumination should be stressed to minimize eye strain. A unidirectional air flow that changes the air 25

times per hour is ideal. Other types of well-filtered air delivery systems may be equally effective.

The need for adequate grounding of electrical devices is of utmost importance. Macroshock occurs whenever an electrical current enters the body through the intact skin and can be avoided by proper grounding. Microshock begins beneath the cutaneous barrier and can be caused by currents from poorly grounded electrical devices. These currents are below the threshold of sensation and can cause cardiac irregularities. Scheduled maintenance and routine safety checks are vital. It is important that the operating room be of adequate size so electrical cables are not crowded into a small area. The electric cables should be shielded.

Mishaps involving operating room gases can occur when cylinders containing gases have nonfunctional relief valves or have been mislabeled or relabeled. Anesthetic gases, which have been found to alter both physical and mental skills in the operating room, can be collected and released through a secondary system to lower the contamination level in the operating room environment.

Contact dermatitis and eczema can occur from excessive contact with irritating detergents and compounds used in the operating room. Alcohol and iodine are frequent irritants. Constant exposure to water and soap may also cause problems with contact dermatitis and eczema.

A sterile environment is essential in the operating room. Full consideration must be given to establishing a routine cleaning procedure. Careful technique must be used in the operating room to minimize the transmission of contaminants and pathogens to the patient. The operating room personnel must strive to maintain an aseptic environment.

OPERATING ROOM SPACE ENGINEERING

A graphic layout should be available for the operating room personnel. The personnel can refer to this graphic depiction when they are setting up the room for arthroscopy of the knee, shoulder, elbow, ankle, and wrist, for example. The graphic diagram should illustrate the location of the overhead lights and the operating room table. There are different positions for the operating table, depending on the joint to be addressed. The location of the anesthesiologist, the monitoring equipment, the back table, the Mayo stand, and the arthroscopy video equipment should be well documented (Fig. 3.2). In many arthroscopy suites, built-in cabinets have been constructed to house much of this equipment.

For most arthroscopic procedures, one Mayo stand and one back table are used. The Mayo stand holds the arthroscopy equipment that is used for the diagnostic procedure. Some commonly used operative arthroscopy equipment may also be placed on the Mayo stand. The back table usually holds the remainder of the appropriate instruments for the type of operative arthroscopy being performed.

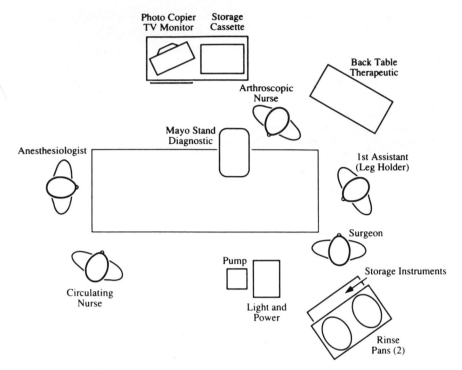

FIGURE 3.2 A graphic layout of the operating room environment.

For knee arthroscopy, the anesthesiologist is usually positioned at the head of the table. For shoulder arthroscopy, the anesthesiologist sometimes assumes a different position when the patient is in the lateral decubitus position.

Draping techniques can vary, but it is important to avoid any contamination from the head of the table toward the operative site. Specialized draping for arthroscopy is preferred. Most arthroscopy drapes incorporate pouches that collect the fluid overflow.

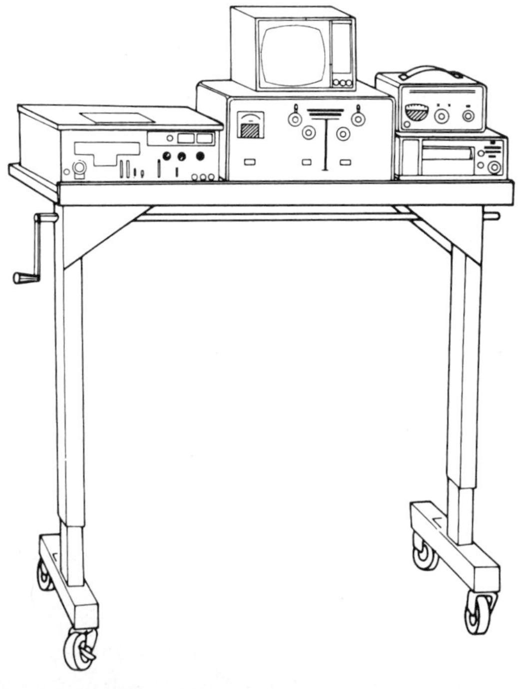

The video monitor, motorized suction shaver unit, copying equipment, and other large arthroscopy items are usually positioned either on the contralateral side of the table or at the foot or head of the table. Instrument tables that actually fit over the operating room table are available (Fig. 3.3).

STAFFING THE OPERATING ROOM

Ideal staffing for the arthroscopy operating suite includes an arthroscopy nurse, a first assistant, and a circulating nurse, in addition to the anesthesiologist and the surgeon. Ideally, the arthroscopy nurse and the first assistant should have extensive experience in arthroscopic surgery.

Arthroscopy nurses have many roles. At various times, they function as manager, teacher, video specialist, instrument technician, and purchasing agent. These nurses must possess management skills because they often function as a coordinator for the arthroscopy team. The arthroscopy nurse should be able to delegate responsibility and to supervise other personnel. The nurse should be able to anticipate the surgeon's needs. Ideally, this nurse should have a working knowledge of surgical anatomy, types of pathologic processes encountered, and methods of treatment. Familiarity with the equipment is mandatory. Most nurses experienced in this area are able to troubleshoot minor problems that may arise. The arthroscopy nurse should also be able to explain the use of the equipment to other members of the arthroscopy team. Because of the complicated video equip-

FIGURE 3.3 Arthroscopic instrument table from Instrument Makar, Okemos, MI. Dimensions: length, 40 inches; width, 13 inches. The table's legs are adjustable from a low height of 41 inches to a maximum of 61 inches.

ment used in arthroscopy, the arthroscopy nurse should have a working knowledge of how to set up this equipment.

The arthroscopy nurse is also responsible for the care of all arthroscopy equipment. This includes the cleaning and inspection of equipment after each use. This person is usually responsible for purchasing instruments on a routine replacement basis and for evaluating new arthroscopy equipment for the hospital or ambulatory surgery center.

OPERATING ROOM STAFF RESPONSIBILITIES FOR OPERATIVE ARTHROSCOPY

Preoperative Routine

Preoperatively, the arthroscopy nurse assembles all the instruments and video equipment while the other team members open supplies and gather the remaining equipment. The video equipment is readied. The microphone is assembled and connected. If video recording is anticipated, a new videotape is labeled with patient information and is inserted in the videocassette recorder. The monitor is calibrated using color bars and white balance. The camera is connected, and all the equipment is tested. The camera is then placed in glutaraldehyde solution (Cidex; Johnson & Johnson Medical, Inc., Arlington, TX) along with the arthroscopes and light cable. The remaining instruments are autoclaved or soaked in Cidex, as deemed appropriate. The remaining equipment is then tested. This includes the light source, shaver, tourniquet, and suction device.

The arthroscopy nurse also assists the surgeon and circulating nurse in positioning the patient and applying the tourniquet. During this time, the first assistant begins setting up the back table and Mayo stand while the circulating nurse prepares the patient's extremity. It is important that the back table and Mayo stand be set up in exactly the same manner for every case. This makes it easier to notice when an instrument is missing. It also enables the surgeon to find a needed instrument quickly when necessary. Once the circulating nurse has finished the surgical preparation, the arthroscopy nurse and the first assistant can then drape the patient. Drapes are now available with pouches attached to prevent excessive leaking and to keep the floor dry. The surgeon is assisted with gown and gloves. The appropriate tubes are then attached to the pouches and drapes. The Mayo stand is pulled over toward the patient or, in some situations, over the top of the supine patient.

Intraoperative Routine

The circulating nurse maintains the fluid and adjusts the arthroscopy infusion pump if needed. The assistant helps with gowning and gloving, draping the patient, and gathering instruments. During surgery, the assistant holds the patient's leg for the surgeon. It is important to hold the patient's leg very still and yet to move it with adequate control

when required during the procedure. The assistant pays close attention to the video monitor. The assistant should be able to anticipate the surgeon's needs.

The arthroscopy nurse hands the instruments to the surgeon. Each time the surgeon uses an instrument, it is important for the nurse to check for missing parts that may have been broken off or may remain in the joint. To perform this task, one must maintain effective overhead lighting. The arthroscopy nurse may on occasion hold the camera, to free both hands for the surgeon. Knowledge of the surgical anatomy and treatment of different types of pathologic processes are useful in anticipating the surgeon's needs and in manipulating the camera. During the entire procedure, the nurse should be constantly aware of the status of all equipment in the room and should be able to direct other team members. The staff should be able to rectify any situation that could lead to potential problems. The arthroscopy nurse or assistant can assist in maintaining adequate joint fluid distention. This distention can be controlled by pinching the suction tubing to the degree necessary to maintain an adequate balance of inflow and outflow. This is especially important when a motorized suction shaving or cutting system is used.

Postoperative Routine

After each procedure, the arthroscopy nurse washes the instruments in soapy water. The camera, arthroscope, and light cable are then placed in Cidex. The other instruments are autoclaved or soaked in Cidex appropriately for the next case. During this time, the first assistant helps to clean and ready the room for the next arthroscopic procedure.

At the end of the surgery day, it is the responsibility of the arthroscopy nurse to clean all the instruments and to put them away in a storage cart. The arthroscopes are prepared for gas sterilization. At this time, all the instruments are checked. A magnifying lens is useful for detecting small defects in the instruments. The instruments should be properly packaged when they are sent out for repair.

BRIEF SUMMARY OF STAFF RESPONSIBILITIES

Arthroscopy Nurse

1. Assemble all instruments and video equipment.
2. Assemble and connect microphone; label and insert videotape.
3. Calibrate monitor using color bars and white balance.
4. Connect camera and test all equipment.
5. Soak camera in Cidex.
6. Test remaining equipment: light source, shaver, tourniquet, and suction device.
7. Assist circulating nurse in positioning the patient.
8. Scrub and set up instrument tables.
9. Drape patient.

10. During procedure, hand instruments to surgeon, and check all instruments after removal from joint for broken pieces.
11. Assist with closing and dressings.
12. After procedure, wash instruments and sterilize for next procedure; soak arthroscope, camera, and light cable.
13. Autoclave instruments.
14. At end of day, place instruments in storage cabinet.

Arthroscopy Assistant

1. Scrub and set up Mayo stand and instrument table.
2. Hold patient's leg during surgical procedure.
3. Assist surgeon in closing and applying dressings.
4. Remove drapes from patient and tables, strip room, and wipe down furniture for next procedure.

Circulating Nurse

1. Help check and assemble equipment and open supplies.
2. Identify patient and bring patient into room.
3. Position patient on operating table with patient's knee over break; maintain adequate support for "well" leg; position appropriately for arthroscopy of the particular joint.
4. Apply tourniquet as high as possible on patient's thigh, to allow room for leg holder.
5. Position leg holder if this is surgeon's preference.
6. Prepare patient's leg.
7. After patient is anesthetized and draped, connect light cable, video equipment, and fluid ingress.
8. Keep close watch on ingress solution and replace when necessary.
9. At conclusion of procedure, assist with applying dressings or splint.
10. Transfer patient to gurney cart and then to recovery room.

CARE OF EQUIPMENT

The task of caring for the equipment rests mainly in the hands of the arthroscopy nurse. It is vital that the equipment be adequate to cover all areas of need. The nurse should be familiar with this equipment and should communicate closely with the arthroscopic surgeon. Knowledge of equipment can come from the following:

1. Review of commercial literature available from companies and their representatives
2. Direct contact with company representatives
3. Textbooks on arthroscopy
4. Arthroscopy videos (both diagnostic and operative)
5. Attendance at orthopaedic meetings (particularly those directed toward the training of the arthroscopy nurse)

When equipment is purchased, a list should be maintained at all times so replacements may be ordered properly. There should be at least one backup for each instrument that plays an important role in diagnostic and therapeutic procedures.

During the procedure, the equipment should be laid out in an identical manner each time. This not only pertains to the arthroscopic equipment but also to the other instruments, such as the scalpel, manual, electrical, or mechanically powered equipment, and other items.

Postoperatively, instruments should be carefully inspected, preferably with a magnifying system, to rule out wear and tear and to observe for possible impending breakage. Instruments that show an impending defect or need repair should be properly packaged and sent out for repair. It is a good idea to call the manufacturer to find out how long the repair will take. Sometimes one may borrow an instrument for use while the original instrument is out for repair.

The following techniques for instrument cleaning are recommended:

1. Arthroscope: wash in soapy water and clean ocular lenses with cotton-tipped applicator dipped in alcohol.
2. Light cable: wash in soapy water and clean cable ends with alcohol.
3. Camera: wash in soapy water and wash and dry pin connector carefully (Cidex can accumulate on pins and can affect picture quality).
4. Shaver: wash in soapy water and pass brush through suction port; flush with water.
5. Hand instruments: clean in soapy water using a soft brush; pay particular attention to working tips; inspect for damage.

Several additional precautionary measures should be taken, as follows:

1. Avoid contacting the lenses with povidone–iodine (Betadine) solutions because such contact will have an erosive effect on the lens system.
2. If normal saline solution is employed, clean the instruments abundantly with tap water after the surgical procedure to avoid saline corrosion.
3. Remember that repeated steam sterilization will affect the sealing of the instruments and may necessitate instrument repair.
4. Always examine the arthroscope; it should be held up to the light to be certain that the image will be properly transmitted.

Proper instrument storage is very important. A portable storage cabinet is helpful. Backup instruments should be available.

STERILIZATION

Arthroscopy equipment can be sterilized using gas sterilization, steam sterilization, or Cidex soaking. Gas sterilization should not be used for any article that can be appropriately steam sterilized. An example of this is the sterilizer used at Northwest Community Hospital in Arlington Heights, Illinois. This is the Amsco Medallion Series combination steam and gas sterilizer with cryotherm gas control. The maximum temperature is 140°F for a maximum total of 26 1/2 hours. The maximum vacuum is 20 inches of mercury for 20 minutes as part of the preconditioning cycle. The type of gas is 12% ethylene oxide, 88% Freon-12. The concentration is 780 mg/L at 8 lb/in^2. The time of exposure is 1 hour and 50 minutes standard run. The aeration time is 12 hours for standard items and 24 hours for implantable items. The aeration chamber is an Amsco chamber and has four to six air changes per minute at a temperature of 140°F. Materials that are impermeable to ethylene oxide, such as metals and glass, require no aeration if they are unwrapped. The sterile wrapped article is placed in an aeration cabinet at 50°C (122°F) for 12 hours or 60°C (140°F) for 8 hours.

Specific aeration requirements for gas-sterilized items should be followed to avoid contamination and the hazards of toxic residues. For ethylene oxide sterilization, the personnel involved oversee the preparation and sterilization. These techniques include decontamination, cleaning, and packaging. The ethylene oxide tape, which is a chemical indicator, indicates only exposure to ethylene oxide, not sterility. Biologic testing for *Bacillus subtilis* is incorporated in each sterilizing cycle. Records should be made of all items tested and approved. Therefore, the following are important records to keep:

1. Identification of the sterilizer
2. Sterilizing conditions
3. Temperature
4. Time
5. Gas concentration
6. Humidity
7. Date of cycle
8. Signature

There must be a close working relationship between the staff using the sterilizer and the manufacturer. The American Sterilizer Dart Test (Erie, PA) is performed monthly on each sterilizer, and results are logged in the sterilizer record book. This test is performed by the American Sterilizer maintenance technician. A record is kept for 7 years of each ethylene oxide sterilization, including all the items mentioned earlier. Loading procedures and precautions when using the gas sterilizer are identical to those used for steam sterilization. Aeration times of ethylene oxide–sterilized items are determined by the content of the item. The manufacturer's recommendations are to be kept on file. At Northwest Community Hospital, the standard time of 12 hours at 130°F with four air changes per minute is used for all items unless recommendations exceed that limit.

For steam sterilization, it is generally agreed that the survival kill data indicate the following protocols:

1. Saturated steam at 120°C (250°F): gravity unit survival time, 5 minutes; kill time, 15 minutes
2. Saturated steam at 132°C (270°F): prevacuum unit survival time, 1 minute; kill time, 3 minutes

It is recommended that instruments other than arthroscopes be steam sterilized. With repeated steam sterilization, arthroscopes will deteriorate because the sealant is susceptible. For the arthroscopes themselves, overnight ethylene oxide gas sterilization followed by Cidex sterilization between cases is appropriate. The arthroscope and camera are soaked in the Cidex solution for at least 10 minutes between cases. The items are then carefully rinsed in two consecutive saline washes.

Before sterilization, all items must be readied for the sterilization procedure. Specific items that are to be gas sterilized are listed with the manufacturer's recommendations. These recommendations contain content of the item, construction, materials, exposure times for sterilization, and aeration time. This listing is kept on file. When wrapping materials are used, it must be determined that the wrapping materials are able to withstand the conditions in the gas sterilizer. Damage may be caused to items constructed of Tenite, Styron, Lucite, and Plexiglas (10).

The infection rate for routine arthroscopic surgery is 0.2% (one in 500 procedures). With appropriate attention to preoperative detail, staff education, patient preparation, and sterilization techniques, this infection rate can, one hopes, be lowered even further.

DOCUMENTATION

In the past, the basic level of documentation of the arthroscopy procedure consisted of a dictated operative report describing the pathologic process and the treatment. Hand drawn illustrations of the pathologic features were added to the text report. The appearance of the articular cartilage as well as the meniscal and ligament findings were usually described with text. The site, size, and depth of the articular lesion were noted. This information was found to be invaluable in the follow-up of the patient, months or years later. The difficulty was in sharing the information with another physician. One surgeon's text description of a pathologic process may not be interpreted in the same way by another physician. Because a picture is worth a thousand words, digital imaging of the pathologic features both before and after arthroscopic treatment became the standard of care. The hard copy of the prints can be stored in the patient's file, and the electronic copy can be stored on the server. What is digital imaging? This is the process of transferring an image into a computer without the use of traditional photographic film. The main methods used to ac-

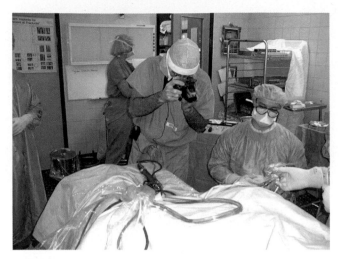

FIGURE 3.4 Using a digital camera to document the patient's pathologic features in the operating room.

quire digital images are digital still cameras, digital still capture units for the arthroscopic cameras, and scanners (Figs. 3.4 and 3.5).

Digital cameras are the easiest way to shoot photographs in the operating room, to record patients' examination findings in the clinical setting, and to view radiographs. I use a megapixel camera to capture radiographs on the view box, to do close-up images in the operating room, and to record clinical examinations of patients. The high-resolution image of the camera is sufficient to print photographs for publication, at least 300 dots per inch (dpi). The camera has a memory card and a compact flash card, and I carry several of them to give me sufficient storage for several days of shooting high-resolution photographs. The card then fits into a personal computer card adapter, which one opens on the computer as another removable drive. The photographs

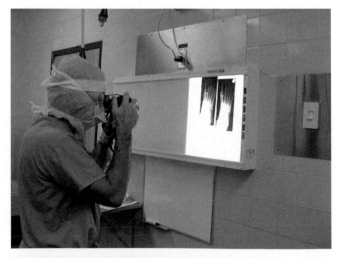

FIGURE 3.5 Recording the radiograph with a digital camera in the operating room.

are dragged and dropped into a folder on the hard disk. These photographs are opened onto an editing program called PhotoShop and are then cropped, adjusted for brightness, sized, named, saved as a compressed jpeg file, and placed in suitable folders on the hard drive. Image Access Pro can catalog the folder with an album of thumbnail images and suitable key words to search the folder. This allows easy retrieval of the images when you go to this folder again. The most frustrating thing is to spend hours looking for that picture one took a year ago. Window ME and Windows 2000 also provide the thumbnail and catalog feature without additional software.

What Other Cameras Are Suitable?

The Kodak, Nikon, and Sony are all cameras with similar resolution. Other options available are the digital video cameras (Canon or Sony) that capture both video and still images. These images may be downloaded quickly with firewire (IEEE 1394) connection to the computer. Software is available that allows capture and editing of the images. The pictures from the video camera are not as a high in resolution as from the still camera. If one needs 35-mm high-quality pictures to publish at 4×6 inch size, one will need to have at least a $2,000 \times 3,000$ pixel image at 300 dpi.

The essentials that one needs in a digital camera are as follows:

- High resolution
- Close-up or macro capabilities
- Zoom lens
- Removal flash cards or high-speed transfer with firewire

Is the picture quality the same as that of a slide from a 35-mm camera? No, but it is sufficient for most orthopaedic applications. Figures 3.6 and 3.7 are examples of an intraoperative photograph and a radiograph, respectively, both taken with the Olympus digital camera.

Scanners

I use a flatbed scanner to scan large photographs. The photograph is acquired by PhotoShop, is manipulated by the program, and is saved as a jpeg. For most applications, I scan at 75 dpi. If I am going to a printer, then 300 dpi is necessary.

I also use a Canon slide scanner to scan my favorite clinical slides into the same PhotoShop program. These slides are named and saved in the appropriate folder on my server hard drive. The Nikon slide scanner is faster, but more expensive. The Canon connects on a fast scsi connection. The parallel port connection scanners are too slow. Again, I use the same scan rates as with the flatbed scanner. The higher scan rates make a large file, such as 15 megabytes. These are difficult to manipulate and to send to other users.

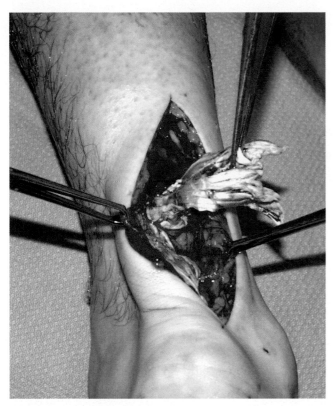

FIGURE 3.6 A digital photograph of an Achilles tendon tear taken during the operative procedure.

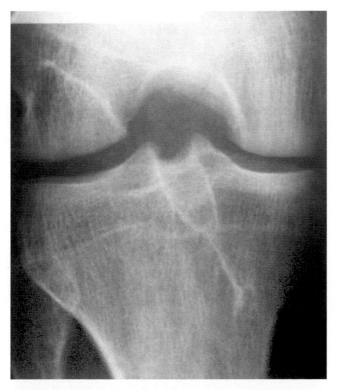

FIGURE 3.7 A digital anteroposterior radiographic photograph taken from the view box of a follow-up anterior cruciate ligament reconstruction with semitendinosus. These images are of sufficient detail to visualize the pathologic features.

Printers

The high quality of photographs from the inexpensive ink jet printers is hard to beat. The current recommendation is the Hewlett Packard ink jet printer. The ink jet printer is very versatile, printing out thumbnail images, 4 × 6 inch prints for publication, or high-resolution 8 × 10 inch color prints (Fig. 3.8).

The photographic representation of chondral disorders is much more dramatic than a text description. This hard copy can be inserted into the patient's chart for easy reference in follow-up.

The dye sublimation printer from Olympus allows one to print a 4 × 6 inch glossy print directly from the camera or the computer. The prints cost about $1 each.

To print a photograph larger than 4 × 6 inches, one will need to have a high-resolution image, at least 300 dpi. The image size and resolution can be checked with photographic editing programs such as PhotoShop.

File Formats

Many file formats can be used for still digital photos. The compressed jpeg format is the most versatile. It produces a small file size. One can use it on Web pages, word documents, and PowerPoint; however, the quality of the image is hard to distinguish on computer monitors. If printing large 4 × 6 inch or even 8 × 10 inch prints is desired, then one should save the file in .bmp or .tiff format at high resolution—300 dpi.

Arthroscopy Image Capture

The capture of still images and video is controlled by the buttons on the arthroscopy camera head. The surgeon is able to acquire and to edit the images on the fly during the procedure (Fig. 3.9).

A Linvatec (Linvatec Corp., Largo, FL) digital capture system can be used to acquire photographs from the arthroscopic camera at the time of the surgical procedure. These photographs are saved in bmp format on a zip drive, which is then transferred to the computer in the same fashion as the camera flash cards. Both Linvatec and Stryker offer systems to integrate the capture of arthroscopy images from their digital camera systems. These images may also be dropped into a templated operative note. The printers that come with most arthroscopy systems can be used to print the arthroscopy images from the computer.

What Are Some Uses for these Digital Images?

- Insert them in electronic files of the operative report, such as Notematic electronic chart (Fig. 3.10).
- Print a hard copy for the patient file (see the RecRoom file in Fig. 3.8).

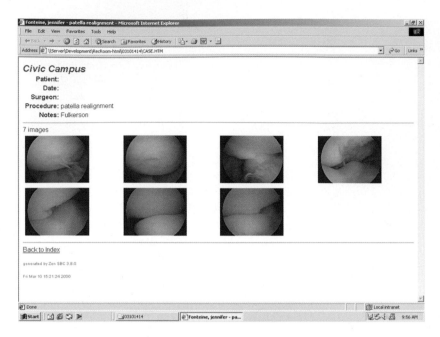

FIGURE 3.8 This is the print sheet using RecRoom for the patient with patellofemoral disease.

- Use them in presentations such as PowerPoint.
- Insert them in FrontPage for a Web site.
- Post the images to Web sites for discussion of orthopaedic problems.
- E-mail the image to colleagues for opinions and exchange of ideas.
- Use them to illustrate articles (in Word documents).
- Make a slide show using an LCD projector for rounds.

File System

The first step is to have a well-organized computer hard drive. After one starts to collect some images, one will want to retrieve them easily. It is best to start by giving the image a name that identifies the slide. For example, with the arthroscopy slides, one can name the images, acl_chronic_tear_1. This is then put it in a folder called arthroscopy and a subfolder called ACL. When one opens the folder, all the photographs of chronic tears appear in the same position. More temporary folders, called "new," are used to download digital images that are collected during the day and require editing. After these images are edited, they are moved to the appropriate folder.

This file directory is the mirror of a LAN server, where the pictures are ultimately stored. The other storage mediums, such as zip and jaz disks, as well as CD-ROMs, are fine initially, but they quickly run out of space. It is difficult to wade through many disks to find the appropriate image. A good solution is to connect all the computers together with a local area network using PCMCIA cards on the laptop and internal cards on the desktop. A large 100-gigabyte NT server, with a tape backup, then becomes the final storage bin.

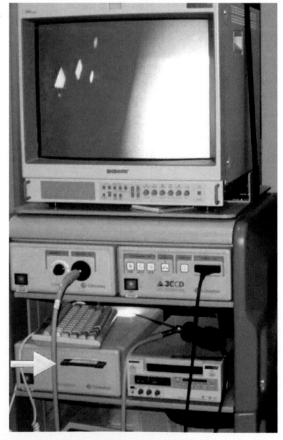

FIGURE 3.9 The arthroscopy stack with the still image capture on the *second row left* and the video capture on the *second row right.*

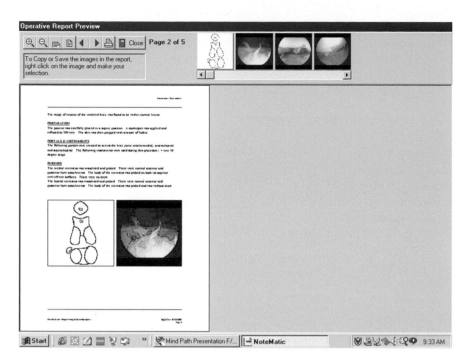

FIGURE 3.10 This is an example of a Notematic electronic chart with a text description of the procedure with images and drawings inserted into the appropriate sites.

File Directory

The file directory for the arthroscopy images and the radiographs are mirrored on the laptop and the server. In Windows 2000 and Windows ME, the images in the folder can be viewed as thumbnails. With earlier versions of windows, one should use ACDSee (ACD Systems, Ltd.) to view the thumbnail images quickly. For more detailed cataloging of images with key words to search the folder, one should use Image Access Pro (Fig. 3.11).

Digital Video

What are we trying to do and where are we trying to go? The ultimate is to have one box (CPU) that captures still arthroscopy images, arthroscopy video, outside still images, and outside video. The download from the cameras should be fast, and firewire fits the specifications. The digital images are processed, edited, and stored for use in presentations and patient–physician education CDs. Several new innovations are on the market. The ideal is to have a turnkey box with all

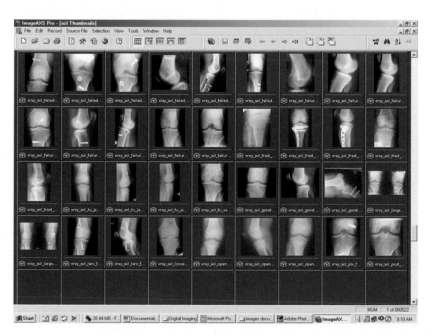

FIGURE 3.11 The contents of the radiographic anterior cruciate ligament folder displayed with Image Access Pro.

the peripherals and accessories configured and ready to go. The most complex topic is the video capture. The old analog VHS worked well compared with the glitches encountered with digital video acquisition and editing.

Sony Notebooks and Cameras

The ultraslim notebook allows one to input the still digital photographs and video into the Sony laptop. Sony has made a commitment to the consumer market with this digital studio capture and editing program loaded on a desktop computer. With firewire, one can capture both still images and digital video. This can be edited with the software, Adobe Premier, which is already loaded onto the computer. The advantages of this system are that the firewire card is factory installed, hence IRQ conflicts are avoided, and the software is compatible. With the Sony system, the digital video can be recorded from the outside view in the room with the Sony TRV900 triple-chip video camera. This camera can also be connected to the arthroscopy camera with a S-video cable to the input of the camera. Now everything can be digitally recorded (both outside and inside view). With the Sony Viao desktop PC, video clips can be produced in both .avi and mpeg compression for use in PowerPoint presentations. Adobe Premier is the editing program that requires one more learning curve. In spite of the time commitment needed to learn how to use the software, this is the most cost-effective method for digital editing. This is labor intensive and not the for the casual video production to give to the patient. The mpeg format is a compression of the large files: mpeg 2 is full-screen DVD-quality video; mpeg 4 is compression for streaming on the Internet.

REFERENCES

1. Johnson LL. Creating the proper environment for arthroscopic surgery. *Orthop Clin North Am* 1982;13:283.
2. McGinty JB. *Operative arthroscopy.* New York: Raven Press, 1991.
3. Wetchler BV. *Anesthesia for ambulatory surgery.* Philadelphia: JB Lippincott, 1985.
4. Jackson RW. Memories of the early days of arthroscopy: 1965–1975. The formative years. *Arthroscopy* 1987;3:1–3.
5. Rosenberg TD, Wong HC. Arthroscopic knee surgery in a free-standing outpatient surgery center. *Orthop Clin North Am* 1982;13:277.
6. Davis JE, Detmer DE. The ambulatory surgical unit. *Ann Surg* 1972;175:856–859.
7. Small NC. *Office operative arthroscopy.* New York: Raven Press, 1994.
8. Small NC, Glogau AI, Berezin MA, et al. Office operative arthroscopy of the knee: technical considerations and a preliminary analysis of the first one-hundred patients. *Arthroscopy* 1994;10:534–539.
9. LoCicero J III, Nichols RL. Environmental health hazards in the operating room. American College of Surgeons director's memo, May 1982 bulletin.
10. *Procedures for operation of steam autoclave.* Northwest Community Hospital, Arlington Heights, IL.

Operative Arthroscopy, third edition. Edited by John B. McGinty, Stephen S. Burkhart, Robert W. Jackson, Donald H. Johnson, and John C. Richmond.
Lippincott Williams & Wilkins © 2003.

ARTHROSCOPIC INSTRUMENTATION

E. MARLOWE GOBLE
SUMANT G. KRISHNAN

In open surgical procedures, properly designed instruments enable the surgeon to complete the surgical mission successfully. Surgical implants usually demand the most professional attention, and implants represent the greatest cost. Indeed, implant manufacturers often give the instruments as a gift to the hospital and recover their costs in the sale of the implant.

Conversely, minimally invasive surgery, such as arthroscopy, is as dependent on sophisticated instrumentation as it is on the design of the implants. If one considers a bullet as an implant and the rifle as the instrument responsible for implanting the bullet, then the metaphor will explain the arthroscopic relation of instrument to implant.

INSTRUMENTATION

The use of an arthroscope enables the surgeon to complete minimally invasive surgical procedures. Many of these arthroscopic and endoscopic procedures will, in time, replace conventional open operative techniques. For example, anterior cruciate ligament (ACL) and posterior cruciate ligament reconstructions have become outpatient procedures because of the development of instrumentation that, in concert with the arthroscope, permits precise surgery, with minimal insult to surrounding soft tissues. Similarly, repair of osteochondral defects, resection or repair of menisci, synovectomy, removal of osteophytes and loose bodies, and meniscal transplantation are knee procedures performed with minimal iatrogenic invasion through the use of the arthroscope and its instrumentation. Bankart repair for anterior instability of the shoulder, rotator cuff repair, and chondral and labral resection or repair are now often completed as arthroscopic procedures, each with its own unique instrumentation.

E. M. Goble: Department of Orthopedic Surgery, University of Utah—SLC, Salt Lake City, Utah.

S. G. Krishnan: Shoulder Service, W. B. Carrell Memorial Clinic, Dallas, Texas.

Afflictions of the small joints of the body are increasingly approached by arthroscopy. Arthroscopic carpal ligament repair and fusion are becoming increasingly popular. Endoscopic carpal tunnel release is now standard. Arthroscopic ankle fusion is an alternative to conventional open surgical procedures. These minimally invasive procedures optimize the advantages of arthroscopy and its associated specialized instrumentation, with a minimum of skin, soft tissue, and vascular insults.

Arthroscopic visualization into otherwise inaccessible space only serves to define the problem; it is left to the design of procedure-specific instrumentation to permit surgical success.

This chapter introduces those arthroscopic instruments required to complete successfully most arthroscopic procedures requiring debridement or repair of intraarticular disease. Procedures demanding ligament reconstruction, soft tissue transplantation, or osteochondral fixation require implants highly dependent on sophisticated arthroscopic instrumentation.

ARTHROSCOPIC PROCEDURES

Arthroscopic procedures either (a) resect soft tissue or bone or (b) repair soft tissue or bone. The former is accomplished with arthroscopic instruments; the latter involves the installation of implants within the joint.

Because the instruments associated with implants are often more important and more sophisticated than the implant they leave behind, it is as pointless to discuss the implant without the instruments as it is to explain the bullet without the rifle. The greatest development of advanced arthroscopic instrumentation (instrument-implant systems) has occurred in association with the knee and shoulder joints. Similar smaller and larger systems have been developed for the elbow, wrist, ankle, and hip, respectively. The shoulder and knee are addressed preferentially.

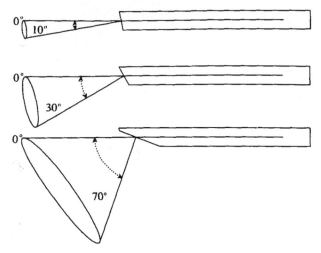

FIGURE 4.1 Varying angles of inclination commonly found in arthroscopes.

ARTHROSCOPES

Fiberoptic technology, the use of magnifying lenses, and television monitor advancements have allowed for the development and expansion in use of the modern arthroscope. Arthroscopes are currently available in various diameters, lengths, and angles of inclination. Arthroscopic diameters range from 2.7 to 7.5 mm and find their appropriate use depending on the size of space to be visualized. The inclination angle of the distal arthroscopic lens, which varies from 10 to 120 degrees, allows for a greater ranger of visualization, through rotation of the arthroscope within a joint space (Fig. 4.1). For example, a 70-degree scope allows for examination of 140 degrees of the operative field when the arthroscope is rotated 180 degrees. However, more than 90% of all arthroscopic procedures are performed using the 30-degree arthroscope (Fig. 4.2).

PROBES

Perhaps the most commonly used arthroscopic instrument is the simple probe. A curved tip at the distal end of a probe allows for evaluation of the extent of meniscal damage, the laxity of ligamentous structures, and the grading and sizing of chondromalacia.

SHOULDER INSTRUMENTATION

Acromial and soft tissue impingement, shoulder instability, and rotator cuff tears are primarily approached arthroscopically by today's advanced shoulder surgeon. Arthroscopic shoulder instrumentation enables the surgeon to perform this minimally invasive, yet precise, surgical objective.

It is more meaningful to relate the surgical objective to arthroscopic instrument and implant design than simply to discuss an instrument or implant. Therefore, the surgical procedures and the instruments are discussed in relation to each other.

Subacromial Decompression

This procedure requires uniquely designed (a) instrument cannulas and (b) bone resection burs and cannulas.

Shoulder Cannulas

Arthroscopic cannulas are plastic or metal sleeves of varying diameter (4 to 8 mm) that are designed to create and maintain an instrument portal (access from skin to joint) (Fig. 4.3). Cannulas are forced through the layers of soft tissue by the penetrating action of a pointed trocar inserted inside the cannula. The trocar is removed. A fluid-impenetrable plastic or silicone dam prevents loss of fluid and permits the introduction of instruments equal to the size of the inside diameter of the cannula. Unique threads or extruding shelves prevent "pushout" of these cannulas.

Bone Resection Burs

Metal burs, containing rotating cutting edges, are used to remove bone from the underside of the acromion (Fig. 4.4). These burs are either round or oval. They vary in diameter from 4 to 6 mm. Cutting speed is adjustable from 1,500 to

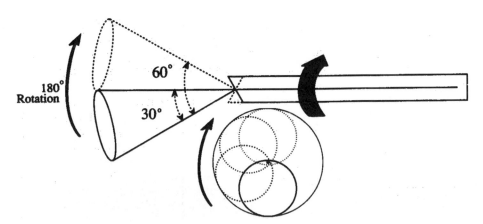

FIGURE 4.2 Increasing field of view with rotation in a 30° arthroscope. (Scope rotation, axial view.)

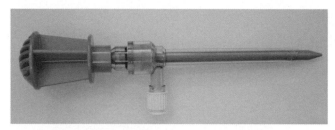

FIGURE 4.3 A shoulder cannula providing easy insertion and removal of instruments, while damming intraarticular (distention) fluids. (Courtesy of Arthrex, Inc.)

6,000 rpm. Removal of acromion bone usually requires an oval-shaped bur 4 to 6 mm in diameter, applied to the bone at high speed. The round bur is used for bone site preparation or osteophyte removal.

Treatment of Glenohumeral Instability and Rotator Cuff Injuries

These shoulder procedures may each require reattachment of soft tissue to bone. Suture anchors and their instrumentation have made repairs from soft tissue to bone arthroscopically possible.

Suture Anchors

The first suture anchor used to treat shoulder instability was developed in 1985 (Statac, Zimmer, Inc.). Today, suture anchors can be divided into four general categories: threaded, barbed, expanding, and rotating.

An example of a threaded suture anchor is the Statac (Fig. 4.5). This "screw" with attached suture is driven into bone by a long screwdriver, the center of which contains the free ends of the suture. The driver (a long, cannulated screwdriver) is removed, leaving the free ends of the sutures exiting the mouth of the cannula. The suture is now fitted with a curved needle and is inserted through the avulsed soft tissue. The soft tissue is reattached to its exact bony origin, that is, the location of the suture anchor.

The Mitek (Johnson & Johnson) suture anchor represents the barbed-type suture anchor (Fig. 4.6). The bone is predrilled, and the nitinol-barbed anchor is pressed into the predrilled hole. The attached sutures are then used in the same manner as described earlier for the threaded suture anchor. The ROC by Mitek represents an expanding, osseous compression suture anchor (Fig. 4.7). This plastic anchor is bioabsorbable.

Stryker has developed a bioabsorbable rotation suture anchor (Fig. 4.8). The anchor is inserted into a predrilled hole. A tug on the suture rotates and secures the anchor into the sidewalls of the 3.5-mm hole. Pullout of this simple design exceeds suture strength by a factor of ten. All suture anchor insertion depends on protective cannulas, disposable drivers or inserters, and arthroscopic needle drivers or suture punches, the design of which is at least as sophisticated as the implant.

The Caspari suture punch (Fig. 4.9) leads the field of jaw and teeth–type soft tissue punches. These soft tissue punches deliver a suture through the punched-out hole. The suture can then be tied to the suture anchor site.

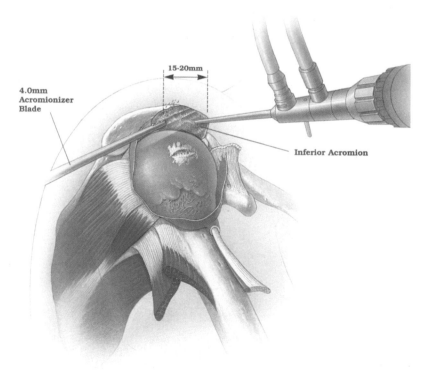

4.0mm
Acromionizer
Blade

15-20mm

Inferior Acromion

FIGURE 4.4 Acromionizer blade. (Courtesy of Smith & Nephew, Inc.)

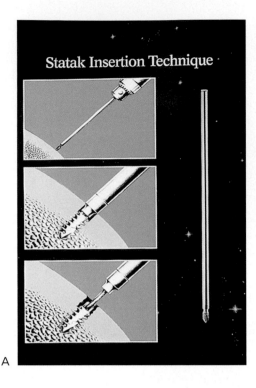

Statak Insertion Technique

A

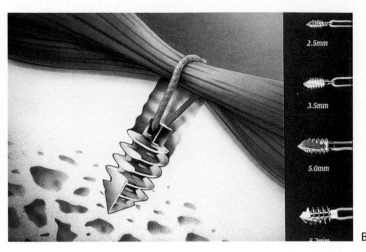

2.5mm

3.5mm

5.0mm

B

FIGURE 4.5 Threaded suture anchor. This self-tapping screw is driven into bone by a disposable driver. Only sutures are exposed from bone. These sutures are fitted with needles, to permit soft tissue reattachment to bone. (Courtesy of Zimmer, Inc.)

Knot pushers are required to advance slipknots and half-hitches through a cannula to the repair site (Fig. 4.10). Typically, a throw of a knot is made outside the joint. The throw is then pushed down to the attachment site by a cupped trocar inside a long, narrow tube. The surgeon holds tension on one arm of the suture as numerous throws are pushed to the repair site to create a compound, nonreleasing knot. The de-

velopment of knot pushers has permitted a minimally invasive surgical approach to target areas of the body.

Thermal Instrumentation

Hippocrates first documented the use of thermal energy in an orthopaedic procedure during treatment of gleno-

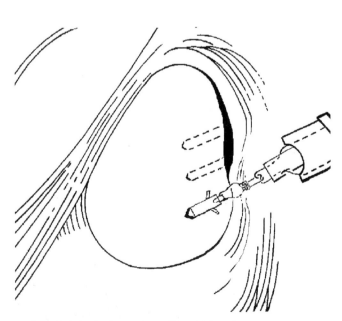

FIGURE 4.6 Barbed suture anchor. Nitinol barbs secure the suture anchor to bone. (Courtesy of Mitek, Inc.)

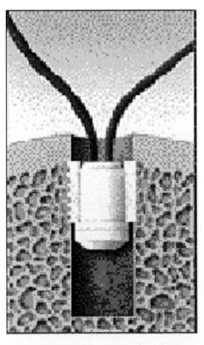

FIGURE 4.7. Expanding suture anchor. The ROC expands to provide compression within the predrilled bone hole. (Courtesy of Mitek, Inc.)

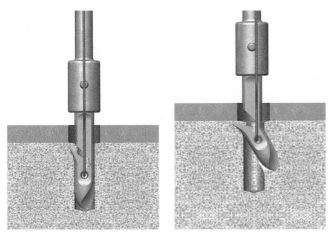

FIGURE 4.8 Rotating suture anchor. The implant rotates when the suture is tensioned, thus securing the anchor within cancellous bone. (Courtesy of Stryker, Inc.)

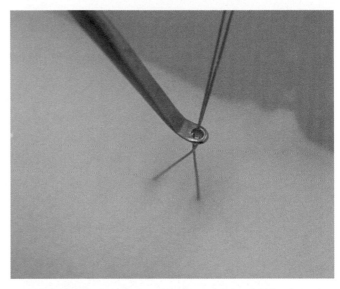

FIGURE 4.10 Knot pushers. After the suture anchor has been implanted, and the soft tissue is penetrated by the suture, a knot pusher delivers any number of throws of a knot through the barrel of the soft tissue cannula. (Courtesy of Arthrex, Inc.)

humeral instability with a heated iron in the axillae (1). Today, the use of thermal energy in the form of lasers, radiofrequency, and electrical thermal devices has provided yet another means for arthroscopic treatment of soft tissue and articular cartilage injuries.

The holmium:yttrium-aluminum-garnet (Ho:YAG) laser, Oratec Vulcan (Oratec Interventions), Mitek VAPR (Mitek Products, Johnson & Johnson), and Arthrocare Arthrowand (Arthrocare Corp.) are several of the current commercially available arthroscopic instruments. These involve laser (Ho:YAG), monopolar radiofrequency (Oratec),

monopolar electrical (Arthrocare), or bipolar electrical (Mitek) thermal energy.

KNEE INSTRUMENTATION

Advanced instrumentation and implant systems have made the arthroscopic approach the surgical method of choice for meniscal repair, meniscal resection, meniscal transplantation, ACL and posterior cruciate ligament reconstruction, cartilage repair, and osteochondral graft transplantation.

Anterior Cruciate Ligament Reconstruction

Modern ACL instrumentation sets include the following:

1. A tibial drill guide: anteromedial tibia to tibial ACL footprint (Fig. 4.11A and B)
2. Notchplasty gouges to resect up to 12 mm of bone from the superior and lateral notch of the femur
3. Cannulated tunnel drills (Fig. 4.11C)

A characteristic of all drills designed for use in arthroscopic surgery is cannulation. Drill points and shafts are gun-drilled (center core removed) to accommodate a guide wire. A guide wire (usually 00.030 to 0.060 inch in diameter) can be precisely drilled within the intraarticular space. This precision permits exact targeting of osteochondral fragments, origins of ligaments, and other bony drilling requirements within a joint.

The preplaced guide wire is overdrilled with the cannulated drill, thus tracking the drill in a predetermined path.

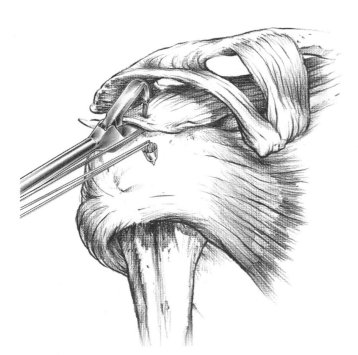

FIGURE 4.9 Suture punch. When loaded with a suture, this instrument implants the suture through a needle hole in soft tissue. (Courtesy of Linvatec, Inc.)

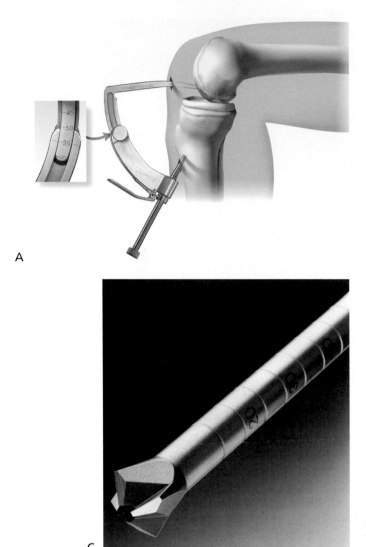

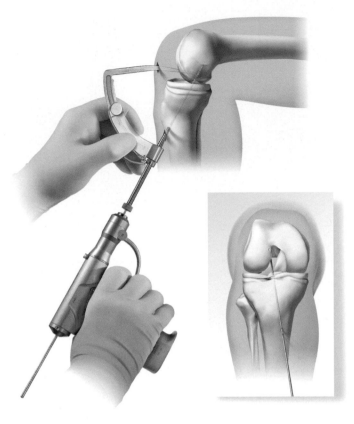

FIGURE 4.11 A–C: Tibial drill guide. This guide delivers a Kirschner wire from the anteromedial tibia to the tibial insertion site of the anterior cruciate ligament. The Kirschner wire will then be overdrilled by cannulated drills. (Courtesy of Linvatec, Inc.)

This controlled system of intraarticular drilling avoids errors, by preventing drill "walking,' magnification distortion (by the scope), and uncontrolled migration of the drill, which may occur as the drill point engages different bone densities along the intended path.

Bone drills may be categorized into one of three designs:

1. Fluted or auger drills
2. End reamers
3. Spade drills

Fluted drills have an end-cutting relief angle, which cuts off bone fragments that are in contact with the point angle. A fluted groove spirals down the drill shaft, beginning at the drill point. The functions of the spiral flute are to unload bone chips from cutting tip and to funnel those chips down the flute, thus keeping the cutting tip free of bone. Without the fluting, bone chips fill the tip of the drill and prevent further cutting of bone. Impacted bone chips at the cutting tip of a drill cause increased friction and heat generation, which may result in bone necrosis. If a drill becomes excessively heated while drilling, one should check the flutes for impacted bone and ensure that the cutting edge of the drill point is sharp. A potential problem with the fluted design is that the spiral flutes may self-advance the drill if not resisted, and drill point contact with osteoporotic bone or soft tissue will allow unmeasured penetration of the drill with each clockwise rotation.

An end reamer (4.11C) is an end-cutting drill point without flutes. Bone chips are ground up and are pushed forward, ahead of the drill. It is much easier to "load up" the cutting points of the reamer than a fluted drill or head indicates a loaded tip and the reamer must be cleared of bone chips before continuing.

The advantage of a reamer is that shaft diameter can be reduced significantly. A reduced diameter drill shaft (e.g., 5 mm) carrying a full-sized reamer head (e.g., 11 mm) can drill through both bones of a joint and can maintain the ability to deviate the axis of a second tunnel relative to the first. A reamer does not self-advance, and it must be pushed forward with force supplied by the surgeon.

A spade drill is an efficient drill design used commonly in a machine shop. The drill tip cuts very efficiently and manages to unload bone chips because of the rectangular spade shape of the drill head. The sides of the spade and the drill point itself are less prone to injure soft tissue, unlike the fluted drill. Additionally, clockwise (right-handed) drilling does not self-advance the drill. The shaft of the spade drill can be reduced similar to an end reamer. The efficiency of the bone cutting, the effective removal of bone chips from the cutting edge, the non–self-advancing design, the atraumatic (to soft tissue) cutting tip and skirts of the spade, and the ability to reduce the shaft diameter make the spade drill a popular arthroscopic drill.

1. Femoral drill guides are inserted through the tibial tunnel, pass across the joint, and reference the posterior cortex between the femoral condyles (Fig. 4.12). A femoral guide wire can then be drilled into the femur by accessing this guide.
2. The U-shaped cross-pin drill guide (Fig. 4.13) references the femoral tunnel to permit a right-angle approach to the femoral tunnel for insertion of a cross pin or set screw.
3. In cannulated interference (Fig. 4.14), the ACL graft is most commonly secured within the recipient tunnel with

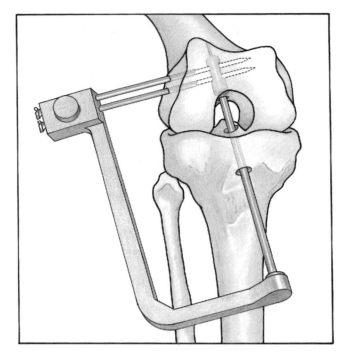

FIGURE 4.13 Cross-pin drill guide. This guide permits a right-angle approach to the anterior cruciate ligament (ACL) femoral tunnel. Cross pins or set screws can be inserted to secure the ACL graft. (Courtesy of Arthrotec, Inc.)

a cannulated interference screw. This threaded screw follows a Kirschner wire alongside the ACL graft within the bony tunnel. The threads of the screw compress and purchase both graft and tunnel wall and secure the ACL graft to bone.

4. The cross-pinned interference screw (Fig. 4.15) guide references standard interference screw to permit right-angle cross pinning of interference screw and adjacent bone block.
5. With the cannulated cross-pin screw (Fig. 4.16), hamstring ACL grafts are looped over the right-angle inserted, proximally threaded screw, to secure the ACL graft within the femoral tunnel.
6. The tensioning device (Fig. 4.17) measures tension applied to the graft at the tibial tunnel exit; it maintains graft tension while the tibial fixation device is applied to graft.

An interference screw fixes a graft to the (opposite) walls of the tunnel by cutting a "flight-of-thread" path between the graft and the tunnel and in line with the long axis of the graft (Fig. 4.14). The guide wire inserted along the side of the graft predetermines the insertion path of the screw. The guide pin, which the screw must follow once it is inserted through its central cannulation, prevents deviation of the screw into the softer bone of the tunnel wall. The guide pin also allows blind connection between the screw and the cannulated driver.

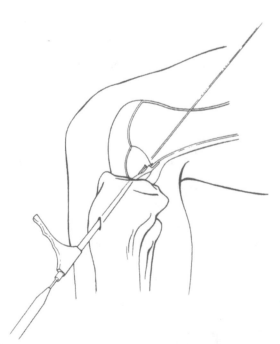

FIGURE 4.12 Femoral drill guide. The Kirschner wire is delivered into the posterior femur through this cannulated guide, which references the posterior cortex of the femur. (Courtesy of Arthrex, Inc.)

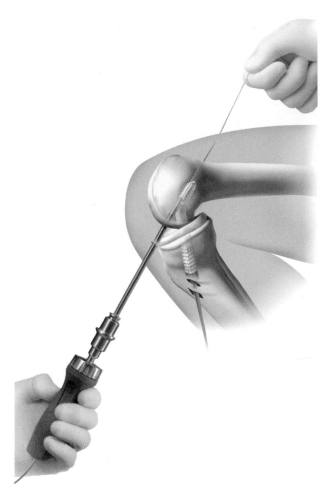

FIGURE 4.14 Cannulated interference screw. This anterior cruciate ligament (ACL) fixation screw is inserted alongside the ACL graft in line with the axis of the graft. (Courtesy of Linvatec, Inc.)

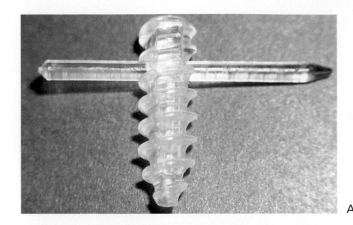

A

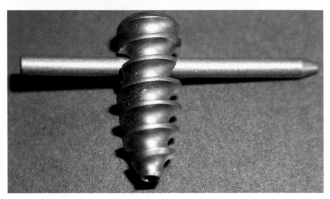

B

FIGURE 4.15 Cross-pinned interference screw: an interference screw with a right-angle hole through the midbody of the screw. A pin can be inserted (by use of a special guide) across the tunnel wall, screw, and anterior cruciate ligament (ACL) graft. This cross pinning further secures the ACL graft to bone in the presence of "less-dense" tibial bone. (Courtesy of Stryker, Inc.)

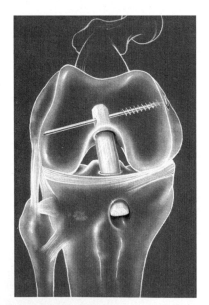

FIGURE 4.16 Cannulated cross-pin screw. This hamstring anterior cruciate ligament graft fixation screw has a smooth distal barrel that allows the graft to loop over within the femoral tunnel. (Courtesy of E. Marlowe Goble, MD)

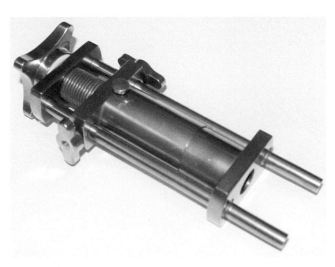

FIGURE 4.17 Anterior cruciate ligament (ACL) ligament tensioning device. This tension-measuring machine is attached to two pins at the exit to the tibial tunnel. The tibial end of the ACL graft is attached to this machine (with sutures). From 10 to 20 lb of tension is applied to the ACL graft before the graft is fixed to the tibia. (Courtesy of Stryker, Inc.)

The cannulated cross pin depends on its instrument, that is, the guide wire, to permit proper position of this ACL fixation device. This cross pin secures the ACL graft at a right angle to the long axis of the graft (Fig. 4.16).

Microfracture Awl

Articular cartilage may avulse from its underlying subchondral bone. If the lesion is less than 3 × 2 cm, an osteochondral transplant can be performed. If a larger lesion exists, the bone can be "picked" or drilled to elicit a subchondral repair process resulting in a fibrocartilage covering (Fig. 4.18). Sharp-pointed (ice) picks have been developed to create lesions about 3 mm apart.

Osteochondral Graft Transplant

Arthex and Mitek have developed similar kits for removal of bone and cartilage plugs (from the edge of the lateral femoral sulcus) to be pressed into holes prepared at the subchondral defect (Fig. 4.19). The 15-mm long bone and cartilage plugs, varying from 5 to 9 mm in diameter, are removed with sharp, round cutting tubes. After the recipient defect site is prepared by removing a bone plug of similar size, the graft is tapped into the hole to a level equal to the surrounding normal cartilage. The disposable cutting tubes come in 1-mm increments, from 5 to 9 mm in diameter.

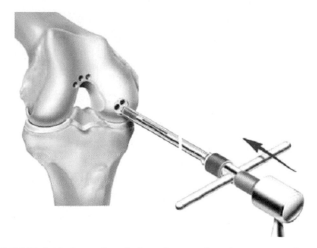

FIGURE 4.19 Osteochondral graft transplant instruments. Bone and cartilage plugs are transferred from a less critical donor site to a weight-bearing recipient site devoid of cartilage. (Courtesy of Arthrex, Inc.)

Meniscal Instrumentation

Meniscal Repair

Suture repair remains the most reliable and least abrasive (to articular cartilage) method to repair a meniscal tear. Many resorbable plastic darts, arrows, and screws have been developed to overcome the significant problem of suture repair, that is, the need to penetrate all soft tissue planes from skin to meniscus, to tie a secure knot, thus joining both surfaces of the meniscal tear.

The zone-specific (Fig. 4.20) cannulated needle driver system consists of various curved cannulas, each shape de-

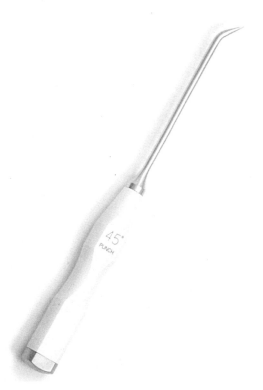

FIGURE 4.18 Microfracture awl. Exposed subchondral bone is "injured" to induce fibroblasts to repair the cartilage defect. (Courtesy of Linvatec, Inc.)

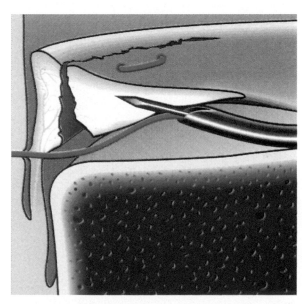

FIGURE 4.20 Zone-specific meniscal repair system, the most popular method of delivering "inside-out" sutures to a torn meniscus. The disadvantage of full-penetration sutures is fixation of tissue planes peripheral to the meniscus. (Courtesy of Linvatec, Inc.)

signed to approach a specific zone of meniscus. The curved tubular cannula is introduced through a parapatellar portal. Under arthroscopic visualization, the beveled tip of the cannula is guided to the central edge of the meniscal tear. One arm of a pair of long, slender needles, joined by a suture, is urged through the curving cannula. The sharp tip of the needle penetrates the two parts of the torn meniscus and then exits through the skin adjacent to the tear. The second arm of the needle pair is now passed through the same cannula and is inserted through the meniscal tear about 10 mm distal from the first. Both needles are pulled firm, thus advancing the horizontal mattress suture. The sutures are tied over deep fascia, to secure the tear.

Meniscal Resection

Meniscal tears not amenable to repair can be resected with handheld meniscal punches (Fig. 4.21) and power shavers. Hand cutting forceps systems contain seven basic direction instruments varying in size between 3 and 5 mm (cross section). A typical kit contains the following necessary forceps and graspers:

1. Small (3 mm) and large (5 mm) straight forceps
2. Small (3 mm) and larger (5 mm) 30-degree up-biter forceps (This instrument is useful to negotiate under the curvature of the femoral condyle or humeral head to reach the meniscus of labrum without injuring the articular cartilage within the joint.)

3. Right and left curved forceps (4 or 5 mm)
4. Right- and left-angle basket cutter (5 mm)
5. Back biter (5 mm) (This allows one to cut back 180 degrees. This instrument is especially designed for debriding the anterior horn region.)
6. Suction grasper and basket cutter
7. Grabber-graspers

Knives

The use of knives is often essential in the completion of an arthroscopic procedure (Fig. 4.22). These arthroscopic knives can be divided into three basic styles featuring side-cutting, forward-cutting, or backward-cutting blades. This diversity allows for resection or division of tissue from nearly all angles of access. Currently, disposable knives constitute the most dependable and economical cutting instruments.

Power Tools

Power shavers consist of a rotating knife housed within a close tolerance tube. The end of the tube has a window, round or oval, which permits exposure of the knife. Suction pulls tissue into the window. The rotation knife amputates the soft tissue at the interface of the tube and the knife. Dyonics first introduced this handheld power shaver. Dyonics 4.5-mm Orbit Incision (Fig. 4.23) is an example of a shaver designed for cutting meniscus. The Orbit Synovator is a nonserrated edged cutter used for the removal of synovium.

Power shavers vary in size from 3.5 to 5 mm. The blades are usually disposable and come in straight or curved designs. The speed of resection varies from 80 to 1,500 rpm or more. The slower speeds are often more useful for resecting soft tissues, and oscillation of the blade is a good feature of some shavers. Both single-use and multiuse blades are available, but blades do become dull with use and must be replaced at intervals. Shaver and bur reusability is an issue in

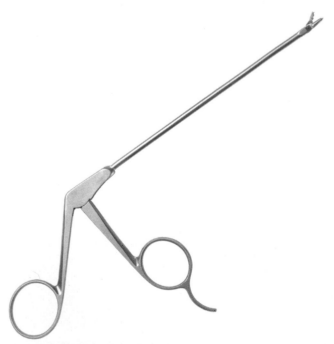

FIGURE 4.21 Meniscal punches. These hard instruments vary in size from 4 to 6 mm. The barrel can be curved lateral or upward. The sharp cutting edge of each punch permits precise cutting of all meniscal borders. (Courtesy of Linvatec, Inc.)

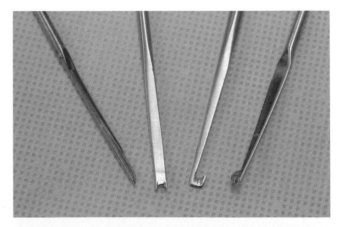

FIGURE 4.22 Arthroscopic knives. Each knife is designed to cut different types of intraarticular soft tissue. This soft tissue includes menisci, synovium, capsule, and articular cartilage.

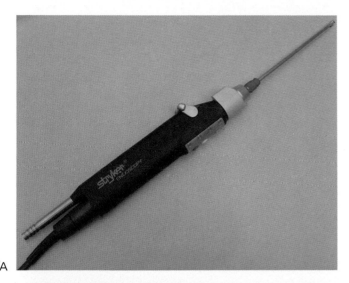

A

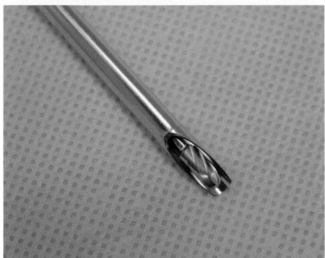

B

FIGURE 4.23 A and **B:** A sharp-edged rotating knife cuts soft tissue as it is sucked into the window of a closely toleranced stationary housing. The rotating knife is controlled by a power source. This power source causes the knife to rotate clockwise or counterclockwise or to oscillate back and forth. (Courtesy of Stryker, Inc.)

cost containment. Most commercially available shavers and burs are not recommended by their manufacturer for multiple use, although it is common knowledge that they are frequently used for more than one procedure. Some companies have stated that their shavers may be resterilized and used up to a recommended maximum of five times.

Burs are generally operated at higher speeds and are used for removing bony osteophytes, for performing notchplasties, and for decompressing the subacromial space. The performance of a specific shaver-bur-pump system largely depends on its intended use and on the skill of the surgeon. Not all shaver-bur instrumentation systems are identical in performance or cost; a thorough evaluation of each system should be made before purchase.

Meniscal Transplantation

Meniscal transplantation instruments permit anatomic installation of the two horns of an allograft meniscus into a meniscal deficient recipient. Arthrex supplies a keyhole design, and Cryolife supplies a precision gouge instrumentation set (Fig. 4.24). Each is equally effective in assisting in the proper positioning of the transplant in this demanding surgical exercise.

SPECIALTY INSTRUMENTATION

Several procedure-specific instruments are now commonplace within the practice of arthroscopic surgery, and they include zone-specific meniscal repair suture cannulas, suture punches (Fig. 4.5), arthroscopic suture tying sheaths, arthroscopic cautery extensions and thermal devices, soft tissue rasps, and various suture anchor devices. A critical review of each of these devices is beyond the scope of this chapter; however, one should become familiar with the differences, uses, and capabilities of each design before the purchase of a specialty item. For example, multiple types of arthroscopic knot pushers have been developed, including slotted, single-hole, double-hole, and mechanical spreader designs. Single-hole and slotted knot pushers have the disadvantage of hiding a twist in the suture ends, which could interfere with knot seating. This problem may be eliminated through the use of a two-hole knot pusher.

Leg Holders

Leg holders have become a useful and time-honored device in knee arthroscopy. Holding the thigh well secured in the leg holder and applying varus or valgus stress allow for visualization of what is, in many cases, an important additional few millimeters in both the medial and lateral compartments of the knee. Currently, several well-designed and functional leg holders are commercially available. No matter what type of leg holder is selected, one must pay attention to establishing a well-padded leg–thigh holder interface, to distribute pressure over a larger area and to prevent tissue damage.

Pumps

Commercially available pump systems greatly enhance the surgeon's ability to carry out many arthroscopic procedures. The advantages of a fluid pump over a gravity-controlled system include a greater ability to control the intraarticular pressure, as well as an increased capacity for high fluid flow rates. For example, during a ligamentous reconstruction of the knee, a low volume pressure is preferable to decrease excessive fluid, losses through bone tunnels, or enlarged arthroscopic portals. Conversely, subacromial decompression may require increased pressure to visualize the subacromial com-

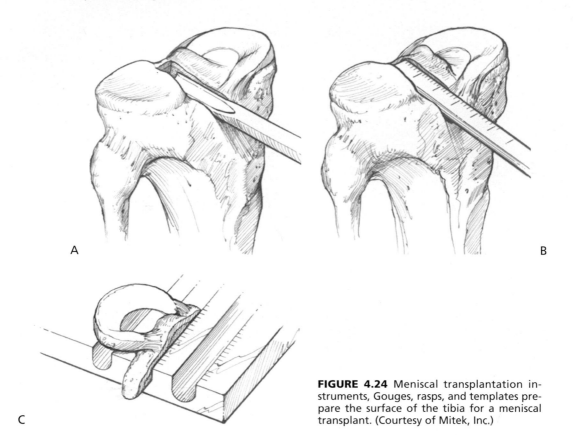

A

B

C

FIGURE 4.24 Meniscal transplantation instruments, Gouges, rasps, and templates prepare the surface of the tibia for a meniscal transplant. (Courtesy of Mitek, Inc.)

partment effectively. Virtually all pump systems currently available are adept at such variations of volume or pressure management, but systems differ, and these differences may or may not be beneficial to an orthopaedic surgeon. For example, some systems are simply designed to function as a fluid pump, whereas others provide both inflow pressure and outflow suction. Some systems, during use of a shaver, automatically cut off a preestablished outflow and reroute suction through the shaver. Any pump system chosen must include a safety mechanism to prevent extremes of pressures from occurring within the arthroscopic space and thus avoid extravasation of large amounts of fluid into the soft tissues.

Some of the differences that can be objectively evaluated among the various pumps available are the initial expense in purchasing the system and the cost per case in tubing setup charges. The cost of each pump varies, depending on the manufacturer and the available options.

In some instances, a handheld remote device is offered with a pump system, which allows the surgeon or scrub nurse to alter flow and pressure rates depending on case necessity. On the operative field, this handheld remote allows the additional convenience of freeing the circulation nurse from controlling pump flow dynamics during the procedure.

Tubing costs per case represent a major portion of the setup fee, and, again, prices vary, depending on the system selected. They range from a minimal charge up to more than $100. Prices listed for both pumps and tubing are subject to

large variations in actual cost to each institution, depending on contractual agreements frequently made between manufacturers and health care organizations. Additionally, as technological advances and product changes are made, cost changes will be inevitable.

Thermal Instrumentation

Lasers

In 1960, Maiman (2) developed the first practical laser. Since that time, various crystals, gases, and other materials have served as laser beam emitters. Currently, those lasers that are commercially available for use in arthroscopic surgery include the carbon dioxide, neodymium:YAG (Nd:YAG), Ho:YAG, and excimer lasers. Other types of lasers including the KPT (potassium-titanyl-phosphate) and ER:YAG are also being used experimentally.

Carbon dioxide lasers have been plagued by problems such as the inability to regulate the depth of thermal transmission, the necessity to operate within a gaseous environment, postoperative effusions, and subcutaneous emphysema. Despite modifications to the carbon dioxide laser system, most surgeons find it cumbersome.

Excimer lasers function through excitation of gases such as xenon chloride, argon fluoride, or krypton fluoride. The xenon chloride laser is currently used in orthopaedics and operates in air, saline, or other fluids.

The Ho:YAG and Nd:YAG lasers operate within a saline solution and can be delivered by a fiberoptic cable. Contact Nd:YAG lasers are used to avoid extensive thermal injury, which has been associated with the use of free-beam Nd:YAG lasers. Ceramic tips have replaced sapphire crystal tips, which are easily broken within the joint. As a general rule, the Ho:YAG laser system probably delivers the most cutting energy to the laser–tissue interface.

Currently, the uses for lasers are within the practice of arthroscopic surgery include meniscectomy (partial or total), chondroplasty, lateral retinacular release, cautery, plica resection, decompression acromioplasty, and possible tissue welding or controlled soft tissue contraction (3,4). Because laser instrumentation is considerably smaller in diameter than conventional mechanical arthroscopic devices, laser use is particularly attractive in small joints or poorly accessible areas of the knee or shoulder, and it has been associated with less scuffing of the articular surfaces.

Nonetheless, the advent of arthroscopic laser surgery has not been without its complications and detractors. Reports of thermally induced soft tissue and bony injury have become available (5–7; Rosenberg TD, *personal communication,* 1994). Additional concerns about the toxicity of gases produced at the laser–tissue interface, the danger of high-voltage instrumentation in the operation suite, and the possibility of a mutagenic potential in laser use have led critics to question the necessity of lasers in arthroscopic procedures. Furthermore, there remains a lack of conclusive studies confirming the beneficial effect of laser-dependent techniques and their increased expense over mechanically assisted methods.

However, as newer and more comprehensive scientific studies are completed evaluating the uses of arthroscopic lasers, it is likely that, like many of the past advances in surgery, lasers will also find a niche within arthroscopic and orthopaedic surgery. This likelihood, coupled with the probable decrease in laser production costs resulting from technical advances, makes investigational studies into the areas of laser attractive.

Radiofrequency and Electrical Thermal Devices

Basic science work has demonstrated that both laser energy and radiofrequency thermal energy produce similar tissue modifications (8–10). Radiofrequency and electrical thermal devices add an easy-to-use weapon to the armamentarium of the arthroscopic surgeon. Oratec advocates the use of its radiofrequency probe for soft tissue procedures, such as the reduction of capsular laxity during arthroscopic glenohumeral instability surgery. Similar uses have been advised with the Mitek and Arthrocare electrical thermal products. In addition, the electrical thermal products have been used to treat articular cartilage lesions.

Peer-reviewed publications are lacking regarding the long-term clinical outcomes of soft tissue and articular cartilage treated with thermal energy. Consequently, the use of these instruments during arthroscopic procedures must continue to be evaluated critically. As with laser instruments, until such long-term outcomes demonstrate successful clinical application, surgeons must temper their initial enthusiasm for these devices.

CONCLUSION

As specialized arthroscopic instrumentation systems have been developed and perfected, the practice of arthroscopy has advanced from primarily a diagnostic procedure to its current position as an interventional and therapeutic science. The future of arthroscopic surgery is bright, and advances in instrumentation and technique will eventually lead to an ever-increasing role of arthroscopy in the practice of orthopaedic surgery.

REFERENCES

1. Adams F, ed. *The genuine works of Hippocrates.* New York: William Wood, 1886.
2. Maiman TH. Stimulate optical radiation in ruby [Letter]. *Nature* 1960:187:493–494.
3. Dillingham MF. Lasers: current status. Presented at the 13th annual fall course of the American Association of Arthroscopy, Palm Springs, CA, December 1–4, 1994.
4. Sherk HH. Current concepts review: the use of lasers in orthopaedic procedures. *J Bone Joint Surg Am* 1993:75:768–776.
5. Arthroscopy Association of North America. Advisory statement, September 4, 1993.
6. *Bull Am Acad Orthop Surg* 1993;41:4.
7. Thal R. Correspondence [Letter]. *J Bone Joint Surg Am* 1994:76:632–633.
8. Hayashi K, Markel MD. Thermal modification of joint capsule and ligamentous tissues. *Oper Tech Sports Med* 1998;6:120–125.
9. Hayashi K, Thabit G, Bigdanske JJ, et al. The effect of nonablative laser energy on the ultrastructure of joint capsular collagen. *Arthroscopy* 1996;12:474–481.
10. Hayashi K, Thabit G, Massa KL, et al. The effect of thermal heating on the length and histologic properties of the glenohumeral joint capsule. *Am J Sports Med* 1997;25:107–112.

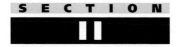

SECTION

II

BASIC SCIENCE

STRUCTURE AND FUNCTION OF DIARTHRODIAL JOINTS

IAN K.Y. LO
GAIL THORNTON
ANTHONY MINIACI
CYRIL B. FRANK
JEROME B. RATTNER
ROBERT C. BRAY

Diarthrosis means movable articulation (1). Diarthrodial joints are defined by the presence of a synovial cavity enclosing physically discrete articulating surfaces (2). Further motion occurs between noncontiguous articular surfaces that contact each other directly, rather than through any deformable intermediary tissue. These properties are derived from the complex interplay of structurally discrete connective tissues (i.e., synovium, ligament, cartilage, meniscus) that are placed throughout the joint.

In this chapter describes some of the basic anatomy, physiology, and functions of articular connective tissues and how they act together in complex, multicomponent organs known as diarthrodial joints. Our purpose is to broaden the arthroscopic surgeon's understanding of connective tissue structure and function, and to provide relevant information on the basic composition of diarthrodial joints.

CLASSIFICATION AND DEVELOPMENT OF DIARTHRODIAL JOINTS

Diarthrodial joints are required to perform a wide range of functions under a wide range of loads. Each of these joints has developed specific adaptations to optimize these functions. The following is a brief review and classification of diarthrodial joints and a summary of their development.

I. K. Y. Lo, G. Thornton, A. Miniaci: Department of Surgery, University of Toronto, Toronto Hospital, Toronto, Ontario, Canada.

C. B. Frank: Department of Surgery, The University of Calgary, Calgary, Alberta, Canada.

J. B. Rattner, R. C. Bray: Department of Surgery, Faculty of Medicine, University of Calgary, Calgary, Alberta, Canada.

Classification of Diathrodial Joints and Joint Motion

Functional demands on diarthrodial joints appear to dictate structural adaptations to motion. Joints with a wide range of motion, such as the shoulder, have limited intrinsic geometric stability and rely heavily on soft tissues to accommodate forces during loading. Other joints, such as the sacroiliac, have less motion but maximal stability, with large, flat articulating surfaces to dissipate forces. In general, joint structures are designed to transfer load so that force is accommodated within a physiologically tolerable range. This is accomplished by specific joint geometries that allow increasing contact area with increasing load; transfer of load to surrounding soft tissues; and compliance of the cartilaginous, cancellous bone unit forming the articulation (3).

As mentioned, diarthrodial joints are distinguished structurally by the presence of a synovial cavity (Fig. 5.1A). This synovial cavity permits physical separation of contact surfaces. Movement takes place by rotational and translational displacements that occur between opposing, freely mobile surfaces. Nondiarthrodial joints (synarthroses) are characterized by the presence of some continuous intervening (intraarticular) fibrous or fibrocartilaginous material. If this intervening material is deformable, motion is accomplished through structural deformation of the whole joint complex (Fig. 5.1B).

Diarthrodial joint motion is complicated, and most would agree that simple terms such as *hinge, saddle,* or *ball and socket* fail to describe complex movement patterns. Joint motion is perhaps better understood in terms of how structures are "coupled" during normal movement (4). From a practical standpoint, joint motion occurs between coupled components, each constrained by other coupled components in the system. In the knee, for example, extension motion is

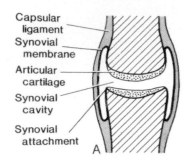
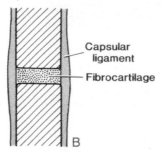

Capsular ligament
Synovial membrane
Articular cartilage
Synovial cavity
Synovial attachment

Capsular ligament
Fibrocartilage

FIGURE 5.1 Characteristic features found in diarthrodial joints (**A**) and nondiarthrodial joints (**B**).

linked to tibial rotation. As the knee extends, an obligatory tibial rotation occurs as a result of geometric constraints of femorotibial topography and other intrinsic soft tissue restraints (4). Load is dissipated by the contacting surfaces, as well as by the restraining forces provided statically in ligament tension or dynamically in muscle–tendon force. Tibial extension and rotation are therefore coupled as determined by joint geometry, loading environment, and the manner in which soft tissues and articular surfaces share the various loads applied.

Classification schemes have traditionally been based on anatomic and functional features of joints and their respective motion properties. This approach is limited by a tremendous diversity of structure and function in the locomotor apparatus. A useful classification scheme should be simple and should convey a practical understanding of how diarthrodial joints achieve motion and distribute forces under normal (or pathologic) conditions. The classification scheme in Table 5.1 differentiates among broad types of joint motion. This scheme is by no means complete, but it does offer practical utility in defining various skeletal joints.

Developmental Biology of Diathrodial Joints

In early development, shortly after the appearance of limb buds (26 to 28 days), a discernible mass of mesenchymal cells coalesces within the limb to form a blastema (5). The blastema represents a growing mass of tissue that is destined to form skeletal structures where no recognizable structures yet exist. Blastemal mesenchymal cells begin to secrete sul-

fated intercellular substances. Gradually the blastema, through the process of chondrification of the extracellular matrix (ECM), is replaced with the cartilaginous *anlagen* (6,7). As the anlagen grow, peripheral cells differentiate into perichondrial tissue layers and a multilayered cartilaginous model of the future bone appears.

At approximately 6 weeks, segmentation of anlagen begins in areas where joints are formed (5). In these putative joint regions, "interzonal" mesenchyme condenses between articulating anlagen. The interzone becomes distinctive as an avascular, homogenous, intensely cellular area, which stains positively for polysaccharides (probably chondroitin sulfate) and can be divided into three layers (8) (Fig. 5.2). Adjacent perichondrial membranes, continuous with the adjacent cartilage models of bones, surround peripheral interzonal mesenchyme layers. The central interzonal layer differentiates at the periphery of the primitive joint to form primordial synovial mesenchyme (8,9). This pluripotent tissue forms the synovial lining, capsule, ligaments, and menisci of the joint, while the central-most portion of the interzone undergoes a process known as *cavitation,* ultimately forming the synovial cavity proper.

Cavitation occurs at 10 weeks of development. Although the exact mechanisms responsible for cavitation are largely unknown, it has been suggested that matrix is destroyed by enzymes released from interzonal cells in this region (10). Multiple interzonal cavities coalesce to form a single, large synovial cavity that physically separates adjacent cartilaginous anlagen. As the cavitation phase proceeds, further differentiation of peripheral mesenchyme forms the joint capsule proper. Vascular invasion results in the arrival in the

TABLE 5.1 SIMPLE CLASSIFICATION SCHEME FOR SKELETAL JOINTS THAT DISTINGUISHES DIARTHRODIAL (SYNOVIAL) JOINTS FROM OTHER MAJOR TYPES OF SEMIMOBILE OR RIGID ARTICULATIONS

Joint Type	Motion Pattern	Common Terms	Examples
Diarthroidal	Freely mobile	Diarthrodial (synovial)	Knee, shoulder, wrist
Synarthroidal	Semimobile	Symphysis (fibrocartilaginous)	Pubic symphysis, intervertebral disk
	Syndesmosis (fibrous)	Distal tibiofibular joint	
	Semirigid	Synchondrosis (cartilaginous)	Sternomanubrial joint, growth plate
	Rigid	Synostosis (ankylosis)	Skull sutures

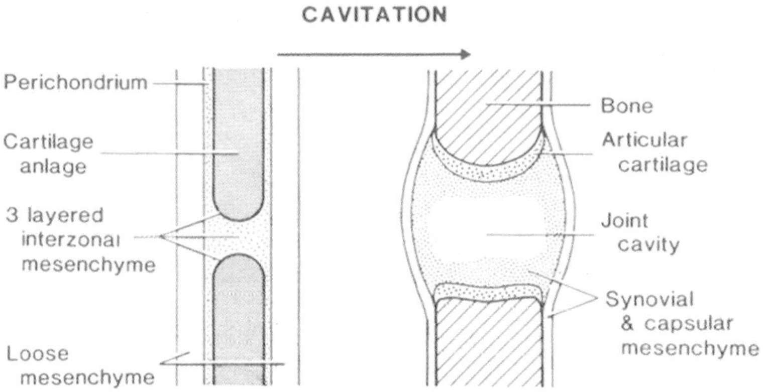

CAVITATION

FIGURE 5.2 Schematic diagram of the early developmental sequence of diarthrodial joints. Trilayered interzonal mesenchyme eventually cavitates to form a typical diarthrodial joint cavity.

tissue of other cell types (e.g., macrophages, monocytes), some of which could potentially differentiate and participate in further development of joint structures (10). Primitive synovial lining cells form a smooth surface over subjacent vascular mesoderm but do not cover the articulating bone ends. The absence of any true epithelial tissue on the synovial lining layer is a major determinant of this tissue's unique physiologic properties and distinguishes diarthrodial cavities from all other mesothelial body cavities (10).

The entire process of development from blastema to recognizable skeletal elements occurs in the human embryo between 4 and 10 weeks of gestation. Because of spatial gradients of differentiation, cranial or proximal structures develop ahead of caudal or distal structures. Specialized connective tissue known as the *apical ectodermal ridge* (AER), located at the outgrowing ectoderm tip of the limb bud (11), is necessary for proper proximodistal differentiation (12). The gradient theory suggests that certain diffusible growth factors are important for proper differentiation of anlagen (13). Another mechanism that is important for proper limb development is the inhibitory effect of certain substances on tissue growth, most notably hyaluronic acid (14).

Among many determinants of development, movement appears to be a critical factor (15,16). Movement can occur through extrinsic hydrodynamic forces acting *in utero* or by intrinsic activity of developing muscle tissue in the limb (5). Animal experiments have shown interruption of the cavitation phase in the absence of movement, but conflicting views exist on developing human joints (17). Most likely, a combination of biologic and biomechanical mechanisms is responsible for normal development, and these mechanisms are probably enhanced by force transmission and displacement of discrete joint structures during movement.

The practical importance of developmental processes in synovial joints is emphasized by the appearance of certain congenital anomalies in mature joint structure and by the remarkable similarity in behavior between "injured" or "healing" connective tissues and the developmental processes these tissues undergo.

CONNECTIVE TISSUE COMPOSITION

Diarthrodial tissues are composed of cells and ECM. Although much of the research to date has focused on the composition and biomechanics of the ECM (i.e., collagen), it has become increasingly evident that it is the interaction between cells and the matrix that is integral in furthering our understanding of diarthrodial tissues and ultimately improving patient care. In the following sections, the cells and the basic building blocks of the ECM are briefly discussed. However, it is the tissue-specific distribution, organization, and interaction of these elements that provides diarthrodial tissues which such a diverse group of functional connective tissues.

Connective Tissue Components

Cells can be considered as either resident or migratory. Resident cells (chondrocytes in cartilage, fibrocytes in ligament and capsule, synoviocytes in synovium) control synthesis, secretion, and degradation of their own ECM. Mast cells, macrophages, mononuclear cells, and polymorphonuclear cells, as well as vascular cells (endothelial, perivascular, smooth muscle) and nerve cells, are found in most articular tissues, excluding cartilage and some areas of fibrocartilage (ligament insertions). Dynamic interactions among resident cells, their ECM, and the variable population of migratory cells account for the normal physiology and function of organized connective tissues.

Connective tissues perform specific biomechanical functions, and, in contrast to other tissues (liver, spleen, kidney), they generally have a large volume excess of ECM over cells. This arrangement is typical of both force-transmitting structures (tendon) and force-dissipating and restraining structures (articular cartilage, ligament, meniscus). The ECM accounts in part for many of the fundamental biomechanical properties that are responsible for normal function of joints. Elaboration and maintenance of this ECM, however, is primarily controlled by cellular mechanisms that presumably are responsive to both genetic and environmental influences.

Collagen and Elastin

Collagen is the most ubiquitous and abundant protein in the animal world, constituting approximately one third of total body proteins (18). Collagen appears in virtually every tissue, but it is most abundant in fibrous connective tissues. It occurs as fibrillar or fibrous structures ranging from 16 to 1,500 nm in diameter (19). These fibrils provide reinforcement to the ECM of ligaments by forming longitudinal tensile-resistant elements in the tissue. In other tissues, loosely woven sheets of collagen form covering layers such as skin, synovium, and fascia. Collagen also acts to reinforce structures that are largely composed of "ground substances" such as articular cartilage or bone (18). In one sense, collagen and ground substances act together, similar to manmade "fiber-reinforced composite materials" (20).

The term *collagen* generally represents a series of related but chemically distinct macromolecular structures derived from collagen molecules (21–29). A protein is defined as collagen if it consists primarily of a triple-chain helix (α chains). However, one or more nonhelical domains may interrupt this chain. Each chain possesses a characteristic tripeptide sequence of the form glycine-x-y, in which every third residue is glycine, x is frequently proline, and y is frequently hydroxyproline. Various types and families of collagen have been categorized on the basis of common physicochemical properties (Table 5.2). Each type of collagen is a genetically distinct species, presumably evolved to perform specific mechanical functions in the ECM (18).

The definitive property of all collagens is their triple-helical structure (18). Three separate α chains of collagen form a right-handed superhelix with a rod-like conformation and a diameter of approximately 1.4 nm (25). Each α chain is composed of amino acids, numbering some 1,050 residues per chain and giving a total chain length of approximately 300 nm (18). The hierarchical structure of collagen is shown in Fig. 5.3.

TABLE 5.2 CLASSES OF COLLAGEN MOLECULES

Group	Physicochemical Properties	Type
1	Chain M, mol wt = 95,000 Continuous helical domain of ~300 nm	I
		II
		III
		V
2	k (1α, 2α, 3α) Chain M, mol wt = 95,000 Helical domains separated by nonhelical segments	IV
		VI
		VII
		VIII
3	Chain M, mol wt <95,000	IX
		X

From Miller EJ. The structure of fibril-forming collagens. *Ann N Y Acad Sci* 1985;460:1–13, with permission.

The type of collagen is determined by the molecular formula of its triple-helical chains (Table 5.3). These macromolecular structures in turn associate into the visible fibers and fiber bundles that can be observed with an electron microscope (see Figs. 5.31 and 5.34).

Biosynthesis of collagen occurs in cellular organelles known as the *rough endoplasmic reticulum* (31,32). The first product of synthesis, the procollagen α chain, is subsequently modified by posttranslational events such as hydroxylation of proline and lysine residues and glycosylation with oligosaccharide side chains (33,34). These and other modifications are required before triple-helical structures can associate normally in the ECM.

Collagen processing also continues in the extracellular space. Further modification through cleavage of amino-terminal and carboxyl-terminal peptide units (35–37) and the formation of specific crosslinks between collagen triple helices occurs before they can associate into laterally packed linear aggregations (38). These collagen microfibrils in turn coalesce to form the fibrils, fibers, and fiber bundles that are typically observed with the electron microscope (see Figs. 5.31 and 5.34). Ultrastructural data suggest that fibril assembly occurs near cell surfaces, particularly within peripheral indentations (see Fig. 5.33).

Proper extracellular aggregation requires the presence of specific enzymes presumably secreted from indigenous matrix cells. When enzyme processing of collagen reactions is blocked, as in lathyrism (absence of crosslinking), connective tissues exhibit deficiencies in their normal mechanical function, particularly if collagen is acting to resist tensile force (39).

The distribution of collagen types is highly tissue specific (Table 5.3). Most noncartilaginous tissues contain collagen types I and III with small quantities of minor types, including types V and VI (40). Tendon and ligament, for example, contain primarily type I collagen (95%), with a small amount of type III (less than 5%) normally present (41). The proportion of these minor fibrillar collagens may be particularly relevant in these tissues. Evidence has demonstrated that collagen fibrils seen on transmission electron microscopy (TEM) are not composed of one type of collagen but rather are heterotypic—that is, composed of two or more types of collagen. The relative proportions of these collagens in part regulate the final collagen fibril diameter. For example, an increased proportion of type V collagen decreases the final collagen fibril diameter during *in vitro* self-assembly assays (42).

Articular cartilage collagen is primarily type II, with fibrocartilage containing type II as well as variable amounts of type I collagen (43). Small amounts of types IX and XI collagen also occur in cartilage (44,45), with the latter apparently functioning in maintenance of the matrix. Bone contains only type I collagen, and studies indicate that in this tissue collagen fibers are organized to facilitate an orderly process of mineralization (46). Collagen in bone is also a

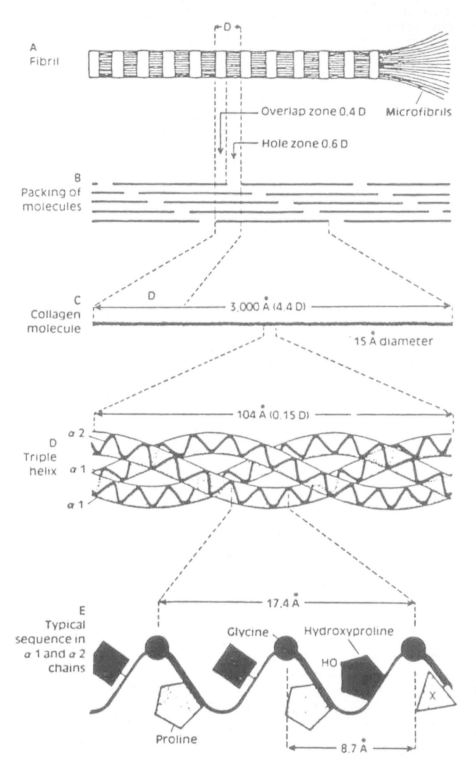

FIGURE 5.3 Hierarchical organization of mature collagen, showing relationship of single-strand proteins (α chains), triple helix, and fully formed fibril. (From Prockop DJ, Kivirikko KI, Tuderman L, et al. Biosynthesis of procollagen and its disorders [Parts 1 and 2]. *N Engl J Med* 1979;301: 13–23,77–85, with permission.)

structural fiber. Collagen's structural function in bone is illustrated most dramatically in osteogenesis imperfecta. In this disease, extreme fragility of bone is associated with molecular defects in the chemical structure of type I collagen (47).

Elastin is another fibrous protein commonly found in ECM tissue. Variable amounts of elastin are present in liga- ment (41), but concentrations are extremely low in tendon and bone (48,49). Elastin is important where reversible elongation of tissue is necessary; hence, extensible tissues and large blood vessels have high elastin contents (50).

Elastin can be seen on electron micrographs to have an amorphous structure (see Fig. 5.33). The chemical structure of elastin is somewhat reminiscent of collagen in that it has

TABLE 5.3 TYPES OF COLLAGEN

Type	Tissue	Polymeric Form
Class 1 (300-nm triple helix)		
Type I	Skin, bone, other	Banded fibril
Type II	Cartilage, disk	Banded fibril
Type III	Skin, blood vessels	Banded fibril
Type V	With type I	Banded fibril
Type XI (1α, 2α, 3α)	With type II	Banded fibril
Class 2 (basement membranes)		
Type IV	Basal lamina	Three-dimensional network
Type VII	Epithelial basement membrane	Anchoring fibril
Type VIII	Endothelial basement membrane	Unknown
Class 3 (short-chain)		
Type VI	Widespread	Microfilaments, 110-nm banded aggregates
Type IX	Cartilage (with type II)	Crosslinked to type II
Type X	Hypertrophic cartilage	Unknown
Type XII	Tendon, other?	Unknown
Type XIII	Endothelial cells	Unknown

From Mankin HJ, Mow VC, Buckwalter JA, et al. Articular cartilage structure, composition, and function. In: Buckwalter JA, Einhorn TA, Simon SR (eds). *Orthopaedic basic science,* 2nd ed. Rosemont, IL: American Academy of Orthopaedic Surgeons, 2000:447, with permission.

high glycine and proline contents. However, the hydroxyproline content is extremely low, and hydroxylysine is virtually absent (51). Other constituent amino acids (valine, leucine) are highly apolar, making elastin one of the most insoluble proteins in nature (50). Posttranslational modification of elastin also occurs. In fact, elastin has considerably more crosslinks than collagen, and the crosslinks are also chemically distinct from those of collagen (52).

Matrix Glycoproteins

The second major protein fraction of the ECM is made up of complex glycoproteins. Matrix glycoproteins occupy interfibrillar spaces, forming the so-called ground substance of connective tissues (53–56). Glycoproteins contain covalently bound carbohydrates. They can be classified as structural glycoproteins, proteoglycans, and glycosylated collagens (56). Depending on their protein and carbohydrate structure, vastly different functional properties are possible.

Because glycoproteins have particular relevance to cartilage and fibrocartilaginous connective tissue, most of what is known of their structure–function relationships is derived from studies in cartilage. Less is known about their functional importance in ligament and synovium.

Proteoglycans

Proteoglycans are a diverse group of macromolecules defined by a protein core with at least one or more specialized carbohydrate side chains, known as *glycosaminoglycans,* attached to it (57,58). An older term was *mucopolysaccharides* because of their highly viscous consistency and high water content (53). The proteoglycan superfamily contains more

than 30 full- or part-time molecules with a broad range of functions. Because of this broad definition, proteoglycans are found almost everywhere in the body; their size and shape vary enormously, and they may be found within cells, on the surface of cells, and in the ECM. Their diversity in structure suggests that proteoglycans play numerous biologic roles, which are now only beginning to be elucidated.

Glycosaminoglycans

Glycosaminoglycans are essentially linear chains consisting of repeating disaccharide units; one sugar is an amino sugar

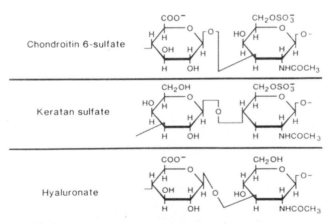

FIGURE 5.4 Molecular models of disaccharides: chondroitin-6-sulfate, keratan sulfate, and hyaluronate. These disaccharides form long chains of glycosaminoglycans in the ground substance of connective tissues. (From Buckwalter JA, Hunziker E, Rosenberg L, et al. Articular cartilage: composition and structure. In: Woo SL-Y, Buckwalter JA, eds. *Injury and repair of the musculoskeletal soft tissues.* Park Ridge, IL: American Academy of Orthopaedic Surgeons, 1987, with permission.)

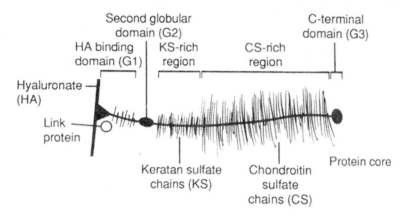

FIGURE 5.5 A schematic diagram of the aggrecan molecule and its binding to hyaluronate. The protein core has several globular domains (G1, G2, and G3); other regions contain the keratan sulfate and chondroitin sulfate glycosaminoglycan chains. The amino-terminal G1 domain is able to bind specifically to hyaluronate. This binding is stabilized by link protein. (From Mankin HJ, Mow VC, Buckwalter JA, et al. Articular cartilage structure, composition, and function. In: Buckwalter JA, Einhorn TA, Simon SR, eds. *Orthopaedic basic science,* 2nd ed. Rosemont, IL: American Academy of Orthopaedic Surgeons, 2000:449, with permission.)

(*N*-acetylglucosamine or *N*-acetylgalactosamine), and the other is usually a uronic acid or a galactose. Four major classes of glycosaminoglycan chains have been identified: hyaluronan, chondroitin sulfate, keratan sulfate, and heparan sulfate (Fig. 5.4). These glycosaminoglycans have the distinctive feature of being highly negatively charged and capable of becoming extremely hydrated (57).

Hyaluronan (formerly also known as hyaluronic acid or hyaluronate) is the only glycosaminoglycan chain that is not covalently bound to a protein core (56). It is abundant in skin, hyaline cartilage, and body fluids. A single strand of hyaluronan can consist of 100 to 100,000 repeating disaccharides and may serve as a scaffold for matrix–matrix and cell–matrix interactions (see later discussion). The chondroitin, keratan, and heparin sulfates, on the other hand, bind to an extended, nonhelical polypeptide known as the *core protein* (53–55). Core proteins have regions that are keratan sulfate–binding and others that are chondroitin sulfate–binding.

Proteoglycan Functional Groupings

The proteoglycans can be loosely grouped into four major categories: the large extracellular proteoglycans, the small leucine-rich repeat proteoglycans, the cell-associated proteoglycans, and the basement membrane proteoglycans. It is not the purpose of this chapter the review each of the proteoglycans extensively, but some that may have important functions in connective tissues are highlighted here.

Large Extracellular Proteoglycans

Aggrecan represents 80% to 90% of all proteoglycans in cartilaginous tissue and is the best-known proteoglycan. Aggrecan contains a core protein with glycosaminoglycan chains (chondroitin and keratan sulfate) attached to it. However, it has other noncovalent binding regions that allow it to attach to hyaluronan through specific interaction with another protein called *link* protein (Fig. 5.5). This allows aggrecan to form large aggregates, which have been likened to a "test tube brush" model (Fig. 5.6). Link protein appears to be im-

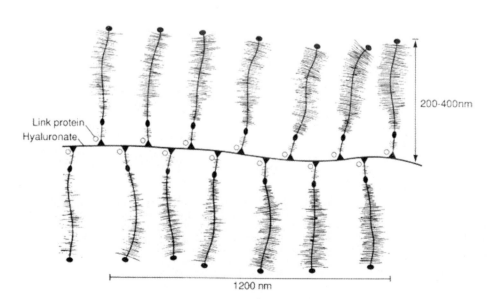

FIGURE 5.6 A diagram of aggrecan molecules arranged as a proteoglycan aggregate. Many aggrecan molecules can bind to a chain of hyaluranon, forming a macromolecular complex that effectively immobilizes the collagen network. (From Mankin HJ, Mow VC, Buckwalter JA, et al. Articular cartilage structure, composition, and function. In: Buckwalter JA, Einhorn TA, Simon SR, eds *Orthopaedic basic science,* 2nd ed. Rosemont, IL: American Academy of Orthopaedic Surgeons, 2000: 449, with permission.)

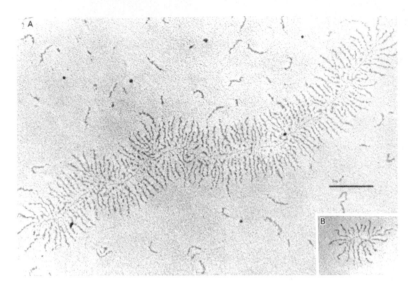

FIGURE 5.7 Transmission electron micrographs showing proteoglycan aggregates from bovine articular cartilage. Note the thin filament of hyaluronic acid acting as a central core (scale = 500 μm). (From Buckwalter JA, Hunziker E, Rosenberg L, et al. Articular cartilage: composition and structure. In: Woo SL-Y, Buckwalter JA, eds. *Injury and repair of the musculoskeletal soft tissues.* Park Ridge, IL: American Academy of Orthopaedic Surgeons, 1987, with permission.)

portant in stabilizing the hyaluronate-binding region and protecting it against enzymatic attack (58–60). Link protein binds aggrecan in a 1:1 stoichiometric fashion and further binds to hyaluronan, locking these three constituents together. In the presence of link protein, one hyaluronan molecule can bind three times more aggrecan than in its absence (61,62). Through the aggregation of many aggrecans with hyaluronate, large aggregate complexes are formed, some visible with the electron microscope (Fig. 5.7).

Proteoglycan aggregation helps entrap individual proteoglycans within the collagen meshwork of the ECM (63). Age-specific changes in these molecules have been demonstrated (64,65), suggesting that significant alterations occur with time. With advancing age, keratan sulfate and protein content increase, chondroitin sulfate chains become shorter, and chondroitin sulfate content decreases in articular cartilage. Although the functional significance of these age-related changes remains unknown, they are quite possibly related to an altered ability of aging cells to restore normal matrix (62).

Other members of this family include versican, neurocan, brevican, and collagen types IX, XII, and XIV, which normally do not contain glycosaminoglycan chains but can carry them and are thus "part-time" or facultative proteoglycans.

Small Leucine-Rich Repeat Proteoglycans

The family of small leucine-rich repeat proteoglycans (SLRPs) comprises currently nine proteoglycans (67,68), including decorin, biglycan, keratocan, fibromodulin, lumican, 3 PG-Lb/epiphycan, and osteoglycin (Fig. 5.8). They are grouped together because of their presence in the ECM and the fact that their central domain consists of a leucine-rich repeat (LRR) motif that dominates the core protein and may function in protein-to-protein interactions.

It is this interaction that may be integral during matrix formation (69). Collagen fibrillogenesis is in part a self-

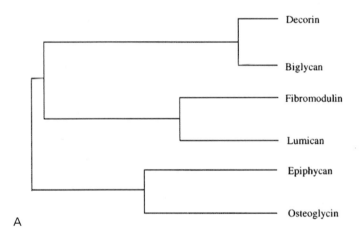

A

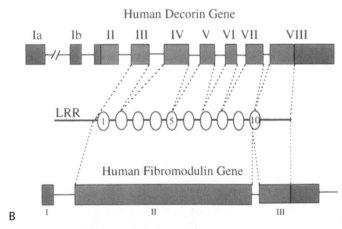

B

FIGURE 5.8 The family of small leucine-rich repeat proteoglycans. The consensus sequence for the leucine rich repeat is shown in the rectangle. A key to the various structural components is given in the bottom panel. (From Iozzo RI, Murdoch AD. Proteoglycans of the extracellular environment: clues from the gene and protein side offer novel perspectives in molecular diversity and function. *FASEB J* 1996;10:598–614, with permission.)

assembly process, however, several of the SLRPs may regulate or modulate this process (70). Several SLRPs have been demonstrated to bind to the surface of fibrillar collagens, including types I, II, III, V, VI, and XIV, and some molecules have demonstrated a delay in fibril formation and a reduction in final fibril diameter *in vitro* (71,72). The role of the SLRPs in collagen fibrillogenesis has been further exemplified *in vivo* in knockout mice, which have demonstrated abnormal collagen fibrillogenesis, abnormal collagen fibrils, and biomechanical alterations (73–76).

The SLRPs may have other effects, including interactions with transforming growth factor β (TGF-β) (77) and effects on cellular proliferation (78–82).

Cell-Associated Glycoproteins

Fibronectin, chondronectin, and anchorin CII are specialized structural glycoproteins that are responsible for cellular adherence. Fibronectin is an adhesive, cell surface glycoprotein and matrix component that serves as an opsonin and a chemoattractant (55,83,84). It plays an important role in cell migration in connective tissues and is considered to act as a substrate to which matrix cells involved in tissue repair can adhere (83,85–87). Fibronectin mediates the attachment of fibroblasts and chondrocytes to their matrix collagen (58).

Chondronectin is a cartilage matrix molecule that mediates the adhesion of chondrocytes to type II collagen and appears to stabilize the chondrocyte in its surrounding matrix (88). Anchorin CII is found only in the pericellular space directly adjacent to chondrocytes, and not in the remaining ECM. Studies suggest that anchorin CII specifically mediates the binding of type II collagen to chondrocytes (89).

The biosynthesis of glycoproteins, like that of the collagens, involves a stepwise assembly through both intracellular and extracellular compartments (90,91). Protein components of glycoproteins are synthesized in the rough endoplasmic reticulum of matrix cells (53–55,90). Attachment of oligosaccharide side chains begins there and continues during passage to the Golgi apparatus. Factors that regulate posttranslational modification include the amounts and types of enzymes present, the concentrations of substrate molecules (disaccharides and sulfates), and the rates at which components move through cellular and extracellular spaces (56). In the ECM, proteoglycans associate with hyaluronic acid filaments and link proteins to form larger aggregate complexes (Figs. 5.6 and 5.7). Extracellular modifications include change in length of the core protein as well as changes in carbohydrate side chains.

THE JOINT AS AN ORGAN

Diarthrodial joints are complex structures composed of many biologic components (ligament, meniscus, synovial fluid, muscle), all working together to maintain the normal function of the joint. After injury, the restoration of such function is a fundamental goal of musculoskeletal treatment. Much of the conceptual thinking to date has focused on the isolated structural and biomechanical alterations of injury and treatment. However, joints and joint structures are complex systems whose components are interdependent on one another and are constantly altering their cellular and molecular mechanisms to maintain and restore tissue homeostasis (92).

For example, both animal and clinical studies have demonstrated that after transection of the anterior cruciate ligament (ACL) there is an increased incidence of meniscal injury and osteoarthritis (93–103). In some fashion, normal ACL function is fundamentally important in maintaining tissue homeostasis of other structures such as the meniscus and cartilage. In addition, restoration of static knee stability with ACL reconstruction is inadequate in preventing osteoarthritis (i.e., restoring tissue homeostasis) (99). Interactions among joint structures may also be more subtle. For example, an important concept in ligament function is the fact that ligaments work together to share loads across a joint (104,105) and that they work with other joint structures (cartilage, bones, muscles, tendon units) to define the normal mechanical environment of that joint and its function. When one ligament is damaged, the tensile load across that joint must be borne by other structures (tendons or ligaments), resulting in a cascade of secondary events. In the case of the ACL, this ligament functions in concert with all other structures in and around the knee to maintain static and dynamic joint equilibrium. When the ACL is injured, other structures, such as the posterolateral corner, may also serve to control anterior tibial translation and anterolateral tibial rotation relative to the femur (106–111). In an attempt to maintain knee function and tissue homeostasis, these abnormal stresses on the compensating joint structures can then result in their adaptation or their failure (112). This may be one factor responsible for the variability in outcome after joint injury (99).

These concepts have led some authors to propose that there exists for each joint and for each individual an envelope of function or a range of loading that is compatible with overall tissue homeostasis (113,114). Loads above or below this "zone of homeostasis" may lead to pathologic changes. For example, loads beyond the upper limit of the zone of homeostasis, which are not enough to cause macrostructural failure, initiate injury, inflammation, and repair (i.e., early stress fracture), whereas loads below the zone of homeostasis (e.g., prolonged bed rest), in the "zone" of subphysiologic load, may lead to muscle atrophy.

In the following sections, each of the knee components is described and evaluated in detail, including synovial membranes, ligaments, articular cartilage, and menisci. This approach was chosen to emphasize the importance of each of these structures as well as their unique physiologic and functional biomechanical properties. However, it is important to consider that a diarthrodial joint must conceptually be evaluated not as individual components but as a complex, dynamic, interdependent system or organ.

SYNOVIAL MEMBRANE

Synovial membranes have been detected only in vertebrate animals (115). They are distinct from the mesothelial membranes that line other body cavities because they line a closed space in the body but lack true epithelial tissue or basement membrane (116). The following sections describe the major histologic classes of synovium (areolar, fibrous, and adipose), as well as their cells, ECM composition, innervation, vascular supply, and function, including the production of synovial fluid. It will become clear that the cellular and matrix architecture of synovium is a continuum between surface and deep layers. Similarly, synovial function arises from a continuum of structural and physiologic properties of the various membrane components.

Classification of Synovium

The structural organization of synovial tissue has been addressed in several detailed reviews (117–120). By light microscopy, this tissue is approximately 25 μm in thickness and highly cellular. The most superficial layer of synovium, called synovial intima, is a unique cellular lining one to three cells thick. Cells within the synovial intima are called synoviocytes although they are also present in deeper tissues. Underneath the synovial intima lies the subsynovial tissue, which, depending on its anatomic position, may be composed of areolar, fibrous, or adipose connective tissue. This distinction forms the basis for the most widely accepted histologic classification, that described by Key (117) (Fig. 5.9). These categories are based on differences not only in the deep tissue structure but also in the surface lining cells (i.e., the synoviocytes) and in the relative abundance of blood vessels. Key suggested that, although these are the main types present, mixed types (muscular and periosteal) also occur.

Areolar Synovium

Areolar synovium is characterized by a surface compact zone composed of collagen bundles and surface lining cells, the synoviocytes (Fig. 5.9A). Deeper zones contain synoviocytes that appear to send cytoplasmic processes toward the surface. Deeper zones exhibit a fibrous ECM containing blood vessels, nerves, and migratory cells such as mast cells and mononuclear cells. Synovial collagen is most likely a mixture of types I and III (120). Interfibrillar ground substance is partially composed of dermatan sulfate proteoglycan and hyaluronic acid (120). Areolar tissue has complex surface projections covered with lining cells and often surrounding

a central core of collagen and, occasionally, blood vessels (121). These projections increase the synovial surface area by forming numerous spaces or folds in the lining layer, and they also facilitate motion through expansion of the membrane complex.

Fibrous Synovium

Fibrous surfaces usually cover capsular and ligamentous structures. The synovial intima differs from the deeper zones by being more cellular (Fig. 5.9B). Surface synoviocytes are somewhat flattened and are aligned with a thin, dense collagenous sheet adjacent to the synovial cavity. Lining cells bear little resemblance histologically to the lining cells of areolar or adipose synovial membranes. Often the surface exhibits discontinuous regions not lined by regular cellular arrays. The cells from deeper zones sometimes appear semiencapsulated, although distinct lacunae are not formed. Fibrous lining regions have also been described in ligament surfaces on the inner and outer aspects of the joint cavity (122). These epiligamentous membranes may be important to ligamentous and capsular physiology in that nerves and blood vessels from this tissue often give rise to intraligamentous neurovascular networks (123). Key (117) postulated that transition zones between areolar and fibrous linings reflect the different stresses at different sites in diarthrodial joints, although he did not describe how this could be ascertained *in vivo*.

Adipose Synovium

Adipose synovium is found in regions where fat predominates, such as the anterior part of the knee. Adipose tissue is covered by a layer of synovium containing synovial cells, dense collagen bundles (Fig. 5.9C), and some neurovascular elements (120). The synovial cells form a uniform and continuous array. It is unlikely that adipocytes are ever in direct contact with the synovial cavity. Gaps between surface lining cells are infrequent and never more than a few microns wide. The lining cells tend to be flattened or polyhedral, and in the deeper layers a few synovial cells are found between larger adipocytes and within fibrous septations and crevices, often in association with blood vessels. Mast cells are occasionally found, but not as commonly as in areolar or fibrous surfaces. Adipose synovium fills potential spaces, and its deformability allows it to function as a mobile "packing" tissue during movement.

Synovial Cells: Ultrastructural Morphology and Function

Lining cells are distinguished from cells in deeper layers only by their position and arrangement (117). Although there is some controversy as to how many distinct cell types truly exist, two major morphologies are commonly identified with

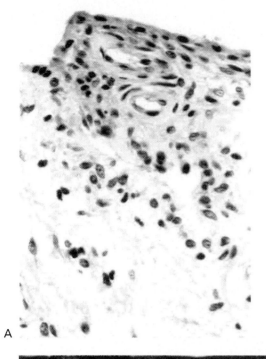

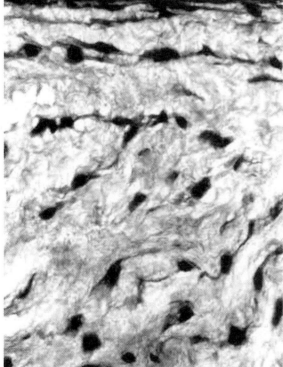

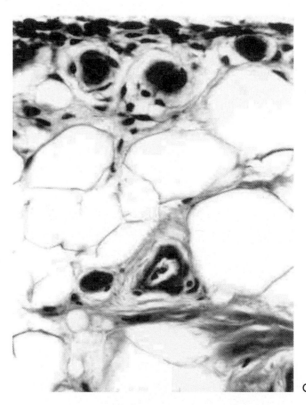

FIGURE 5.9 Characteristic types of human synovial membrane found in diarthrodial joints (150× magnification). **A:** Areolar synovium. **B:** Fibrous synovium. **C:** Adipose synovium. (After Key JA. The synovial membrane of joints and bursae. In: Hoeber PB, ed. *Special cytology II,* 2nd ed. New York: Paul B. Hoeber, 1932: 1055:76.)

the electron microscope. Type A synoviocytes share similarities with macrophages, whereas type B synoviocytes appear similar to fibroblasts or fibrocytes (124). Estimates of the ratio of type A to type B cells vary (125–127), with some studies suggesting that type A cells tend to line the surface of the synovium while type B cells lie deeper (128).

Type A cells have nuclei with a relatively dense chromatin pattern, but nucleoli are not a common feature (Fig.

5.10). Type A cells typically contain intracellular vacuoles, Golgi complexes, and smaller amounts of rough endoplasmic reticulum and free ribosomes (120). Rough endoplasmic reticulum rarely accounts for more than half of the cytoplasm, and it is usually loosely arranged rather than densely packed into stacked arrays.

Type A cells may have multiple functions depending on environmental stimuli (129). They have been shown to syn-

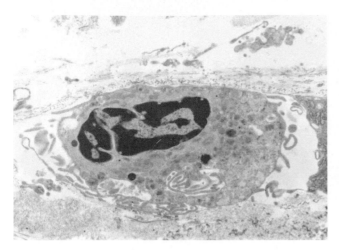

FIGURE 5.10 Transmission electron micrograph of human type A synoviocyte (15,000× magnification). Type A cells show ultrastructural features typical of tissue macrophages.

thesize hyaluronic acid (130), but they are primarily responsible for phagocytosis (131–133). On the basis of electron microscopy, these cells can reasonably be considered "surface macrophages" (115).

Type B cells have prominent nucleoli and an open nuclear chromatin pattern (Fig. 5.11). Type B cells are characterized by long cytoplasmic processes, often larger than the cytoplasm surrounding the nucleus. These processes typically contain regular stacked arrays of rough endoplasmic reticulum and rarely other types of organelles. Type B cytoplasmic processes frequently extend to synovial surfaces and may even be longer than the cell body itself (115). Type B cells secrete proteins and enzyme such as collagens, fibronectin, hyaluronan, and other glycosaminoglycans, implicating them in ECM remodeling (134–137). Some cells may also be capable of immune responses, such as synthesis

of molecules derived from the major histocompatibility complex (MHC) (115).

In addition to these morphologic characteristics, type A cells can be distinguished from type B cells based on their similarity to macrophages. Type A cells exhibit cross-reactivity to antibodies specific for macrophages, and they are positive for receptors for the Fc component of antibodies. They also express major Ia antigens and MHC class II molecules that play roles in antigen presentation in the initial stages of the immune response (138,139). Type B cells lack these macrophage markers but stain for the presence of uridine diphosphoglucose dehydrogenase, which is the rate-limiting enzyme for hyaluronan synthesis (140). A monoclonal antibody (Mab67) may be specific for type B synoviocytes (141).

Whereas many normal cells of the synovial intima can usually be described as type A or type B, other cellular morphologies can be distinguished deeper within the tissue, and particularly during development (129) or disease (142). Two that have been reported are a type C cell, which has morphologic characteristics between those of type A and type B, and a "dendritic" or "stellate" cell type (143), which has variable amounts of endoplasmic reticulum, Golgi complexes, and intracellular vacuoles (129). It is unclear whether these intermediary morphologies represent a unique population of synoviocytes or whether the differences in cell morphology reflect the function they are performing at a given moment. (133). However, the possible existence of intermediate cell types is not surprising, because morphologic characteristics such as nuclear and cytoplasmic patterns change with cell activity (115). In addition, it appears that the stellate cell morphology may be mediated by prostaglandin E_2 and cyclic adenosine monophosphate (cAMP) (144,145). Evidence suggests that the cells within normal synovium commonly contain long cytoplasmic processes and that the majority of cells are stellate shaped (146,147).

Synoviocytes show diverse functions, including phagocytosis, protein secretion, and remodeling of the synovial membrane ECM (142). With the use of cell culture techniques, synoviocytes have been shown to synthesize collagen (types I and III predominantly), enzymes (proteinases, activators, and inhibitors of proteinases), glycoproteins, hyaluronan, fibronectin, and many other minor and possibly as yet unidentified matrix constituents (129, 131,137,142, 148–150).

Type B synoviocytes in particular synthesize a significant amount of hyaluronan, as reflected by the high activity of uridine diphosphoglucose dehydrogenase, a key enzyme in hyaluronan synthesis (140). Hyaluronon levels are approximately 3 mg/mL in the normal synovial fluid. Synoviocytes also produce lubricin, a glycoprotein that contributes to the lubricating properties of synovial fluid (151,152).

Normal synovial tissue in culture can be induced to secrete substances, such as interleukin-1 or nitric oxide, that stimulate chondrocyte-mediated articular cartilage degradation and may be mediators of disease (153–157). Such

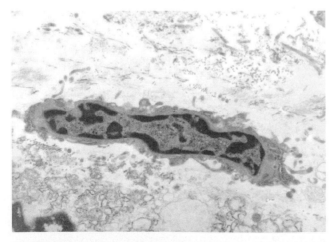

FIGURE 5.11 Transmission electron micrograph of human type B synoviocyte (17,500× magnification). Type B cells show ultrastructural features typical of tissue fibroblasts.

properties of synoviocytes, particularly under conditions of inflammation, suggest that these cells play an active role in joint homeostasis and are also important in the pathophysiology of many joint diseases.

Synovial Extracellular Matrix

As suggested by Key (117), the structure of synovial membrane reflects, in part, its mechanical function. However, the control mechanisms responsible for changing this structure in response to various conditions are unknown. Synovial ECM is also more than simply a scaffolding to anchor synoviocytes. Synovium plays a role in cell migration and in differentiation (17); additionally, synovial ECM can entrap autoantigens such as DNA, thus contributing to immune responses in diarthrodial joints (158).

Synovial membrane architecture is distinct from that of capsular or ligamentous tissue (Fig. 5.12). Membrane constituents include collagens, glycosaminoglycans (proteoglycans and special glycoproteins such as fibronectin, laminin, and lubricin), hyaluronic acid, and various amounts of lipids, electrolytes, and serum proteins (142). Rather than being arranged into discrete layers, synovial tissue represents a continuum from surface to deep zones, with ECM that is variable in content and composition through these zones. Because the synovial lining is so thin, biochemical characterization of its composition has been difficult and many studies have relied on immunohistochemistry to identify tissue constituents. This section reviews the major components and briefly describes special constituents that are important in the synovial matrix.

Collagen types I, III, and VI have been immunolocalized in synovium, and their distribution varies across the tissue (159–162). The literature however, is contradictory regarding the presence of type IV or type V collagen (159,160,

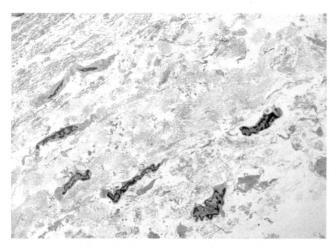

FIGURE 5.12 Transmission electron micrograph of human synovial extracellular matrix (4,500× magnification). Note the relatively loosely organized matrix and varying cell morphologies typical of areolar synovium.

161,163,164). Collagen from synovial matrix was quantified in one study by assessment of hydroxyproline and cyanogen bromide peptide analysis (162). Collagen content ranged from 25% to 50% of the dry weight of various synovial membranes, with type I and III collagens present in approximately equal amounts.

Elastin is a minor component of synovial ECM, amounting to less than 1% of the dry weight (165). Dermal elastin content, by contrast, is higher than that of the synovium (approximately 4% of dry weight of skin) (166). This difference is puzzling in view of the apparent extensibility of synovial membranes, although it is possible that certain membrane constituents may be compartmentalized in various tissue types. Global estimates may give inaccurate information about the distribution of elastin in synovium, and, in the absence of appropriate biomechanical studies relating tissue composition to mechanical behavior, it is difficult to draw simple relationships between composition and function. The relatively low content of elastin at least suggests that synovium might be subject to a different set of mechanical stresses and strains than skin is (115).

The distribution of glycoproteins also varies according to location, particularly between the surface lining layers and subintimal tissue, and in the matrix regions adjacent to cells (167,168). With the use of ruthenium red, an electron-dense dye that binds to acid glycoproteins and various proteoglycans, areas of densely stained ground substance are seen to surround synoviocytes in the lining layers. Within the subintimal tissue, ruthenium red–staining material is associated with collagen fibers or possibly with hyaluronic acid as large proteoglycan aggregates (169). Biochemical analysis suggests that chondroitin sulfate, dermatan sulfate, and hyaluronic acid are constituents of this ground substance (168).

Hyaluronic acid surrounds cells in synovial lining and is also distributed generally in the ECM (167,168, 170,171). Canine synovial cell cultures produce link protein, suggesting that at least some of the hyaluronic acid present is in the form of complex proteoglycan aggregate molecules (169). Although hyaluronic acid was long thought to be important for joint lubrication, this may not be the case (172). Rather, its main role remains obscure and, although hyaluronan is an important synovial membrane proteoglycan, other functions have been suggested, including its influence on healing of connective tissues (173). Exactly how hyaluronic acid is partitioned between synovial tissue and synovial fluid, as well as many other questions about the control of hyaluronic acid turnover, remain to be answered.

Several other structural glycoproteins are important constituents of synovium. One of these, fibronectin, is found in a variety of connective tissues and has important effects on cell adhesion and cell migration (174,175). Fibronectin is distributed in a fibrillar meshwork on top of synovial cells as well as between and around synoviocytes in the lining layer (176). Fibronectin also appears to be associated with hyaluronic acid, and this association has led some to speculate that such complexes might help control fluid and protein exchange between synovial lining and synovial fluid (164,176).

Blood Supply, Lymphatics, and Innervation

Hunter (177), in 1743, described a vascular plexus common to joints, which he called the "circulus articuli vasculosus." This plexus was described in detail by Davies and Edwards (178) in 1948. Together with the geniculate arteries, this plexus has been shown to contribute to much of the synovial microvasculature. Vessels typically appear as venules and arterioles in deeper tissue, giving rise to a branching anastomotic capillary network in the more superficial layers of the membrane (179). This arrangement has been confirmed by morphometric analysis of rabbit synovium: a high frequency of capillaries was found within 25 μm of the synovial surface, with a peak density between 6.2 and 11.2 μm deep (179). The proximity of the vessels to the joint space predisposes the joint to hemarthrosis after vessel rupture. The density of blood vessels also varies according to tissue type. Fibrous synovium has very few vessels, adipose synovium shows an intermediate amount, and areolar synovium demonstrates the greatest number of vessels. Capillaries are always covered by lining cells and synovial ECM. Some synovial capillaries demonstrate numerous fenestrae or pores, particularly those vessels facing the joint cavity (180,181), and are probably involved in the production of plasma filtrates (182).

Lymphatic tissue in synovium appears as blind sacs that pass from the subintimal vascular plexus toward the surface. Unlike capillaries, synovial lymphatic sacs or channels do not pass between surface lining cells (183). Lymphatics are also absent from smaller synovial projections. Lymphatic channels in the deeper synovial vascular plexus typically appear larger than blood vessels and tend to occur in groups of two or three to each set of vessels (115). Larger channels form lymphatic plexuses that eventually drain into deep regional lymph nodes.

Synovial innervation occurs chiefly through vascular-associated, unmyelinated nerves, principally autonomic in character (184). Some myelinated nerve bundles also give rise to free nerve endings in synovial ECM (185) and may provide free nerve endings in the vicinity of blood vessels (186). In general, however, synovium is considered a less "sensitive" tissue than other joint structures (ligaments and capsule) (187). Certain regions of the joint capsule, and especially discrete articular ligaments, are richly supplied with myelinated and unmyelinated nerves, some ending as free terminals in the ECM and others ending in what appear to be specialized encapsulated structures (186). The functions of synovial nerves therefore potentially include proprioceptive, nociceptive, and vasomotor actions. Undoubtedly,

neurovascular elements will be shown to have many important physiologic actions and homeostatic roles in synovial tissue as well as many other joint connective tissues. The importance of diarthrodial joint innervation is also apparent in light of studies indicating altered peripheral innervation patterns of diseased synovium between osteoarthritis and rheumatoid arthritis (188).

SYNOVIAL FLUID

All diarthrodial joints contain a small volume of synovial fluid. The exact relationship between joint fluid and synovial membrane, is complex but in general synovial membrane appears to be a passive, selective barrier rather than an active transport system (115). Several classic studies of synovial fluid composition, formation, and resorption are relevant to this subject (189–191).

If synovial lining were similar to other soft connective tissues, synovial fluid would be rapidly "pumped" away by lymphatics during joint movement. This would be expected to leave the tissue "moist" but not "wet" (115). Since this does not occur, the synovial membrane is uniquely responsible for maintaining a small but constant pool of fluid within the joint. Synovial tissue somehow prevents rapid fluid exit across its surface without impeding diffusional exchange of small molecules and water.

Synovial membrane does not produce fluid *de novo* and has no natural point of exit in the sense of a true exocrine gland. It does not truly resorb fluid in the manner that kidney tubules do, nor does it behave like other connective tissues which rely on hydrostatic and osmotic forces transmitted through capillaries and lymphatics to clear excess fluid (192). It does appear however, that both the synovial capillaries and the synovial matrix both contribute to the final composition of the synovial fluid (193) (Fig. 5.13). Approximately 50% of the synovial capillaries contain fenestrations along their length, which are arranged to face the intraarticular space. These fenestrations, which are approximately 5 to 10 μm in circumference, are the major routes for flow of water and hydrophilic molecules from the capillary to the synovium (194, 195). Because the functional pore size of these fenestrae is less than 52 nm, they act as a sieve, restricting larger molecules from leaving the plasma (195). Thus synovial membrane, with its inherent properties of permeability to water and certain solutes, in combination with the cellular ability to secrete glycoproteins, acts collectively with other hydrostatic and osmotic forces to control the volume and composition of synovial fluid (115). On the contrary, the flow of synovial fluid out of the joint is not restricted by size but is removed via the lymph (196–199).

Synovial fluid composition reflects its derivation from plasma and the additional solutes provided by synovial cells. The electrolyte concentration is similar to that of plasma, as are the concentrations of other small molecules (200). Al-

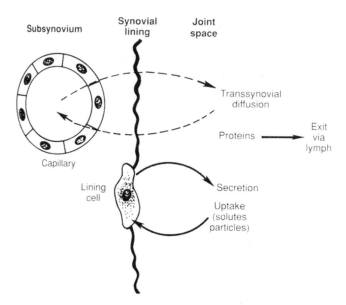

FIGURE 5.13 Diagram demonstrating how synovium helps regulate the intraarticular biochemical environment. Materials are added to synovial fluid by diffusion from the synovial capillaries or by secretion from the synovial lining cells. Solutes may leave the joint space by diffusion into the capillaries, by uptake by the synovial lining, or through the lymph. Proteins leave the joint through the lymphatics. The contributions of cartilage and chondrocytes are excluded from this diagram. (From Evans CH. Response of synovium to mechanical injury. In: Finerman G, Noyes FR, eds. *Biology and biomechanics of the traumatized synovial joint: the knee as a model.* Park Ridge, IL: American Academy of Orthopaedic Surgeons 1993:17–26, with permission.)

though the glucose concentration would normally be similar to that of plasma, glucose appears to enter the joint cavity more rapidly than expected by diffusion alone; therefore, it is considered to have "facilitated transport" (200). Plasma proteins show an inverse relationship between size and concentration in synovial fluid (201). The restriction of protein passage through synovial ECM is thought to depend on hyaluronic acid and presumably on proteoglycan aggregates in the matrix, which exclude large solute molecules from the fluid (202).

Additional proteins include the glycoproteins that are important for joint lubrication. In a fascinating study of the lubricating ability of synovial fluid, Linn and Radin (172) showed that boundary lubrication was destroyed by trypsin (a serine proteinase) but not by hyaluronidase (hyaluronate-cleaving enzyme), suggesting that hyaluronic acid is not primarily responsible for lubrication. This work stimulated the discovery of two glycoproteins, termed *lubricating glycoproteins I and II* (LGP-I and -II) (203,204). Most of the lubricating activity resides in LGP-I, which is also referred to as *lubricin* (205). Lubricin appears to be an unusual glycoprotein with some similarities to proteoglycan monomers. It is a long, thin, fiber-like molecule with numerous oligosaccharide side chains (206). Little is known about how lubricin acts to lower the coefficient of friction at joint sur-

faces (207–209). In addition, there is some controversy as to whether lubricin or a carrier for surface-active phospholipid is the actual lubricant (210,211).

Although the volume of fluid normally present in diarthrodial joints is quite small, it nonetheless has an extremely important influence on "packing" of the synovial membrane (212). The resting joint cavity is at a pressure just below atmospheric. If joints contained less fluid, normal movement could create high enough vacuums to impair tissue deformation. As discussed by Edwards (182), "moving a limb [without synovial fluid] would be like trying to bend a pack of vacuum-packed bacon."

Functions of Synovial Lining

Many functional properties of synovium have already been discussed. In summary, the most important and commonly cited properties include provision of membrane surface nonadherence and very low surface friction coefficients; a very compliant membrane forming a deformable soft tissue packing within the joint; an abundant blood supply that nourishes avascular cartilage chondrocytes; and a controlled volume of normal synovial fluid for joint lubrication and possibly nourishment of other connective tissues (115). In particular, the main biologic advantages of synovial tissue and synovial fluid appear to be facilitation of diarthrodial joint motion and the provision of a source of nourishment for avascular chondrocytes.

SYNOVIAL DISEASES

The following is a brief summary of the more common disorders related to the synovium. These include pigmented villonodular synovitis (PVNS), hemosiderotic synovitis, synovial chondromatosis, crystal-induced synovitis, osteoarthritis, and rheumatoid arthritis.

Pigmented Villonodular Synovitis

PVNS is a localized or diffuse, proliferative nodular thickening of the synovium (213–216). Localized PVNS has only a single mass within the synovium. Diffuse PVNS alters the majority of the synovium from a smooth to a nodular appearance with thin, finger-like projections and rounded nodules (0.5 to 2.0 cm) (Fig. 5.14). Microscopically, PVNS is characterized by villous, papillary, and nodular enlargement of the synovial membrane. The synovium contains mononuclear rounded and epithelioid cells, multinucleated giant cells, and lipid-rich cells that are arranged in either a lobular or a sheet-like pattern and are covered by surface synovial cells. Hemosiderin is commonly seen in mononuclear cells and appears in aggregates (Fig. 5.15) (213,214,217). PVNS can also result in erosion of the adjacent articulating bones.

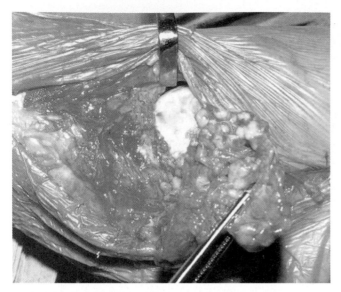

FIGURE 5.14 The synovial surface of this knee joint (intraoperative photograph) is diffusely nodular, tan-gold, and thickened—the typical appearance of pigmented villonodular synovitis. (From O'Connell JX. *Am J Clin Pathol* 2000;114:773–784, with permission.)

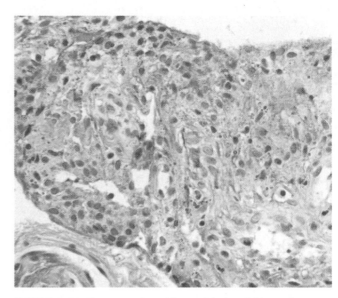

FIGURE 5.16 Fine granules of hemosiderin within surface synovial cells and macrophages. There are no nodules or sheets of proliferative synovial cells (hematoxylin and eosin stain, 200× magnification). (From O'Connell JX. *Am J Clin Pathol* 2000;114: 773–784, with permission.)

Hemosiderotic Synovitis

Hemosiderotic synovitis commonly occurs in the knees of male hemophiliac patients secondary to chronic intraarticular hemorrhage (218–220). With chronic hemarthrosis, pain and stiffness are common complaints because secondary osteoarthritis typically develops (218–221). Hemosiderotic synovium is brown or rust colored and early on may have fine villous projections similar to PVNS but smaller. Late

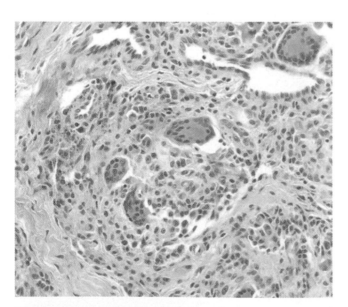

FIGURE 5.15 A cluster of multinucleated giant cells with an adjacent aggregate of hemosiderin-laden cells (hematoxylin and eosin stain, 200× magnification). (From O'Connell JX. *Am J Clin Pathol* 2000;114:773–784, with permission.)

hemosiderotic synovium is characterized by thickening and fibrosis of the synovium and subsynovial tissue.

Microscopically, cuboidal, synovial cells containing hemosiderin granules line the surface synovial membrane (219,222) (Fig. 5.16). Additional hemosiderin-laden macrophages lie within the subsynovial connective tissue. In contrast to PVNS, there are no sheets of mononuclear synovial cells, lipid-laden cells, or multinucleated giant cells.

Synovial Chondromatosis

Synovial chondromatosis results from a metaplastic production of multiple hyaline cartilage nodules by subsynovial cells (223–225). This disorder can affect patients at any age, with an equal male-to-female distribution. Macroscopically, synovial chondromatosis nodules may be 2.0 mm to 1.0 cm in size and appear as glistening blue-gray nodules in the synovium (Fig. 5.17). The nodules can calcify or undergo enchondral ossification.

Microscopically, the nodules are more cellular than articular cartilage and commonly form clusters. Although individual cells may display some atypical features, the clinical and radiographic features of synovial chondromatosis help distinguish it from low-grade intraosseous chondrosarcoma (223–227).

In addition to primary synovial chondromatosis, secondary synovial chondromatosis may occur when loose bodies from disorders such as osteochondritis dissecans or osteochondral fracture embed themselves within the folds of the synovium. In secondary chondromatosis, the nodules are larger (1.5 cm), are less frequent, and contain a central

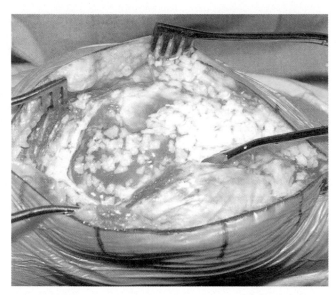

FIGURE 5.17 Knee arthrotomy. Innumerable nodules of glistening blue hyaline cartilage are demonstrated throughout the synovial surface. (From O'Connell JX. *Am J Clin Pathol* 2000;114: 773–784, with permission.)

cartilaginous or osteocartilaginous nidus. Microscopically, there is no cellular atypia or clustering (223,228,229).

Crystal-Induced Synovitis

Monosodium urate, calcium pyrophosphate dihydrate, and calcium hydroxyapatite crystals may all be deposited in the synovium and other articular tissues, resulting in a spectrum of clinical conditions (230,231).

Monosodium urate deposition disease, or gout, results in the deposition of monosodium urate crystals in the synovium. These deposits, known as tophi, appear cream-white or tan and result in thickening and opacification of the synovial membrane (231,232). Under red-compensated polarized light microscopy, the crystals appear needle-shaped and negatively birefringent (Fig. 5.18). There is usually an associated histiocytic and giant cell reaction.

Deposition of calcium pyrophosphate dihydrate within tissues results in the disease of pseudogout. Grossly, the crystals appear as chalky deposits on the surface of the synovium and other periarticular tissues, including cartilage and menisci. Microscopic examination reveals dark blue or purple rhomboid crystals (233,234). Usually there is an absence of histolytic cells or foreign body giant cell reaction.

Hydroxyapatite crystal deposition is most commonly seen around the shoulder in the syndrome of calcific tendonitis (235–237). Although deposition is commonly seen in tendon and synovial sheaths, it may also occur intraarticularly and may be associated with a rapidly destructive arthritis known as "Milwaukee shoulder" (238,239). Hydroxyapatite crystal disease leads to creamy-white deposits, which may coalescence and form larger structures. Synovial deposition

usually leads to papillary and fibrous thickening of the membrane. Microscopically, the individual crystals are very small (75 to 250 nm) and can be detected only by TEM or x-ray diffraction (237–239). However, large deposits may be seen as blue-purple aggregates by hematoxylin and eosin staining before decalcification and palely eosinophilic or basophilic after decalcification (235,237).

Osteoarthritis

Historically, osteoarthritis was assumed to be a mechanical problem of the material properties of cartilage that resulted in passive erosion of the joint cartilage. However, it now appears that osteoarthritis is the results of biologic processes with significant changes in the metabolism of chondrocytes (240). The degree of synovial involvement in the pathogenesis of ostearthritis remains controversial (241,242). Most investigators suggest that the synovium becomes involved only late into the process, when osteoarthritis is severe (241,242). Synovial changes including synovial lining hyperplasia, sublining mononuclear infiltration, and other inflammatory changes can occur, but to a lesser degree than rheumatoid arthritis. In addition, synovial changes may develop in response to cartilaginous or osteocartilaginous fragments and have been correlated with the onset of clinical symptoms (243–246).

Rheumatoid Arthritis

Synovitis a major component of chronic inflammatory diseases such as rheumatoid arthritis. Although the etiology of rheumatoid arthritis remains unknown, the pathologic

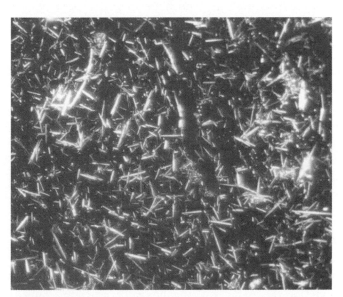

FIGURE 5.18 Intensely birefringent, needle-shaped crystals from a smear preparation of unfixed tissue viewed with polarized light (200× magnification). (From O'Connell JX. *Am J Clin Pathol* 2000; 114:773–784, with permission.)

changes within the synovium are well described. Grossly, rheumatoid synovium appears hypertrophic and edematous, with redundant folds and villi. Synovial tissue is rich in blood vessels, and it appears that angiogenesis is a key feature in synovial inflammation (247,248–253). Angiogenesis results from endothelial cell proliferation and migration from existing synovial blood vessels, with the eventual creation of anastomoses and blood flow. Although rheumatoid synovium has a rich vascular network, it is more disorganized than normal tissue, and there is relative ischemia of the synovial tissue.

There is marked hyperplasia of the intimal layer, with accumulation of T cells, plasma cells, macrophages, B cells, neutrophils, mast cells, natural killer (NK) cells, and dendritic cells in the subsynovial tissue (249). In the synovial lining there is a proliferation of type B synoviocytes and migration of new, macrophage-like type A synoviocytes. An inadequate rate of apoptosis also probably plays a role in the increased cellularity of the synovial lining layer (250).

The lymphocytes, particularly CD4-positive memory T cells, organize into lymphocyte aggregates in 50% to 60% of rheumatoid patients. Aggregates may be surrounded by plasma cells, and between aggregates there is usually an infiltrate of macrophages and lymphocytes. Some intervening areas may also be characterized by granulomatous necrobiosis, with fibrinoid necrosis lined by an area of epithelioid histiocytes and granulation tissue (251). Other T cells may form perivascular lymphocyte aggregates with B cells or as a diffuse infiltrate throughout the synovium.

Synovial tissue adjacent to areas of cartilage (synovial pannus) are often involved in the disease process; the rheumatoid synovium can erode into cartilage and also bone and ligament. Typically this area contains type B synoviocytes and macrophages, which are seen at the leading edge of the degrading cartilage. Degradation of adjacent tissue is mediated by enzymes from the serine, cysteine (cathepsin B, L) and metalloproteinase (MMP-1, -2, and -3) families. It also appears that osteoclasts play a critical role in bone erosion at adjacent sites (252).

LIGAMENTS

Skeletal ligaments are anatomically discrete, dense connective tissue structures that connect bones and serve a number of important functions. These functions include kinematic (254,255), biomechanical (256–259), and possibly neurosensory (260) roles in both guiding and protecting joint movements (254–263).

This section reviews current understanding of skeletal ligaments—in particular the medial collateral ligament (MCL), the ACL, and the posterior cruciate ligament (PCL)—at gross, light microscopic, and ultrastructural levels, as well as their function. It should be understood that very few ligaments have been studied intensively, and infor-

mation most likely cannot be extrapolated simply from structure to structure or from species to species. Except where indicated, the descriptions of normal ligament structure refer to the rabbit MCL model.

General Ligament Structure
Gross Appearance

Skeletal ligaments have been defined most commonly on the basis of their gross appearance (263). More specifically, they have usually been named by their points of bony attachment (e.g., coracoacromial), their relationship to the joint that they serve (e.g., collateral, superficial, deep), their shape (e.g., deltoid), or their relationship to other ligaments (e.g., cruciate). Further classification of skeletal ligaments on biologic or functional grounds has never seemed worthwhile, because their homogeneity was rarely questioned. Although there is evidence to suggest that such indiscriminate grouping may not be appropriate (264), at the present time there is insufficient information to propose any reasonable alternative subclassifications of ligaments.

In general, skeletal ligaments are distinguished by their appearance as short bands of dense, white, tough but flexible, fibrous connective tissue that are attached at both ends to bone (265–267). Whereas some ligaments are very distinct and cord-like (Fig. 5.19), and thus are grossly similar

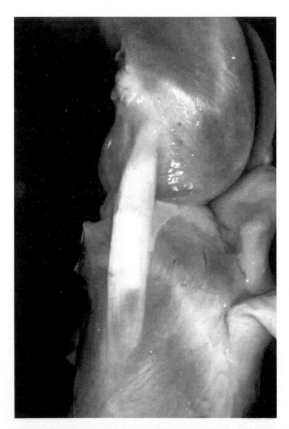

FIGURE 5.19 Gross appearance of normal rabbit medial collateral ligament.

to tendons, the majority of ligaments are not as discrete. Instead, most (e.g., the glenohumeral ligaments of the shoulder) consist of less distinct bands of tissue running between specific, but often hidden, sites of bony attachment. In many areas, these ligamentous bands merge into one another or overlap, making specific definition even more difficult. This is particularly true of so-called "capsular" ligaments, in which individual identification by dissection can be extremely difficult (268).

A further contribution to the definition of ligaments is made by a simple modification of these observations. The ability to alter tension in various parts of ligaments by changing the position of the joint has introduced the concept that apparently homogeneous ligaments actually have less obvious functional "parts." This organization has been recognized mainly in the ACL, where one part of the ligament is generally tighter near extension of the knee joint and another is tighter in flexion (269). It is probably also true for a variety of other ligaments. If confirmed, these functional separations will almost certainly have important implications for interpretation of *in vitro* biomechanical tests of many ligament complexes (270) and may ultimately influence their clinical treatments as well. For the purposes of this review, however, it is important to recognize that many presently defined "normal ligament structures" are unlikely to be completely homogeneous when examined more closely.

The final important gross feature of normal ligaments is their relative hypovascularity. When compared with other musculoskeletal tissues, ligaments have a modest blood supply, contributing to their white appearance. Vascular patterns are, nonetheless, well documented for more than one ligament complex (271), showing some vessels lying near (but not passing through) bony insertions, more in overlying or surrounding ligament sheaths, and fewer distributed in ligament midsubstance (186). The general vascular anatomy of the MCL is shown in (Figs. 5.20 and 5.21). The MCL derives its blood supply from the overlying epiligamentous tissue. Within the epiligament, numerous vascular plexuses are found randomly dispersed. These vessels give rise to a smaller number of well-organized vessels that branch off into the deeper ligament tissue and assume a more longitudinal orientation. The vascularity of ligament tissue is often found in patterns with nerves, which suggest that these neurovascular structures probably have physiologic significance.

Dissecting Microscopy

Under low-power magnification, the fibrous nature of isolated ligaments becomes more obvious. Nearly parallel col-

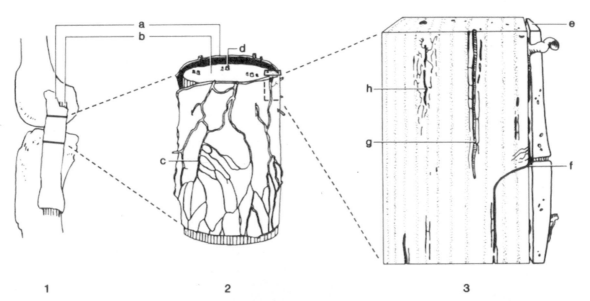

FIGURE 5.20 Diagram of proposed fine vascular anatomy of adult rabbit model medial collateral ligament (MCL). Model of knee joint medial view (1) shows MCL and epiligamentous tissue covering it: a, epiligamentous tissue layer; b, ligament proper. Midsubstance region (2) shows relationship between epiligament and ligament: c, vascular plexuses in epiligamentous tissue (note the abundant blood supply and typical pattern of arborization into small vascular channels); d, intraligamentous vessels (deep ligament tissues typically have fewer vessels, with a very different pattern and distribution from the epiligament). Thin-section model of MCL (3) shows details of microvascular anatomy: e, epiligament at peripheral border of ligament proper (note the relative abundance of vessels here, compared with ligament substance); f, blood vessels entering ligament from epiligamentous plexus; g, typical linear anastomotic vessels deep in ligament substance (vessels usually run parallel to ligament collagen bundles); h, glomus-like anastomosis found (infrequently) in ligament substance. (From Bray R, Fisher AWF, Frank C. Fine vascular anatomy of adult rabbit knee ligaments. *J Anat* 1990;172:69–79, with permission.)

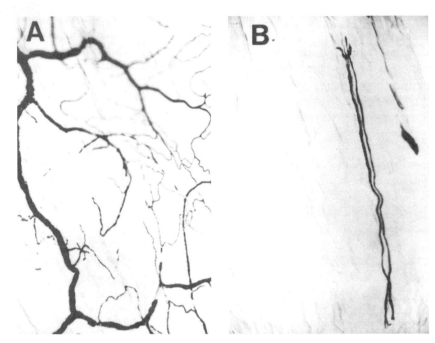

FIGURE 5.21 Photomicrographs of ink-injected epiligament covering normal medial collateral ligament (MCL) (A) and ink-injected ligament tissue from normal MCL (B) (bar = 50 μm). (From Bray RC. Blood supply of ligaments: a brief overview. *Orthopaedics International Edition* 1995;39–48, with permission.)

lagen fibers run between bony attachments, usually deviating only to accommodate underlying bony contours. The ligament is surrounded by a very thin external sheath, the epiligament (265,272). This tissue is more cellular and contains more vessels than ligamentous tissue (Fig. 5.22). The epiligament is continuous with the endoligament, which has septal divisions that extend deep into ligaments, forming bundles of collagen fibers (Fig. 5.23). Some structures may also have gross structural separations (e.g., two bands of an ACL) (268).

When ligaments are cut with a blade, other features of their gross internal architecture can be seen. Transverse cuts can reveal longitudinal grouping of collagen fiber bundles within some ligaments, consistent with the functional subdivisions noted previously. This is noticeably true in the hu-

man ACL, where septa can divide substance into bands that are reminiscent of tendon fascicles. This is not true of all ligaments, however, and may be a reflection of their varying functional complexities. Alternatively, such differences in ligament architecture may reflect location, size, or varying tissue composition among ligaments.

Light Microscopy

Matrix and Cells

Polarized light microscopy is one of the techniques most commonly employed to examine ligament microstructure. With this technique, collagen bundles appear aligned along the longitudinal axis of the ligament. However, there can be also seen to be seen an underlying "waviness" or crimp along

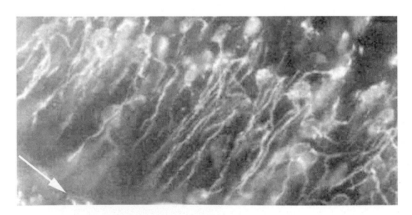

FIGURE 5.22 Histologic section of the epiligament demonstrating increased cellularity and long, branching, cytoplasmic projections perpendicular to the long axis of the ligament (1,500× magnification). Sections were immunolabeled for vimentin; arrow denotes axis of ligament.

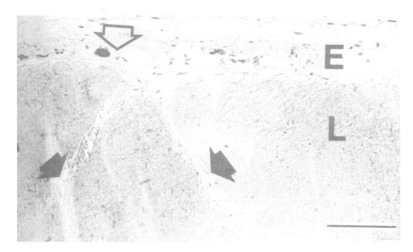

FIGURE 5.23 Low-power view of junction between medial-side epiligament (E) and ligament (L) sectioned in the transverse plane. Note the connective tissue septa *(solid arrows)*, which are continuous with epiligament at the epiligament–ligament junction. These septa (endoligament) subdivide the medial collateral ligament into discrete fascicles. Open arrow indicates neuroascular bundle. (Partly-polarized illumination with Nomarski optics; hematoxylin and eosin stain; bar = 100 μm.) (From Chowdhury P, Matyas JR, Frank CB. The "epiligament' of the rabbit medial collateral ligament: a quantitative morphological study. *Connect Tissue Res* 1991;27:33–50, with permission.)

its length (Fig. 5.24). The nonhomogeneity and significance of this crimp has been reviewed by others (263,273–275), and its possible biomechanical function remains a subject of ongoing investigation (276). In paraffin-embedded, formalin-fixed rabbit MCL, for example, the crimp wavelength varies from 40 to 85 μm depending on a number of factors, including sampling location, animal age, strain state of the tissue during fixation, type of fixative, and time of fixation. Crimp periods and angles (273) probably have important functional implications, but more work is required to define these implications more clearly.

Historically, thin sections of ligament tissue stained with hematoxylin and eosin have provided an overview of both matrix and cellular morphology. In general, as suggested at the gross level, ligaments appear to be made up of nearly parallel arrangements of collagen. However, individual collagen fibrils usually cannot be seen at these magnifications. Embedded within the pink-staining collagen mass are dark-staining cells which have been called either fibroblasts or fi-

brocytes by various investigators (261,263). These ovoid or spindle-shaped cells are sparse and are usually oriented longitudinally along the long axis of the structure. Even in the midsubstance, however, not all of these ligament cells look the same (264). The rabbit MCL, for example, contains cells that have larger boundary dimensions compared with those of patellar ligament or other cruciate ligaments from the same animal. The cruciate ligaments are unique in having longitudinal chains of more ovoid cells, whereas the patellar ligament (the structure connecting the patella to the tibia; often called the patellar tendon) appears to have more sparsely distributed, very long, thin cells. A similar pattern is seen in the adult human homologs of these ligaments (Fig. 5.25), suggesting ligament-specific rather than species-specific differences in tissue development, maintenance, or function (265).

The cellular morphology of these cells has been clarified. Although these cells may appear functionally and physically isolated, evidence from immunohistochemical studies demonstrated that this is not the case (277). With the use of indirect immunofluorescence of thick ligament sections and antibodies to cytoskeletal proteins, the full extent of ligament cells was demonstrated. Normal ligaments contained fusiform cells arranged in rows parallel to the collagen fiber orientation. Normal ligament cells exhibited prominent cytoplasmic extensions that extended for long distances through the ECM and were connected to cytoplasmic processes from adjacent cells (Fig. 5.26) to form an elaborate three-dimensional architecture. Gap junctions were detected in association with these cell connections, forming the basis for potential cell-to-cell communication (Fig. 5.27) (277). These new findings suggest that ligament cells similar to cells in other tissue types (e.g., those involved in spread of excitation in the heart) (278) may have the potential to coordinate their cellular and metabolic responses throughout the entire length of the ligament (Fig. 5.28). These findings require further investigation to understand their significance.

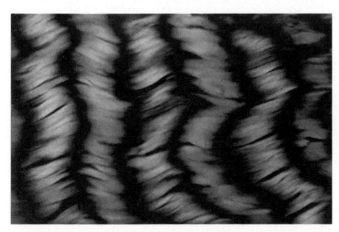

FIGURE 5.24 Wavy crimp in the midsubstance of a rabbit medial collateral ligament seen with polarized light. Note distinct superficial epiligament (E) on surface of ligament (L) (hematoxylin and eosin stain, 125× magnification).

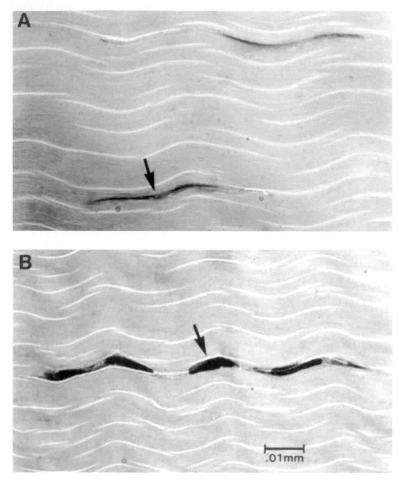

FIGURE 5.25 Cells in midsubstance of adult human ligaments. **A:** Medial collateral ligament. **B:** Anterior cruciate ligament (hematoxylin and eosin stain, 310× magnification).

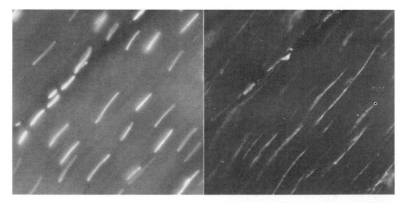

FIGURE 5.26 Histologic sections of normal medial collateral ligament. When sectioned along the long axis of the ligament, the cells were found to have long cytoplasmic processes connecting cells within rows. Left figure is stained with DAPI for cell nuclei; right figure is immunolabeled for vimentin (1,000× magnification). (From Lo IKY, et al. The cellular networks of normal ovine medial collateral and anterior cruciate ligaments are not accurately recapitulated in scar. J Anatomy *[in press]*, with permission.)

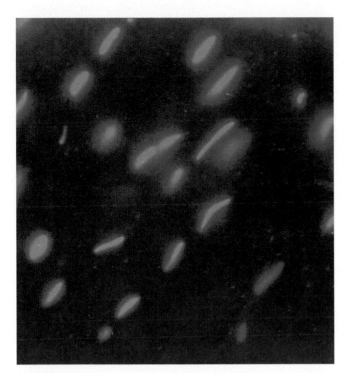

FIGURE 5.27 Gap junctions between adjacent cells within the normal medial collateral ligament demonstrated in sections immunolabeled for connexin-43 (red) and counterstained with DAPI (false-colored green) (600× magnification). (From Lo IKY, et al. The cellular networks of normal ovine medial collateral and anterior cruciate ligaments are not accurately recapitulated in scar. *J Anatomy [in press]*, with permission.)

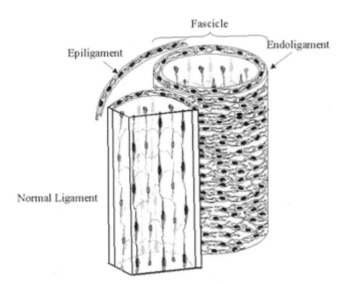

FIGURE 5.28 Schematic representation of the three-dimensional array of cells in a normal ligament. Cells are organized into parallel sheets in which the cells are arranged in adjacent rows. Within each row, the cells are spindle-shaped and have long cytoplasmic projections connected by gap junctions. Cells between sheets are also connected by long projections and gap junctions. Each fascicle, containing multiple sheets of cells, is enveloped by the endoligament. The cellular projections of the epiligament cells are oriented perpendicular to ligament cells. The fascicles are then surrounded by epiligament.

Insertions

Insertions of ligaments into bone are unique, with varying fiber orientations, cell shapes, and dimensions. At most ligament insertions, there are characteristic zones of cellular change, which have been well described by others (279). Thin midsubstance ligament cells gradually merge into more round "cartilaginous" cells. Near the surface of the bone, this cartilage becomes calcified and merges finally into compact bone (Fig. 5.29). The entire area over which this differentiation occurs has been called the *ligament insertion* and corresponds with the gross area at which ligament fibers appear to end in bone.

Although this arrangement is considered typical of all ligament insertions, it is not universal. The tibial insertion of the rabbit MCL, for example, is less typical in the sense that its zonal arrangement is less distinct (280–282), and this arrangement changes dramatically with growth and maturation.

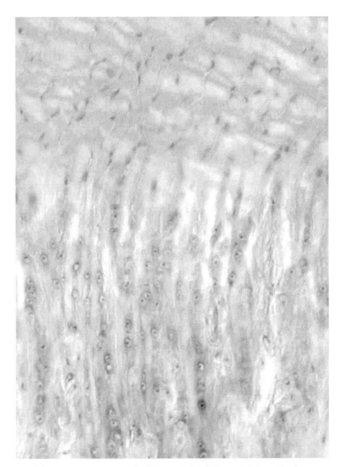

FIGURE 5.29 Femoral insertion of rabbit medial collateral ligament. Note ligament substance, characterized by fibroblasts *(top)* merging into round cartilaginous cells *(bottom)*. Zones from top to bottom would be: ligament, fibrocartilage, and mineralized fibrocartilage approaching bone (250× magnification).

Electron Microscopy

Scanning Microscopy

The scanning electron microscope provides higher-power perspectives of ligament surfaces. In frozen-fractured ligaments, undulating collagen fibers are again seen along the long axis of the ligament. High-power micrographs show only fractions of these undulations and therefore are more useful for studying individual collagen fibrils. A specific image analysis method showed that "average" fibril orientations can be quantified (283–285) and statistically compared from area to area within a single ligament or between several ligaments. A typical plot shows that collagen fibrils in the midsubstance of these fractured samples of normal MCL undulate within 30 degrees of their long axis (Fig. 5.30).

Transmission Microscopy

TEM offers another perspective on ligament structure. With glutaraldehyde fixation and postfixation in osmium tetroxide, cross sections of MCL matrix show a very com-

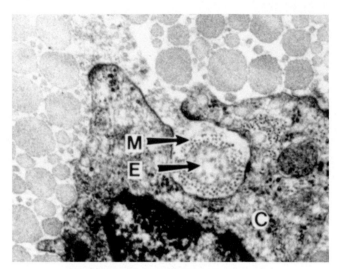

FIGURE 5.31 Elastic fiber, within a pocket of a cell (C), is made up of an amorphous core (E) and small microfibrils (M) (37,000× magnifcation).

plex, heterogeneous architecture. Roughly circular collagen fibrils of many different sizes are seen in cross section. As with other dense connective tissues (286–290), these fibril sizes can be quantified and compared statistically. With the use of such methods, collagen fibril diameter distributions in the rabbit MCL have been shown to vary with age and also with location within the ligament (286). At this time, the ligament collagen hierarchy is speculated to be analogous to the previously proposed structure of some tendons (274).

In addition to collagen fibrils, TEM sections of ligaments demonstrate a relatively small number of elastic fibers, characterized by an electron-translucent elastin core surrounded by 10- to 15-nm microfibrils (289,290). In many MCL sections, these fibers qualitatively appear to be more concentrated in juxtacellular areas (Fig. 5.31).

The main body of ligament cells observed in TEM micrographs can be seen to contain a nucleus that is separated from the surrounding cell membrane by a thin layer of cytoplasm. Most ligament cell cytoplasm is contained within the cell processes (Fig. 5.32). These thin, lamellar, cytoplasmic extensions ramify through the matrix fibrils over great distances from the cell body. Junctions between these cell processes can be seen, confirming the light microscopic findings. Thus it has been demonstrated that ligament cells are interconnected and therefore are not as isolated as previously thought.

Cationic stains applied before TEM embedding can also be used to gain a qualitative appreciation of dense connective tissue matrix and cells (291). Cuprolinic blue–stained granules are seen adjacent to D-bands of ligament collagen fibrils, consistent with the presence of small dermatan sulfate proteoglycans (probably decorin) demonstrated at these locations in other connective tissues (291). Ruthenium

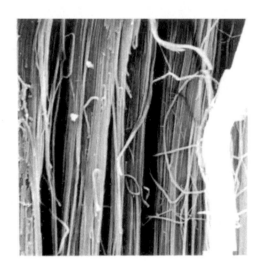

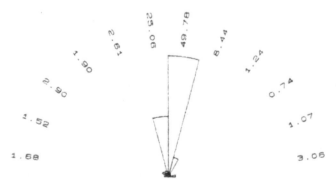

FIGURE 5.30 Collagen fibrils in normal rabbit medial collateral ligament midsubstance seen with scanning electron microscopy (4,000× magnification). Rose diagram below shows relative distribution of fibril directions in this area and demonstrates that fibril orientation varies within about 30 degrees of the long axis of the ligament.

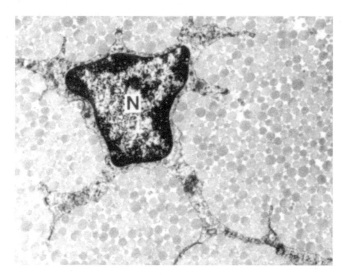

FIGURE 5.32 Collagen fibrils adjacent to ligament cell containing a nucleus (N). Note long lateral cytoplasmic processes which interconnect cells (10,000× magnification).

staining further suggests that the MCL midsubstance may be separated longitudinally by 20- to 100-nm wide "seams" of granular, anionic material (Fig. 5.33). This material also interconnects the processes of adjacent cells and is found in abundance near cells (Fig. 5.34). When specimens are treated with glycosaminoglycan-degrading enzymes, much

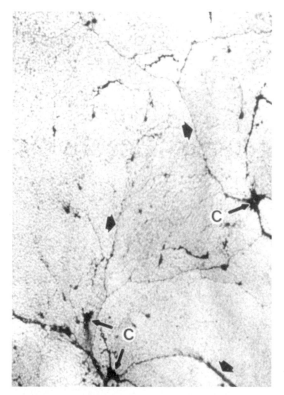

FIGURE 5.33 Low-magnification cross section showing subdivision of rabbit medial collateral ligament midsubstance by "seams" *(broad arrowheads)* of anionically charged material, which is also interconnecting cells (C) (3,000× magnification).

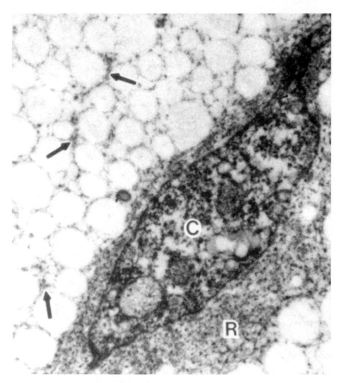

FIGURE 5.34 High magnification of cell process (C) surrounded by ruthenium-stained material (R), containing both granules and filaments (40,000× magnification). Note that ruthenium-stained granules *(arrows)* are also seen in interfibrillar locations. Extraction with the enzyme chondroitinase ABC suggests that this granular material consists, in part, of glycosaminoglycans.

of this granular material is removed from seams, suggesting that a major seam component is proteoglycan. When these proteoglycans are removed, a beaded filamentous network is revealed, consistent with the appearance of type VI collagen (292,293). Another microfilamentous network, most likely elastic in origin, is also seen in these seams. If the seams are, in fact, rich in proteoglycan, they potentially represent hydrophilic zones, which could serve either biomechanical or biologic roles in a functioning ligament. Further quantification of these areas is clearly required before such speculations can be tested (293).

Anterior Cruciate Ligament

Anatomy

The ACL is an intraarticular ligament that originates from the medial aspect of the lateral femoral condyle and inserts distally on the anterior tibial plateau (265,294). The ACL is enveloped by a synovial sheath together with the PCL and is thus intraarticular yet extrasynovial. The synovial membrane is an important source of blood supply and may aid in sheltering the ACL from the intraarticular environment (295,296). The mean length of the structure varies from 31 to 38 mm (294,297).

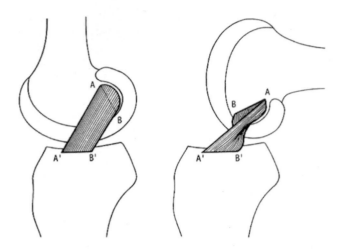

FIGURE 5.35 Schematic drawing representing changes in shape and tension of anterior cruciate ligament components in flexion and extension. In flexion, there is lengthening of the small medial band (A–A') and shortening of the bulk of the ligament (B–B'). (From Girgis FG, Marshall JL, Monajem ARS. The cruciate ligaments of the knee joint: anatomical, functional and experimental analysis. *Clin Orthop* 1975;106:216–231, with permission.)

The ACL has been described classically as containing two functional bundles, the anteromedial and the posterolateral bundles, referring to the anatomic position of their tibial insertions (265,294,298–300) (Fig. 5.35). The posterolateral component comprises the bulk of the ACL; the anteromedial bundle is smaller. Many investigators have reported that the bundles have differential tensions during knee motion, with the anteromedial bundle taut in flexion and the posterolateral bundle taut in extension. Although others have described a third (intermediate) bundle (294), the ACL is best thought of conceptually as a continuum of fibers that are tight at different angles of knee flexion, with no true "isometric" point.

Insertional Anatomy

Several authors have described the insertional anatomy of the ACL (294,297,301). Their studies demonstrated that the femoral attachment circumscribes an oval or circular segment of approximately 18 to 23 mm in maximal diameter on the medial aspect of the lateral femoral condyle (Fig. 5.36). The tibial insertion has also been described as oval in shape, with a maximal diameter of 17 mm and minimal diameter of 11 mm (294,297,301) (Fig. 5.37). The cross-sectional areas of the insertions is more than 3.5 times greater than the cross-sectional area of the midsubstance, emphasizing the manner in which the ACL attachments spread widely over their bony insertions.

Microscopic Anatomy

The cellular morphology and ultrastructure of the ACL are in general similar to those of other ligaments (302). The

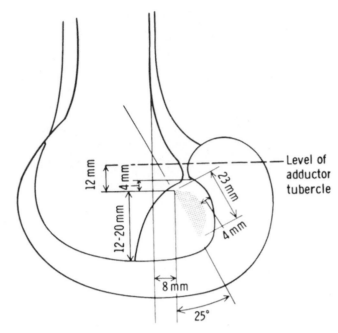

FIGURE 5.36 Drawing of the medial surface of the right lateral femoral condyle showing the average measurement and bony relations of the femoral attachment of the anterior cruciate ligament. (From Girgis FG, Marshall JL, Monajem ARS. The cruciate ligaments of the knee joint. *Clin Orthop* 1975;105:216–231, with permission.)

cells of the ACL appear to be a unique population of fibroblasts, which are in the early stages of characterization (303–305). Some differences have been noted in the cellular morphology and behavior of cells of the ACL compared with those of the MCL, but further research is necessary to understand the implications of such findings (303–313).

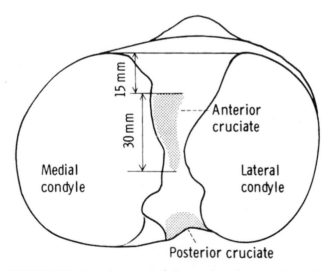

FIGURE 5.37 Superior view of the cruciate ligament insertion sites on the tibia. The anterior cruciate ligament inserts on the anterior aspect of the intercondylar eminence. The posterior cruciate ligament inserts on the posterior tibia well below the joint line. (From Girgis FG, Marshall JL, Monajem ARS. The cruciate ligaments of the knee joint. *Clin Orthop* 1975;105:216–231, with permission.)

Histologically, the cells of the ACL are surrounded by a matrix consisting mainly of type I and type III collagen.

The ECM consists of a range of small-diameter (20 to 30 nm) and large-diameter (155 to 175 nm) fibrils (314–316). The fibril diameters vary over the length of the ACL and match the changes in cross-sectional area. That is, the cross-sectional area and the mean fibril diameters increase from the femoral to the tibial insertion. Since the percentage area occupied by collagen is similar throughout the length of the ACL, this suggests that the increase in cross-sectional area is primarily secondary to the changes in collagen fibril diameter.

Neurovascular Anatomy

During development, there is a significant vascular contribution from the bony insertions of the ACL. However, this decreases with maturation (317,318). The main blood supply of the ACL in skeletally mature individuals is from the middle genicular artery and secondarily from smaller vessels of the lateral inferior genicular artery (265,319). These vessels are the primary supply to the periligamentous vessels within the enveloping synovial sheath, and they extend transversely into the ACL, branching into a meshwork of longitudinal vessels that run parallel between collagen bundles (265). After injury, the synovial membrane and the infrapatellar fat pad are the structures primarily responsible for the vascular response, again suggesting little contribution from the bony attachments (265,319,320).

The neural anatomy of the ACL closely follows the course of the synovial vessels. The origin of the nerve supply to the ACL is through the tibial nerve posteriorly (321,322). Several studies have now documented mechanoreceptors within the human ACL (322), including Gogli tendon organs, Ruffini's corpuscles, pacinian corpuscles, and free nerve endings, suggesting a neurosensory function of the human ACL. In addition, the paravascular neural elements may be involved in vasomotor control (323).

Posterior Cruciate Ligament

Anatomy

The PCL is named for both its spatial orientation and its insertion site on the posterior aspect of the tibia. Like the ACL, the PCL is enveloped by a fold of synovium from the posterior capsule, leading to its intraarticular yet extrasynovial structure.

Traditionally, the PCL has been described as having three major components: the anterolateral bundle, the posteromedial bundle, and the meniscofemoral ligaments (Fig. 5.38) (324–327). Although other investigators have suggested that the PCL is not composed of anatomically distinct bundles but rather is a continuum of fibers that slacken and tighten with knee motion (328–331), these traditional

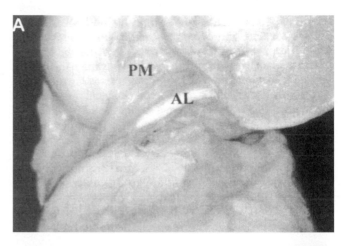

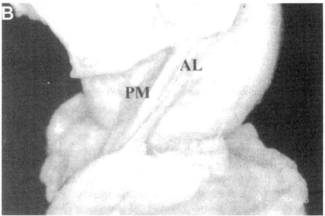

FIGURE 5.38 Lateral view of the right knee with the lateral femoral condyle removed, showing anatomy of the posterior collateral ligament and its components. **A:** Knee in extension. **B:** Knee in 80 degrees of flexion. AL, anterolateral component; PM, posteromedial component. (From Harner CD, Hoher J. Evaluation and treatment of posterior cruciate ligament injuries. *Am J Sports Med* 1998;26:471–482, with permission.)

subdivisions allow an easy discussion of basic anatomy. The anterolateral bundle is thicker than the posteromedial bundle, and each of them has distinct anatomic characteristics, insertion sites, and biomechanical properties (332). The two bundles were named based on their positions at their femoral and tibial insertions (i.e., the anterolateral bundle is more anterior on the femur and more lateral on the tibia than the posteromedial bundle), and they have different tensioning patterns during knee motion (332,333). The anterolateral bundle is tight in flexion and relatively lax in extension. Conversely, the posteromedial bundle is tight in extension and relatively lax in flexion (327,333–336). The anterolateral bundle is larger than the posteromedial bundle, and its structural properties are also superior (325,332). For this reason, the anterolateral bundle is commonly reconstructed during one-bundle PCL reconstruction.

The meniscofemoral ligaments originate from the posterior horn of the lateral meniscus, pass anterior or posterior to the PCL, and insert onto the medial femoral condyle near the origin of the PCL. There are two meniscofemoral ligaments which are variably present anterior and posterior to the PCL (the ligament of Humphry and the ligament of Wrisberg, respectively). These ligaments are present in approximately 71% of knees with equal frequency; however, only 6% of knees have both meniscofemoral ligaments (337). Although these two ligaments have largely been ignored, their biomechanical properties (stiffness, ultimate load) are at least equal to if not greater than those of the posteromedial bundle (332,338). This suggests that the meniscofemoral ligaments may have important functional implications, including increasing the congruity between the meniscus and femoral condyle during knee flexion or as secondary restraints to posterior translation (337,339).

Insertional Anatomy

Several investigators have revealed that the PCL has a broad femoral origin, attaching in a semicircular outline on the medial femoral condyle (333,340) (Fig. 5.39). The PCL has an average length of 32 mm and a femoral insertion site that is approximately 14 mm at its greatest proximal–distal dimension (range, 12 to 17 mm), with an anteroposterior dimension of approximately 33 mm (range, 29 to 39 mm) (333,341).

The tibial insertion site lies within a depression 1 cm posterior and inferior to the articular surface of the tibial

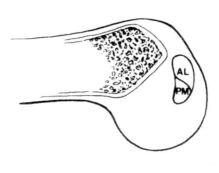

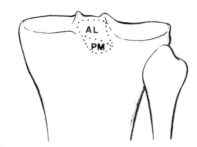

FIGURE 5.39 Schematic of posterior cruciate ligament femoral and tibial insertion site areas. AL, anterolateral component; PM, posteromedial component. (From Harner CD, Hoher J. Evaluation and treatment of posterior cruciate ligament injuries. *Am J Sports Med* 1998;26:471–482, with permission.)

plateau (Figs. 5.37 and 5.39). The mean dimension of the tibial attachment is approximately 24 by 25 mm.

Microscopic Anatomy

Like other ligaments, the PCL comprises multiple collagen fascicles containing primarily type I collagen, although types III, IV, and VI collagen are also found distributed throughout the matrix. (342,343). When placed under polarized light microscopy, the typical sinusoidal pattern of collagen crimp can be demonstrated; it has less amplitude than that of the MCL (344).

Ultrastructural studies of the collagen fibrils demonstrated that their diameters varied along the PCL length, ranging from approximately 20 to 175 nm (314–316) and increasing from the tibial to the femoral insertion opposite to the ACL. The cross-sectional area of the PCL also increased from the tibial to the femoral insertion (341). As with the ACL, the change in cross-sectional area was most likely secondary to the increase in fibril diameters. The meniscofemoral ligaments demonstrated the largest collagen fibrils and did not vary over their length. These studies highlight the intricate structural and ultrastructural morphologies of the PCL and may be important characteristics to reproduce during ligament reconstruction.

Neurovascular Anatomy

The vascular supply to the PCL is predominantly through a branch of the popliteal artery, the middle genicular artery (345). The bony attachments of the PCL (origin and insertion) do not significantly contribute to the overall vascularity. The middle genicular artery also supplies the synovium overlying the PCL and is itself a contributor to the vascularity of the PCL (346). Vessels within the synovial sheath of the PCL arborize and form a plexus of vessels, which penetrate the ligament and anastomose with longitudinal endoligamentous vessels (347). In addition to the popliteal artery, the medial and lateral inferior genicular arteries may supply a portion of the blood supply to the distal PCL.

The primary nerve supply to the PCL is via the posterior articular nerve and from terminal branches of the obturator nerve (323). Several authors have also identified Golgi-like tendon organs, Ruffini's corpuscles, Vater–Pacini corpuscles, and free nerve endings within the PCL (321,323,348). These receptors may relay important sensory information centrally, concerning noxious stimuli, joint position, or motion sense (349).

NORMAL LIGAMENT FUNCTIONS
Passive Joint Stabilizers

Skeletal ligaments are uniquely positioned on bones to passively stabilize joints and to help guide those joints through

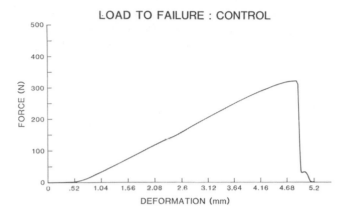

FIGURE 5.40 Load–deformation curve of normal rabbit medial collateral ligament complex showing nonlinear behavior. Note increasing stiffness up to a linear region before yield and tensile failure.

their normal range of motion. As noted previously, different parts of an otherwise homogeneous-appearing ligament can become tight in different positions of the joint that they serve, or under different loading conditions. Ligaments thus act collectively as a series of stabilizing elements during joint function.

Of particular importance to this stabilizing function of ligaments is their nonlinear, anisotopic mechanical behavior (Fig. 5.40). Under low-load conditions, ligaments are relatively compliant. With increasing tensile loads, ligaments become increasingly stiff until they reach a range in which they exhibit almost linear stiffness. Beyond that range, ligaments continue to absorb energy up to the point of tensile failure. This low-load, nonlinear behavior results, in part, from recruitment of "crimped" collagen fibers (262,276,350), and also from the viscoelastic behaviors and interactions of collagen and other matrix materials. Not all parts of a ligament are under the same conditions of strain at any point in time (259,270,276), and loads may be distributed across or along the structure, depending on the conditions under which it is loaded. Failures may therefore occur in various ways across the width of a ligament, along its length, or in combined configurations—all dependent on the boundary conditions of how loads are applied to the joint in question. Clinical grades of ligament injuries can be correlated with increasing degrees of structural failure. A grade I injury to a ligament probably represents the failure of a small number of its elements. A grade II injury represents the failure of a significant portion of the ligamentous structure, but with some elements remaining intact. A grade III injury probably correlates with complete structural disruption of the ligament.

Viscoelastic Behaviors for Joint Homeostasis

In addition to their obviously important protective resistance against high joint loads, ligaments serve several other functions. Under low-load conditions, ligaments provide low resistances. They do, nonetheless, offer some tensile resistance across a joint, and the amount of that resistance probably varies with specific factors such as age and gender. Possibly the most important factor determining the low-load resistance of ligaments is their loading history (259). As with other viscoelastic materials, ligaments alter their mechanical behaviors depending on the manner in which they have been loaded (loading rate, loading limits, loading history) and on their environments (e.g., temperature, water content). The detailed evidence for these characteristics is beyond the scope of this chapter, but it can be reviewed by those who are interested (261–263,257–259,266,270).

The first of these low-load behaviors of ligaments is that of cyclic load relaxation. With an increasing number of cycles under similar conditions of displacement, ligaments reach progressively lower peak loads. Ultimately, they appear to reach an optimum, or at least a repeatable peak load, suggesting that they adapt structurally when being cycled to achieve a new biomechanical equilibrium (Fig. 5.41).

An analogous ligament behavior is that of static load relaxation (Fig. 5.42). Again, the rate at which this relaxation takes place is almost certainly specific to the conditions under which the relaxation is occurring (261) and the age of the individual from whom the ligament was taken (351,352). As with cyclic relaxation, the ability of a ligament to adjust its load-carrying capacity to suit a particular set of environmental circumstance indicates that ligaments are adaptable. This probably represents one of the "fine-tuning" mechanisms of joint loading that helps to control tissue behaviors.

Although these two low-load behaviors were previously evaluated in detail (353–359), more recent evidence suggests that ligaments (360) and tendons (361,362) may func-

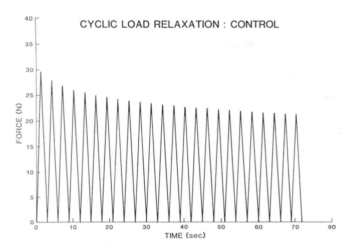

FIGURE 5.41 Cyclic load relaxation behavior of normal control medial collateral ligament, showing decreasing peak load with repeated similar deformations over time. Note the nonlinear pattern and the tendency for the ligament to reach a new equilibrium as the number of cycles increases.

STATIC LOAD RELAXATION : CONTROL

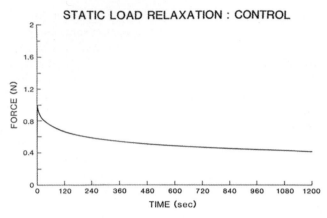

FIGURE 5.42 Static load relaxation of normal medial collateral ligament. A fixed deformation causes nonlinear load relaxation through the ligament complex over time.

tion in normal daily activity under repeated low loads (cyclic creep) (Fig. 5.43) or sustained low loads (static creep) (Fig. 5.44). For example, the same step repeated in walking requires the same acceleration and deceleration of the limbs and therefore the same loads at the joint. Ligaments under this environment would respond through creep rather than relaxation. Creep is defined as deformation (or elongation) under a constant or cyclically repetitive load. This type of behavior is particularly relevant clinically, because excessive ligament creep could result in laxity of a joint after joint injury or reconstructive surgery.

Creep results cannot be predicted from stress relaxation tests, suggesting that a fundamental difference exists in the way ligaments respond to creep versus relaxation conditions (363). Under conditions of stress relaxation, the viscoelastic response probably results from an unchanging subset of fibers within a ligament, whereas under conditions of creep the viscoelastic properties are a result of progressive recruitment of fibers (364,365). With progressive

fiber recruitment, there is an increase in the load-bearing area of the ligament over time. Therefore, the initial stress is redistributed, reducing stress on the fibers initially loaded. Ligaments seem to be uniquely designed to resist creep and excessive ligament elongation through fiber recruitment (366–371).

A final viscoelastic behavior of ligament complexes is that of strain-rate sensitivity. *In vitro* failure tests have shown that ligaments themselves are relatively strain-rate insensitive, while bone is more sensitive (262). At higher strain rates, ligaments do become slightly more stiff and can absorb slightly more energy than when strained slowly. Bone, on the other hand, such as the bone at the insertion of the ligaments, is more strain-rate dependent, exhibiting even more strength and stiffness when strained more quickly. The implications of these responses are that bone–ligament–bone complexes can adapt, to some extent, to high strain rates in a way that would help to minimize their injury. Further, at high loading rates, ligament substance will be the "weak link" in the bone–ligament–bone complex, because it is somewhat less strain-rate responsive than bone.

Ligament viscoelastic recovery is an entirely different subject that has been studied incompletely but clearly has equally important implications. The rate at which ligaments return to prestrained states is obviously critical to joint recovery from various loading states and may be important in resistance to injury. These rates of recovery are not well documented, but under *in vitro* conditions they appear to be in the order of hours to days.

Neurosensory Function of Ligaments

In addition to these mechanical functions, ligaments may serve a role in joint proprioception. Proprioception is now generally referred to as the conscious perception of limb po-

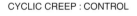

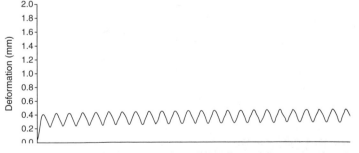

FIGURE 5.43 Cyclic creep behavior of normal control medial collateral ligament, showing increasing deformation with repeated similar stresses over time. Note the nonlinear pattern and the tendency for the ligament to reach a new equilibrium as the number of cycles increases.

STATIC CREEP : CONTROL

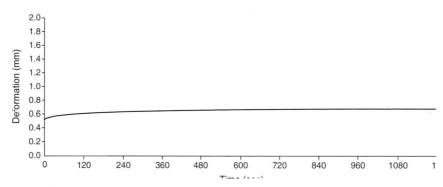

FIGURE 5.44 Static creep behavior of normal medial collateral ligament. A sustained stress causes a nonlinear creep (deformation) through the ligament complex over time.

sition in space (372). The central nervous system receives input from several sources of stimuli, which ultimately define the perception and sensation of joint movement and position. These stimuli—visual, auditory, vestibular, cutaneous, joint, and muscle—provide proprioceptive information to three distinct levels of motor control: the spine, the brainstem, and the higher centers (e.g., cerebellum, basal ganglia, motor cortex) (373–377).

Although the visual, auditory, and vestibular systems aid in keeping body balance, providing visual cues and references points for orientation, in joints such as the knee proprioception is provided primarily by joint, muscle, and cutaneous receptors (373,378–381).

Within ligament, at least four different types of proprioceptors have been identified, including bare nerve endings, Ruffini endings, pacinian corpuscles, and Golgi tendon organs (260,380,382,383). In essence, what has been suggested is that this innervation, although relatively sparse, may be critical to joint physiology; this idea has supplied the impetus for an explosion of investigations of ligament neurophysiology.

An involuntary reaction in response to a stimulus applied to the periphery and transmitted to the nervous centers in the brain or spinal cord is termed a neural reflex. Such a reflex, a ligamentomuscular protective reflex, was demonstrated in ligaments of the knee (380,384). Several studies have now demonstrated that ligament strains or stimuli do evoke afferent nerve traffic in periarticular nerves, with some spinal cord connections and muscle feedback loops (380,384–390), creating a type of neural reflex. For example, Palmer (390) demonstrated that excessive valgus force placed on the knee is resisted not only by the MCL but also by contraction of the semimembanosus, sartorius, and vastus medialis muscles.

Similarly, Solomonow et al. (384) demonstrated that when the ACL is placed under loads that are beyond the physiologic strain limits of the normal ligament, receptors

within the ACL are stimulated and there is a reflex contraction of the hamstring musculature. Therefore, any abnormal anterior translation of the tibia is detected by the receptors within the ACL and is resisted by hamstring muscle contraction (384,387,388).

These finding were supported by Sjolander et al. (389), who observed that direct deformation of the ACL intraoperatively elicited activity in the neural arcs of the muscle spindles in the hamstring muscles, presumably to decrease anterior translation of the knee. Although the ligamentomuscular protective reflex presumably functions during excessively high loads, other reflexes, including those with receptors in the joint capsule and muscle, may be relevant at lower loads (380,391).

However, the significance of these connections and a feedback system of proprioceptors and nociceptors in ligaments to potentially "protect" joints remains controversial. It does appear, however, that proprioception and neuromuscular control can be affected by a number of factors, including training, fatigue, injury, surgery, and rehabilitation. These factors have been reviewed extensively (374,375,392).

Function of the Anterior Cruciate Ligament

The primary mechanical role of the ACL is to carry loads across the knee and to resist forces that may cause abnormal translation or rotation throughout the normal physiologic range of motion (393–399). The ACL is particularly designed to resist anterior tibial translation (394,400–403). Several investigators have demonstrated that the ACL accounts for approximately 86% of the primary restraint to anterior tibial translation. In addition, the ACL resists forces that may cause abnormal tibial rotation or abduction (404–406). The unique gross (i.e., bundles) and microscopic (i.e., fiber orientation) anatomy of the ACL allows for differential fiber recruitment to resist loads during knee motion and during subtle changes in the position of the tibia relative to the femur (407).

However, the ACL does not function in isolation. For example, cadaveric studies have demonstrated that division of the MCL significantly increases the forces borne by the ACL in external rotation of the tibia (408). In addition, MCL transection significantly increases anterior tibial translation in an ACL-deficient knee (409). These findings suggest that an incompetent MCL may increase the resultant forces and loads on the ACL or after ACL reconstruction. Several other *in vitro* studies have demonstrated that the ACL works in concert with other structures, such as the LCL, posterolateral structures, menisci, and muscles of the knee, to maintain stability (410–415). This further emphasizes the importance of evaluating and treating the entire knee joint.

Like other ligaments, the normal daily loads encountered by the ACL are probably only small (360,416–418). Attempts have estimated such loads to be approximately 400 to 500 N (360,419,420), representing only about 20% of the ligament's failure load (2,500 N in young specimens) (421,422). Only during cutting and sudden acceleration and deceleration activities does the magnitude of the load approach its failure capacity (420). Furthermore, estimates and *in vivo* measurements show that the strain of the ACL is approximately only 5% during any rehabilitation exercise (400,418,419,423–425). These strains represent only 25% of the maximal failure strain of a normal ACL (407,426).

Although the vast majority of investigations have focused on high-load properties of the ACL (i.e., failure loads, failure strains), the ACL, like all ligaments, possess viscoelastic behaviors that allow it to dissipate energy and adjust its length and internal load distribution according to its load history (426–429). In this way the ACL is able to constantly adapt to internal stresses over time, altering laxity, stresses, and kinematics of the joint. The role of these properties in normal function of ligaments and during ligament healing and reconstruction are continuing to be investigated (363–371).

With the identification of specific mechanoreceptors within the ACL, there has been increasing interest in the role of proprioception within the knee joint. Damage to the ACL probably likely disrupts the mechanoreceptor function of the ACL and therefore the pathways involved in joint position sense and kinesthesia (threshold to detection of passive motion). Several investigators have demonstrated alterations in proprioception in patients with ACL insufficiency (430–432). In addition, ACL deficiency may result in deficiencies in the ligamentomuscular protective reflex (431,432). For example, Beard et al. (431) demonstrated a significant delay in reflex activation of the hamstring muscles after a 100 N anterior shear force in ACL-insufficient patients. Although ACL reconstruction appears to partly restore proprioceptive abilities, measurable deficits still are detectable between normal and ACL-reconstructed patients. (430,433).

Function of the Posterior Cruciate Ligament

Several authors have demonstrated *in vitro* that the strain of fibers within the PCL is altered during knee motion. Collectively these studies have suggested that the degree and pattern of change of ligament fibers or modeled ligament fibers is more sensitive to the position in the femoral origin than in the tibial insertion (434–438). In addition, the most isometric portion of the PCL is represented only by a small, posterior oblique fiber region (439,440); the bulk of the PCL, including those fibers represented traditionally as the anterolateral bundle, are nonisometric.

The PCL provides the primary restraint to posterior tibial translation and a secondary restraint to external rotation (401,441–444). After complete PCL transection, as *in vitro* studies have demonstrated, there is an increase in posterior tibial translation with the application of a posterior tibial load. This translation is greatest at 90 degrees of flexion (401,445), reflecting the fact that the PCL carries approximately 85% to 100% of the load at that angle (401, 441, 446). Only small degrees of rotatory or varus/valgus laxities are obtained by isolated PCL transection (401,445). The PCL, however, is not a functionally isolated ligament. In particular, there is a close interrelationship between the PCL and the posterolateral structures of the knee (441–444,447–452). Injury to these structures can significantly increase the posterior laxity and rotatory stability of the knee and therefore may be critical in restoring normal joint function after injury.

Injury to the PCL alters the normal kinematic function of the knee. *In vitro* studies have demonstrated that after isolated or combined section of the PCL and posterolateral structures there is an increase in the medial and patellofemoral contact pressures in the knee (453,454). These finding are also consistent with long-term clinical outcome studies, which have demonstrated a high incidence of arthrosis in the medial femoral condyle and patellofemoral joint (456–458). This has been postulated to occur secondary to a shift in the joint's center of rotation medially and a relative positioning of the tibial tubercle posteriorly. Other *in vivo* studies have demonstrated (455) that rupture of the PCL results in posterior tibial subluxation during activities of daily living in which the knee is positioned in high flexion angles (i.e., using stairs). These findings stress the importance of the PCL at higher flexion angles. More than 85% to 90% of the PCL becomes tight at higher flexion angles, and this may act as a checkrein to prevent posterior tibial subluxation when other secondary structures (posteromedial capsule, posterolateral complex, posterior oblique ligament, MCL) become lax.

The role of the PCL as a neurosensory organ has not been as extensively studied as in the ACL. One study suggested that PCL-deficient knees have alterations in kinesthesia (the threshold to detect passive motion) and joint-position sense, indicating a role of the PCL in proprioception (459).

CONNECTIVE TISSUE RESPONSE TO INJURY

Diarthrodial joints are injured commonly in people of all ages, but from the relatively low incidence of subsequent joint destruction it might be inferred that joint tissues have some mechanisms for healing. Each tissue component of a joint probably undergoes either macroscopic or microscopic changes in structure or function in response to injuries, depending on the forces involved, the amount of physical disruption of the joint, and a number of factors peculiar to the tissues themselves. Collectively, these variables determine the ability of a joint to heal after an injury.

Empirically, however, compared with some organs within the body (e.g., skin), joint tissues probably do not heal well. Their healing appears to be more comparable to that of certain specialized organs (e.g., brain, kidney, heart), where an incomplete or minimal healing response takes place. In such circumstances, compensation by undamaged tissue or by other tissues is required. With the more microscopic injuries (such as those which may be occurring during normal activities), these joint tissues may actually respond very effectively. Such responses (i.e., their capacity for intrinsic repair to microscopic damage) are not well documented for most joint tissues and therefore cannot be discussed with much data. Healing responses to macroscopic injuries, on the other hand, are relatively well documented in both humans and animal models and form the bulk of our understanding of the ability of joint tissue to repair itself.

Injury and Healing of Ligaments

Again, relatively few ligaments have been studied with regard to their mechanisms of injury and repair. Knee ligaments have been studied most extensively and may serve as models for the healing of all others (460). As with subtle variations in normal ligament structure and function, however, some variations in ligament healing between ligaments and between joints can probably be expected and remain to be defined. This review of ligament injury and repair is restricted to what is currently known about damage and healing of the ACL and MCL of the knee. In addition, we review the current methods of altering the healing response of ligaments.

Anterior Cruciate Ligament

The ACL of the knee is thought to heal particularly poorly (Fig. 5.45), based on a number of clinical (461) and experimental (462) studies. Complete midsubstance disruptions of the ACL have been suggested in particular to have a very limited healing potential (462), and several potential causes have been proposed.

First, it is clear that the ACL is unique in spanning a joint space. Although extrasynovial, both the ACL and its surface layer of synovium are often totally disrupted, leaving free ends exposed to the space and relative vacuum of the joint

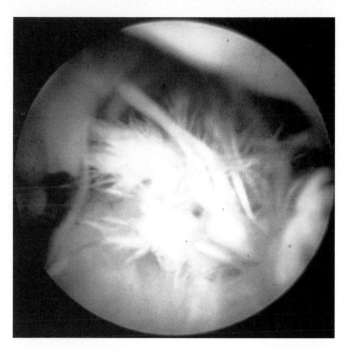

FIGURE 5.45 Chronic tear of human anterior cruciate ligament seen arthroscopically. Note resorption of torn ends, in this case, to fibrillated stumps.

cavity. The simple lack of any anatomic scaffolding or enclosure of torn ends (which prevents the formation of an organizing hematoma and vascular bed of soft tissue) may disrupt the initiation of healing. Further, this anatomic separation may be aggravated by joint movement, which might easily disrupt any connections that do form. The second explanation of poor ACL healing, therefore, may be attributed to mechanical causes. The lack of the ACL itself may destabilize the joint to a point beyond which healing is impossible. Forces on healing tissue may exceed the limits required for a "scar" to form. A third possibility, which has been proposed for many years but remains unproven, is a potential inhibitory property of synovial fluid (463). Exposure of torn ligament ends to synovial fluid may be directly inhibitory, or it may interfere with other factors required to initiate scar formation (e.g., blood clotting).

It is important to differentiate "no" healing response from "some" healing response: the latter implies that this intrinsic response may be augmented or improved in some fashion. Several studies have now demonstrated that after injury human ACLs can exhibit some signs of a healing response. For example, when observed arthroscopically, many torn ACLs do exhibit some signs of healing by which the torn ACL ends reattach to something new in the joint and may even provide some stability to the knee (Fig. 5.46) (464–467). Although the healing potential of such injuries may be species specific (rabbits and dogs seem to have less potential to heal), this healing response does in some ways seem to be similar to that described in extraarticular ligament healing (468).

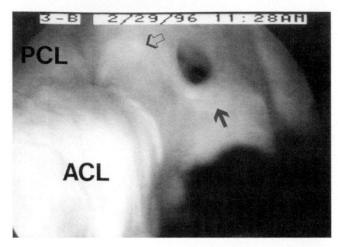

FIGURE 5.46 Arthroscopic appearance of the tibial remnant of an anterior cruciate ligament (ACL) disruption reattached to the roof of the notch and the posterior cruciate ligament (PCL) *(open arrow)*. The femoral end of the ACL *(solid arrow)* is also seen to be attached to the convergence of the ACL stump and the PCL. (From Lo IKY, de Matt GHR, Valk JW, et al. The gross morphology of torn human anterior cruciate ligaments in unstable knee. *Arthroscopy* 1999;15:301–306, with permission.)

Further, whereas complete injuries to the ACL result in little healing response, partial ACL injuries may enjoy more success (469–471). Although the fate of such "partial injuries" in clinical circumstances is not well known, animal experiments suggest that some healing potential of the ACL may exist and that the presence of a synovial sheath around the healing area may facilitate repair (469,470). The extent and limiting variables of this response, if proven, may be of utmost importance. At this point in time, however, the limited healing response of the ACL has necessitated other reconstructive measures, including ACL reconstruction, which are beyond the scope of this review.

Medial Collateral Ligament

Clinical studies on MCL healing have suggested that isolated MCL injuries heal quite well (472). In fact, these conclusions are based not so much on actual healing of that ligament as on the relative lack of functional disability that results from MCL injuries, compared with injuries to the ACL. Some degree of such successful healing of the MCL may actually relate to successful compensation for MCL function by other knee structures; structures that may become stiffer or stronger after MCL injury and help to stabilize the joint.

Experimental studies of the MCL have been carried out in a number of different animal models (261,263,473,474), providing a varied impression of its healing capabilities. Several multidisciplinary studies of healing-MCL structure and function have provided data on the mechanisms of MCL healing processes (473–496).

As noted in previous reviews (261,263,485–489), the healing process of the MCL can be subdivided into three phases: hemorrhage with inflammation, proliferation, and re-

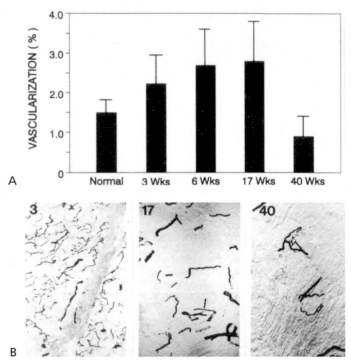

FIGURE 5.47 A: Plot of percent vascularization in the healed scar of medial collateral ligament (MCL) gap injury site at various intervals of healing. B: Photomicrographs of ink-injected, healing MCL scar from three distinct healing intervals. Note the progressive vascular regression as healing continues (bar = 50 μm). Injection of a scar in an MCL shows multiple vessels *(arrows)*. (From Bray RC. Blood supply of ligaments: a brief overview. *Orthopaedics International Edition* 1995;39–48, with permission.)

modeling. In the inflammatory phase, an initial blood clot is resorbed as torn ligament ends are filled by a heavy cellular infiltrate. Both degradative processes (to remove damaged material) and reparative processes (to replace material) are initiated by cellular and vascular factors. These changes may take place throughout the entire ligament substance and may even reach its insertions (490). A considerable hypertrophic vascular response then takes place in the gap between disrupted lig-

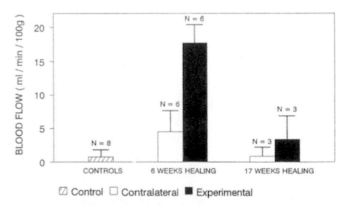

FIGURE 5.48 Blood flows to normal and healing medial collateral ligament tissues. Blood flow was determined with the use of colored microspheres. (From Bray RC. Blood supply of ligaments: a brief overview. *Orthopaedics International Edition* 1995;39–48, with permission.)

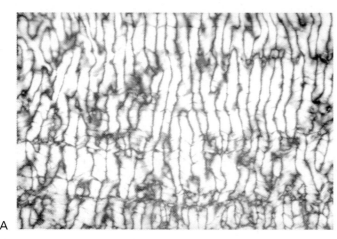 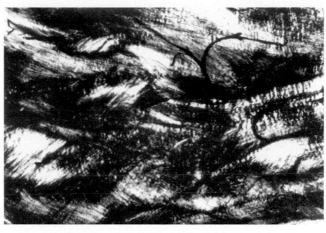

A   B

FIGURE 5.49 Polarized histologic appearance of rabbit medial collateral ligament (MCL) scar (A) compared with normal MCL (B) at the same magnification, showing differences in organization.

ament ends. This vascular response has been quantified and demonstrates increases in both vascularity and blood flow (Figs. 5.47 and 5.48) that decrease with time (492,493).

The proliferative phase of both adult and immature rabbit MCL healing involves the production of what appears to be "scar tissue." Hypertrophic fibroblastic cells produce a dense, cellular, collagenous connective tissue matrix that bridges torn MCL ends. This matrix is initially quite disorganized if the joint is allowed movement during the healing

process, and it has a histologic appearance that is different from the organization of normal ligament matrix (Fig. 5.49). Specific examination of scar ultrastructure during this phase, and even more chronically in the healing process, reveals that the types of collagen are probably abnormal (475,477,491) and that the collagen fibrils have smaller diameters in the proliferating tissue. This collagen is initially disorganized but does realign quite well along the ligament axis with time (497) (Fig. 5.50).

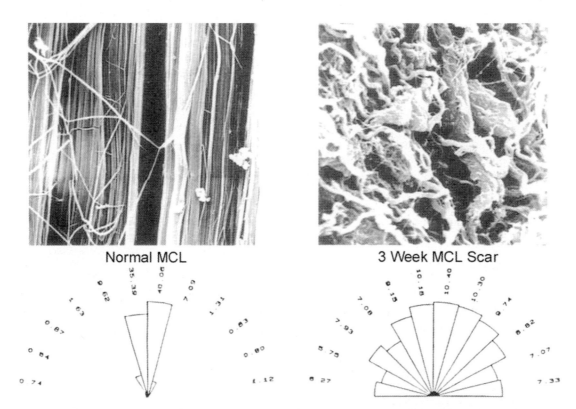

FIGURE 5.50 Scanning electron micrographs of a normal medial collateral ligament (MCL) **(right)** and a 3-week MCL scar **(left)** showing the differences in fibril alignment (4,000× magnification). Below each micrograph is the corresponding rose diagram that illustrates fibril orientation. Each petal of the rose diagram represents the relative number of fibrils in each of the 15-degree bands from 0 to 180 degrees. The ligament longitudinal axis is vertical.

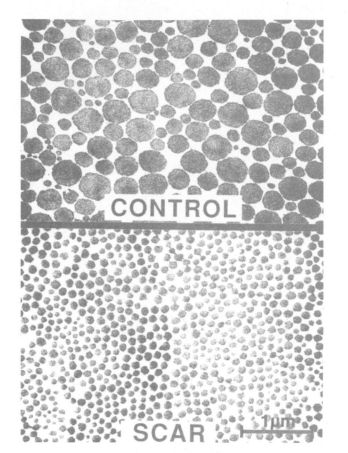

FIGURE 5.51 Transverse transmission electron micrographs of a control rabbit medial collateral ligament (MCL) and a 40-week MCL scar, demonstrating differences in collagen fibril diameters. (From Frank C, McDonald D, Bray D, et al. Collagen fibril diameters in the healing adult rabbit medial collateral ligament. *Connect Tiss Res* 1992,;27:251–263, with permission.)

As healing progresses, MCL scar components change their character and their orientation. Cellularity and vascularity decrease, but both remain abnormal (i.e., higher than in normal MCLs) for months to years. Scar components are modified and apparently mature to a new structural and functional baseline. Although some matrix components do

recover to within normal ligament baselines, several distinct abnormalities of healing scars appear to be chronic in nature (483–489) and may be responsible for the inferior mechanical properties of scar tissue. There appear to be differences in proteoglycan types (481), collagen types (474,477,491), collagen crosslinks (480), collagen fibril diameters (478,479; Fig. 5.51) and "flaws" (Fig. 5.52) (482). Although some of these discrepancies have been correlated with biomechanical outcomes, the role each plays in the normal day-to-day function of ligaments remains unclear.

The functional recovery of rabbit MCL scars over these same phases of healing has also been studied, at least in terms of specific biomechanical measures of integrity. As compared with normal MCL tissue, healing MCLs demonstrate a slow recovery of many properties. Prefailure viscoelastic properties of MCLs show an early relative increase in viscosity (Figs. 5.53 and 5.54), because the scar tends to stress-relax to a greater extent than normal ligament tissue. During cyclic loading or during a single static load, the healing MCL complex therefore maintains a load less efficiently than a normal ligament, thereby relying on other tissues to compensate by carrying more load. During the remodeling phase of MCL healing, these viscoelastic properties are recovered to within about 10% to 20% of normal (473).

Similar investigations have also been performed to analyze the response of healing ligaments to cyclic and static creep (366,367). It appears that ligament scars have inferior creep properties and creep more than twice as much as a normal MCL complex when subjected to cyclic and static loads that are only a fraction of their failure loads (Figs. 5.55 and 5.56).

Interestingly, ligament length ("laxity") is reasonably well reestablished during this remodeling, possibly as the MCL scar contracts. This suggests that for specific cyclic activities (i.e., daily activities), the MCL can adapt very well under some circumstances (473).

Failure behaviors of the healing rabbit MCL complex do not recover as well. Early in the healing process, the injured complex is weaker, is less stiff, and absorbs much less energy

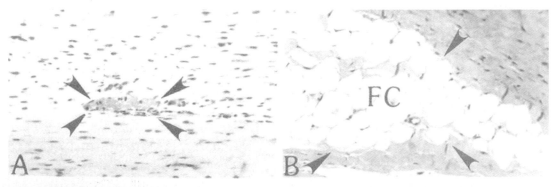

FIGURE 5.52 Histologic appearances of midsubstance "flaws" within rabbit medial collateral ligament scars, showing different types of defects within the new matrix: **A**, blood vessels; **B**, fat cells; *continued*

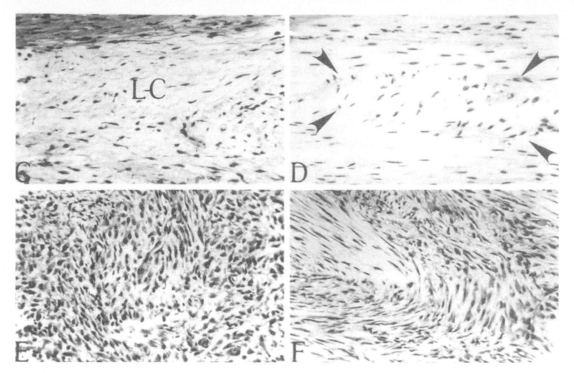

FIGURE 5.52 *Continued* **C**, loose collagen; **D**, disorganized collagen; **E**, inflammatory site with little matrix; **F**, a combination of all (hematoxylin and eosin stain, 125× magnification). (From Shrive N, Chimich D, Marchuk L, et al. Soft-tissue flaws are associated with the material properties of the healing rabbit medial collateral ligament. *J Orthop Res* 1995;13:923–929, with permission.)

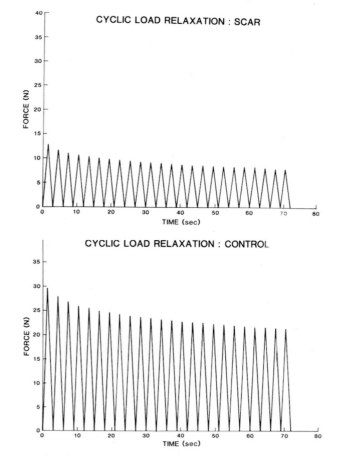

FIGURE 5.53 Comparison of normal control medial collateral ligament (MCL) cyclic relaxation with scar MCL cyclic relaxation under equal amounts of deformation. Note decreased peak loads in the scar.

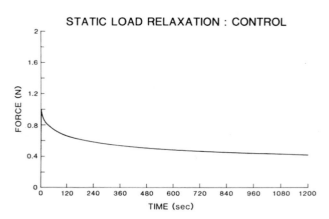

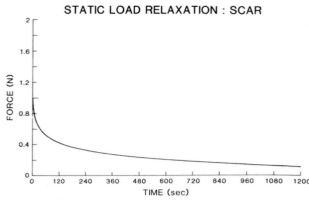

FIGURE 5.54 Comparison of static load relaxation of normal control medial collateral ligament (MCL) and 6-week scar MCL showing different amounts of relaxation and different relaxation rates over time.

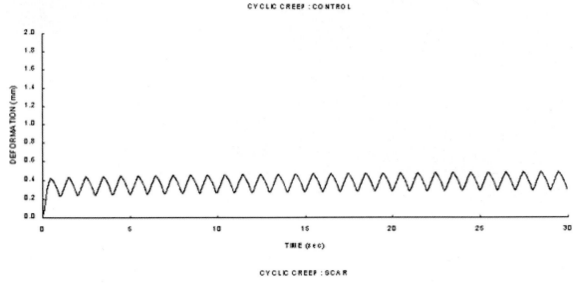

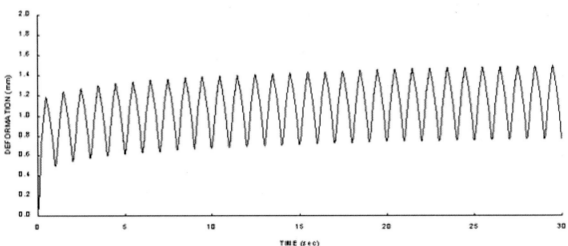

FIGURE 5.55 Comparison of normal control medial collateral ligament (MCL) cyclic creep with that of a 6-week scar under equal amounts of stress. Note increased deformation in the scar.

before failure than the normal MCL complex (Fig. 5.57). On a longer term, the MCL scar may continue to recover depending on a number of factors—the size of the gap to be filled, the presence of contact between torn ligament ends, and the degree of joint movement (473,474)—that appear to contribute to the rate and possibly the endpoint of MCL biomechanical recovery (Fig. 5.58).

Improving Ligament Healing

With the recent advances in the biotechnology field, investigators have begun to study the molecular aspects of healing with particular interest in determining the possible mechanisms leading to compositional and structural differences in scar tissue (483–489). These studies have demonstrated collectively that there is a cascade of specific molecular changes that occurs after injury (494–496). Alterations in messenger RNA (mRNA) levels for proteinases, proteinase inhibitors, growth factors, growth factor receptors, and ECM molecules have been demonstrated and may contribute to the altered composition and structure of ligament scar. These findings, along with the structural and compositional changes, have led to attempts to improve ligament healing.

Altering the Mechanical Environment

It has long been held that cells may respond to their local mechanical environment (498–500). Indeed, there is significant body of knowledge with respect to chondrocytes and their response to changes in their local mechanical environment (498–506). The use of ligament or tendon fibroblasts

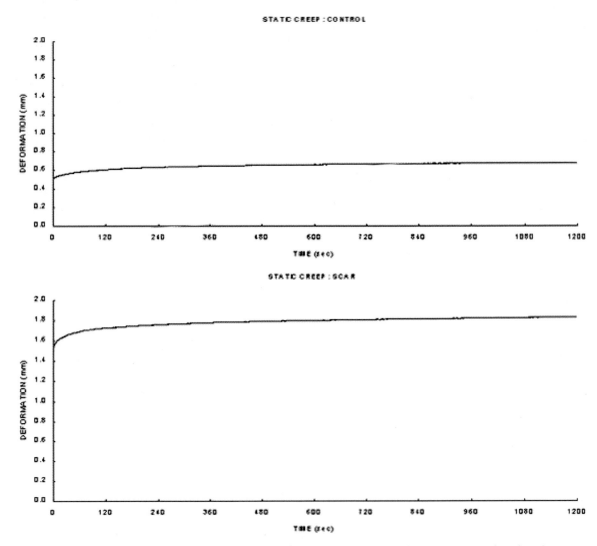

FIGURE 5.56 Comparison of static creep of normal control medial collateral ligament (MCL) and 6-week scar MCL showing different amounts of creep over time.

has only recently gained attention (507) and has demonstrated that mRNA levels for type I collagen are increased in ACL monolayers while type III collagen mRNA levels are increased in MCL fibroblast monolayers subjected to cyclic strain. Other investigators have used bone–ligament–bone complexes and have demonstrated load-dependent alterations in mRNA levels. Collectively, these results suggest that it is possible to selectively alter mRNA levels for some genes by subjecting cells and ligament tissues to mechanical stimuli *in vitro* (508,509).

Many researchers have examined the influence of mechanical stimuli on ligaments *in vivo* (510–518). Most studies have used immobilization, exercise, or combined ligament injuries (i.e., MCL with or without ACL) to create a presumed spectrum of ligament load (510–518). Investigations have focused on biomechanical outcomes of such experiments and have demonstrated that there exists a window

of mechanical stimulus within which joint motion optimizes the return of ligament mechanical properties. Few studies, however, have quantified or evaluated how the biologic response to healing is altered (497,519).

Growth Factors

The use of exogenous growth factors as a strategy to improve ligament healing has been investigated (520–531). A number of transcripts for growth factors and growth factor receptors have been documented within ligaments, including TGF-β_1, epidermal growth factor (EGF), ET-1, basic fibroblast growth factor (bFGF), insulin-like growth factor 1 (IGF-1), hepatocyte growth factor (HGF), IGF-2, vascular endothelial growth factor (VEGF), c-met, and insulin and IGF-2 receptors (489,496). After injury, mRNA and protein levels for a number of these growth factors are elevated

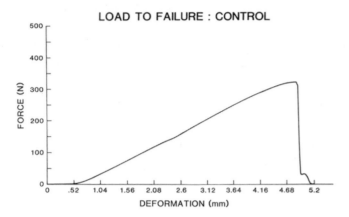

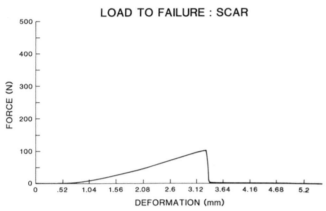

FIGURE 5.57 Comparison of load deformation to failure curves of normal medial collateral ligament (MCL) and 6-week healing MCL. Note decreased stiffness *(slope)*, decreased energy absorption *(area under curve)*, and lower peak strength of the healing complex.

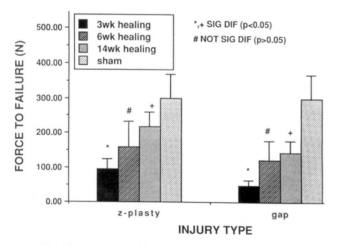

FIGURE 5.58 Bar graph of loads at failure in two models of adult rabbit medial collateral ligament (MCL) healing. Note the inferiority of the 4-mm, sharply cut "gap" as compared with the Z-plasty "contact" model. A decreased gap between cut ends may improve either the rate or the endpoint of MCL healing.

at least transiently (532–534). These studies and others (520–531) collectively suggest that healing ligaments are particularly responsive to these growth factors.

Several studies have used growth factors or a combination of growth factors (platelet-derived growth factor BB [PDGF-BB], EGF, TGF-β_1) and dosages to enhance ligament healing (531,535–540). One study (537) used growth factors suspended within fibrin glue that was interposed between the ends of the injured MCL. After 6 weeks of healing, PDGF-BB–treated ligaments demonstrated improved biomechanical (structural) properties that were 1.6 to 2.4 times greater than in the fibrin glue control group. The cross-sectional area was also increased, suggesting that at least some of the improvement in structural properties related to PDGF-BB treatment may be attributable to increased "scar tissue" alone and not to improvement in the quality of the scar material.

Although the strategy of exogenous addition of growth factors to healing ligaments seems feasible, several authors have now reported that the effect of these growth factors is dependent on the timing, dosages, combinations, and methods of administration (535–540). Although the most consistent results appear to have been obtained with PDGF-BB, these variables, in addition to the short half-life of most growth factors, have led to investigations of other techniques of optimizing ligament healing.

Gene Therapy

Gene therapy involves the transfer of a gene or genes to tissues within an individual for a therapeutic purpose. This technique was originally conceived as a means of compensating for heritable genetic diseases, but it has also been shown to be potentially very useful in treating acquired disease. Gene therapy could be used to augment or inhibit factors that are involved in biologic reactions such as those involved in healing.

Much of the research to date has focused on optimization of gene delivery to ligament or tendon, either directly or through cell-mediated gene transfer (541–552). Some studies have claimed gene transfer efficiencies approaching 100% into ligament or tendon, even with nonviral gene delivery methods (552). Few, however, have transferred biologically active genes within ligament or tendon and measured a functional improvement as an outcome (553,554). Some recent results have been promising (555,556), demonstrating functional improvements in biomechanical properties, although they were still significantly lower than in normal ligament.

ARTICULAR CARTILAGE

Articular cartilage is a smooth, low-friction surface that covers the articular ends of bones at diarthrodial joints. Grossly, cartilage does not appear to be structurally complex, and it is characterized by overall low metabolic activity and the absence of neural, lymphatic, and vascular structures. Histologically, however, cartilage can be divided into four zones (superficial, middle, deep, and calcified), which extend from the surface to the cartilage–bone interface. Each zone has its own characteristic cellular composition, biochemistry, and ECM. Together, these zones function to produce a durable, low-friction bearing surface ideally designed for joint motion and loading. No synthetic material has approached the level of performance of articular cartilage in terms of its frictionless movement and longevity.

This section reviews the basic cellular and ECM organization of articular cartilage. In addition, we examine how this organization supports many vital biologic and biomechanical functions. Some effects of aging, injury, and chronic wear on the composition, structure, and ultimate function of articular cartilage are examined.

Cartilage Composition

Articular cartilage is a complex structure composed of both cells (557–559) and ECM. The ECM is composed primarily of tissue fluid (70% to 80%) and structural macromolecules (20% to 30%), which consist mainly of collagen (50%), proteoglycans (35%), and noncollagenous proteins and glycoproteins (15% to 20%) (560–563).

Articular cartilage has traditionally been subdivided into four distinct histologic zones (Fig. 5.59): the superficial (tangential) zone, the middle (transition) zone, the deep (radial) zone, and the zone of calcified cartilage. Each zone has been further characterized by both scanning and electron microscopy (564–567). From superficial to deep, these regions vary in cell size, shape, density, and metabolic activity; proteoglycan and collagen content; and collagen fiber alignment (565,566,568). The structural differences in these regions imply variability of specific functions (568,569).

Superficial (Tangential) Zone

This tangential zone has also been referred to as the gliding zone; it is the thinnest and most superficial layer of cartilage. At the very surface is a layer known as the *lamina splendens* that is approximately 200 μm thick, cell free, and composed mainly of randomly oriented flat bundles of fine collagen fibrils (564,565,570). Deep to this layer are more densely packed collagen fibers interspersed with elongated, oval chondrocytes that are oriented parallel to the articular surface. Cells in this region are small, resemble fibroblasts, and are relatively inactive metabolically; they contain little endoplasmic reticulum, few Golgi bodies, and few mitochondria. Cells within this layer are flatter and more densely packed than those found deeper in matrix substance. The parallel arrangement of collagen fiber bundles in this zone is reflected by the undulating contour of the articular surface that runs parallel to the plane of joint motion (571,572).

This zone has little hyaluronic acid content, and few if any proteoglycan aggregates, but the highest concentration of water. Proteoglycans present here are usually found in the monomeric form that is strongly linked to the collagen fibers. The collagen fibrils are primarily responsible for providing the increased tensile stiffness and strength to this zone, and they may provide increased resistance to the high shear stresses that are encountered. The superficial tangential zone may also act as a barrier by limiting the penetration of large molecules such as antibodies into the deeper zones or preventing the loss of molecules (e.g., aggrecan) from the cartilage to the synovial fluid.

Middle (Transitional) Zone

The transitional zone contains collagen fibrils with an orientation parallel to the plane of joint motion, although obliquely coursing bundles can be identified. Characteristi-

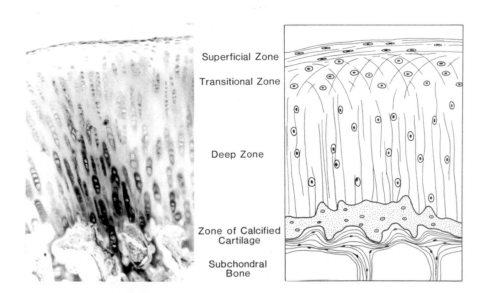

Superficial Zone

Transitional Zone

Deep Zone

Zone of Calcified Cartilage

Subchondral Bone

FIGURE 5.59 Electron micrographs of chondrocytes from articular cartilage from the medial femoral condyle of a skeletally mature rabbit: superficial zone, transitional zone, middle (radial) or deep zone, calcified cartilage zone (bar = 3 μm). (From Buckwalter JA, Hunziker EB, Rosenberg LC, et al. Articular cartilage: composition and structure. In: Woo SLY, Buckwalter JA. *Injury and repair of the musculoskeletal soft tissues*. Park Ridge, IL: American Academy of Orthopaedic Surgeons, 1998:415, with permission.)

cally, the proteoglycan content is increased and water content is decreased, compared with the superficial zone. Chondrocytes become more spherical and have much more endoplasmic reticulum, Golgi bodies, and mitochondria and occasional intracytoplasmic filaments, suggesting increased matrix synthesis function.

Deep (Radial) Zone

The deep zone is also referred to as the radial zone because collagen bundles are arranged perpendicular to the surface. Collagen bundles were originally thought to form continuous arcades (570,573), called the "arcades of Benninghoff," and were presumed to have some structural significance. These bundles, however, are not continuous and the collagen orientation is actually more random.

Proteoglycan concentration is highest, water content is lowest, and collagen fiber size and content are highest in this zone. Chondrocytes are round and are arranged in a columnar pattern perpendicular to the joint surface. These cells have many intracytoplasmic filaments, glycogen granules, and abundant endoplasmic reticulum and Golgi bodies, suggesting a very active zone with respect to protein synthesis.

Calcified Cartilage

The zone of calcified cartilage acts as a zone of transition from the soft articular cartilage to stiffer subchondral bone. Cells in this zone are usually smaller and are surrounded in a cartilaginous matrix encrusted with apatitic salts. The tidemark region marks an area of transition from the deep zone to the zone of calcified cartilage. It is an undulating, hematoxophilic line approximately 2 to 5 μm in width. Collagen fibers from the deep zone penetrate this line directly into the calcified cartilage. The number of tidemark lines may increases with age as the cartilage remodels.

Together, these zones function to form the basis of articular cartilage. Each of its two major components—the chondrocytes and the ECM—is discussed separately in the next section, to highlight some of their more importance characteristics.

CHONDROCYTES AND CHONDRONS

The chondrocyte and its associated ECM can also be divided structurally into different regions depending on the proximity to chondrocytes. These regions are termed the *pericellular, territorial,* and *interterritorial* matrices (Fig. 5.60). These specific regions differ in their collagen content, fibril diameter, and orientation as well as proteoglycan and noncollagenous protein content and organization (574–576). The *pericellular matrix* completely surrounds cells and contains small

amounts of collagen, proteoglycans, and glycoproteins such as anchorin CII and chondronectin (577,578). In this region, the chondrocytes appear to contain cytoplasmic projections that extend through the pericellular matrix, assisting in cell-matrix adhesion and providing some protection for the chondrocyte during physiologic loading.

The pericellular matrix and the chondrocyte represent a *chondron,* a possible functional unit of the cartilage (573). There has been renewed interest in the study of chondrons and the microenvironment in which they lie (579–583). These structural units can be isolated from cartilage and con-

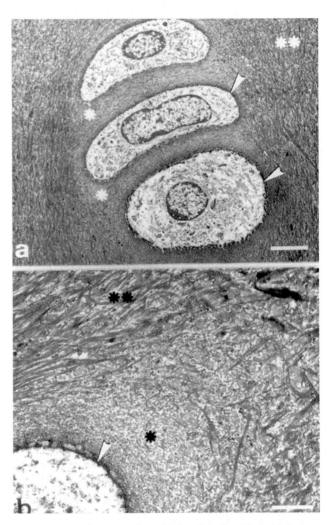

FIGURE 5.60 Electron micrographs showing the matrix compartments of the articular cartilage of the medial femoral condyle of an 8-month-old rabbit. **A:** The image shows the pericellular matrix *(arrowheads),* the territorial matrix *(asterisk),* and the interterritorial matrix *(double asterisk)* (bar = 3 μm). **B:** Higher-magnification view of the compartments of the matrix, showing the relationship between the cell membrane and the pericellular matrix (bar = 1 μm). Note the short cell processes that extend through the pericellular matrix (From Buckwalter JA, Hunziker EB, Rosenberg LC, et al. Articular cartilage: composition and structure. In: Woo SLY, Buckwalter JA. *Injury and repair of the musculoskeletal soft Tissues.* Park Ridge, IL: American Academy of Orthopaedic Surgeons, 1988:416, with permission.)

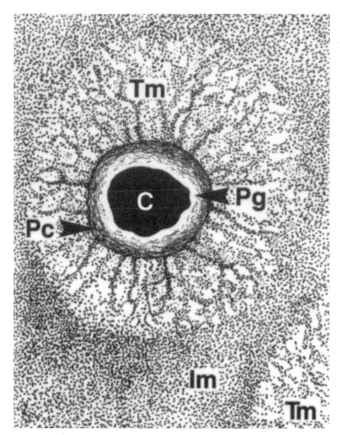

FIGURE 5.61 Horizontal view of circumferential collagen organization in the deep layer, showing chondrocyte (C), pericellular glycocalyx (Pg), pericellular capsule (Pc), territorial matrix (Tm), and interterritorial matrix (Im). (From Poole CA, Flint MH, Beaumont BW. Morphological and functional interrelationships of articular cartilage matrices. *J Anat* 1984;138:113–138, with permission.)

sists of a single, double, or columns of chondrocytes together with a pericellular glycocalyx and fibrillar pericellular capsule (Fig. 5.61). Chondrons appear to be compression-resistant, fluid-filled bladders that dampen mechanical, osmotic, and

physicochemical changes induced by dynamic loading and therefore may act as a mechanical and metabolic functional unit of cartilage.

The *territorial matrix* surrounds the pericellular matrix of the chondrocytes. Fibrillar collagen is present in this region and adheres to the pericellular matrix, spreading and intersecting at some distance from cells and forming "nests" about the chondrocytes, thus presumably protecting cells during cartilage deformation (576). The transition between the territorial and the *interterritorial matrix* regions is marked by an increase in collagen fibril diameter and transition of these fibers to a more parallel arrangement. This region is generally responsible for the structural properties of cartilage as a whole, and it makes up the majority of the matrix in mature articular cartilage. Collagen fibrils in this region are large, and their orientation changes from parallel to perpendicular, in relation to the articular cartilage surface, as one moves from the superficial to the deep zone.

Chondrocytes contribute approximately 1% of the total volume of articular cartilage in humans, although this figure varies among species (584,585). Their apparent paucity, however, should not minimize their importance to cartilage. The chondrocyte is the master architect of articular cartilage and is primarily responsible for its production and maintenance. Although there appears to be only one major cell type within cartilage (i.e., chondrocytes), the cells vary considerably in size, shape, and density (569,586).

Structurally, chondrocytes have short, branched cytoplasmic processes (Fig. 5.62). Although chondrocytes appear to have the machinery to produce cell-to-cell contacts (by demonstrating connexin-43 proteins), they do not appear to form functional gap junctions, although some debate exists on this point (557,558,574,587,588). Many chondrocytes demonstrate short cilia (primary cilia), which project into the extracellular/pericellular matrix and may be involved in sensing mechanical changes within the matrix (Fig. 5.63).

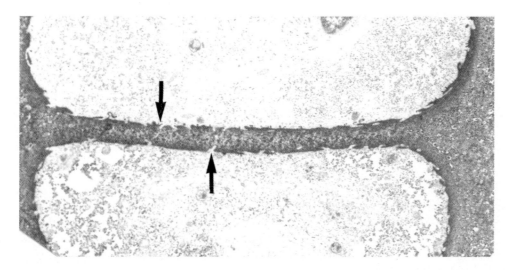

FIGURE 5.62 Electron micrograph of superficial zone chondrocytes from the medial femoral condyle of a skeletally mature rabbit. Note the cytoplasmic extensions between cells *(arrows)*.

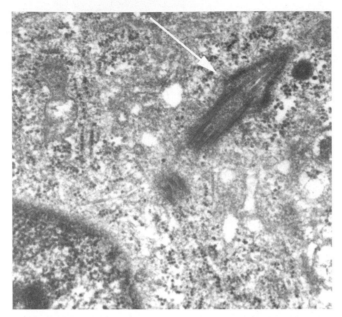

FIGURE 5.63 Electron micrograph of superficial zone chondrocytes from the medial femoral condyle of a skeletally mature rabbit, demonstrating a primary cilium *(arrow)* that extends from the cell into the extracellular matrix.

Chondrocytes are mesenchymal cells that differentiate during development; after growth has ceased, there is little if any detectable cell division in healthy adult articular cartilage (584,589,590). In mature cartilage, chondrocytes are embedded within an avascular and hypoxic matrix and therefore derive most of their energy through anaerobic metabolism. Chondrocytes derive the majority of their nutrition from the synovial fluid. The cartilage matrix acts as a barrier to nutrient flow and restricts the nutrients, which reach the cell by size, charge, and other characteristics (591).

The primary role of the chondrocyte has been understood to be the synthesis and maintenance of the ECM.

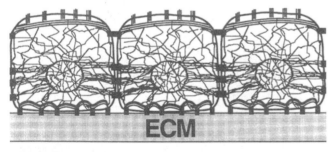

FIGURE 5.64 The intracellular cytoskeleton interconnects with the underlying extracellular matrix and with neighboring cells through, respectively, focal adhesion complexes at the cell base and specialized junctional complexes at the lateral cell border. Because of the presence of this molecular continuum, distant molecules in the extracellular matrix (ECM), cytoplasm, and nucleus may be mechanically coupled. (From Ingber DE. Tensegrity: the architectural basis of cellular mechanotransduction. *Annu Rev Physiol* 1997;59:575–599, with permission.)

Metabolically, although the overall activity of articular cartilage appears to be low, individual cell metabolism is quite high (592,593), emphasizing its active role in maintaining tissue homeostasis. To produce articular cartilage that can support the normal function of a diarthrodial joint, chondrocytes must not only synthesize the appropriate amounts and types of molecules but also assemble and organize them into a supportive, hierarchal architecture. Further, maintenance of such a structure requires the continual replacement and turnover of individual components and possibly alterations in the structure in response to joint use and mechanical loads. In order for the cell to sense and respond to such changes, there is probably an interaction or connection between the ECM and the internal chondrocyte cytoskeleton (Fig. 5.64) (594).

Extracellular Matrix

Tissue Fluid

ECM fluid comprises approximately 75% of the wet weight of cartilage (595); 94% is unbound and freely diffusible (596). This fluid is composed mainly of water with some dissolved gases and metabolites such as lactic acid. Extracellular fluid contributes to chondrocyte nutrition, mechanical properties of the matrix, and joint lubrication mechanisms. Because articular cartilage lacks a vascular and lymphatic supply, the flux of fluid between cartilage and joint cavity is the only means by which nutrients and metabolites can be transported to and from chondrocytes. This fluid flow also augments joint lubrication mechanisms. Finally, interaction of extracellular fluid with structural macromolecules, particularly the large aggregating proteoglycans, provides articular cartilage with its resiliency and ability to withstand repeated compressive loads (568,597–601).

Macromolecules

ECM macromolecules comprise 20% to 30% of the wet weight of articular cartilage and consist of collagen, proteoglycan, glycoproteins, and noncollagenous proteins (568). These have been discussed in detail in the preceding sections.

Collagen forms a fibrillar meshwork and gives cartilage its tensile strength (602–604). The collagens are highly concentrated in the superficial tangential zone but are more uniformly distributed through rest of the cartilage. The superficial tangential zone, with its high concentration of collagen, has been described as a tension-resisting diaphragm (605). This is demonstrated by the tendency of articular cartilage to curl when released from the subchondral bone (606).

The majority (90%) of the collagen is type II, although other types, including types V, VI, IX, X, and XI, have all been identified (607–609). The role of the minor collagens within cartilage continues to be investigated. The fibrillar collagens II, IX, and XI form the fibrous meshwork that provides cartilage its shape, strength, and tensile stiffness but little resistance to compression. Type XI collagen is found within type II collagen fibrils and copolymerizes with type II collagen to form heterotypic fibrils (610). Type IX collagen can be demonstrated covalently linked to the surface of type II collagen fibrils; it assists in binding together the collagen fibril meshwork and in connecting the collagen meshwork to the proteoglycans (607,608,611–613). Type VI collagen probably plays a role in chondrocyte to matrix attachment and is concentrated in the pericellular matrix (614). Type X collagen may play a role in the mineralization of cartilage, because it has been identified in the underlying calcified zone of articular cartilage (615). Collagen within the articular cartilage has a slow rate of turnover and a proposed half-life in tissue of longer than 3 months (616).

Proteoglycans contribute significantly to the structural properties of cartilage, providing resilience, elasticity, and resistance to compression. Proteoglycans also contribute to the fluid dynamics of lubrication. Articular cartilage contains two major proteoglycan types: the large aggregating proteoglycans (aggrecans) and the small proteoglycans (decorin, biglycan, fibromodulin) (613,617–621). The most abundant proteoglycan in cartilage is aggrecan (622,623). An aggrecan monomer consists of a central core protein with many glycosaminoglycan side chains (up to 100 chondroitin sulfate side chains. Proteoglycan monomers are commonly attached to long hyaluronic acid filaments through a specialized link protein, forming a large aggregate (624).

Proteoglycan aggregates are so large that they are immobilized within the collagen network and occupy most of the interfibrillar space of the matrix. Each aggrecan molecule also has many negative charges arising from the glycosaminoglycan sidechains. Adjacent side chains tend to repel one another and therefore attempt to assume an expanded "bottle brush" form, which is restricted by the associated collagen meshwork. Proteoglycans are highly hydrophilic, and water is attracted to them by electrostatic and osmotic forces. Their ability to imbibe water and swell is similarly restricted by the collagen meshwork (625); therefore, they remain only partially hydrated. This swelling pressure contributes to the unique mechanical properties of cartilage. Fluid flow is also regulated by other factors, including loading, motion, and ultrastructural damage to the cartilage matrix (626,627).

The other proteoglycans—the small proteoglycans biglycan, decorin, and fibromodulin—have been identified in cartilage and are distinct from aggrecan. Decorin has one dermatan sulfate side chain attached to its core protein, and biglycan has two.

Fibromodulin contains keratan sulfate side chains. Although on a mass basis these proteoglycans are only minor components (compared to aggrecan), there are as many molecules of small proteoglycans as there are large aggrecan molecules. Therefore they may play important roles in tissue architecture and function.

Cartilage Biomechanics

Viscoelastic behavior in cartilage (Figs. 5.65 and 5.66) is attributable to tissue fluid, fluid flow (628–631), and the structural macromolecules that are present (632–635).

Glycosaminoglycan side units of the proteoglycan aggregates have sulfate and carboxyl groups with fixed negative charges that result in strong repulsive forces between chains as well as between proteoglycan aggregates. These repulsive forces cause proteoglycan aggregates to expand and stiffen. The negative charges also attract mobile cations such as Na^+ and Ca^{++} (636–639), creating an osmotic swelling pressure (Donnan osmotic pressure) and further attracting water molecules. This tendency to swell is resisted by the fibrillar collagen network, which provides strength in tension (640).

With an applied external load there is deformation of the matrix macromolecules and an increase in the interstitial fluid pressure, causing net flow of fluid out of the ECM. This fluid flow is resisted by the low permeability of the matrix, which slows the rate of flow from the site of compression. This prevents the fluid from leaving too quickly and thus provides cushioning for the matrix, chondrocytes, and subchondral bone (629,641,642). The eventual efflux of fluid increases proteoglycan density, which subsequently increases negative charge density and elevates the osmotic swelling pressure until it balances the applied external load (Fig. 5.67). It is estimated that up to 75% of the compressive stress is absorbed by the fluid within the matrix during the initial application of a load. However, during periods of sustained loading (up to 2.5 to 6 hours), most of the fluid is squeezed out of the matrix and the compressive stress is gradually transferred from the fluid phase to the solid phase (i.e., absorbed by matrix macromolecules) (629,642). However, these sustained conditions are unlikely to occur during normal conditions, since joints are almost always dynamically loaded.

In addition to contributing to the biomechanical properties of articular cartilage, fluid flow within the cartilage is primarily responsible for nutrient delivery to chondrocytes. Thus water, collagen, and proteoglycans all contribute to the biomechanical behavior of articular cartilage as well as to chondrocyte nutrition and joint lubrication.

Joint Lubrication

Diarthrodial joint surfaces move together with a remarkably low coefficient of friction. This is accomplished by an effective system of joint lubrication combined with a smooth

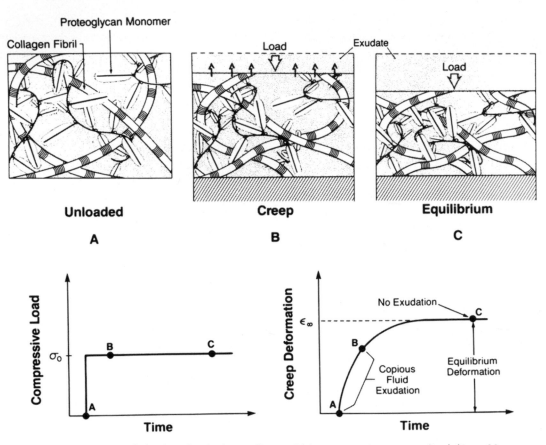

FIGURE 5.65 Creep behavior of articular cartilage, which occurs under constant load. (From Mow V, Rosenwasser M. Articular cartilage: biomechanics. In: Woo SL-Y, Buckwalter JA, eds. *Injury and repair of the musculoskeletal soft tissues.* Park Ridge, IL: American Academy of Orthopaedic Surgeons, 1987:434, with permission.)

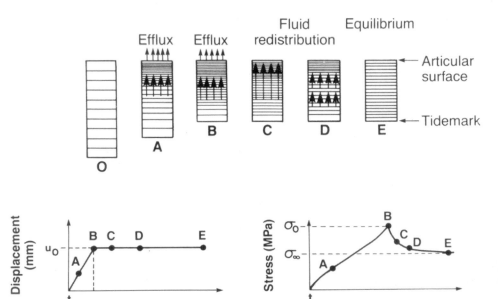

FIGURE 5.66 With controlled displacement, cartilage undergoes stress relaxation. (From Mow V, Rosenwasser M. Articular cartilage: biomechanics. In: Woo SL-Y, Buckwalter JA, eds. *Injury and repair of the musculoskeletal soft tissues.* Park Ridge, IL: American Academy of Orthopaedic Surgeons, 1987:438, with permission.)

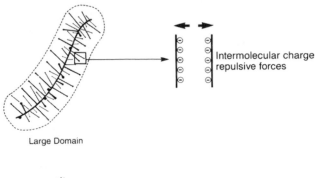

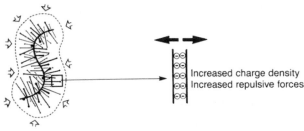

FIGURE 5.67 Proteoglycan aggregate domain. The carboxyl and sulfate groups on the glycosaminoglycans have negative charges that result in repulsive forces *(top)*. With compression and efflux of fluid from the cartilage matrix, there is a net increase in intermolecular repulsive forces and osmotic swelling pressure. (From Mow V, Rosenwasser M. Articular cartilage: biomechanics. In: Woo SL-Y, Buckwalter JA, eds. *Injury and repair of the musculoskeletal soft tissues.* Park Ridge, IL: American Academy of Orthopaedic Surgeons, 1987:439, with permission.)

gliding surface. Articular cartilage, by way of its intrinsic material properties and the ease of fluid flow through its matrix, contributes significantly to joint lubrication. Diarthrodial joints can be compared with other load-bearing structures with regard to lubrication. In bearings, two main types of lubrication theory have been proposed. These are known as the boundary theory and the fluid film theory.

Boundary Lubrication

Boundary lubrication occurs because a boundary lubricant, lubricin (205,643), is adsorbed as a monolayer to each articulating surface. This monolayer ranges from 1 to 100 nm in thickness and prevents direct surface-to-surface contact, thereby reducing surface wear and friction. This form of lubrication is independent of joint motion, viscosity of the lubricant, or stiffness of the bearing surface but is wholly dependent on the chemical properties of the lubricant (644–647) and its ability to adsorb to the articulating surface. This type of lubrication is most important in prolonged loading conditions in which there is relatively little or no joint motion or velocity (Fig. 5.68).

Fluid Film Lubrication

In fluid film lubrication, a thin layer of lubricating fluid is present between the bearing surfaces but is not adsorbed to them. The hydrodynamic pressure developed in this fluid layer keeps surfaces separated, thereby reducing contact and minimizing friction. This type of lubrication, in contrast to boundary lubrication, is affected by the physical properties of the bearing surface and the lubricant. Fluid film lubrication theory assumes relative motion between the joint surfaces. Two types of fluid film lubrication have been described: hydrodynamic lubrication and squeeze film lubrication (Fig. 5.69).

Hydrodynamic Lubrication

This form of fluid film lubrication occurs when two nonparallel bearing surfaces move on each other tangentially. Tangential motion results in a converging wedge of fluid that is drawn between the moving surfaces. The fluid drawn into these gaps creates a lifting pressure, thereby separating the two articulating surfaces at the point of joint contact.

Squeeze Film Lubrication

Squeeze film is a form of fluid film lubrication that occurs when bearing surfaces move perpendicularly toward each other. Joint loading creates fluid pressure between the articulating surfaces, forcing the fluid out from between them. The rate at which the fluid is forced out depends on the viscosity of the lubricant. This type of lubrication is time limited and therefore is most effective for high loads that are applied over a short period of time.

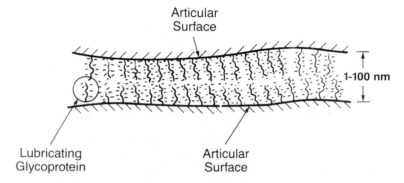

FIGURE 5.68 Boundary lubrication of articular cartilage with a lubricating glycoprotein, lubricin. A monolayer of this glycoprotein adsorbs to each articulating surface so that direct contact is avoided. (From Mow V, Rosenwasser M. Articular cartilage: biomechanics. In: Woo SL-Y, Buckwalter JA, eds. *Injury and repair of the musculoskeletal soft tissues.* Park Ridge, IL: American Academy of Orthopaedic Surgeons, 1987:446, with permission.)

Rigid Bearings

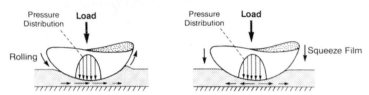

Thin Fluid Film and High Pressures

Deformable Bearings

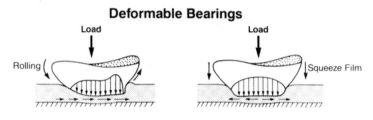

Thick Fluid Film and Low Pressures

FIGURE 5.69 Fluid film lubrication with both hydrodynamic *(right)* and squeeze film *(left)* mechanisms illustrated. With hydrodynamic lubrication, the joint motion results in fluid's being drawn into the space between the articulating surfaces; this creates a fluid pressure which separates the surfaces. Squeeze film lubrication occurs with joint loading; fluid from between the articulating surfaces is gradually "squeezed" out. In deformable bearings *(bottom)* such as articular cartilage, regular fluid film lubrication is augmented, since surface deformation results in increased surface contact area. (From Mow V, Rosenwasser M. Articular cartilage: biomechanics. In: Woo SL-Y, Buckwalter JA, eds. *Injury and repair of the musculoskeletal soft tissues.* Park Ridge, IL: American Academy of Orthopaedic Surgeons, 1987:447, with permission.)

A variation of fluid film lubrication, known as *elastohydrodynamic lubrication,* occurs in diarthrodial joints because the bearing surface, articular cartilage, is also deformable. This deformability allows normal asperities present in articular cartilage surfaces to be compressed with applied loads. This surface deformation increases the surface area of contact, resulting in a longer lasting fluid film and increased the load-carrying capacity (646–651).

Two additional theoretical modes of lubrication have been proposed and are based on the ability of fluid to flow in and out of cartilage matrix. These forms of lubrication,

termed *weeping* and *boosted* lubrication, occur in addition to the typical fluid film lubrication.

Weeping lubrication occurs in conjunction with the elastohydrodynamic mechanism in situations in which articular surfaces are moving tangentially to each other. Loaded articular cartilage exudes fluid from its matrix into the joint cavity between the leading halves of the contact areas, which generates an increase in fluid pressure. As the cartilage is unloaded, fluid is once again resorbed into the cartilage matrix (649,652–654) (Fig. 5.70).

Boosted lubrication is thought to occur in conjunction

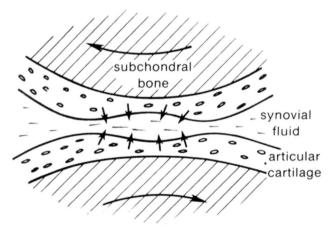

FIGURE 5.70 Weeping lubrication in articular cartilage. As the cartilage is compressed extracellular fluid moves into the joint space, separating articulating surfaces. (From Brand RA. Joint lubrication. In: Albright JA, Brand RA, eds. *The scientific basis of orthopedics.* New York: Appleton-Century-Crofts, 1979:360, with permission.)

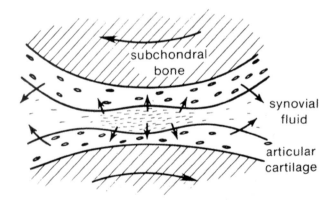

FIGURE 5.71 Boosted lubrication as it occurs with articular cartilage loading. The applied load creates an increase in fluid pressure between the areas of joint contact. This pressure increase results in a net fluid flux out of synovial fluid into articular cartilage, so that the viscosity of the lubricating fluid is increased during squeeze film lubrication. (From Brand RA. Joint lubrication. In: Albright JA, Brand RA, eds. *The scientific basis of orthopedics.* New York: Appleton-Century-Crofts, 1979:361, with permission.)

with squeeze film lubrication (655–658). As the loaded joint surfaces move toward each other, the increase in fluid pressure forces fluid into the cartilage matrix. This dynamic fluid flow results in increased fluid viscosity, which slows lateral movement from between the loaded areas. This increased viscosity augments the effectiveness of squeeze film as a lubricating mechanism (Fig. 5.71).

CARTILAGE WEAR

Despite its overall durability and resiliency, cartilage can become damaged. This section reviews some of the more theoretical aspects of cartilage wear. Mechanical wear results in the loss of small particles from articular surfaces and occurs to some degree in all joints despite their low friction state. As opposed to articular cartilage injury, wear can occur after repetitive submaximal stresses by interfacial or fatigue mechanisms or by impact loading. However, as the knowledge of disease processes such as osteoarthritis grows, it is becoming understood that this process is not just mechanical but also has a biologic basis.

Interfacial Wear

Interfacial wear is thought to be caused by direct contact of bearing surfaces with one another. It can occur by one of two mechanisms—abrasion or adhesion. As the surfaces make contact, they can adhere, resulting in damage due to the shear created by motion, or they can abrade each other at areas of contact. Although it is unlikely that this sort of wear occurs in normal joints, there is some evidence to suggest that it may be more prevalent in joints with damaged or diseased cartilage (646–649).

Fatigue Wear

Fatigue wear is thought to result from the accumulation of repetitive stresses resulting in microscopic damage. Fatigue can occur either with high loads for a short period or with low loads over a prolonged period. With repetitive loading, the ECM fluid is in a continuous flux in and out of articular cartilage (651–654,659). Because the structural macromolecules are constantly being stressed, fatigue damage can occur to solid matrix components through accumulation of these stresses. Another possible mechanism of matrix damage is secondary to "washout" of proteoglycans, caused by repetitive flux of tissue fluid through ECM.

Impact Loading

This type of wear occurs with repetitive impact loading that does not allow sufficient time for stress relaxation.

The result may be articular cartilage wear and damage (660–663).

CARTILAGE INJURY, HEALING, AND REPAIR

The healing response of cartilage to injury is significantly different from the healing of other connective tissues because of two major features of cartilage: its avascularity and its intricate structure (664). The absence of a vascular system limits the inflammatory and reparative response of cartilage and also limits the migration of new pluripotent or phagocytic cells to the area of healing. In addition, chondrocytes are entrapped by a dense network of collagen and proteoglycan, restricting their ability to migrate from adjacent healthy cartilage to an injury site. This section reviews the cartilage response to injury and then recent advances in the augmentation of this response.

Cartilage Injury and Healing

In general, injury to articular cartilage can occur as a result of loss of matrix macromolecules or secondary to mechanical trauma. Perhaps most important, however, is the depth of injury to cartilage, which seems to be a crucial determinant of the type of healing response mounted.

Generalized partial-thickness injury is commonly found in inflammatory arthritis and results in superficial chondrocyte death and depletion of proteoglycans. Providing that there is no significant disruption of the structural matrix, chondrocytes can divide and increase their rate of synthesis so that proteoglycan is restored (665,666). This type of repair is often seen with destructive arthritis, where the insult is continuous and repair is incomplete. Despite this continuous insult, however, the chondrocytes continue to divide and produce collagen and proteoglycan at increased rates (667,668).

For localized injuries that are superficial, chondrocytes in the adjacent area die (669) and a wedge-shaped matrix defect is formed. Partial-thickness injuries appear to be the same whether they are perpendicular or tangential to the articular cartilage surface (664,670,671). Chondrocytes in the surrounding regions that do not die are often seen to proliferate and form cell clusters (670,672–674). However, they do not migrate into the defect. An inflammatory response is not seen in these types of injury. The increased matrix that is synthesized is transient and usually is not sufficient to fill the defect (664,670,671,675–678). Several studies have demonstrated that isolated partial-thickness injuries do not show significant healing over time but nevertheless appear stable and rarely progress to osteoarthritis (664,670,679–681).

If the injury is full thickness, extending into subchondral bone, there is access to the vascular supply of the bone, an inflammatory response is stimulated, and marrow cells and bone matrix become involved (682,683). These defects initially fill with fibrin clot and allow infiltration of undifferentiated mesenchymal cells of the marrow (684). These cells eventually differentiate along a chondroblast lineage. The deeper portion of the injury is reconstituted with bone, and the subchondral plate is restored. The cartilage defect, however, fills with fibrocartilage that is biomechanically inferior to regular articular cartilage (685,686). This tissue has a higher concentration of type I collagen (670,686) and less proteoglycan than normal articular cartilage, and the tangential collagen layers of the superficial zone fail to regenerate (687). Several other studies have demonstrated a failure of the fibrocartilage to integrate with the residual cartilage, possibly creating vertical shear stresses at the interface. Long-term studies have demonstrated that this healing fibrocartilage undergoes fibrillation and degeneration (670, 674,686,688–690).

Several factors may also modulate the cartilage response to injury. Continuous passive motion has been demonstrated to augment the ability of full-thickness cartilage defects to heal, with some improvements in the tissue quality morphologically and histochemically (691–696). Chondrocytes from skeletally immature animals have also demonstrated a greater ability to proliferate and synthesize proteoglycan (697,698). In addition, small defects (less than 3 mm) may have a better ability to heal than larger defects (699).

Methods of Augmenting Cartilage Healing

Significant lesions of articular cartilage do not heal adequately; therefore, intense effort has been directed at discovering methods to augment cartilage healing. Several approaches have been used, including altering the loads on the articular cartilage, improving the vascularity to the area of repair, delivering reparative cells to the area of injury, and augmenting the natural healing response.

Debridement of Articular Lesions

Shaving of fibrillated cartilage has been advocated as a useful method in the treatment of cartilage injuries. Cartilage shaving may help alleviate symptoms by eliminating unstable chondral flaps, thereby reducing mechanical symptoms, or by removing fragmented and loose cartilage that could elicit synovitis and joint effusion (700). However, there is no experimental evidence suggesting that this procedure stimulates significant repair (701–703), and adjacent hyaline cartilage may become fibrillated and necrotic (702,704). Recent studies have questioned the usefulness of this procedure for the treatment of osteoarthritis of the knee (705).

Subchondral Bone Penetration

Perforation or abrasion of subchondral bone has been shown to be effective in healing partial or full-thickness cartilage defects both clinically (706–708) and experimentally (709–716). Various techniques have been used, including drill holes (707,714), microfracture (717,718), spongialization (711), and abrasion (712,715,719–722), but all function by facilitating access to the vascular system. The reparative response that is stimulated with drilling is similar to that seen with full-thickness cartilage lesions involving subchondral bone. There is an initial appearance of fibrocartilage, but it degenerates with time (670,672,687,710).

Altering Cartilage Loading

Osteotomies theoretically function by realigning the joint to move the joint reaction force from the diseased articular cartilage to more normal, articular cartilage. Osteotomies have been performed primarily on the lower extremity (hip and knee joint) and are commonly combined with subchondral bone penetration. The clinical results of osteotomy have been mixed (722–726). Most results tend to deteriorate with time. Although most of the symptom relief is probably a result of the shift in joint contact, there is some evidence that changing the loading conditions associated with osteotomy may allow diseased areas to fill in more readily with fibrocartilage (672,726–731).

Osteochondral Grafting

Osteochondral grafting can be an effective method for replacing isolated areas of damaged articular cartilage, and it does not rely on the stimulation or formation of an effective repair tissue. This procedure can restore joint contour, the subchondral bone and can integrate within the host defect. Several factors are associated with success of osteochondral transplantation. Because the cartilage matrix is exceptionally dense, transplanted cartilage cannot act as a scaffold for migrating host chondrocytes. Therefore, a high chondrocyte survival rate within the osteochondral graft is essential for long-term maintenance of the articular cartilage. In addition, because bonding of graft cartilage to the host cartilage is difficult, success with osteochondral grafting relies on the success of bone-to-bone engraftment and healing. Both allogeneic and autogenous tissues have been used for osteochondral transplantation.

Allograft

The concept of osteochondral grafting by segmental replacement is not new. Clinical experience with both fresh and frozen allografts suggests that these grafts can integrate to the host tissue and functionally restore articular surfaces (672, 732–736). Lexer, in 1908, reported on the use of fresh allografts for segmental replacement (672). More recently results have demonstrated long-term survival for 76%, 69%, and 67% at 5, 10, and 14 years after engraftment (736). The primary advantage of allograft transplantation is the ability to harvest large portions of articular cartilage and bone from a donor site that is identical to the defect to be replaced. This allows for a graft that which closely matches the surrounding cartilage thickness and contour.

Several factors are important in determining the success for osteochondral allografting, including the use of younger donors, perfect restoration of the surface of the cartilage (i.e., no mismatch), and the avoidance of bone resorption leading to cartilage collapse (737). However, the risks of allograft use—including the potential for disease transmission and the difficulty in the procurement of fresh, unirradiated osteochondral grafts—have limited its clinical application. In addition, allogeneic tissue is associated with an immune response within the graft. Although chondrocytes within their dense, avascular ECM appear to be immunologically privileged, the cells within the subchondral bone are subject to an immune reaction that can result in graft rejection (738,739). Freezing of the graft before implantation can reduce the immunogenicity of the tissue, but there is also a significant loss in chondrocyte viability (740–742).

Autografts

The use of osteochondral autografts has recently gained widespread attention. In this technique, small osteochondral autografts are harvested from "nonessential" areas of the articular cartilage and transplanted as plugs into a larger defect (Fig. 5.72) (743,744). The use of osteochondral autografts eliminates the risk of disease transmission and immune reaction, and the chondrocyte survival rate is high. However, there is a limited supply of autogenous sources, the age of the implanted tissue is fixed, there is potential morbidity from graft harvest, and technically it is difficult to match the graft to the repair site. Although several clinical and experimental studies have demonstrated promising early results with healing of the osteochondral grafts (744–754), in most cases the border between the grafts and native cartilage is easily demarcated and the tissue between the grafts becomes filled with fibrocartilage (747,751). The clinical success of these grafts appears to be closely associated with the degree to which the osteochondral grafts closely

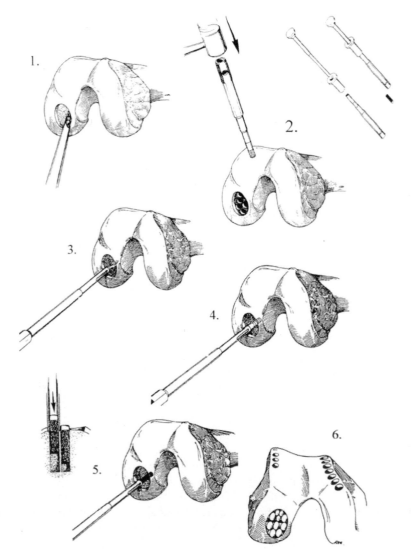

FIGURE 5.72 Technique of Hangody's mosaicplasty. This schematic diagram demonstrates the six steps: 1, preparation of donor site; 2 through 5, procurement and placement of donor graft and transplantation of osteochondral graft; and 6, the final results showing the osteochondral grafts in the recipient defect. (From Mandelbaum BR, Browne JE, Fu F, et al. Articular cartilage lesions of the knee. *Am J Sports Med* 1998;26:853–861, with permission.)

mirror the contour and height of the surrounding cartilaginous tissue (743,752–754).

Pharmacologic Therapies

Several studies have been performed to understand the influence of various molecules (e.g., growth factors, cytokines) on cartilage synthesis and degradation. Many of these molecules, such as bFGF (755–758), IGF (755,757, 759–764), TGF-β (765–774), and bone morphogenic proteins (BMPs), can affect cartilage metabolism and development (672,775–777). Some studies have determined the potential to augment the restoration of articular cartilage (672,778,779). There have been promising effects where some protease inhibitors (780), growth factors (TGF-β) (781–783), or chondroprotective agents (782,784–786) potentiated the regeneration of the articular surface or prevented progression of degeneration. However, careful evaluation *in vivo* is necessary before these techniques can be used clinically. Several cytokines may have pleotropic effects that are often not evident in the simplistic conditions that pertain during *in vitro* culture studies. For example TGF-β stimulates matrix synthesis *in vitro*, but *in vivo* they could also stimulate inflammation and fibrosis in the synovium and the production of osteophytes (787–789).

Periosteum and Perichondrium Grafts

Both periosteum and perichondrium may have the potential to facilitate repair of large cartilage defects (790–796), especially if combined with the use of continuous passive motion (794,795). Periosteum and perichondrium grafts have been used both clinically and experimentally to repair articular cartilage defects (794,795,797–812) with variable success. It appears that the biologic environment in which these tissues are placed determines the phenotypic expression of the graft (809,813–815). An environment with low oxygen tension favors the production of cartilage-like tissue, whereas one with high oxygen tension favors the formation of bone. Several experimental studies have demonstrated hyaline-like cartilage repair tissue within these defects (794,795,797,800,801,803); however, differences in comparison with normal articular cartilage persist, including abnormalities in the distribution and arrangement of type II collagen, chondrocyte clustering, and chondrocyte death (808). Type II collagen production is more promising when grafts are taken from immature animals (808).

Early clinical reports suggested that good clinical results with hyaline-like cartilage are produced; however, longer-term follow-up up at 5 years demonstrated production of type X collagen and endochondral ossification or calcification of the cartilage in 66% of the patients (816–819). The presence of calcification resulted in failure of the transplant and poor clinical results.

Synthetic and Biologic Matrices

Because there is a limited supply of both autogenous and allogeneic tissue, several investigators have attempted to use synthetic materials, with or without cells, as a "tissue-engineered" cartilage replacement. A synthetic matrix can be fabricated and shaped to permit filling and initial stabilization of the defect. This decreases the need for donor tissue, provides a three-dimensional matrix within which cells can adhere and organize, provides initial mechanical properties (which may change over time), acts as a carrier for bioactive materials (i.e., growth factors), and allows biomechanical manipulation of the tissue-engineered graft. Many substances have been used for such matrices, including fibrinogen-based materials, collagen gels, carbon fiber pads, and polylactic and polyglycolic acid meshes (686,797,812,820–826).

There is only limited clinical experience with the use of synthetic scaffolds. Most reports on the use of carbon fiber implants have demonstrated filling in of the defects with fibrocartilage similar to that of abrasion arthroplasty (825–828).

Cell Transplantation

Autologous Chondrocyte Transplantation

In an effort to increase the numbers of chondrocytes within the defect, Grande et al. combined the use of a periosteal graft with cultured autologous chondrocytes (829), which were injected underneath the periosteal graft. The rationale for this technique was that these chondrocytes would redifferentiate and produce more hyaline-like cartilage. Grande et al. demonstrated improved healing with this method, which was supported by others (830), and the technique was subsequently commercialized.

In this procedure, full-thickness cartilage (200 to 300 mg) is initially harvested from the outer edge of the condyle or intercondylar notch (Fig. 5.73). The cells are then extracted and expanded in a commercial facility. The surgical procedure involves debriding the lesion without penetration of the subchondral bone and suturing a flap of periosteum over the top of the lesion. The periosteum–host cartilage interface is then sealed with fibrin glue, leaving only a small opening. Condensed chondrocytes are injected through the opening and sealed (831,832). Continuous passive motion is used postoperatively.

Initial clinical results on 23 patients were promising, with 87% of femoral condyle lesions yielding good or excellent results, although patellar lesions did not fare as well (833). In a larger study, Peterson (818) reported on 100 patients who had a mean articular defect of 5.2 cm^2 with 2 to 9 years of follow-up. Patients with isolated femoral condyle lesions demonstrated 96% good or excellent results, those with osteochondritis dissecans had 89% good or excellent results, and those with an associated ACL tear showed 76% good to excellent results. A subset of these patients (30 pa-

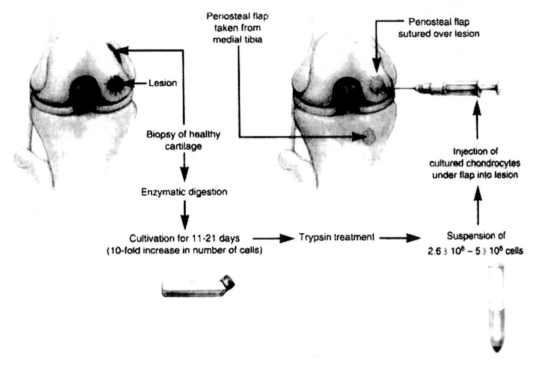

FIGURE 5.73 Autologous chondrocyte implantation procedure. This schematic diagram demonstrates the steps of the procedure, including articular cartilage biopsy procurement, growing of the chondrocyte cells over a 21-day period, graft site preparation, procurement of the periosteal graft from the proximal and medial tibias, and implantation of chondrocytes under the "watertight" periosteal flap that is then sealed with fibrin glue. (From Mandelbaum BR, Browne JE, Fu F, et al. Articular cartilage lesions of the knee. *Am J Sports Med* 1998;26:853–861, with permission.)

tients) underwent a second-look arthroscopy and biopsy that revealed the presence of hyaline-like cartilage repair, as well as some integration at the repair site (19 of 25 biopsies). The overall benefit of this procedure is unclear and may become more evident as an increasing number of patients receive the treatment (818,834).

Mesenchymal Stem Cells

As cells differentiate, their phenotype becomes more specialized to their microenvironment and they become less able to adapt to other circumstances. For example, as explained earlier, the cells of the various zones of articular cartilage are significantly different in cell morphology, metabolism, and matrix production. The use of undifferentiated mesenchymal stem cells is theoretically advantageous because it would allow cells to adapt to their microenvironment, resulting in a structure more closely resembling normal tissue.

Mesenchymal stem cells have been isolated from periosteum and bone marrow and expanded in culture (835–837). These cells have been demonstrated to be capable of a broader range of chondrogenic expression (838,839) and may be able to replicate normal cartilage microarchitecture and composition better than chondrocytes derived from mature cartilage.

Some very early studies demonstrated that these cells could be isolated, expanded *in vitro*, seeded onto type I collagen gels, and transplanted into full-thickness cartilage defects *in vivo* (837). They appeared to differentiate into chondrocytes and to form cartilage on the surface of the defect while other cells formed bone at the base of the defect. The repair tissue, however, became thinner and demonstrated some fibrillation and surface irregularities at longer follow-up.

Gene Therapy

With the advent of new technologies there has been increasing interest in the use of genes that may encode for a chondroprotective or chondroregenerative product. These genes may be delivered to cells within cartilage directly, where the gene product is produced and responded to, or indirectly into the synovium, where the product is produced by synoviocytes and then must diffuse into the cartilage. Several investigators have demonstrated gene transfer into the synovium (840,841), and clinical trials are already in progress (842). The transfer of a gene encoding interleukin-1 receptor antagonist (IL-1Ra) has been demonstrated to be chondroprotective in animal models of osteoarthritis (843–845) and rheumatoid arthritis (846). Delivery of growth factors by this method has been less successful (847,848).

Gene transfer has also been demonstrated in chondrocytes and cartilage through a variety of vectors and methodologies (849–859). Several genes encoding growth factors (IGF-1, BMP-2, TGF-β_1) have been transferred *in vitro* and demonstrated increases in collagen and proteoglycan production without alterations in the phenotype (849, 859–861). In addition, genetically modified chondrocytes have been implanted in animal models and have demonstrated sustained expression of marker genes for 1 to 2 months (852,855,857,862). The transfer of a gene encoding BMP-7 was demonstrated to improve osteochondral defect healing (862), suggesting that these methodologies, used alone or in combination with other technologies, may prove useful in restoring or protecting articular cartilage.

MENISCUS

Menisci are intraarticular, fibrocartilaginous structures located between the articular surfaces of some diarthrodial joints. Typically, menisci are wedge-shaped, with the wider, outer portion of the wedge attached to the peripheral joint margins and the internal, thinner portion located centrally (Fig. 5.74). The following discussion is based on information about knee menisci. However, as knowledge of knee meniscal structure and function is expanded, a better understanding of the roles played by menisci in other joints will undoubtedly emerge.

In the knee, menisci were once though to represent functionless remnants of an evolutionarily redundant muscle (863). In fact, meniscectomy was once performed almost indiscriminately because the meniscus was considered as superfluous as the intestinal appendix (864). Recently, much interest has been focused on the meniscus, partly because of the observed clinical relationship of degenerative joint dis-

ease with meniscectomy (865–870) and partly because experimental evidence has elucidated an indisputable association of meniscectomy with eventual articular cartilage degeneration in the knee joint (871–876).

It should be noted that, although knee menisci are found in all mammals, their shape and insertional anatomy vary considerably. Several animals models, including rabbit (877–880), canine (881–883), ovine (884,885), and bovine (886–888) have been commonly studied. The differences in anatomy, and presumably in function, may reflect major differences in limb use and joint mechanics and somewhat limit the validity of these models in application to humans.

In this section, a general overview of meniscal structure and function is given. A brief discussion of cellular and matrix characteristics and of normal tissue anatomy (neurovascular and structural organization) and function is presented. The reader is advised to consult other discussions of these topics for more details (889–896). The complex chemical composition (897–903), as well as the well-organized structural heterogeneity of cells (120,904) and matrix tissue in the meniscus (905–909) underscores its many important biologic and mechanical roles in normal diarthrodial joint physiology.

Gross and Microscopic Anatomy

Within the knee, a pair of menisci, the medial and lateral menisci, are interposed between the femoral condyle and the tibial plateau. These menisci assume their characteristic shape within the first 4 months of gestation (910). The medial and lateral menisci cover the tibial plateaus by approximately 60% and 80%, respectively, and this proportion remains relatively constant throughout growth.

The human medial meniscus is crescent-shaped and has been divided anatomically into a central "body" region and anterior and posterior "horn" attachments (911). The posterior horn of the medial meniscus is wider than the anterior horn. The attachments consist of tissue that is very fibrous,

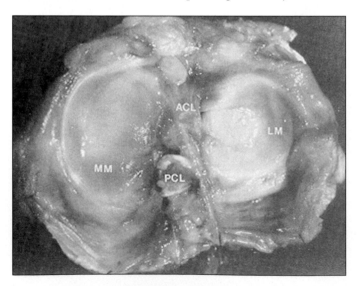

FIGURE 5.74 Human knee disarticulated to show gross anatomy of medial (MM) and lateral (LM) menisci. Cut tibial stumps of anterior cruciate (ACL) and posterior cruciate (PCL) ligaments are shown. (From Warren R, Arnoczky S, Wickiewicz T. Anatomy of the knee. In: Nicholas JA, Hershman EB, eds. *The lower extremity and spine in sports medicine.* St. Louis: CV Mosby, 1986:657, with permission.)

resembling ligamentous tissue in composition and histologic structure (911). The anterior horn attaches in the intercondylar fossa of the tibia, just in front of the ACL (912,913). The posterior horn attaches to the tibia in the posterior intercondylar fossa, between the lateral meniscus (laterally) and the PCL. The peripheral attachment of the main body of the meniscus to the tibia and femur is through short ligaments that blend with the joint capsule and collateral ligaments. The meniscotibial ligaments are distinct and have been called coronary ligaments. The medial meniscus has a somewhat longer radius of curvature than the lateral meniscus (appearing more open centrally). The central portion of the medial meniscus does not extend as far under the condyle as does the lateral meniscus, and the peripheral border is also firmly attached to the deep portion of the MCL, rendering the medial meniscus less mobile than the lateral meniscus (913,914).

The lateral meniscus appears more circular than the medial, and the anterior and posterior horns are of similar widths. The anterior horn attaches to the tibia in front of the intercondylar eminence and behind the attachment of the ACL. The posterior horn attaches to the tibia behind the intercondylar eminence and in front of the posterior attachment of the medial meniscus. In some cases the lateral meniscus may also have two unique attachments to the intercondylar notch of the femur. These attach the posterior horn of the lateral meniscus to the lateral aspect of the medial femoral condyle adjacent to the PCL. The ligament of Humphry attaches anterior to the PCL, and the ligament of Wrisberg attaches posterior to the PCL (912,913).

Meniscal Cells and Matrix

Light microscopy reveals a fibrocartilaginous tissue made up of cells interspersed in matrix composed of collagen bundles and various other noncollagenous proteins and proteoglycans. Superficially, meniscal tissue may at first seem relatively homogeneous; however, the microscopic appearance of meniscal tissue is characterized by marked microheterogeneity (915). This heterogeneity can be demonstrated with cationic stains such as Safranin-O (which stains proteoglycan) (Fig. 5.75). Some areas show rich staining for proteoglycan, while other show almost none (916,917). Tissue heterogeneity is further demonstrated by the complex but organized orientations of collagen bundles and cells in the matrix (889). These apparent regional differences probably reflect the tissue's adaptation to local loads, indicating important functional roles for each region of the meniscus.

Historically, two cell types have been identified in the meniscus, a fusiform or fibroblastic cell type and a rounded or chondrocytic cell type (120). These cell types have specific regional variations and cell distribution within the meniscus, which probably reflects the differing loads of each region (Fig. 5.29).

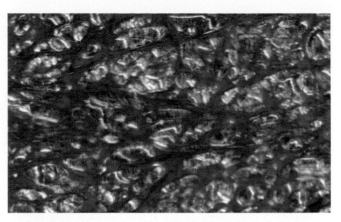

FIGURE 5.75 Canine medial meniscus stained with Safranin-O staining (600× magnification). Meniscal cells embedded in matrix stain positively for proteoglycans.

Recently, the cellular organization and cytoarchitecture of meniscal cells has been clarified in the rabbit model (918). This study demonstrated that there are four morphologically distinct cellular phenotypes within the rabbit meniscus, which are related to the basic architecture and functional domains of the meniscus (Fig. 5.76). These include two classes of cells present within the fibrocartilaginous region of the meniscus that have long cellular projections extending from the cell body. A third cell type in the inner, hyaline-like region of the meniscus has a rounded morphology and no cellular projections, and a fourth cell type with a fusiform shape and no cytoplasmic projections is seen along the superficial regions of the meniscus. This fourth cell type has a similar morphology to that observed in the superficial (tangential) zone of cartilage (120,904). These morphologically distinct cell types are strikingly similar to those found in other tissues. For example, cells of the peripheral meniscus are similar to cells of ligament and tendon, and the cells of the central meniscus are similar to hyaline cartilage. These similarities suggest that specific cellular phenotypes may be associated with specific types of connective tissue function. These findings need to be investigated further, particularly in human menisci (904).

Meniscal cells are embedded in an ECM that is composed primarily of collagen, noncollagenous proteins such as elastin and proteoglycan molecules, and water. Approximately 72% of the human meniscus is water, while the dry weight is 75% collagen, 8% to 13% noncollagenous protein, and 1% hexosamine (919).

Although meniscal tissue contains several different molecular species of collagen, type I collagen is most abundant, accounting for about 90% of the total collagen present (898). Types II, III, V, and VI are also present in small amounts (898,920) and demonstrate regional differences. For example, in the bovine meniscus, the majority of colla-

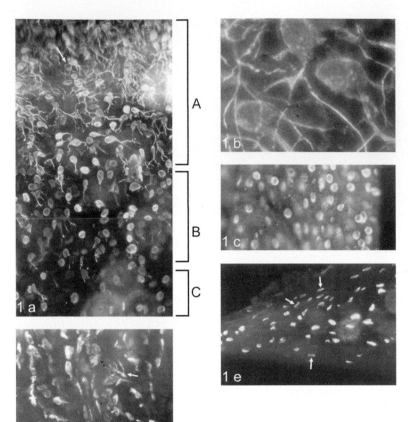

FIGURE 5.76 A: Montage of an oblique 75-μm section of the meniscus stained with an antibody to vimentin. Cells with distinct morphologies are found in each of the three zones. The arrow denotes a row of cells found in zone A (600× magnification). **B:** High-magnification view of cells from zone A as shown in (A). Each cell has a large cell body and several branched cell processes (2,500× magnification). **C:** A 75-μm section stained for vimentin showing the spherical cells that occupy zone C (700× magnification). **D:** A 75-μm section through zone A. In regions where rows of cells are cut obliquely, cell projections can be seen passing between the rows *(arrow)* (700× magnification). **E:** Section through the inner tip of the meniscus showing the fusiform cells *(arrows)* that line the superficial layer of the tissue (600× magnification). (From Hellio LE, Graverand MP, Ou YC, et al. The cells of the rabbit meniscus: their arrangement, interrelationship, morphological variations and cytoarchitecture. *J Anat* 2001 *(in press)*, with permission.)

gen in the peripheral two thirds of the meniscus is type I, with trace amounts of type III and V. However, in the inner third, type II collagen represents 60% of the total collagen, with type I collagen representing 40% (888). In addition, the amount of type II collagen appears to change with maturation. In the rabbit fetus, types I, III, and V collagen are detectable in the meniscus; however, type II collagen can be detected only at 3 weeks after birth, increasing with further maturation (921). Therefore, the appearance of type II collagen may be associated with the increase in joint loading during postnatal development.

Type I meniscal collagen shows greater posttranslational chemical differences compared with bone, tendon, and skin type I collagen, having higher hydroxylysine and hydroxylysine glycoside content (898). Meniscal collagen is also heavily crosslinked by hydroxylysine-based aldehydes and has a high level of mature hydroxypyridinium crosslinking residues (905,922), making it one of the most heavily crosslinked type I collagens found in connective tissues.

The organization and microanatomic orientation of collagen bundles in meniscal matrix is most likely related to its function as a load-bearing structure. In Bullough's classic study of collagen orientation in menisci (889), the principal direction of these bundles was circumferential, with a few radially (outwardly) disposed bundles (Fig. 5.77). It is hypothesized that these radial "tie" fibers provide structural rigidity and help resist splitting forces that arise with compressive loading (Fig. 5.78). Subsequent studies using scanning electron microscopy (923) and x-ray diffraction (890) have revealed three different collagen orientations, depending on which tissue layer is sampled. In these studies, surface layers are composed of a network of irregularly oriented collagen bundles, but deeper layers are primarily circumferentially aligned.

In addition to collagen, elastin is present in small amounts, but little information is available on the ultrastructural localization of this molecule in meniscal tissue. The content of elastin is estimated to be less than 0.6% in human meniscus (897).

Proteoglycan content of meniscal tissue is also site-specific, showing variation in hexosamine levels depending on whether tissue is sampled from thick (outer) regions, from thinner (inner) regions (905), or from attachment sites (908). Meniscal proteoglycan content appears to be only about one eighth that of articular cartilage proteoglycan content (in canine knee menisci) (906,907).

Aggrecan has been found to be the major proteoglycan in the bovine meniscus (900), as in cartilage, although other,

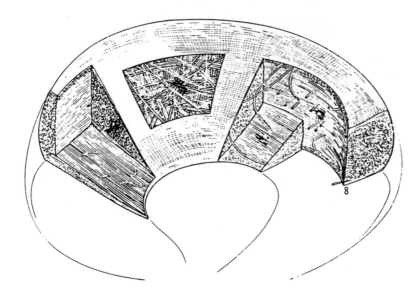

FIGURE 5.77 Schematic of a meniscus illustrating various collagen bundle orientations. (From Bullough P, Munuera L, Murphy J, et al. The strength of the menisci of the knee as it relates to their fine structure. *J Bone Joint Surg Br* 1970;52:564, with permission.)

smaller proteoglycans are also found, including decorin, biglycan, and fibromodulin (924,925). Similarly, tissue explant cultures predominantly produce aggrecan. However, tissue explants from the inner and middle thirds of the menisci produce more aggrecan, whereas the outer third of the meniscus produces less proteoglycan and more small proteoglycans (926).

In a detailed study of meniscal glycosaminoglycan composition in adult canines (based on chondroitinase digestion products), a relatively constant distribution of 60% chondroitin-6-sulfate, 25% chondroitin-4-sulfate, 10% chondroitin, and 5% dermatan sulfate was found

(906–908). These glycosaminoglycans also demonstrate regional differences: the inner third is approximately 8% glycosaminoglycans, and the outer third is only 2% glycosaminoglycans. Chondroitin sulphate accounts for 80% of the total glycosaminoglycans in the inner third and 50% to 56% of the outer third of the meniscus. In addition, the dermatan/chondroitin sulfate ratio was found to be 1:5 to 1:6 in the inner third of the meniscus and approximately 1:1.5 in the outer third. Hyaluronic acid also accounts for approximately 4% to 5% of the total glycosaminoglycans in the inner third and for approximately 10% in the peripheral third.

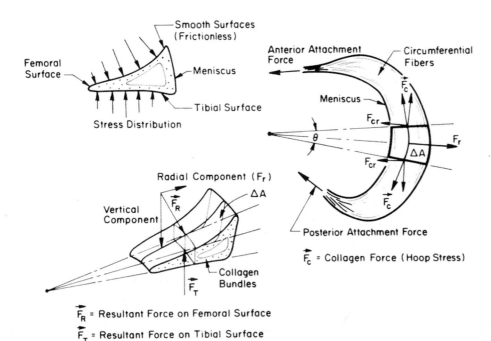

FIGURE 5.78 Schematic diagrams depicting meniscal forces with load bearing. (From Arnoczky S, Adams M, DeHaven K, et al. Meniscus. In: Woo SL-Y, Buckwalter JA, eds. *Injury and repair of the musculoskeletal soft tissues.* Park Ridge, IL: American Academy of orthopaedic Surgeons, 1987:509, with permission.)

These regional differences collectively suggest that there have been significant adaptations of the meniscal tissue to the different loads seen by each of the regions of the meniscus. Moreover, the complex interaction between proteoglycans, collagen, and water probably accounts for the complex biphasic mechanical behavior of this tissue in response to compressive loads (927).[IQ]

Neurovascular Anatomy

Like other fibrous articular connective tissues, menisci appear to be relatively avascular at the macroscopic level. However, some areas of menisci show an organized and relatively extensive microvasculature after ink injection (Fig. 5.79) (928–930). Knee menisci, both medial and lateral, demonstrate a common pattern and distribution of blood vessels that arise from the medial and lateral geniculate arteries, respectively (both superior and inferior branches). Within the synovial and capsular tissues of the knee, anastomotic vessels known as the perimeniscal capillary plexus (928), which are mainly oriented in a circumferential fashion, branch extensively into smaller vessels and supply the peripheral border of the meniscus throughout its attachment to the joint capsule. These vessels terminate before reaching the central (avascular) portion of the tissue (Fig. 5.80), limiting the internal (intrameniscal) microvasculature to the peripheral 10% to 25% of the meniscus. In addition, the surface layers of menisci sometimes are covered by a synovial fringe of vessels, particularly in regions where direct contact with articular cartilage is limited (outer periphery) (Fig. 5.81).

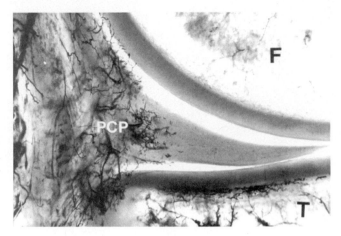

FIGURE 5.80 Perimeniscal capillary plexus (PCP) after ink injection and clearing with the Spaltholz technique. Coronal, 5-mm-thick section of the medial compartment of the knee. F, femur, T, tibia. (From Arnoczky SP, Warren RF. Microvasculature of the human meniscus. *Am J Sports Med* 1982;10:90, with permission.)

Because only the peripheral 10% to 25% of the meniscus is well vascularized, the bulk of the meniscus must receive its nutrition through other mechanisms, such as passive diffusion of nutrients (931) or mechanical pumping of nutrients by intermittent compression of the tissue during loading. Because of the dense, fibrous nature of the ECM, diffusion of nutrients into the central meniscus is thought to be limited (932,933); therefore, mechanical pumping may be an important source of nutrients (931). Some studies have demonstrated "openings" on the articular surfaces of menisci (934,935), which are theorized to connect to a system of canals running between the collagen fibers of the meniscus (Fig. 5.82). These openings and canals may allow nutrients to pass through the meniscus to cells within the central zones. Direct cell-to-cell communication may be another source of nutrients in some meniscal cells (Fig. 5.76).

Less is known about the innervation patterns in meniscal tissue, but several studies have shown nerves and specialized end receptors in the tissue (936–940). The most densely innervated areas appear to be the anterior and posterior horns of both menisci; however, nerve fibers have been identified in the body of the meniscus also. Similar to the vascular anatomy of the meniscus, the nerve fibers originate in the perimeniscal tissue and radiate into the peripheral 30% of the meniscus.

Three distinct neuroreceptors have been identified in the human meniscus (930,940). Ruffini endings, Golgi tendon organs, and pacinian corpuscles have all been identified within human tissue and are particularly prevalent in the horns of the menisci. Some authors have hypothesized a proprioceptive role for these nerves, speculating that meniscally derived sensory signals (during deformation and stretching under loaded conditions) may be important to joint-position sense and to protective neuromuscular reflex

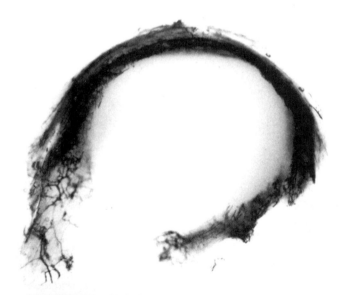

FIGURE 5.79 Blood supply to meniscus after vascular injection with ink and tissue clearing with a modified Spaltholz technique. Vessels are limited to the peripheral aspect of the meniscus. (From Arnoczky SP, Warren RF. Microvasculature of the human meniscus. *Am J Sports Med* 1982;10:90, with permission.)

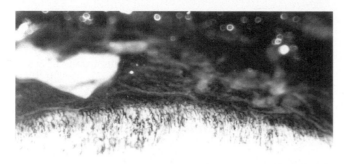

FIGURE 5.81 Synovial fringe vessels on the peripheral border of a meniscus after injection with ink. (From Arnoczky S, Adams M, Dehaven K, et al. Meniscus. In: Woo SL-Y, Buckwalter JA, eds. *Injury and repair of the musculoskeletal soft tissues.* Park Ridge, IL: American Academy of orthopaedic Surgeons, 1987:499, with permission.)

control of joint motion and loading (930,936,938–940). Other potential roles include pain sensation and vasomotor actions such as regulation of blood flow, plasma extravasation, and inflammation (186). The juxtaposition of many small, unmyelinated nerves with blood vessels from menisci (as well as ligamentous and capsular tissues) supports these additional physiologic roles for articular nerves and their termini (185,186). Until more detailed information about the structure and function of neurovascular elements in the meniscal tissue is available, most of these speculations remain unproven.

Meniscal Function

In the human knee, the menisci are located medially and laterally, giving the tibial plateaus a more concave contour to

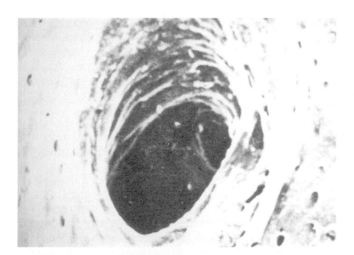

FIGURE 5.82 Scanning electron micrograph of the surface of a calf meniscus showing the opening of a canal. (From Bird MD, Sweet MBE. A system of canals in semilunar menisci. *Ann Rheum Dis* 1987;46:670–673, with permission.)

accept the rounded femoral condyles. This geometry enhances static joint stability (941–948) and situates the meniscal fibrocartilage for load bearing and shock absorption (892–894,949–951) within the diarthrodial joint cavity. This relationship is also maintained during knee flexion and rotation, because the menisci move and deform to follow the motion of the opposing joint surfaces (952–954). The lateral meniscus translates approximately 10 mm during knee flexion and extension, while the medial meniscus translates only half as much (954,955). In addition, the anterior horns are displaced more than the posterior horns, leading to some deformation of the shape of the meniscus (955).

Repeated compression and unloading of menisci is also thought to create a natural circulation pathway that is speculated to be important for tissue nourishment as well as for fluid film lubrication in diarthrodial joints (649,896).

Meniscal function is thought to depend, in part, on the biphasic nature of its mechanical response under compression (652,956,957). When a material is loaded and shows a time-dependent mechanical response to the applied load, it is said to be viscoelastic. In menisci, this viscoelastic response is characterized by creep and by stress relaxation of the tissue. The significance of this behavior is that when the joint is loaded for long periods, the contact area greatly increases, spreading the compressive load over an increasing surface area and thereby reducing the load per unit area of that tissue (958). It is probable that such viscoelasticity arises from the intrinsic properties of the tissue components (e.g., collagen, proteoglycans) and the frictional drag exerted by fluid as it flows through the porous permeable matrix of the meniscus.

Beyond the material behaviors of the tissue are the complex and as yet incompletely understood functions of menisci as anatomic structures. King (892) first proposed that the meniscus was involved in force transmission across the knee joint. More recently, Ahmed and Burke (951,959) showed that at least 50% of compressive loads in the knee are shared by the meniscus in extension, and this figure rises to 85% with 90 degrees of knee flexion. After complete meniscectomy, the tibial–femoral contact areas decrease by approximately 50% (951,959), leading to increased contact stresses and cartilage degeneration. Even partial meniscectomy of as little as 15% to 34% of the meniscus can increase contact pressures by more than 350% (960,961). These studies have emphasized the important role of the meniscus in force transmission and have been supported by long-term clinical studies of complete and partial meniscectomy (962–972).

Shrive and associates proposed a model for how compressive loads are converted into radially directed forces by the meniscus (894). During normal joint loading, it was hypothesized that the anterior and posterior insertions of the meniscus are tensioned along with the circumferential fibers of the meniscus. This tension is subsequently converted into hoop stresses at the meniscal periphery. Thus, the compressive loads are resisted by the anterior and posterior attachments of the meniscus, and the radial forces are balanced by tensile stresses developed in the circumferentially oriented collagen bundles of the matrix (894). Both the circumferential fibers of the meniscus and the strong anterior and posterior insertions into bone are critical for this function. A radial transection through the entire meniscal body disrupts the load-converting function of the meniscus, as does transection of the anterior and posterior meniscal insertions (973–976). Further work directed at relating the material and structural behaviors of meniscal tissue is necessary to better understand the complex mechanisms of load bearing as well as the reasons why certain patterns of injury are common in meniscal tissue. More rational approaches to treatment will be predicated on a better understanding of these properties.

Another important function of menisci is absorption of the shock waves generated by impulse loading of the knee with normal gait (961,977,978). The inability to absorb shock waves has been implicated in the development of degenerative arthritis (979), and the mechanical properties of menisci, which are softer and less permeable to fluid than articular cartilage (980), appear to help dissipate and absorb this mechanical energy and attenuate forces experienced by articular cartilage. A normal knee is estimated to have a 20% higher shock-absorbing capacity than a knee after meniscectomy (981). More work is necessary to determine the role of meniscal tissue in this process, because few studies have actually attempted to characterize the nature of energy dissipation under repeated impulse loading conditions before and after partial or total removal of menisci.

Menisci are also thought to contribute additional stability to the knee by maintaining proper alignment of the femoral condyles on the tibial plateaus (944–946,952,982). This function is apparently most important if other joint structures are damaged (i.e., ligaments and capsular restraints), and some investigators question the importance of meniscal contributions to static stability under normal conditions (942,943,947,983). However, if meniscectomy is added to ACL disruption, joint instability is considerably increased (942–944,947,948,983). With respect to the medial meniscus, the posterior horn is particularly important in providing this stability (947).

The various functions of menisci are underscored by the effects of meniscectomy. In his classic article, Fairbank (865) proposed that meniscectomy leads to considerable degenerative changes in the knee, including joint space narrowing, marginal osteophytes, and flattening of the external half of the opposing femoral condyle in the involved knee compartment. Several studies subsequently confirmed his observations in patients (866,984).

Experimental studies have confirmed that load bearing in the knee is adversely affect by meniscectomy. A reduction in contact area after meniscectomy has been documented, and

significant alterations in proximal tibial strain distributions have been measured *in vivo* (951,978,985). Furthermore, animal models of meniscectomy have shown histologic (875,986) and biochemical (987,988) alterations in articular cartilage. Thus, the long-term mechanical, radiologic, and clinical sequelae of meniscectomy are also accompanied by substantial deterioration of many biologic mechanisms responsible for normal diarthrodial joint homeostasis.

Meniscal Healing and Repair

With increased understanding of meniscal function coupled with the poor long-term results of meniscectomy, there has been a shift toward meniscal preservation and meniscal repair (989). King (892) was the first to propose that the healing response after meniscal injury is closely correlated with communication of the meniscus with the peripheral blood supply. Subsequent studies, both experimental and clinical, confirmed that injuries in regions vascularized by the peripheral meniscal blood supply are capable of producing a healing response similar to that of other connective tissues, comprising hemorrhage, proliferative, and remodeling phases (990–996). This section briefly reviews the healing response after injury to the meniscus and also various methods of augmenting this response.

Meniscal Healing

Injuries in the peripheral vascularized zone of the meniscus initially fill with a highly cellular (inflammatory cells) fibrin clot (Fig. 5.83). The fibrin clot functions as a meshwork or

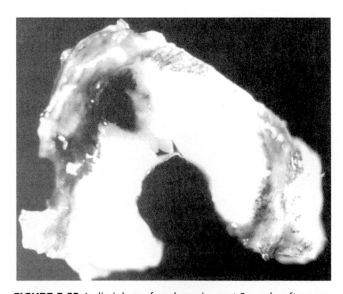

FIGURE 5.83 India ink–perfused meniscus at 2 weeks after complete transection. Note the proliferation of vessels from the perimeniscal capillary plexus into the fibrous clot. (From Arnoczky SP, Warren RF. The microvasculature of the meniscus and its response to injury: an experimental study in the dog. *Am J Sports Med* 1983;11:131–141, with permission.)

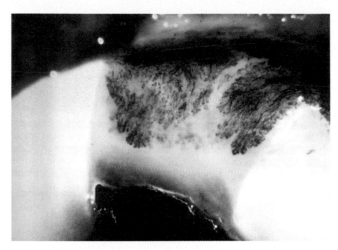

FIGURE 5.84 India ink–perfused specimen showing the fibrovascular scar at 6 weeks after complete transection of the medial meniscus. Notice the proliferation of vascular synovial tissue over the fibrovascular scar. (From Arnoczky SP, Warren RF. The microvasculature of the meniscus and its response to injury: an experimental study in the dog. *Am J Sports Med* 1983;11:131–141, with permission.)

scaffold for proliferating capillary buds to infiltrate from the adjacent perimeniscal plexus. These new vessels from the perimeniscal plexus and a proliferative vascular pannus from the synovial fringe penetrate and infiltrate into the fibrin clot and support the healing process (Fig. 5.84). Concurrently, there is migration and proliferation of undifferentiated mesenchymal cells into this cellular, fibrovascular scar (Fig. 5.85) (990). Although the meniscal injury appears to be completely healed within 10 weeks (990,991), scar tissue remodeling most likely requires months and may never be complete. The strength of this scar tissue is now being investigated (997–1000). Although several differences exists

in these experiments regarding the animal model, injury model, repair techniques, and mechanical testing protocols, these studies have collectively demonstrated that the scar tissue is still mechanically inferior despite 3 to 4 months of healing (997–1000).

The understanding that vascularity is an important determinant in the healing response after injury has led to the clinical classification of meniscal injuries in relation to the blood supply and the vascular appearance of the surfaces of the tear. Meniscal tears can be divided into red–red tears, red–white tears, and white–white tears (Fig. 5.86). Red–red tears are injuries to the peripheral capsular attachment of the meniscus; they have a rich blood supply on both the peripheral and central surfaces of the tears and therefore have a excellent prognosis for healing. Red–white tears are injuries through the peripheral meniscal rim; they have an active peripheral blood supply from the perimeniscal capillary plexus, but the central surface has no blood supply. These lesions have an intermediate prognosis and should have a sufficient blood supply to support the healing process. White–white tears occur in the avascular zone and are completely devoid of blood supply on both surfaces (peripheral and central). These lesions theoretically cannot support a healing response and this has provided the rationale for partial meniscectomy for lesions in this zone. Although vascularity has been presumed to be the cause of the varying healing responses and forms the basis of this clinical classification, it is important to remember other differences in these zones exist, including differences in cell morphology, organization, and metabolism; matrix composition and organization; and possibly meniscal function.

Augmenting the Meniscal Healing Response

In an attempt to extend the indications for meniscal preservation and repair, several techniques have emerged to aug-

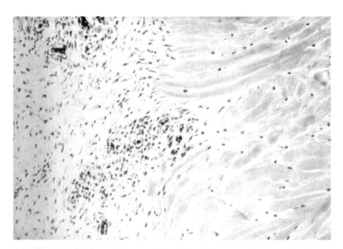

FIGURE 5.85 Photomicrograph of healing meniscus at the junction of the fibrovascular scar and the normal adjacent meniscal tissue (hematoxylin and eosin stain, 100× magnification). (From Arnoczky SP, Warren RF. The microvasculature of the meniscus and its response to injury: an experimental study in the dog. *Am J Sports Med* 1983;11:131–141, with permission.)

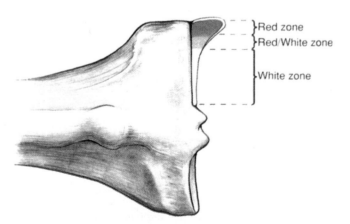

FIGURE 5.86 Schematic drawing indicating the various zones of the meniscus. Note that red–red and red–white zones are capable of healing, and repair is recommended. (From Miller MD, Warner JJP, Harner CD. Meniscal repair. In: Fu FH, Harner CD, Vince KG. *Knee surgery.* Baltimore: Williams & Wilkins, 1994: 613–630, with permission.)

ment the vascularity or healing response to these injuries. Synovial abrasion, trephination (i.e., the development of vascular access channels), and the addition of a exogenous fibrin clot have been used (1001–1003). The rationale for synovial abrasion (1004) originated from the observation of a proliferative vascular pannus, which originated from the meniscal synovial junction and infiltrated the fibrovascular scar in lesions in the periphery of the meniscus. The technique of synovial abrasion, when used in central tears, attempts to augment this response by stimulating the synovial fringe (through rasping or abrasion) adjacent to the tibial and femoral surfaces of the torn meniscus. Some experimental studies using this technique have demonstrated promising results, with improvements of the healing response in the avascular zone (1005,1006).

Trephination, or the creation of vascular access channels from the avascular zone of the meniscus to the peripheral blood supply, can result in healing of the meniscus (990, 1007). Although this simple technique may improve meniscal healing, the creation of access channels large enough to permit vascular ingrowth may disrupt the normal, complex organization of the meniscus and further disrupt its function (1004). Therefore, other techniques, such as the use of an exogenous fibrin clot, have been proposed (1008,1009). The use of a fibrin clot, initially studied in canines, interposes an exogenous fibrin clot within a lesion in the avascular zone of the meniscus (1008,1009). This provides a scaffold for the healing process as well as potential mitogenic and chemotactic stimuli. Early clinical results of this technique are mixed (1010–1012).

In the future, the use of fibrin glue (1013,1014), growth factors (1014,1015), gene therapy (1016,1017), and drugs (hyaluronic acid) (1018,1019) will require further investigations. Although these approaches and other methods of meniscal repair or enhancement techniques continue to be important areas of research, the prevention of articular degeneration remains to be proven. Specifically, restoration of the peripheral circumferential collagen fiber arrangement and the biomechanical functions of menisci (particularly with radial tears) remains to be seen. Some authors have reported in experimental studies that, even with successful gross and histologic healing, the ability of a repaired meniscus to transmit load was no different than after total meniscectomy (997).

REFERENCES

1. *Dorland's illustrated medical dictionary*, 28th ed. Philadelphia: WB Saunders, 1994.
2. Simkin PA. Joints: structure and function. In: Schumacher R, Klippel JH, Robinson OR, eds. *Primer on the rheumatic diseases*, 9th ed. The Arthritis Foundation, 1988.
3. Kelly WN, Harris ED, Ruddy S, et al. *Textbook of rheumatology*, 3rd ed. Philadelphia: WB Saunders; 1989.
4. Daniel DM, Biden EN. The language of knee motion. In: Jackson DW, Drez D, eds. *The anterior cruciate deficient knee: new concepts in ligament repair.* St. Louis: CV Mosby, 1987.
5. Moore KL. The articular and skeletal systems. In: *The developing human,* 2nd ed. Philadelphia: WB Saunders, 1977.
6. Thorogood PV, Hinchcliffe JR. An analysis of the condensation process during chondrogenesis in embryonic chick hind limb. *J Embryol Exp Morphol* 1975;33:581.
7. O'Rahilly R. The development of joints. *Irish J Med Sci* 1957;6:456.
8. Anderson H, Bro-Rasmussen F. Histochemical studies on the histogenesis of the joints in human fetuses with special reference to the development of the joint cavities in the hand and foot. *Am J Anat* 1961;108:111.
9. Warsilev W. Elektronenmikroskopische und histochemische unter suchungen zur entwicklung des kniegelenkes der ratte. *Anat Entwicklungsgest* 1972;137:221.
10. Sledge CB, Zaleske DJ. Developmental anatomy of joints. In: Resnick D, Niwayama G, eds. *Diagnosis of bone and joint disorders,* 2nd ed. Philadelphia: WB Saunders, 1988.
11. O'Rahilly R, Gardner E, Gray DJ. The ectodermal thickening and ridge in the limbs of staged human embryos. *J Embryol Exp Morphol* 1956;4:254.
12. Saunders JW Jr. The experimental analysis of chick limb bud development. In: Ede DA, Hinchliffe JR, Balls M, eds. *Vertebrate limb and somite morphogenesis.* Cambridge: Cambridge University Press, 1977:1.
13. MacCabe JA, Saunders JW Jr, Pickett M. The control of the antero-posterior and dorso-ventral axes in embryonic chick limbs constructed of dissociated and reaggregated limb bud mesoderm. *Dev Biol* 1973;31:323.
14. Toole BP, Jackson G, Gross J. Hyaluronate in morphogenesis: inhibition of chondrogenesis in vitro. *Proc Natl Acad Sci U S A* 1972;69:1384.
15. Drachman DB, Sokoloff L. The role of movement in embryonic joint development. *Dev Biol* 1966;14:401.
16. Murray PDF, Drachman DB. The role of movement in the development of joints and related structures: the head and neck in the chick embryo. *J Embryol Exp Morphol* 1969;22:349.
17. Yasuda Y. Differentiation of human limb buds in vitro. *Anat Rec* 1973;175:561.
18. Eyre DR. Collagen: molecular diversity in the body's protein scaffold. *Science* 1980;207:1315–1322.
19. Miller EJ. The structure of fibril-forming collagens. *Ann N Y Acad Sci* 1985;460:1–13.
20. Hukins DWL, Aspden RM. Composition and properties of connective tissues. *Trends Biochem Sci* 1985;10:260.
21. Gay S, Miller EJ. What is collagen, what is not. *Ultrastruct Pathol* 1983;4:365–377.
22. Miller EJ, Gay S. Collagen: an overview. *Methods Enzymol* 1982;82A:3–32.
23. Miller EJ. Chemistry of the collagens and their distribution. In: Piez KA, Reddi AH. *Extracellular matrix biochemistry.* New York: Elsevier, 1984.
24. Miller EJ. Recent information on the chemistry of the collagens. In: Butler WT, ed. *The chemistry and biology and mineralized tissues,* Birmingham, AL: Ebasco Media, 1985:80–93.
25. Ramachandran GN, Reddi AH, eds. *Biochemistry of collagen.* New York: Plenum, 1976.
26. Miller EJ. Biochemical characteristics and biological significance of the genetically distinct collagen. *Mol Cell Biochem* 1976;13:165–192.
27. Prockop DJ, Kivirikko KI, Tuderman L, et al. Biosynthesis of procollagen and its disorders [Parts 1 and 2]. *N Engl J Med* 1979;301:13–23,77–85.

28. Fessler JH, Fessler LI. Biosynthesis of procollagen. *Annu Rev Biochem* 1979;47:129.

29. Piez KA, Reddi AH, eds. *Extracellular matrix biochemistry.* Amsterdam: Elsevier, 1984.

30. Eikenberry E, Brodsky B, Cassidy K. Does the genetic type of collagen determine fibril structure? *Biophys J* 1980;32:221.

31. Graves PN, Olsen BR, Fietzerk PP, et al. Comparison of the NH₂-terminal sequences of chick type I procollagen chains synthesized in an mRNA-dependent reticulocyte lysate. *Eur J Biochem* 1981;118:363–369.

32. Palmiter RD, et al. NH2-terminal sequence of the chick proalpha 1(I) chain synthesized in the reticulocyte lysate system: evidence for a transient hydrophobic leader sequence. *J Biol Chem* 1979;254:1433.

33. Bornstein P. The biosynthesis of collagen. *Annu Rev Biochem* 1974;43:567.

34. Myllyla R, Risteli L, Kivirikko KI. Assay of collagen galactosyltransferase and collagen glucosyltransferase activities and characterization of enzyme reactions with transferases from chick embryo cartilage. *Eur J Biochem* 1975;52:40.

35. Leung MKK, Fessler LI, Greenberg DB, et al. Separate amino acid carboxyl procollagen peptidases in chick embryo tendon. *J Biol Chem* 1979;254:224.

36. Gallop PM, Blumenfield OO, Seifter S. Structure and metabolism of connective tissue proteins. *Annu Rev Biochem* 1972;41:617.

37. Tanzer ML. Cross-linking (of collagen). In: Ramachandran GN, Reddi AH, eds. *Biochemistry of collagen.* New York: Plenum Press, 1976.

38. Trelstad RL, Birk DE, Silver FH. Collagen fibrillogenesis in tissues, in solutions, and from modeling: a synthesis. *J Invest Dermatol* 1982;79:109.

39. Gross J. Collagen biology: structure, degradation and disease. *Harvey Lect* 1974;68:351.

40. Epstein EH, Munderloh NH. Isolation and characterization of CNBr peptides of human [α1(IV)]₃ collagen and tissue distribution of [α1(I)]₂ and [α1(III)]₃ collagens. *J Biol Chem* 1975;250:9304.

41. Frank C, McDonald D, Sabiston P, et al. Biochemical heterogeneity along the length of the rabbit medial collateral ligament. *Clin Orthop Rel Res* 1988;236:279–288.

42. Birk DE, Fitch JM, Babiarz JP, et al. Collagen fibrillogenesis in vitro: interaction of types I and V collagen regulates fibril diameter. *J Cell Sci* 1990;95:649–657.

43. Miller EJ. A review of biochemical studies on the genetically distinct collagens of the skeletal system. *Clin Orthop* 1973;92:260.

44. Olsen BR, Niomiya Y, Lozano G, et al. Short-chain collagen genes and their expression in cartilage. *Ann N Y Acad Sci* 1986;460:141.

45. Gay S, Miller EJ. Distribution and disposition of the collagens in connective tissues. In: Gasy S, Miller EJ, eds. *Collagen in the physiology and pathology of connective tissue.* New York: Gustav Fisher, 1978:57–62.

46. Glimcher MJ, Krane SM. The organization and structure of bone and the mechanism of calcification. In: Gould BS, Ramachandran GN, eds. *A treatise on collagen,* vol 2. New York: Academic Press, 1968.

47. McKusick VA. *Heritable disorders of connective tissue.* St. Louis: CV Mosby, 1972:412.

48. Sandberg LB, Soskel NJ, Wolt MS. Structure of the elastin fiber: an overview. *J Invest Dermatol* 1982;79:128.

49. Foster JA, Rubin L, Kagen HM, et al. Isolation and characterization of cross-linked peptides from elastin. *J Biol Chem* 1974;249:6191.

50. Franzblau C, Farris B. Elastin. In: Hay ED, ed. *Cell biology of extracellular matrix.* New York: Plenum, 1981:65.

51. Urry DW. Molecular perspectives of vascular wall structure and disease-elastin component. *Perspect Biol Med* 1978;21:265.

52. Burnett W, Yoon K, Finnigan-Burnick A, et al. Control of elastin synthesis. *J Invest Dermatol* 1982;79:138.

53. Fransson LA. Mammalian glycosaminoglycans. In: Aspinal GO, ed. *The polysaccharides,* vol 3. New York: Academic Press, 1985:337–415.

54. Hardingham TE. Structure and biosynthesis of proteoglycans. In: Kuhn K, Krieg T, eds. *Connective tissue: biological and clinical aspects.* Basel: S Kargcr, 1986:143–183.

55. Poole AR. Changes in the collagen and proteoglycan of articular cartilage in arthritis. In: Kuhn K, Krieg T, eds. *Connective tissue: biological and clinical aspects.* Basel: S Karger, 1986:316–371.

56. Trelstad RL. Glycosaminoglycans: mortar, matrix, mentor. *Lab Invest* 1985;53:1.

57. Poole AR. Proteoglycan in health and disease: structures and functions. *Biochem J* 1986;236:1.

58. McDevitt CA. The proteoglycans of cartilage and the intervertebral disc in aging and osteoarthritis. In: Glynn LE, ed. *Handbook of inflammation, tissue repair and regeneration,* vol 3. New York: Elsevier/North-Holland Biomedical Press, 1981:111–143.

59. Faltz LL, Caputo CB, Kimura JH, et al. Structure of the complex between hyaluronic acid: the hyaluronic acid-binding region and the link protein of proteoglycan aggregates from the swarm rat chondrosarcoma. *J Biol Chem* 1979;254:1381–1387.

60. Manicourt DH, Pita JC. Quantification and characterization of hyaluronic acid in different topographical areas of normal articular cartilage from dogs. *Coll Relat Res* 1988;8:39–48.

61. Buckwalter JA, Rosenberg LC, Tang LH. The effect of link protein on proteoglycan aggregate structure. *J Biol Chem* 1984;259:5391–5393.

62. Tang LH, Buckwalter JA, Rosenberg LC. Effect of link protein concentration on articular cartilage proteoglycan aggregation. *J Orthop Res* 1996;14:334–339.

63. Hascall VC. Interaction of cartilage proteoglycans with hyaluronic acid. *J Supramol Struct* 1977;7:101–120.

64. Buckwalter JA, Kuettner KE, Thonar EJM. Age-related changes in articular cartilage proteoglycans: electron microscopic studies. *J Orthop Res* 1985;3:251–257.

65. Thonar EJ, Buckwalter JA, Kuettner KE. Maturation-related differences in the structure and composition of proteoglycans synthesized by chondrocytes from bovine articular cartilage. *J Biol Chem* 1986;261:2567–2574.

66. Buckwalter JA, Hunziker E, Rosenberg L, et al. Articular cartilage: composition and structure. In: Woo SL-Y, Buckwalter JA, eds. *Injury and repair of the musculoskeletal soft tissues.* Park Ridge, IL: American Academy of Orthopaedic Surgeons, 1987.

67. Iozzo RV. The family of small leucine-rich proteoglycans: key regulators of matrix assembly and cellular growth. *Critical Rev Biochem Mol Biol* 1997;32:141–174.

68. Hocking AM, Shinomura T, McQuillan DJ. Leucine-rich repeat glycoproteins of the extracellular matrix. *Matrix Biol* 1998;17:1–19.

69. Iozzo RV. The biology of the small leucine-rich proteoglycans. *J Biol Chem* 1999;274:18843–18846.

70. Kadler KE, Holmes DF, Trotter JA, et al. Collagen fibrillogenesis. *Biochem J* 1996;316:1–11, 1996.

71. Vogel KG, Koob TJ, Fisher LW. Characterizations and inter-

actions of a fragment of the core protein of the small proteo-glycan (PGII) from bovine tendon. *Biochem Biophys Res Commun* 1987;148:658–663.

72. Rada JA, Carnuet Pk, Hassell JR. Regulation of corneal collagen fibrillogenesis in vitro by corneal proteoglycan (lumican and decorin) core proteins. *Exp Eye Res* 1992;56:635–648.

73. Danielson KG, Baribault H, Holmes DF, et al. Targeted disruption of decorin leads to abnormal collagen morphology and skin fragility. *J Cell Biol* 1997;136:729–743.

74. Xu T, Bianco P, Fisher LW, et al. Targeted disruption of the biglycan gene leads to an osteoporosis phenotype in mice. *Nat Genet* 1998;20:78–82.

75. Svensson L, Aszodi A, Reinholt FP, et al. Fibromodulin null mice have abnormal collagen fibrils, tissue organization, and altered lumican deposition in tendon. *J Biol Chem* 1999;274:9636–9647.

76. Chakravarti S, Magnuson T, Lass JH, et al. Lumican regulates collagen fibril assembly: skin fragility and corneal opacity in the absence of lumican. *J Cell Biol* 1998;141:1277–1286.

77. Hildebrand A, Romaris M, Rasmussen, et al. Interaction of the small proteoglycans biglycan, decorin and fibromodulin with transforming growth factor beta. *Biochem J* 1994;302:527–534.

78. Coppock DL, Kopman C, Scandali S, et al. Preferential gene expression in quiescent human lung fibroblasts. *Cell Growth Differ* 1993;4:483–493.

79. Asundi VK, Dreher KL. Molecular characterization of vascular smooth muscle decorin: deduced core protein structure and regulation of gene expression. *Eur J Cell Biol* 1992;59:314–321.

80. De Luca A, Santra M, Baldi A, et al. Decorin-induced growth suppression is associated with up-regulation of p21, an inhibitor of cyclin-dependent kinases. *J Biol Chem* 1996;271:18961–18965.

81. Santra M, Mann DM, Mercer EW, et al. Ectopic expression of decorin protein core causes a generalized growth supresion in neoplastic cells of various histogenetic origin and requires endogenous p21, an inhibitor of cyclin-dependent kinases. *J Clin Invest* 1997;100:149–157.

82. Santra M, Skorski T, Calabretta B, et al. De novo decorin gene expression suppresses the malignant phenotype in human colon cancer cells. *Proc Natl Acad Sci U S A* 1995;92:7016–7020.

83. Humphries MJ, Yamada K. Non-collagenous glycoproteins. In: Kuhn K, Krieg T, eds. *Connective tissue: biological and clinical aspects,* vol 10. Basel: S Karger, 1986:104–142.

84. Albini A, Allavena G, Gabriella A, et al. Chemotaxis of 3T3 and SV3T3 cells to fibronectin is mediated through the cell attachment site in fibronectin and a fibronectin cell surface receptor. *J Cell Biol* 1987;105:1867.

85. Hynes R. Molecular biology of fibronectin. *Annu Rev Cell Biol* 1985;1:67.

86. Cohen J, Burne JF, McKinlay, et al. The role of laminin and the laminin and laminin/fibronectin receptor complex in the outgrowth of retinal ganglion cell axons. *Dev Biol* 1987;122:407.

87. Culp LA, Laterra J, Lark MW, et al. Heparan sulphate proteoglycan as mediator of some adhesive responses and cytoskeletal reorganization of cells on fibronectin matrices: independent versus cooperative functions. Functions of proteoglycans at the cell surface. *Ciba Found Symp* 1986;124:158.

88. Hewitt AT, Varner HH, Silver MH, et al. The role of chondronectin and cartilage proteoglycan in the attachment of chondrocytes to collagen. In: Kelley RO, Goetinck PF, MacCabe JA, eds. *Limb development and regeneration,* part B. New York: Alan R Liss, 1982:25–33.

89. von der Mark K, Mollenhauer J, Pfaffle M, et al. Role of anchorin CII in the interaction of chondrocytes with extracellu-lar collagen. In: Kuettner KE, Schleyerback R, Hascall VC, eds. *Articular cartilage biochemistry.* New York: Raven Press, 1986:125–141.

90. Kaplan HA, Welply JK, Lennarz WJ. Oligosaccharyl transferase: the central enzyme in the pathway of glycoprotein assembly. *Biochim Biophys Acta* 1987;906:161.

91. Farquhar MG. Progress in unraveling pathways of Golgi traffic. *Annu Rev Cell Biol* 1985;1:447.

92. Guyton AC, ed. *Textbook of medical physiology,* 7th ed. Philadelphia: WB Saunders, 1986.

93. Andersson C, Odensten M, Gillquist J. Knee function after surgical or nonsurgical treatment of acute rupture of the anterior cruciate ligament: a randomized study with a long-term follow-up period. *Clin Orthop* 1991;264:255–263.

94. Arnold JA, Coker TP, Heaton LM, et al. Natural history of anterior cruciate tears *Am J Sports Med* 1979;7:305–313.

95. Feagin JA Jr, Curl WW. Isolated tear of the anterior cruciate ligament: 5-year follow-up study. *Am J Sports Med* 1976;4:95–100.

96. Fetto JF, Marshall JL. The natural history and diagnosis of anterior cruciate ligament insufficiency. *Clin Orthop* 1980;147:29–38.

97. McDaniel WJ Jr, Damerson TB Jr. Untreated ruptures of the anterior cruciate ligament: a follow-up study. *J Bone Joint Surg Am* 1980;62:696–705.

98. Noyes FR, Bassett RW, Grood ES, et al. Arthroscopy in acute traumatic hemarthrosis of the knee: incidence of anterior cruciate tears and other injuries. *J Bone Joint Surg Am* 1980;62:687–695.

99. Daniel DM, Stone ML, Dobson BE, et al. Fate of the ACL-injured patient: a prospective outcome study. *Am J Sports Med* 1994;22:632–644.

100. McDevitt C, Gilbertson E, Muir M. An experimental model of osteoarthritis: early morphological and biomechanical changes. *J Bone Joint Surg Br* 1977;59:24–35.

101. Marshall JL. Periarticular osteophytes: Initiation and formation in the knee of the dog. *Clin Orthop* 1969;62:37–47.

102. Marshall JL, Olsson SE. Instability of the knee: a long-term experimental study in dogs. *J Bone Joint Surg Am* 1971:53:1561–1570.

103. Bohr H. Experimental osteoarthritis in the rabbit knee joint. *Acta Orthop Scand* 1976;47:558–565.

104. Markolf KL, Mensch JS, Amstutz HC. Stiffness and laxity of the knee: the contributions of the supporting structures. *J Bone Joint Surg Am* 1976;58:583–594.

105. Andriacchi TP, Mikosz RP, Hampton SJ, et al. Model studies of the stiffness characteristics of the human knee joint. *J Biomech* 1983;16:23–29.

106. Markolf KL, Wascher DC, Finerman GAM. Direct in vitro measurement of forces in the cruciate ligaments: part II: The effect of section of the posterolateral structures. *J Bone Joint Surg Am* 1993;75:387–394.

107. Terry GC, Norwood LA, Hughston JC, et al. How iliotibial tract injuries of the knee combine with acute anterior cruciate ligament tears to influence abnormal anterior tibial displacement. *Am J Sports Med* 1993;21:55–60.

108. Wroble RR, Grood ES, Cummings JS, et al. The role of the lateral extraarticular restraints in the anterior cruciate ligament-deficient knee. *Am J Sports Med* 1993;21:257–262.

109. Sakane M, Fox RJ, Woo SL, et al. In situ forces of the anterior cruciate ligament and its bundles in reponse to anterior tibial loads. *J Orthop Res* 1997;15:285–293.

110. Kanamori A, Sakane M, Zeminski J, et al. In-situ force of the medial and lateral structures of intact and ACL deficient knees. *J Orthop Sci* 2000;5:567–571.

111. Sakane M, Livensay GA, Fox RJ, et al. Relative contribution of

the ACL, MCL and bony contact to the anterior stability of the knee. *Knee Surg Sports Traumatol Arthrosc* 1999;7:93–97.

112. Lo IKY, Leatherbarrow K, Marchuk L, et al. MCL/Partial ACL transection leads to molecular changes in other periarticular ligaments. *Trans Orthop Res Soc* 2001;26:68.

113. Dye SF. The knee as a biologic transmission with an envelope of function: a theory. *Clin Orthop* 1996;325:10–18.

114. Dye SF, Wojtys EM, Fu FH, et al. Factors contributing to function of the knee joint after injury or reconstruction of the anterior cruciate ligament. *Instr Course Lect* 1999;48:185–198.

Synovium References

115. Henderson B, Edwards JCW. *The synovial lining in health and disease.* London: Chapman and Hall, 1987.

116. Collins DH. *The pathology of articular and spinal disease.* London: Arnold, 1949.

117. Key JA. The synovial membrane of joints and bursae. In: Hoeber PB, ed. *Special cytology II,* 2nd ed. New York: Paul B. Hoeber, 1932:1055:76.

118. Barnett CH, Davies DV, MacConnaill MA. *Synovial joints.* London: Longman, 1961:131.

119. Castor CW. The microscopic structures of normal human synovial tissue. *Arthritis Rheum* 1960;3:140.

120. Ghadially FN. *Fine structure of synovial joints.* London: Butterworths, 1983.

121. Edwards JCW, Mackay A, Moore AR, et al. The mode of formation of synovial villi. *Ann Rheum Dis* 1983;42:585–590.

122. Chowdhury P, Matyas JR, Frank CB. The "epiligament" of the rabbit MCL: a quantitative morphological study. *Connect Tissue Res* 1991;274:33–50.

123. Bray RC, Fisher AWF, Frank CB, et al. Fine vascular anatomy of adult rabbit knee ligaments. *J Anat* 1990;172:69–79.

124. Barland P, Novikoff AB, Hamerman D. Electron microscopy of the human synovial membrane. *J Cell Biol* 1962;14:207.

125. Barratt MEJ, Fell HB, Coombs RRA, et al. The pig synovium: II. Some properties of isolated intimal cells. *J Anat* 1977;123:47–66.

126. Jilani M, Ghadially FN. An ultrastructural study of age: associated changes in the rabbit synovial membrane. *J Anat* 1987;146:201–215.

127. Levick JR, McDonald JN. Ultrastructure of transport pathways in stressed synovium of the knee in anaesthetized rabbits. *J Physiol* 1989;419:493–508.

128. Revell PA. Synovial lining cells. *Rheumatol Int* 1989;9:49–51.

129. Krey PR, Cohen AS, Smith CB, et al. The human fetal synovium: histology, fine structure and changes in organ culture. *Arthritis Rheum* 1971;14:319.

130. Roy S, Ghadially FN. Synthesis of hyaluronic acid by synovial cells. *J Pathol Bacteriol* 1967;93:555.

131. Werb Z, Reynolds JJ. Stimulation by endocytosis of the secretion of collagenase and neutral proteinases from rabbit synovial fibroblasts. *J Exp Med* 1976;140:1482.

132. Norton WL, Lewis DC, Ziff M. Electron-dense deposits following injection of gold sodium thiomalate and thiomalic acid. *Arthritis Rheum* 1968;11:436.

133. Ghadially FN, Ailsby RL, Yong NK. Ultrastructure of the hemophilic synovial membrane and electron-probe x-ray analysis of haemosiderin. *J Pathol* 1976;120:201.

134. Mapp PI, Revell PA. Fibronectin production by synovial intimal cells. *Rheumatol Int* 1985;5:229–237.

135. Yielding KL, Tomkins GM, Bunim JJ. Synthesis of hyaluronic acid by human synovial tissue slices. *Science* 1957;125:1300.

136. Matsubara T, Spycher MA, Ruttner JR, et al. The ultrastructural localization of fibronectin in the lining layer of the rheumatoid arthritis synovium: the synthesis of fibronectin by type B lining cells. *Rheumatol Int* 1983;3:75–79.

137. Roy S, Ghadially FN. Synthesis of hyaluronic acid by synovial cells. *J Pathol Bact* 1967;93:555–557.

138. Athanasou NA. Synovial macrophages. *Ann Rheum Dis* 1995;54:392–394.

139. Nazawa-Inoue K, Takagi R, Kobayashi T, et al. Immunocytochemistry demonstration of synovial membrane in experimentally induced arthritis of the rat temporomandibular joint. *Arch Histol Cyto* 1998;61:451–466.

140. Wilkinson LS, Pitsillides AA, Worrall JG, et al. Light microscopic characterization of the fibroblast-like synovial intial cell (synoviocyte). *Arthritis Rheum* 1992;35:1179–1184.

141. Stevens CR, Mapp PI, Revell PA. A monoclonal antibody (MAB 67) marks type B synoviocytes. *Arthritis Rheum* 1998;10:1179–1184.

142. Hirohata K, Kobayashi I. Fine structure of the synovial tissue in rheumatoid arthritis. *Kobe J Med Sci* 1964;10:195.

143. Winchester RJ, Burmester GM. Demonstration of Ia antigens on certain dendritic cells and on a novel elongate cell found in human synovial tissue. *Rheumatol Int* 1987;7:13–22.

144. Gadher SJ, Woolley DE. Comparative studies of adherent rheumatoid synovial cells in primary culture: characterization of the dendritic (stellate) cell. *Rheumatol Int* 1987;7:13–22.

145. Clarris BJ, Leizer T, Fraser JRE, et al. Diverse morphological responses of normal human synovial fibroblasts to mononuclear leukocyte products: relationship to prostaglandin production and plasminogen activator activities, and comparison to the effects of purified interleukin-1. *Rheumatol Int* 1987;7:35.

146. McDonald JN, Levick JR. Morphology of surface synoviocytes in situ at normal and raised joint pressure, studied by scanning electron microscopy. *Ann Rheum Dis* 1988;47:232–240.

147. Frizziero L, Georgountzos A, Zizzi F, et al. Microarthroscopic study of the morphologic features of normal and pathological synovial membrane. *Arthroscopy* 1992;8:504–509.

148. Scott DL, Wainwright AC, Walton KW, et al. Significance of fibronectin in rheumatoid arthritis and osteoarthritis. *Ann Rheum Dis* 1981;40:142.

149. Lavietes BB, Carson S, Diamond HS, et al. Synthesis, secretion and deposition of fibronectin in cultured human synovium. *Arthritis Rheum* 1985;28:1016.

150. Hynes RO. Cell surface proteins and malignant transformation. *Biochim Biophys Acta* 1976;458:73.

151. Swann DA, Hendren RB, Radin EL, et al. The lubricating activities of synovial fluid glycoproteins. *Arthritis Rheum* 1981;24:22–30.

152. Swann DA, Silver FH, Slayter HS, et al. The molecular structure and lubricating activity of lubricin isolated from bovine and human synovial fluids. *Biochem J* 1985;225:195–201.

153. Fell HB, Jubb RW. The effect of synovial tissue on the breakdown of articular cartilage in organ culture. *Arthritis Rheum* 1977;20:1359.

154. Dingle JT, Saklatvata J, Hembry R, et al. A cartilage catabolic factor from synovium. *Biochem J* 1979;184:177.

155. Von Rechenberg B, McIlwraith CW, Akins MK, et al. Spontaneous production of nitric oxide (NO), prostaglandin (PGE2) and neutral metalloproteinases (NMPs) in media of explant cultures of equine synovial membrane and articular cartilage from normal and osteoarthritic joints. *Equine Vet J* 2000;32:140–150.

156. Saklatvala J, Pilsworth LMC, Sarsfield SJ, et al. Pig catabolin is a form of interleukin-1. *Biochem J* 1984;224:461–466.

157. Stefanovic-Racic M, Stadler J, Georgescu HI, et al. Synovial production of nitric oxide and its modulation by cytokines. In: Moncada S, Marletta MA, Hibbs JB, et al., eds. *Biology of nitric oxide.* Colchester, England: Portland Press, 1992:179–182.

158. Lake RA, Morgan A, Henderson B, et al. A key role for fi-

bronectin in the sequential binding of native dsDNA and monoclonal anti-DNA antibodies to components of the extracellular matrix: its possible significance in glomerulonephritis. *Immunology* 1985;54:389.

159. Okada Y, Naka K, Minamoto T, et al. Localization of type VI collagen in the lining cell layer of normal and rheumatoid synovium. *Lab Invest* 1990;63:647–656.

160. Ashurst DE, Bland YS, Levick JR. An immuohistochemical study of the collagen of rabbit synovial instertition. *J Rheumatol* 1991;18:1669–1672.

161. Wolf J, Carson SE. Distribution of type VI collagen expression in synovial tissue and cultured synoviocytes: relation to fibronectin expression. *Ann Rheum Dis* 1991;50:493–496.

162. Eyre DR, Muir H. Type III collagen: a major constituent of rheumatoid and normal human synovial membrane. *Connect Tissue Res* 1975;4:11–16.

163. Pollock LE, Lalor O, Revell PA. Type IV collagen and laminin in the synovial intimal layer: an immunohistochemical study. *Rheumatol Int* 1990;9:277–280.

164. Linck G, Stocker S, Grimaud J-A, et al. Distribution of immunoreactive fibronectin and collagen (type I, III, IV) in mouse joints. *Histochemistry* 1983;77:323.

165. Lovell CR, Nicholls AC, Jayson MIV, et al. Changes in collagen of synovial membrane in rheumatoid arthritis and effect of D-penicillamine. *Clin Sci Mol Med* 1978;55:31.

166. Smith LT, Holbrook KA, Byers PH. Structure of the dermal matrix during development and in the adult. *J Invest Dermatol* 1982;79[Suppl 1]:93s.

167. Highton TC, Myers DB. Ruthenium red positive material at the surface of normal human synovial cells. *Proc Otago Med School* 1973;51:28.

168. Myers DB, Highton TC, Rayns DG. Acid mucopolysaccharides closely associated with collagen fibrils in normal human synovium. *J Ultrastruct Res* 1969;28:203.

169. Fife RS, Caterson B, Myers SL. Identification of link proteins in canine synovial cell cultures and canine articular cartilage. *J Cell Biol* 1985;100:1050.

170. Yielding KL, Tomkins GM, Bunim JJ. Synthesis of hyaluronic acid by human synovial tissue. *Science* 1957;125:1300.

171. Hamerman D, Ruskin J. Histologic studies on human synovial membrane: 1. Metachromatic staining and the effects of streptococcal hyaluronidase. *Arthritis Rheum* 1959;2:546.

172. Linn FC, Radin EL. Lubrication of animal joints: III. The effect of certain chemical alterations of the cartilage and lubricant. *Arthritis Rheum* 1968;11:674.

173. Wiig ME, Amiel D, Van de Berg J, et al. The early effect of high molecular weight hyaluronan (hyaluronic acid) on anterior cruciate ligament healing: an experimental study in rabbits. *J Orthop Res* 1990;8:425–434.

174. Kleinman HK, Klebe RJ, Martin GR. Role of collagenous matrices in the adhesion and growth of cells. *J Cell Biol* 1981;88:473.

175. Hynes RO. Fibronectin and its relation to cellular structure and behavior. In: Hay ED, ed. *Cell biology of extracellular matrix.* New York: Plenum Press, 1981:295.

176. Clemmenson I, Holund B, Andersen RB. Fibrin and fibronectin in rheumatoid synovial membrane and rheumatoid synovial fluid. *Arthritis Rheum* 1983;26:479.

177. Hunter W. Of the structure and diseases of articulating cartilages. *Philos Trans R Soc Lond* 1743;42:514.

178. Davies DV, Edwards DAW. The blood supply of the synovial membrane. *Ann R Coll Surg Engl* 1948;2:142–156.

179. Knight AD, Levick JR. The density and distribution of capillaries around a synovial cavity. *Q J Exp Physiol* 1983;68:629–644.

180. Levick JR, Synovial fluid and trans-synovial flow in stationary and moving normal joints. In: Helminen H, ed. *Articular cartilage and other intra-articular structures.* Wright, Potters Bar, 1987.

181. Suter ER, Majno G. Ultrastructure of the joint capsule in the rat: presence of two kinds of capillaries. *Nature* 1964;202:920.

182. Edwards JCW. Synovial structure and function. *Reports on rheumatic diseases (series 2).* UK: The Arthritis and Rheumatism Council, January 1988.

183. Davies DV. The lymphatics of the synovial membrane. *J Anat* 1946;80:21–23.

184. Samuel EP. The autonomic and somatic innervation of the articular capsule. *Anat Rec* 1952;113:53–70.

185. Gardner E. Physiology of moveable joints. *Physiol Review* 1950;30:127–176.

186. Bray RC, Fisher AW, Hennenfent BW, et al. Neurovascular anatomy of collateral knee ligaments as revealed by vascular injection and metallic impregnation techniques. *Trans Orthop Res Soc* 1990;1512:526.

187. Dee R. The innervation of joints. In: Sokoloff L, ed. *The joints and synovial fluid.* New York: Academic Press, 1978.

188. Gronblad M, Konttinen YT, Korkala O, et al. Neuropeptides in synovium of patients with rheumatoid arthritis and osteoarthritis. *J Rheumatol* 1988;15:1807.

189. Bauer W, Short CL, Bennett GA. The manner of removal of proteins from normal joints. *J Exp Med* 1933;57:419–433.

190. Ropes MW, Bauer W. *Synovial fluid changes in joint disease.* Cambridge, MA: Harvard University Press, 1953.

191. Levick JR. Synovial fluid dynamics. In: Holborrow EJ, Maroudas A, eds. *Studies in joint disease.* London: Pitman Medical, 1983.

192. Guyton AC, Scheel K, Murphree D. Interstitial fluid pressure: III. Its effect on resistance to tissue fluid mobility. *Circ Res* 1966, 19:412–420.

193. Levick JR, Synovial fluid exchange: a case of flow through fibrous mats. *New Physiol Soc* 1989;4:198–202.

194. Levick JR, Smaje LM. An analysis of the permeability of a fenestra. *Microvasc Res* 1987;33:233–256.

195. Knight AD, Levick JR. The density and distribution of capillaries around a synovial cavity. *Q J Exp Physiol* 1983;68:629–644.

196. Sliwinski AF, Zvaifler NJ. The removal of aggregated and nonaggregated autologous gamma globulin from rheumatoid joints. *Arthritis Rheum* 1979;12:504–514.

197. Brown DL, Cooper AG, Bluestone R. Exchange of IgM and albumin between plasma and synovial fluid in rheumatoid arthritis. *Ann Rheum Dis* 1979;20:644–651.

198. Wallis WJ, Simkin PA, Nelp WB. Protein traffic in human synovial effusions. *Arthritis Rheum* 1987;30:57–63.

199. Rodnan GP, MacLaughlin ML. The absorption of serum albumin and gamma globulin from the knee joint of man and rabbit. *Arthritis Rheum* 1970;3:152–157.

200. Simkin PA, Pizzoro JE. Transsynovial exchange of small molecules in normal human subjects. *J Appl Physiol* 1974;36:581.

201. Kushner I, Somerville JA. Permeability of human synovial membrane to plasma proteins. *Arthritis Rheum* 1971;14:560.

202. Nettelbladt E, Sundblad L, Jonsson E. Permeability of the synovial membrane to proteins. *Acta Rheum Scand* 1963;9:28.

203. Swann DA, Radin EL. The molecular basis of articular lubrication: I. *J Biol Chem* 1972;274:8069–8073.

204. Swann DA, Sotman S, Dixon M, et al. The isolation and partial characterization of the major glycoprotein (LGP-1) from the articular lubricating fraction from bovine synovial fluid. *Biochem J* 1977;161:473–485.

205. Swann DA, Silver FH, Slayter HS, et al. The molecular structure and lubricating activity of lubricin isolated from bovine and human synovial fluids. *Biochem J* 1985;225:195.

206. Swann DA, Radin RL. The molecular basis of articular lubrication: I. Purification and properties of a lubricating fraction from bovine synovial fluid. *J Biol Chem* 1972;247:8069.

207. Jay GD, Britt DE, Cha CH. Lubricin is a product of megakaryocyte stimulating factor gene expression by human synovial fibroblasts. *J Rheumatol* 2000;27:594–600.

208. Swann DA, Silver FH, Slayter HS, et al. The molecular struc-

ture and lubricating activity of lubricin isolated from bovine and human synovial fluids. *Biochem J* 1985;225:195–201.

209. Jay GD, Haberstroh K, Cha CH. Comparison of the boundary-lubricating ability of bovine synovial fluid, lubricin, and Healon. *J Biomed Mater Res* 1998;40:414–418.

210. Schwarz IM, Hills BA. Surface-active phospholipid as the lubricating component of lubricin. *Br J Rheumatol* 1998;37:21–26.

211. Hills BA. Boundary lubrication in vivo. *Proc Inst Mech Eng [H]* 2000;214:83–94.

212. Levick JR. Synovial fluid and trans-synovial flow in stationary and moving normal joints. In: Heliminen H, ed. *Articular cartilage and other intra-articular structures*. Wright, Potters Bar, 1987.

213. Jaffe JL, Lichtenstein L, Sutro CJ. Pigmented villonodular synovitis, bursitis and tenosynovitis. *Arch Pathol* 1984;31:731–765.

214. Dorwart RH, Genant HK, Johnston WH, et al. Pigmented villonodular synovitis of synovial joints: clinical, pathologic and radiologic features. *AJR Am J Roentgenol* 1984;143:877–885.

215. Myers BW, Masi AT, Feigenbaum SL. Pigmented villonodular synovitis and tenosynovitis: a clinical epidmiologic study of 166 cases and literature review. *Medicine (Baltimore)* 1980;59;223–238.

216. Schwartz HS, Unni KK, Pritchard DJ. Pigmented villonodular synovitis: a retrospective review of affected large joints. *Clin Orthop* 1989;247:243–255.

217. Rao AS, Vigority VJ. Pigmented villonodular synovitis (giant cell tumor of tendon sheath and synovial membrane): a review of eighty-one cases. *J Bone Joint Surg Am* 1984;66:76–94.

218. Luck JV, Kasper CK. Surgical management of advanced hemophilic arthropathy: an overview of 20 years experience. *Clin Orthop* 1989;242:60–82.

219. Mainardi CL, Levine PH, Werb Z, et al. Proliferative synovitis in hemophilia: biochemical and morphologic observations. *Arthritis Rheum* 1978;21:137–144.

220. Stein H, Duthie RB. The pathogenesis of chronic haemophilic arthropathy. *J Bone Joint Surg Br* 1981;63:601–609.

221. Rippey JJ, Hill RRH, Lurie A, et al. Articular cartilage degradation and the pathology of hemophiliac arthropathy. *S Afr Med J* 1978;54:345–351.

222. Devaney K, Vinh TN, Sweet DE. Synovial hemangioma: a report of 20 cases with differential diagnostic considerations. *Hum Pathol* 1993;24:737–745.

223. Villacin AB, Brigham LN, Bullough PG. Primary and secondary synovial chondrometaplasia: histopathologic and clinicoradiologic differences. *Hum Pathol* 1979;10:439–451.

224. Apte SS, Athanasou NA. An immunohistological study of cartilage and synovium in primary synovial synovial chondromatosis. *J Pathol* 1992;166:277–281.

225. Leu J, Matsubara T, Hirohata K. Ultrastructural morphology of early cellular changes in the synovium of primary synovial chondromatosis. *Clin Orthop* 1992;272:299–306.

226. Sim FH, Dahlin DC, Ivins JC. Extra-articular synovial chondromatosis. *J Bone Joint Surg Am* 1977;59:492–495.

227. Sviland L, Malcolm AJ. Synovial chondromatosis presenting as painless soft tissue mass: a report of 19 cases. *Histopathology* 1995;27:275–279.

228. Milgram JW. The classification of loose bodies in human joints. *Clin Orthop* 1977;24:282–291.

229. Milgram JW. The development of loose bodies in human joints. *Clin Orthop* 1977;24:292–303.

230. Fox IH. Crystal induced synovitis. In: Kelley WN, ed. *Textbook of internal medicine*, 3rd ed. Philadelpia: Lippincott-Raven, 1996:1130–1136.

231. Schumacher HR. Pathology of crystal deposition diseases. *Rheum Dis Clin North Am* 1988;14:269–288.

232. Schumacher HR. Pathology of the synovial membrane in gout:

233. Ishikawa K, Masuda I, Ohira T, et al. A histological study of calcium pyrophosphate dihydrate crystal-deposition disease. *J Bone Joint Surg Am* 1989;71:875–886.

234. Keen CE, Crocker PR, Brady K, et al. Calcium pyrophosphate dihydrate deposition disease: morphological and microanalytical features. *Histopathology* 1991;19:529–536.

235. Gravanis MG, Gaffney EF. Idiopathic calcifying tenosynovitis: histopathologic features and possible pathogenesis. *Am J Surg Pathol* 1983;7:357–361.

236. Uhtoff HK. Calcifying tendonitis, an active cell mediated calcification. *Virchows Arch A Pathol Anat Histol* 1975;366:51–58.

237. Uhtoff HK, Sarkar K, Maynard JA. Calcifying tendonitis: a new concept of its pathogenesis. *Clin Orthop* 1976;118:164–168.

238. Halverson PB, Garancis JC, McCarty DJ. Histopathological and ultrastructural studies of synovium in Milwaukee shoulder syndrome: a basic calcium phosphate crystal arthropathy. *Ann Rheum Dis* 1984;43:734–742.

239. Dieppe PA, Huskisson EC, Crocker P, et al. Apatite deposition disease: a new arthropathy. *Lancet* 1976;1:266–269.

240. Hamerman D: The biology of osteoarthritis. *N Engl J Med* 1989;320:1322.

241. Revell PA, Mayson V, Lalor P, et al. The synovial membrane in osteoarthritis: a histological study including the characterization of the cellular infiltrate present in inflammatory osteoarthritis using monoclonal antibodies. *Ann Rheum Dis* 1988;47:300.

242. Soren A, Cooper NS, Waugh TR. The nature and designation of osteoarthritis determined by its histopathology. *Clin Exp Rheum* 1988;6:41.

243. Chang RW, Falconer J, Stulberg SD, et al. A randomized, controlled trial of arthroscopic surgery versus closed-needle joint lavage for patients with osteoarthritis of the knee. *Arthritis Rheum* 1993;36:289–296.

244. Evans CH, Mazzocchi RA, Nelson DD, et al. Experimental arthritis induced by the intra-articular injection of allogenic cartilaginous particles into rabbit knees. *Arthritis Rheum* 1984;27:200.

245. Evans CH, Mears DC, McKnight JL. A preliminary ferrographic survey of the wear particles in human synovial fluid. *Arthritis Rheum* 1981;24:912.

246. Evans CH, Mears DC, Stanitski CL. Ferrographic analysis of wear in human joints: evaluation by comparison with arthroscopic examination of symptomatic knee joints. *J Bone Joint Surg Br* 1982;64:572.

247. Koch AE. Angiogenesis: implications for rheumatoid arthritis [Review]. *Arthritis Rheum* 1998;41:951–962.

248. Walsh DA. Angiogenesis and arthritis. *Rheumatol* 1999;38:103–112.

249. Tak PP. Examination of the synovium and synovial fluid. In: Firestein GS, Panayi GS, Panayi GS, et al., eds. *Rheumatoid arthritis: frontiers in pathogenesis and treatment*. New York: Oxford University Press, 2000:55–68.

250. Tak PP, Firestein GS. Apoptosis in rheumatoid arthritis. In: Winkler JD, ed. Apoptosis and inflammation. Basel: Birkhauser, 1999:149–162.

251. Klimiuk PA, Goronzy JJ, Bjornsson J, et al. Tissue cytokine patterns distinguish variants of rheumatoid synovitis. *Am J Pathol* 1997;151:1311–1319.

252. Goldring SR, Gravallese EM. Pathogenesis of bone erosions in rheumatoid arthritis. *Curr Opin Rheumatol* 2000;12:195–199.

253. Tak PP, Bresnihan B. The pathogenesis and prevention of

joint damage in rheumatoid arthritis. *Arthritis Rheum* 2000;42: 2619–2633.

Ligament References

254. Andriacchi TP, Mikosz RP, Hampton SJ, et al. Model studies of the stiffness characteristics of the human knee joint. *J Biomech* 1983;16:23–29.

255. Blacharski PA, Somerset JH, Murray DG. A three-dimensional study of the kinematics of the human knee. *J Biomech* 1975;8:375–384.

256. Butler DL, Noyes FR, Grood ES. Ligamentous restraints to anterior-posterior drawer in the human knee. *J Bone Joint Surg Am* 1980;62:259–270.

257. Grood ES, Noyes FR, Butler DL. Ligamentous and capsular restraints preventing straight medial and lateral laxity in intact human cadaver knees. *J Bone Joint Surg Am* 1981;63:1257–1269.

258. Markolf KL, Mensch JS, Amstutz HC. Stiffness and laxity of the knee: the contributions of the supporting structures. *J Bone Joint Surg Am* 1976;58:583–594.

259. Woo SL-Y, Gomez MA, Woo YK, et al. Mechanical properties of tendons and ligaments. *Biorheology* 1982;19:385–396.

260. Brand RA. Knee ligaments: a new view. *J Biomech Eng* 1986; 108:106–110.

261. Akeson WH, Frank C, Amiel D, et al. Ligament biology and biomechanics. In: Funk FJ, Hunter LY, eds. *AAOS symposium on sports medicine: the knee.* St. Louis: CV Mosby, 1985: 93–148.

262. Butler DL, Grood ES, Noyes FR, et al. Biomechanics of ligaments and tendons. In: Hutton RS, ed. *Exercise and sports sciences reviews.* Washington, DC: Franklin Institute Press, 1978:125–181.

263. Frank C, Amiel D, Woo SL-Y, et al. Normal ligament properties and ligament healing. *Clin Orthop* 1985;196:15–25.

264. Amiel D, Frank C, Harwood F, et al. Tendons and ligaments: a morphological and biochemical comparison. *J Orthop Res* 1984;1:257–265.

265. Arnoczky SP. Anatomy of the anterior cruciate ligament. *Clin Orthop* 1983;172:19–25.

266. Kennedy JC, Weinberg HW, Wilson AS. The anatomy and function of the anterior cruciate ligament. *J Bone Joint Surg Am* 1974;56:223–225.

267. Furman W, Marshall JL, Girgis FG. The anterior cruciate ligament: a functional analysis based on postmortem studies. *J Bone Joint Surg Am* 1976;58:179–185.

268. Warren RF, Marshall JL. The supporting structures and layers of the medial side of the knee: an anatomical analysis. *J Bone Joint Surg Am* 1979;61:56–62.

269. Jackson RW. Anterior cruciate ligament injuries. In: Casscells SW, ed. *Arthroscopy: diagnostic and surgical practice,* Philadelphia: Lea and Febiger, 1984:52–63.

270. Woo SL-Y, Hollis JM, Roux RD, et al. Effects of knee flexion on the structural properties of the rabbit femur–anterior cruciate ligament–tibia complex (FATC). *J Biomech* 1987;20:447–453.

271. Scapinelli R. Studies on the vasculature of the human knee joint. *Acta Anatomica* 1968;70:305–331.

272. Chowdhury P, Matyas JR, Frank CB. The "epiligament" of the rabbit medial collateral ligament: a quantitative morphological study. *Connect Tissue Res* 1991;27:33–50.

273. Diamant J, Keller A, Baer E, et al. Collagen: ultrastructure and its relation to mechanical properties as a function of ageing. *Proc R Soc Lond B Biol Sci* 1972;180:293–315.

274. Kastelic J, Palley I, Baer E. A structural mechanical model for tendon crimping. *J Biomech* 1980;13:887–893.

275. Stouffer DC, Butler DL, Hosney D. The relationship between crimp pattern and mechanical response of human patellar tendon-bone units. *J Biomech Eng* 1985;107:158–165.

276. Butler DL, Grood ES, Noyes FR, et al. Effects of structure and strain measurement technique on the materials properties of young human tendons and fascia. *J Biomech* 1984;17:579–596.

277. Lo IKY, Randle JR, Ou Y, et al. Ligament cells are organized in a 3-dimensional network that is disrupted during healing. *Trans Orthop Res Soc* 2001;26:701.

278. Evans WH. Intercellular communication: the roles and structure of gap junctions. In: Bittar EE, Bittar N, eds. *Principles of medical biology: vol 7B. Membranes and cell signalling.* New York: Jai Press, 1997:609–628.

279. Cooper RR, Misol S. Tendon and ligament insertion: a light and electron microscopic study. *J Bone Joint Surg Am* 1970;52: 1–21.

280. Matyas J, Bodie D, Andersen M, et al. The developmental morphology of a periosteal ligament insertion: growth and maturation of the tibial insertion of the rabbit medial collateral ligament. *J Orthop Res* 1990;8:412–424.

281. Matyas J. *Tendon and ligament insertions* [Master's dissertation]. Ithaca, NY: Cornell University, 1985.

282. Hurov JR. Soft tissue bone interface: how do attachments of muscles, tendons and ligaments change during growth. A light microscopic study. *J Morphol* 1986;189:313–325.

283. Chaudhuri S. *Digital image processing techniques for quantitative analysis of collagen fibrial alignment in ligaments* [Master's dissertation]. Calgary, Alberta, Canada; University of Calgary, 1987.

284. Chaudhuri S, Nguyen H, Rangayyan R, et al. A Fourier domain directional filtering method for analysis of collagen alignment in ligaments. *IEEE Trans Biomech Eng* 1987;34:509–518.

285. Frank C, MacFarlane B, Edwards P, et al. A quantitative analysis of matrix alignment in ligament scars: a comparison of movement versus immobilization in an immature rabbit model. *J Orthop Res* 1991;9:219–927.

286. Frank CB, Bray DF, Rademaker A, et al. Electron microscopic quantification of collagen fibril diameters in the rabbit medial collateral ligament: a baseline for comparison. *Connect Tissue Res* 1989;19:11–25.

287. Frank CB, McDonald D, Bray DF, et al. Collagen fibril diameters in the healing adult rabbit medial collateral ligament. *Connect Tissue Res* 1992;27:251–263.

288. Frank CB, McDonald D, Shrive NG. Collagen fibril diameters in the rabbit medial collateral ligament scar: a longer-term assessment. *Connect Tissue Res* 1997;36:261–263.

289. Parry DAD, Craig AS, Barnes GRG. Tendon and ligament from the horse: an ultrastructural study of collagen fibrils and elastic fibers as a function of age. *Proc R Soc Lond B Biol Sci* 1978;203:293–303.

290. Parry DAD, Barnes GRG, Craig AS. A comparison of the size distribution of collagen fibril size distribution and mechanical properties. *Proc R Soc Lond B Biol Soc* 1978;203:305–321.

291. Scott JE, Orford CR. Dermatan sulphate-rich proteoglycan associates with rat-tail tendon collagen at the D-band in the gap region. *Biochem J* 1981;197:213–216.

292. Bray DF, Frank CB, Bray RC. Cytochemical evidence for a proteoglycan-associated filamentous network in ligament extracellular matrix. *J Orthop Res* 1990;8:1–12.

293. Bray DF, Bray RC, Frank CB. Ultrastructural immunolocalization of type-VI collagen and chondroitin sulphate in ligament. *J Orthop Res* 1993;11:677–685.

294. Girgis FG, Marshall JL, Al Monajem ARS. The cruciate ligaments of the knee joint: anatomical and experimental analysis. *Clin Orthop* 1975;106:216–231.

295. Andrish J, Holmes R. Effects of synovial fluid on fibroblasts in tissue culture. *Clin Orthop* 1979:138;279–283.

296. Amiel D, Billings E Jr, Harwood FL. Collagenase activity in the anterior cruciate ligament: protective role of the synovial sheath. *J Appl Physiol* 1990;69:902–906.

297. Odensten M, Gillquist J. Functional anatomy of the anterior cruciate ligament and a rationale for reconstruction. *J Bone Joint Surg Am* 1985;67:259–261.

298. Clark JM, Sidles JA. The interrelation of fiber bundles in the anterior cruciate ligament. *J Orthop Res* 1988;8:180–188.

299. Danylchuk KD, Finlay JB, Krcek JP. Microstructural organization of human and bovine cruciate ligament. *Clin Orthop* 1978;131;294–298.

300. Fuss FK. Anatomy of the cruciate ligaments and their function in extension and flexion of the human knee joint. *Am J Anat* 1989;184:165–176.

301. Harner CD, Baek GH, Vogrin TM, et al. Quantitative analysis of human cruciate ligament insertions. *Arthroscopy* 1999;15:741–749.

302. Lyon RM, Akeson WH, Amiel D, et al. Ultrastructural differences between the cells of the medial collateral and anterior cruciate ligaments. *Clin Orthop* 1991;272:279–286.

303. Amiel D, Kuiper SD, Wallace CD, et al. Age-related properties of medial collateral ligament and anterior cruciate ligament: a morphologic and collagen maturation study in the rabbit. *J Gerontol B Psychol Sci Soc Sci* 1991;46:159–165.

304. Nagineni CN, Amiel D, Green MH, et al. Characterization of the intrinsic properties of the anterior cruciate and medial collateral ligament cells: an in vitro cell culture study. *J Orthop Res* 1992;10:465–475.

305. Yoshida M, Fujii K. Differences in cellular properties and responses to growth factors between human ACL and MCL cells. *J Orthop Sci* 1999;4:293–298.

306. Hung CT, Allen FD, Pollack SR, et al. Intracellular calcium response of ACL and MCL ligament fibroblasts to fluid-induced shear stress. *Cell Signal* 1997;9:587–594.

307. Scherping SC Jr, Schmidt CC, Georgescu HI, et al. Effect of growth factors on the proliferation of ligament fibroblasts from skeletally mature rabbits. *Connect Tissue Res* 1997;36:1–8.

308. Sung KL, Yang L, Whittemore DE, et al. The differential adhesion forces of anterior cruciate and medial collateral ligament fibroblasts: effects of tropomodulin, talin, vinculin and alpha-actinin. *Proc Natl Acad Sci U S A* 1996;93:9182–9187.

309. Amiel D, Nagineni CN, Choi SH, et al. Intrinsic properties of ACL and MCL cells and their responses to growth factors. *Med Sci Sports Exerc* 1995;27:844–851.

310. Sung KL, Kwan MK, Maldonado F, et al. Adhesion strength of human ligament fibroblasts. *J Biomech Eng* 1994;116:237–242.

311. Geiger MH, Green MH, Monosov A, et al. An in vitro assay of anterior cruciate ligament (ACL) and medial collateral ligament (MCL) cell migration. *Connect Tissue Res.* 1994;30:215–224.

312. Murphy PG, Hart DA. Plasminogen activators and plasminogen activator inhibitors in connective tissues and connect tissue cells: influence of the neuropeptide substance P on expression. *Biochim Biophys Acta* 1993;1182:205–214.

313. Murphy PG, Frank CB, Hart DA. Characterization of the plasminogen activators and plasminogen activator inhibitors expressed by cells isolated from rabbit ligament and synovial tissues: evidence for unique cell populations. *Exp Cell Res* 1993;205:16–24.

314. Baek GH, Carlin GJ, Vogrin TM, et al. Quantitative analysis of collagen fibrils of human cruciate and meniscofemoral ligaments. *Clin Orthop* 1998;357:205–211.

315. Neurath M, Stofft E. Fascicular and sub-fascicular architecture of the cruciate ligament. *Unfallchirurg* 1992;18:125–132.

316. Oakes BW. Collagen ultrastructure in the normal ACL and ACL graft. In: Jackson DW, ed. *The anterior cruciate ligament: current and future concepts.* New York: Raven Press, 1993: 209–217.

317. Gray DJ, Gardner E. Prenatal development of the knee joint. *Am J Anat* 1950;86:235–287.

318. Ellison AE, Berg EE. Embryology, anatomy, function of the anterior cruciate ligament. *Orthop Clin North Am* 1985;16:3–14.

319. Marshall JL, Warren RF, Wickiewicz TL. The anterior cruciate ligament: a technique of repair and reconstruction. *Clin Orthop* 1979;143:97–106.

320. Arnoczky SP, Rubin RM, Marshall JL. Microvasculature of the cruciate ligaments and its response to injury: an experimental study in dogs. *J Bone Joint Surg Am* 1979;61:1221–1229.

321. Schultz RA, Miller DC, Kerr CS, et al. Mechanoreceptors in human cruciate ligaments: a histological study. *J Bone Joint Surg Am* 1984;66:1072–1076.

322. Schutte MJ, Dabezies EJ, Zimny ML, et al. Neural anatomy of the human anterior cruciate ligament. *J Bone Joint Surg Am* 1987;69:243–247.

323. Kennedy JC, Alexander IJ, Hayes KC. Nerve supply of the human knee and its functional importance. *Am J Sports Med* 1982;10:329–335.

324. Harner CD, Xerogeanes JW, Livesay GA, et el. The human posterior cruciate ligament complex: an interdisciplinary study. Ligament morphology and biomechanical evaluation. *Am J Sports Med* 1995;23:736–745.

325. Race A, Amis AA. The mechanical properties of the two bundles of the human posterior cruciate ligament. *J Biomech* 1994;27:13–24.

326. Barton TM, Torg JS, Das M. Posterior cruciate ligament insufficiency: a review of the literature. *Sports Med* 1984;1:419–430.

327. Hughston JC, Bowden JA, Andrews JR, et al. Acute tears of the posterior cruciate ligament: results of operative treatment. *J Bone Joint Surg Am* 1980;62:438–450.

328. Covey DC, Sapega AA, Sherman GM. Testing for 'isometry' during posterior cruciate ligament reconstruction: anatomic and biomechanical considerations. *Am J Sports Med* 1996;24:740–746.

329. Kannus P, Bergfeld J, Jarvinen M, et al. Injuries to the posterior cruciate ligament of the knee. *Sports Med* 1991;12:110–131.

330. Kurosawa H, Yamakoshi K-I, Yasuda K, et al. Simultaneous measurement of changes in length of the cruciate ligaments during knee motion. *Clin Orthop* 1991;265:233–240.

331. Fuss FK. The restraining function of the cruicate ligaments on hyperextension and hyperflexion of the human knee joint. *Anat Rec* 1991;230:283–289.

332. Harner CD, Zerogeanes JW, Livesay GA, et al. The human posterior cruciate ligament complex: an interdisciplinary study. Ligament morphology and biomechanical evaluation. *Am J Sport Med* 1995;23:736–745.

333. Girgis FG, Marshall JL, Monjem A. The cruciate ligaments of the knee joint: anatomical, functional and experimental analysis. *Clin Orthop* 1975;106:216–231.

334. Brantigan OC, Voshell AF. The mechanics of the ligaments and menisci of the knee joint. *J Bone Joint Surg* 1941;23:44–66.

335. Johnson CJ, Back BR. Current concepts review: posterior cruciate ligament. *Am J Knee Surg* 1990;3:143–153.

336. Van Dommelen BA, Fowler PJ. Anatomy of the posterior cruciate ligament: a review. *Am J Sports Med* 1989;17:24–29.

337. Heller L, Langman J. The menisco-femoral ligaments of the human knee. *J Bone Joint Surg* 1964;46:307–313.

338. Kusayama T, Harner CD. Anatomical and biomechanical characteristics of the human meniscofemoral ligaments. *Knee Surg Sports Traumatol Arthrosc* 1994;2:234–237.

339. Cooper DE, Warren RF, Warner JJP. The posterior cruciate ligament and posterolateral structures of the knee: anatomy, function and patterns of injury. *Instr Course Lect* 1991;40:249–270.

340. Harner CD: Insertion site anatomy of the human ACL and PCL. *Trans Orthop Res Soc* 1993;18:340.

341. Harner CD, Livesay GA, Kashiwaguchi S, et al. Comparative study of the size and shape of human anterior and posterior cruciate ligaments. *J Orthop Res* 1995;13:429–434.

342. Covey DC, Sapega AA. Anatomy and function of the posterior cruciate ligament. *Clin Sports Med* 1994;13:509–518.

343. Neurath M, Stofft E. Faszikulare und subfazikulare Architektur der Ligamenta cruciatea. *Unfallchirurg* 1992;18:125–132.

344. Amiel D, Billings E Jr, Akeson WH. Ligament structure, chemistry, and physiology. In: Daniel DM, Akeson WH, O'Connor JJ, eds. Knee ligaments: structure, function, injury and repair. New York: Raven Press, 1990:77–91.

345. Vladimirow B. Arterial sources of blood supply of the knee joint in man. *Acta Med* 1968;47:1–10.

346. Scapinelli R. Studies on the vasculature of the human knee joint. *Acta Anat* 1968;70:305–331.

347. Arnoczky SP. Blood supply to the anterior cruciate ligament and supporting structures. *Orthop Clin North Am* 1985;16:15–28.

348. Katonis PG, Assimakopoulos AP, Agapitos MV, et al. Mechanoreceptors in the posterior cruciate ligament: histologic study on cadaver knees. *Acta Orthop Scand* 1991;62:276–278.

349. Johansson H, Sjolander P, Sojka P. A sensory role for the cruciate ligaments. *Clin Orthop* 1991;268:161–178.

350. Kastelic J, Galeski A, Baer E. The multicomposite structure of tendon. *Connect Tissue Res* 1978;6:11–23.

351. Woo SL-Y, Orlando CA, Frank CB, et al. Tensile properties of medial collateral ligament as a function of age. *J Orthop Res* 1986;4:133–141.

352. Lam TC. *The mechanical properties of the maturing medial collateral ligament* [Doctoral thesis]. Calgary, Alberta, Canada: University of Calgary, 1988.

353. Bray RC, Shrive NG, Frank CB, et al. The early effects of joint immobilization of medial collateral ligament healing in an ACL-deficient knee: a gross anatomic and biomechanical investigation in the adult rabbit model. *J Orthop Res* 1992; 10:157–166.

354. Chimich D, Frank C, Shrive N, et al. The effects of initial end contact on medial collateral ligament healing: a morphological and biomechanical study in a rabbit model. *J Orthop Res* 1991;9:37–47.

355. Frank C, Woo SL, Amiel D, et al. Medial collateral ligament healing: a multidisciplinary assessment in rabbits. *Am J Sports Med* 1983;11:379–389.

356. Akeson WH, Frank CB, Amiel D, et al. Ligament biology and biomechanics. In: Finerman G, ed. *Symposium on sports medicine: the knee.* 1985:111–151.

357. Woo SLY, Chan SS, Yamaji T. Biomechanics of knee ligament healing, repair and reconstruction. *J Biomech* 1997;30:431–439.

358. Woo SLY, Debski RE, Withrow JD, et al. Biomechanics of knee ligaments. *Am J Sports Med* 1999;27:533–543.

359. Daniel DM, Akeson WH, O'Connor JJ. In: Daniel DM, Akeson WH, O'Connor JJ, eds. *Knee ligaments: structure, function, injury and repair.* New York: Raven Press, 1990.

360. Holden JP, Grood ES Korvick DL, et al. In vivo forces in the anterior cruciate ligament: direct measurements during walking and trotting in a quadruped. *J Biomech* 1994;27:517–526.

361. Butler DL, Malaviya P, Awad H, et al. A multidisciplinary approach to analyzing tendon fibrocartilage mechanics, structure and chemistry. *Abstracts of the Third World Congress of Biomechanics,* 1998:213.

362. Yamamoto N, Takauchi M. In vivo measurement of patellar tendon force in rat during running on a treadmill. *Abstracts of the Third World Congress of Biomechanics,* 1998:461.

363. Thornton GM, Oliynyk A, Frank CB, et al. Ligament creep cannot be predicted from stress relaxation at low stress: a biomechanical study of the rabbit medial collateral ligament. *J Orthop Res* 1997;15:652–656.

364. Thornton GM, Frank CB, Shrive NG. The effect of fibre recruitment during creep of ligaments. In: Middleton J, Jones ML, Shrive NG, et al., eds. *Computer methods in biomechanics and biomedical engineering* 2000 *(in press).*

365. Thornton GM, Frank CB, Shrive NG. Ligament creep behavior can be predicted from stress relaxation by incorporating fiber recruitement. *J Rheol* 2001;45:493–507.

366. Thornton GM, Frank CB, Shrive NG. Creep mechanics of normal and healing ligaments. *Applied Mechanics of the Americas* 1999;6:45–48.

367. Thornton GM, Leask GP, Shrive NG, et al. Early medial collateral ligament scars have inferior creep behaviour. *J Orthop Res* 2000;18:238–246.

368. Thornton GM, Shrive NG, Frank CB. Altering ligament water content affects ligament pre-stress and creep behaviour. *J Orthop Res* 2001;19:845–851.

369. Thornton GM, Frank CB, Shrive NG. Ligament creep recruits fibres at low stresses and can lead to modulus-reducing fibre damage at higher creep. *J Orthop Res* 2000 *(submitted).*

370. Thornton GM, Frank CB, Shrive NG. Medial collateral ligament autografts have increased creep response for at least two years and early immobilization makes this worse. *J Orthop Res* 2000 *(submitted).*

371. Boorman RS, Shrive NG, Frank CB. Immobilization increases the vulnerability of rabbit medial collateral ligament autografts to creep. *J Orthop Res* 1998;16:682–689.

372. Skinner HB, Wyatt MP, Stone ML, et al. Exercise-related knee joint laxity. *Am J Sports Med* 1986;14:3–34.

373. Burgess PR, Yu WJ, Clark F, et al. Signaling of kinaesthetic information by peripheral sensory receptors. *Annu Rev Neurosci.* 1982;5:171–187.

374. Lephart SM, Fu FH. *Proprioception and neuromuscular control in joint stability.* Champaign, IL: Human Kinetics, 2000.

375. Lephart SM, Fu FH. The role of proprioception in the treatment of sports injuries. *Sports Exerc Inj.* 1995;1:96–102.

376. Lephart SM, Henry TH. Functional rehabilitation for the upper and lower extremity. *Orthop Clin North Am* 1995;26:579–592.

377. Lephart SM, Henry TJ. The physiological basis for open and closed kinetic chain rehabilitation for the upper extremity. *J Sports Rehab* 1992;1:188–196.

378. McCloskey DI. Kinesthetic sensibility. *Physiol Rev* 1978;58:763–820.

379. Skinner HB, Barrack RL. In: Daniel D. *Knee ligaments: structure, function, injury and repair.* New York: Raven Press, 1990:95–114.

380. Solomonow M, D'Ambrosia R. *The knee,* vol 1. New York: Mosby–Year Book, 1994.

381. Tyldesley B, Griences JI. *Muscle, nerves and movement: kinesi-*

ology in daily living. Cambridge, MA: Blackwell Scientific, 1989.

382. Kennedy JC, Alesander IJ, Hayes KC. Nerve supply of the human knee and its functional importance. *Am J Sports Med* 1982;10:329–335.

383. Zimmy ML, Wink CS. Neuroreceptors in the tissues of the knee joint. *J Electromyogr Kinesiol* 1991;1:148–157.

384. Solomonow M, Baratta R, Zhou BH, et al. The synergistic action of the anterior cruciate ligament and thigh muscle in maintaining joint stability. *Am J Sports Med* 1987;15:207–212.

385. Marshall KW, Tatton WG. Joint receptors modulate short and long latency muscle responses in the awake cat. *Exp Brain Res* 1983;1:137–150.

386. Beard DJ, Kyberd PJ, Fergusson CM, et al. Proprioception after rupture of the anterior cruciate ligament. *J Bone Joint Surg Br* 1993;75:311–315.

387. Baratta R, Solomonow M, Zhou BH, et al. Muscular coactivation: the role of the antagonist musculature in maintaining knee stability. *Am J Sports Med* 1988;16:113–122.

388. Pitman MI, Mainzadeh N, Menche D, et al. The intraoperative evaluation of the neurosensory function of the anterior cruciate ligament in humans using somatosensory evoked potentials. *Arthroscopy* 1992;8:442–447.

389. Sjolander P. *A sensory role for the cruciate ligaments* [Dissertation]. Umea, Sweden: Wmea University, 1989.

390. Palmer I. Pathophysiology of the medial ligament of the knee joint. *Acta Chiropractica Scandinavia* 1958;115:312–318.

391. Jennings AB, Seedhom BB. Proprioception in the knee and reflex hamstring contraction latency. *J Bone Joint Surg Br* 1994;76:491–494.

392. Lephart SM, Pincivero DM, Giraldo JL, et al. The role of proprioception in the management and rehabilitation of athletic injuries. *Am J Sports Med* 1997;25:130–137.

393. Butler DL. Anterior cruciate ligament: its normal response and replacement. *J Orthop Res* 1989;7:910–921.

394. Smith BA, Livesay GA, Woo SLY. Biology and biomechanics of the anterior cruciate ligament. *Clin Sports Med* 1993;12:637–670.

395. Blankevoort L, Huiskes R, de Lange A. Recruitment of knee joint ligaments. *J Biomech Eng* 1991;113:94–103.

396. Dodds JA, Arnoczky SP. Anatomy of the anterior cruciate ligament: a blueprint for repair and reconstruction. *Arthroscopy* 1994;10:132–139.

397. Fuss FK. The restraining function of the cruciate ligaments on hyperextension and hyperflexion of the human knee joint. *Anat Rec* 1991;230:283–289.

398. Hollis JM, Woo SLY. The estimation of anterior cruciate ligament loads in situ: indirect methods. In: Jackson DW, Arnoczky SP, Woo SLY, et al., eds. *The anterior cruciate ligament: current and future concepts.* New York: Raven Press, 1993:85–93.

399. Xerogeanes JW, Takeda Y, Livesay GA, et al. Effect of knee flexion on the in situ force distribution in the human anterior cruciate ligament. *Knee Surg Sports Traumat Arthrosc* 1995;3:9–13.

400. O'Connor JJ, Zavatsky A. Anterior cruciate ligament function in the normal knee. In: Jackson DW, Arnoczky SP, Woo SLY, et al., eds. *The anterior cruciate ligament: current and future concepts.* New York: Raven Press, 1993:39–52.

401. Butler DL, Noyes FR, Grood ES. Ligamentous restraints to anterior-posterior drawer in the human knee. *J Bone Joint Surg Am* 1980;62:259–270.

402. Grood ES, Suntay WJ, Noyes FR, et al. Biomechanics of the knee-extension exercise: effect of cutting the ACL. *J Bone Joint Surg Am* 1984;66:725–734.

403. Fukibayashi T, Torzilli PA, Sherman MF, et al. Medial restraints to anterior-posterior motion of the knee. *J Bone Joint Surg Am* 1982;64:258–264.

404. Ahmed AM, Burke DL, Duncan NA, et al. Ligament tension pattern in the flexed knee in combined passive anterior translation and axial rotation. *J Orthop Res* 1992;10:854–867.

405. Hefzy MS, Grood ES. Knee motions and their relations to the function of the anterior cruciate ligament. In: Jackson DWS, Arnoczky SP, Woo SLY, et al., eds. *The anterior cruciate ligament: current and future concepts.* New York: Raven Press, 1993;141–151.

406. Markolf KL, Wascher DC, Finerman GAM. Direct in vitro measurement of forces in the cruciate ligaments: part II. The effect of section of the posterolateral structures. *J Bone Joint Surg Am* 1993;75:387–394.

407. Butler DL, Guan Y, Kay MD, et al. Location-dependent variations in the material properties of the anterior cruciate ligament. *J Biomech* 1992;25:511–518.

408. Shapiro MS, Markolf KL, Finerman GA, et al. The effect of section of the MCL on force generated in the ACL. *J Bone Joint Surg Am* 1991;73:248–256.

409. Sullivan D, Levy IM, Shesker S, et al. Medial restraints to anterior-posterior motion of the knee. *J Bone Joint Surg Am* 1984;66:930–936.

410. Kanamori A, Sakane M, Zeminski J, et al. In-situ force in the medial and lateral structures of intact and ACL-deficient knees. *J Orthop Sci* 2000;5:567–571.

411. Sakane M, Livesay GA, Fox RJ, et al. Relative contribution of the ACL, MCL and bony contact to the anterior stability of the knee. *Knee Surg Sports Traumatol Arthrosc* 1999;7:93–97.

412. More RC, Karras BT, Neiman R, et al. Hamstrings: an anterior cruciate ligament protagonist. An in vitro study. *Am J Sports Med* 1993;21:231–237.

413. Li G, Rudy TW, Sakane M, et al. The importance of quadriceps and hamstring muscle loading on knee kinematics and in-situ forces in the ACL. *J Biomech* 1999;32:395–400.

414. Allen CR, Wong EK, Livesay GA, et al. Importance of the medial meniscus in the anterior cruciate ligament-deficient knee. *J Orthop Res* 2000;18:109–115.

415. Shoemaker SC, Markolf KL. The role of the meniscus in the anterior-posterior stability of the loaded anterior cruciate-deficient knee: effects of partial versus total excision. *J Bone Joint Surg Am* 1986;68:71–79.

416. Beynnon BD, Fleming BC, Pope MH, et al. The measurement of anterior cruciate ligament strain in vivo. In: Jackson DW, Arnoczky SP, Woo SLY, et al., eds. *The anterior cruciate ligament: current and future concepts.* New York: Raven Press, 1993:101–111.

417. Lewis JL, Lew WD, Markolf K. The measurement of anterior cruciate ligament loads: direct methods. In: Jackson DW, Arnoczky SP, Woo SLY, et al., eds. *The anterior cruciate ligament: current and future concepts.* New York: Raven Press, 1993:95–100.

418. O'Connor JJ, Zavatsky A. Anterior cruciate ligament forces in activity. In: Jackson DW, Arnoczky SP, Woo SLY, et al., eds. *The anterior cruciate ligament: current and future concepts.* New York: Raven Press, 1993:131–140.

419. Beynnon BD, Fleming BC, Johnson RJ, et al. Anterior cruciate ligament strain behavior during rehabilitation exercises in vivo. *Am J Sports Med* 1995;23:24–34.

420. Butler DL, Grood ES, Noyes FR, et al. An interpretation of our data. *Clin Orthop* 1985;196:26–34.

421. Kasperczyk WJ, Rosocha S, Bosch U, et al. Age, activity and loading capacity of knee ligaments. *Unfallchirurg* 1991;94:372–375.

422. Woo SLY, Blomstrom GL. The tensile properties of the anterior cruciate ligament as a function of age. In: Jackson DW, Arnoczky SP, Woo SLY, et al., eds. *The anterior cruciate ligament: current and future concepts.* New York: Raven Press, 1993:53–61.

423. Beynnon BD, Johnson RJ, Fleming BC. The mechanics of anterior cruciate ligament reconstruction. In: Jackson DW, Arnoczky SP, Woo SLY, et al., eds. *The anterior cruciate ligament: current and future concepts.* New York: Raven Press, 1993:259–272.

424. Beynnon B, Howe JG, Pope MH, et al. The measurement of anterior cruciate ligament strain in vivo. *Int Orthop* 1992; 16:1–12.

425. Piziali RL, Rastegar J, Nagel DA, et al. The contribution of the cruciate ligaments to the load-displacement characteristics of the human knee joint. *J Biomech Eng* 1980;102:277–283.

426. Haut RC. The mechanical and viscoelastic properties of the anterior cruciate ligament and of ACL fascicles. In: Jackson DW, Arnoczky SP, Woo SLY, et al., eds. *The anterior cruciate ligament: current and future concepts.* New York: Raven Press, 1993:63–73.

427. King GJW, Edwards P, Brant RF, et al. Intraoperative graft tensioning alters viscoelastic but not failure behaviors of rabbit medial collateral ligament autografts. *J Orthop Res* 1995;13: 915–922.

428. Kwan MK, Lin TH, Woo SLY. On the viscoelastic properties of the anteromedial bundle of the anterior cruciate ligament. *J Biomech* 1993;26:447–452.

429. Ng GY, Oakes BW, McLean ID, et al. The long-term biomechanical and viscoelastic performance of repairing anterior cruciate ligament after hemitransection injury in a goat model. *Am J Sports Med* 1996;24:109–117.

430. Barrack RL, Skinner HB, Buckley SL. Proprioception in the anterior cruciate deficient knee. *Am J Sports Med* 1989;17:1–6.

431. Beard DJ, Kyberd PJ, O'Connor JJ, et al. Reflex hamstring contraction latency in anterior cruciate ligament deficiency. *J Orthop Res* 1994;12:219–228.

432. Solomonow M, Baratta R, Zhou BH, et al. The synergistic action of the anterior cruciate ligament and thigh muscles in maintaining joint stability. *Am J Sports Med* 1987;15:207.

433. Lephart SM, Kocher MS, Fu FH, et al. Proprioception following ACL reconstruction. *J Sport Rehab* 1992;1:186–196.

434. Bradley J, Fitzpatrick D, Daniel D, et al. Orientation of the cruciate ligament in the saggital plane: a method of predicting its length change with flexion. *J Bone Joint Surg* 1988;70: 94–99.

435. Grood ES, Hefzy MS, Lindenfield TL. Factors affecting the region of most isometric femoral attachments: I. The posterior cruciate ligament. *Am J Sports Med* 1989;17:197–207.

436. Ogata K, McCarthy JA. Measurements of length and tension patterns during reconstruction of the posterior cruciate ligament. *Am J Sports Med* 1992;20:351–355.

437. Ogata K, McCarthy JA, Dunlap J, et al. Pathomechanics of posterior sag of the tibia in posterior cruciate deficient knees: an experimental study. *Am J Sports Med* 1998;16:630–636.

438. Sidles JA, Llarson RV, Garbini JL, et al. Ligament length relationships in the moving knee. *J Orthop Res* 1988;6:593–610.

439. Covey DC, Sapega AA, Torg JS, et al. Intra-operative isometry testing for posterior cruciate ligament reconstruction: a biomechanical study. *Orthop Trans* 1993;17:224–225.

440. Covey DC, Sapega AA. Current concepts review: injuries to the posterior cruciate ligament. *J Bone Joint Surg Am* 1993; 75;1376–1386.

441. Gollehon DL, Torzilli PA, Warren RF. The role of the posterolateral and cruciate ligaments in the stability of the human knee: a biomechanical study. *J Bone Joint Surg Am* 1987;69: 233–242.

442. Grood ES, Stowers SF, Noyes FR. Limits of movement in the human knee: effect of sectioning posterior cruciate ligament and posterolateral structures. *J Bone Joint Surg* 1988;174:527–530.

443. Veltri DM, Deng X-H, Torzilli PA, et al. The role of the popliteofibular ligament in stability of the human knee: a biomechanical study. *Am J Sports Med* 1996;24:19–27.

444. Veltri DM, Deng X-H, Torzilla PA, et al. The role of the cruciate and posterolateral ligaments in stability of the knee: a biomechanical study. *Am J Sports Med* 1995;23:436–443.

445. Fox RJ, Harner CD, Sakane M, et al. Determination of in situ forces in the human posterior cruciate ligament using robotic technology: a cadaveric study. *Am J Sports Med* 1998;26: 395–401.

446. Piziali RL, Seering WP, Nagel DA, et al. The function of the primary ligaments of the knee in anterior-posterior and medial-lateral motions. *J Biomech* 1980;13:777–784.

447. Harner CD, Vogrin TM, Hoher J, et al. The effects of loading the popliteus muscle on the intact and PCL deficient knee. *Trans Orthop Res Soc* 1997;43:863.

448. Muller W. *The knee: form, function, and ligament reconstruction.* Berlin: Springer-Verlag, 1983:246–248.

449. Staubli HU. Posteromedial and posterolateral capsular injuries associated with posterior cruciate ligament insufficiency. *Sport Med Arthrosc Rev* 1994;2:146–164.

450. Staubli HU, Birrer S. The popliteus tendon and its fascicles at the popliteal hiatus: gross anatomy and functional arthroscopic evaluation with and without anterior cruciate ligament deficiency. *Arthroscopy* 1990;6:209–220.

451. Maynard MJ, Deng X, Wickiewicz TL, et al. The popliteofibular ligament: rediscovery of a key element in posterolateral stability. *Am J Sports Med* 1996;24:311–316.

452. Baker CL, Jr, Norwood LA, Hughston JC. Acute combined posterior cruciate and posterolateral instability of the knee. *Am J Sports Med* 1984;12:204–208.

453. Skyhar MJ, Warren RF, Ortiz GJ, et al. The effects of sectioning of the posterior cruciate ligament and the posterolateral complex on the articular contact pressures within the knee. *J Bone Joint Surg Am* 1993;75:694–699.

454. MacDonald P, Miniaci A, Fowler P, et al. A biomechanical analysis of joint contact forces in the posterior cruciate deficient knee. *Knee Surg Sports Traumatol Arthrosc* 1996;3:252–255.

455. Castle TH, Noyes FR, Grood ES. Posterior tibial subluxation of the posterior cruciate deficient knee. *Clin Orthop* 1992; 284:193–202.

456. Clancy WG Jr, Shelbourne KD, Zoellner GB, et al. Treatment of knee joint instability secondary to rupture of the posterior cruciate ligament: report of a new procedure. *J Bone Joint Surg Am* 1983;65:310–322.

457. Dejour H, Walch G, Peyrot J, et al. The natural history of rupture of the posterior cruciate ligament. *Fr J Orthop Surg* 1988;2:112–120.

458. Keller PM, Shelbourne KD, McCarroll JR, et al. Nonoperatively treated isolated posterior cruciate ligament injuries. *Am J Sports Med* 1993;21:846–849.

459. Safran MR, Allen AA, Lephart SM, et al. Proprioception in the posterior cruciate ligament deficient knee. *Knee Surg Sports Traumatol Arthrosc* 1999;7:310–317.

460. Frank C, Woo SL-Y, Andriacchi T, et al. Normal ligament: structure, function and composition. In: Woo SL-Y, Buckwalter JA, eds. *Injury and repair of the musculoskeletal soft tissues.* Park Ridge, IL: American Academy of Orthopaedic Surgeons, 1987;45–101.

461. O'Donoghue DH. An analysis of end results of surgical treatment of major injuries to the ligaments of the knee. *J Bone Joint Surg Am* 1955;37:1–13.

462. O'Donoghue DH, Frank GR, Jeter GL, et al. Repair and reconstruction of the anterior cruciate ligament in dogs: factors influencing long term results. *J Bone Joint Surg Am* 1971; 53:710–718.

463. Andrish J, Holmes F. Effects of synovial fluid on fibroblasts in tissue culture. *Clin Orthop* 1979;138:279.

464. Lo IKY, de Matt GHR, Valk JW, et al. The gross morphology of torn human anterior cruciate ligaments in unstable knee. *Arthroscopy* 1999;15:301–306.

465. Crain EH, Fithian DC, Daniel DM. Variation in ACL scar pattern: does this contribute to anterior stability in ACL efficient knees? Presented at the Annual Meeting of the Arthroscopy Association of North America, San Diego, CA, 1997.

466. Ihara H, Miwa M, Deya K, et al. MRI of anterior cruciate ligament healing. *J Comput Assist Tomogr* 1995;20:317–321.

467. Fowler PJ, Regan WD. The patient with symptomatic chronic anterior cruciate ligament insufficiency: results of minimal arthroscopic surgery and rehabilitation. *Am J Sport Med* 1987;15:321–325.

468. Neurath MF, Printz H, Stofft E. Cellular ultrastructure of the ruptured anterior cruciate ligament: a transmission electron microscopic and immunohistochemical study in 55 cases. *Acta Orthop Scand* 1994;65:71–76.

469. Hefti FL, Cress A, Fasel J, et al. Healing of the transected anterior cruciate ligament in the rabbit. *J Bone Joint Surg Am* 1991;73:373–383.

470. Kleiner JB, Roux RD, Amiel D, et al. Primary healing of the anterior cruciate ligament. Presented at the 32nd Annual Meeting of the Orthopaedic Research Society, New Orleans, LA, 1986.

471. O'Donoghue DH, Rockwood CA, Frank GR, et al. Repair of the anterior cruciate ligament in dogs. *J Bone Joint Surg Am* 1966;48:503–519.

472. Hastings DE. The non-operative treatment of collateral ligament injuries of the knee joint. *Clin Orthop* 1980;147:22–28.

473. Chimich D, Frank C, Shrive N, et al. The effects of initial end contact on medial collateral ligament healing: a morphological and biomechanical study in a rabbit model. *J Orthop Res* 1991;9:37–47.

474. Woo SL-Y, Inoue M, McGurk-Burleson E, et al. Treatment of the medial collateral ligament injury: II. Structure and function of canine knees in response to differing treatment regimens. *Am J Sports Med* 1987;15:22–29.

475. Frank C, Woo SL-Y, Amiel D, et al. Medial collateral ligament healing: a multidisciplinary assessment in rabbits. *Am J Sports Med* 1983;11:379–389.

476. Frank C, Schachar N, Dittrich D. Natural history of healing in the repaired medial collateral ligament. *J Orthop Res* 1983;1: 179–188.

477. Amiel D, Frank CB, Harwood FL, et al. Collagen alteration in medial collateral ligament healing in a rabbit model. *Connect Tiss Res* 1987;16:357–366.

478. Frank CB, McDonald D, Shrive NG. Collagen fibril diameters in the rabbit medial collateral ligament scar: a longer-term assessment. *Connect Tiss Res* 1992;36:261–263.

479. Frank C, McDonald D, Bray D, et al. Collagen fibril diameters in the healing adult rabbit medial collateral ligament. *Connect Tiss Res* 1992;27:251–263.

480. Frank C, McDonald D, Wilson J, et al. Rabbit medial collateral ligament scar weakness is associate with decreased collagen pyridinoline cross link density. *J Orthop Res* 1995;13:157–165.

481. Plaas AHK, Wong-Palms S, Koob T, et al. Proteoglycan metabolism during repair of the ruptured medial collateral ligament in skeletally mature rabbits. *Arch Biochem Biophys* 2000;374:35–41.

482. Shrive N, Chimich D, Marchuk L, et al. Soft-tissue flaws are associated with the material properties of the healing rabbit medial collateral ligament. *J Orthop Res* 1995;13:923–929.

483. Akeson WH, Frank CB, Amiel D, et al. Ligament biology and biomechanics. In: Finerman G, ed. *Symposium on sports medicine: the knee.* St. Louis: CB Mosby 1985:111–151.

484. Woo SLY, Chan SS, Yamaji T. Biomechanics of knee ligament healing, repair and reconstruction. *J Biomechanics* 1997;30: 431–439.

485. Daniel DM, Akeson WH, O'Connor JJ. In: Daniel DM, Akeson WH, O'Connor JJ, eds. *Knee ligaments: structure, function, injury and repair.* New York: Raven Press 1990.

486. Frank CB, Hart DA, Shrive NG. Molecular biology and biomechanics of normal and healing ligaments: a review. *Osteoarthritis Cartilage* 1999;7:130–140.

487. Hildebrand KA, Frank CB. Scar formation and ligament healing. *Can J Surg* 1998;41:425–429.

488. Loitz BJ, Frank CB. Biology and mechanics of ligament and ligament healing. *Exer Sport Sci Rev* 1993;21:33–64.

489. Frank C, Shrive N, Hiraoka H, et al. Optimization of the biology of soft tissue repair. *J Sci Med Sport* 1999;2:190–210.

490. Frank C, Schachar N, Dittrich D. The natural history of healing the repaired medial collateral ligament: a morphological assessment in rabbits. *J Orthop Res* 1983;1:179–188.

491. Niyibizi C, Kavalkovich K, Yamaji T, et al. Type V collagen is increased during rabbit medial collateral ligament healing. *Knee Surg Sports Trauamatol Arthrosc* 2000;8:281–285.

492. Bray RC. Blood supply of ligaments: a brief overview. *Orthopaedics International Edition* 1995;39–48.

493. Bray RC, Rangayyan RM, Frank CB: Normal and healing ligament vascularity: a quantitative histological assessment in the rabbit medial collateral ligament. *J Anat* 1996;188:87–95.

494. Boykiw R, Sciore P, Reno C, et al. Altered levels of extacellular matrix molecule mRNA in healing rabbit ligaments. *Matrix Biol* 1998;17: 371–378.

495. Reno C, Boykiw R, Martinez ML, et al. Temporal alterations in mRNA levels for proteinases and inhibitors and their potential regulators in the healing medial collateral ligament. *Biochem Biophys Res Comm* 1998;252:757–763.

496. Sciore P, Boykiw R, Hart DA. Semiquantitative reverse transcription-polymerase chain reaction analysis of mRNA for growth factors, and growth factor receptors from normal and healing rabbit medial collateral ligament tissue. *J Orthop Res* 1998;16:429–437.

497. Frank C, MacFarlane B, Edwards P, et al. A quantitative analysis of matrix alignment in ligament scars: a comparison of movement versus immobilization in an immature rabbit model. *J Orthop Res* 1991;9:219–227.

498. Banes A, Tsuzaki M, Yamamoto J, et al. Mechanoreception at the cellular level: the detection, interpretation and diversity of responses to mechanical signals. *Biochem Cell Biol* 1995;73: 349–355.

499. Grodzinsky AJ, Kim YJ, Buschmann MD, et al. Response of the chondrocyte to mechanical stimuli. In: Brandt KD, Doherty M, Lohmander LS, eds. *Osteoarthritis.* Oxford: Oxford Medical Publishing, 1998:123—136.

500. Guilak F, Sah RL, Setton L. Physical regulation of cartilage metabolism. In: Mow VC, Hayes WC, eds. *Basic Orthopaedic Biomechanics,* Philadelphia: Lippincott-Raven 1997:179–207.

501. Benya PD, Shaffer JD. Dedifferentiated chondrocytes reex-

press the differentiated collagen phenotype when cultured in agarose gels. *Cell* 1982;30:215–224.

502. Knight MM, Lee DA, Bader DL. The influence of elaborated pericellular matrix on the deformation of isolated articular chondrocytes cultured in agarose. *Biochim Biophys Acta* 1998; 1405:67–77.

503. Buschmann MD, Gluzband YA, Grodzinsky AJ, et al. Mechanical compression modulates matrix biosynthesis in chondrocyte agarose culture. *J Cell Science* 1995;108: 1497–1508.

504. Buschmann MD, Hunziker E, Kim YJ, et al. Altered aggrecan synthesis correlates with cell and nucleus structure in statically compressed cartilage. *J Cell Science* 1996;109:499–508.

505. Lee DA, Noguchi T, Knight MM, et al. Response of chondrocyte subpopulations cultured within unloaded and loaded agarose. *J Orthop Res* 1998;16:726–733.

506. Ragan PM, Badger AM, Cook M, et al. Down-regulation of chondrocyte aggrecan and type II collagen gene expression correlates with increases in static compression magnitude and duration. *J Orthop Res* 1999;17:836–842.

507. Hsieh AH, Tsai CM, Ma QJ, et al. Time-dependent increases in type-III collagen gene expression in medial collateral ligament fibroblasts under cyclic strain. *J Orthop Res* 2000;18: 220–227.

508. Majima T, Marchuk LL, Sciore P, et al. Compressive versus tensile loading of medial collateral ligament scar in vitro uniquely influences mRNA levels for aggrecan, collagen type II and collagenase. *J Orthop Res* 2000;18:524–531.

509. Majima T, Marchuk LL, Shrive NG, et al. In vitro cyclic tensile loading of an immobilized and mobilized ligament autograft selectively inhibits mRNA levels for collagenase (MMP-1). *J Orthop Sci* 2000;5:503–510.

510. Bray RC, Shrive NG, Frank CB, et al. The early effects of joint immobilization on medial collateral ligament healing in an anterior cruciate ligament-deficient knee: a gross anatomic and biomechanical investigation in the adult rabbit model. *J Orthop Res* 1992;10:157–166.

511. Engle CP, Noguchi M, Ohland KJ, et al. Healing of the rabbit medial collateral ligament following an O-Donoghue triad injury: effects of anterior cruciate ligament reconstruction. *J Orthop Res* 1994;12:357–365.

512. Yamaji T, Levine RE, Woo SLY, et al. Medial collateral ligament healing one year after a concurrent medial collateral ligament and anterior cruciate ligament injury: an interdisciplinary study in rabbits. *J Orthop Res* 1996;14:223–227.

513. Inoue M, McGurk-Burleson E, Hollis JM, et al. Treatment of the medial collateral ligament injury: I. The importance of anterior cruciate ligament on the varus-valgus knee laxity. *Am J Sports Med* 1987;15:15–21.

514. Inoue M, Woo SL-Y, Gomez MA, et al. Effects of surgical treatment and immobilization on the healing of the medial collateral ligament: a long-term multidisciplinary study. *Connect Tiss Res* 1990;25:13–26.

515. Ohno K, Pomaybo AS, Schmidt CC, et al. Healing of the medial collateral ligament after a combined medial collateral and anterior cruciate ligament injury and reconstruction of the anterior cruciate ligament: comparison of repair and nonrepair of medial collateral ligament tears in rabbits. *J Orthop Res* 1995; 13:442–449.

516. Woo SL-Y, Inoue M, McGurk-Burleson E, et al. Treatment of the medial collateral ligament injury: II. Structure and function of canine knees in response to differing treatment regimens. *Am J Sports Med* 1987;15:22–29.

517. Woo SL-Y, Young EP, Ohland KJ, et al. The effects of transection of the anterior cruciate ligament on healing of the me-

dial collateral ligament: a biomechanical study of the knee in dogs. *J Bone Joint Surg Am* 1990;72:382–392.

518. Burroughs P, Dahners L. The effect of enforced exercise on the healing of ligament injuries. *Am J Sports Med* 1990;18:376–378.

519. Majima T, Randle JA, Lo IKY, et al. Collagen type I mRNA expression in ACL deficient MCL scars versus ACL intact scars. Poster presentation at the Canadian Orthopaedic Research Society Annual Meeting, Edmonton, June, 2000.

520. Murphy PG, Loitz BJ, Frank CB, et al. Influence of exogenous growth factors on the synthesis and secretion of collagen types I and III by explants of normal and healing rabbit ligaments. *Biochem Cell Biol* 1994;72:403–409.

521. Murphy PG, Hart DA. Influence of exogenous growth factors on the expression of plasminogen and plasminogen activator inhibitors by cells isolated from normal and healing rabbit ligaments. *J Orthop Res* 1994;12:564–575.

522. Woo SL-Y, Smith DW, Hildebrand KA, et al. Engineering the healing of the rabbit medial collateral ligament. *Med Biol Eng Comput* 1998;36:359–364.

523. Woo SL-Y, Suh JK, Parsons IM, et al. Biological intervention in ligament healing effect of growth factors. *Sports Med Arthrosc Rev* 1998;6:74–82.

524. Spindler KP, Imro AK, Mayes CE, et al. Patellar tendon and anterior cruciate ligament have different mitogenic responses to platelet-derived growth factor and transforming growth factor β. *J Orthop Res* 1996;14:542–546.

525. Scherping SC JR, Schimidt CC, Georgescu HI, et al. Effect of growth factors on the proliferation of ligament fibroblasts from skeletally mature rabbits. *Connect Tissue Res* 1997;36:1–8.

526. Schmidt CC, Georgescu HI, Kwoh CK, et al. Effect of growth factors on the proliferation of fibroblasts from the medial collateral and anterior cruciate ligaments. *J Orthop Res* 1995;13: 184–190.

527. Marui T, Niyibizi C, Georgescu HI, et al. The effect of growth factors on matrix synthesis by ligament fibroblasts. J Orthop Res 1997;15:18–23.

528. Weiss JA, Beck CL, Levine RE, et al. Effects of platelet-derived growth factor on early medial collateral ligament healing. *Trans Orthop Res Soc* 1995;20:159.

529. Duffy FJJ, Seiler JG, Gelberman RH, et al. Growth factors and canine flexor tendon healing: initial studies in uninjured and repair models. *J Hand Surg Am* 1995;20:645–649.

530. Kobayashi D, Kurosaka M, Yoshiya S, et al. Effect of basic fibroblast growth factor on the healing defects in the canine anterior cruciate ligament. *Knee Surg Sports Traumatol Arthrosc* 1997;5:189–194.

531. Hart DA, Nakamura N, Marchuk L, et al. Complexity of determining cause and effect in vivo after antisense gene therapy. *Clin Orthop* 2000;379:S242–S251.

532. Lee J, Harwood FL, Akeson WH, et al. Growth factor expression in healing rabbit medial collateral and anterior cruciate ligaments. *Iowa Orthop J* 1998;18:19–25.

533. Panossian V, Liu SH, Lane JM, et al. Fibroblast growth factor and epidermal growth factor receptors in ligament healing. *Clin Orthop* 1997;342:173–180.

534. Chang J, Most D, Thunder R, et al. Molecular studies in flexor tendon wound healing: the role of basic fibroblast growth factor gene expression. *J Hand Surg* 1998;23:1052–1058.

535. DesRosiers EA, Yahia L, Rivard C-H. Proliferative and matrix synthesis response of canine anterior cruciate ligament fibroblasts submitted to combined growth factors. *J Orthop Res* 1996;14:200–208.

536. Letson AK, Dahners LE. The effect of combinations of growth factors on ligament healing. *Clin Orthop* 1994;308:207–212.

537. Hildebrand KA, Woo SLY, Smith DW, et al. The effects of

platelet-derived growth factor-BB on healing of the rabbit medial collateral ligament. *Am J Sports Med* 1998;26:549–554.

538. Batten ML, Hansen JC, Dahners LE. Influence of dosage and timing of application of platelet-derived growth factor on early healing of the rat medial collateral ligament. *J Orthop Res* 1996;14:736–741.

539. Yasuhiro Y, Abrahamssom S. Dose-related cellular effects of platelet derived growth factor-BB vary between different types of rabbit tendons in vitro. *Trans Orthop Res Soc* 2000;25:801.

540. Woo SL-Y, Taylor BJ, Schimidt CC, et al. The effect of dose levels of growth factors on the healing of the rabbit medial collateral ligament. *Trans Orthop Res Soc* 1996;21:97.

541. Nakamura N, Horibe S, Matsumoto N, et al. Transient introduction of a foreign gene into healing rat patellar ligament. *J Clin Invest* 1996;97:226–231.

542. Nakamura N, Timmermann SA, Hart DA, et al. A comparison of in vivo gene delivery methods for antisense therapy in ligament healing. *Gene Ther* 1998;5:1455–1461.

543. Nakamura N, Frank CB, Hart DA. Gene therapy in joint repair. *Curr Opin Orthop* 1998;9:25–30.

544. Gerich TG, Kang R, Fu FH, et al. Gene transfer to the rabbit patellar tendon: potential for genetic enhancement of tendon and ligament healing. *Gene Ther* 1996;3:1089–1093.

545. Gerich TG, Kang R, Fu FH, et al. Gene transfer to the patellar tendon. *Knee Surg Sports Traumatol Arthrosc* 1997;5:118–123.

546. Martinek V, Lattermann C, Pelinkovic D, et al. Ex-vivo gene transfer for preconditioning of ACL tendon grafts *Trans Orthop Res Soc* 2000;25:811.

547. Day CS, Kasemkijwattana C, Menetrey J, et al. Myoblast-mediated gene transfer to the joint. *J Orthop Res* 1997;15:893–903.

548. Menetrey J, Kasemkijwattana C, Day CS, et al. Direct-, fibroblast- and myoblast-mediated gene transfer to the anterior cruciate ligament. *Tissue Eng* 1999;5:435–442.

549. Hildebrand KA, Deie M, Allen CR, et al. Early expression of marker genes in the rabbit medial collateral and anterior cruciate ligaments: the use of different viral vectors and the effects of injury. *J Orthop Res* 1999;17:37–42.

550. Latterman C, Clatworthy M, Weiss KR, et al. Targeting of gene therapy in ligament insertions: bone or tendon? *Trans Orthop Res Soc* 1999;24.

551. Lou J, Manske PR, Aoki M, et al. Adenovirus-mediated gene transfer into tendon and tendon sheath. *J Orthop Res* 1996;14:513–517.

552. Gommer R, Silva M, Boyer M, et al. Direct non-viral gene delivery during surgery to repair canine flexor tendons resulted in surprisingly high fraction of transfected cells. *Trans Orthop Res Soc* 2000;25:1058.

553. Lou J, Kubota H, Hotokezaka S, et al. In vivo gene transfer and overexpression of focal adhesion kinase [pp125 FAK] mediated by recombinant adenovirus-induced tendon adhesion formation and epitenon cell change. *J Orthop Res* 1997;15:911–918.

554. Tu Y, Lou J, Burns M, et al. BMP 12 gene transfer augmentation of injured tendon repair. *Trans Orthop Res Soc* 2000;5:812.

555. Nakamura N, Hart DA, Boorman RS, et al. Decorin antisense gene therapy improves functional healing of early rabbit ligament scar with enhanced collagen fibrillogenesis in vivo. *J Orthop Res* 2000;18:517–523.

556. Hart DA, Nakamura N, Boorman R, et al. Functional improvement in ligament scar tissue following antisense gene therapy: a model system for in vivo engineering of connective tissues. *Gene Ther Mol Biol* 2000;4:85–90.

Cartilage References

557. Hamerman D, Rosenberg LC, Schubert M. Diarthrodial joints revisited. *J Bone Joint Surg Am* 1970;52:725–774.

558. Stockwell RA. Chondrocytes. *J Clin Pathol* 1978;12[Suppl]:7–13.

559. Stockwell RA. The cell density of human articular and costal cartilage. *J Anat* 1967;101:753–763.

560. Muir IHM. The chemistry of the ground substance of joint cartilage. In: Sokoloff L, ed. *The joints and synovial fluid,* vol 2. New York: Academic Press, 1980:27–94.

561. Muir IHM. Biochemistry. In: Freeman MAR, ed. *Adult articular cartilage,* 2nd ed. Tunbridge Wells: Pitman Medical, 1979:145–214.

562. Buckwalter JA. Articular cartilage. *Instr Course Lect* 1983;32:349–370.

563. Muir H, Bullough P, Maroudas A. The distribution of collagen in human articular cartilage with some of its physiological implications. *J Bone Joint Surg Br* 1970;52:554–563.

564. Maroudas A. Physiochemical properties of articular cartilage. In: Freeman MAR, ed. *Adult articular cartilage,* 2nd ed. Tunbridge Wells: Pitman Medical, 1979:215–290.

565. Clark JM. The organization of collagen in cryofractured rabbit articular cartilage: a scanning electron microscopic study. *J Orthop Res* 1985;3:17–29.

566. Meachim G, Denham D, Emery IH, et al. Collagen alignments and artificial splits at the surface of human articular cartilage. *J Anat* 1974;118:101.

567. Clarke IC. Articular cartilage: a review and scanning electron microscope study. II: the territorial fibrillar architecture. *J Anat* 1974;118:261.

568. Buckwalter JA, Rosenberg LC, Hunziker EB. Articular cartilage: composition, structure, response to injury, and methods of facilitation repair. In Ewing JW, ed. *Articular cartilage and knee joint function: basic science and arthroscopy.* New York: Raven Press, 1990:19–56.

569. Aydelotte MB, Schumacher BL, Kuettner KE. Heterogeneity of articular chondrocytes. In: Kuettner KE, Schleyerback R, Peyron JG, et al., eds. *Articular cartilage and osteoarthritis.* New York: Raven Press, 1992:237–249.

570. Hunter JA, Finley B. Scanning electron microscopy of connective tissues: articular cartilage. *Int Rev Connect Tissue Res* 1973;6:615.

571. Clarke IC. The microevaluation of articular surface contours. *Ann Biochem Eng* 1972;1:31.

572. Wright V, Dowson D, Kerr J. The structure of joints: IV. Articular cartilage. *Int Rev Connect Tissue Res* 1973;6:109.

573. Benninghoff A. Form und bau der gelenkknorpel in ihren bezienunger zur funktion II: Der aufbau des gelenkknorpels in seimen bezlehurgen zur funktion. *Z Zellforsch Mikrosk Anat* 1925;2:783.

574. Schenk RK, Eggli PS, Hunziker EB. Articular cartilage morphology. In: Kuettner KE, Schleyerback R, Hascall VC, eds. *Articular cartilage biochemistry.* New York: Raven Press, 1986:3–22.

575. Poole AR, Pidoux I, Reiner A, et al. An immunoelectron microscope study of the organization of proteoglycan monomer, link protein, and collagen in the matrix of articular cartilage. *J Cell Biol* 1982;93:921–937.

576. Poole CA, Flint MH, Beaumont BW. Morphological and functional interrelationships of articular cartilage matrices. *J Anat* 1984;138:113–138.

577. Mollenhauer J, Bee JA, Lizarbe MA, et al. Role of anchorin CII, a 31,000-mol-wt membrane protein, in the interaction of chodrocytes with type II collagen. *J Cell Biol* 1984;98:1572–1579.

578. Pfaffle M, Borcher M, Deutzmann R, et al. Anchorin CII, a collagen-binding chondrocyte surface protein of the calpactin family. *Prog Clin and Biol Res* 1990;349:147–157.

579. Szirmair JA. Structure of cartilage. In: Engel A, Larsson T, eds. *Ageing of Connective and Skeletal Tissue* 1969;163–184.

580. Poole CA. Articular cartilage chondrons: form, function and failure. *J Anat* 1997;191:1–13.

581. Lee GM, Poole CA, Kelley SS, et al. Isolated chondrons: a viable alternative for studies of chondrocyte metbolism in vitro. *Osteoarthritis Cartilage* 1997;5:261–274.

582. Poole CA, Flint MH, Beaumont BE. Chondrons in cartilage: ultrastructural analysis of the pericelliular microenvironment in adult human articular cartilage. *J Orthop Res* 1987;5:509–522.

583. Poole CA, Flint MH, Beaumont BW. Chondrons isolated from canine tibial cartilage: preliminary report on their isolation and structure. *J Orthop Res* 1988;6:408–419.

584. Stockwell RA. The cell density of human articular and costal cartilage. *J Anat* 1967;101:753–763.

585. Stockwell RA. Chondrocytes. *J Clin Pathol* 1978;12:7–13.

586. Aydelotte MB, Michal LE, Reid DR, et al. Chondrocytes from the articular surface and deep zones express different but stable phenotypes in alginate gel culture. *Trans Orthop Res Soc* 1996:21:317.

587. Ghadially FN. Fine structure of joints. In: Sokoloff L, ed. *The joints and synovial fluid,* vol 1. New York: Academic Press, 1978:105–176.

588. Stockwell RA. Cellular aspects: the chondrocyte population and the chondrocyte. In: Ali, Elves, Leaback, eds. *Normal and osteoarthrotic articular cartilage.* London: University of London, 1974.

589. Mankin HJ. Localisation of tritiated thymidine in articular cartilage of rabbits: III. Mature aritcular cartilage. *J Bone Joint Surg Am* 1963;45:529–540.

590. Stockwell RA, Meachim G. The chondrocytes. In: Freeman MAR, ed. *Adult articular cartilage,* 2nd ed. Turnbridge Wells: Pitman Medical, 1979:69–144.

591. Fischer AE, Carpenter TA, Tyler JA, et al. Visualisation of mass transport of small organic molecules and metal ions through articular cartilage by magnetic resonance imaging. *Magnet Res Imag* 1995;13:819–826.

592. Mankin HJ. The metabolism of articular cartilage in health and disease. In: Burleigh PMC, Poole AR, eds. *Dynamics of connective tissue macromolecules.* New York: Elsevier, 1975:327–355.

593. Brower TD, Wan-YI H. Normal articular cartilage. *Clin Orthop* 1969;64:9.

594. Ingber DE. Tensegrity: the architectural basis of cellular mechanotransduction. *Annu Rev Physiol* 1997;59:575–599.

595. Mankin HJ, Thrasher AZ. Water content and binding in normal and osteoarthritic human cartilage. *J Bone Joint Surg Am* 1975;57:76.

596. Mankin HJ. Water binding in articular cartilage. *J Bone Joint Surg Am* 1974;56:1031.

597. Lai WM, Mow VC, Roth V. Effects of nonlinear strain-dependent permeability and rate of compression on the stress behavior of articular cartilage. *J Biomech Eng* 1981;103:61–66.

598. Linn FC, Sokoloff L. Movement and composition of interstitial fluid of cartilage. *Arthritis Rheum* 1965;8:481–494.

599. Mankin HJ. The water of articular cartilage. In: Simoin WH, ed. *The human joint in health and disease.* Philadelphia: University of Pennsylvania Press, 1978:37–42.

600. Maroudas A, Schneiderman R. "Free" and "exchangeable" or "trapped" and "non-exchangeble" water in cartilage. *J Orthop Res* 1987;5:133–138.

601. Mow VC, Rosenwasser MP. Articular cartilage. Biomechanics.

In: Woo SLY, Buckwalter JA. *Injury and repair of the musculoskeletal soft tissues.* Park Ridge, IL: The American Academy of Orthopaedic Surgeons, 1988:427–463.

602. Harris ED Jr, Parker HG, Radin EL, et al. Effects of proteolytic enzymes on structural and mechanical properties of cartilage. *Arthritis Rheum* 1972;15:497–503.

603. Kempson GE. The mechanical properties of articular cartilage. In: Sokoloff L, ed. *The joints and synovial fluid,* vol 2. New York: Academic Press, 1980:177–238.

604. Kempson GE, Muir H, Pollard C, et al. The tensile properties of the cartilage of human femoral condyles related to the content of collagen and glycosaminoglycans. *Biochim Biophys Acta* 1973;297:456–472.

605. Meachim G, Stockwell RA. The matrix. In: Freeman MAR, ed. *Adult articular cartilage,* 2nd ed. Tunbridge Wells: Pitman Medical, 1979:1–67.

606. Broom ND, Poole CA. A functional morphological study of the tidemark region of articular cartilage maintained in a nonviable physiological condition. *J Anat* 1982;135:65–82.

607. Eyre DR. Collagen structure and function in articular cartilage: metabolic changes in the development of osteoarthritis. In: Kuettner KE, Goldberg VM, eds. *Osteoarthritic disorders.* Rosemont, IL: American Academy of Orthopaedic Surgeons, 1995:219–229.

608. Eyre DR, Wu JJ, Woods P. Cartilage-specific collagens: structural studies. In: Kuettner KE, Schleyerbach R, Peyron JG, et al. *Articular cartilage and osteoarthritis.* New York: Raven Press, 1992:119–131.

609. Sandell LJ. Molecular biology of collagens in normal and osteoarthritic cartilage. In: Kuettner KE, Goldberg VM, eds. *Osteoarthritic disorders.* Rosemont, IL: American Academy of Orthopaedic Surgeons, 1995:131–146.

610. Mendler M, Eich-Bender SV, Vaughan L, et al. Cartilage contains mixed fibrils of collagen types II, IX and XI. *J Cell Biol* 1989;108:191–197.

611. Bruckner P, Mendler M, Steinmann B, et al. The structure of human collagen type IX and its organization in fetal and infant cartilage fibrils. *J Biol Chem* 1988;263:16911–16917.

612. Diab M, Wu JJ, Eyre DR. Collagen type IX from human cartilage: a structural profile of intermolecular cross-linking sites. *Biochem J* 1996;314:327–332.

613. Roughley PJ, Lee ER. Cartilage proteoglycans: structure and potential functions. *Microsc Res and Tech* 1994;28:385–397.

614. Eyre DR, Wu JJ, Woods PE. The cartilage collagens: structural and metabolic studies. *J Rheumatol* 1991;27:S49–S51.

615. Schmid TM, Lisenmayer F. Immunohistochemical localization of short chain cartilage (type X) in avian tissue. *J Cell Biol* 1985;100:598.

616. Nimni M, Desmukh K. Differences in collagen metabolism between normal and osteoarthritic human articular cartilage. *Science* 1973;181:751.

617. Hardingham TE, Fosang AJ, Dudhia J. Aggrecan: the chondroitin/keratan sulfate proteoglycan from cartilage. In: Kuettner KE, Schleyerbach R, Peyron JG, et al. eds. *Articular cartilage and osteoarthritis.* New York: Raven Press, 1992:5–20.

618. Poole AR, Rosenberg LC, Reiner A, et al. Contents and distributions of the proteoglycans decorin and biglycan in normal and osteoarthritic human articular cartilage. *J Orthop Res* 1996;14:681–689.

619. Rosenberg LC. Structure and function of dermatan sulfate proteoglycan in articular cartilage. In: Kuettner KE, Schleyerbach R, Peyron JG, et al. *Articular cartilage and osteoarthritis.* New York: Raven Press, 1992:45–63.

620. Rosenberg LC, Buckwalter JA. Cartilage proteoglycans. In: Kuettner KE, Schleyerback R, Hascall VC. *Articular cartilage biochemistry.* New York: Raven Press, 1986:39–57.

621. Sandell LJ, Chansky H, Zaniparo O, et al. Molecular biology of cartilage proteoglycans and link protein. In: Kuettner KE, Goldberg VM, eds. *Osteoarthritic disorders.* Rosemont, IL: American Academy of Orthopaedic Surgeons, 1995:117–130.

622. Buckwalter JA, Mankin HJ. Articular cartilage: tissue design and chondrocyte-matrix interactions. *Instr Course Lect* 1998; 47:477.

623. Naeme PJ. Extracellular matrix of cartilage: proteoglycans. In: Woessner JF, Howell DS, eds. *Joint cartilage degradation: basic and clinical aspects.* New York: Marcel Dekker, 1993:109.

624. Mow VC, Zhu W, Lai WM, et al. The influence of link protein stabilization on the viscometric properties of proteoglycan aggregate solution. *Biochim Biophys Acta* 1989;992:201.

625. Evans CH. Cartilage and synovium. In: Baratz ME, Watson AD, Imbriglia JE, eds. *Orthopedic surgery: the essentials.* New York: Theime Medical Publishers, 1999:33.

626. Hardingham TE, Muir H, Kwan MK, et al. Viscoelastic properties of proteoglycan solutions with varying proportions present as aggregates. *J Orthop Res* 1987;5:36–46.

627. Mow VC, Mak AF, Lai WM, et al. Viscoelastic properties of proteoglycan subunits and aggregates in varying solution concentrations. *J Biomech* 1984;17:325–338.

628. Mow VC, Kwan MK, Lai WM, et al. A finite deformation theory for nonlinearly permeable soft hydrated biological tissues. In: Schmid-Schonbein GW, Woo SL-Y, Zweifach BE, eds. *Frontiers in biomechanics.* New York: Springer-Verlag, 1986: 153–179.

629. Mow VC, Kuei SC, Lai WM, et al. Biphasic creep and stress relaxation of articular cartilage in compression: theory and experiments. *J Biomech Eng* 1980;102:73–84.

630. Holmes MH. A theoretical analysis for determining the nonlinear hydraulic permeability of a soft tissue from a permeation experiment. *Bull Math Biol* 1985;47:669–683.

631. Holmes MH. Finite deformation of soft tissue: analysis of a mixture model in uni-axial compression. *J Biomech Eng* 1986; 108:372–381.

632. Mow VC, Lai WM, Holmes MH. Advanced theoretical and experimental techniques in cartilage research. In: Huiskes R, van Campen DH, de Wijn JR, eds. *Biomechanics: principles and applications.* The Hague: Martinus Nijhoff, 1982:47–74.

633. Hayes WC, Bodine AJ. Flow-independent viscoelastic properties of articular cartilage matrix. *J Biomech* 1978;11:407–419.

634. Roth V, Schoonbeck JM, Mow VC. Low frequency dynamic behaviour of articular cartilage under torsional shear. *Trans Orthop Res Soc* 1982;7:150.

635. Zhu WB, Lai WM, Mow VC. Intrinsic quasi-linear viscoelastic behaviour of the extracellular matrix of cartilage. *Trans Orthop Res Soc* 1986;11:407.

636. Maroudas A. Biophysical chemistry of cartilaginous tissues with special reference to solute and fluid transport. *Ann Rheum Dis* 1975;12:233–248.

637. Maroudas A. Physicochemical properties of articular cartilage. In: Freeman MAR, ed. *Adult articular cartilage,* 2nd ed. Tunbridge Wells: Pitman Medical, 1979:215–290.

638. Maroudas A. Physicochemical properties of cartilage in the light of ion exchange theory. *Biophys J* 1968;8:575–595.

639. Schubert M, Hamerman D. *A primer on connective tissue biochemistry.* Philadelphia: Lea & Febiger, 1968.

640. Nimni ME. Collagen: structure, function, and metabolism in normal and fibrotic tissues. *Semin Arthritis Rheum* 1983;13: 1–86.

641. Cohen NP, Foster RJ, Mow VC. Composition and dynamics of articular cartilage: structure, function and maintaining healthy state. *J Orthop Sports Phys Ther* 1998;28:203.

642. Mow VC, Holmes NH, Lai WM. Fluid transport and mechanical properties of articular cartilage: a review. *J Biomech* 1984;17:377.

643. Swann DA, Radin EL, Hendren RB. The lubrication of articular cartilage by synovial fluid glycoproteins. *Arthritis Rheum* 1979;22:665–666 (abst).

644. Swann DA, Silver FH, Slayter HS, et al. The molecular structure and lubricating activity of lubricin isolated from bovine and human synovial fluids. *Biochem J* 1985;225:195–201.

645. McCutchen CW. Boundary lubrication by synovial fluid: demonstration and possible osmotic explanation. *Fed Proc* 1966;25:1061–1068.

646. Dowson D. Modes of lubrication in human joints. *Proc Inst Mech Eng* 1967;1813J:45.

647. Dowson D, Wright V, eds. *An introduction to the biomechanics of joints and joint replacement.* London: Institute of Mechanical Engineering, 1981:120–145.

648. Armstrong CG, Mow VC. Friction, lubrication and wear of synovial joints. In: Owen R, Goodfellow J, Bullough P, eds. *Scientific foundations of orthopaedics and traumatology.* London: William Heinemann, 1980:223–232.

649. Mow VC, Mak AF. Lubrication of diarthrodial joints. In: Skalak R, Chien S, eds. *Handbook of bioengineering.* New York: McGraw-Hill, 1987:5.1–5.34.

650. Higginson GR, Litchfield MR, Smaith J. Load-displacement-time characteristics of articular cartilage. *Int J Mech Sci* 1976; 18:481.

651. Higginson GR, Unsworth T. The lubrication of natural joints. In: Dumbleton JH, ed. *Tribology of natural and artificial joints.* Tribology Series 3. Amsterdam: Elsevier, 1981:47–73.

652. Mow VC, Lai WM: Recent developments in synovial joint biomechanics. *SIAM Rev* 1980;22:275–317.

653. Lai WM, Mow VC. Stress and flow fields in articular cartilage. In: *Advances in civil engineering through engineering mechanics.* American Society of Civil Engineers, 1979:202:205.

654. Mow VC, Lai WM. The optical sliding contact analytical rheometer (OSCAR) for flow visualization at the articular surface. In: Wells MK, ed. *Advances in bioengineering.* New York: American Society of Mechanical Engineers, 1979:97–99.

655. Walker PS, Dowson D, Longfield MD, et al. "Boosted lubrication" in synovial joints by fluid entrapment and enrichment. *Ann Rheum Dis* 1968;27:512–520.

656. Walker PS, Sikorski J, Dowson D, et al. Behaviour of synovial fluid on surfaces of articular cartilage: a scanning electron microscope study. *Ann Rheum Dis* 1969;28:1–14.

657. Walker PS, Unsworth A, Dowson D, et al. Mode of aggregation of hyaluronic acid protein complex on the surface of articular cartilage. *Ann Rheum Dis* 1970;29:591–602.

658. Maroudas A. Hyaluronic acid film. *Proc Inst Mech Eng* 1967; 181:122.

659. Kwan MK, Lai WM, Mow VC. Fundamentals of fluid transport through cartilage in compression. *Ann Biomed Eng* 1984;12:233–248.

660. Radin EL, Martin RB, Burr DB, et al. Effects of mechanical loading on the tissues of the rabbit knee. *J Orthop Res* 1984;2: 221–234.

661. Radin EL, Parker HG, Pugh JW, et al. Response of joints to impact loading: III. Relationship between trabecular microfractures and cartilage degeneration. *J Biomech* 1973;6: 51–57.

662. Radin EL, Paul IL, Lowy M. A comparison of the dynamic force transmitting properties of subchondral bone and articular cartilage. *J Bone Joint Surg Am* 1970;52:444–456.

663. Radin EL, Paul IL. Response of joints to impact loading: I. In vitro wear. *Arthritis Rheum* 1971;14:356–362.

664. Mankin HJ. The response of articular cartilage to mechanical injury. *J Bone Joint Surg Am* 1982;64:460–466.

665. Behrens F, Shepard N, Mitchell N. Metabolic recovery of articular cartilage after intra-articular injections of glucocorticoid. *J Bone Joint Surg Am* 1976;58:1157.

666. Edwards CC, Michael R. The effect of intra-articular amphotericin-B on articular cartilage. *Trans Orthop Res Soc* 1977;2:29.

667. Mankin HJ, Baron PA. The effect of aging on protein synthesis in articular cartilage of rabbits. *Lab Invest* 1965;14:658.

668. Lippiello L, Hall D, Mankin HJ. Collagen synthesis on normal and OA human cartilage. *J Clin Invest* 1977;59:593.

669. Ghadially FN, Thomas I, Oryschak AF, et al. Long-term results of superficial defects in articular cartilage: a scanning electron-microscope study. *J Pathol* 1977;121:213–217.

670. Buckwalter JA, Wossenbery L, Coutts R, et al. Articular cartilage: injury and repair. In: Woo SLY, Buckwalter JA, eds. *Injury and repair of the musculoskeletal soft tissues.* Park Ridge, IL, The American Academy of Orthopaedic Surgeons, 1988:465–482.

671. Ghadially FN, Thomas I, Oryschak AF, et al. Long term results of superficial defects in articular cartilage: a scanning electron-microscope study. *J Pathol* 1977;121:213–217.

672. Buckwalter JA, Hankin HJ. Articular cartilage: part II: Degeneration and osteoarthritis, repair, regeneration and transplantation. *J Bone Joint Surg Am* 1997;79:612–632.

673. Mankin HJ. The reaction of articular cartilage to injury and osteoarthritis [Second of two parts]. *N Engl J Med* 1974;291:1335–1340.

674. Mankin NH. The reaction of articular cartilage to injury and osteoarthritis [First of two parts]. *N Engl J Med* 1974;291:1285–1292.

675. Campbell CJ. The healing of cartilage defects. *Clin Orthop* 1969;64:45–63.

676. DePalma AF, McKeever CD, Subin DK. Process of repair of articular cartilage demonstrated by histology and autoradiography with tritiated thymidine. *Clin Orthop* 1966;48:229–242.

677. Fuller JA, Ghadially FN. Ultrastructural observations on surgically produced partial-thickness defects in articular cartilage. *Clin Orthop* 1972;86:193–205.

678. Mankin HJ, Boyle CJ. The acute effects of lacerative injury on DNA and protein synthesis in articular cartilage. In: Bassett CAL, ed. *Cartilage degradation and repair.* Washington, DC: National Research Council, National Academy of Sciences, National Academy of Engineering, 1967:185–199.

679. Meachim G. The effect of scarification on articular cartilage in the rabbit. *J Bone Joint Surg Br* 1963;45:150–161.

680. Meachim G, Roberts C. Repair of the joint surface from sub-articular tissue in the rabbit knee. *J Anat* 1971;109:317–327.

681. Thompson RC. An experimental study of surface injury to articular cartilage and enzyme responses within the joint. *Clin Orthop Orthop Res* 1975;107:239–248.

682. Reddi AH. Role of subchondral bone matrix factors in the repair of articular cartilage. In: Verbruggen G, Veys EM, eds. *Degenerative joints,* vol 2. Amsterdam: Excerpta Medica, 1985:271–274.

683. Reddi AH. Extracellular bone matrix dependent local induction of cartilage and bone. *J Rheumatol* 1983;10[Suppl 11]:67–69.

684. Shapiro F, Koide S, Glimcher MJ. Cell origin and differentiation in the repair of full-thickness defects of articular cartilage. *J Bone Joint Surg Am* 1993;75:532–553.

685. Whipple RR, Gibbs MC, Lasi WM, et al. Biphasic properties of repaired cartilage at the articular surface. *Trans Orthop Res Soc* 1985;10:340.

686. Furukawa T, Eyre DR, Koide S, et al. Biochemical studies on repair cartilage resurfacing experimental defects in the rabbit knee. *J Bone Joint Surg Am* 1980;62:79–89.

687. Mitchell N, Shepard N. The resurfacing of adult rabbit articular cartilage by multiple perforations through the subchondral bone. *J Bone Joint Surg Am* 1976;58:230–233.

688. Coletti JM Jr, Akeson WH, Woo SLY. A comparison of the physical behavior of normal articular cartilage and the arthroplasty surface. *J Bone Joint Surg Am* 1972;54:147–160.

689. Shapiro F, Koide S, Glimcher MJ. Cell origin and differentiation in the repair of full-thickness defects of articular cartilage. *J Bone Joint Surg Am* 1993;75:532–553.

690. Mankin HJ. Localization of tritiated thymidine in articular cartilage of rabbits: II. Repair in immature cartilage. *J Bone Joint Surg Am* 1962;44:688–698.

691. Moran ME, Kim HK, Salter RB. Biological resurfacing of full-thickness defects in patellar articular cartilage of the rabbit: investigation of autogenous periosteal grafts subjected to continuous passive motion. *J Bone Joint Surg Br* 1992;74:659–667.

692. O'Driscoll SW, Kelley FW, Salter RB. Durability of regenerated articular cartilage produced by free autogenous periosteal grafts in major full-thickness defects in joint surfaces under the influence of continuous passive motion: a follow-up report at one year. *J Bone Joint Surg Am* 1988;70:595–606.

693. O'Driscoll SW, Salter RB. The repair of major osteochondral defects in joint surfaces by neochondrogenesis with autogenous osteoperiosteal grafts stimulated by continuous passive motion. *Clin Orthop* 1986;208:131–140.

694. O'Driscoll SW, Salter RB. The induction of neochondrogenesis in free intra-articular periosteal autografts under the influence of continuous passive motion: an experimental investigation in the rabbit. *J Bone Joint Surg Am* 1984;66:1248–1257.

695. Rubak JM, Poussa M Ritsila V. Effects of joint motion on the repair of articular cartilage defects by free periosteal grafts. *Acta orthop Scand* 1982;53:187–191.

696. Salter RB, Simmonds DF, Malcolm BW, et al. The biological effect of continuous passive motion on the healing of full-thickness defects in articular cartilage: an experimental investigation in the rabbit. *J Bone Joint Surg Am* 1980;62:1232–1251.

697. Kerder HJ, Moran M, Keeley FW, et al. Biologic resurfacing of a major joint defect with cryopreserved allogeneic periosteum under the influence of continuous passive motion in a rabbit model. *Clin Orthop* 1994;300:288–296.

698. Nevo Z, Robinson D, Halperin H, et al. Culturing chondrocytes for implantation. In: Maroudas A, Kuettner K, eds. *Methods in cartilage research.* London: Academic Press, 1990:98–100.

699. Convery FR, Akeson WH, Keown GH. The repair of large osteochondral defects: an experimental study in horses. *Clin Orthop* 1972;82:253–262.

700. Evans CH, Mazzocchi RA, Nelson DD, et al. Experimental arthritis induced by intraarticular injection of allogenic cartilaginous particles into rabbit knees. *Arthritis Rheum* 1984;27:200–207.

701. Mitchell N, Shepard N. Effect of patellar shaving in the rabbit. *J Orthop Res* 1987;5:388–392.

702. Kim HKW, Moran ME, Salter RB. The potential for regeneration of articular cartilage in defects created by chondral shaving and subchondral abrasion: an experimental investigation in rabbits. *J Bone Joint Surg Am* 1991;73:1301–1315.

703. Mitchell N, Shepard N. Effect of patellar shaving in the rabbit. *J Orthop Res* 1987;5:388–392.

704. Schmid A, Schmid F. Results after cartilage shaving studied by electron microscopy. *Am J Sports Med* 1987;15:386–387.

705. Moseley JB, Wray NP, Kuykendall D, et al. Arthroscopic treatment of osteoarthritis of the knee: a randomized, double-glind, placebo controlled trial: two year follow-up of 180 patients. Presented at the 68th Annual Meeting of the American Association of Orthopaedic Surgeons, San Francisco, CA, 2001: 563.

706. Haggart GE. The surgical treatment of degenerative arthritis of the knee joint. *J Bone Joint Surg* 1940;22:717–729.

707. Insall J. The Pridie debridement operation for osteoarthritis of the knee. *Clin Orthop* 1974;101:61–67.

708. Magnuson PB. Joint debridement: surgical treatment of degenerative arthritis. *Surg Gynecol Obstet* 1941;73:1–9.

709. Mitchell N, Shepard N. The resurfacing of adult rabbit articular cartilage by multiple perforations through the subchondral bone. *J Bone Joint Surg Am* 1976;58:230–233.

710. Buckwalter JA, Lohmander S. Operative treatment of osteoarthritis: current practice and future development. *J Bone Joint Surg Am* 1994;76:1405–1418.

711. Ficat RP, Ficat C, Gedeon P, et al. Spongialization: a new treatment for diseased patellae. *Clin Orthop* 1979;144:74–83.

712. Johnson LL. Arthroscopic abrasion arthroplasty—historical and pathological perspective: Present status. *Arthroscopy* 1976; 2:54–69.

713. Pridie KH. A method of resurfacing osteoarthritic knee joints. *J Bone Joint Surg Br* 1959;41:618–619.

714. Rae PJ, Noble J. Arthroscopic drilling of ostechondral lesions of the knee. *J Bone Joint Surg Br* 1989;71:534.

715. Rand JA. Role of arthroscopy in osteoarthritis of the knee. *Arthroscopy* 1991;7:358–363.

716. Insall J. The Pridie debridement operation for osteoarthritis of the knee. *Clin Orthop* 1974;101:61–67.

717. Rodrigo JJ, Steadman JR, Silliman JF, et al. Improvement of full-thickness chondral defect healing in the human knee after debridement and microfracture using continuous passive motion. *Am J Knee Surg* 1994;7:109–116.

718. Steadman JR, Rodkey WG, Briggs KK, et al. The microfracture technic in the management of complete cartilage defects in the knee joint. *Orthopade* 1999;28:26–32.

719. Bert JM. Role of abrasion arthroplasty and debridement in the management of osteoarthritis of the knee. *Rheum Dis Clin North Am* 1993, 19:725–739.

720. Bert JM, Maschka K. The arthroscopic treatment of unicompartmental gonarthrosis: a five-year follow-up study of abrasion arthroplasty plus arthroscopic debridement and arthroscopic debrdement alone. *Arthroscopy* 1989;5:25–32.

721. Friedman MJ, Berase CC, Fox JM, et al. Preliminary results with abrasion arthroplasty in the osteoarthritic knee. *Clin Orthop* 1984;182:200–205.

722. Akizuki S, Yasukawa Y, Takizawa T. Does arthroscopic abrasion arthroplasty promote cartilage regeneration in osteoarthritic knees with eburnation? A prospective study of high tibial osteotomy with abrasion arthroplasty versus high tibial osteotomy alone. *Arthroscopy* 1997;13:9–17.

723. Coventry MB, Ilstrup DM, Wallrich SL. Proximal tibial osteotomy: a critical long-term study of eighty-seven cases. *J Bone Joint Surg Am* 1993;75:196–201.

724. Insall JN, Joseph DM, Msika C. High tibial osteotomy for varus gonarthrosis: a long-term follow-up study. *J Bone Joint Surg Am* 1984;66:1040–1048.

725. Reigstad A, Gronmark T. Osteoarthritis of the hip treated by intertrochanteric osteotomy: a long-term follow-up. *J Bone Joint Surg Am* 1984;66:1–6.

726. Weisl H. Intertrochanteric osteotomy for osteoarthritis: a long-term follow-up. *J Bone Joint Surg Br* 1980;62:37–42.

727. Radin EL, Burr DB. Hypothesis: joints can heal. *Semin Arthritis Rheum* 1984;13:293–302.

728. Fujisawa Y, Masuhara K, Shiomi S. The effect of high tibial osteotomy on osteoarthritis of the knee. *Orthop Clin North Am* 1979;10:585.

729. Byers PD. The effect of high femoral osteotomy on osteoarthritis of the hip: an anatomical study of six hip joints. *J Bone Joint Surg Br* 1974;56:279–290.

730. Itoman M, Yamamoto M, Yonemoto K, et al. Histological examination of surface repair tissue after successful osteotomy for osteoarthirtis of the hip joint. *Int Orthop* 1992;16:118–121.

731. Odenbring S, Egund N, Lindstrand A, et al. Cartilage regeneration after proximal tibial osteotomy for medial gonarthrosis: an arthroscopic, roentgenographic, and histologic study. *Clin Orthop* 1992;277:219–216.

732. Bayne O, Langer F, Pritzker KP, et al. Osteochondral allografts in the treatment of osteonecrosis of the knee. *Orthop Clin North Am* 1985;16:727–740.

733. Beaver RJ, Mahomed M, Backstein D, et al. Fresh osteochondral allografts for post-traumatic defects in the knee: a survivorship analysis. *J Bone Joint Surg Br* 1992;74:105–110.

734. Convery FR, Meyers MH, Akeson WH. Fresh osteochondral allografting of the femoral condyle. *Clin Orthop* 1991;273:139–145.

735. Gross AE, Beaver RJ, Majomed MH. Gresh small fragment osteochondral allografts used for posttraumatic defects in the knee joint. In: Finerman GAM, Noyes FR, eds. *Biology and biomechanics of the traumatized synovial joint: the knee as a model.* Rosemont, IL: American Academy of Orthopaedic Surgeons, 1992:123–141.

736. Mahomed MN, Beaver RJ, Gross AE. The long-term success of fresh, small fragment osteochondral allografts used for intraarticular post-traumatic defects in the knee joint. *Orthopedics* 1992;15:1191–1199.

737. Newman AP. Articular cartilage repair. *Am J Sports Med* 1998;26:309–324.

738. Langer F, Czitrom A, Pritzker KP, et al. The immunogenicity of fresh and frozen allogeneic bone. *J Bone Joint Surg* 1975; 57:216.

739. Langer F, Gross AE. Immunogenicity of allograft articular cartilage. *J Bone Joint Surg* 1974;56:297.

740. Schachar N, McAllister D, Stevenson M, et al. Metabolic and biochemical status of articular cartilage following cryopreservation and transplantation: a rabbit model. *J Orthop Res* 1992; 10:603.

741. Schachar NS, McGann LE. Investigations of low-temperature storage of articular cartilage for transplantation. *Clin Orthop* 1986;208:146.

742. Tomford WW, Duff GP, Mankin HJ. Experimental freeze-preservation of chondrocytes. *Clin Orthop* 1985;197:11.

743. Bobic V. Arthroscopic osteochondral autograft transplantation in anterior cruciate ligament reconstruction: a preliminary clinical study. *Knee Surg Sports Truamatol Arthrosc* 1996;3: 262–264.

744. Matsusue Y, Yamamuro T, Hama H. Arthroscopic multiple osteocondral transplantation to the chondral defect in the knee associated with anterior cruciate ligament disruption. *Arthroscopy* 1993;9:318–321.

745. Yamashita F, Sakakida K, Suzu F, et al. The transplantation of an autogeneic osteochondral fragment for osteochondritis dissecans of the knee. *Clin Orthop* 1985;201:43–50.

746. Outerbridge KK, Outerbridge AR, outerbridge RE. The use of a lateral patellar autogenous graft for the repair of a large osteochondral defect in the knee. *J Bone Joint Surg Am* 1995; 66:65–72.

747. Hangody L. Autogenous osteochondral graft technique for replacing knee cartilage defects in dogs. *Orthopedics Int* 1997; 5:175–181.

748. Takahashi S, Oka M, Kotoura Y, et al. Autogenous callo-osseous grafts for the repair of osteochondral defects. *J Bone Joint Surg Br* 1995;77:194–204.

749. Hangody L. Mosaicplasty for repair of articular cartilage defects. Proceedings of the 2nd Freibourg International Sympo-

sium on Cartilage Repair, Freibourg, Switzerland, October, 1997.

750. Garrett JC. Fresh osteochondral allografts for treatment of articular defects in osteochondritis dissecans of the lateral femoral condyle in adults. *Clin Orthop* 1994;303:33–37.

751. Desjardins MR, Hurtig MB, Palmer NC. Heterotoopic transfer of fresh and cryopreserved autogenous articular cartilage in the horse. *Vet Surg* 1991;20:434–445.

752. Hangody L, Kish G, Karpati Z, et al. Treatment of osteochondritis dissecans of the talus: use of the mosaicplasty technique-a preliminary report. *Foot Ankle Int* 1997;18:628.

753. Hangody L, Kish G, Karpati Z, et al. Arthroscopic autogenous osteochondral mosaicplasty for the treatment of femoral condylar articular defects. A preliminary report. *Knee Surg Sports Traumatol Arthrosc* 1997;5:262.

754. Minas T, Nehrer S. Current concepts in the treatment of articular cartilage defects. *Orthopedics* 1997;20:525.

755. Osborn KD, Trippel SB, Mankin HJ. Growth factor stimulation of adult articular cartilage. *J Orthop Res* 1989;7:35–42.

756. Sachs BL, Goldberg VM, Moskowitz RW, et al. Response of articular chondrocytes to pituitary fibroblast growth factor (FGF). *J Cell Physiol* 1982;112:51–59.

757. Sah RL, Chen AC, Grodzinsky AJ, et al. Differential effects of bFGF and IGF-I on matrix metabolism in calf and adult boine cartilage explants. *Arch Biochem Biophys* 1994;308:137–147.

758. Chin JE, Hatfield CA, Krzesicki RF, et al. Interactions between interleukin-1 and basic fibroblast growth factor on articular chondrocytes: effects on cell growth, prostanoid production and receptor modulation. *Arthritis Rheum* 1991;34: 314–324.

759. Luyten FP, Hascall VC, Nissley SP, et al. Insulin-like growth factors maintain steady-state metabolism of proteoglycans in bovine articular cartilage explants. *Arch Biochem Biophys* 1988;267:416–425.

760. Tyler JA. Insulin-like growth factor 1 can decrease degradation and promote synthesis of proteglycan in cartilage exposed to cytokines. *Biochem J* 1989;260:543–548.

761. Barone-Varelas J, Schnitzer TJ, Meng Q, et al. Age-related differences in the metabolism of proteoglycans in bovine articular cartilage explants maintained in the presence of insulin-like growth factors 1. *Connect Tissue Res* 1991;26:101–120.

762. Morales TI, Roberts AB. Transforming growth factors-beta regulates the metabolism of proteoglycans in bovine cartilage organ cultures. *J Biol Chem* 1988;263:12828–12831.

763. Florini JR, Roberts SB. Effect of rat age on blood levels of somatomedin-like growth factors. *J Gerontol* 1980;35:23–30.

764. Kumar N. Unresponsiveness of cartilage to serum somatomedins: furher observations. *Indian J Exp Biol* 1979;17: 571–573.

765. Morales TIK, Joyce ME, Sobel ME, et al. Transforming growth factor-beta in calf articular cartilage organ cultures: synthesis and distribution. *Arch Biochem Biophys* 1991;288: 397–405.

766. Guerne PA, Sublet A, Lotz M. Growth factor responsiveness of human articular chondrocytes: distinct profiles in primary chondrocytes, subcultured chondrocytes, and fibroblasts. *Cell Physiol* 1994;158:476–484.

767. Hill DJ, Han VK. Paracrinology of growth regulation. *J Dev Physiol* 1991;15:91–104.

767. Ignotz RA, Massague J. Transforming growth factor-beta stimulates the expression of fibronectin and collagen and their incorporation into the extracellular matrix. *J Biol Chem* 1986; 261:4337–4345.

768. Schonfeld HJ, Poschl B, Wessner B, et al. Altered differentiation of limb bud cells by transforming growth factors-beta isolated from bone matrix and from platelets. *Bone Miner* 1991; 13:171–189.

769. Laiho M, Saksela O, Andreasen PA, et al. Enhanced production and extracellular deposition of the endothelial-type plasminogen activator inhibitor in cultured human luing fibroblasts by transforming growth factor-beta. *J Cell Biol* 1986; 103:2403–2410.

770. Rosen DM, Stempien SA, Thompson AY, et al. Transforming growth factor-beta modulates the expression of osteoblast and chondroblast phenotypes in vitro. *J Cell Physiol* 1988;134: 337–346.

771. Rosier RN, O'Keefe RJ, Crabb ID, et al. Transforming growth factor-beta: an autocrine regulator of chondrocytes. *Connect Tissue Res* 1989;20:295–301.

772. Gelb DE, Rosier RN, Puzas JE. The production of transforming growth factor-beta by chick growth plate chondrocytes in short term monolayer culture. *Endocrinology* 1990;127–1941–1947.

773. Carrington JL, Reddi AH. Temporal changes in the response of chick limb bud mesodermal cells to transforming growth factor beta-type 1. *Exp Cell Res* 1990;186:368–373.

774. van der Kraan PM, Vitters EL, van den Berg WB. Inhibition of proteoglycan synthesis by transforming growth factor beta in anatomically intact articular cartilage of murine patellae. *Ann Rheum Dis* 1992;51:643–647.

775. Reddi AH. Regulation of cartilage and bone differentiation by bone morphogenetic proteins. *Curr Opin Cell Biol* 1992;4: 850–855.

776. Chen P, Carrington JL, Hammonds RG, et al. Stimulation of chondrogenesis in limb bud mesoderm cells by recombinant human bone morphogenetic protein 2B (BMP-2B) and modulation by transforming growth factor-beta 1 and beta 2. *Exp Cell Res* 1991, 195:509–515.

777. Lotz M, Blanco FJ, von Kempis J, et al. Cytokine regulation of chondrocytes functions. *J Rheumatol* 1995;43[Suppl]:104–108.

778. Brittberg M. *Cartilage repair: on cartilaginous tissue engineering with the emphasis on chondrocyte transplantation* [Thesis]. Goetburg, Sweden. Institute of Laboratory Medicine, Vasatdens Bokbinderi, 1996.

779. Hunziker EB, Rosenberg LC. Repair of partial thickness defects in articular cartilage: cell recruitment from synovial membrane. *J Bone Joint Surg Am* 1996;78:721–733.

780. Howell DS, Altman RD. Cartilage repair and conservation in osteoarthritis: a brief review of some experimental approaches to chondroprotection. *Rheum Dis Clin North Am* 1993;19: 713–724.

781. Hunziker EB, Rosenberg L. Induction of repair in partial thickness articular cartilage lesions by timed release of TGF-beta. *Trans Orthop Res Soc* 1994;19:236.

782. Rosenberg L, Hunziker EB. Cartilage repair in osteoarthritis: the role of dermatan sulfate proteoglycans. In: Kuettner KE, Goldberg VM, eds. *Osteoarthritic disorders*. Rosemont, IL: American Academy of Orthopaedic Surgeons, 1995:341–356.

783. Hunziker EB, Rosenberg LC. Repair of partial-thickness defects in articular cartilage: cell recruitment from the synovial membrane. *J Bone Joint Surg Am* 1996;78:721–722.

784. Altman RD, Gottlief NL, Howell DS. Cartilage degradation: is there a place for chondroprotective agents? *Semin Arthritis Rheum* 1990;19:1–30.

785. Howell DS, Altman RD. Cartilage repair and conservation in osteoarthirits: a brief review of some experimental approaches to chondroprotection. *Rheum Dis Clin North Am* 1993;19: 713–724.

786. Howell DS, Altman RD, Pelletier JP, et al. Disease modifying antirheumatic drugs: current status of their application in animal models of osteoarthritis. In: Kuettner KE, Goldberg VM, eds. *Osteoarthritic disorders*. Rosemont, IL: American Academy of Orthopaedic Surgeons, 1995:365–377.

787. Allen JB, Manthey CL, Hand AR, et al. Rapid onset synovial inflammation and hyperplasia induced by transforming growth factor beta. *J Exp Med* 1990;171:231.

788. Elford PR, Graeber M, Ohtsu H, et al. Induction of swelling, synovial hyperplasia and cartilage proteoglycan loss upon intra-articular injection of transforming growth factor beta-2 in the rabbit. *Cytokine* 1992;4:232.

789. Van Beuningen HM, Glansbeek HL, van der Kraan PM, et al. Differential effects of local application of BMP-2 or TGF-beta 1 on both articular cartilage composition and osteophyte formation. *Osteoarthritis Cartilage* 1998;6:306.

790. Salter RB, Minster RR, Bell RS, et al. Continuous passive motion and the repair of full-thickness articular cartilage defects: a one-year follow-up. *Trans Orthop Res Soc* 1982;7:167.

791. Salter RB, Simmonds DF, Malcolm BW, et al. The biological effect of continuous passive motion on healing of full-thickness defects in articular cartilage: an experimental study in the rabbit. *J Bone Joint Surg Am* 1980;62:1232–1251.

792. Kleiner JB, Coutts RD, Woo SL-Y, et al. The short term evaluation of different treatment modalities upon full thickness articular cartilage defects: a study of rib perichondrial chondrogenesis. *Trans Orthop Res Soc* 1986;11:282.

793. Kwan MK, Woo SL-Y, Amiel D, et al. Neocartilage generated from rib perichondrium: a long-term multidisciplinary evaluation. *Trans Orthop Res Soc* 1987;12:277.

794. O'Driscoll SW, Keeley FW, Salter RB. The chondrogenic potential of free autogenous periosteal grafts for biological resurfacing of major full-thickness defects in joint surfaces under the influence of continuous passive motion: an experimental study in the rabbit. *J Bone Joint Surg Am* 1986;68:1017–1035.

795. O'Driscoll SW, Salter RB. The induction of neochondrogenesis in free intra-articular periosteal antografts under the influence of continuous passive motion: an experimental study in the rabbit. *J Bone Joint Surg Am* 1984;66:1248–1257.

796. Zarnett R, Delaney JP, O'Driscoll SW, et al. Cellular origin and evolution of neochondrogenesis in major full-thickness defects of a joint surface treated by free autogenous periosteal grafts and subjected to continuous passive motion in rabbits. *Clin Orthop* 1987;222:267–274.

797. Coutts RD, Woo SL, Amiel D, et al. Rib perichondrial autografts in full-thickness aritcular cartilage defects in rabbits. *Clin Orthop* 1992;275:263–273.

798. O'Driscoll SW. Articular cartilage regeneration using periosteum. *Clin Orthop* 1999;367:S186–S203.

799. Engkvist O, Johansson SH. Perichondrial arthroplasty: a clinical study in twenty-six patients. *Scand J Plast Reconstr Surg* 1980;14:71–87.

800. Homminga GN, Bulstra SK, Kuijer R, et al. Repair of sheep articular cartilage defects with rabbit costal perichondrial graft. *Acta Orthop Scand* 1991;62:415–418.

801. Homminga GN, van der Linden TJ, Terwindt-Rouwenhorst EAW, et al. Repair of articular defects by perichondrial grafts: experiments in the rabbit. *Acta Orthop Scand* 1989;60:326–329.

802. Ohlsen L. Cartilage formation from free perichondrial grafts: an experimental study in rabbits. *Br J Plast Surg* 1976;29:262–267.

803. Skoog T, Ohlsen L, Sohn SA. Perichondrial potential for cartilaginous regeneration. *Scand J Plast Reconstr Surg* 1972;6:123–125.

804. Argun M, Baktir A, Turk CY, et al. The chondrogenic potential of free autogenous periosteal and fascial grafts for biological resurfacing of major full-thickness defects in joint surfaces (an experimental investigation in the rabbit). *Tokai J Exp Clin Med* 1993;18:107–116.

805. Curtin WA, Reville WJ, Brady MP. Quantitative and morphological observations on the ultrastructure of articular tissue generated from free periosteal grafts. *J Electron Microsc (Toyko)* 1992;41:82–90.

806. Korkala O, Kuokkanen H. Autogenous osteoperiosteal grafts in the reconstruction of full-thickness joint surface defects. *Int Orthop* 1991;15:233–237.

807. Kreder HJ, Moran M, Keeley FW, et al. Biologic resurfacing of a major joint defect with cryopreserved allogeneic periosteum under the influence of continuous passive motion in a rabbit model. *Clin Orthop* 1994;300:288–296.

808. Moran ME, Kim HK, Salter RB. Biological resurfacing of full-thickness defects in patellar articular cartilage of the rabbit: investigation of autogenous periosteal grafts subjected to continuous passive motion. *J Bone Joint Surg Br* 1992;74:659–667.

809. Ritsila VA, Santavirta S, Alhopura S, et al. Periosteal and perichondral grafting in reconstructive surgery. *Clin Orthop* 1994;302:259–265.

810. Rubak JM. Reconstruction of articular cartilage defects with free periosteal grafts: an experimental study. *Acta Orthop Scand* 1982;53:175–180.

811. Rubak JM, Poussa M, Ritsila V. Effects of joint motion on the repair of articular cartilage defects by free periosteal grafts. *Acta Orthop Scand* 1982;53:187–191.

812. Von Schroeder HP, Kwan M, Amiel D, et al. The use of polylactic acid matrix and periosteal grafts for the reconstruction of rabbit knee articular defects. *J Biomed Mater Res* 1991;25:329–339.

813. Bassett CAL. Current concepts of bone formation. *J Bone Joint Surg Am* 1962;44:1217–1244.

814. Gospodarowicz D, Delgado D, Vlodavsky I. Permissive effects of the extracellular matrix on cell proliferation in vitro. *Proc Natl Acad Sci U S A* 1980;77:4094–4098.

815. Italy S, Abramovici A, Nevo Z. Use of cultured embryonal chick epiphyseal chondrocytes as grafts for defects in chick articular cartilage. *Clin Orthop* 1987;220:284–303.

816. Skoog T, Johansson SH. The formation of articular cartilage from free perichondrial grafts. *Plast Reconstr Surg* 1976;57:59–75.

817. Homminga GN, Bulstra SK, Bouwmeester PS, et al. Perichondral grafting for cartilage lesions of the knee. *J Bone Joint Surg Br* 1990;72:1003–1007.

818. Newman AP. Articular cartilage repair. *Am J Sports Med* 1998;26:309–324.

819. Minas T, Nehrer S. Current concepts in the treatment of articular cartilage defects. *Orthopedics* 1997;20:525–538.

820. Robinson D, Halperin H, Nevo Z. Regenerating hyaline cartilage in articular defects of old chickens using implants of embryonal chick chondrocytes embedded in a new natural delivery substance. *Calcif Tissue Int* 1990;46:246–253.

821. Freed LE, Marquis JC, Nohria A, et al. Neocartilage formation in vitro and in vivo using cells cultured on synthetic biodegradable polymers. *J Biomed Mater Res* 1993;27:11–23.

822. Freed LE, Grande DA, Lingbin Z, et al. Joint resurfacing using allograft chondrocytes and synthetic biodegradable polymer scaffolds. *J Biomed Mater Res* 1994;28:891–899.

823. Freed LE, Vunjak-Novakovic G. Microgravity tissue engineering. *In Vitro Cell Dev Biol Anim* 1997;33:381–385.

824. Chu CR, Coutts RD, Yoshioka M, et al. Articular cartilage repair using allogeneic perichondrocyte-seeded biodegradable porous polylactic acid (PLA): a tissue-engineering study. *J Biomed Mater Res* 1995;29:1147–1154.

825. Muckle DS, Minns RJ. Biological response to woven carbone fibre pads in the knee: a clinical and experimental study. *J Bone Joint Surg Br* 1990;72:60–62.

826. Muckle DS, Minns RJ, Sunter JP. The synovium before and after intra-articular implantation of woven carbon fibre patches into osteochondral defects. *J Bone Joint Surg Br* 1988;70:152.

827. Brittberg M, Faxen E, Peterson L. Carbon fiber scaffolds in the treatment of early knee osteoarthritis: a prospective 4-year follow-up of 37 patients. *Clin Orthop* 1994;307:155–164.

828. Hemmen B, Archer CW, Bentley G. Repair of articular cartilage defects by carbon fibre plugs loaded with chondrocytes. *Trans Orthop Res Soc* 1991;16:278.

829. Grande DA, Pitman MI, Peterson L, et al. The repair of experimentally produced defects in rabbit articular cartilage by autologous chondrocyte implantation. *J Orthop Res* 1989;7:208:218.

830. Brittberg M, Nilsson A, Lindahl A, et al. Rabbit articular cartilage defects treated with autologous cultured chondrocytes. *Clin Orthop* 1996;326:270–283.

831. Gillogly SD, Voight M, Blackburn T. Treatment of articular cartilage defects of the knee with autologous chondrocyte implantation. *J Orthop Sports Phys Ther* 1998;28:241.

832. Minas T, Peterson L. Advanced techniques in autologous chondrocyte transplantation. *Clin Sports Med* 1999;18:13.

833. Brittberg M, Lindahl A, Nilsson A, et al. Treatment of deep cartilage defects in the knee with autologous chondrocyte transplantation. *N Engl J Med* 1994;331:889–895.

834. Mandelbaum BR, Brown JE, Fu F, et al. Articular cartilage lesions of the knee. *Am J Sports Med* 1998;26:853–861.

835. Caplan AL, Goto T, Wakitani S, et al. Cell-based technologies for cartilage repair. In: Finerman GAM, Noyes FR, eds. *Biology and biomechanics of the traumatized synovial joint: the knee as a model.* Rosemont, IL: American Academy of Orthopaedic Surgeons, 1992:111–122.

836. Nakahara H, Goldberg VM, Caplan AL. Culture-explanded human periosteal-derived cells exhibit osteochondral potential in vivo. *J Orthop Res* 1991;9:465–476.

837. Wakitani S, Goto T, Pineda SJ, et al. Mesenchymal cell-based repair of large, full-thickness defects of articular cartilage. *J Bone Joint Surg Am* 1994;76:579–592.

838. Caplan AI. Mesenchymal stem cells. *J Orthop Res* 1991;9:641–650.

839. Wakitani S, Kimura T, Hirooka A, et al. Repair of rabbit articular surfaces with allograft chondrocytes embedded in collagen gel. *J Bone Joint Surg Br* 1989;71:74–80.

840. Bandara G, Robbins PD, Georgescu HI, et al. Gene transfer to synoviocytes: prospects for gene treatment for arthritis. *DNA Cell Biol* 1992;11:227–231.

841. Evans CH, Ghivizzani SC, Kang R, et al. Gene therapy for rheumatic diseases. *Arthirtis Rheum* 1999;42:1–19.

842. Evans CH, Robbins PD, Ghiviani SC, et al. Clinical trial to assess the safety, feasibility and efficacy of transferring a potentially anti-arthritic cytokine gene to human joints with rheumatoid arthritis. *Hum Gene Ther* 1996;7:1261–1280.

843. Fernandes JL, Tradif G, Martel-Pelletier J, et al. In vivo transfer of interleukin-1 receptor antagonist gene in osteoarthritic rabbit knee joints: prevention of osteoarthritic progression. *Am J Pathol* 1999;154:1159–1169.

844. Frisbie DD, McIlwraith CW. Evaluation of gene therapy as a treatment for equine tramatic arthritis and osteoarthritis. *Clin Orthop* 2000;379S:S273–S287.

845. Pelletier P, Caron JP, Evans CH, et al. In vivo suppression of early experimental osteoarthritis by IL-1Ra using gene therapy. *Arthritis Rheum* 1997;40:1012–1019.

846. Otani K, Nita I, Macaulay W, et al. Suppression of antigen-induced arthiritis by gene therapy. *J Immunol* 1996;156:3558–3562.

847. Bakker AC, Beuningen H, Van Lent P, et al. Adenoviral-mediated transfer of active transforming growth factor-β1 in the murine knee joint induces fibrosis and osteophyte formation. *Trans Orthop Res Soc* 1999;45:411.

848. Evan CH, Chivizzani SC, Smith P, et al. Using gene therapy to protect and restore cartilage. *Clin Orthop* 2000;379S:S214–S219.

849. Arai Y, Kubo T, Kobayashi K, et al. Adenovirus-vector mediated gene transduction to chondrocytes: in vitro evaluation of therapeutic efficiency of transforming growth factor-β1 and heat shock protein 70 gene transduction. *J Rheumatol* 1997;24:1787–1795.

850. Baragi VM, Renkiewicz RR, Jordan H, et al. Transplantation of adenovirally transduced allogeneic chondrocytes into articular cartilage defects in vivo. *Osteoarthritis Cartilage* 1997;5:275–282.

851. Doherty PJ, Zhang H, Tremblay L, et al. Resurfacing of articular cartilage explants with genetically modified human chondrocytes in vitro. *Osteoarthritis Cartilage* 1998;6:153–159.

852. Kang R, Marui T, Ghivizzani SC, et al. Ex vivo gene transfer to chondrocytes in full-thickness articular cartilage defects: a feasibility study. *Osteoarthritis Cartilage* 1997;5:139–143.

853. Madry H, Trippel SB. Efficient lipid-mediated gene transfer to articular chondrocytes. *Gene Ther* 2000;7:286–291.

854. Tomita T, Hashimoto H, Tomita N, et al. In vivo direct gene transfer into articular cartilage by intraarticular injection mediated by HVJ (sendai) virus and liposomes. *Arthritis Rheum* 1997;40:901–906.

855. Baragi VM, Renkiewicz RR, Qiu L, et al. Transplantation of adenovirally transduced allogeneic chondrocytes into articular cartilage defects in vivo. *Osteoarthritis Cartilage* 1997;5:275–282.

856. Ikeda T, Kubao T, Arai Y, et al. Adenovirus mediated gene delivery to the joints of guinea pigs. *J Rheumatol* 1998;25:1666–1673.

857. Mason JM, Grande DA, Barcia M, et al. Expression of human bone morphogenentic protein 7 in primary rabbit periosteal cells: potential utility in gene therapy for osteochondral repair. *Gene Ther* 1998;5:1098–1104.

858. Oyama M, Tatlock A, Fukuta S, et al. Retrovirally transduced bone marrow stromal cells isolated from a mouse model of human osteogenesis imperfecta (oim) persists in bone and retains the ability to form cartilage and bone after extended passaging. *Gene Ther* 1999;6:321–329.

859. Shuler FD, Georgescu HI, Niyibizi C, et al. Increased matrix synthesis following adenoviral transfer of transforming growth factor-β1 gene into articular chondrocytes. *J Orthop Res* 2000;18:585–592.

860. Nixon AJ, Brower-Toland BD, Bent SS, et al. Insulin-like growth factor-1 gene therapy in cartilage repair and degenerative joint diseases. *Clin Orthop* 2000;379:S201–S213.

861. Smith P, Shuler FD, Georgescu HI, et al. Genetic enhancement of matrix synthesis by articular chondrocytes: comparison of different growth factors in the presence or absence of interleukin-1. *Arthritis Rheum* 2000;43:1156–1164.

862a. Breinan HA, Minas T, Barone L, et al. Histological evaluation of the course of healing of canine articular cartilage defects treated with cultured autologous chondrocytes. *Tissue Eng* 1998;4:101–114.

862b. Mason JM, Breitbart AS, Barcia M, et al. Cartilage and bone regeneration using gene enhanced tissue engineering. *Clin Orthop* 2000;379:S171–S178.

Meniscus References

863. Sutton JB. *Ligaments. their nature and morphology.* London: MK Lewis & Co., 1897.

864. Unnecessary meniscectomy [Editorial]. *Lancet* 1976;1:235–236.

865. Fairbank TJ. Knee joint changes after meniscectomy. *J Bone Joint Surg Br* 1948;30:664–670.

866. Jackson JP. Degenerative changes in the knee after meniscectomy. *Br Med J* 1968;2:525–527.

867. Johnson RJ, Kettelkamp DB, Clark W, et al. Factors affecting late results after meniscectomy. *J Bone Joint Surg Am* 1974; 56:719–729.

868. McGinty JB, Geuss LF, Marvin RA. Partial or total meniscectomy: a comparative analysis. *J Bone Joint Surg Am* 1 977;59: 763–766.

869. Smillie IS. *Injuries of the knee joint,* 4th ed. Edinburgh: E and S Livingstone, 1970;61.

870. Tapper EM, Hoover NW. Late results after meniscectomy. *J Bone Joint Surg Am* 1969;51:517–526.

871. Cox JS, Cordell LD. The degenerative effects of medial meniscus tears in dogs' knees. *Clin Orthop* 1977;125:236–242.

872. Korkala O, Karaharju E, Gronblad M, et al. Articular cartilage and meniscectomy: rabbit knees studied with the scanning electron microscope. *Acta Orthop Scand* 1984;55:273–277.

873. Lufti AM. Morphological changes in the articular cartilage after meniscectomy: an experimental study in the monkey. *J Bone Joint Surg Br* 1975;57:525–528.

874. Shapiro F, Glimcher MJ. Induction of osteoarthrosis in the rabbit knee. *Clin Orthop* 1980;147:287–295.

875. Cox JS, Nye DE, Schaefer WW, et al. The degenerative effects of partial and total resection of the medial meniscus in dog's knees. *Clin Orthop* 1975;109:178–183.

876. Floman Y, Eyre DR, Glimcher MJ. Induction of osteoarthrosis in the rabbit knee joint: biochemical studies on the articular cartilage. *Clin Orthop* 1980;147:278.

877. Gao J, Oqvist G, Messner K. The attachment of the rabbit medial meniscus: a morphological investigation using image analysis and immunohistochemistry. *J Anat* 1994;185:663–667.

878. Ghadially FN, Thomas I, Yong N, et al. Ultrastructure of rabbit semilunar cartilages. *J Anat* 1978;125:499–517.

879. Moon NS, Kim JM. Ok IY. The normal and regenerated meniscus in rabbits: morphologic and histologic studies. *Clin Orthop* 1982;182:264–269.

880. Webber RJ, Harris MG, Hough Jr AJ. Cell culture of rabbit mesnical fibrochondrocytes: proliferative and synthetic response to growth factors and ascorbate. *J Orthop Res* 1985; 3:36–42.

881. O'Connor BL. The histological structure of dog knee menisci with comments on its possible significance. *Am J Anat* 1976; 147:407–418.

882. O'Connor BL. The mechanoreceptor innervation of the posterior attachments of the lateral meniscus of the dog knee joint. *J Anat* 1984;1:15–26.

883. Adams ME, Muir H. The glycoaminoglycans of canine menisci. *Biochem J* 1981;197:385–389.

884. Swiontkowski MF, Schlehr F, Sanders R. Direct, real time measurement of meniscal blood flow: an experimental investigation in sheep *Am J Sports Med* 1988;16:429–433.

885. Ghadially FN, Wedge JH, Lalonde J-MA. Experimental methods of repairing injured menisci. *J Bone Joint Surg Br* 1976; 68:106–110.

886. Proctor CS, Schmidt MR, Whipple RR, et al. Material properties of the normal medial bovine meniscus. *J Orthop Res* 1989;7:771–782.

887. Skaggs DL Warden WH, Mow VC. Radial tie fibers influence the tensile properties of the bovine medial meniscus. *J Orthop Res* 1994;12:176–185.

888. Cheung HS. Distribution of type I, II, III and V in the pepsin solubilized collagen in bovine menisci. *Connect Tissue Res* 1987;16:343–356.

889. Bullough PG, Munuera L, Murphy J, et al. The strength of the menisci of the knee as it relates to their fine structure. *J Bone Joint Surg Br* 1970;52:564–570.

890. Aspden RM, Yarker YE, Hukins DWL. Collagen orientations in the meniscus of the knee joint. *J Anat* 1985;140:371–380.

891. Mow VC, Whipple RR. Biology and mechanical properties of cartilage and menisci. In: *AAOS Committee on Basic Sciences: Williamsburg Seminar, 1984. Resource for basic science educators.* Park Ridge, IL: American Academy of Orthopaedic Surgeons, 1984;165–197.

892. King D. The function of semilunar cartilages. *J Bone Joint Surg* 1936;18:1069–1076.

893. Walker PS, Erkman MJ. The role of the menisci in force transmission across the knee. *Clin Orthop* 1975;109:184–192.

894. Shrive NG, O'Connor JJ, Goodfellow JW. Load-bearing in the knee joint. *Clin Orthop* 1978;131:279–287.

895. Seedholm BB, Hargreaves DJ. Transmission of the load in the knee joint with special reference to the role of the menisci. *Eng Med* 1979;8:220–228.

896. MacConaill MA. The function of intra-articular fibrocartilages, with special reference to the knee and inferior radio-ulnar joints. *J Anat* 1932;66:210–227.

897. Peters TJ, Smillie IS. Studies on the chemical composition of the menisci of the knee joint with special reference to the horizontal cleavage lesion. *Clin Orthop* 1972;86:245–252.

898. Eyre DR, Wu JJ. Collagen of fibrocartilage: a distinctive molecular phenotype in bovine meniscus. *FEBS Lett* 1983; 158:265–270.

899. Habuchi H, Yamagata T, Iwata H, et al. The occurrence of a wide variety of dermatan sulfate-chondroitin sulfate copolymers in fibrous cartilage. *J Biol Chem* 1973;248:6019–6028.

900. McNicol D, Roughley PJ. Extraction and characterization of proteoglycan from human meniscus. *Biochem J* 1980;185: 705–713.

901. Roughley PJ, McNicol D, Santer V, et al. The presence of a cartilage-like proteoglycan in the adult human meniscus. *Biochem J* 1981,;197:77–83.

902. Norby DP, Goldberg VM, Malemud CJ, et al. Proteoglycans from pig menisci: major differences from proteoglycans of articular cartilage. *Trans Orthop Res Soc* 1982;7:116.

903. Fife RS. Identification of link proteins and a 116,000-dalton matrix protein in canine meniscus. *Arch Biochem Biophys* 1985;240:682–688.

904. Ghadially FN, Thomas I, Yong N, et al. Ultrastructure of rabbit semilunar cartilages. *J Anat* 1978;125:499–517.

905. Nakano T, Thompson JR, Aherne FX. Distribution of glycosaminoglycans and the nonreducible collagen crosslink, pyridinoline in porcine menisci. *Can J Vet Res* 1986;50: 532–536.

906. Adams ME, Muir H. The glycosaminoglycans of canine menisci. *Biochem J* 1981;197:385–389.

907. Adams ME, McDevitt CA, Ho A, et al. Isolation and characterization of high-buoyant-density proteoglycans from semilunar menisci. *J Bone Joint Surg Am* 1986;68:55–64.

908. Adams ME, Ho YA. Localization of glycosaminoglycans in human and canine menisci and their attachments. *Connect Tissue Res* 1987;16:269–279.

909. Fife RS, Hook GL, Brandt KD. Topographic localization of a 116,000-dalton protein in cartilage. *J Histochem Cytochem* 1985;33:127–133.

910. Clark CR, Ogden JA. Development of the menisci of the human knee joint: morphological changes and their potential role in childhood meniscal injury. *J Bone Joint Surg Am* 1984;65: 538–547.

911. O'Connor BL. Histological structure of dog knee menisci with comments on its possible significance. *Am J Anat* 1976;147: 407–417.

912. Bullough PG, Vosburg F, Arnoczky SP, et al.: The menisci of the knee. In: Insall JN, ed. *Surgery of the knee.* New York: Churchill Livingstone, 1984;135–146.

913. Warren R, Arnoczky SP, Wickiewicz TL. Anatomy of the knee. In: Nicholas JA, Hershman EB, eds. *The lower extremity and spine in sports medicine.* St. Louis: CV Mosby, 1986;657–694.

914. Arnoczky SP. Gross and vascular anatomy of the meniscus and its role in meniscal healing, regeneration, and remodelling. In: Mow VC, Arnoczky SP, Jackson DW, eds. *Knee meniscus: basic science and clinical foundations.* New York: Raven Press, 1992;177–190.

915. Hough AJ, Sokoloff L. Tissue sampling as a potential source of error in experimental studies of cartilage. *Connect Tissue Res* 1975;3:27–31.

916. Rosenberg L. Chemical basis for the histological use of safranin O in the study of articular cartilage. *J Bone Joint Surg Am* 1971;53:69.

917. Kiviranta I, Jurvelin J, Tammi M, et al. Microspectrophotometric quantification of glycosaminoglycans in articular cartilage sections stained with safranin O. *Histochemistry* 1985;82:249.

918. Hellio Le Graverand MP, Ou YC, et al. The cells of the rabbit meniscus: their arrangement, interrelationship, morphological variations and cytoarchitecture. *J Anat* 2001 *(in press).*

919. Herwig J, Egner E, Buddecke E. Chemical changes of human knee joint menisci in various stages of degeneration. *Ann Rheum Dis* 1984;43:635–640.

920. Wu JJ, Eyre DR, Slatter HS. Type VI collagen of the intervertebral disc: biochemical and electron microscopic characterization of the native protein. *Biochem J* 1987;248:373–381.

921. Bland YS, Ashhurst DE. Changes in the content of the fibrillar collagens and the expression of their mRNAs in the menisci of the rabbit knee joint during development and ageing. *Histochemical J* 1996;28:265–274.

922. Eyre DR, Oguchi H. The hydroxypyridinium crosslinks of skeletal collagens: their measurement, properties and a proposed pathway of formation. *Biochem Biophys Res Commun* 1980;92:403–410.

923. Yasui K. Three dimensional architecture of human normal menisci. *J Jpn Orthop Assoc* 1978;52:391–399.

924. Nakano T, Dodd CM, Scott PG. Glycosaminoglycans and proteoglycans from different zones of the porcine knee meniscus. *J Orthop Res* 1997;15:213–222.

925. Scott PG, Nakano T, Dodd CM. Isolation and characterization of small proteoglycans from different zones of the porcine knee meniscus. *Biochimica et Biophysica Acta* 1997;1336:254–262.

926. Collier S, Ghosh P. Effect of transforming growth factor beta on proteoglycan synthesis by cell and explant cultures derived from the knee joint meniscus. *Osteoarthritis Cartilage* 1995;3:127–138.

927. Favenesi JA, Shaffer JC, Mow VC. Biphasic mechanical properties of knee meniscus. *Trans Orthop Res Soc* 1983;8:57.

928. Arnoczky SP, Warren RF. Microvasculature of the human meniscus. *Am J Sports Med* 1982;10:90–95.

929. Danzig L, Resnick D, Gonsalves M, et al. Blood supply to the normal and abnormal menisci of the human knee. *Clin Orthop* 1983;172:271–276.

930. Day B, MacKenzie WG, Shim SS, et al. The vascular and nerve supply of the human meniscus. *Arthroscopy* 1985;1:58–62.

931. Arnoczky SP, Marshall JL, Joseph A, et al. Meniscal diffusion: an experimental study. *Trans Orthop Res Soc* 1980;5:42.

932. Noble J, Hamblen DL. The pathology of the degenerative meniscus lesions. *J Bone Joint Surg Br* 1975;57:180–186.

933. Peters TJ, Smillie IS. Studies on the chemical composition of the menisci of the knee joint with special reference to the horizontal cleavage lesions. *Clin Orthop* 1972;86:245–252.

934. Bird MDT, Sweet MDBE. A system of canals in semilunar menisci. *Ann Rheum Dis* 1987;46:670–673.

935. Bird MDT, Sweet MDE. Canals in the semilunar meniscus: brief report. *J Bone Joint Surg Br* 1988;70:839.

936. O'Connor BL, McConnaughey JS. The structure and innervation of cat knee menisci, and their relation to a "sensory hypothesis" of meniscal function. *Am J Anat* 1978;153:431–442.

937. Wilson AS, Legg PG, McNeur JC. Studies on the innervation of the medial meniscus in the human knee joint. *Anat Rec* 1969;165:485–492.

938. Kennedy JC, Alexander IJ, Hayes KL. Nerve supply of the human knee and its functional importance. *Am J Sports Med* 1982;10:329–335.

939. O'Connor BL. The mechanoreceptor innervation of the posterior attachment of the lateral meniscus of the dog knee joint. *J Anat* 1984;138:15–26.

940. Zimny ML, Albright DL, Dabeziew E. Mechanoreceptors in the human medial meniscus. *Acta Anat* 1988;133:35–40.

941. Brantigan OC, Voshell AF. The mechanics of the ligaments and menisci of the knee joint. *J Bone Joint Surg* 1941;23:44–66.

942. Wang C-J, Walker PS. Rotary laxity of the human knee joint. *J Bone Joint Surg Am* 1974;56:161–170.

943. Hsieh H-H, Walker PS. Stabilizing mechanisms of the loaded and unloaded knee joint. *J Bone Joint Surg Am* 1976;58:87–93.

944. Markolf KL, Bargar WL, Shoemaker SC, et al. The role of joint load in knee stability. *J Bone Joint Surg Am* 1981;63:570–585.

945. Markolf KL, Mensch JS, Amstutz HC. Stiffness and laxity of the knee: the contributions of the supporting structures. *J Bone Joint Surg Am* 1976;58:583–593.

946. Fukubayashi T, Torzilli PA, Sherman MF, et al. An in vitro biomechanical evaluation of anterior-posterior motion of the knee: tibial displacement, rotation, and torque. *J Bone Joint Surg Am* 1982;64:258–264.

947. Levy IM, Torzilli PA, Warren RF. The effect of medial menisectomy on anterior-posterior motion of the knee. *J Bone Joint Surg Am* 1982;64:883–888.

948. Shoemaker SC, Markholf KL. The role of the meniscus in the anterior-posterior stability of the loaded anterior cruciate-deficient knee. *J Bone Joint Surg Am* 1986;68:71–79.

949. Kettlekamp DB, Jacobs AW. Tibiofemoral contact area-determination and implications. *J Bone Joint Surg Am* 1972;54:349–356.

950. Fukubayashi T, Kurosawa H. The contact area and pressure distribution pattern of the knee: a study of normal and osteoarthrotic knee joints. *Acta Orthop Scand* 1980;51:871–879.

951. Ahmed AM, Burke DL. In-vitro measurement of static pressure distribution in synovial joints: part 1. Tibial surface of the knee. *J Biomech Eng* 1983;105:216–225.

952. Brantigan OC, Voshell AF. The mechanics of the ligaments and menisci of the knee joint. *J Bone Joint Surg Am* 1941;23:44–66

953. Bylski-Austrow DI, Ciarelli MR, Kayner DC, et al. Displacement of the menisci under joint load: an in vitro study in human knees. *J Biomechanics* 1994;27:421–431.

954. Kapandji IA. *The physiology of joints,* 5th ed, vol 2. Edinburgh: Livingstone, 1987:94–96.

955. Thompson WO, Thaete FL, Fu FH, et al. Tibial meniscal dynamics using three-dimensional reconstruction of magnetic resonance images. *Am J Sports Med* 1991;19:210–216.

956. Mow VC, Holmes MH, Lai WM. Fluid transport and me-

chanical properties of articular cartilage: a review. *J Biomech* 1984;17:377–394.

957. Mow VC, Kuei SC, Lai WM, et al. Biphasic creep and stress relaxation of articular cartilage in compression: theory and experiments. *J Biomech Eng* 1980;102:73–84.

958. Mow VC, Fithian DC, Kelly MA. Fundamentals of articular cartilage and meniscus biomechanics. In: Ewing JW ed. *Articular cartilage and knee joint function.* New York: Raven Press, 1990:12.

959. Ahmed AM. The load-bearing role of the knee mesnici. In: Mow VC, Arnoczky SP, Jackson DW, eds. *Knee meniscus: basic and clinical foundations.* New York: Raven Press, 1992:59–73.

960. Baratz ME, Fu FH, Mengato R. Meniscal tears: the effect of meniscectomy and repair on intra-articular contact areas and stresses in the human knee. *Am J Sports Med* 1986;14:270–275.

961. Seedholm BB, Hargreaves DJ. Transmission of the load in the knee joint with special reference to the role of the menisci: II. *Eng Med* 1979;8:220–228.

962. Higuchi H, Kimura M, Shirakura K, et al. Factors affecting long-term results after arthroscopic partial meniscectomy. *Clin Orthop* 2000;377:161–168.

963. Schimmer RC, Brulhart KB, Duff C, et al. Arthroscopic partial meniscectomy: a 12-year follow-up and two-step evaluation of the long-term course. *Arthroscopy* 1998;14:136–142.

964. Covall DJ, Wasilewski SA. Roentgenographic changes after arthroscopic meniscectomy: five-year follow-up in patients more than 45 years old. *Arthroscopy* 1992;8:242–246.

965. Abdon P, Turner MS, Pettersson H, et al. A long-term follow-up study of total meniscectomy in children. *Clin Orthop* 1990;257:166—1170.

966. McNicholas MJ, Rowley DI, McGurty D, et al. Total meniscectomy in adolescence: a thirty-year follow-up. *J Bone Joint Surg Br* 2000;82:217–221.

967. Rockborn P, Messner K. Long-term results of meniscus repair and meniscectomy: a 13-year functional and radiographic follow-up study. *Knee Surg Sports Traumatol Assoc* 2000;8:2–10.

968. Kruger-Franke M, Siebert CH, et al. Late results after arthroscopic partial medial meniscectomy. *Knee Surg Sports Traumatol Arthrosc* 1999;7:81–84.

969. Dai L, Zhang W, Xu Y. Meniscal injury in children: long-term results after meniscectomy. *Knee Surg Sports Traumatol Arthrosc* 1997;5:77–79.

970. Matsusue Y, Thomson NL. Arthroscopic partial medial meniscectomy in patients over 40 years old: a 5- to 11-year follow-up study. *Arthroscopy* 1996;12:39–44.

971. Rangger C, Klestil T, Gloetzer W, et al. Osteoarthritis after arthroscopic partial meniscectomy. *Am J Sports Med* 1995;23:240–244.

972. Benedetto KP, Rangger C. Arthroscopic partial meniscectomy: 5- year follow-up. *Knee Surg Sports Traumatol Arthrosc* 1993;1:235–238.

973. Seedhom BB, Hargreaves DJ. Transmission of the load in the knee joint with special reference to the role of the menisci: part II: Experimental results, discussion and conclusions. *Eng Med* 1979;4:220–228.

974. Gao J, Messner K. Natural healing of anterior and posterior attachments of the rabbit meniscus. *Clin Orthop* 1996;328:276–284.

975. Paletta GA Jr, Manning T, Snell E, et al. The effect of allograft meniscal replacement on intraarticular contact area and pressures in the human knee: a biomechanical study. *Am J Sports Med* 1997;25:692–698.

976. Sommerlath K, Gillquist J. The effect of a meniscus prosthesis on knee biomechanics and cartilage: an experimental study in rabbits. *Am J Sports Med* 1992;20:73–81.

977. Krause WR, Pope MH, Johnson RJ, et al. Mechanical changes in the knee after meniscectomy. *J Bone Joint Surg Am* 1976;58:599–604.

978. Kurosawa H, Fukubayashi T, Nakajima H. Load-bearing mode of the knee joint: physical behavior of the knee joint with or without menisci. *Clin Orthop* 1980;149:283–290.

979. Radin EL, Rose RM. Role of subchondral bone in the initiation and progression of cartilage damage. *Clin Orthop* 1986;213:34–40.

980. Woo SL-Y, Mow VC, Lai WM. Biomechanical properties of articular cartilage. In: Skalak R, Chein S, eds. *Handbook of bioengineering.* New York: McGraw-Hill, 1987;4.1–4.41.

981. Voloshin AS, Wosk J. Shock absorption of meniscectomized and painful knees: a comparative in vivo study. *J Biomed Eng* 1983;5:157–161.

982. Oretorp N, Gillquist J, Liljedahl S-0. Long term results of surgery for non-acute anteromedial rotatory instability of the knee. *Acta Orthop Scand* 1979;50:329–336.

983. Bargar WL, Moreland JR, Markolf KL, et al. In vivo stability testing of post-meniscectomy knees. *Clin Orthop* 1980;150:247–252.

984. Dandy DJ, Jackson RW. The diagnosis of problems after meniscectomy. *J Bone Joint Surg Br* 1975;57:349–352.

985. Bourne RB, Finlay JB, Papadopoulos P, et al. The effect of medial meniscectomy on strain distribution in the proximal part of the tibia. *J Bone Joint Surg Am* 1984;66:1481–1437.

986. Korkala O, Karaharju E, Gronblad M, et al. Articular cartilage after meniscectomy: rabbit knees studied with the scanning electron microscope. *Acta Orthop Scand* 1984;55:273–277.

987. Moskowitz RW. Osteoarthritis: studies with experimental models. *Arthritis Rheum* 1977;20:S104–SIO8.

988. Moskowitz RW, Howell DS, Goldberg VM, et al. Cartilage proteoglycan alterations in an experimentally induced model of rabbit osteoarthritis. *Arthritis Rheum* 1979;22:155–163.

989. Arnoczky SP, Cooper DE. Meniscal repair. In: Goldberg VM, ed. *Controversies of total knee arthroplasty.* New York: Raven Press, 1991:291–302.

990. Arnoczky SP, Warren RF. The microvasculature of the meniscus and its response to injury: an experimental study in the dog. *Am J Sports Med* 1983;11:131–141.

991. Cabaud HE, Rodkey WB, Fitzwater JE. Medial meniscus repairs: an experimental and morphologic study. *Am J Sports Med* 1981;9:129–134.

992. Heatley FW. The meniscus: can it be repaired? An experimental study in the rabbit. *J Bone Joint Surg Br* 1980;62:397–402.

993. Cassidy RE, Shaffer AJ. Repair of peripheral meniscus tears: a preliminary report. *Am J Sports Med* 1981;9:209–214.

994. DeHaven KE. Peripheral meniscus repair: an alternative to meniscectomy. *Orthop Trans* 1981;5:399–400.

995. Hamberg P, Gillquist J, Lysholm J. Suture of new and old peripheral meniscus tears. *J Bone Joint Surg Am* 1983;65:193–197.

996. Wirth CR. Meniscus repair. *Clin Orthop* 1981;157:153–160.

997. Newman AP, Anderson DR, Daniels AU, et al. Mechanics of the healed meniscus in a canine model. *Am J Sports Med* 1989;17:164–175.

998. Okuda K, Ochi M, Shu N, et al. Meniscal rasping for repair of meniscal tear in the avascular zone. *Arthroscopy* 1999;15:281–286.

999. Kawai Y, Fukubayashi T, Nishino J. Meniscal suture: an experimental study in the dog. *Clin Orthop* 1989;243:286–293.

1000. Roeddecker K, Muennich U, Nagelschmidt M. Meniscal healing: a biomechanical study. *J Surg Res* 1994;56:20–27.

1001. Port J, Jackson DW, Lee TQ, et al. Meniscal repair supplemented with exogenous fibrin clot and autogenous cultured marrow cells in the goat model. *Am J Sports Med* 1996;24:547–555.

1002. DeHaven K, Arnoczky SP. Meniscal repair: part I. Basic science, indications for repair, and open repair. *J Bone Joint Surg Am* 1994;76:140–152.

1003. McAndrews PT, Arnoczky SP. Meniscal repair enhancement techniques. *Clin Sports Med* 1996;15:499–510.

1004. Henning CE, Lynch MA, Clark JR. Vascularity for healing of mesnicus repairs. *Arthroscopy* 1987;3:13–18.

1005. Ritchie JR, Miller MD, Bents RT, et al. Meniscal repair in the goat model: the use of healing adjuncts on central tears and the role of magnetic resonance arthrography in repair evaluation. *Am J Sports Med* 1998;26:278–284.

1006. Nakhostine M, Gershuni DH, Anderson R, et al. Effects of abrasion therapy on tears in the avascular region of the sheep menisci. *Arthroscopy* 1990;6:280–287.

1007. Fox JM, Rintz KG, Ferkel RD. Trephination of incomplete meniscal tears. *Arthroscopy* 1993;9:451–455.

1008. Nakhostine M, Gershuni DH, Danzig LA. Effects of an insubstance conduit with injection of a blood clot on tears in the avascular region of the meniscus. *Acta Orthop Belg* 1991;57: 242–246.

1009. Arnoczky SP, Warren RF, Spivak J. Meniscal repair using an exogenous fibrin clot: an experimental study in the dog. *J Bone Joint Surg Am* 1988;70:1207–1217.

1010. Van Trommel MF, Simonian PT, Potter HG, et al. Arthroscopic meniscal repair with fibrin clot of complete radial tears of the lateral meniscus in the avascular zone. *Arthroscopy* 1998;14:360–365.

1011. Henning CE, Lynch MA, Yearout KM, et al. Arthroscopic meniscal repair using an exogenous fibrin clot. *Clin Orthop* 1990;252:64–72.

1012. Henning CE, Yearout KM, Vequist SW, et al. Use of the fascia sheath coverage and exogenous fibrin clot in the treatment of meniscal tears. *Am J Sports Med* 1991;19:626–631.

1013. Ishimura M, Ohgushi H, Habata T, et al. Arthroscopic meniscal repair using fibrin glue: part I. Experimental study. *Arthroscopy* 1997;13:551–557.

1014. Hashimoto J, Kurosaka M, Yoshiya, et al. Meniscal repair using fibrin sealant and endothelial cell growth factors: an experimental study in dogs. *Am J Sports Med* 1992;20:537–541.

1015. Bhargava MM, Attia ET, Murrell GA, et al. The effect of cytokines on the proliferation and migration of bovine meniscal cells. *Am J Sports Med* 1999;27:636–643.

1016. Goto H, Shuler FD, Lamsam C, et al. Transfer of lacZ marker gene to the meniscus. *J Bone Joint Surg Am* 1999;81:918–925.

1017. Goto H, Shuler FD, Niyibizi C, et al. Gene therapy for meniscal injury: enhanced synthesis of proteoglycan and collagen by mesnical cells transduced with a TGFbeta(1) gene. *Osteoarthritis Cartilage* 2000;8:266–271.

1018. Sonoda M Harwood FL, Amiel ME, et al. The effects of hyaluronan on tissue healing after meniscus injury and repair in a rabbit model. *Am J Sports Med* 2000;28:90–97.

1019. Ishima M, Wada Y, Sonoda M, et al. Effects of hyaluronan on the healing of rabbit meniscus injured in the peripheral region. *J Orthop Sci* 2000;5:579–584.

CARTILAGE REPAIR AND REGENERATION

TOM MINAS
JULIE GLOWACKI

CARTILAGE STRUCTURE AND FUNCTION

Chondrocyte as an Anabolic and Catabolic Cell

Chondrocytes are highly specialized cells that differentiate from clusters of mesenchymal cells during skeletal embryogenesis. The chondrocyte synthesizes and secretes the components of the extracellular matrix, primarily proteoglycans and collagen type II. Most of the immature cartilage is temporary, to be replaced by bone during epiphyseal development, whereas the regions nearest the synovial cavity remain as the permanent articular cartilage of the adult. During growth and development, immature cartilage undergoes cellular replication in both the superficial and deep zones. However, as skeletal maturity approaches, replication occurs only in the deep zone. It is rare to see cell replication after skeletal maturity. The cell content of articular cartilage is low, occupying no more than 10% of the tissue volume in humans. Cell density has been estimated as 10^5 cells/mm^3 in newborns and one-tenth of that in adult cartilage. Values are higher in the superficial zones than in the deeper zones. Experimental animals have far greater cellularity; adult rabbits, for example, have nearly tenfold greater cell density than human cartilage, and mice have 25-fold greater cell density (1). The general cellular morphology ranges from flattened and discoidal in the most superficial zones to ovoid in the deeper regions. The ovoid cells display enlarged Golgi bodies, a characteristic of cells actively secreting proteins, and cellular processes that extend into the adjacent pericellular matrix.

Chondrocytes are normally long-lived cells, not replaced by new cells as occurs as part of the turnover of other tissues. The capacity for cell division is manifest however, when the integrity of the matrix is compromised, as in osteoarthritis.

Cartilage fibrillation is associated with necrosis in the superficial zone and clusters of cells in deep zones. Metabolic studies show increased sulfate incorporation by the cells in the clusters surrounded by proteoglycan-poor matrix. If viewed as an attempt to repair, the cells in clusters are active in matrix synthesis, but they are not capable of replacement of matrix at distances from the clusters. Thus, the overall content of proteoglycan is low in fibrillated cartilage.

Chondrocytes are embedded in an avascular matrix in which nutrients and waste products must diffuse. Oxygen tension is approximately one-third that measured between capillaries in soft tissues. On a per cell basis, oxygen uptake is one-fiftieth that of kidney, but the rate of glycolysis is comparable. Thus, chondrocytes engage in relatively anaerobic metabolism.

Chondrocytes are dynamic cells with both anabolic and catabolic activity; they mediate both the synthesis and the degradation of the matrix. Proteoglycan metabolism has been studied extensively. As is typical for other cells, the protein components are synthesized in the cytoplasmic rough endoplasmic reticulum, and sulfation of the polysaccharides occurs in the Golgi bodies. *Ex vivo* studies with radioactive tracer isotope of sulfur-35 sulfate show incorporation into glycosaminoglycans by intermediate and deep cells and subsequent movement into the matrix. Type II collagen is synthesized and secreted as separate procollagen chains with extensions on their ends, is converted to tropocollagen, and is organized into fibrils with small amounts of collagen IX and XI. In contrast to the dense, thick, and highly oriented collagen fibers of bone, cartilage fibrils are thin and are crosslinked into an open meshwork. The fibrils contain variable amounts of noncollagenous macromolecules, notably decorin. The half-life of collagen II is more than 200 years in humans. Thus, the major component of the native fibrils does not appear to be renewed or reparable in the normal setting. The collagen fibrillar network is under tension and serves to contain the glycosaminoglycans in a compressed state. It is difficult to imagine how that network could be turned over without compromising the mechanical integrity

T. Minas: Brigham Orthopedic Associates, Inc., Boston, Massachusetts.

J. Glowacki: Orthopedic Surgery, Harvard Medical School; Skeletal Biology, Orthopedic Surgery, Brigham and Women's Hospital, Boston, Massachusetts.

of the tissue or how denatured foci could be mended. Evidence shows damage to the fibrillar network in osteoarthritis. Osteoarthritis drastically affects the mechanical properties of cartilage: excessive swelling of osteoarthritic samples in dilute salt solution is taken as evidence of the loss of resistance afforded by the fibrillar net to absorption of water by the polysaccharides. Although there appears to be little turnover of the fibrillar network, the entrapped proteoglycans undergo turnover that can be accelerated by local cytokines.

Chondrocytes are responsible for maintaining the matrix environment in which they are encased and hence ensure the tissue's mechanical characteristics (2). They are protected from osmotic and mechanical damage by the rigid pericellular matrix, called the chondron. Maintenance of the matrix involves degradation by proteinases and free radicals generated by the chondrocyte. Matrix metalloproteinases and aggrecanase catalyze the turnover of cartilage matrix in normal cartilage as well as in diseased cartilage. Because many of the matrix components in cartilage are specific to that tissue, there is great interest in developing and validating assays for their degradation products in plasma or synovial fluid as markers for turnover (3).

The modern view of osteoarthritis is that it results from an imbalance between dynamic anabolic and catabolic activities that are normally well balanced. The chondrocyte functions as the agent of these two processes. This is in contrast to bone tissue, for example, in which anabolic activities are ascribed to the osteoblast and catabolic or osteolytic activities are ascribed to the osteoclast. Although normally interaction occurs between those two cell types to maintain skeletal mass constant within the remodeling process, imbalance occurs with aging, osteoporosis, and infection. The situation in cartilage is distinct. Evidence suggests that the earliest stages of osteoarthritis are balanced by an upregulation of the biosynthetic processes. Synovial fluid collects a byproduct of procollagen II processing, called chondrocalcin or C-properide; its levels are elevated in traumatic and primary osteoarthritis.

Previously, cartilage was regarded to be immunologically privileged because of either the absence of transplantation antigens or the protective effect of the matrix. These features were invoked to explain the endurance of allografts in heterotopic sites. It is now appreciated that chondrocytes do display major transplantation antigens, and components of the matrix are weakly antigenic. In healthy, intact cartilage, these determinants are probably shielded from antibodies because of steric hindrance resulting from the proteoglycans in the matrix. Preservation of matrix integrity appears to be essential to prevent exposure of the cells and rejection of the tissue.

The heterogeneous group of inflammatory joint diseases involves underlying disturbances in immune regulation. In rheumatoid arthritis, the synovial lining is the initial target of inflammatory disease. Proliferation of synovial lining cells and infiltration by lymphocytes and activated macrophages produce the tissue mass called the pannus. The pannus can invade and destroy the integrity of the articular cartilage. Products of the pannus act as cytokine mediators of both chondrolysis and osteolysis. The major agents are interleukin-1 (IL-1) and tumor necrosis factor-α. These agents signal the cascade of release of IL-6, IL-8, IL-17, cyclooxygenase-2, and nitric oxide, all of which are actual or potential targets of pharmacologic management. *In vitro* models have been useful to describe the mechanisms by which these immunomodulatory cytokines change gene expression in chondrocytes and promote chondrolysis.

Mechanical Properties of Articular Cartilage

Articular cartilage is a hypocellular, viscoelastic tissue that lines synovial joints and provides them with a nearly frictionless environment. It is said that synovial cartilage articulations provide a coefficient of friction for joint motion that is less than one-fifth of ice on ice (4). The mechanical properties of articular cartilage depend on its composition and its architecture. Normally, the hydrophilic proteoglycans and collagen constitute 30% of the tissue mass, the remainder being water. Cartilage matrix can be viewed as a biphasic material, in which the fluid phase flows on mechanical deformation of its solid phase. Although the water is constrained by the proteoglycan molecules, the fluid phase can also be called the porosity of the cartilage. The tissue's high water content also generates its high viscoelasticity. Its elastic modulus is low at slow rates of loading, but is two orders greater at physiologic rates.

The surface cartilage layer or "skin" is resistant to compressive loads or penetration. The vertically arranged collagen fibers of the radial and calcified zones are resistant to shear. On application of pressure to articular cartilage through weight bearing, the water contained within the cartilage exudes on pressure. With diminished pressure, water is drawn back to the aggrecan. A surface protein, dermatan sulfate, also acts as an antiadhesion substance. The fine filaments of the superficial zone combine with water so articulation with the opposite joint surface is also with combined water and superficial zone filaments (2). The lubricating barrier between joint surfaces is therefore mostly water. Water is released during weight-bearing pressure from hyperhydrated, negatively charged proteoglycans in articular cartilage. With damage or degeneration, loss of proteoglycans and water results in impaired mechanical properties and joint function.

Incidence of Cartilage Lesions

The true incidence of cartilage lesions and their natural history are unknown. It has been proposed that between 5% and 10% of acute knee hemarthroses after a work-related or sports injury are associated with an acute chondral injury (5). In a retrospective review of 31,516 knee arthroscopies, the prevalence of chondral lesions was 63%. Isolated unipolar chondral defects in patients younger than 40 years of age, however, were rare. Only 5% of chondral defects occurred in this young patient population (6). Clinical and experimental evidence shows that, with time, focal cartilage injuries enlarge and progress to osteoarthritis (7).

Mechanical injury to articular cartilage during sporting injuries may occur with shearing forces secondary to disruption of the anterior cruciate ligament. At the time of ligament disruption, shearing osteochondral fractures have been noted. Blunt injury to the joint surfaces may also cause injury to and death of articular chondrocytes. If the articular chondrocyte is not able to continue to synthesize and remodel its matrix macromolecules, eventual degeneration of pericellular matrix will occur. This may account for the high incidence of osteoarthritis encountered with anterior cruciate ligament injuries. Acutely, the incidence of chondral injuries is approximately 2%, but this may approach 20% in the long run (8).

In a study performed by Repo and Finlay (9), blunt force to articular chondrocytes in excess of 25 megapascals reproducibly resulted in death of articular chondrocytes. Hence there appears to be a threshold to which articular chondrocytes can withstand blunt trauma. This may be an important factor in understanding articular cartilage degeneration after injury, as well as an important technical factor during new repair techniques, such as osteochondral graft transfers. Large impaction forces needed to introduce osteochondral grafts to recipient sites may result in injury and cell death to the cartilage cap of the osteochondral grafts. This may result in failed long-term results.

Magnetic resonance imaging scans demonstrated bone bruises after blunt injuries during work-related and sporting activities. Arthroscopic biopsy studies of cartilage overlying bone bruises demonstrated superficial chondrocyte death and matrix dehydration (10). It is proposed that cartilage cell death arises directly from the blunt trauma exceeding this threshold.

The natural history of osteoarthritis itself is unknown. A Swedish longitudinal study (11), however, notes that in the knee, radiographic progression of osteoarthritis occurs over a 20-year time course when greater than 50% joint space narrowing is present at the initial evaluation (Ahlback stages II to V). In only 60% of patients, however, will disease progress radiographically if patients have Ahlback stage 0 (peripheral osteophytes and a normal joint space) or Ahlback stage 1 (more than 50% joint space narrowing) at initial presentation. Not all cases of radiographic osteoarthritis will progress.

In the United States, more than 250,000 total knee replacements are performed annually. The disability and economic hardship caused by osteoarthritis are substantial, especially when a cartilage injury occurs at a young age when socioeconomic productivity and recreational activities are strongly affected. The problem arises from the unique structure, function, and repair mechanisms of articular cartilage.

Cartilage Injuries and Repair

Articular cartilage is devoid of a nerve supply. Cartilage covers and protects the richly innervated subchondral bone plate from being stimulated. Once articular cartilage is damaged, pain can result from contact of the subchondral bone plate. If a healing response does not develop, the load will be borne by the shoulders of the chondral defects in addition to the exposed subchondral bone. This situation will result in overload and breakdown of the shoulders of the defect, with progressive enlargement of the defect. The opposing articulation would be exposed to a bare bone surface with resultant erosive degradation of its cartilage surface. The resultant bone-on-bone articulation is, by definition, osteoarthritis. Symptoms may occur from direct stimulation of the subchondral bone plate or from indirect stimulation to the bone through an attached cartilage flap. Breakdown products from the cartilage along with liberated enzymes may cause effusions in the joint, capsular distention, synovitis, and other mechanisms of pain. As the subchondral bone plate hardens, secondary vascular venous congestion in the medullary cavity results and may cause deep, aching pain.

Cartilage repair would be beneficial in the short term to alleviate symptoms and in the long term to prevent progressive breakdown of the articulations of the joint and the development of osteoarthritis. Thus, the goal of cartilage repair is to produce a tissue that will fill the defect, integrate with the adjacent articular cartilage and subchondral bone plate, have the same viscoelastic mechanical properties, and maintain its matrix over time without breakdown. The goal is to restore the osteochondral functional unit with a repair tissue that approaches regeneration.

Clinical and experimental evidence shows that damage involving the articular cartilage surface and confined to the cartilage undergoes little restoration. Cartilage has little intrinsic ability to heal. Chondrocytes in mature articular cartilage rarely divide, and their density declines with age. In contrast, lesions that extend to the subchondral bone marrow may heal clinically (12). Therefore, a cell source for cartilage regeneration or repair must arise from the underlying subchondral bone marrow, from the adjacent synovial tissue, or from an exogenous source.

Absence of blood supply and endogenous source of new cells contribute to cartilage's incapacity for repair. The typical wound healing response of hemorrhage, fibrin clot formation, and mobilization of cells and growth factors is absent. The only spontaneous repair reaction that may occur is at the edge of superficial articular cartilage lesions. Articular cartilage is isolated from the subchondral bone marrow cells by the dense subchondral bone and cartilage matrix.

Cartilage repair depends on the mobilization of cells derived from the subchondral bone marrow, including multipotential cells, osteoblasts, chondroblasts, fibroblasts, and hematopoietic progenitor cells (13). The repair tissue that results may therefore be variable, depending on the predominant cell line that proliferates and its modulation by local growth factors, cytokines, and the local mechanical environment.

Clinical Repair for Full-Thickness Cartilage Defects

The spectrum of repair tissue is variable clinically, depending on the clinical technique used, as well as intrinsic and local factors. Repair tissue may be fibrous tissue, transitional tissue, fibrocartilage, hyaline cartilage, articular cartilage, or bone, or a mixture of any of these (14). Fibrous tissue consists of fibrocytes and a type I collagen fibrous matrix. Transitional tissue consists of ovoid cells that may produce proteoglycans as well as a fibrous matrix. The matrix may stain positively with safranin 0 for proteoglycan production. Fibrocartilage consists of round chondrocyte-appearing cells with a type I collagen fibrous matrix. Hyaline cartilage con-

sists of chondrocytes in a matrix of type II collagen and proteoglycans, with a hyaline, ground-glass appearance by light microscopy. The cellular and matrix organization may be different from that of normal articular cartilage. Articular cartilage resembles normal articular cartilage. Articular cartilage is essentially a regenerating tissue with articular chondrocytes, arranged in the usual palisading columns found in normal articular cartilage, with markers of normal articular cartilage matrix including type II collagen and proteoglycans, for example. There may be a mixture of all these components in a single repair site. The predominant repair tissue type determines the long-term outcome for the patient. If the majority of the repair tissue is hyaline or articular cartilage, then the viscoelastic properties found with a type II collagen framework and proteoglycans will give a durable repair and usually a superior clinical result. Fibrocartilage and fibrous repairs consist of type I collagen, which is usually not as strong as type II collagen and often contains short-chain proteoglycans. Fibrocartilage and fibrous repairs do not maintain a high negative charge density, they are soft, and they break down.

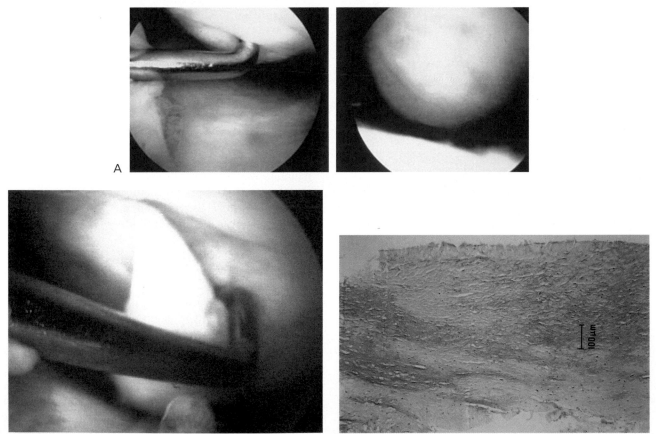

FIGURE 6.1 **A:** Arthroscopic appearance of a symptomatic fibrocartilage repair after drilling. Repair tissue is evident from native articular cartilage. Complete fill of defect with white repair tissue is evident. However, its mechanical properties are insufficient and soft, with resultant symptoms. **B:** Arthroscopic appearance of a symptomatic fibrocartilage flap after drilling. Poor integration and mechanically soft tissue have resulted in a poor clinical result. **C:** Low-power photomicrograph of retrieved fibrocartilage repair stained with safranin O for proteoglycans. Alternating layers of fibrous and fibrocartilage repair tissue, with a porous appearance and a degenerating surface. This is a human retrieval resulting from a failed arthroscopic abrasion arthroplasty with resultant filled defect and a soft repair tissue, as in A.

TABLE 6.1 EVALUATION OF TISSUE RETRIEVED AFTER FAILED ARTICULAR CARTILAGE REPAIR PROCEDURES: A HISTOLOGIC AND IMMUNOHISTOCHEMICAL COMPARATIVE ANALYSIS[a]

Treatment Follow-up	ABR (n = 12) 21±4	PCH (n = 4) 31±8 mo	ACI (n = 6) 3±1 mo	$p < .05$ ANOVA
Tissue Types				
Articular cartilage	2±1%	3±2	0	Not significant
Hyaline cartilage	30±10	47±7	2±1	Significant
Fibrocartilage	28±7	15±4	6±2	Not significant
Transition tissue	18±2	12±3	31±7	Not significant
Fibrous tissue	22±9	4±2	61±9	Significant
Bone	0	19±6	0	Significant

[a] Notice variable quantities of tissue types in each failed cartilage repair procedure in a human series of arthroscopic abrasion arthroplasty (ABR), perichondrial rib grafting (PCH), and autologous chondrocyte implantation (ACI), at various time intervals after treatment (in months).
Modified from Nehrer S, Spector M, Minas T. Histological analysis of failed cartilage repair procedures. *Clin Orthop* 1999;365:149–162, with permission.

Factors that may influence the quality of the repair tissue noted clinically include acuteness of injury, age, size of defect, ligament stability, axial alignment, and presence or absence of the meniscus (12,15). In a study conducted by Nehrer and associates (14) (Table 6.1), failed repair tissues were analyzed after three techniques of marrow stimulation: drilling, abrasion, and microfracture. The repair tissues retrieved were composed predominantly of fibrous and fibrocartilaginous tissues. The tissues were soft and degenerating. They had poor mechanical viscoelastic properties, even though they filled the defects. The repair tissues clinically failed by 2.5 years after treatment, with an average defect size of greater than 3 cm². Cartilage defects that were treated by perichondrial grafting had an excellent clinical result early postoperatively. By 4 to 5 years postoperatively, however, the repair tissue had undergone enchondral ossification. The perichondrial chondrocytes had features of hypertrophic chondrocytes, notably type X collagen, a precursor to mineralization (Fig. 6.2). Although those grafts had a high percentage of hyaline cartilage, they also contained bone. The autologous chondrocyte implantation grafts that failed did so early, less than 6 months after implantation, as a result of trauma as the grafts were growing. At this early stage of repair, a high percentage of the repair tissue was fibrous or transitional. Mature autologous chondrocyte implant grafts, more than 2 years after implantation, may have excellent clinical outcomes, with hyaline cartilage repair with firm viscoelastic properties (Fig. 6.3).

Intrinsic repair in the acute situation is possible by marrow stimulation repair, if chondral injury involves the underlying subchondral bone. However, appropriate rehabilitation after injury is critical (Table 6.2). The factors previously described delineating the possibility of a successful repair are important. Rehabilitation after such an injury

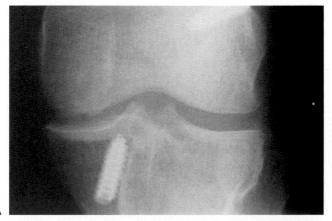
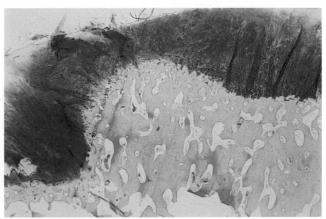

A   B

FIGURE 6.2 A: Radiographic appearance of medial femoral condyle autologous perichondrial graft undergoing ossification. Ossification developed 3 years after cartilage repair with initial excellent clinical result. Revision cartilage repair with autologous chondrocyte implantation graft resulted in a successful clinical outcome. Retrieval of the failed perichondrial graft specimen allowed histologic analysis (see B–D). **B:** Low-power photomicrograph of retrieved perichondrial autograft undergoing enchondral ossification stained with safranin O. Notice the excellent proteoglycan production as demonstrated by red staining. However, the advancing front of bone formation *(blue stain)* will eventually ossify the entire cartilage graft without stabilization with a tidemark.

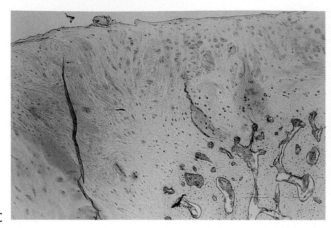
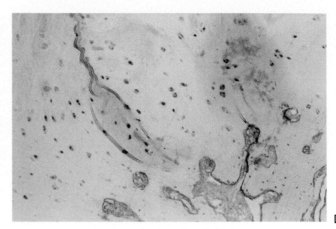

C   D

FIGURE 6.2 *(continued)* **C:** Antibody staining to type X collagen, low-power photomicrograph, demonstrating intracellular production of type X collagen as expressed by hypertrophic chondrocytes undergoing enchondral ossification. **D:** High-power photomicrograph demonstrating intracellular antibody staining to type X collagen of hypertrophic chondrocytes. This is a common mechanism of failure of perichondrial autografts clinically.

is also important. There may be a critical size of subchondral bone involvement, however, that will result in cystic degeneration rather than repair. This occurs specifically in osteochondritis dissecans or when lesions are deep. One study with experimental deep osteochondral defects greater than 8 mm in diameter in adult goats demonstrated cystic enlargement of the defects rather than repair (16). Repair of an osteochondral defect is therefore more complex. A staged reconstruction using autogenous tissues is required. Other options include allogeneic osteochondral reconstruction

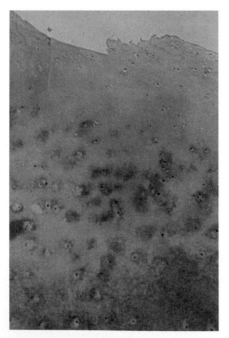

FIGURE 6.3 High-power photomicrograph of a biopsy specimen stained with safranin O of autologous chondrocyte implantation in a human. Note the homogeneous ground-glass appearance of matrix and abundant chondrocyte formation.

and autologous-derived tissue engineering solutions (Fig. 6.4).

Experimental Models and Usefulness

Selection of an appropriate animal model to assess mechanisms and outcomes of procedures for cartilage repair has been problematic. The ideal is a skeletally mature animal with anatomic morphologic similarities to the human clinical situation. Inclusion of multiple control groups is essential to assess the hypothesis that a certain treatment is superior. In this way, the relative value of a therapy can be assessed but with limited translation to the human. This, however, is not always practically feasible in that bilateral simultaneous treatments may not be ethically or physiologically sound for the repair model. The duration of the experiment to confirm endurance of cartilage repair and the prevention of osteoarthritis is usually cost-prohibitive.

The use of periosteum to treat full-thickness chondral defects under the influence of continuous passive motion has been investigated in a rabbit model (17). An elegant experiment demonstrated that periosteum was capable of undergoing neochondrogenesis and that, under the influence of continuous passive motion, the quality of the repair tissue was similar to that of hyaline cartilage.

The translation of this model to demonstrate proof of principle in the human, however, has not been fully realized (18,19). It is not known whether the rabbit is capable of an unusually robust healing response or whether technical differences in the experimental method account for unpredictable results in patients.

The technique of autologous chondrocyte implantation has also been controversial (20–23). Much of the controversy has apparently been caused by the conflicting results with two different animal models. The Swedish model was

TABLE 6.2 TIMELINE FOR HEALING[a]

Time	0–6 weeks	7–12 weeks	>13 weeks–3 years
Stage	Proliferation	Transition	Remodeling and Maturation
Histologic features	Rapid proliferation of spindle-shaped cells with defect fill; mostly type I collagen with early formation of colonies of chondrocytes forming type II collagen	Matrix formation, mostly chondrocytes producing type II collagen and proteoglycans; poor integration to underlying bone and cartilage	Ongoing remodeling of matrix with reorganization and quantity of collagen type II, with integration to bone (arcades of Benninghoff), and adjacent host cartilage; large chain aggregates of proteoglycans, with increased water content of cartilage
Viscoelastic arthroscopic appearance	Filled, soft, white tissue	Jelly-like firmness, with "wave-like" motion when probed, not yet firm and integrated to underlying bone	Firm "indentable", but not "wave-like", when probed by 4–6 months after ACT, graft whiter than host cartilage, may demonstrate periosteal hypertrophy (20%); equal firmness to host cartilage 9–18 months after ACT
Activity level	Continuous passive motion starts 6 hours after surgery for 6–8 hours/day for 6 weeks Touch weight bearing Isometric muscle exercices and range of motion	Discontinue continuous passive motion Active range of motion Partial graduated to full weight bearing by 12 weeks Functional muscle usage, stationary bicycle, treadmill	Discontinue assistive devices 4–5 months postoperatively if free of pain, catching, swelling Distance walking, resistance walking Nonpivoting running 9–12 months 14–18 months pivoting allowed

[a] Clinical recommendations made for a careful rehabilitation after autologous chondrocyte implantation (ACI) based on correlative observations on the basic science repair process learned from the canine model, and arthroscopic evaluations in humans (with biopsies) at various stages of repair to understand the viscoelastic mechanical maturation over time so as to not prematurely overload the healing grafts. From Minas T, Peterson L. Autologous chondrocyte transplantation. *Oper Tech Sports Med* 2000;8:144–157, with permission.

based on a pilot study performed in patellar chondral defects in rabbits (24). The rabbit model showed that the implanted *in vitro*–labeled chondrocytes were largely responsible for the repair tissue that developed to fill chondral defects. The repair tissue was superior to that of periosteum alone.

The quality and quantity of repair tissues remained consistently higher in the rabbit model when compared with empty defects, periosteum, periosteum plus autologous chondrocytes, and carbon fiber pads plus autologous chondrocytes (25). A similar study was performed in a rabbit model with bilateral patellar chondral defects, unlike the human situation, in which defects are most commonly found on the femoral condyles.

When the experiment was completed in a canine model using the femoral sulcus, comparing empty defect, periosteum, and periosteum plus autologous chondrocytes, the results were similar in the early postoperative period (less than 6 months), but the long-term results (12 to 18 months) were uniformly osteoarthritic (13,26). No treatment difference could be detected. There was clearly a species difference at 12 months between rabbit and dog (Figs. 6.5 to 6.12).

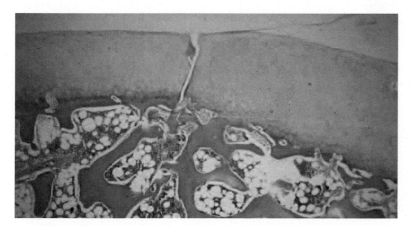

FIGURE 6.4 Low-power photomicrograph of a human biopsy specimen at the junction of osteochondral graft transfer and native cartilage margin. Note the persistent cleft without integration at the cartilage–cartilage junctures and the differing thicknesses of articular cartilage with the differing tidemark junctures. Excellent bony remodeling is noted in the subchondral bone marrow. (Courtesy of Laszlo Hangody, M.D., Budapest. Hungary.)

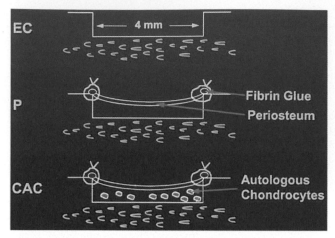

FIGURE 6.5 Schematic representation of a canine experiment to evaluate the effect of autologous chondrocyte implantation using cultured articular chondrocytes (CAC), versus periosteal resurfacing alone (P), versus empty control (EC); 4-mm defect. The periosteum was microsutured with absorbable suture to the native articular margins with the canbium layer of periosteum facing the bony surface, and the margins were then sealed with autologous fibrin glue. The animal and was then protected with an external fixation device for 10 days and was then allowed to bear weight as tolerated. Two chondral defects were made per knee, in the femoral sulcus or trochlea, as seen in Fig. 6.6.

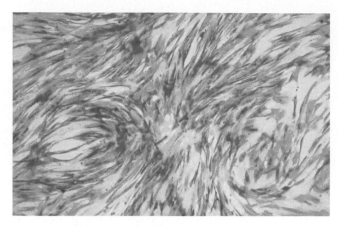

FIGURE 6.7. High-power photomicrograph of a β-galactosidase–labeled reporter gene in chondrocyte culture in monolayer approaching confluence. The reporter gene will allow tracking of implanted chondrocytes over time. It was found that the label was no longer effective after 3 months *in vivo*.

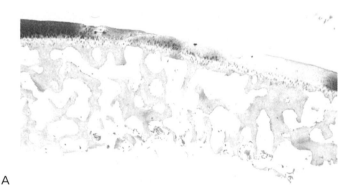

A

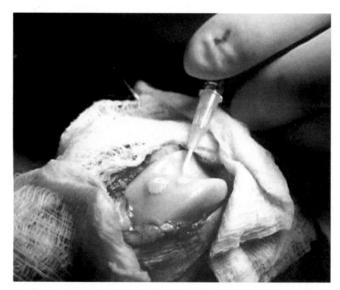

FIGURE 6.6 Gross appearance of periosteal patches sutured to chondral defects undergoing autologous chondrocyte implantation on the femoral sulcus in a canine model. The chondral defects measured 4 mm in diameter.

B

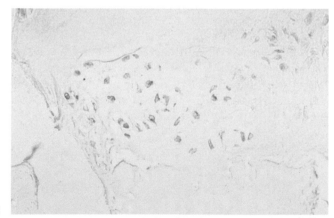

FIGURE 6.8 A: Three-month histologic section at low power with hematoxylin and eosin (H&E) staining of a canine defect treated by autologous chondrocyte implantation. The defect appears filled but has poor staining characteristics, although the repair tissue appears to be predominantly composed of cellular chondrocytes. **B:** High-power photomicrograph of the area that is poorly staining in A, demonstrates the persistence of β-galactosidase reporter gene labeling of implanted chondrocytes 3 months after implantation. This demonstrates that the implanted chondrocytes constitute the repair tissue.

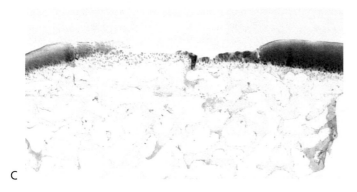

C

FIGURE 6.8 *(continued)* **C:** Three-month histologic section at low power with H&E staining of a canine defect, as a control defect. Note the lack of repair tissue fill, except around the margins.

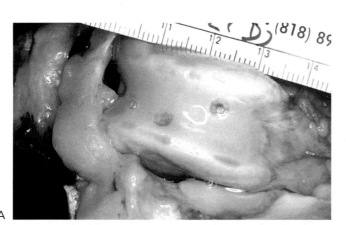

A

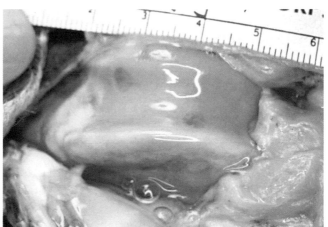

B

FIGURE 6.9 **A:** Gross appearance of empty canine defects 6 months after treatment. There is minimal repair tissue around the margins. **B:** Gross appearance of defects in a canine model 6 months after treatment with autologous chondrocytes. Note the complete fill and smoothness of the surface.

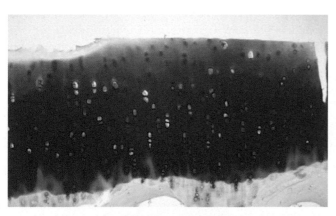

A

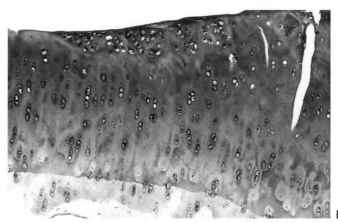

B

FIGURE 6.10 **A:** High-power photomicrograph with safranin O staining of retrieved tissue from Fig. 6.9B. This demonstrates a hyaline cartilage repair tissue, with deep proteoglycan staining, palisading chondrocyte arrangement, and excellent subchondral bone integration with tidemark formation. However, note the cleft to the far right of the cartilage–cartilage integration. This is a common finding after autologous chondrocyte implantation grafting, early after treatment. **B:** Same specimen stained with antibody to type II collagen. Note the uniform density of staining.

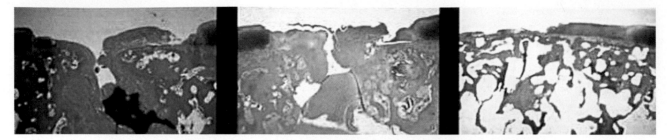

FIGURE 6.11 Low-power photomicrographs of an empty defect *(left)*, periosteum alone *(center)*, and autologous chondrocyte implantation of canine experiment at 12 months after treatment *(right)*. The worst-case situation demonstrates collapse of the subchondral bone plate with fibrous tissue formation in an empty defect in both the empty-control and periosteum-alone groups. The group receiving autologous chondrocyte implantation similarly has a poor repair tissue that is delaminating with the subchondral bone intact. Independent observation by a histologist could not grade the difference among the three treatments.

Translational Research

Perhaps no perfect animal model exists with similar repair characteristics to the human species. However, new technologies and treatment options can be evaluated in an animal model with control groups In this way, assessment of the efficacy of repair may be established. In general, proof of principle involves the progression of scientific method from *in vitro* methods, small animal experimentation, and larger animal validation before human clinical trials. The hypotheses for the scientific methods are derived from clinical problems or failures of existing techniques. The method of pursuing a hypothesis rendered from a clinical situation taken to the basic science laboratory is the basis of translational research. The topic of cartilage repair is an especially difficult clinical problem to model experimentally. The concept of translational research is especially suited in the field of cartilage repair.

STATE-OF-THE-ART

Tissue Engineering

Because cartilage is a relatively simple tissue with respect to its cellular homogeneity and avascularity, it has been a model for research of *in vitro*–engineered tissues (27). Progress has been slow and obstructed on several levels. The adult chondrocyte has limited capacity for proliferation and has both catabolic and anabolic functions. These metabolic features must be optimized and controlled for engineered tissue to endure. The motivation for tissue engineering is to promote biologic repair or regeneration. The conceptual approaches include implantation of inert substitutes for discontinuities or missing parts, drug or matrix treatments to stimulate tissue regeneration, autogenous cell or tissue transfer, or *in vitro* production of tissues or tissue equivalents for implantation. There are three considerations in designing a construct for engineered tissue: the source of cells, if any; the nature of the carrier or scaffold; and the use, if any, of genes, factors, or adjuvants.

Cell-Based Techniques

Theoretically, cartilage tissue appears well-suited for transplantation; it lacks a blood supply, is nourished by diffusion, and has a low cell-to-matrix ratio. There are sites for donor tissue, especially for pediatric patients. Transplanted autogenous cartilage has been used successfully for construction of ears in children with congenital microtia or atresia, with

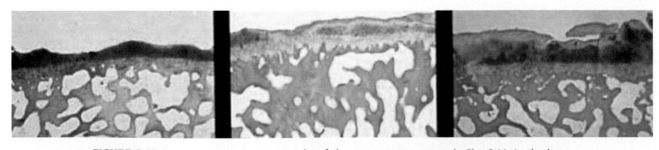

FIGURE 6.12 Low-power photomicrographs of the same treatments as in Fig. 6.11. In the best-case situation, repair tissue in all three treatment arms could not be graded as different. There did not seem to be a difference in treatment effect. The canine model for cartilage repair for periods longer than 12 months demonstrated spontaneous repair or degeneration to a similar treatment endpoint. However, autologous chondrocyte implantation at less than 6 months demonstrated a superior repair.

excellent long-term maintenance. Long-term results of osteochondral shell allograft resurfacing of knees indicate better function in unipolar than bipolar cases. Segments of cartilage, however, are less suitable for repair of articular surfaces or intracartilaginous defects in which bonding to the tissue bed is important. Autogenous cells, often expanded *in vitro,* have been useful for cartilage tissue engineering. Precursor and progenitor cells derived from bone marrow, perichondrium, periosteum, and other sources also have potential for cartilage repair. It has also been shown that human dermal fibroblasts can be induced to differentiate to chondrocytes and to produce cartilage matrix by culture in the presence of demineralized bone powder (28). Whether chondrocytes that are differentiated *in vitro* will maintain the articular phenotype or will develop into hypertrophic chondrocytes may depend on the site into which they are implanted or the mediators in their microenvironment. More information about the plasticity of chondrocytes and their potential for developing endochondral bone will be needed for clinical applications.

Gene Therapy

Advances in gene transfer technology have been translated into clinical applications. Proof of principle has been demonstrated for *in vivo* and *ex vivo* transfection of genes into articular chondrocytes. Efficient transfection requires vectors, materials, or methods to promote the uptake and expression of the gene of interest. In principle, different methods may result in transient or more enduring expression of the gene product. For chondrocytes, some of the useful genes include insulin-like growth factor I, transforming growth factor-α, and IL-1 receptor antagonist.

Materials

Delivery of simple cell suspensions is of limited value in musculoskeletal applications because of the requirement that the cells be retained at the desired site. Isolated chondrocytes lack adherence to the lesion sites, and suspensions may produce fibrocartilage or small foci of cartilage. Fluid carriers or three-dimensional scaffolds can be used for delivery and retention of cells. Popular natural hydrogels are alginates, fibrin, denatured collagen gels, hyaluronan, or admixtures useful to contain or immobilize cell suspensions. In addition to the important function as a carrier of cells, three-dimensional scaffolds are useful to define the space for the new tissue and, potentially, to enhance the maturation and function of the regenerated tissue. Candidate scaffolds include natural polymeric materials such as collagen lattices, synthetic polymers, biodegradable polymers, and polymers with adsorbed proteins (29) or immobilized functional groups.

The key requirements of bioresorbable materials are that (a) their rates of degradation must be compatible with the intended use and (b) the products of their degradation must be nontoxic. Of the synthetic materials, polyglycolic acid, polylactic acid, and their copolymers are most widely studied.

FUTURE DIRECTIONS

Widespread discourse about the early experiments with tissue and organ engineering has generated public demand and expectations that engineered tissues will be available before long. However, critical hurdles need to be overcome. In the case of engineered cartilage, it would seem desirable to avoid harvesting of normal tissue and to have a single operation for implantation of engineered tissue. Mature chondrocytes are exceptional in their ability to serve catabolic as well as anabolic functions. Control to inhibit the chondrolytic activities of chondrocytes would seem important for maintaining engineered tissues. Consideration of the limited proliferative and regenerative capacity of adult chondrocytes and the of potential for dedifferentiation on expansion also leads to the goal of alternate source of cells. Use of xenogeneic or allogeneic cells requires selective shattering of the immunogenicity barrier in transplantation. There remain difficulties in incorporation of neocartilage with adjacent healthy tissue. We have incomplete understanding of the relationship between cartilage and vascular response to wounding. Engineered cartilage needs to attach to the implantation site without evoking an angiogenic response. It is conceivable that genetically modified cells could be grown on a biocompatible scaffold with internal signals for programmed histogenesis. Advances in materials design may generate "smart" scaffolds that will control tissue topology and will have surface modifications to stimulate cell attachment, differentiation, and growth.

REFERENCES

1. Stockwell RA, Meachim G. The chondrocytes. In: Freeman MAR, ed. *Adult articular cartilage.* Kent, UK: Pitman Medical, 1979:69–144.
2. Mankin HJ, Mos VW, Buckwalter JA, et al. Articular cartilage structure, composition and function. In: Buckwalter JA, Einhorn TA, Simon SR, eds. *Orthopaedic basic science.* Rosemont, IL: American Academy of Orthopaedic Surgeons, 2000.
3. Seibel MJ, Robbins SP, Bilezikian JP, eds. *Dynamics of bone and cartilage metabolism.* San Diego: Academic Press, 1999.
4. Mow VC, Ratcliffe A. Structure and function of articular cartilage and meniscus. In: Mow VC, Hayes WC, eds. *Basic orthopaedic biomechanics.* Philadelphia: Lippincott–Raven, 1997.
5. Noyes FR, Bassett RW, et al. Arthroscopy in acute traumatic hemarthrosis of the knee: incidence of anterior cruciate tears and other injuries. *J Bone Joint Surg Am* 1980;62:687–695.
6. Curl W, Krome J, et al. Cartilage injuries: a review of 31,516 knee arthroscopies. *Arthroscopy* 1997;13:456–460.
7. Messner K, Maletius W. The long-term prognosis for severe damage to weight-bearing cartilage in the knee: a 14-year clinical and radiographic follow-up in 28 young athletes. *Acta Orthop Scand* 1996;67:165–168.

8. Minas T, Nehrer S. Current concepts in the treatment of cartilage defects. *Orthopedics* 1997;20:525–538.

9. Repo RU, Finlay J. Survival of articular cartilage after controlled impact. *J Bone Joint Surg Am* 1977;59:1068–1076.

10. Johnson DL, Urban WP, Caborn NNM, et al. Articular cartilage pathology associated with MRI detected "bone bruises" after ACL rupture. Presented at the American Academy of Orthopaedic Surgeons Society for Sports Medicine Specialty Day, Atlanta, 1996.

11. Sahlström A, Johnell O, Redlund-Johnell I. The natural course of arthrosis of the knee. *Clin Orthop* 1997;40:152–157.

12. Dzioba RB. The classification and treatment of acute articular cartilage lesions. *Arthroscopy* 1988;4:72–80.

13. Breinan H, Minas T, Hsu HP, et al. Effect of cultured articular chondrocytes on repair of chondral defects in a canine model. *J Bone Joint Surg Am* 1997;79:1439–1451.

14. Nehrer S Spector M, Minas T. Histological analysis of failed cartilage repair procedures. *Clin Orthop* 1999;365:149–162.

15. Friedman MJ, Berasi CC, Fox JM, et al. Preliminary results with abrasion arthroplasty in the osteoarthritic knee. *Clin Orthop* 1984;182:200–205.

16. Jackson DW, Lalor PA, Aberman HM, et al. Spontaneous repair of full-thickness defects of articular cartilage in a goat model: a preliminary study. *J Bone Joint Surg Am* 2001;83:53.

17. O'Driscoll SW, Salter R. The induction of neochondrogenesis in free intra-articular periosteal autografts under the influence of continuous passive motion. *J Bone Joint Surg Am* 1984;66:1248–1257.

18. Angermann P, Riegels-Nielsen P, Pedersen H. Osteochondritis dissecans of the femoral condyle treated with periosteal transplantation: poor outcome in 14 patients followed for 6–9 years. *Acta Orthop Scand* 1998;69:595–597.

19. Madsen BL, Noer HH, Carstensen JP, et al. Long-term results of periosteal transplantation in osteochondritis dissecans of the knee. *Orthopedics* 2000; 23:223–226.

20. Brittberg M, Lindahl A, Nilsson A, et al. Treatment of full-thickness cartilage defects in the human knee with cultured autologous chondrocytes. *N Engl J Med* 1984;331:889–895.

21. Messner K, Gillquist J. Cartilage repair: a critical review. *Acta Orhop Scand* 1996;67:523–529.

22. Brittberg M. A critical analysis of cartilage repair. *Acta Orthop Scand* 1999;88:186–191.

23. Jackson DW, Simon T. Current concepts: chondroctye transplantation. *Arthroscopy* 1996;12:732–738.

24. Grande DA, Pitman ML, et al. The repair of experimentally produced defects in the rabbit articular cartilage by autologous chondrocyte transplantation. *J Othop Res* 1989;7:208–218.

25. Brittberg M, Nilsson A., Lindahl A, et al. Rabbit articular cartilage defects treated with autologous cultured chondroctye. *Clin Orthop* 1995;326:270–283.

26. Breinan H, Minas,T, Barone L, et al. Histological evaluation of the course of healing of canine articular cartilage defects treated with cultured chondrocytes. *Tissue Eng* 1998;4:101–114.

27. Glowacki J. *In vitro* engineering of cartilage. *J Rehabil Res Dev* 2000;37:171–177.

28. Mizuno S, Glowacki J. Chondroinduction of human dermal fibroblasts by demineralized bone in three-dimensional culture. *Exp Cell Res* 1996;227:89–97.

29. Eid K, Chen E, Griffith L, Glowacki J. Effect of RGD coating on osteocompatibility of PLGA-polymer disks in a rat tibial wound. *J Biomed Mater Res* 2001;57:224–231.

APPROACHING JOINT PROPRIOCEPTION: A MULTIDISCIPLINARY INVESTIGATION

WAYNE K. AUGÉ, II
PATRICIA A. VELÁZQUEZ

Arthroscopy has generated extraordinary advances in musculoskeletal care since the 1970s. This phenomenon has attracted and stimulated many research disciplines to join orthopaedic investigators in pursuing additional innovation. Within these endeavors, the role of the nervous system in musculoskeletal function is becoming increasingly apparent. Insight that disease, injury, and treatment interact with this system to determine outcome is now well accepted. Clinical examples such as pain distribution patterns for diagnosis (1,2), anesthesia techniques for surgical treatment (3,4), reflex inhibition or dystrophy during rehabilitation (5,6), chronic pain syndromes (7), and other neurologic sequelae of injury and disease (8,9) reinforce its importance for musculoskeletal care. However, the nervous system is perhaps the last and most difficult frontier for the orthopaedist to surmount and to integrate into clinical practice.

Traditionally, orthopaedic investigators have followed two general research approaches. *Orthopaedic neurologists (or neuroepidemiologists)* have sought to explain the functional disparity observed among patients as a means of improving musculoskeletal function. Characterizing the disruption of motor control observed in cerebral palsy (10), the frustration of workers' compensation care (11), and the wonder of motor ability in the elite athlete (12) are examples that have revealed biologic principles about the nervous system that may be amenable to new treatment methods. Equally important is the work of *orthopaedic neurobiologists,* who focus on the neurologic component of joint injury. Many investigators in this area have adopted a conceptual framework from which to explore the disruption of neural structures

that occurs during the disruption of tissue integrity (13). In this manner, joint injury induces an altered neurologic state that also requires treatment. These two orthopaedic approaches have been complementary and serve as the foundation for further investigation.

The prevailing view of this chapter is that the nervous system is an orthopaedic tissue, much like cartilage, ligament, and bone, and, as such, also requires a level of attention and integration during musculoskeletal care. The nervous system demonstrates significant *plasticity* whereby neural processes can be manipulated—both in the prevention and in the treatment of disease and injury. Whether the orthopaedist is treating the sequelae of neurologic disorders or the neurologic sequelae of injury, general principles that guide care need to be developed through investigation. The purpose of this chapter is to review some investigative approaches into the nervous system and to encourage further interaction among research disciplines that expands arthroscopy's innovative momentum into new areas.

SCOPE OF INVESTIGATION

The task of investigating the nervous system is quite daunting because of its sheer complexity. Investigators estimate that the brain contains approximately 10^{12} nerve cells encompassing about 10,000 different types of cells (14). It expresses more of the genetic information encoded in DNA than does any other organ system (15). Considering the recent accomplishment of detailing the *static* human genome of 10^5 genes, a *functional* 10^{12} cytologic diverse nerve cell population presents a much higher level of complexity not currently accessible to even today's supercomputers. Neural information is transmitted by billions of transient electrical and chemical signals that are exquisitely timed to provide coordinated and deliberate movements within the environment. *Activation thresholds* at each nerve ending control this flow of infor-

W. K. Augé: Center for Orthopaedic and Sports Performance Research; Northern New Mexico Orthopaedic Center; Department of Orthopaedic Surgery, Los Alamos Medical Center, Espanola-Presbyterian Medical Center, and the United States Department of Health and Human Services, Santa Fe, New Mexico.

P. A. Velázquez: Center for Orthopaedic and Sports Performance Research, Santa Fe, New Mexico.

mation and, in turn, are governed by nanoscale molecular processes. Reconciling this intricacy will require the work of many research disciplines including neuroanatomy, neurophysiology, neuropharmacology, behavioral science, computer sciences, theoretical mathematics, epidemiology, cell biology, quantum mechanics, molecular genetics, neural imaging, and others. The neurobiologist seeks to integrate these disciplines by reducing neural function into cohesive and understandable elemental processes.

To facilitate this research integration, *principles of organization* have been developed to partition investigative approaches and biologic elements into manageable components. This partitioning is based on levels of function within the nervous system. For example, simply classifying nerve cell function into afferent and efferent fibers provides a level of organization that interfaces well with clinical practice. Afferent nerve fibers transmit sensory signals from neural end organs to the central nervous system; efferent nerve fibers transmit motor signals to the peripheral muscular system to control movement. Placing such a classification of nervous system divisions next to investigative approaches can assist in creating manageable topics for inquiry (Fig. 7.1).

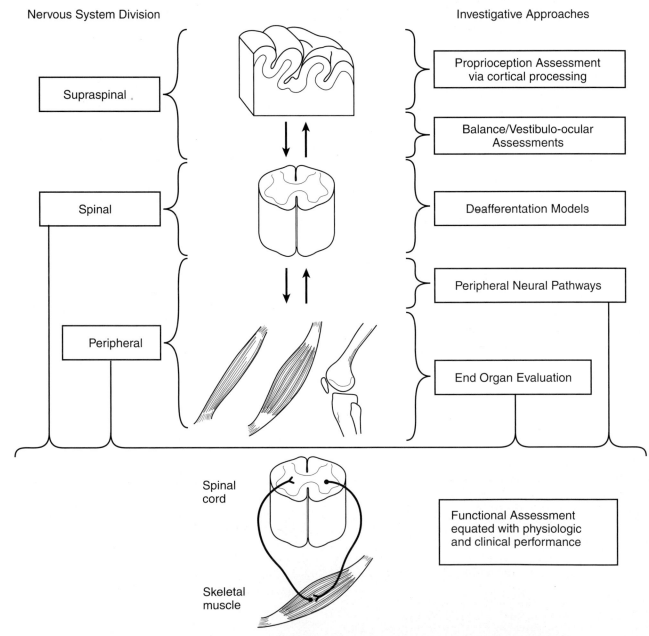

FIGURE 7.1 Principles of organization. A representative example of nervous system divisions and investigative approaches toward neuromotor evaluation. Partitioning investigative disciplines and biologic elements into manageable components can facilitate research inquiry. SSR, spinal stretch reflex. (Redrawn from Augé WK II, Morrison DS. Assessment of the infraspinatus spinal stretch reflex in the normal, athletic, and multidirectionally unstable shoulder. *Am J Sports Med* 2000;28:206–213, with permission.)

DEFINITIONS

Because of the complexity of the nervous system, many terms have been used to describe neural observations and have led to some confusion. The *neuromotor (or neuromuscular) system* refers to all processes mediated by the nervous system by which the motor system functions. This includes all anatomic structures such as the cerebral cortex, cerebellum, thalamus, brainstem, and spinal cord, as well as all levels of organ system interaction including the neuroendocrine, neuroimmune, and neurosensory axes. These levels of organ system structure and interaction hold wide implications for orthopaedic care but are beyond the scope of this chapter.

The *sensorimotor system* more specifically refers to mechanisms involved in receiving sensory information and converting that information into appropriate motor responses. It provides the ability to *read* the afferent environment within which the body resides. Within the sensorimotor system, three broad categories of neural faculties provide sensory information that allows interaction within the environment: exteroception, proprioception, and nociception. *Exteroception* is the ability to sense the spatial coordinates of environmental objects and is mediated by peripheral sense organs such as the retina, cochlea, and olfactory bulbs. *Proprioception* is the ability to sense the position and movement of the body in space and is mediated by mechanoreceptors typically located in muscles, joints, ligaments, tendons, and skin (16). *Nociception* is the ability to sense pain in the form of heat or strong mechanical stimuli and is mediated by structures such as free nerve endings. The sensorimotor system provides information regarding actions and consequences of actions that contributes to neuromotor development, learning, and behavior. These neural sensory processes can be *perceived* by cerebral cortex awareness (i.e., conscious) or can be *received* by lower central nervous system centers without awareness (i.e., subconscious). The central nervous system serves to integrate these neural faculties as the ultimate arbiter of function.

For the purposes of this chapter, the investigative approaches to be discussed are divided into categories that deal predominately with the *proprioceptive sensorimotor system,* outlining different vantage points of the neuromotor system. In this manner, the chapter should be viewed as a description of one system with integrating principles attempting to reconcile all findings. The order of presentation follows historical perspectives, from early observations detailing the presence of neural elements in tissue to more sophisticated neural imaging and computer modeling techniques that can characterize disease and injury.

INVESTIGATIVE APPROACHES

Afferent Receptor Characterization

Sensory acquisition is the process by which information is collected from sensory organs that allows neural processing. Historically, soft tissues such as ligament, joint capsule, and fibrocartilage were not considered sensory organs like the retina or cochlea, but rather they were regarded as static bricks-and-mortar structural material. However, these tissues are true sensory organs and play a fundamental role in the function of the neuromotor system (17,18).

Soft tissue structures receive stimuli by afferent receptors during interaction with the environment. Afferent receptors populate all soft tissue structures and all types of connective tissue (Table 7.1). The function of specific receptors, such as muscle spindles (19–21) and Golgi tendon organs (22), is quite complex and often is not fully understood (23). Afferent receptors are activated by changes in their environment such as alteration of osmotic and electrolyte gradients, chemical transmitter concentrations, active and passive electrical properties, temperature, and mechanical deformation such as pressure and stretch. This activation can then be transmitted to the central nervous system for processing. The orchestration between afferent receptor stimulation and the induction of neuronal activation thresholds is controlled by the flux of inhibitory and stimulatory connections within the central nervous system. This process is extremely complex and is an active area of research (24).

Environmental and endogenous stimuli that induce neural activity are segregated into specific sensory channels through the filtering properties of the various *afferent receptor fields.* This level of sensory acquisition is the first point at which stimuli are transformed by the nervous system into coding signals that characterize a particular afferent environment. Various sensory profiles are generated for each set of afferent circumstances and serve as the *language* for *sensorimotor reading.* This language is transmitted to the central nervous system by nerve fibers designed for specific receptor function and receptor field (Table 7.2). The ability to encode afferent information into a language that the central nervous system can use is critical for neuromotor function.

Neurohistologic evaluations have profiled afferent receptor populations in various tissues types and serve as the anatomic basis by which neural mechanisms can be evaluated. The pattern of neural elements observed within a specific tissue is not random and correlates well with specific tissue function. For example, the shoulder retains all types of receptors listed in Table 7.1, but the distribution of these receptors is varied among ligamentous, capsular, tendonous, muscular, skin, and labral tissue, based on the tissue's physical properties (25–30). Likewise, in the knee, meniscal tissue afferent receptor profiles vary considerably from cruciate ligament profiles because of the different types of forces typically observed in each instance (31–33). Afferent receptor function follows their residence tissue function; yet their populations have been observed to decrease with age (28) and to demonstrate senescence (34,35).

Joint injury and repair can alter afferent receptor populations and are good examples of neural plasticity. Biopsies of untreated anterior cruciate ligament (ACL) tears show morphologically normal mechanoreceptors within the ligament 3 months after injury; however, this population gradually

TABLE 7.1 TYPE AND FUNCTION OF PREDOMINATE SOFT TISSUE NEURAL RECEPTORS

Ruffinian corpuscles (Golgi-Mazzoni bodies, spray endings)
  Slowly adapting mechanoreceptors that respond to low mechanical thresholds
  Static or dynamic receptors that respond to joint position, intraarticular pressure, movement amplitude and velocity
  Possibly tonically active at intermediate joint angles (i.e., midrange afferents)
  Parent axon diameter 5–9 μm
Merkel receptors
  Slowly adapting mechanoreceptors
  Located primarily in the superficial portion of dermis
  Small receptor fields for tactile discrimination
  Interposed synapse between membrane and parent axon
Pacinian corpuscles (Meissner corpuscles, Vater-Pacinian corpuscles, Krause's endkörpechen, bulbous corpuscles)
  Rapidly adapting mechanoreceptor that responds to low mechanical thresholds
  Dynamic receptors that respond to acceleration and deceleration
  Inactivity with joint immobilization and constant velocity movement
  Parent axon diameter 8–12 μm
Free nerve endings
  Nociceptor system (group III and IV afferents)
  Active during abnormal circumstances such as mechanical deformation, temperature, inflammation
  Spot-like receptive fields
  Chemical (seratonin, bradykinin, histamine, prostaglandins) and osmotic (ion activation) mediators
Golgi tendon–like organs (stretch receptors, spray endings)
  Slowly adapting mechanoreceptors that respond to high mechanical thresholds
  Inactive in immobile joints
  Sensitive to small changes in tension
  Parent axon diameter 13–17 μm
Muscle spindles (stretch receptors)
  Specialized encapsulated intrafusal muscle fibers arranged in parallel with extrafusal muscle fibers
  Innervated by γ motor neurons
  Types of intrafusal muscle fibers:
    Nuclear bag fibers produce slow contractions
    Nuclear chain fibers produce fast contractions
  Types of afferent terminals:
    Primary innervate all intrafusal fibers
    Secondary innervate nuclear chain fibers

TABLE 7.2 TYPES OF AFFERENT AND EFFERENT NERVE FIBERS

Nerve		Afferent Nerve Fibers		
Muscle	Cutaneous	Fiber Diameter (μm)	Conduction Velocity (m/sec)	Afferent Receptors
Ia	[Aα]	12–20	70–120	Muscle spindle
Ib	[Aα]	12–20	70–120	Golgi tendon organ
II	Aβ	5–12	25–75	Spindles, mechanoreceptor
III	Aδ	1–5	5–30	Free nerve endings
IV	C	0.2–1.5	0.5–2	Free nerve endings

Efferent Nerve Fibers	
Motor Neuron Type	Motor Unit Innervated
α	Innervates extrafusal skeletal muscle fibers (motor)
β	Innervates both intrafusal and extrafusal skeletal muscle fibers (skeletofusimotor)
γ	Innervates intrafusal skeletal muscle fibers (fusimotor)
γ-dynamic	Innervates nuclear bag fibers
γ-static	Innervates nuclear chain fibers

decreases toward zero by 1 year (36). Disuse neuronal atrophy typically parallels loss of ligament function after injury. Conversely, regeneration of viable afferent receptors occurs between 2 and 4 weeks after ACL reconstruction with normalization toward controls by 8 weeks (36–40). Sensory reinnervation typically parallels the graft remodeling processes of revascularization, collagen reorganization, and fibroblast repopulation (37). Although the function of these injured or regenerated neural elements is unclear, reconstruction of altered neuromotor function may be possible based on neurohistologic evidence. Indeed, preserving ACL fiber remnants containing afferent receptors during reconstruction can improve clinical outcome (41,42).

Because information from afferent receptors projects to many areas of the nervous system including supraspinal centers such as the cerebral cortex (43), *somatosensory evoked potentials* (SSEPs) have been used as a means to detect altered afferent receptor function after tissue injury. SSEP evaluations are a measure of central nervous system function with deviations indicating changes in neural circuitry or conduction. In the case of the ACL, SSEPs are consistently altered after ligament disruption indicating a compensatory central nervous system remodeling response to the loss of ligament afferent receptors (44). Normalization of the SSEP responses can occur parallel with the sensory reinnervation observed after ACL reconstruction (45), further detailing the clinical and functional importance of afferent receptors within the neuromotor system (46,47).

End-Organ Evaluation

End-organ evaluations typically involve investigation of the macroscopic anatomic effectors of the musculoskeletal system—the skeletal muscles, tendons, and bones—and their relation to function and injury. This series of components is designed to modulate energy encountered during interaction within the environment from both voluntary and reactionary movement. The design is a product of evolutionary development within *global gravitational fields*. Researchers in these areas have focused on physiologic parameters that confer differences among subject populations. For instance, the structural properties of bone (48), tendon (49), and the myotendinous junction (50) can impart variations in function (i.e., energy modulation, force generation, and movement synchronization) that correlate well with clinical observation.

Within this research area, skeletal muscle examination has been the most productive because its clinical variation and adaptation responses are quite readily apparent. All biologic tissue morphology and composition can be modified by habitual local conditions through a process called *mechanotransduction*. This is the process whereby physiologic forces induce changes in gene expression that lead to phenotypic modification. This mechanotransductive response is an important physiologic basis of tissue homeostasis, exercise, training, and rehabilitation. Because of the

wide variation observed with skeletal muscle, the intrinsic metabolic, architectural, and developmental adaptations to various loading and contraction patterns have provided good estimates of motor ability that characterize subject populations (51,52).

These studies have revealed intrinsic properties of skeletal muscle that allow for limb segment protection, injury prevention, and economy of movement. Intrinsic muscle properties are generated by contractile elements such as actin–myosin interaction and by noncontractile elements (series elastic component) that provide energy transforming mechanical properties to limb segments (53). The predominance of *eccentric-mode* contraction patterns displayed during physiologic activity reflects the importance of these elements for energy dissipation. Eccentric contraction, when compared with other contraction modes, allows energy dissipation with marked efficiency, that is, low oxygen requirements and myoelectric activity, short electromechanical delays, the ability to generate high peak forces, and low perceived exertion ratings (54). Skeletal muscle contraction also generates joint reactive forces that directly contribute to joint protection and stability (55–57). Cocontraction of musculature with opposing force vectors creates a muscular sling that controls joint displacement and translation (58), thus *limiting the demand on other joint tissues for energy dissipation.* Animal models used to assess skeletal muscle function have further detailed these processes (59), providing a strong rationale for strength training regimens.

Neural factors also influence and coordinate musculoskeletal function (60,61). Traditionally, neural influence on muscle function has been considered unidirectional. For example, neural drive induces motor unit health, activation state, fiber recruitment order, and coding rate. Diseases such as poliomyelitis, amyotrophic lateral sclerosis, and myasthenia gravis provide clinical insight into these influences. However, skeletal muscle activity also influences and maintains the properties of the motor neuron (62) and, based on activity pattern, can induce variations in afferent neural outflow (63). Whereas the affect of skeletal muscle fatigue on motor function is well known (64), the effect of *neural fatigue* on motor function has only recently become clear (65,66). These reciprocal influences retain functional significance for proprioceptive sensorimotor function.

Intrinsic muscle properties are the first line of defense to imposed environmental perturbations and therefore have been a useful means for testing. Isokinetic measurements of muscle function have provided a method for controlled evaluation and for limiting testing-induced injury that can occur with other types of physiologic (eccentric) assessment. Muscle testing has been used successfully as a criterion for return to activity by many practitioners (67,68) even though the relevance to physiologic function remains questionable (i.e., skeletal muscle generally functions in a nonisokinetic fashion during normal physiologic activities) (69,70). Gait assessments with high-speed cineography have further contributed to understanding the role of these intrinsic muscle properties during normal and altered musculoskeletal function.

Despite such testing shortcomings, gross muscle recruitment and coordination pattern alterations reflect functional changes and adaptations in neuromotor function of a compensatory or protective nature after injury. Evaluation of these changes by skeletal muscle testing has contributed to the design of successful rehabilitative programs. For instance, the increase in quadriceps activity observed after an acute ACL tear is generally followed by a compensatory augmentation of hamstring activity indicative of the chronically ACL-deficient knee (71,72). The quadriceps-avoidance gait illustrates the aversion to those force couples that may further induce injury and have guided rehabilitative therapeutics (73,74). Characterizing changes in limb segment movement through end-organ evaluation provides clinical details of the neuromotor response to injury and treatment.

Perceived Proprioception

Kinesthesia is the conscious perception of movement in space by cerebral cortex function. This perception can be of active or passive movements, voluntary or reactionary movements, or conditioned or novel movements. Because information from afferent receptors projects to supraspinal centers, evaluating kinesthesia has a sound physiologic basis (75,76) and has been a popular research approach for orthopaedic investigation. Because joint injury or disease can affect local neural elements, researchers have sought to develop clinical testing methods than can assess treatment outcome relative to these neural structures. Joint kinesthesia, joint position sense, muscle activation sense, and postural evaluations have become the most accepted perceived proprioception approaches.

Joint kinesthesia is evaluated by determining the threshold to detection of movement of particular limb segments. Subjects are typically asked to determine the angle or position of the limb joint at which movement is detected in a controlled setting. This estimate is recorded as the outcome value. *Joint position sense* is evaluated by reproduction of an index position set by study parameters. Visual analog scales or comparative limb segment positioning may be used to match this index position as a measure of the ability to reproduce position. Measures of *muscle activation sense* such as muscle magnitude estimation or muscle magnitude reproduction have also been used as outcome parameters for various clinical states and follow similar controlled study design as used with joint kinesthesia or joint position sense evaluations. These senses have been evaluated in healthy persons (77,78), as well as in patients with injury and after treatment (79–82), and they have generated useful kinesthetic data regarding neuromotor response to injury and treatment.

Postural (or balance) evaluations provide assessments of vestibular, visual, and sensorimotor influences on the lower extremity. Customarily, these methods are not considered true perceived proprioception evaluations, but they are included here because of the complex interplay of these influences in the central nervous system. These assessments measure static, dynamic, or functional abilities designed to maintain equilibrium. Alterations in force plate measurement, single-limb agility, and single- or double-limb postural sway (i.e., sway amplitude, speed and number of sway amplitudes) are parameters that have been correlated with injury-induced changes in balance (83,84). Even though elimination of the vestibulooccular influences has been difficult during these assessments, correlation with functional outcome during musculoskeletal care as been successful.

Normalization of perceived proprioception as demonstrated by these testing methods has been used in many settings to determine neurologic treatment outcome (85). However, validation of these testing methods has been the subject of much debate as a result of the many experimental techniques, methods, and styles of data analysis. Parameters and values studied are often subject participant estimates whose sensations are composed of afferent information from many types of peripheral receptors (86). Activation of these receptors is quite variable among subjects and is difficult to standardize. Generally, joint kinesthesia has been the most repeatable perceived proprioceptive parameter, even though further standardization is required for intrastudy comparisons (87).

Received Proprioception

Most perceived proprioception evaluations rely on measurements through the cerebral cortex. Subject differences are determined by evaluating cortical processing of passive, voluntary, or reactionary movement. This approach has been criticized because of the difficulty in controlling and measuring *cerebral cortex impressionability* (88,89). Cerebral cortex processing is often subjective and can be influenced by many variables including emotion, attention, experience, and environment. These concerns have generated a vast body of research directed toward understanding peripheral neural pathways that can be assessed "independent" of conscious participant expression.

Afferent receptor stimulation induces nerve transmission that ultimately evokes changes in motor neuron activity (90,91). These effects are mediated largely by the α-γ muscle spindle or *fusimotor system* (Fig. 7.2). Afferent receptor information is integrated by the fusimotor neurons and is processed to provide appropriate and coordinated muscle tension and function. This process results from both the excitatory and inhibitory influences of afferent receptor information that is exerted on both the agonist and antagonist muscles around a joint. This "reflex-mediated" muscle stiffness combined with intrinsic muscle properties and descending supraspinal neural pathways adds to the control of joint movement.

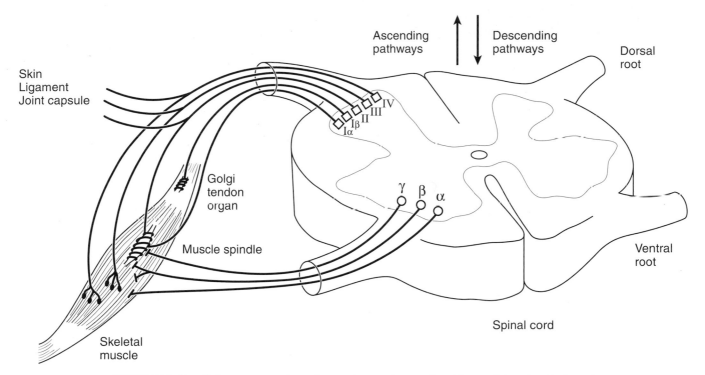

FIGURE 7.2 Simplistic representation of sensorimotor integration. The peripheral, spinal, and supraspinal nervous systems interact at many levels to coordinate receipt of afferent information and subsequent neural processing. Specifically, the proprioceptive sensorimotor system functions to gather afferent information so central neural processing can generate appropriate motor responses. This function of reciprocal processing allows coordination within the environment. Ia, Ib, II, III, IV refer to afferent nerve fibers; α, β, γ refer to efferent nerve fibers; IN, interneurons.

Peripheral neural reflex pathways have been characterized around the knee and shoulder joint and have contributed significantly to our understanding of this process (92,93). Electrical or mechanical stimulation of joint tissues induces muscle spindle afferent discharge within the muscles that control joint function. The anterior cruciate ligament (94,95), posterior cruciate ligament (96,97), collateral ligaments (98), and skin receptors (99) all project neural pathways that can influence knee joint muscle activity through the fusimotor system. In the shoulder, the capsule reflex (100–102), the glenohumeral-biceps reflex (103), and the infraspinatus spinal stretch reflex (104) have also demonstrated the effect afferent receptors can exert on muscle control of the joint.

Soft tissue afferent receptors provide information from all situations, not just in response to injurious stimuli such as extremes of motion. Small loads on joint tissues such as occur during normal physiologic activity provide afferent information that affects muscular control of the joint. Tissue forces as low as 5 to 10 N (comparable to 1.5% to 5% of ligament ultimate tensile strength) generate afferent information that can alter muscular function (97). Additionally, afferent receptors induce "midrange" neural responses at all positions of joint movement (105). This wide range of afferent information provides good evidence that the proprioceptive nervous system garners a canvassing-like land-

scape of detail. In its entirety, this information has been termed the *joint afferent profile,* and its composition is continuously updated through all phases of joint movement and function. The joint afferent profile is but one reflection of the proprioceptive sensorimotor system interface between subject and environment.

Characterization of these neural pathways retains clinical relevance. Injury to joint structures induces an altered joint afferent profile that affects neuromotor function. Altered muscle recruitment or coordination patterns (106,107), biomechanically related changes in muscle latency (108), and muscle latency response (reaction time) to imposed perturbations (109) have been useful clinical evaluation techniques. For instance, ankle injury has demonstrated prolonged reaction times and slowing of peripheral nerve conduction velocity (110–112). Hamstring muscle reaction times are slowed in ACL-deficient knees (72,113,114), whereas shoulder instability is associated with altered muscle coordination and activity patterns (115). Early treatment methods have been developed to address these alterations in neural conductivity and muscular synchronization because it is clear that neural influences are driving these changes.

The *spinal stretch reflex* has been used to evaluate elements of dynamic joint stability and function from both a physiologic and a clinical perspective (104). The spinal stretch reflex is the simplest and fastest stimulus–response paradigm in the vertebrate nervous system (i.e., a two-neuron arc). It is an innate spinal segmental pathway whose evaluation provides a reproducible method of testing subject populations that display clinical differences in neuromotor characteristics, development, and maturation. The normal spinal stretch reflex evolves from a hyperexcitable and prominent state during infancy to a less-prominent or quiescent state during adulthood. Disruption of this process occurs in subjects with cerebral palsy who demonstrate significant spasticity that interferes with normal motor function (116–118). Skeletal muscle activity level such as inactivity or exercise can also alter spinal stretch reflex characteristics and provides a means to discriminate subject populations with clinical differences in motor ability.

The spinal stretch reflex is reliably elicited in the infraspinatus muscle, and this phenomenon has been used to evaluate the neuromotor sequelae of various shoulder conditions. Reflex parameters (i.e., percentage of elicitation, latency, and amplitude) of normal subjects serve as control data that allow for comparison of groups of patients who display various clinical characteristics (104). For instance, patients with multidirectional shoulder instability demon-

strate a prominent reflex response indicative of decreased supraspinal reflex control processes when they are compared with normal subjects (119). Conversely, athletic persons demonstrate a quiescent reflex response indicative of enhanced reflex control mechanisms (119). The regulation of *reflex activation threshold* as measured with the spinal stretch reflex profile can serve as a window into the attributes of neuromotor performance between subject populations (Fig. 7.3).

The role of the proprioceptive sensorimotor system within this process has become clearer through the reflex evaluation of shoulder outlet impingement syndrome. Patients with acute shoulder outlet impingement syndrome exhibit pronounced rotator cuff reflex inhibition typical of *muscular dyskinesia* (120). This pain-induced neuromuscular imbalance leads to disruption of normal glenohumeral and scapulothoracic rhythm that, in turn, leads to changes in extremity function. As this process continues, the neuromotor system adapts to the pain-related joint afferent profile by altering its normal local relationship between sensory acquisition and motor control. Patients with chronic untreated shoulder outlet impingement syndrome display the

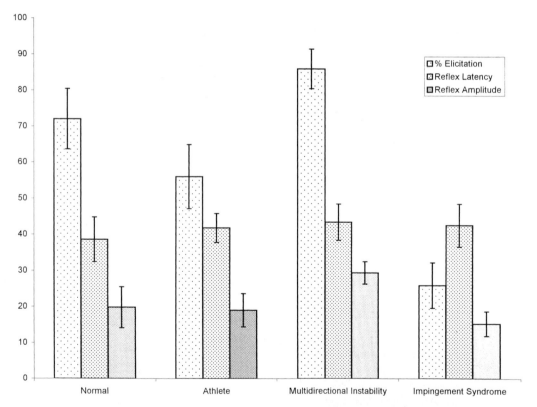

FIGURE 7.3 Graphic representation of the infraspinatus spinal stretch reflex profile. This profile is composed of the reflex percentage of elicitation, latency, and amplitude. These parameters together create a neuromotor profile that may be used to discriminate subject populations before, during, and after treatment. In this example, patients who exhibit particular clinical shoulder characteristics, such as athletic disposition, instability, or outlet impingement, can be profiled, thus allowing assessment of the neuromotor sequelae of particular conditions. Although control of reflex activation threshold by the central nervous system depends on many variables, this technique has been a useful first step in neuromotor profiling of clinical conditions. Adapted from references 119 and 120.

inability to use complex sensory information effectively to execute accurate arm movements in space characteristic of *kinesthetic apraxia* (120). In this manner, the process of *sensorimotor integration* is disrupted. These findings provide an explanation for the improved outcome observed clinically with the early treatment of shoulder outlet impingement syndrome (121).

Trends in evaluating the neurologic outcome of musculoskeletal treatment have been geared toward normalizing received proprioceptive responses. For instance, after successful ACL reconstruction, hamstring muscle latency responses can be improved toward more normal reaction times (122). In patients with multidirectional shoulder instability, physical therapy and biofeedback techniques can decrease spinal stretch reflex prominence and can provide symptomatic improvement without surgical treatment (123). Likewise, successful arthroscopic subacromial decompression can normalize the pain-induced reflex inhibition and muscular dyskinesia of acute outlet impingement syndrome (124). These examples have been some of the first studies to apply received proprioceptive evaluation to clinical treatment outcome.

Neuromotor Modeling of the Injury Scenario

Neuromotor modeling techniques characterize principles that incorporate anatomic neural framework into motor programming theories. The concept of the *motor program* has been a fruitful construct borrowed from computer sciences to facilitate the understanding of more elaborate neural circuitry (125). The purpose of neuromotor modeling is not only to explain proprioceptive phenomena such as kinesthesia but also to describe neuromotor programming, learning, and development as it relates to sensory acquisition. The function of the global organism is characterized within specific controlled afferent environments, typically in terms of injury prevention, to determine neuromotor response strategies that are developed in reaction to the afferent scenarios. Two general categories of *neuromotor modeling of the injury scenario* have been described: feedback and feed-forward theories.

Linear *feedback models* have focused on the natural link between afferent receptors and reflex muscle activity. In this theory, afferent receptors provide information to the central nervous system that induces reflex motor responses designed to correct for the encountered perturbations characterized by the afferent receptors. Reflex responses can be linked together by the central nervous system to form more complex behaviors representative of normal function. This feedback modeling approach, however, has lost favor as result of various physiologic constraints when it is used to explain injury prevention.

The most notable constraint for feedback modeling is electromechanical delay (126–128). *Electromechanical delay*

is the time necessary from stimulation to muscle contraction and includes nerve conduction, synaptic transmission, muscle activation, and mechanical force development. The fastest peripheral nerve conduction velocities approximate 80 to 120 m per second, with the quickest neural arc approximating 25 to 50 milliseconds (the spinal stretch reflex). Injury can occur much too fast for a feedback-only system to accommodate all environmental perturbation (129–132). Further, reflex activity can be modified by voluntary intentions (129,133,134) or can occur before specific voluntary movement (35). Intentions occurring less than 100 milliseconds from kinesthetic input can dissociate linked reflex and voluntary motor activity (135,136). Reflex changes can be learned (137) and movement modification can occur without sensory input (138). These constraints and others have forced researchers to consider feed-forward modeling approaches to explain the injury scenario.

A significant amount of research provides a physiologic basis for *feed-forward modeling* because of the link between afferent information and motor programming (139). Even though feed-forward muscle activity can be generated centrally without the need for peripheral feedback (140), afferent information is used to determine movement accuracy. This allows fine tuning of responses by updated environmental perceptions to achieve the desired control of movement more precisely (89,141–146). Because motor activity is tailored by more detailed afferent information, the timing of neuromotor events becomes more specific, and the need for subjects to concentrate decreases (141,147,148). In this manner, afferent information has been linked to the development of central motor programs (142,144,146).

Epidemiologic and behavioral studies indicate that injury often occurs when unexpected environmental perturbations are encountered with forces that overcome the preparedness of subjects to dissipate those forces (149). The neuromotor strategies involved in learning to *prevent* such occurrences of energy mismatch are important for injury prevention. Based on the function of the neuromotor system to modulate environmental energy, an elemental parameter by which motor control and learning develop is the ability to manage forces in an anticipatory feed-forward fashion (Fig. 7.4). This ability as a skill acquisition has been equated with injury avoidance and has been termed *neuromotor programming by energy management* (150).

The learned response of recognizing an impending perturbation that may retain injury potential through afferent input and enlisting motor activity to accommodate that perturbation before it is encountered allows dissipation of energy that may induce injury. The unexpected perturbations associated with injury would become expected through learning to recognize particular situations before particular perturbations are encountered. In an anticipatory feed-forward system, situational afferent cues would alert subjects to the impending forces in a meaningful manner. Exteroception, proprioception, and nociception allow receipt of these cues;

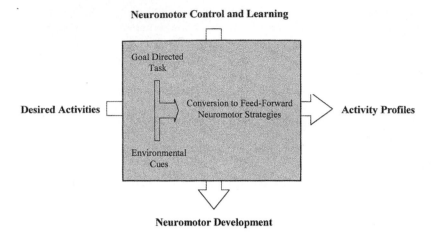

Neuromotor Control and Learning

Goal Directed Task

Desired Activities

Conversion to Feed-Forward Neuromotor Strategies

Activity Profiles

Environmental Cues

Neuromotor Development

FIGURE 7.4 Neuromotor programming by energy management. Neuromotor control, learning, and development can occur by similar processes through environmental energy management. This process of sensorimotor integration is especially important for injury prevention and is the basis for anticipatory feed-forward central motor programming through environmental interaction. (From Augé II WK. Response strategies for injury prevention: confirmation of neuromotor learning during acquisition of motor control. *COSPR* 2000;5:97–106, with permission.)

the central nervous system processes this input to develop appropriate profiles of specific anticipatory feed-forward neuromotor responses during skill acquisition (150). This process of sensorimotor integration is a basis of neuromotor learning and development important for injury prevention.

Correlations between motor skill acquisition and the incidence of injury have been difficult to clarify, even though the intuitive conclusion infers that as greater motor skill develops, injury decreases (151). Defining, measuring, and quantifying motor skill in the context of neuromotor learning certainly holds wide implications for injury prevention (152). Anticipatory feed-forward ability can be limited by the capacity of subjects to recognize and process afferent cues that statistically telegraph impending perturbations. As the afferent complexity of environmental scenarios increase, sensorimotor integration aptitude has demonstrated significant variation among participant groups (152). These findings partially explain the epidemiologic injury pattern disparity observed between physiologically similar subject populations. As an example, athletes develop neuromotor responses to controlled environmental scenarios much quicker and more efficiently than do control populations. Such neuromotor responses characterize sensorimotor integration aptitude and have been a useful clinical and physiologic assessment of athletic ability (Fig. 7.5).

Other modeling techniques related to energy management have been developed to characterize neuromotor control, learning, and development (153–155). For instance, the observations that energy expenditure is minimized during locomotion (156), that activity can be governed by specific internal muscle properties (157), that motor unit recruitment can change with skill acquisition (158), and that the ability to dissipate loads may affect reflex activity (159) reflect aspects of neuromotor programming by energy management. Mathematic representations (160–163) and concepts of pattern generators (164) have characterized neuromotor control through energy modulation. Researchers in other disciplines have contributed theories of motor skill acquisition that have sought to unify investigative observations of neuromotor control and learning (165–173). These approaches have not been previously applied to the injury scenario but may assist in further elucidating those parameters that may be manipulated to assist in injury avoidance.

Functional Neural Imaging

Various neural imaging techniques have been developed that provide additional insight into nervous system structure and function. These techniques are being integrated into multimodal neural imaging evaluations designed to

FIGURE 7.5 Assessment of athletic ability through neuromotor response strategies. Comparison of athlete versus nonathlete in the ability to learn motor control during skill acquisition in response to a novel environmental scenario. Environmental scenario I is controlled for one afferent stimulus, a random perturbation force that induces a spinal stretch reflex response; Environmental scenario II is controlled for two linked afferent stimuli, an auditory stimulus followed by the same random perturbation force. Subjects were instructed to resist the perturbation force but had no knowledge of the presence or significance of the auditory stimulus before testing. The size of the perturbation area reflects the subjects' ability to resist the perturbation force whereby a small area reflects successful neuromotor strategy development for the goal-directed task. Voluntary muscle activity occurs in an anticipatory feed-forward manner only when the auditory stimulus is present, thus allowing subjects to telegraph the onset of the perturbation force through stimulus linking. The athlete can rapidly fine tune the onset of voluntary activity to correspond with the onset of the perturbation force. (From Augé II WK. Assessment of athletic ability through neuromotor response strategy. *COSPR* 2001;6:49–57, with permission.)

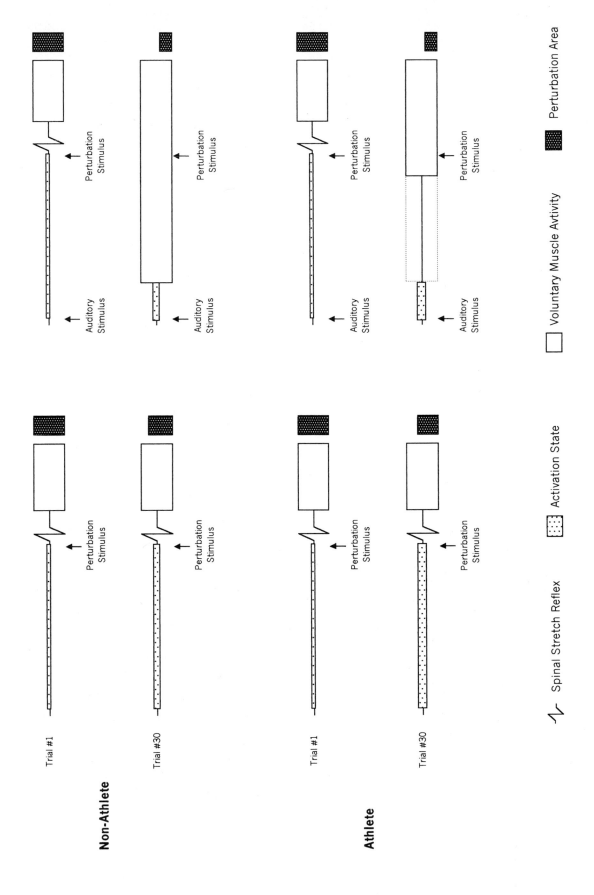

improve our understanding of normal neural processes and adaptive responses to injury and disease (174–176). These methods provide both static and dynamic spatial–temporal maps of neural activation patterns that reflect neural circuitry.

Anatomic magnetic resonance imaging (MRI) is clinically the most common imaging modality for the nervous system. It provides high-resolution images that characterize tissue geometry and composition. Three-dimensional volume imaging (177), brain warping (178), and cortical unfolding (179) techniques are examples of more sophisticated methods that can provide significant anatomic detail. *Functional MRI (fMRI)* evaluations record hemodynamic and electromagnetic neural activation patterns that occur in response to various neural processes (180,181). Sensory stimulation, cognition, or motor tasks can be mapped to specific central nervous system locations. *Electromagnetic* evaluations, such as magnetoencephalography (MEG), which directly measures the magnetic fields produced by the brain, provide more accurate temporal recordings of neurologic systems in response to similar stimulation modes (182).

Neurophysiologic studies demonstrate that neurons in the motor cortex receive strong topographically organized input from peripheral afferent receptors that is similar to the input arriving at the sensory cortex. This input occurs through direct contributions from both the thalamus and the somatosensory cortex (i.e., through corticocortical connections) and is very effective in altering motor cortex neuronal activity (183). These findings provide the neurophysiologic basis for use of multimodal functional imaging technologies for assessing the changes in motor function that result from injury-induced disruption of the normal receipt of afferent information by the central nervous system.

By using multimodal neural imaging techniques (i.e., combined fMRI, EEG, and MEG), cerebral cortical activity can be localized and assessed in response to afferent information (Fig. 7.6) (184–186). In one example, median nerve stimulation was used to monitor the integrity of tissue in the motor and somatosensory cortex (187–189). Peaks of evoked magnetic responses after electrical median nerve stimulation provide an assessment of the temporal dynamics and geographic locations of nerve fiber connectivity. The neurophysiologic changes that occur after sensorimotor ischemic stroke have been evaluated in this manner (190,191), and they provide a means to assess motor function in patients

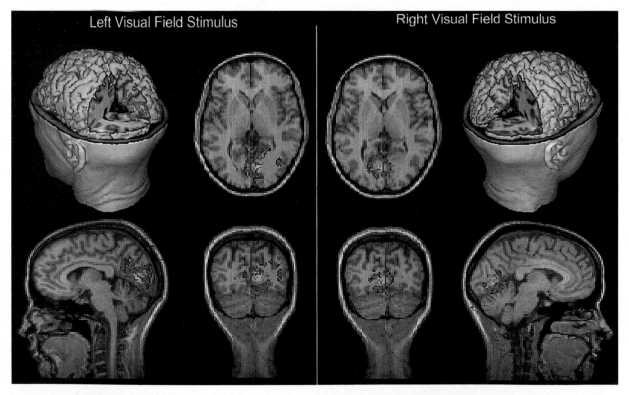

FIGURE 7.6 Source probability maps estimated for visual evoked response data. This figure displays multimodal neural imaging techniques to define brain cortex activation sites. Four views of a region found to contain activity at a 95% probability level demonstrates interactive visualization of spatial–temporal source probability maps that coregister with anatomic magnetic resonance imaging. (From ref. 232: Schmidt DM, George JS, Wood CC. Bayesian inference applied to the electromagnetic inverse problem. *Human brain mapping*, vol 7. New York: John Wiley, 1999:195–212, with permission.)

who are unable to perform sensorimotor tasks (191). Similar applications may be developed for assessing the changes evoked by injury-induced joint deafferentation.

Other techniques, such as functional electrical impedance tomography for assessing cranial conductivities (192,193), transcranial magnetic stimulation for mapping sensory stimulation and endogenous control processes (194), and somatosensory evoked optical intensity changes in neural tissues (195), are examples of other innovative techniques for investigating the nervous system. Optical illumination imaging (196,197) can even track the electrical and hemodynamic processes of neural tissue through the changes in neuron osmotic gradients typically observed with activation (198). Imaging at this level is generating remarkable detail of neural processes.

Computer Modeling of Neurobiologic Systems

The first attempts at mathematic modeling of neural systems were made in the 1930s. *The ionic theory of nervous conduction* was based on ionic motion around neurons as a description of electrical pulse conduction. Properties of axon membranes were represented by electrical circuits that allowed calculation of the shape and velocity of propagating action potentials using differential mathematic equations (i.e., Hodgkin-Huxley) (199–202). The *extended cable theory* was introduced to explain the electrochemical properties of a neuron among neurons (203–207). Within this theory, the nerve cell functions simply as a cable, like an electrical cord. *Single-compartment cable models* assume a single membrane potential can characterize the whole neuron, whereby an equation for the temporal change of membrane potential and a set of kinetic equations for the gating variables can be applied (208). *Multicompartment models* allow the solution of the cable equation with nonlinear voltage-dependent membrane and time-dependent synaptic conductance (209). Sophisticated differential equation sets have since been developed that can imitate the behavior of most known neuron types (210).

More recent advances, however, in neural recordings and molecular probe staining are revealing the details of microarchitectural neural circuitry. This is the level believed to hold the secret of how the nervous system performs complex functions such as sensory integration and motor control. Some highly detailed computer models of neurobiologic systems have been developed that mimic *in vivo* network behavior to determine what contributions various aspects of structure make to function.

In vivo neural systems retain a great deal more structure than that captured by traditional neural network modeling *(neural nets)*. Neurons demonstrate a variety of cell types (i.e., pyramidal, Purkinje, amacrine, bushy, Martinotti) that exhibit diverse shapes, structures, distributions, and spatial arrangements. Dynamic neural responses also vary; some cells react in a classic Hodgkin–Huxley fashion, whereas others react through an assortment of ion currents that generate bursting, graded, or more complex response patterns. Neural tissue demonstrates a highly intricate connectivity matrix, rather than the all-to-all relationship assumed with most neural nets. Even more complex is cellular and synaptic plasticity that itself changes over time with experience, learning, and memory.

This seemingly inaccessible complexity has been addressed through the development of comprehensive neural simulators (211,212). Neural simulators attempt to capture various aspects of microarchitectural neural circuitry by incorporating as many *in vivo* features as possible. Simulations can be as simple as a single neuron's response to a controlled stimulus to very large systems consisting of multiple nuclei each consisting of layers of neurons of various types, dynamics, and connectivities. Neural simulators allow experimentation of a type that has long been used in physics and various engineering fields—building a system model to compute its responses to various stimuli and stresses, ultimately to gain a better understanding of *in vivo* relationships and functions. The steps in a neural tissue simulation consist of the following: (a) specifying the numbers, types, spatial distributions, spatial dimensions, and conductive properties of neurons; (b) determining the connectivity matrix based on sizes and locations of dendritic trees and axonal projections; (c) computing the state of each neuron at each sequence of time in response to a given input stimulation pattern; and (d) analyzing graphic and statistical simulation data results.

Auditory (213–215), visual (216–218), cortical processing (219), and cerebellar (220) systems have been modeled in this fashion with the BioSENSE neural simulator developed and located at Los Alamos National Laboratory in Los Alamos, New Mexico. BioSENSE provides highly detailed models of sensory organs, stimuli, and neural responses. Versions of the simulator are taking advantage of parallel development of massive computer architectures occurring at the Laboratory. Newer applications of the simulator will likely uncover additional insight into the proprioceptive sensorimotor system. Investigations focusing on the role of synchronicity within the brain for object recognition may clarify afferent information processing methods. Integrated brain system models that include neural signal processing from a sensory organ to the thalamus to the cerebral cortex with feedbacks from higher and lower levels may also generate greater understanding of nervous system function.

This technology allows further integration among research disciplines. BioSENSE data can be compared with other larger-scale brain functioning data such as MEG and fMRI. Other experimental biologic data can be tested against the predicted simulation outcomes. This integration provides a good example of the multidisciplinary approach necessary for nervous system investigation.

Other Areas

Other research disciplines have much to offer investigation of the proprioceptive sensorimotor system. Three additional disciplines are active research areas and worth brief review in this chapter: neuroinformatics, the endocrine–immune–neural axes, and evolutionary–comparative–developmental neurobiology.

Informatics is the study of information. Complexity models, quantum mechanics, and chaos theory are techniques that have been used to address the overwhelming amount of information that exists within the universe (221). Neuroinformatics may allow the opportunity to access the complexity of the nervous system during environmental interaction and overlaps with other computer simulation approaches. For example, the reduction of neural processes to elemental binary probabilities that detail atomic behavior may be translated to higher levels of function through further statistical assimilation. Supercomputers not yet conceived may allow organized reading of the information gathered by the sensorimotor system and may allow prediction of motor phenomena within complex environmental scenarios. These methods may mimic brain information-processing techniques and, once characterized, may provide additional clues into the brain's integrative functions (222).

The *immune and endocrine systems* interact with the nervous system at all levels to maintain homeostasis (223,224). Endocrine and immune influences are equally important to neural function as nerve cell transmission is for muscle function. The hypothalamic–pituitary–adrenal axis and the nervous system interact with immune surveillance and inflammatory process at many levels (225). Simple examples such as the affects of anesthetic agents placed within an inflamed joint (226) or the hormonal influence on ligament injury (227) provide entry-level evidence of these influences. Studies detailing neurovascular coupling provide characterization of the interface among these systems (228). Endocrine, immune, and neural mediators, often the same compound, modulate sensory acquisition, processing, and neuromotor function and will become a productive area for musculoskeletal inquiry.

Learning and development research will have direct implications on the proprioceptive sensorimotor system. Growth and development are governed largely by the control of gene expression. From this expression, motor learning occurs through environmental interaction, itself governed by sensory acquisition, leading to profiles of motor activity. Ultimately, behavior and social dealings arise through changes in the structure of neural circuits and synaptic activity. These processes further induce higher levels of cerebral integration such as cultural development. Evolutionary, comparative, and developmental neurobiologies describe genetic drift and ecologic influences on these processes and provide additional characterization of our interaction with our surroundings (229–231).

SUMMARY

The *spectrum of neuromotor sensibility* describes the variation in the ability to sense, as observed among patient groups. We are familiar with the spectrum of sensibility in the evaluation of exteroceptors such as vision and hearing. Eyeglasses and hearing aids are prostheses that are used to enhance these particular sensory faculties by drawing more information from the body and environment to assist in functional improvement. Yet what about proprioceptors? Can the fusimotor system be augmented to allow better processing of afferent information to induce further performance improvements? What prostheses can be developed for the proprioceptive sensorimotor system? Does a limit exist in proprioceptive function or sensorimotor integration aptitude?

The nervous system demonstrates significant plasticity in its response to activity level, injury, disease, and treatment. It responds at all times to all circumstances regardless of situation during its life span. This chapter has reviewed many instances of these properties as related to musculoskeletal care. The nervous system is attentive to all of life's circumstances, and these properties are immensely fertile grounds for musculoskeletal innovation.

Arthroscopic techniques limit alteration of joint afferent profiles by limiting iatrogenic joint damage. Rehabilitative physical therapy after injury or surgical reconstruction is a process of sensory reeducation whereby patients learn the new afferent profile of particular limb segments. Aggressive rehabilitation programs induce early development of neuromotor activity that provides appropriate functional adaptations and improvements. Athletes practice and train as a means to improve function within particular sensory environments. Learning situational afferent cues typical of a specific environment allows subjects to excel within that environment. In each instance, activity pattern repetition leads to neural circuitry synaptic changes that induce improvements in performance, ability, and skill. This neuromotor plasticity at both the conscious and subconscious level holds immediate implications for musculoskeletal care.

Perhaps additional means exist to improve proprioceptive sensorimotor reading. Such may be a way to improve environmental awareness for injury prevention, to combat age-related afferent neuronal loss, or even to restore the relative deafferentiation induced by joint injury. Subsequent innovation may allow improvements in sensorimotor integration such as fine neural control of limb prosthesis by self-contained processing of afferent information, restoration of spinal cord function after injury, or even neuromotor robotics. An understanding of neurologic injury, disease, and rehabilitative states can further uncover the processes that govern the musculoskeletal system and can shape ideas toward additional treatment avenues that optimize reconstitution of function. Assimilation of the nervous system in musculoskeletal care is our next great challenge.

ACKNOWLEDGMENTS

We wish to acknowledge many persons for providing research updates of their respective fields included in this chapter: Cheryl J. Aine, Ph.D. and Ming-Xiong Huang, Ph.D., Center for Functional Brain Imaging, New Mexico Veterans Affairs Health Care System, Albuquerque, New Mexico; John S. George, Ph.D., Biophysics Group, Los Alamos National Laboratory, Los Alamos, New Mexico; Antonio Redondo, Ph.D., Theoretical Chemistry and Molecular Physics, Theoretical Division, Los Alamos National Laboratory, Los Alamos, New Mexico; and Bryan J. Travis, Ph.D.; Earth and Environmental Services Division, Center for Nonlinear Studies, Los Alamos National Laboratory, Los Alamos, New Mexico.

REFERENCES

1. Hilton J. Joint innervation: reflex control of muscles activating joints. In: *Rest and pain,* 6th ed. London: Bell, 1950:156–167.
2. Augé WK II. The trapped shoulder: clinical characterization and results of four treatment approaches. *Arthroscopy* 1999;15:S61–S62.
3. Cappellino A, Jokl P, Rowe PA. Regional anesthesia in knee arthroscopy: a new technique involving femoral and sciatic nerve blocks in knee arthroscopy. *Arthroscopy* 1996;12:120–123.
4. Augé WK II, Griffin JA. ACL reconstruction performed under 3-in-1 nerve block: results using newer generation surgical techniques. *Arthroscopy* 2000;16:433.
5. Snyder-Mackler L, DeLuca PF, Williams PR, et al. Reflex inhibition of the quadriceps femoris muscle after injury or reconstruction of the anterior cruciate ligament. *J Bone Joint Surg Am* 1994;76:555–560.
6. Pawl RP. Controversies surrounding reflex sympathetic dystrophy: a review article. *Curr Rev Pain* 2000;4:259–267.
7. Reuler JB, Girard DE, Nardone DA. The chronic pain syndrome: misconceptions and management. *Ann Intern Med* 1980;93:588–596.
8. Pitman MI, Nainzadeh N, Ergas E, et al. The use of somatosensory evoked potentials for detection of neuropraxia during shoulder arthroscopy. *Arthroscopy* 1988;4:250–255.
9. Augé WK II, Velázquez PA. Parsonage-Turner syndrome in the Native American Indian. *J Shoulder Elbow Surg* 2000;9:99–103.
10. Sussman MD. *The diplegic child: evaluation and management.* Rosemont, IL: American Academy of Orthopaedic Surgeons, 1992.
11. Nackley JV. *Primer on workers' compensation.* Washington, DC: Bureau of National Affairs, 1999.
12. Schenck RC. *Athletic training and sports medicine,* 3rd ed. Rosemont, IL: American Academy of Orthopaedic Surgeons, 2000.
13. Lepart SM. Preface. In: Lepart SM, Fu FH, eds. *Proprioception and neuromuscular control in joint stability.* Champaign, IL: Human Kinetics, 2000:xv–xvi.
14. Kandel ER. Nerve cells and behavior. In: Kandel ER, Swartz JH, eds. *Principles of neural science,* 2nd ed. New York: Elsevier Science, 1985:13–24.
15. Swartz JH. Synthesis and distribution of neural proteins. In: Kandel ER, Swartz JH, eds. *Principles of neural science,* 2nd ed. New York: Elsevier Science, 1985:37–48.
16. Sherrington CS. *The integrative action of the nervous system.* New Haven, CT: Yale University Press, 1906.
17. Johansson H, Sjölander P, Sojka P. A sensory role for the cruciate ligaments. *Clin Orthop* 1991;268:1161–178.
18. Kennedy JC, Alexander IJ, Hayes KC. Nerve supply of the human knee and its functional importance. *Am J Sports Med* 1982;10:329–335.
19. Burke D, Hagbarth KE, Lofsedt L. Muscle spindle activity in man during shortening and lengthening contractions. *J Physiol (Lond)* 1978;277:131–142.
20. Houk JC. An assessment of stretch reflex function. *Prog Brain Res* 1976;44:303–413.
21. Loeb GE. The control and responses of mammalian muscle spindles during normally executed motor tasks. *Exerc Sport Sci Rev* 1984;12:157–204.
22. Jami L, Petit J. Frequency of tendon organ discharges elicited by the contraction of motor units in cat leg muscles. *J Physiol (Lond)* 1976;261:633–645.
23. Matthews PBC. The 1989 James A. Stevenson Memorial Lecture. The knee jerk: still an enigma? *Can J Physiol Pharmacol* 1990;68:347–354.
24. Levin MF, Feldman AG. The role of stretch reflex threshold regulation in normal and impaired motor control. *Brain Res* 1994;657:23–30.
25. Guanche CA, Noble J, Solomonow M, et al. Periarticular neural elements in the shoulder joint. *Orthopedics* 1999;22:615–617.
26. Hashimoto T, Hamada T, Sasaguri Y, et al. Immunohistochemical approach for the investigation of nerve distribution in the shoulder joint capsule. *Clin Orthop* 1994;305:273–282.
27. Ide K, Shirai Y, Ito H, et al. Sensory nerve supply in the human subacromial bursa. *J Shoulder Elbow Surg* 1996;5:371–382.
28. Morisawa Y. Morphological study of mechanoreceptors on the coracoacromial ligament. *J Orthop Sci* 1998;3:102–110.
29. Soifer TB, Levy HJ, Soifer FM, et al. Neurohistology of the subacromial space. *Arthroscopy* 1996;12:182–186.
30. Vangsness CT, Ennis M, Taylor JG, et al. Neuroanatomy of the glenohumeral ligaments, labrum, and subacromial bursa. *Arthroscopy* 1995;11:180–184.
31. Assimakipoulos AP, Katonis PG, Agapitos MV, et al. The innervation of the human meniscus. *Clin Orthop* 1992;275:232–236.
32. Schultz RA, Miller DC, Kerr CS, et al. Mechanoreceptors in human cruciate ligaments. *J Bone Joint Surg Am* 1984;66:1072–1076.
33. Schutte MJ, Dabezies EJ, Zinny ML, et al. Neural anatomy of the human anterior cruciate ligament. *J Bone Joint Surg Am* 1987;69:243–247.
34. Cavna N. The effects of aging on the receptor organs of the human dermis. In: Montagna W, ed. *Advances in biology of the skin.* New York: Pergamon Press, 1965:63–96.
35. Burke JR, Kamen G. Changes in spinal reflexes preceding a voluntary movement in young and old adults. *J Gerontol A Biol Sci Med Sci* 1996;51:17–22.
36. Denti M, Monteleone M, Berardi A, et al. Anterior cruciate ligament mechanoreceptors: histologic studies on lesions and reconstruction. *Clin Orthop* 1994;308:29–32.
37. Aune AK, Hukkanen M, Madsen JE, et al. Nerve regeneration during patellar tendon autograft remodeling after anterior cruciate ligament reconstruction: an experimental and clinical study. *J Orthop Res* 1996;14:193–199.
38. Goertzen M, Gruber J, Dellmann A, et al. Neurohistological findings after experimental anterior cruciate ligament allograft transplantation. *Arch Orthop Trauma Surg* 1992;111:126–129.
39. Shimizu T, Takahashi T, Wada Y, et al. Regeneration process of mechanoreceptors in the reconstructed anterior cruciate ligament. *Arch Orthop Trauma Surg* 1999;119:405–409.

40. Wada Y, Takahashi T, Michinaka Y, et al. Mechanoreceptors of patellar tendon used for ACL reconstruction: rabbit experiments. *Acta Orthop Scand* 1997;68:559–562.

41. Adachi N, Ochi M, Uchio Y, et al. Anterior cruciate ligament augmentation under arthroscopy: a minimum 2-year follow-up in 40 patients. *Arch Orthop Trauma Surg* 2000;120:128–133.

42. Augé II WK. Radio frequency induced thermal modification for treatment of single bundle anterior cruciate ligament rupture. In: Proceedings of the International Society of Arthroscopy, Knee Surgery, and Orthopaedic Sports Medicine, Montreux, Switzerland. *Arthroscopy* 2001;17[Suppl].

43. Macefield G, Gandevia SC, Burke D. Perceptual responses to microstimulation of single afferents innervating joints, muscles, and skin of the human hand. *J Physiol (Lond)* 1990;429:113–129.

44. Valeriani M, Restuccia D, Di Lazzaro V, et al. Central nervous system modifications in patients with lesion of the anterior cruciate ligament of the knee. *Brain* 1996;119:1751–1762.

45. Ochi M, Iwasa J, Uchio Y, et al. The regeneration of sensory neurones in the reconstruction of the anterior cruciate ligament. *J Bone Joint Surg Br* 1999;81:902–906.

46. Gandevia SC, Macefield G, Burke D, et al. Voluntary activation of human motor axons in the absence of muscle afferent feedback: the control of the deafferented hand. *Brain* 1990;113:1563–1581.

47. Grigg P. The role of capsular feedback and pattern generators in shoulder kinematics. In: Madsen FA, Fu FH, Hawkins RJ, eds. *The shoulder: a balance of mobility and stability.* Rosemont, IL: American Academy of Orthopaedic Surgeons, 1993:173–183.

48. Kaplan FS, Hayes WC, Keaveny TM, et al. Form and function of bone. In: Simon SR, ed. *Orthopaedic basic science.* Rosemont, IL: American Academy of Orthopaedic Surgeons, 1994:127–184.

49. Renström PA, Leadbetter WB. Epidemiology of tendon injuries in sports. *Clin Sports Med* 1992;11:493–504.

50. Tidball JG. Myotendinous junction injury in relation to junction structure and molecular composition. *Exerc Sport Sci Rev* 1991;19:419–445.

51. Costill DL, Coyle EF, Fink WF, et al. Adaptations in skeletal muscle following strength training. *J Appl Physiol* 1979;46:96–99.

52. Newham DJ, McPhail G, Mills KR, et al. Ultrastructural changes after concentric and eccentric contractions of human muscle. *J Neurol Sci* 1983;61:109–122.

53. Asmussen E, Bonde-Peterson F. Storage of elastic energy in skeletal muscles in man. *Acta Physiol* 1974;91:385–392.

54. Albert M. Physiologic and clinical principles of eccentrics. In: Albert M. *Eccentric muscle training in sports and orthopaedics.* New York: Churchill Livingstone, 1991:11–23.

55. Baratta R, Solononow M, Zhou BH, et al. Muscular coactivation: the role of the antagonist musculature in maintaining knee stability. *Am J Sports Med* 1988;16:113–122.

56. Goldfuss AJ, Morehouse CA, LeVeau BF. Effect of muscular tension on knee stability. *Med Sci Sports Exer* 1973;5:267–271.

57. Hirokawa S, Solomonow M, Luo Y, et al. Muscular co-contraction and control of the knee stability. *J Electromyogr Kinesiol* 1991;1:199–208.

58. Draganich LF, Jaeger RJ, Kralj AR. Coactivation of the hamstrings and quadriceps during extension of the knee. *J Bone Joint Surg Am* 1989;71:1075–1081.

59. Hecht RW, McKeever KH, Alway SE, et al. Resistance training—induced increases in muscle mass and performance in ponies. *Med Sci Sports Exerc* 1996;28:877–883.

60. Ghez C, Gordon J, Ghilardi MF, et al. Roles of proprioceptive input in the programming of arm trajectories. *Cold Spring Harb Symp Quant Biol* 1990;55:837–847.

61. Moritani T, deVries HA. Neural factors versus hypertrophy in the time course of muscle strength gain. *Am J Phys Med* 1979;58:115–130.

62. Czeh G, Gallego R, Kudo N, et al. Evidence for the maintenance of motoneurone properties by muscle activity. *J Physiol (Lond)* 1982;281:239–252.

63. Burke D, Hagbarth KE, Löfstedt L. Muscle spindle activity in man during shortening and lengthening contractions. *J Physiol (Lond)* 1977;277:131–142.

64. Wojtys EW, Wylie BB, Huston LJ. The effects of muscle fatigue on neuromuscular function and anterior tibial translation in healthy knees. *Am J Sports Med* 1996;24:615–621.

65. Edgerton VR, Hutton RS. Nervous system and sensory adaptation. In: Bouchard C, Shepard RJ, Stephens T, et al. eds. *Exercise, fitness, and health: a consensus of current knowledge.* Champaign, IL: Human Kinetics, 1990:363–376.

66. Leisman G, Zenhausern R, Ferenty A, et al. Electromyographic effects of fatigue and task repetition on the validity of estimates of strong and weak muscles in applied kinesiological muscle-testing procedures. *Percept Mot Skills* 1995;80:963–977.

67. Scoville CR, Arciero RA, Taylor DC, et al. End range eccentric antagonist/concentric agonist strength ratios: a new perspective in shoulder strength assessment. *J Orthop Sports Phys Ther* 1997;25:203–207.

68. Greenberger HB, Paterno MV. Relationship of knee extensor strength and hopping test performance in the assessment of lower extremity function. *J Orthop Sports Phys Ther* 1995;22:202–206.

69. Murphy AJ, Wilson GJ. The ability of tests of muscular function to reflect training-induced changes in performance. *J Sports Sci* 1997;15:191–200.

70. Wilson G, Murphy A. The efficacy of isokinetic, isometric and vertical jump tests in exercise science. *Aust J Sci Med Sport* 1995;27:20–24.

71. Walla DJ, Albright JP, McAuley E, et al. Hamstring control and the unstable anterior cruciate ligament-deficient knee. *Am J Sports Med* 1985;13:34–39.

72. Wojtys EM, Huston LJ. Neuromuscular performance in normal and anterior cruciate ligament–deficient lower extremities. *Am J Sports Med* 1994;22:89–104.

73. Berchuck M, Andriacchi TP, Bach BR, et al. Gait adaptations by patients who have a deficient ACL. *J Bone Joint Surg Am* 1990;72:871–879.

74. McNair PJ, Marshall RN, Matheson JA. Gait of subjects with anterior cruciate ligament deficiency. *Clin Biomech* 1989;4:243–248.

75. Goodwin GM, McCloskey DI, Matthews PBC. The contribution of muscle afferents to kinesthesia shown by vibration induced illusions of movement and by the effects of paralyzing joint afferents. *Brain* 1972;95:705–748.

76. Inglis JT, Frank JS, Inglis B. The effect of muscle vibration on human position sense during movements controlled by lengthening muscle contraction. *Exp Brain Res* 1991;84:631–634.

77. Fu FJ, Lephart SM, Warner JJP. Normal shoulder proprioception measurements in college are individuals. *Orthop Trans* 1992;16:759–760.

78. Hall LA, McCloskey DI. Detections of movements imposed on finger, elbow, and shoulder joints. *J Physiol (Lond)* 1983;335:519–533.

79. Barrack RL, Skinner HB, Buckley SL, et al. Proprioception in the anterior cruciate deficient knee. *Am J Sports Med* 1989;17:1–6.

80. Blasier RB, Carpenter JE, Huston LJ. Shoulder proprioception: effects of joint laxity, joint position, and direction of motion. *Orthop Rev* 1994;23:45–50.

81. Lephart SM, Warner JJP, Borsa PA, et al. Proprioception of the

shoulder in healthy, unstable, and surgically repaired shoulders. *J Shoulder Elbow Surg* 1994;3:371–380.

82. Smith RL, Brunolli J. Shoulder kinesthesia after anterior glenohumeral joint dislocation. *Phys Ther* 1989;69:106–112.

83. Aniss AM, Diener HC, Hore J, et al. Behavior of human muscle receptors when reliant on proprioceptive feedback during standing. *J Neurophysiol* 1990;64:661–670.

84. Leanderson J, Eriksson E, Nilsson C, et al. Proprioception in classical ballet dancers: a prospective study of the influence of ankle sprain on proprioception in the ankle joint. *Am J Sports Med* 1996;24:370–374.

85. Iwasa J, Ochi M, Adachi N, et al. Proprioceptive improvement in knees with anterior cruciate ligament reconstruction. *Clin Orthop* 2000;381:168–176.

86. Martin JH. Receptor physiology and submodality coding in the somatic sensory system. In: Kandel ER, Swartz JH, eds. *Principles of neural science,* 2nd ed. New York: Elsevier Science, 1985:287–300.

87. Beynnon BD, Renström PA, Konradsen L, et al. Validation of techniques to measure knee proprioception. In: Lepart SM, Fu FH, eds. *Proprioception and neuromuscular control in joint stability.* Champaign, IL: Human Kinetics, 2000:127–138.

88. Gandevia SC, McCloskey DI, Burke D. Kinesthetic signals and muscle contraction. *Trends Neurosci* 1992;15:62–65.

89. Leplow B, Schluter V, Fersti R. A new procedure for assessment of proprioception. *Percept Mot Skills* 1992;74:91–98.

90. Bergenheim M, Johansson H, Pedersen J, et al. Ensemble coding of muscle stretches in afferent populations containing different types of muscle afferents. *Brain Res* 1996;734:157–166.

91. Miyatsu M, Atsuta Y, Wantakabe M. The physiology of mechanoreceptors in the anterior cruciate ligament: an experimental study in decerebrate-spinalized animals. *J Bone Joint Surg Br* 1993;75:653–657.

92. Ferrell WR, Baxendale RH, Carnachan C, et al. The influence of joint afferent discharge on locomotion, proprioception, and activity in conscious cats. *Brain Res* 1985;347:41–48.

93. Johansson H, Sjölander P, Sojka P. Fusimotor effects in triceps surae muscle elicited by natural and electrical stimulation of joint afferents. *Neuroorthopaedics* 1988;6:670–680.

94. Johansson H, Lorentzon, R, Sjölander P, et al. The anterior cruciate ligament: a sensor acting on the gamma muscle spindle systems of muscles around the knee joint. *Neuroorthopedics* 1990;9:1–23.

95. Tsuda E, Okamura Y, Otsuka H, et al. Direct evidence of the anterior cruciate ligament-hamstring reflex arc in human. *Am J Sports Med* 2001;29:83–87.

96. Johansson H, Sjölander P, Sojka P, et al. Reflex actions of the gamma-muscle spindle systems of muscles acting at the knee joint elicited by stretch of the posterior cruciate ligament. *Neuroorthopaedics* 1989;8:9.

97. Sojka P, Johansson H, Sjölander P, et al. Fusimotor neurons can be reflexively influenced by activity in receptor afferents from the posterior cruciate ligament. *Brain Res* 1989;483:177–183.

98. Sojka P, Sjölander P, Johansson H, et al. Influence from stretch-sensitive receptors in the collateral ligaments of the knee joint on the gamma-muscle-spindle systems of flexor and extensor muscles. *Neurosci Res* 1991;11:55–62.

99. Johansson H, Sojka P. Actions on gamma-motorneurons elicited by electrical stimulation of cutaneous afferent fibers in the hind limb on the cat. *J Physiol (Lond)* 1985;366:343–363.

100. Guanche CA, Knatt T, Solomonow M, et al. The synergistic action of the capsule and the shoulder muscles. *Am J Sports Med* 1995;23:301–306.

101. Jerosch J, Steinbeck J, Schrode M, et al. Intraoperative EMG: Ableitung bein Reizug der glenohemeralen Gelenkkapsel. *Unfallchirurgie* 1995;98:580–585.

102. Solomonow M, Guanche CA, Wink CA, et al. Shoulder capsule reflex arc in the feline shoulder. *J Shoulder Elbow Surg* 1996;5:139–146.

103. Knatt T, Gaunche CA, Solomonow M, et al. The glenohumeral-biceps reflex. *Clin Orthop* 1995;314:247–252.

104. Augé WK II, Morrison DS. A new investigational technique examining the neural circuitry of normal, athletic, and unstable shoulders. In: *Proceedings of the American Orthopaedic Society for Sports Medicine interim meeting, New Orleans, 1998.* American Orthopaedic Society for Sports Medicine, 1998.

105. Ferrell WR. The adequacy of stretch receptors in the cat knee joint for signaling joint angle throughout a full range of movement. *J Physiol (Lond)* 1980;299:85–99.

106. Huston LJ, Wojtys EM. Neuromuscular performance characteristics in elite female athletes. *Am J Sports Med* 1996;24:427–436.

107. Sinkjr T, Toft E, Arendt-Nielsen L. Knee stability and muscle coordination in patients with anterior cruciate ligament injuries: an electromyographic approach. *J Electromyogr Kinesiol* 1991;1:209–217.

108. Fellows SJ, Thilmann AF. The role of joint biomechanics in determining stretch reflex latency at the normal ankle. *Exp Brain Res* 1989;77:135–139.

109. Lynch SA, Eklund U, Gottlieb D, et al. Electromyographic latency changes in the ankle musculature during inversion moments. *Am J Sports Med* 1996;24:362–369.

110. Johnson MB, Johnson CL. Electromyographic response of peroneal muscles in surgical and nonsurgical injured ankles during sudden inversion. *J Sports Phys Ther* 1993;18:497–501.

111. Kleinrensink GJ, Stoeckart R, Meulstee J, et al. Lowered motor conduction velocity of the peroneal nerve after inversion trauma. *Med Sci Sports Exerc* 1994;26:877–883.

112. Löfvenberg R, Kärrholm J, Sundelin G. Prolonged reaction time in patients with chronic lateral instability of the ankle. *Am J Sports Med* 1995;23:414–417.

113. Beard DJ, Kyberd PJ, O'Connor JJ, et al. Reflex hamstring contraction latency in anterior cruciate ligament deficiency. *J Orthop Res* 1994;12:219–228.

114. Kålund S, Sinkjær T, Arendt-Nielsen L, et al. Altered timing of hamstring muscle action in anterior cruciate ligament-deficient patients. *Am J Sports Med* 1990;18:245–248.

115. Kronberg M, Bröstrom LA, Nemeth G. Differences in shoulder muscle activity between patients with generalized joint laxity and normal controls. *Clin Orthop* 1991;269:181–192.

116. Myklebust BM, Gottlieb GL, Penn RD, et al. Reciprocal excitation of antagonist muscles as a differentiating feature in spasticity. *Ann Neurol* 1982;12:367–374.

117. Myklebust BM. A review of myotactic reflexes and the development of motor control and gait in infants and children: a special communication. *Phys Ther* 1990;70:188–203.

118. Pierrot-Deseilligny E. Pathophysiology of spasticity. *Triangle* 1983;22:165–174.

119. Augé WK II, Morrison DS. Assessment of the infraspinatus spinal stretch reflex in the normal, athletic, and multidirectionally unstable shoulder. *Am J Sports Med* 2000;28:206–213.

120. Augé II WK. Evaluation of the neuromotor sequelae of outlet impingement syndrome: rotator cuff reflex inhibition. In: Proceedings of the International Congress on Surgery of the Shoulder. Cape Town, South Africa. April, 2001.

121. Morrison DS, Frogameni AD, Woodworth P. Non-operative treatment of subacromial impingement syndrome. *J Bone Joint Surg Am* 1997;79:732–737.

122. Beard DJ, Dodd CA, Simpson HA. Sensorimotor changes after anterior cruciate ligament reconstruction. *Clin Orthop* 2000;372:205–216.

123. Augé II WK. Nonsurgical treatment for multidirectional shoulder instability through normalization of reflex characteristics. Submitted for publication, 2001.

124. Augé II WK. Neuromotor sequelae of arthroscopic subacromial decompression for treatment of outlet impingement syndrome. Submitted for publication, 2001.

125. MacKay WA. The motor program: back to the computer. *Trends Neurosci* 1980;3:284–287.

126. Bell DG, Jacobs IRS. Electromechanical response times and rate of force development in males and females. *Med Sci Sports* 1986;18:31–36.

127. Dunn TG, Gillig SE, Ponser SE, et al. The learning process in biofeedback: is it feedfoward or feedback? *Biofeedback Self Reg* 1986;11:143–155.

128. Norman RW, Komi PV. Electro-mechanical delay in skeletal muscle under normal movement conditions. *Acta Physiol Scand* 1979;106:241–248.

129. Evarts EV, Granit R. Relations of reflexes and intended movements. *Prog Brain Res* 1976;44:1–14.

130. Ramos CF, Hacisalihzade SS, Stark LW. Behavior space of a stretch reflex model and its implications for the neural control of voluntary movement. *Med Biol Eng Comput* 1990;28:15–23.

131. Weeks DL, Aubert MP, Feldman AG, et al. One-trial adaptation of movement to changes in load. *J Neurophysiol* 1996;75:60–74.

132. Yamashita N, Nakabayashi T, Moritani T. Inter-relationships among anticipatory EMG activity, Hoffman reflex amplitude and EMG reaction time during voluntary standing movement. *Eur J Appl Physiol* 1990;60:98–103.

133. Evarts EV, Tanji J. Reflex and intended responses in motor cortex pyramidal tract neurons of monkey. *J Neurophysiol* 1976;39:1069–1080.

134. Tanji J, Evarts EV. Anticipatory activity of motor cortex neurons in relation to direction of an intended movement. *J Neurophysiol* 1976;39:1062–1068.

135. Hasan Z, Stuart DG. Animal solutions to problems of movement control: the role of proprioceptors. *Annu Rev Neurosci* 1988;11:100–223.

136. Lee RG, Lucier GE, Mustard BE, et al. Modification of motor output to compensate for unanticipated load conditions during rapid voluntary movements. *Can J Neurol Sci* 1986;13:97–102.

137. Wolpaw JR. Acquisition and maintenance of the simplest motor skill: investigation of CNS mechanisms. *Med Sci Sports Exerc* 1994;26:1475–1479.

138. Ivry R. Representative issues in motor learning: phenomena and theory. In: Keel S, ed. *Handbook of perceptions and action: motor skills.* New York: Academic Press.

139. Easton TA. On the normal use of reflexes. *Am Sci* 1972;60:591–599.

140. Forget R, Lamarre Y. Anticipatory postural adjustment in the absence of normal peripheral feedback. *Brain Res* 1990;508:176–179.

141. Bard C, Paillard J, Lajoie Y, et al. Role of afferent information in the timing of motor commands: a comparative study with a deafferented patient. *Neuropsychologia* 1992;30:201–206.

142. Cordo P, Bevan L, Gurfinkel V, et al. Proprioceptive coordination of discrete movement sequences: mechanism and generality. *Can J Physiol Pharmacol* 1995;73:305–315.

143. Gandevia SC, Burke D. Does the nervous system depend on kinesthetic input to control natural limb movements? *Behav Brain Sci* 1992;15:615–633.

144. Ghez C, Gordon MF, Ghilardi MF, et al. Roles of proprioceptive input in the programming of arm trajectories. *Cold Spring Harbor Symp Quant Biol* 1990;55:837–847.

145. Ghez C, Sainburg R. Proprioceptive control of interjoint coordination. *Can J Physiol Pharmacol* 1995;73:273–284.

146. Sanes JN, Shadmehr R. Sense of muscular effort and somesthetic afferent information in humans. *Can J Physiol Pharmacol* 1995;73:223–233.

147. Bard C, Fleury M, Teasdale N, et al. Contribution of proprioception for calibrating and updating the motor space. *Can J Physiol Pharmacol* 1995;73:246–254.

148. LaRue J, Bard C, Fleury M, et al. Is proprioception important for the timing of motor activities? *Can J Physiol Pharmacol* 1995;73:255–261.

149. Van Mechelen W, Hlobil H, Kemper HC. Incidence, severity, aetiology, and prevention of sports injuries: a review of concepts. *Sports Med* 14:82–89, 1992.

150. Augé II WK. Response strategies for injury prevention: confirmation of neuromotor learning during acquisition of motor control. *COSPR* 2000;5:97–106.

151. MacKenzie CL, Marteniuk RG. Motor skill: feedback, knowledge, and structural issues. *Can J Psychol* 1985;39:313–317.

152. Augé II WK. Assessment of athletic ability through neuromotor response strategy. COSPR 2001;6:49–57.

153. Dugas C, Marteniuk RG. Strategy and learning effects on perturbed movements: an electromyographic and kinematic study. *Behav Brain Res* 1989;35:181–193.

154. Jeannerod M. *The neural and behavioral organization of goal-directed movements.* Oxford: Clarendon Press, 1988.

155. Shiffrin RM, Schneider W. Controlled and automatic human information processing: part II. Perceptual learning, automatic attending, and a general theory. *Psychol Rev* 1977;76:127–190.

156. Saibene F. The mechanisms for minimizing energy expenditure in human locomotion. *Eur J Clin Nutr* 1990;44[Suppl 1]:65–71.

157. Gottlieb GL. Muscle compliance: implications for the control of movement. *Exerc Sport Sci Rev* 1996;24:1–34.

158. Bernardi M, Solomonow M, Nguyen G, et al. Motor unit recruitment strategy changes with skill acquisition. *Eur J Appl Physiol* 1996;74:52–59.

159. Lacquaniti F, Borghese NA, Carrozzo M. Functional characteristics of reflex coactivation in man. *Soc Neurosci Abstr* 1990;16:69.

160. Feldman AG, Orlovsky GN. The influence of different descending systems on the tonic stretch reflex in the cat. *Exp Neurol* 1972;37:481–494.

161. Feldman AG. Once more on the equilibrium-point hypothesis (δ model) for motor control. *J Mot Behav* 1986;18:17–54.

162. Feldman AG. Fundamentals of motor control, kinesthesia, and spinal neurons: in search of a theory. *Behav Brain Sci* 1992;15:735–737.

163. Feldman AG, Levin ML. Control variables and related concepts in motor control. *Concepts Neurosci* 1993;4:25–51.

164. Smith JL, Zernicke RF. Predictions for neural control based on limb dynamics. *Trends Neurosci* 1987;10:123–128.

165. Fleishman EA. On the relationship between abilities, learning, and human performance. *Am Psychol* 1972;27:1017–1032.

166. Kerr R. Movement control and maturation in elementary-grade children. *Percept Mot Skills* 1975;41:151–154.

167. Kerr R, Booth B. Specific and varied practice of motor skill. *Percept Mot Skills* 1978;46:395–401.

168. Kerr R, Boucher JL. Knowledge and motor performance. *Percept Mot Skills* 1992;74:1195–1202.

169. Paillard J. Apraxia and the neurophysiology of motor control. *Philos Trans R Soc Lond B Biol Sci* 1982;298:111–134.

170. Paillard J. The cognitive penetrability of sensorimotor mechanisms: a key problem in sport research. *Int J Sport Psychol* 1991;22:244–250.

171. Proteau L, Marteniuk RG, Lévesque L. A sensorimotor basis for motor learning: evidence indicating specificity of practice. *Q J Exp Psychol A* 1992;44:557–575.

172. Ripoll H. The understanding-acting process in sport: the relationship between the semantic and the sensorimotor visual function. *Int J Sport Psychol* 1991;22:221–243.

173. Schmidt RA. A schema theory of discrete motor skill learning. *Psychol Rev* 1975;82:225–260.

174. George JS, Aine CJ, Mosher JC, et al. Mapping function in the human brain with MEG, anatomical MRI, and functional MRI. *J Clin Neurophysiol* 1995;12:406–431.

175. Kleinschmidt A, Obrig H, Requardt M, et al. Simultaneous recording of cerebral blood oxygenation changes during human brain activation by magnetic resonance imaging and near-infrared spectroscopy. *J Cereb Blood Flow Metab* 1996;16:817–826.

176. Paus T, Jech R, Thompson CJ, et al. Transcranial magnetic stimulation during position emission tomography: a new method for studying connectivity of the human cerebral cortex. *J Neurosci* 1997;17:378–3184.

177. MacDonald D, Kabani N, Avis D, et al. Automated 3-D extraction of inner and outer surfaces of cerebral cortex from MRI. *Neuroimage* 2000;12:340–356.

178. Ghanei A, Soltanian-Zadeh H, Jacobs MA, et al. Boundary-based warping of brain MR images. *J Magn Reson Imaging* 2000;12:417–429.

179. Zeineh MM, Engel SA, Bookheimer SY. Application of cortical unfolding techniques to functional MRI of the human hippocampal region. *Neuroimage* 2000;11:668–683.

180. Kwong KK, Belliveau JW, Chesler DA, et al. Dynamic magnetic resonance imaging of human brain activity during primary sensory stimulation. *Proc Natl Acad Sci USA* 1992;89:5675–5679.

181. Stehling MK, Turner R, Mansfield P. Echo-planar imaging: magnetic resonance imaging in a fraction of a second. *Science* 1991;254:43–50.

182. Hamalainen MS, Hari R, Ilmoniemi RJ, et al. Magnetoencephalography: theory, instrumentation, and applications to noninvasive studies of the working human brain. *Rev Mod Phys* 1993;65:413–497.

183. Asanuma H, Arissian K. Experiments on functional role of peripheral input to motor cortex during voluntary movements in the monkey. *J Neurophysiol* 1984;52:212–227.

184. Dale A, Serano M. Improved localization of cortical activity by combining EEG and MEG with MRI cortical surface reconstruction: a linear approach. *J Cog Neurosci* 1993;5:162–176.

185. George JS, Sanders JS, Lewine JD, et al. Comparative studies of brain activation with MEG and functional MRI. In: Baumgartner C, et al. eds. *Biomagnetism: fundamental research and clinical applications.* Amsterdam: Elsevier/IOS, 1995:60–65.

186. Sanders JA, Lewine JD, Orrison WW. Comparison of primary motor cortex localization using functional magnetic resonance imaging and magnetoencephalography. *Hum Brain Mapping* 1996;4:47–57.

187. Aine C, Huang M, Stephen J, et al. Multi-start algorithms for MEG empirical data analysis reliably characterize locations and time-courses of multiple sources. *Neuroimage* 2000;12:159–172.

188. Huang M, Aine CJ, Supek S, et al. Multi-start downhill simplex method for spatio-temporal source localization in magnetoencephalography. *Electroencephalogr Clin Neurophysiol* 1998;108:32–44.

189. Huang M, Aine C, Davis L, et al. Source on anterior and posterior banks of the central sulcus identified from magnetic somatosensory evoked responses using multi-start spatio-temporal localization. *Hum Brain Mapping* 2000;11:59–76.

190. Forss N, Hietanen M, Salonen O, et al. Modified activation of somatosensory cortical network in patients with right-hemisphere stroke. *Brain* 1999;22:1889–1899.

191. Huang MX, Davis LE, Aine CJ, et al. Characterizing the recovery process of primary sensorimotor functions of the hand in ischemic stroke magnetoencephalography. *COSPR* 2001;6.

192. Gibson A, Bayford RH, Holder DS. Development of a reconstruction algorithm for imaging impedance changes in the human head. *Ann NY Acad Sci* 1999;873:482–492.

193. Holder DS. Impedance changes during the compound nerve action potential: implications for impedance imaging of neuronal depolarization in the brain. *Med Biol Eng Comput* 1992;30:140–146.

194. Ilmoniemi RJ, Ruohonen J, Karhu J. Transcranial magnetic stimulation: new tool for functional imaging of the brain. *Crit Rev Biomed Eng* 1999;27:241–284.

195. Steinbrink J, Kohl M, Obrig H, et al. Somatosensory evoked fast optical intensity changes detected non-invasively in the adult human head. *Neurosci Lett* 2000;291:105–108.

196. Benaron DA, Hintz SR, Vilringer A, et al. Noninvasive functional imaging of human brain using light. *J Cereb Blood Flow Metab* 2000;20:469–477.

197. Rector DM, Rogers RF, George JS. A focusing image probe for assessing neural activity *in vivo. J Neurosci Methods* 1999;91:135–145.

198. Tasaki I, Byrne PM. Rapid structural changes in nerve fibers evoked by electrical current pulses. *Biochem Biophys Res Comm* 1992;188:559–564.

199. Bell J, Cook LP. A model of the nerve action potential. *Math Biosci* 1979;46:11–36.

200. Hodgkin AL, Huxley AF. The components of membrane conductance in the giant axon of Loligo. *J Physiol (Lond)* 1952;116:473–496.

201. Hodgkin AL, Huxley AF. A quantitative description of membrane current and its application to conduction and excitation in nerve. *J Physiol (Lond)* 1952;117:500–544.

202. Muratov CB. A quantitative approximation scheme for the traveling wave solutions in the Hodgkin-Huxley model. *Biophys J* 2000;79:2893–2901.

203. Jack JJB, Noble D, Tsien RW. *Electrical current flow in excitable cells.* London: Oxford University Press, 1975.

204. Johnston D, Magaee JC, Colbert DM, et al. Active properties of neuronal dendrites. *Annu Rev Neurosci* 1996;19:165–186.

205. Rall W. Electrophysiology of a dendritic neuron model. *Biophys J* 1962;2:145–167.

206. Rall W. Distinguishing theoretical synaptic potentials computed for different soma-dendritic distributions of synaptic inputs. *J Neurophysiol* 1967;30:1138–1168.

207. Rall W. Cable theory for dendritic neurons. In: *Methods in neuronal modeling.* Cambridge, MA: MIT Press, 1989:9–62.

208. Ermentrout GB. Phase-plane analysis of neural activity. In: Arbib MA, ed. *The handbook of brain theory and neural networks.* Cambridge, MA: Bradford Books/MIT Press, 1995:732–738.

209. Traub RD, Jefferys JGR, Miles R, et al. A branching dendritic model of rodent CA3 pyramidal neurons. *J Physiol (Lond)* 1994;481:79–95.

210. Arbib MA, Érdi P, Szentágothai J. *Neural organization, structure, function, and dynamics.* Cambridge, MA: Bradford Books/MIT Press, 1998.

211. Coghlan S, Gremillion MV, Travis BJ. NeuroBuilder: a user interface and network simulator for building neuro-biological networks. In: Eeckman FH, ed. *Analysis and modeling of neural systems I.* Boston: Kluwer Academic, 1992:115–122.

212. Travis BJ. A neural network model of the auditory system. In: *American Institute of Physics conference proceedings: neural networks for computing,* no 151. American Institute of Physics, 1986:432–439.

213. Travis BJ. A computational model of the auditory system. *Proc IEEE Int Conf Neural Networks* 1987;4:67–74.

214. Travis BJ. A computational model of the cat medial geniculate body ventral division. In: Eeckman FH, ed. *Analysis and modeling of neural systems I.* Boston: Kluwer Academic, 1992:293–305.
215. Travis BJ. A computational model of one pathway in the cat sub-cortical auditory system. *Math Comput Simul* 1996;40:81–99.
216. Gremillion MA, Mandell A, Travis BJ. Neural nets with complex structure: a model of the visual system. *Proc IEEE Int Conf Neural Networks* 1987;4:235–246.
217. Gremillion MAV, Travis BJ. Modeling spatiotemporal receptive fields of cat retinal X ganglion cells with realistic population interactions. Submitted for publication, 2001.
218. Kenyon GT, Travis BJ, Marshak DW. Computer model of the primate cone-horizontal cell network. *Soc Neurosci Abstr* 1998;24:1027.
219. Travis BJ. A layered network model of sensory cortex. In: *Proceedings of the International Conference on Computer Simulation in Brain Science.* Cambridge: Cambridge University Press, 1988:119–147.
220. Travis BJ. A computational model of the cerebellum. In: Eeckman FH, ed. *Analysis and modeling of neural systems I.* Boston: Kluwer Academic, 1992:131–137.
221. Zurek WH. Complexity, entropy, and the physics of information: a manifesto. In: Zurek WH ed. *Complexity, entropy, and the physics of information.* Redwood City, CA: Addison–Wesley, 1990:vii–x.
222. Aitken PG, Sauer T, Schiff SJ. Looking for chaos in brain slices. *J Neurosci Methods* 1995;59:41–48.
223. Moynihan JA, Kruszewska B, Brenner GJ, et al. Neural, endocrine, and immune system interactions: relevance for health and disease. *Adv Exp Med Biol* 1998;438:541–549.
224. Tomaszewska D, Przekop F. The immune-neuro-endocrine interactions. *J Physiol Pharmacol* 1997;48:139–158.
225. Papanicolaou DA, Chrousos GP. Interactions of the endocrine and immune systems in children and young adults. *Curr Opin Pediatr* 1995;7:440–444.
226. Gandevia SC, Hall LA, McCloskey, et al. Proprioceptive sensation at the terminal joint of the middle finger. *J Physiol (Lond)* 1983;335:507–517.
227. Slauterbeck J, Clevenger C, Lundberg W, et al. Estrogen level alters the failure load of the rabbit anterior cruciate ligament. *J Orthop Res* 1999;17:405–408.
228. Frostig RD, Lieke EE, Ts'o DY, et al. Cortical functional architecture and local coupling between neuronal activity and the microcirculation revealed by *in vitro* high-resolution imaging of intrinsic signals. *Proc Natl Acad Sci USA* 1990;87:6082–6086.
229. Callahan HS, Pigliucci M, Schlichting CD. Developmental phenotypic plasticity: where ecology and evolution meet molecular biology. *Bioessays* 1997;19:519–525.
230. Striedter GF. Progress in the study of brain evolution: from speculative theories to testable hypotheses. *Anat Rec* 1998;253:105–112.
231. Donald M. The neurobiology of human consciousness: an evolutionary approach. *Neuropsychologia* 1995;33:1087–1102.
232. Schmidt DM, George JS, Wood CC. Bayesian inference applied to the electromagnetic inverse problem. *Hum Brain Mapping* 1999;7:195–212.

ARTHROSCOPIC ANATOMY

ANATOMY AND BIOMECHANICS OF THE SHOULDER

MARIA E. SQUIRE
ADIL N. ESMAIL
LOUIS J. SOSLOWSKY

Normal shoulder kinematics requires the combined efforts of the sternoclavicular joint, scapulothoracic joint, acromioclavicular joint, and glenohumeral joint and associated muscles. An understanding of the biomechanics of the shoulder is important so disorders that affect normal movement can be properly diagnosed and treated. Although all the joints mentioned here contribute to shoulder movement, the acromioclavicular and glenohumeral joints are clinically the most significant. This chapter briefly addresses the biomechanics of the sternoclavicular joint and scapulothoracic joint, discusses the acromioclavicular joint in more detail, and then focuses on the biomechanics of the glenohumeral joint.

STERNOCLAVICULAR JOINT

Anatomy

The *sternoclavicular joint* is a saddle-shaped synovial joint in which the medial clavicle fits into the sternal notch and the cartilage of the first rib (1,2). Approximately one-half of the clavicle articulates with the sternum, and the other half forms the borders of the sternal notch (3). An articular disc is attached to the upper nonarticular medial clavicle superiorly and to the sternum and first ribs inferiorly, in essence dividing the joint into two compartments (1,4). The joint is encompassed by a capsule and is also supported by the costoclavicular, interclavicular, and sternoclavicular ligaments (Fig. 8.1).

Biomechanics

Stability of the sternoclavicular joint depends on the disc, the joint capsule, and the ligaments. The disc is primarily in-

M. E. Squire: McKay Orthopaedic Research Laboratory, University of Pennsylvania, Philadelphia, Pennsylvania.
A. N. Esmail: McKay Orthopaedic Research Laboratory, University of Pennsylvania, Philadelphia, Pennsylvania.
L. J. Soslowsky: Departments of Orthopaedic Surgery and Bioengineering, McKay Orthopaedic Research Laboratory, University of Pennsylvania, Philadelphia, Pennsylvania.

volved in preventing medial dislocation when forces are transmitted along the clavicle to the axial skeleton (4). The capsule is loose but fairly strong and acts as a hinge and a shock absorber on which the clavicle moves during shoulder motion (2,5). Sternoclavicular joint stability through the interclavicular, sternoclavicular, and costoclavicular ligaments depends on the sternal and clavicular position and on loading configuration (3,6) (Fig. 8.2). The interclavicular ligament unites the nonarticular medial ends of the two clavicles with an intermediate attachment to the manubrium. It limits excessive downward movement of the medial end of the clavicle (1,6). The sternoclavicular ligaments run from the anterior and posterior portions of the sternal end of the clavicle to the anterior and posterior portions of the manubrium and function to reinforce the capsule and to limit anteroposterior translation (2). The costoclavicular ligament, which has anterior and posterior portions, runs from the first rib to the undersurface of the medial clavicle. The anterior fibers resist upward displacement, whereas the posterior portions resist downward displacement of the medial clavicle (7).

The movements allowed at the sternoclavicular joint are elevation, depression, protraction, retraction, upward rotation, and downward rotation (6). The relationship between motion and ligament tension is depicted in Fig. 8.2. The range of motion allowed at the sternoclavicular joint is 30 to 35 degrees of elevation, 35 degrees of combined forward and backward movement, and 45 to 50 degrees of rotation around the long axis of the clavicle. The significance of the sternoclavicular joint to shoulder motion is clinically evident. When this joint is fused, shoulder elevation is limited to 90 degrees (8,9).

SCAPULOTHORACIC ARTICULATION

Anatomy

The *scapula* is a flat, triangular bone that is concave on its ventral surface, thus conforming to the convex surface of the

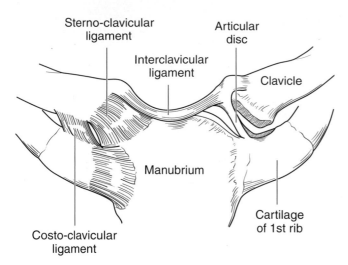

FIGURE 8.1 Anterior view of the sternoclavicular joint.

rib cage (2,10). It has four processes including the scapular spine, the acromion, the coracoid, and the glenoid, and it also has multiple muscle attachments. Two processes that are readily treated arthroscopically are the acromion and the glenoid. The acromion and its anatomic importance are discussed under subacromial impingement, and the glenoid is discussed in the section on the glenohumeral joint.

In addition to the bony anatomy, the scapula has multiple muscle attachments. The two muscles that require mention are the serratus anterior and the trapezius. The serratus anterior holds the medial angle of the scapula against the chest wall. The trapezius is important in rotating and elevating the scapula in synchrony with glenohumeral motion (3).

Clinically, scapulothoracic snapping is treated arthroscopically (11). Although discussion of technique and arthroscopic anatomy is beyond the scope of this chapter, anatomic investigations performed to evaluate the anatomy of the scapulothoracic articulation further allow for safe portal placement and treatment of scapulothoracic disorders (12,13).

Biomechanics

The scapulothoracic articulation is not a true joint. The shape of the scapula and the reciprocal shape of the thorax allow smooth scapulothoracic motion. In the resting position, the scapula lies 30 to 40 degrees anteriorly rotated and 20 degrees anteriorly tilted (3). Three rotatory motions and two translatory movements of the scapula are described. Rotation of the scapula occurs about the sagittal, vertical, and coronal axis (1). The scapula can translate upward or downward and toward or away from the vertebral column (1).

In any discussion of scapulothoracic biomechanics, the description of scapulohumeral rhythm is important. The concept of *scapulohumeral rhythm* was introduced by Codman to describe the smooth, integrated movements of the humerus, scapula, and clavicle (14). Inman reported the contribution ratio between glenohumeral and scapulothoracic motion to be approximately 2:1 during arm elevation (15). This ratio is nonlinear. Poppen and Walker claimed a 4:1 ratio in the first 25 degrees of elevation and 5:4 ratio thereafter (16). They average out at 2:1. It appears that this ratio is variable, depending on shoulder loading and arm position (17,18). In addition, altered scapular kinematics may be clinically important in pathologic conditions such as impingement syndrome and glenohumeral instability (19,20).

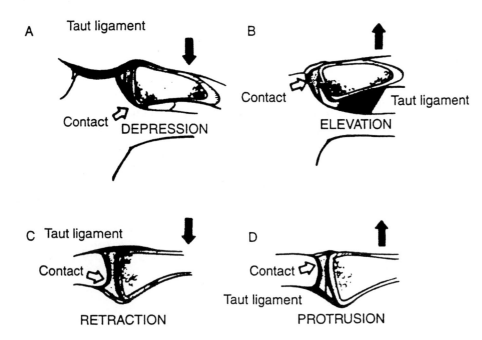

FIGURE 8.2 Contribution of ligaments to the stability of the sternoclavicular joint at different sternal and clavicular positions and loading configurations. (From Dempster WT. Mechanisms of shoulder movement. *Arch Phys Med Rehabil* 1965;46:49–70, with permission.)

ACROMIOCLAVICULAR JOINT

Anatomy

The *acromioclavicular joint* is the junction between the medial tip of the acromion and the lateral clavicle (Fig. 8.3). It is a plane, synovial joint that may have a fibrocartilaginous disc of variable size. A capsule that is thin and lax surrounds the acromioclavicular joint, and, therefore, the acromioclavicular, coracoacromial, and coracoclavicular ligaments must provide the stability for the joint.

Biomechanics

Stability

Stresses at the acromioclavicular joint can be high, and compressive forces act at the joint, especially with horizontal adduction of the arm and internal rotation of the shoulder (21). Because the acromioclavicular capsule is thin and lax, the joint integrity must come from the capsular ligaments (inferior and superior acromioclavicular ligaments), the coracoacromial ligament, and coracoclavicular ligaments (1,22,23) (Fig. 8.3). Although all the ligaments work together to maintain the integrity of the acromioclavicular joint, their individual contributions change with direction and amount of loading (3). Fukuda et al. evaluated the ligamentous contribution to loads and displacements associated with motion at the acromioclavicular joint (23). The acromioclavicular ligaments provide most resistance to small anterior displacements of the clavicle (those corresponding to daily physiologic loads), whereas with larger loads and displacements, the primary restraint comes from the conoid portion of the coracoclavicular ligament. At all loads, the primary restraint to posterior clavicular displacement is provided by the acromioclavicular ligaments. For superior displacements, again with smaller loads, the acromioclavicular ligaments provide restraint, whereas the conoid ligament provides resistance to the larger loads (23). The conoid ligament also provides the primary restraint to anterior clavicular rotation. However, with posterior rotation, the acromioclavicular ligaments and both coracoclavicular ligaments seem to contribute equally. Both the acromioclavicular and conoid ligaments provide combined resistance to small loads in superior clavicular rotation, and then the conoid ligament primarily resists the larger loads. Finally, with axial joint compression, the trapezoid part of the coracoclavicular ligament provides the primary resistance.

Motion

The acromioclavicular joint allows motion about three axes. Codman first described acromioclavicular joint motion in 1934. He said that the joint "swings a little, rocks a little, twists a little, slides a little inward and acts like a hinge when the shoulder is shrugged" (14). Moseley described how the acromioclavicular joint allows movement of the scapula on the clavicle about three axes (24). About the frontal axis, scapular tipping occurs such that the inferior angle tilts away from the chest wall. About the sagittal axis, the inferior angle of the scapula rotates forward and backward to rotate the glenoid fossa upward and downward. Finally, the scapula

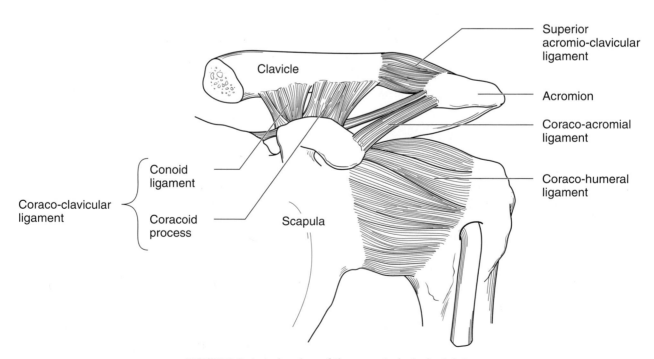

FIGURE 8.3 Anterior view of the acromioclavicular joint.

rotates forward and backward on the clavicle about the vertical axis such that the vertebral border moves away from and back toward the chest wall (i.e., scapular winging and antiwinging) (24). Total range of motion of the acromioclavicular joint is 20 degrees, and it occurs in the first 30 degrees and again after 135 degrees of arm elevation (15).

Acromioclavicular joint motion occurs as a result of the action of muscles with tendinous attachments on the scapula. We previously described the three axes about which motion at the acromioclavicular joint occurs. About the frontal axis, antagonistic muscles act on the scapula to cause motion. The rhomboids, lower trapezius, and serratus anterior maintain the inferior angle of the scapula close to the chest wall, whereas the pectoralis minor pulls the inferior angle of the scapula away from the chest wall to cause scapular tipping. About the sagittal axis, the lower trapezius and the serratus anterior act to rotate the inferior angle of the scapula forward on the chest wall, and this movement rotates the glenoid fossa upward (25). The lower trapezius is more active when the arm is horizontally abducted, and the serratus anterior is more active when the arm is brought into forward flexion (26). Conversely, the levator scapula, the pectoralis minor, and the rhomboids act to rotate the inferior angle of the scapula backward on the chest wall, and this movement rotates the glenoid fossa down (25). Finally, many muscles act to cause joint motion about a vertical axis. The lower trapezius, rhomboids, and levator scapulae apply a medially directed pull on the scapula and maintain the vertebral border of the scapula close to the chest wall (27). The only muscle to pull the vertebral border away from the chest wall and thereby to cause scapular winging is the pectoralis minor.

CLINICAL RELEVANCE

Acromioplasty

Acromioplasty is frequently performed arthroscopically to treat impingement syndrome. However, certain precautions and reported complications must be taken into consideration. In a 5-year follow-up study, both accelerated degeneration and mild instability were observed (28). This could be caused, in part, by the disruption of the inferior acromioclavicular ligament when the acromion is removed. Any interference with the inferior acromioclavicular ligament could compromise its function in stabilizing the acromioclavicular joint, especially in resisting displacements of the clavicle. Other complications from this procedure that can affect shoulder biomechanics include deltoid injury, subacromial calcification, and ossification (29).

Distal Clavicular Resection

Distal clavicular resections are frequently done arthroscopically, especially in patients with acromioclavicular joint osteoarthrosis or osteolysis of the distal clavicle (30). The amount of clavicular bone resected is key to postoperative joint stability, and studies have shown that by resecting 5 to 6 mm, both capsular and ligamentous stability is maintained (21,31). It is also important to preserve the superior and posterior capsular ligaments because they provide 90% of the resistance to posterior clavicular displacement (31,32). In summary, a surgeon performing arthroscopic distal clavicular resections needs to protect both the capsular ligaments and the capsule, to prevent postsurgical weakness and instability at the acromioclavicular joint (30).

SHOULDER IMPINGEMENT

Subacromial impingement can be defined as compression of the tendinous portion of the rotator cuff beneath the components of the coracoacromial arch. The coracoacromial arch consists of the acromion, the coracoacromial ligament, and the coracoid. The bone-to-bone distance between the head of the humerus and the undersurface of the acromion that accommodates the soft tissue contents of the subacromial space has been termed the *acromiohumeral interval*. The normal average interval ranges between 6 and 14 mm (33), and reduction of the acromiohumeral interval to less than 6 mm is considered pathologic (34) although significant variation exists in these measures.

In 1972, Neer stated that subacromial impingement results from compression of the tendons against the undersurface of the anterior one-third of the acromion, the coracoacromial ligament, and the acromioclavicular joint (35). Anatomic variations in the acromion have been associated with subacromial impingement. Bigliani et al. defined three types of acromions, flat, curved and hooked (Fig. 8.4) (36). In a study of 140 cadavers, there was a higher incidence of rotator cuff tears in hooked acromions (type III), in acromions with anterior spurs, and in acromions with a greater angle of anterior slope (36). Another anatomic variation, called os acromiale, and acquired variations of the acromion such as anterior spurs are frequently seen with impingement (36). In addition, osteophytes can form at the insertion site of the coracoacromial ligament or on the undersurface of the acromioclavicular joint and have also been associated with impingement (34). Finally, degenerative changes caused by age and repetitive microtrauma and resulting in inflammation of the rotator cuff tendons could lead to impingement from an increased tendon volume that must pass under the coracoacromial arch (37).

Neer's explanation of subacromial impingement is one of two defined extrinsic causes of rotator cuff injury, the other being glenohumeral or functional scapular instability (38). Glenohumeral instability can be the result of overuse from repetitive motion, which causes the glenohumeral ligaments to become stretched and leads to alterations in static stabilization. Although the rotator cuff muscles compensate for the loss of stabilization from the ligaments, there is a chance

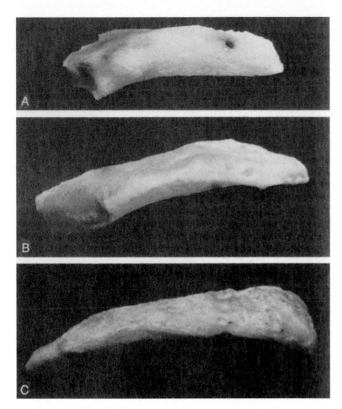

FIGURE 8.4 Variations in the shape of the acromion: flat or type I (A), curved or type II (B), and hooked or type III (C). (From Bigliani LU, Ticker JB, Flatow EL, et al. The relationship of the acromial architecture to rotator cuff disease. *Clin Sports Med* 1991;10:823–838, with permission.)

for impingement because of excessive humeral head translation. Subacromial impingement caused by glenohumeral instability can also occur if there is disruption of the normal elevation force couple, resulting in superior translation of the humeral head with arm movement. If the rotator cuff muscles (specifically the infraspinatus, teres minor, and subscapularis) do not act to depress the humerus with elevation, then the abduction and flexion action of the deltoid will drive the rotator cuff tendons into the acromion process (39). Finally, if there is functional scapular instability and the scapula fails to move synchronously with the humerus, then an increased chance exists that the rotator cuff tendons will become impinged on the coracoacromial arch structures with elevation of the arm (38).

Another type of shoulder impingement recognized in the literature is superior glenoid impingement, or internal impingement. This type of impingement can occur with normal physiologic motion and involves compression of the rotator cuff at its attachment to the greater tuberosity against the posterior superior glenoid and the labrum (40–42) (Fig. 8.5). Contact most frequently occurs with the arm in the throwing position of horizontal extension, in maximal external rotation and abduction (42), or with full elevation as in performing the Neer sign (40,41). If frequent repetitive movements occur in any of these positions, chronic injury

can result. Superior glenoid impingement can be amplified in the presence of hyperangulation of the glenohumeral joint, limited scapular rotation, or an overstretched anterior capsule (40,41). This has been evaluated arthroscopically in overhand-throwing athletes with shoulder pain. The predominant pathologic findings of undersurface rotator cuff fraying and posterosuperior labral fraying are suggestive of internal impingement (43).

Internal impingement and the role of instability are topics that continue to be questioned. When the arm is abducted and is in maximum external rotation, the humeral head normally translates 4 mm posteriorly on the glenoid articular surface (44,45). However, with repetitive microtrauma to the anterior restraints and the inability of the dynamic stabilizers to compensate because of instability, ante-

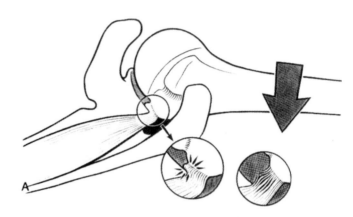

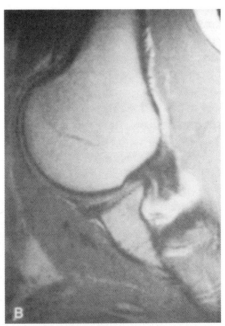

FIGURE 8.5 Illustration (A) and magnetic resonance image (B) of superior glenoid impingement between the rotator cuff at the greater tuberosity and the posterior superior glenoid. (From Walch G, Boileau P. Impingement of the deep surface of the supraspinatus tendon on the posterosuperior glenoid rim: an arthroscopic study. *J Shoulder Elbow Surg* 1992;1:238–245, with permission.)

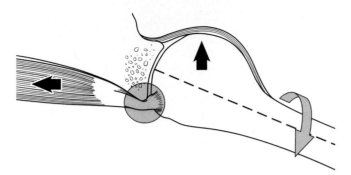

FIGURE 8.6 Compression of the rotator cuff against the posterior glenoid rim with abduction and maximal external rotation as a result of anterior instability.

rior translation of the humeral head occurs in the late cocking phase of throwing and thus contributes to impingement of the rotator cuff along the posterior glenoid rim (Fig. 8.6) (43). As a result, anterior capsular labral reconstruction, which corrects for capsular laxity, has been proposed as a surgical option for impingement-type shoulder pain in the overhead-throwing athlete. It is believed that many athletes who undergo this procedure return to their preinjury level of competition (46). Instability is not believed by some to be a causative factor of internal impingement. Halbrecht et al. used magnetic resonance imaging to evaluate a group of asymptomatic throwers and did not find a correlation of anterior instability and magnetic resonance imaging changes (47). Similarly, during arthroscopy of patients with instability, McFarland et al. placed patients in abduction and external rotation and examined contact between the rotator cuff and the glenoid rim (48). Not all patients with instability demonstrated internal impingement (48). To define more precisely the pathogenesis of internal impingement, further study is necessary.

Mechanics of Rotator Cuff Tendons Associated with Impingement

The soft tissue structure that is most frequently impinged on is the supraspinatus tendon at its insertion to the greater tuberosity of the humerus. This anterior portion of the supraspinatus is the strongest portion of the tendon mechanically and performs the tendon's main functional role (49). In severe cases of impingement, tendinitis and rupture can extend to include both the anterior infraspinatus tendon and the tendon of the long head of the biceps (14). The superior portion of the anterior infraspinatus tendon has been shown to be weaker, thus allowing for this propagation of a tear resulting from subacromial impingement (50).

Rotator cuff injuries can occur on the bursal side, the articular side, and within the tendon itself, and they frequently occur at the insertion site of the tendons. Insult to the articular side of the tendon is more common than to the bursal side, because the articular side of the supraspinatus

tendon is more susceptible to mechanical failure than the bursal side when both are subjected to similar loads (51). Rotator cuff injuries occur when their tendons and the undersurface of the acromion are in closest proximity, between 60 and 120 degrees of elevation (52). In addition, the critical zone of the supraspinatus tendon passes under the acromioclavicular joint at approximately 80 degrees of abduction, and it is at this point that mechanical impingement is most likely to occur (53). Internal tendon injuries and tears occur as a result of contact between the glenoid and the greater tuberosity, which compresses the soft tissues between the two bones. This is most likely to occur with the arm in horizontal extension, maximal external rotation, and between 90 and 150 degrees of abduction or with the arm in full overhead extension (40,41).

Model for Studying Rotator Cuff Injuries

Injuries to the rotator cuff are among the most common soft tissue injuries of the musculoskeletal system. To study the mechanisms of injury, the reparative process, and possible therapeutic interventions, it is ideal to use an animal model so repeatable and controllable alterations can be made, monitored, and evaluated over time (54). The rat, because of its anatomic similarities to the human, has been determined to be an appropriate *in vivo* model to study rotator cuff tendinosis (54). Schneeberger et al. used a rat model to evaluate extrinsic compression (55). In their model, extrinsic compression was provided by bony transplants placed on the scapular spine that resulted in bursal sided tears of the infraspinatus (55). In the senior author's laboratory, we have developed and extensively used a rat model to study rotator cuff tendinosis as an appropriate model to use based on anatomic similarities to the human. The rat model is appropriate because it has a supraspinatus tendon that inserts on the greater tuberosity of the humerus and passes directly under an enclosed arch composed of the coracoid, clavicle, acromion, and acromioclavicular ligament, similar to that in humans (Fig. 8.7). The rat model has been used to study tendinosis and address intrinsic, extrinsic, and overuse injuries as possible causes (56). Studies have shown that the effects of extrinsic compression combined with overuse causes significantly greater injury than either overuse or extrinsic compression alone. This finding supports the multifactorial nature of the etiology of rotator cuff tendinosis. By gaining a better understanding of the mechanisms of injury, this model can be used to develop and assess appropriate treatment modalities.

GLENOHUMERAL JOINT
Anatomy

The *glenohumeral joint* is a synovial joint formed by the head of the humerus articulating with the glenoid cavity of the

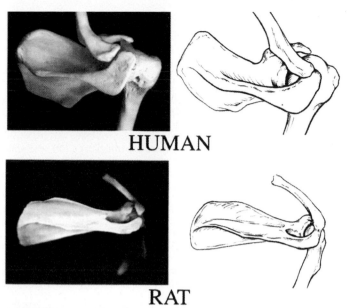

HUMAN

RAT

Photographs and schematics of the bony anatomy of the right human and rat shoulders from a postero-superior view demonstrating the similarity of the acromion projecting anteriorly over the humeral head to the clavicle.

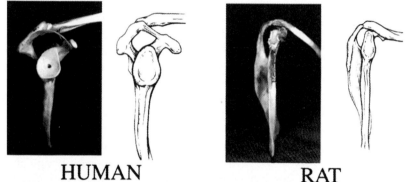

HUMAN **RAT**

Photographs and schematics of the right human and rat shoulders from a lateral or "outlet" view with the humerus removed demonstrating the similar presence of an enclosed arch over the space for the supraspinatus tendon.

FIGURE 8.7 Comparison of the human and rat shoulder bony anatomy demonstrating similarities with the bony enclosed arch over the supraspinatus tendon. (From Soslowsky LJ, Carpenter JE, DeBano CM, et al. Development and use of an animal model for investigations on rotator cuff disease. *J Shoulder Elbow Surg* 1996;5:383–392, with permission.)

scapula. When one compares the dimension of the humeral head to that of the glenoid, the so-called *glenohumeral ratio,* the relationship is 0.8 in the coronal plane and 0.6 in the transverse plane (57). The glenoid has a slight superior tilt of approximately 5 degrees and is retroverted about 7 degrees (57). The humerus has a superior tilt of about 45 degrees and is retroverted approximately 30 degrees (9,58,59). There is also a lateral humeral offset of approximately 56±5.7 mm (60). The joint is surrounded and stabilized by a soft tissue envelope consisting of the joint capsule, the glenohumeral ligaments, the coracohumeral ligament, the rotator cuff, deltoid, and the biceps muscles (Fig. 8.8).

Joint Classification

The glenohumeral joint is classified as a ball-and-socket synovial joint whose center of rotation is the humeral head (16). The joint has three degrees of rotational freedom and three degrees of translational freedom. Rotational movements include flexion and extension, abduction and adduction, and internal and external rotation. Flexion and extension occur about an axis through the frontal plane, abduction and adduction occur through an axis lying in the sagittal plane, and internal and external rotation occur through a vertical axis (2). Relative to the scapula, the humerus can move, on average, 100 degrees (61,62). The translational movements, which occur simultaneously with rotational movements, include superoinferior, anteroposterior, and mediolateral migration of the humeral head on the glenoid. It is difficult to show *in vivo* humeral head translations with normal movement based on the reported results from *in vitro* studies. In general, anterior translations appear to occur with flexion and internal rotations, and posterior translations appear to occur with extension and external rotation (44). Anterior and superior humeral head translations occur when the arm is abducted (63). Finally, a combination of posterior, lateral,

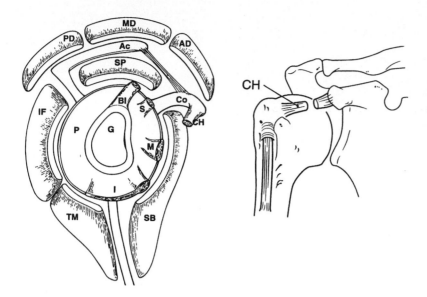

FIGURE 8.8 Lateral view of the glenoid portion of the glenohumeral joint showing muscles and ligaments. The muscles shown are the posterior deltoid (PD), the middle deltoid (MD), the anterior deltoid (AD), the supraspinatus (SP), the infraspinatus (IF), the long head of the biceps (BI), the subscapularis (SB), and the teres minor (TM). The ligaments and capsule shown are the superior glenohumeral ligament (S), the coracohumeral ligament (CH), the middle glenohumeral ligament (M), the inferior glenohumeral ligament (I), and the posterior aspect of the capsule (P). Other structures include the acromion (AC), the glenoid (G), and the coracoid (CO). (From Blasier RB, Soslowsky LJ, Malicky DM, et al. Posterior glenohumeral subluxation: active and passive stabilization in a biomechanical model. *J Bone Joint Surg Am* 1997;79:433–440, with permission.)

and superior migration of the humeral head occurs with combined extension, external rotation, and abduction of the arm (64).

Forces across the Joint, Contact Areas and Patterns, and Movers

Force Couple

Normal shoulder kinematics relies on the coordinated contributions of various muscles. Inman defined a force couple in the frontal plane with the deltoid and supraspinatus muscles as elevators and the infraspinatus, teres minor, and subscapularis as depressors (15). For the deltoid and supraspinatus to act as arm elevators without also jamming the humeral head into the acromion, the depressor mechanism must pull the head down while the arm is abducted. In addition, a force couple in the horizontal plane has also been described, with the stability provided by the subscapularis anteriorly and the infraspinatus and teres minor posteriorly (Fig. 8.9) (65).

Compressive Forces and Contact Patterns

Muscles whose lines of action are nearly perpendicular to the face of the glenoid act to compress the convex humeral head into the concave glenoid fossa. Throughout the entire range of arm abduction except at full abduction, the rotator cuff muscles and the posterior deltoid are properly positioned to press the head of the humerus into the glenoid fossa (16). As the arm is abducted and the muscles act as compressors, the cartilage of the humeral head contacts the cartilage of the glenoid surface, with a maximal contact area of 5.70 cm^2 at 120 degrees of elevation (66). The patterns of contact between the head of the humerus and the glenoid surface change with arm abduction. This variations in the contact patterns between the cartilage surfaces are depicted in Fig. 8.10 (66).

Movers

Muscles that cross the glenohumeral joint act at different times to produce arm abduction, flexion, extension, and rotation. The primary abductor is the deltoid, and more specifically the middle deltoid, reaching peak activity between 90 and 180 degrees of elevation (2,10,15). The supraspinatus muscle also acts as an abductor, but it can work equally well as a flexor. Forward flexion is achieved primarily by a combination of efforts of the anterior deltoid and the clavicular head of the pectoralis major, which reaches peaks in activity at 75 and 115 degrees of elevation (15). Another muscle that contributes to arm elevation is the biceps, which assists with forward flexion and can assist with abduction if the arm is also externally rotated (2).

Normal arm elevation requires that the rotator cuff muscles work as the depressor component of the force couple. Starting with arm abduction, the most active depressor is the subscapularis (2). Both the teres minor and infraspinatus muscles display similar behaviors and have greater activity levels as depressors with forward flexion of the arm than with arm abduction (15).

To return the arm back to the dependent position requires the work of the adductors and the extensors. The primary adductors and extensors are the latissimus dorsi and the pectoralis major (67). These muscles, along with the teres minor, the posterior deltoid, and the long head of the triceps extend the arm, with the posterior deltoid causing hyperextension (39).

Many of the muscles already mentioned also work to cause rotation at the glenohumeral joint. The muscles that cause external rotation about the vertical axis are the infraspinatus, the teres minor, and the posterior deltoid. If working alone, the posterior deltoid will cause not only external rotation but also hyperextension of the arm (39). There are multiple internal rotators, but the subscapularis is

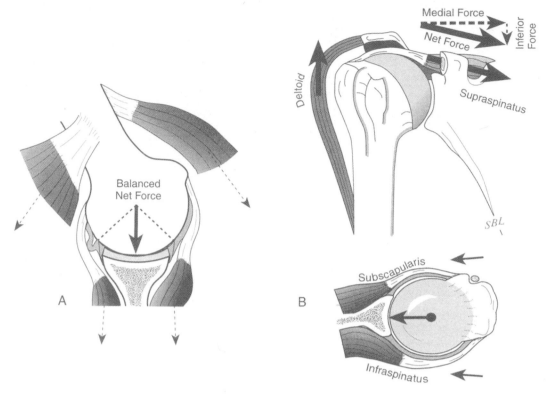

FIGURE 8.9 **A:** The force couple in the frontal plane consists of the deltoid and the supraspinatus as elevators and the inferior rotator cuff as depressors. **B:** The force couple in the horizontal plane consists of the subscapularis anteriorly and the teres minor posteriorly. (From Halder AM, Itoi E, An KN. Anatomy and biomechanics of the shoulder. *Orthop Clin North Am* 2000;31:159–176, with permission.)

the only pure internal rotator. The other muscles combine other actions with internal rotation. The teres major and latissimus dorsi cause internal rotation with extension and adduction, the pectoralis major combines internal rotation with adduction, and the anterior deltoid causes internal rotation with flexion (39).

Stability

The glenohumeral joint is the most mobile joint in the body. Unfortunately, the wide range of mobility comes at the expense of stability. Stability of the glenohumeral joint has historically been divided into two categories: static and

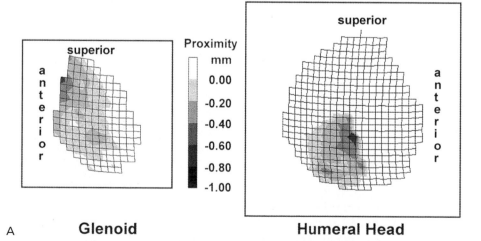

FIGURE 8.10 Glenohumeral contact patterns in a typical shoulder at 60 degrees (**A**) and 20 degrees (**B**) of elevation with external rotation in the scapular plane. (From Soslowsky LJ, Flatow EL, Bigliani LU, et al. Quantitation of *in situ* contact areas at the glenohumeral joint: a biomechanical study. *J Orthop Res* 1992;10:524–534, with permission.) (*continued*)

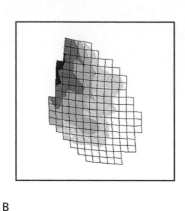
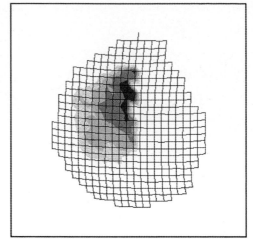

B

FIGURE 8.10 *(continued).*

dynamic. The static stabilizers include the osteoarticular surfaces and labrum, the intraarticular pressure, and the joint capsule, and the ligaments, whereas the muscles that cross the joint act as the dynamic stabilizers (68–72). According to Kent, the primary stabilizer is the capsulolabral complex, and the secondary stabilizer is the rotator cuff (2). However, at all arm positions, stability is the result of a complex interaction of multiple components and is not the result of any one component acting alone (70).

Static Stabilizers

Osteoarticular Geometry

Historically, glenohumeral joint instability was thought to be partly caused by the lack of glenohumeral joint congruence. More recently, however, the congruence of the joint has been studied and recognized using the technique of *stereophotogrammetry.* This technique has shown that the glenohumeral joint is quite congruent and remains this way throughout the entire range of arm motion (66, 73). It has been shown that the cartilage on the humerus is thicker in the center, whereas the cartilage on the glenoid is thicker along the periphery; the result is a convex humeral head sitting on a concave glenoid fossa. This reciprocal geometry and the compression provided by the rotator cuff and deltoid muscles serve as a stabilizing mechanism for the joint. This mechanism, called *concavity compression,* prevents excess translatory movements of the humeral head on the glenoid when elevation occurs (Fig. 8.11) (74).

Labrum

The concavity of the joint is also caused, in part, by the *glenoid labrum.* It has also been proven that the labrum, a ring of fibrous tissue attaching to the rim of the glenoid, provides 50% of the concavity of the glenoid. Therefore, damage to the labrum can cause a decrease in the effectiveness of the concavity compression mechanism (Fig. 8.12). The labrum also helps to contain the humeral head in the glenoid socket by generating hoop stresses (45).

Clinically, the importance of the labrum is recognized when Bankart lesions are encountered. Bankart lesions involve tearing of both the inferior glenohumeral ligament and the anteroinferior labrum from the glenoid (75). *In vitro* studies have analyzed the biomechanics of the shoulder both after a Bankart tear and after the subsequent repair. After an artificially created tear, significant increases in anteroinferior translation (crank test) and posterior translation (drawer test) were reported (76). The maximum anterior translation reported was 4.7 mm in a shoulder with a Bankart tear, as compared with the average anterior translation of 3.8 mm in the normal shoulder (44,77). Bankart repairs are done, in part, to reduce this excess translation and thus provide increased stability.

Intraarticular Pressure

Intraarticular pressure, in combination with a limited joint volume, is also a contributor to static stabilization of the

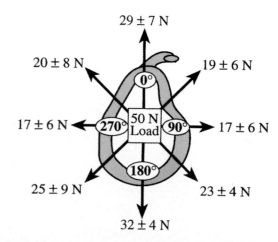

FIGURE 8.11 Average maximum translation resisted in each direction (0, 45, 90, 135, 180, 225, 270, and 315 degrees) by the humeral head compressed into the glenoid cavity with a 50-N load. Note: 0 degrees, superior; 90 degrees, anterior. (From Lippitt S, Matsen F. Mechanisms of glenohumeral joint stability. *Clin Orthop* 1993;291:20–28, with permission.)

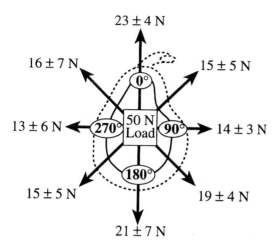

FIGURE 8.12 Average maximum translation resisted in each direction (0, 45, 90, 135, 180, 225, 270, and 315 degrees) by the humeral head compressed with a 50-N load into the glenoid cavity after excision of the labrum. Note: 0 degrees, superior; 90 degrees, anterior. (From Lippitt S, Matsen F. Mechanisms of glenohumeral joint stability. *Clin Orthop* 1993;291:20–28, with permission.)

glenohumeral joint (the role of intraarticular pressure in a joint with dynamic stabilizers active is believed to be minimal). At rest, the intraarticular pressure has been measured to be −67.8 mm Hg (78). With arm movement, the intraarticular pressure becomes more negative and acts like a vacuum as it pulls the capsule inward (79,80). This action has been shown to contribute to anterior, posterior, and inferior stability of the glenohumeral joint (Fig. 8.13). As would be expected, with venting of the joint, the intraarticular pressure's contribution to stability is removed, and the result is an unstable shoulder (80).

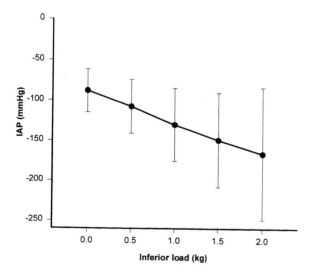

FIGURE 8.13 With increasing inferior loads, the intraarticular pressure becomes more negative. (From Inokuchi W, Sanderhoff Olsen B, Sojbjerg JO, et al. The relation between the position of the glenohumeral joint and the intraarticular pressure: an experimental study. *J Shoulder Elbow Surg* 1997;6:144–149, with permission.)

Joint Capsule

The loose *joint capsule* attaches to the circumference of the glenoid and the anatomic neck of the humerus (2). The contribution of the joint capsule to stability varies greatly and depends on the direction of the applied load and the position of the arm when the load is applied (77). With the arm in the dependent position and the humeral head centered on the glenoid, the capsule carries no force and does not contribute to stability (68). However, with increasing arm abduction and rotation, the capsule increasingly contributes to anterior, posterior, and inferior glenohumeral joint stability. Anteriorly, glenohumeral joint stability is provided by the posterior capsule when the arm is abducted 50 to 90 degrees and by the anterior capsule with 70 and 90 degrees of arm abduction (81,82). Posterior glenohumeral joint stability is primarily provided by the posterior capsule when the arm is between 60 and 90 degrees of abduction (83). Finally, inferior glenohumeral stability is provided by the anterior capsule with 45 degrees of arm abduction and by the posterior capsule with 90 degrees of arm abduction (84).

Reinforcing the joint capsule are the coracohumeral ligament and the glenohumeral ligaments. As with the capsule, the contribution of these ligaments to glenohumeral stability changes with arm movement, because the orientation of the ligaments crossing the joint changes. In investigating the contribution of these ligaments to stability, many studies have been done with parts of the soft tissue envelope excised. These types of models have an inherent weakness in that they are measuring the contribution of the ligament while not taking into account the contribution of the muscles (70,85). However, these studies are still valuable, and they provide some idea of the role of the coracohumeral and glenohumeral ligaments in stability of the joint.

Coracohumeral Ligament

The *coracohumeral ligament* spans from the base of the lateral coracoid to the greater tuberosity (Fig. 8.8) (10). Because of its position, it is able to reinforce the anterior and posterior margins of the rotator interval (49). The reported structural properties of the coracohumeral ligament indicate that it can play a significant role in stabilization at the glenohumeral joint (86). When the arm is at the side in external rotation, the coracohumeral ligament is an important factor in inferior stability and plays some role in superior stability of the joint (49,82,87). Moreover, in external rotation, as anteriorly directed loads are applied to the glenohumeral joint, the coracohumeral ligament acts to stabilize against anterior translations of the humeral head (88). Finally, because the coracohumeral ligament tightens with increasing external rotation, it also functions to check this motion (2,89).

Superior Glenohumeral Ligament

The *superior glenohumeral ligament* attaches at the anterior labrum and runs inferiorly and laterally to insert on the humerus near the lesser tuberosity (Fig. 8.8) (90). Biomechanical studies have shown that the superior glenohumeral ligament, like the coracohumeral ligament, is capable of assisting in stability of the glenohumeral joint (70,86). The superior glenohumeral ligament assists in stabilizing the capsule both anteriorly and inferiorly and also checks external rotation (2,72,88,91). Anteriorly, the superior glenohumeral ligament can stabilize the joint when the arm is externally rotated and abducted. Inferiorly, the superior glenohumeral ligament can stabilize the joint when the arm is in neutral or external rotation at the side, or as the arm is adducted (79, 84). With external rotation, the ligament becomes taut, and this tension allows it to check this motion as well.

Middle Glenohumeral Ligament

The *middle glenohumeral ligament* runs from the anterior labrum to the lesser tuberosity underneath the tendon of the subscapularis (Fig. 8.8) (10). The middle glenohumeral ligament can stabilize the joint anteriorly and inferiorly and can also check external rotation of the arm. When the arm is externally rotated, the middle glenohumeral ligament can stabilize the glenohumeral joint anteriorly in the lower to middle ranges of abduction (68,72,79,92,93). Moreover, in external rotation, the middle glenohumeral ligament acts as a secondary stabilizer of the joint inferiorly when the arm is adducted (82,84).

Inferior Glenohumeral Ligament

The *inferior glenohumeral ligament* consists of three parts: an anterior band, a posterior band, and an interposed axillary pouch (72,94). The inferior glenohumeral ligament spans from the glenoid or labrum to the anatomic neck of the humerus (Fig. 8.8) (10). As a whole, the inferior glenohumeral ligament is considered an anterior and inferior stabilizer of the glenohumeral joint, and it also checks external rotation (70). Anteriorly, the inferior glenohumeral ligament is a most effective stabilizer when the arm is abducted and externally rotated (10,79). In the midranges of abduction, anterior stabilization resulting from the inferior glenohumeral ligament is provided by the anterior band, whereas in the upper ranges of abduction, the axillary pouch stabilizes the joint anteriorly (72,84,94). Inferiorly, the inferior glenohumeral ligament is the most important stabilizer of the joint when the arm is in the dependent position and either neutrally or externally rotated. In addition, in the upper ranges of abduction, the posterior portion of the inferior glenohumeral ligament provides inferior stabilization for the glenohumeral joint (84). Finally, as the arm is externally rotated, all parts of the inferior glenohumeral ligament tighten, thus allowing this ligament to check that movement.

Studies looking at the structural and mechanical properties of the inferior glenohumeral ligament have found that the ligament is more likely to fail at the glenoid insertion (40%) than at the midsubstance (35%) and humeral insertion site (25%) (85). In addition, results have shown that each of the three inferior glenohumeral ligament regions has an ultimate stress of 5.5 MPa (70). Coracohumeral and superior glenohumeral ligament studies report that the prop-

erties of these ligaments are similar to those of the inferior glenohumeral ligament, a finding indicating that none of the glenohumeral ligaments can stabilize the glenohumeral joints alone (86). Each component must work as a part of a static team and with the dynamic muscle stabilizers to keep the humeral head centered on the glenoid (70).

Dynamic Stabilizers

Rotator Cuff

The *rotator cuff* consists of four muscles: supraspinatus, infraspinatus, teres minor, and subscapularis. The supraspinatus, innervated by the suprascapular nerve (C4–6), has its origin in the supraspinatus fossa and its insertion on the greater tuberosity. The infraspinatus, innervated by the suprascapular nerve (C4–6), has its origin on the infraspinatus fossa and scapular spine and inserts onto the middle facet of the greater tuberosity. The teres minor, innervated by the axillary nerve (C5–6), originates from the lateral border of the scapula and infraspinatus fascia and inserts on the inferior facet of the greater tuberosity. Finally, the subscapularis, innervated by the upper and lower subscapular nerve (C5–8), has its origin at the subscapularis fossa and inserts onto the lesser tuberosity.

As a group, the rotator cuff muscles stabilize the joint by providing joint compression and resisting excess humeral head translations. The supraspinatus aids in joint compression (10,95). Anterior humeral head translations are resisted by the subscapularis (10,96). Posterior translations are resisted by both the infraspinatus and teres minor muscles (10,81,83,97). Both these muscles also resist superior translations of the humeral head (10,81,83,97). Finally, inferior translations of the humeral head are resisted by the subscapularis (10,96).

The rotator cuff muscles contribute to stability both passively and dynamically. Passively, the cuff provides anterior and posterior glenohumeral stabilization, but not inferior stabilization. Anterior stabilization is provided by passive muscle tension of the subscapularis in early (0 to 45 degrees) abduction (72). Posterior stabilization of the glenohumeral joint is provided partially by passive muscle tension in the supraspinatus and infraspinatus and teres minor (9,83). Finally, it has been shown that passive tension in the rotator cuff muscles does not contribute significantly to inferior stability of the glenohumeral joint. A comparison humeral head positions relative to the glenoid in cadaveric shoulders with and without a load at different degrees of abduction with sequential dissection of the rotator cuff muscles found the role of the cuff in static inferior stability to be insignificant (49).

Dynamically, the rotator cuff muscles function together in a few ways to provide glenohumeral stability. First, the rotator cuff muscles act as the depressor part of the force couple, as Inman described in 1944 (15). Furthermore, on evaluation of the forces generated by each muscle, the supraspinatus and subscapularis provide higher dynamic stability than the other cuff muscles in the midranges of motion, whereas at the end range, the position of anterior instability, the subscapularis, teres minor, and infraspinatus provide much higher dynamic stability (98). Finally, the role of the cuff in dynamic stabilization of the shoulder has been shown using dynamic shoulder models. There was increased anterior and posterior displacement with a 50% reduction in rotator cuff force. Those authors concluded that the rotator cuff force significantly contributed to the stabilization of the glenohumeral joint during arm motion (63).

Deltoid

The *deltoid,* innervated by the axillary nerve (C4–5), originates from the lateral clavicle, the acromion, and the scapular spine and inserts on the deltoid tubercle of the humerus. Its role in stability has been investigated and is somewhat controversial. Investigations using a model with a pulley effect looked at the forces applied by the deltoid onto the humerus and concluded that the deltoid may prevent upward migration of the humeral head and compresses it against the glenoid (32). However, the role of the deltoid in inferior and posterior stability has been questioned. The deltoid has been shown not to contribute significantly to inferior humeral head stability with arm abduction and adduction because displacement of the humeral head did not change with deltoid removal (99). With regard to the deltoid's role in posterior instability, it appears that the anterior and middle portions of the muscle do not contribute to posterior instability in forward flexion (101).

Biceps

The *biceps muscle* is composed of both a long head and a short head. The long head of the biceps muscle originates from the supraglenoid tubercle, and the short head of the biceps originates from the coracoid process. Both heads insert on the tuberosity of the radius and on the ulnar fascia of the forearm (10). The biceps muscle receives its innervation from the musculocutaneous nerve (C5–6).

The mechanical properties of the long head of the biceps tendon are of the same magnitude as tendons of other joints, a feature implying that it has the ability to support large loads (102). Although the major role of the long head of the biceps is to stabilize the humeral head in the glenoid during elbow flexion and forearm supination (103), it also plays a role in anterior, superior, and posterior shoulder stability. In a dynamic cadaveric model, the long head of the biceps has been found to contribute to anterior stability by increasing the shoulder's resistance to torsional forces (104). Superior shoulder stability is provided by the long head of the biceps when the arm is abducted (105). In a study of seven patients with documented loss of the tendon's proximal attachment, excess superior translation of the humeral head was noted in each patient and in all positions of abduction except 0 degrees, a finding thus supporting the role of the tendon as a superior stabilizer of the humeral head in abduction. Finally, posterior shoulder stability is provided by the long head of the biceps when the arm is in midranges of elevation (106). As expected, lesions in the labrum that destabilize the insertion of the biceps result in significant increases in anteroposterior and superoinferior glenohumeral translations (107).

Thermal Modification of Tissue

Application of thermal energy to a lax or redundant capsule for the treatment of instability has gained substantial interest. The application of nonablative, thermal energy to the anterior capsule has been shown to result in significant decreases in both anterior and posterior translations of the humeral head (108). This process is done clinically using either laser energy or radiofrequency energy. Unfortunately, both processes appear to induce histologic, ultrastructural, and biomaterial alterations of the tissue (109). At approximately 65°C, collagen denaturation and shrinkage occur (109) (Figs. 8.14 and 8.15). As this energy is applied and the

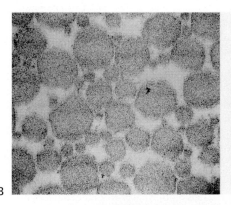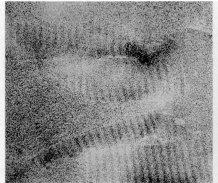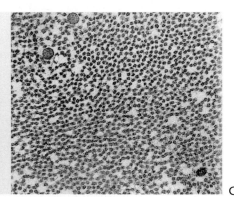

A, B   C

FIGURE 8.14 A: Electron photomicrograph of a cross section of normal rabbit patellar tendon. Note the normal bimodal pattern of large- and small-diameter collagen fibers and the longitudinal orientation of all fibers (34,000× original magnification). **B:** Cross section of rabbit patellar tendon immediately after thermal shrinkage. Note the random orientation of the collagen fibers (34,000× original magnification). **C:** Cross section of a rabbit patellar tendon 8 weeks after thermal modification shows remodeling with small-diameter collagen fibers, indicative of scar tissue (34,000× original magnification). (From Arnoczky SP, Aksan A. Thermal modification of connective tissues: basic science considerations and clinical implications. *J Am Acad Orthop Surg* 2000;8:305–313, with permission.)

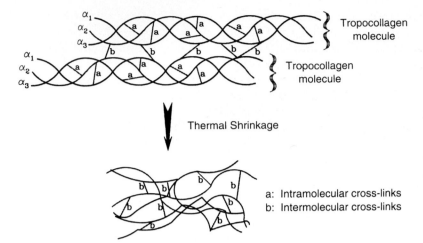

Thermal Shrinkage

a: Intramolecular cross-links
b: Intermolecular cross-links

FIGURE 8.15 Molecular mechanism of collagen shrinkage. The intramolecular crosslinks within the tropocollagen molecules are denatured, but the intermolecular crosslinks between the tropocollagen molecules are maintained. (From Arnoczky SP, Aksan A. Thermal modification of connective tissues: basic science considerations and clinical implications. *J Am Acad Orthop Surg* 2000;8:305–313, with permission.)

tissues shrink, alterations in the mechanical properties of the tissue occur. In a cadaver model, modified glenohumeral capsular tissue exhibited decreased stiffness, although the viscoelastic properties remained the same (110,111). Additionally, in bovine extensor tendons, the cross-sectional area of the tissues increased and the mechanical properties decreased with shrinkage (112). Furthermore, tensile stiffness of rabbit knee capsule significantly decreased after exposure to high levels of thermal energy (110,111). What happens to thermally shrunken tissue postoperatively and the effect of early rehabilitation of tissue with decreased biomechanical properties are still under investigation.

It is unclear why patients improve clinically after thermal modification. Maintenance of initial capsular shrinkage, posttreatment capsular thickening, and loss of afferent sensory stimulation may all play a part in this clinical benefit (109). As mentioned earlier, the shrunken tissue has inferior biomechanical properties. Thus, to maintain the initial shrinkage, there needs to be a balance between the amount of shrinkage and the postoperative protection from undue stresses. As with all insults to the human body, the response is inflammatory and reparative. It is likely that the fibroplasia and collagen deposition in response to the thermal treatment result in a hypertrophied joint capsule, and this condition may also contribute to its stability in a structural manner (109). As the denaturation of the capsule is occurring with treatment, it is likely that the neural receptors that significantly innervate the capsule are also being affected. As a result, this thermal treatment could affect the sensory feedback mechanism and in essence decrease the pain and provide symptomatic relief (109,113). As more information about the mechanism, optimal postoperative rehabilitation, and clinical course of thermal capsulorraphy becomes available through research and long-term clinical follow-up, more light will be shed on this very interesting topic.

REFERENCES

1. Culham E, Peat M. Functional anatomy of the shoulder complex. *J Orthop Sports Phys Ther* 1993;18:342–350.
2. Kent BE. Functional anatomy of the shoulder complex: a review. *Phys Ther* 1971;51:947.
3. Flatow EL. The biomechanics of the acromioclavicular, sternoclavicular, and scapulothoracic joints. *Instr Course Lect* 1993; 42:237–245.
4. Peat M. Functional anatomy of the shoulder complex. *Phys Ther* 1986;66:1855–1865.
5. DePalma A. Surgical anatomy of acromioclavicular and sternoclavicular joints. *Surg Clin North Am* 1963;43:1541.
6. Depmster W. Mechanisms of shoulder movement. *Arch Phys Med Rehabil* 1965;46:49–70.
7. Bearn JG. Direct observations on the function of the capsule of the sternoclavicular joint in clavicular support. *J Anat* 1967;101: 159–170.
8. Rockwood CA Jr, Green DP, eds. *Fractures,* 2nd ed. Philadelphia: JB Lippincott, 1984.
9. Rockwood CA Jr, Matsen FA III, eds. *The Shoulder,* 2nd ed. Philadelphia: WB Saunders, 1998.
10. Halder AM, Itoi E, An KN. Anatomy and biomechanics of the shoulder. *Orthop Clin North Am* 2000;31:159–176.
11. Kuhn JE, Plancher KD, Hawkins RJ. Symptomatic scapulothoracic crepitus and bursitis. *J Am Acad Orthop Surg* 1998;6: 267–273.
12. Ruland LJ 3rd, Ruland CM, Matthews LS. Scapulothoracic anatomy for the arthroscopist. *Arthroscopy* 1995;11:52–56.
13. Williams GR Jr, Shakil M, Klimkiewicz J, et al. Anatomy of the scapulothoracic articulation. *Clin Orthop* 1999;359:237–246.
14. Codman E. *The shoulder: rupture of the supraspinatus tendon and other lesions in or about the subacromial bursa.* Boston: Thomas Todd, 1934.
15. Inman V. Observations on the function of the shoulder joint. *J Bone Joint Surg Am* 1944;26:1–30.
16. Poppen NK, Walker PS. Normal and abnormal motion of the shoulder. *J Bone Joint Surg Am* 1976;58:195–201.
17. McQuade KJ, Smidt GL. Dynamic scapulohumeral rhythm: the effects of external resistance during elevation of the arm in the scapular plane. *J Orthop Sports Phys Ther* 1998;27:125–133.

18. Doody SG, Freedman L, Waterland JC. Shoulder movements during abduction in the scapular plane. *Arch Phys Med Rehabil* 1970;51:595–604.

19. Lukasiewicz AC, McClure P, Michener L, et al. Comparison of 3-dimensional scapular position and orientation between subjects with and without shoulder impingement. *J Orthop Sports Phys Ther* 1999;29:574–583; 584–586.

20. Warner JJ, Micheli LJ, Arslanian LE, et al. Scapulothoracic motion in normal shoulders and shoulders with glenohumeral instability and impingement syndrome: a study using Moire topographic analysis. *Clin Orthop* 1992;285:191–199.

21. Bigliani LU, Nicholson GP, Flatow EL. Arthroscopic resection of the distal clavicle. *Orthop Clin North Am* 1993;24:133–141.

22. Engin AE. On the biomechanics of the shoulder complex. *J Biomech* 1980;13:575–590.

23. Fukuda K, Craig EV, An KN, et al. Biomechanical study of the ligamentous system of the acromioclavicular joint. *J Bone Joint Surg Am* 1986;68:434–440.

24. Moseley HF. The clavicle: its anatomy and function. *Clin Orthop* 1968;58:17–27.

25. Hollinshead WH. *Textbook of anatomy.* New York: Harper and Row, 1967.

26. MacConaill MA, Basmaijin JB. *Muscles and movements: a basis for human kinesiology.* Huntington, NY: Robert E. Krieger, 1977.

27. Kapandji I. *The physiology of the joints: annotated diagrams of the mechanics of the human joints,* vol 1. London: E & S Livingstone, 1970.

28. Kuster MS, Hales PF, Davis SJ. The effects of arthroscopic acromioplasty on the acromioclavicular joint. *J Shoulder Elbow Surg* 1998;7:140–143.

29. Yamaguchi K, Flatow EL. Arthroscopic evaluation and treatment of the rotator cuff. *Orthop Clin North Am* 1995;26:643–659.

30. Corso SJ, Furie E. Arthroscopy of the acromioclavicular joint. *Orthop Clin North Am* 1995;26:661–670.

31. Flatow EL, Cordasco FA, Bigliani LU. Arthroscopic resection of the outer end of the clavicle from a superior approach: a critical, quantitative, radiographic assessment of bone removal. *Arthroscopy* 1992;8:55–64.

32. Klimkiewicz JJ, et al. The acromioclavicular capsule as a restraint to posterior translation of the clavicle: a biomechanical analysis. *J Shoulder Elbow Surg* 1999;8:119–124.

33. Cotton RE, Nottingham, Rideout DF. Tears of the humeral rotator cuff: a radiologic and pathological necropsy. *J Bone Joint Surg Br* 1964;46:314–328.

34. Petersson CJ, Gentz CF. Ruptures of the supraspinatus tendon: the significance of distally pointing acromioclavicular osteophytes. *Clin Orthop* 1983;174:143–148.

35. Neer CS. Anterior acromioplasty for the chronic impingement syndrome in the shoulder: a preliminary report. *J Bone Joint Surg Am* 1972;54:41–50.

36. Bigliani LU, Ticker JB, Flatow EL, et al. The relationship of the acromial architecture to rotator cuff disease. *Clin Sports Med* 1991;10:823–838.

37. Neviaser RJ, Neviaser TJ. Observations on impingement. *Clin Orthop* 1990;254:60–63.

38. Fu F, Harner CD, Klien AH. Shoulder impingement lesions. *Clin Orthop* 1991;269:162–172.

39. Brunnstrom S. *Clinical kinesiology,* 3rd ed. Philadelphia: FA Davis, 1972.

40. Jobe CM. Superior glenoid impingement: current concepts. *Clin Orthop* 1996;330:98–107.

41. Jobe CM. Superior glenoid impingement. *Orthop Clin North Am* 1997;28:137–143.

42. Walch G, Boileau P. Impingement of the deep surface of the supraspinatus tendon on the posterosuperior glenoid rim: an arthroscopic study. *J Shoulder Elbow Surg* 1992;1:238–245.

43. Paley KJ, Jobe FW, Pink MM, et al. Arthroscopic findings in the overhand throwing athlete: evidence for posterior internal impingement of the rotator cuff. *Arthroscopy* 2000;16:35–40.

44. Harryman DT, Sidles JA, Clark JM, et al. Translation of the humeral head on the glenoid with passive glenohumeral motion. *J Bone Joint Surg Am* 1990;72:1334–1343.

45. Howell SM, Galinat BJ, Renzi AJ, et al. Normal and abnormal mechanics of the glenohumeral joint in the horizontal plane. *J Bone Joint Surg Am* 1988;70:227–232.

46. Montgomery WH 3rd, Jobe FW. Functional outcomes in athletes after modified anterior capsulolabral reconstruction. *Am J Sports Med* 1994;22:352–358.

47. Halbrecht JL, Tirman P, Atkin D. Internal impingement of the shoulder: comparison of findings between the throwing and nonthrowing shoulders of college baseball players. *Arthroscopy* 1999;15:253–258.

48. McFarland EG, Hsu CY, Neira C, et al. Internal impingement of the shoulder: a clinical and arthroscopic analysis. *J Shoulder Elbow Surg* 1999;8:458–460.

49. Itoi E., Motzkin NE, Morrey BF, et al. The static rotator cuff does not affect inferior translation of the humerus at the glenohumeral joint. *J Trauma* 1999;47:55–59.

50. Soslowsky LJ, Robinson PS, Reynolds P. Basic science of the rotator cuff. In: Norris T, ed. *Orthopaedic knowledge update: shoulder and elbow,* 2nd ed. Rosemont, IL: American Academy of Orthopaedic Surgeons, 2001.

51. Soslowsky LJ, Carpenter JE, Bucchieri JS, et al.. Biomechanics of the rotator cuff. *Orthop Clin North Am* 1997;28:17–30.

52. Flatow EL, et al. Excursion of the rotator cuff under the acromion: patterns of subacromial contact. *Am J Sports Med* 1994;22:779–788.

53. Neer CS. Impingement lesions. *Clin Orthop* 1983;173:70–77.

54. Soslowsky LJ, Carpenter JE, DeBano CM, et al. Development and use of an animal model for investigations on rotator cuff disease. *J Shoulder Elbow Surg* 1996;5:383–392.

55. Schneeberger AG, Nyffeler RW, Gerber C. Structural changes of the rotator cuff caused by experimental subacromial impingement in the rat. *J Shoulder Elbow Surg* 1998;7:375–380.

56. Soslowsky LJ, Thomopoulos S, Tun C, et al. Neer Award 1999. Overuse activity injures the supraspinatus tendon in an animal model: a histologic and biomechanical study. *J Shoulder Elbow Surg* 2000;9:79–84.

57. Saha AK. Dynamic stability of the glenohumeral joint. *Acta Orthop Scand* 1971;42:491–505.

58. Randelli M, Gambrioli PL. Glenohumeral osteometry by computed tomography in normal and unstable shoulders. *Clin Orthop* 1986;208:151–156.

59. Cyprien JM, Vasey HM, Burdet A, et al. Humeral retrotorsion and glenohumeral relationship in the normal shoulder and in recurrent anterior dislocation (scapulometry). *Clin Orthop* 1983;175:8–17.

60. Iannotti JP, Gabriel JP, Schneck SL, et al. The normal glenohumeral relationships: an anatomical study of one hundred and forty shoulders. *J Bone Joint Surg Am* 1992;74:491–500.

61. Freedman L, Munro RR. Abduction of the arm in the scapular plane: scapular and glenohumeral movements—a roentgenographic study. *J Bone Joint Surg Am* 1966;48:1503–1510.

62. Steindler A. *Kinesiology of the human body under normal and pathological conditions.* Springfield, IL: Charles C Thomas, 1955.

63. Wuelker N, Korell M, Thren K. Dynamic glenohumeral joint stability. *J Shoulder Elbow Surg* 1998;7:43–52.

64. Novotny JE, Nichols CE, Beynnon BD. Normal kinematics of the unconstrained glenohumeral joint under coupled moment loads. *J Shoulder Elbow Surg* 1998;7:629–639.

65. Saha AK. The classic. Mechanism of shoulder movements and a plea for the recognition of "zero position" of glenohumeral joint. *Clin Orthop* 1983;173:3–10.

66. Soslowsky LJ, Flatow EL, Bigliani LU, et al. Quantitation of *in situ* contact areas at the glenohumeral joint: a biomechanical study. *J Orthop Res* 1992;10:524–534.

67. Basmajian JV. *Muscles alive: their functions revealed by electromyography*, 2nd ed. Baltimore: Williams & Wilkins, 1967.

68. Debski RE, Wong EK, Woo SL, et al. *In situ* force distribution in the glenohumeral joint capsule during anterior-posterior loading. *J Orthop Res* 1999;17:769–776.

69. Debski RE, Sakone M, Woo SL, et al. Contribution of the passive properties of the rotator cuff to glenohumeral stability during anterior-posterior loading. *J Shoulder Elbow Surg* 1999; 8:324–329.

70. Bigliani LU, Kelkar R, Flatow EL, et al. Glenohumeral stability: biomechanical properties of passive and active stabilizers. *Clin Orthop* 1996;330:13–30.

71. McMahon PJ, Debski RE, Thompson, WO, et al. Shoulder muscle forces and tendon excursions during glenohumeral abduction in the scapular plane. *J Shoulder Elbow Surg* 1995;4: 199–208.

72. Turkel SJ, Panio MW, Marshall JL, et al. Stabilizing mechanisms preventing anterior dislocation of the glenohumeral joint. *J Bone Joint Surg Am* 1981;63:1208–1217.

73. Soslowsky LJ, Flatow EL, Bigliani LU, et al. Articular geometry of the glenohumeral joint. *Clin Orthop* 1992;285:181–190.

74. Lippitt S, Matsen F. Mechanisms of glenohumeral joint stability. *Clin Orthop* 1993;291:20–28.

75. McMahon PJ, Tibone JE, Cawley PW, et al. The anterior band of the inferior glenohumeral ligament: biomechanical properties from tensile testing in the position of apprehension. *J Shoulder Elbow Surg* 1998;7:467–471.

76. Harryman DT, Ballmer FP, Harris SL, et al. Arthroscopic labral repair to the glenoid rim. *Arthroscopy* 1994;10:20–30.

77. Black KP, Schneider DJ, Yu JR, et al. Biomechanics of the Bankart repair: the relationship between glenohumeral translation and labral fixation site. *Am J Sports Med* 1999;27:339–344.

78. Inokuchi W, Sanderhoff Olsen B, Sojbjerg JO, et al. The relation between the position of the glenohumeral joint and the intraarticular pressure: an experimental study. *J Shoulder Elbow Surg* 1997;6:144–149.

79. Matsen FA, Harryman DT, Sidles JA. Mechanics of glenohumeral instability. *Clin Sports Med* 1991;10:783–788.

80. Gibb TD, Sidles JA, Harryman DT, et al. The effect of capsular venting on glenohumeral laxity. *Clin Orthop* 1991;268:120–127.

81. Ovesen J, Nielsen S. Anterior and posterior shoulder instability: a cadaver study. *Acta Orthop Scand* 1986;57:324–327.

82. Ovesen J, Neilsen S. Stability of the shoulder joint: cadaver study of stabilizing structures. *Acta Orthop Scand* 1985;56:149–151.

83. Ovesen J, Nielsen S. Posterior instability of the shoulder: a cadaver study. *Acta Orthop Scand* 1986;57:436–439.

84. Warner JJ, Deng XH, Warren RF, et al. Static capsuloligamentous restraints to superior-inferior translation of the glenohumeral joint. *Am J Sports Med* 1992;20:675–685.

85. Bigliani L, Pollock RG, Soslowsky LJ, et al. Tensile properties of the inferior glenohumeral ligament. *J Orthop Res* 1992;10:187–197.

86. Boardman ND, Debski RE, Warner JJ, et al. Tensile properties of the superior glenohumeral and coracohumeral ligaments. *J Shoulder Elbow Surg* 1996;5:249–254.

87. Soslowsky LJ, Malicky DM, Blasier RB. Active and passive factors in inferior glenohumeral stabilization: a biomechanical model. *J Shoulder Elbow Surg* 1997;6:371–379.

88. Malicky DM, Soslowsky LJ, Blasier RB, et al. Anterior glenohumeral stabilization factors: progressive effects in a biomechanical model. *J Orthop Res* 1996;14:282–288.

89. Neer CS, Satterlee CC, Dalsey RM, et al. The anatomy and potential effects of contracture of the coracohumeral ligament. *Clin Orthop* 1992;280:182–185.

90. Morrey BE Itoi, E An K. Biomechanics of the shoulder. In: Rockwood CA, Matsen FA III, eds. *The shoulder*. Philadelphia: WB Saunders, 1998.

91. O'Connell PW, Nuber GW, Mileski RA, et al. The contribution of the glenohumeral ligaments to anterior stability of the shoulder joint. *Am J Sports Med* 1990;18:579–584.

92. Debski RE, Wong EK, Woo SL, et al. An analytical approach to determine the *in situ* forces in the glenohumeral ligaments. *J Biomech Eng* 1999;121:311–315.

93. Ferrari DA. Capsular ligaments of the shoulder: anatomical and functional study of the anterior superior capsule. *Am J Sports Med* 1990;18:20–24.

94. O'Brien SJ, Neves MC, Arnoczky SP, et al. The anatomy and histology of the inferior glenohumeral ligament complex of the shoulder. *Am J Sports Med* 1990;18:449–456.

95. Howell SM, Imoberssteg AM, Seger DH, et al. Clarification of the role of the supraspinatus muscle in shoulder function. *J Bone Joint Surg Am* 1986;68:398–404.

96. Tillett F, Smith M, Fulcher M, et al. Anatomic determination of humeral head retroversion: the relationship of the central axis of the humeral head to the bicipital groove. *J Shoulder Elbow Surg* 1993;2:255–256.

97. Colachis SC Jr, Strohm BR, Brechner VL. Effects of axillary nerve block on muscle force in the upper extremity. *Arch Phys Med Rehabil* 1969;50:647–654.

98. Lee SB, Kim KJ, O'Driscoll SW, et al. Dynamic glenohumeral stability provided by the rotator cuff muscles in the mid-range and end-range of motion: a study in cadavers. *J Bone Joint Surg Am* 2000;82:849–857.

99. Gagey O, Hue E. Mechanics of the deltoid muscle: a new approach. *Clin Orthop* 2000;375:250–257.

100. Motzkin N, Itoi E, Morrey BF, et al. Contribution of passive bulk tissues and deltoid to static inferior glenohumeral stability. *J Shoulder Elbow Surg* 1994;3:313.

101. Blasier RB, Soslowsky LJ, Malicky DM, et al. Posterior glenohumeral subluxation: active and passive stabilization in a biomechanical model. *J Bone Joint Surg Am* 1997;79:433–440.

102. McGough RL, Debski RE, Taskiran E, et al. Mechanical properties of the long head of the biceps tendon. *Knee Surg Sports Traumatol Arthrosc* 1996;3:226–229.

103. Kumar VP, Satku K, Balasubramaniam P. The role of the long head of biceps brachii in the stabilization of the head of the humerus. *Clin Orthop* 1989;244:172–175.

104. Rodosky M., Harner CD, Fu FH. The role of the long head of the biceps muscle and superior glenoid labrum in anterior stability of the shoulder. *Am J Sports Med* 1994;22:121–130.

105. Warner JJ, McMahon PJ. The role of the long head of the biceps brachii in superior stability of the glenohumeral joint. *J Bone Joint Surg Am* 1995;77:366–372.

106. Pagnani MJ, Deng XH, Warren RF, et al. Role of the long head of the biceps brachii in glenohumeral stability: a biomechanical study in cadavers. *J Shoulder Elbow Surg* 1996;5:255–262.

107. Pagnani MJ, Deng XH, Warren RF, et al. Effect of lesions of the superior portion of the glenoid labrum on glenohumeral translation. *J Bone Joint Surg Am* 1995;77:1003–1010.

108. Tibone JE, McMahon PJ, Shrader TA, et al. Glenohumeral

joint translation after arthroscopic, nonablative, thermal capsuloplasty with a laser. *Am J Sports Med* 1998;26:495–498.

109. Arnoczky SP, Aksan A. Thermal modification of connective tissues: basic science considerations and clinical implications. *J Am Acad Orthop Surg* 2000;8:305–313.

110. Hayashi K, Markel MD, Thabit G 3rd, et al. The effect of nonablative laser energy on joint capsular properties: an *in vitro* mechanical study using a rabbit model. *Am J Sports Med* 1995; 23:482–487.

111. Hayashi K, Thabit G 3rd, Massa KL, et al. The effect of thermal heating on the length and histologic properties of the glenohumeral joint capsule. *Am J Sports Med* 1997;25:107–112.

112. Wall MS, Deng XH, Torzilli PA, et al. Thermal modification of collagen. *J Shoulder Elbow Surg* 1999;8:339–344.

113. Vangsness CT Jr, Smith CF. Arthroscopic shoulder surgery with three different laser systems: an evaluation of laser applications. *Arthroscopy* 1995;11:696–700.

9

THE KNEE

EDWIN M. TINGSTAD

Watanabe described and illustrated much of the arthroscopic anatomy of knee in an arthroscopic atlas that was first published in 1957 (1), and use of the arthroscope has increased steadily since that time. Learning and improving arthroscopic skills has become one of the mainstays of orthopaedic training. For many orthopaedists, arthroscopy is the most common procedure performed. An understanding and application of arthroscopic anatomy is an essential component of any arthroscopic procedure. This fact and the widespread use of arthroscopy have given rise to arthroscopy training simulators, which attempt to teach basic arthroscopic skills and anatomy (2). Currently, arthroscopy is accepted as the standard against to which all other diagnostic methods are compared for intraarticular derangements of the knee. Standard arthroscopy has a higher sensitivity and specificity than a standard clinical examination and radiographic measures and has decreased the indications for open treatment of many knee conditions (3–11) (Figs. 9.1 and 9.2) This chapter briefly reviews the normal variants of arthroscopic evaluation in a systematic fashion. The knee is divided into four components: the suprapatellar pouch, the medial and lateral compartments, and the intercondylar notch.

SUPRAPATELLAR POUCH

Most arthroscopic procedures of the knee begin in the suprapatellar pouch. The pouch is a synovial-lined area that extends approximately 3 to 5 cm above the superior pole of the patella. The synovium tends to be three to five layers thick and has free nerve endings, as do the anterior fat pad and joint capsule. These structures can produce severe pain when injured (12,13). The pouch often contains an incomplete transverse embryonic remnant called the plica synovialis suprapatellaris (14). This is complete in 4% to 20% of adults and can subdivide the pouch into superior and infe-

rior portions (15,16) (Fig. 9.3). At the apex of the superior portion of the pouch is often noted the genu articularis, which appears reddish in nature. This muscle and its attachments help to maintain the relationship of the suprapatellar pouch with the synovial membrane (Fig. 9.4). Synovial membranes of the knee are most clearly identified in the suprapatellar pouch. These synovial membranes are sometimes referred to as plicae and are normal embryonic remnants (Fig. 9.5). Plicae are the most frequently noted cause of symptoms in the preadolescent knee at the time of arthroscopy (17). The synovial lining throughout the knee has been shown by neurosensory mapping to have a significant sensory component, whereas palpation of the articular cartilage tends to produce little or no sensation (Fig. 9.6). The identification of peripheral opioid receptors and increased understanding of the neurosensory pathways in the knee have improved pain management in the perioperative period, making knee arthroscopy almost exclusively an outpatient procedure (12,13,18,19).

Patellofemoral Joint

The patellofemoral joint is usually the first articulation inspected at the time of knee arthroscopy. Visualization through a variety of portals allows a more complete assessment. The patellofemoral joint consists of the articular surface of the patella, which has seven facets, and the trochlea, which is the anterior notch in the distal femur. The patella appears wider superiorly and narrows inferiorly in a triangular shape. The trochlea exhibits significant variability, and femoral anteversion influences the orientation of the patella in the groove and its subsequent tracking (10).

For practical purposes, the facets of the patella can be divided into three portions: the medial and lateral facets, each subdivided into superior, middle, and inferior parts, and the distally and medially located odd facet. With normal knee flexion, the lateral facet should be contacted first at approximately 30 degrees of flexion; subsequently, at about 45 degrees of flexion, the medial facet should also be contacted (Figs. 9.7 and 9.8). With increasing flexion, there is gradual migration of the contact area from the distal inferior medial

E. M. Tingstad: Orthopaedics and Sports Medicine, University of Washington, Seattle, Washington; Pullman Memorial Hospital, Pullman, Washington.

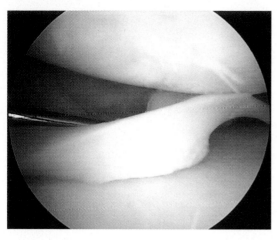

FIGURE 9.1 Bucket handle tear of medial meniscus of left knee.

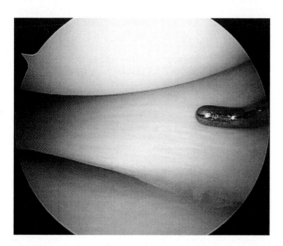

FIGURE 9.2 Medial meniscus with normal thinning of meniscus at its free margin.

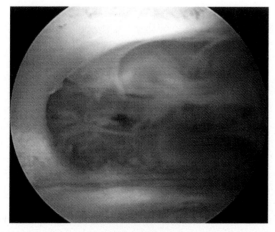

FIGURE 9.3 Incomplete plica synovialis suprapatellaris viewed from anterolateral portal with knee in extension.

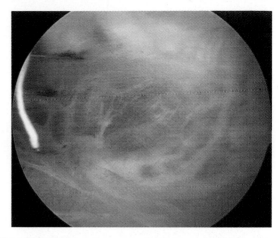

FIGURE 9.4 Portion of genu articularis seen at apex of suprapatellar pouch with knee in extension.

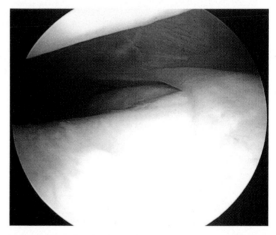

FIGURE 9.5 Slightly thickened medial plica overlying medial femoral condyle viewed through anterolateral portal.

and inferior lateral facets to the proximal superior medial and superior lateral facets. In full extension, there is no articulation between the patella and the femur. The odd facet comes into contact with femur, particularly in near-terminal flexion of 125 to 130 degrees. This is the only position in which the odd facet makes contact (20).

The articular cartilage of the patella is thickest in the body and often does not conform to the underlying bone; therefore, the cartilaginous apex of the patella rarely coincides with its osseous apex (21). The synovium surrounding the patellofemoral joint can often be peeled away to visualize the geniculate vessels. The lateral geniculate in particular can be seen running transversely to the longitudinal axis approximately 1 cm from the proximal edge of the lateral patella (22).

Lateral Gutter

The lateral gutter consists of the lateral femoral condyle and the synovial-lined lateral soft tissues, with the floor being the

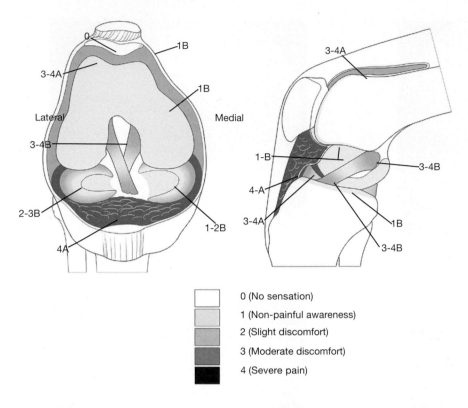

0 (No sensation)
1 (Non-painful awareness)
2 (Slight discomfort)
3 (Moderate discomfort)
4 (Severe pain)

FIGURE 9.6 Neurosensory map of intraarticular structures palpated without anesthesia in conscious patient. A: Coronal view. B: Sagittal view. Pain index: 0 (insensate) to 4 (severe pain). (A) refers to good spatial localization. (B) refers to poor spatial localization. (Courtesy of S. F. Dye, M.D.)

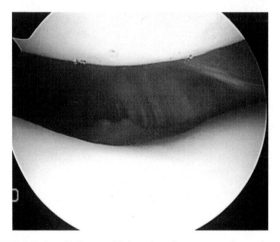

FIGURE 9.7 Patellofemoral joint view from anterolateral portal, with knee extended.

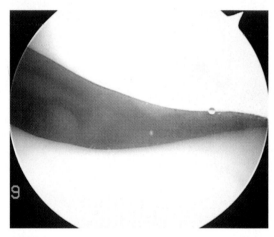

FIGURE 9.8 Patellofemoral joint viewed from superomedial portal with knee flexed 30 to 40 degrees, showing normal initial lateral facet articulation.

tibial plateau, lateral meniscus, and popliteal hiatus (Fig. 9.9). Like its medial counterpart, the lateral gutter has a synovial-lined portion of the lateral femoral condyle and a synovial-lined lateral aspect of the lateral joint capsule. This is often a point of collection of loose bodies. The examination distally in the posterior and forward portion of the lateral gutter shows the sheath around the popliteal tendon, with a consistent synovial fold running transversely between femoral condyle and the lateral capsule of the bottom of the lateral gutter. This fold should not be considered a pathologic plica (23).

Medial Gutter

The medial gutter is similar to the lateral gutter. The medial aspect is a synovial-lined medial joint capsule with the lateral aspect being a synovial-lined portion of the medial femoral condyle (Fig. 9.10). The gutter may be entered from the patellofemoral joint or from the medial compartment. In approximately one third of patients, a thin, smooth synovial shelf or plica is encountered. This runs from the fat pad to the patellar retinaculum; stretching of the medial synovial shelf may cause bowstringing across the femoral condyle (15,16). This medial patellar plica or shelf is the one

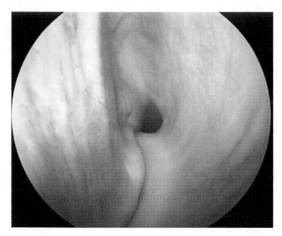

FIGURE 9.9 Lateral gutter viewed with knee extended in anterolateral portal. The cleft posteriorly is the opening of the popliteal hiatus.

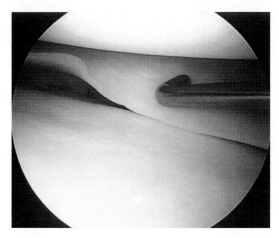

FIGURE 9.11 Medial meniscus viewed through anterolateral portal with 30 degrees of flexion and valgus stress.

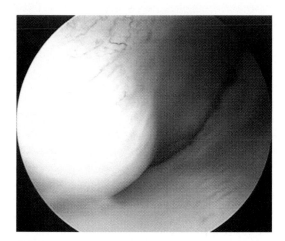

FIGURE 9.10 Medial gutter with normal peripheral meniscocapsular attachments and synovial lining of medial aspect of medial femoral condyle.

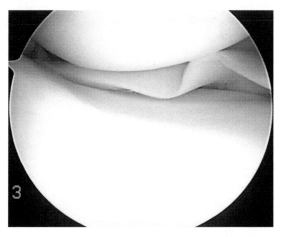

FIGURE 9.12 Normal flounce or ruffled border of medial meniscus, which may be accentuated with external rotation.

that most commonly becomes symptomatic, and resection of the symptomatic plica has been shown to be helpful (24,25). Spurs and loose bodies may also form and be deposited in the medial compartment. With the arthroscope in the posterior aspect of the recess, the meniscocapsular junction and portions of the meniscotibial and mensiscofemoral or coronary ligaments may be assessed.

MEDIAL COMPARTMENT

Following the edge of the medial femoral condyle with gentle flexion of the knee and following the condyle, the medial compartment may be entered with the arthroscope. The medial compartment may be further opened with slight extension and external rotation of the foot with a valgus stress being applied. The normal medial meniscus has a small flounce or ruffle, most typically seen in the posterior horn along its free edge (Figs. 9.11 through 9.13). The medial

meniscus is C-shaped, with a larger posterior horn. The outer 25% to 30% of the meniscus is vascular, and two thirds of the peripheral meniscus has nerve endings. The meniscus is divided into zones based on vascular supply (26,27). The most peripheral portion is the "red–red," the middle portion is the "red–white," and the area out to free margin is the "white–white" zone. Menisci are vital to distributing load across the knee; they transmit 50% of the weight-bearing forces in extension and 85% in flexion. Meniscectomy reduces the load transmission function by 50% to 70% (28,29). The menisci also assist in maintaining joint stability and shock absorption during ambulation (30).

Elevation of the posterior horn of the medial meniscus reveals the meniscotibial ligaments or coronary ligaments (Fig. 9.13). The tibial ligaments function to anchor the slightly mobile meniscus to the tibia and thereby prevent excessive translation. The meniscotibial ligaments tend to be stiffer than those on the femoral side. Prevention of excessive posterior translation by the meniscotibial ligaments is complemented by the meniscofemoral ligaments, which

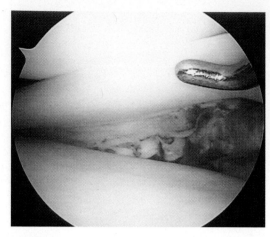

FIGURE 9.13 Meniscocapsular injury in medial compartment in patient with a medial collateral ligament injury.

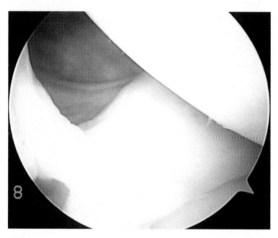

FIGURE 9.14 Posterior head of medial meniscus viewed through intercondylar notch with arthroscope pushed medially past the posterior cruciate ligament.

with the most common site of wear being at the 30- to 45-degree flexion site (10). Visualization of the posterior horn of the medial meniscus may be facilitated by passage of the arthroscope through the intraarticular notch just medial to the posterior cruciate ligament (PCL). This allows visualization of the posterior medial and, on the lateral side, the posterior lateral compartment of the knee and is recommended as a valuable part of routine arthroscopy (36).

THE INTRACONDYLAR NOTCH

The intracondylar notch contains the two cruciate ligaments, the attachment points of both menisci, and several accessory ligamentous structures. The notch typically is entered from the medial compartment or from the patellofemoral joint. The medial and lateral tibial spines are noted on the floor of the intracondylar notch. Proceeding anteriorly to posteriorly with the arthroscope, the intermeniscal ligament, which may be partially obscured by the fat pad, is seen, followed by the anterior horn of the medial meniscus, the tibial insertion of the anterior cruciate ligament (ACL), the anterior horn of the lateral meniscus, the posterior horn of the lateral meniscus, the posterior horn of the medial meniscus, and then, 10 to 15 mm below the plateau surface, the PCL (37) (Fig. 9.15). The ligamentum mucosum or infrapatellar plica extends from the apex of the intracondylar notch to the fat pad anteriorly, lying in front of the ACL. The ligamentum mucosum may interfere with passage of the arthroscope between medial and lateral compartments (Fig. 9.16). The intrameniscal ligament anteriorly typically connects the anterior margin of the lateral meniscus to the anterior end of the medial meniscus. Variable intact insertion patterns of the anterior meniscal ligament

prevent "riding up" of the femoral condyle on the posterior horn of the medial meniscus. This assists in allowing the meniscus to control anterior tibial translation (23,31,32).

The medial meniscus typically is able to translate approximately 5 mm in the anterior–posterior direction, with more motion seen in its anterior horn (33). Identification of increased translation of the anterior horn usually is not pathologic, particularly if it occurs in isolation (34). The anterior and posterior horns of the medial meniscus may have variable attachments (Fig. 9.14). The anterior horn in particular has been noted to have at least four differing patterns of insertion, the most common being on the flat intercondylar region of the tibial plateau (35). The articular surface of the tibia in the medial compartment tends to be more concave than its lateral counterpart. The articular surface typically is firm to probing, with increased softening and fibrillation seen with injury and aging. The articular cartilage of the medial femoral condyle may be examined with progressive flexion, beginning from an extended position,

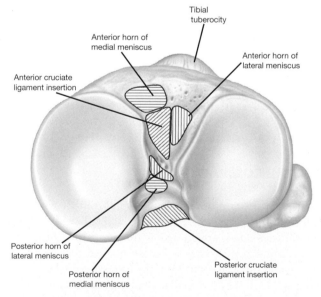

FIGURE 9.15 Axial representation of intraarticular structures of intracondylar notch.

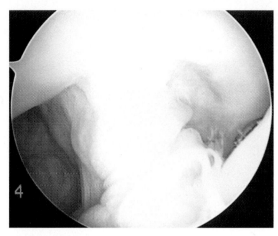

FIGURE 9.16 Ligamentum mucosum (infrapatellar plica) seen originating from apex of intercondylar notch.

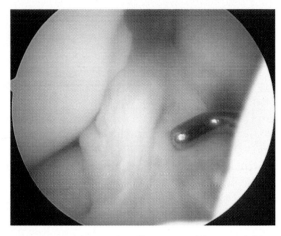

FIGURE 9.18 Anterior cruciate ligament with normal, blood vessel–lined synovium loosely covering.

have been described. These may mimic lateral meniscal tears on magnetic resonance imaging (38).

Anterior Cruciate Ligament

The ACL is approximately 3 to 4 cm long and 11 mm wide; it originates in the most posterior medial aspect of the lateral femoral condyle (Figs. 9.17 and 9.18). The anterior medial bundle of the ACL is tight in flexion, whereas the posterior lateral bundle is tight in extension (39). The ACL contains mechanoreceptors and free nerve endings that are believed to provide some proprioceptive effect and may provide protective and sensory input (12,40,41). The ACL fibers should become taut with an anterior force placed on the tibia. Internal rotation increases the tension on the ACL, and external rotation tends to decrease the tension on the ligament (42). With knee flexion the ACL rotates 90 degrees between its origin and insertion. The posterolateral component is shorter and

makes up more of the ligament; this may partially explain why the Lachman sign is more specific than the anterior drawer test in diagnosing ACL injuries (23).

Complete visualization of the ACL is possible by passing the arthroscope between the lateral femoral condyle and the ACL to view the femoral insertion. The "residents ridge" is a prominence in the lateral condylar wall that can be mistaken for the posterior margin of the lateral femoral condyle and can lead to incorrect placement of the femoral portion of an ACL graft The tibial insertion of the ACL is oval and is longer in the anterior–posterior dimension than in its medial lateral width, much like a footprint. The insertion on the tibial plateau lies just medial to the attachment of the anterior horn of the lateral meniscus, and fibers of the ACL may mingle with the insertion of the lateral meniscus (43–46). The two cruciate ligaments are believed to form a four-bar linkage mechanically and are probably connected via neural conduits that cause them to function as a complex (47,48) (Fig. 9.19).

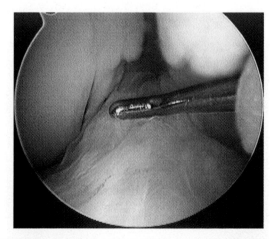

FIGURE 9.17 Anterior cruciate ligament viewed through anterolateral portal with normal footprint insertion on tibia.

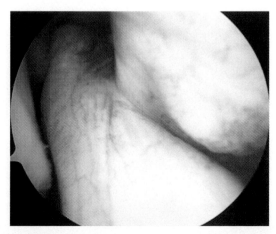

FIGURE 9.19 Anterior *(left)* and posterior *(right)* cruciate ligaments are believed to be linked by neural components that cross between the synovial linings.

Posterior Cruciate Ligament

The PCL, which is often covered with a layer of fatty synovium, inserts approximately 1.5 to 2 cm below the tibial plateau (Fig. 9.20). The ligament is larger and stronger than the ACL; it is approximately 38 mm in length and 13 mm in diameter (47). The PCL has two bands, the posterior medial band and anterior lateral band. The posterior medial band of the PCL is shorter, and it originates from the posterior portion of the intracondylar surface of the medial femoral condyle. The anterolateral band is the stronger of the two bands; it originates more anteriorly on intracondylar surface of the medial femoral condyle and tends to run slightly laterally and posteriorly, inserting on the lateral side of the insertion on the tibia. This band therefore progressively tightens as the knee flexes. The anterolateral band is usually the main focus of PCL reconstructions (49).

The PCL, like the ACL, receives its neural supply from the posterior articular nerve, which arises in the popliteal fossa and penetrates and innervates the posterior capsule (50). The PCL is associated with two meniscofemoral ligaments that share an insertion with the posterior portion of the PCL. The meniscofemoral ligaments, one or both, are present in 80% of knees. The meniscofemoral ligaments may contribute approximately 15% of the strength of the PCL (51). The anterior meniscal femoral ligament (ligament of Humphry) is anterior to the PCL and attaches to the posterior horn of the lateral meniscus. Its counterpart, the posterior meniscal femoral ligament, or ligament of Wrisberg, is found posterior to the PCL from the posterior horn of the lateral meniscus. The ligament of Wrisberg tends to be the larger of the two, obtaining a diameter as great as one-half that of the PCL; the ligament of Humphry may be as large as one-third the diameter of the PCL (23,52–54). Flexion of the knee increases the distance between the PCL and the posterior neurovascular structures, particularly the popliteal artery. This can reduce the risk of arterial injury during arthroscopic procedures such as a PCL reconstruction (55).

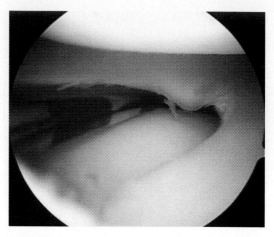

FIGURE 9.21 Normal lateral meniscus viewed from anterolateral portal with knee in figure-of-four position and arthroscope over the anterior horn.

LATERAL COMPARTMENT

The lateral compartment is best visualized arthroscopically with a varus stress and knee flexion in the so-called figure-of-four position (Fig. 9.21). The more circular-shaped lateral meniscus covers more of the articular surface than the medial meniscus does. It translates 10 to 12 mm on the tibial surface with flexion and extension. In full extension, the anterior horn of the lateral meniscus is located in the sulcus terminalis of the lateral femoral condyle. The popliteal artery is located just posterior to the origin of the posterior horn of the lateral meniscus and can be damaged with lateral meniscal repairs (51). Unlike the medial meniscus, the lateral meniscus has no attachment to the collateral ligament, just a loose connection to the capsule. This capsular attachment is lacking at the popliteal hiatus, and a probe may normally be placed between the popliteal tendon and the posterior horn of the lateral meniscus (56).

Fasicles are frequently seen on magnetic resonance imaging and with the arthroscope between the popliteus and the lateral meniscus; they can contribute to instability of the entire meniscus if disrupted (57) (Figs. 9.22 and 9.23). Palpa-

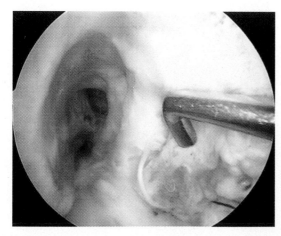

FIGURE 9.20 Synovium covering posterior cruciate ligament in an anterior cruciate ligament–deficient knee with empty lateral wall of intercondylar notch.

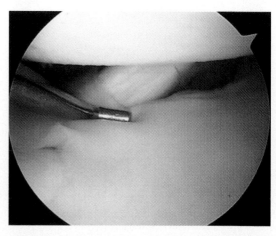

FIGURE 9.22 Popliteus as seen through anterolateral portal.

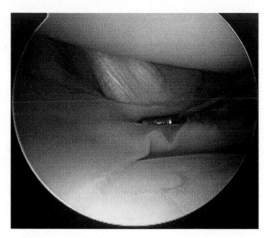

FIGURE 9.23 Lateral meniscus with normal chondral fissures on tibial plateau.

tion below the lateral meniscus at the level of popliteal hiatus may reveal loose bodies. Fraying and calcification of the free edge is commonly seen in the aged lateral meniscus and is considered normal. The presence of chondral fissures parallel to the lateral meniscal rim without evidence of significant articular surface changes is also believed to be a normal variant (10,58). Gentle probing of the articular surfaces is the most reliable means of assessing the integrity of the articular cartilage and may demonstrate separation of the cartilage from the subchondral bone.

CONCLUSION

The arthroscope provides a minimally invasive form of evaluation and treatment that is an invaluable tool in caring for patients with knee problems. Continuing efforts to better understand the anatomy and variability of the components of the knee is a necessity to appropriately diagnose and treat conditions of the knee.

REFERENCES

1. Watanabe M. *Atlas of arthroscopy.* Tokyo: Igaku Shoin, 1957.
2. Muller W, et al. [VRATS—Virtual Reality Arthroscopy Training Simulator.] *Radiologe* 2000;40:290–294.
3. Dandy DJ. Arthroscopic surgery of the knee. *Br J Hosp Med* 1982;27:360,362,365.
4. Dandy DJ. The impact of arthroscopic surgery on the management of disorders of the knee. *Arthroscopy* 1990;6:96–99.
5. Clevers GJ, Haarman HJ. Diagnostic arthroscopy of the knee joint: comparison of the accuracy to physical examination, contract arthrography and arthroscopy. *Neth J Surg* 1988;40:104–107.
6. Guercio H. Arthrography in the study of extra-meniscal pathology of the knee. *Ital J Orthop Traumatol* 1988;14:257–265.
7. Phillips B. In: Canale S, ed. *Campbell's operative orthopaedics,* 9th ed. St. Louis: Mosby, 1998.
8. Fu F, Baratz. In: DeLee J, Drez D, eds. *Orthopaedic sports medicine,* vol 2. Philadelphia: WB Saunders, 1994.
9. Chen MC, et al. MRI of meniscus and cruciate ligament tears correlated with arthroscopy. *J Formos Med Assoc* 1995;94:605–611.
10. Andrews JR. *Diagnostic and operative arthroscopy.* Philadelphia: WB Saunders, 1997.
11. Quinn SF, Brown TF. Meniscal tears diagnosed with MR imaging versus arthroscopy: how reliable a standard is arthroscopy? *Radiology* 1991;181:843–847.
12. Dye SF, Vaupel GL, Dye CC. Conscious neurosensory mapping of the internal structures of the human knee without intraarticular anesthesia. *Am J Sports Med* 1998;26:773–777.
13. Reuben SS. *Pain management in patients who undergo outpatient arthroscopic surgery of the knee.* J Bone Joint Surg Am 2000;82:1754–1767.
14. Fulkerson J. *Disorders of the patellofemoral joint,* 3rd ed. Baltimore: Williams & Wilkins, 1997.
15. Johnson DP, Witherow PJ. Symptomatic synovial plicae of the knee. *J Bone Joint Surg Am* 1993;75:1485–1496.
16. Patel D. *Arthroscopy of the plicae: synovial folds and their significance.* Am J Sports Med 1978;6:217–225.
17. Faraj A., Schilders E, Martens M. *Arthroscopic findings in the knees of preadolescent children: report of 23 cases.* Arthroscopy 2000;16:793–795.
18. Stein C, Haimnerl E, Yassourdis A, et al. Analgesic effect of intraarticular morphine after arthroscopic knee surgery. *N Engl J Med* 1991;325:1123–1126.
19. Beidert RM, Friederich NF. *Occurrence of the nerve endings in the soft tissue of the knee joint.* Am J Sports Med 1992;20:430–433.
20. Goodfellow J, Zindel M. *Patellofemoral joint mechanics and pathology: functional anatomy of the patellofemoral joint.* J Bone Joint Surg Br 1976;58:287–290.
21. Staubli H, Durrenmatt U, Porcellini B, et al. Anatomy and surface geometry of the patellofemoral joint in the axial plane. *J Bone Joint Surg Br* 1999;81:452–458.
22. Schreiber S. *Arthroscopic surgery and the lateral release for patellofemoral disorders.* Op Tech Sports Med 1999;7:69–75.
23. Olson EJ. In: Fu FH, Vince KG, Miller MD, eds. *Arthroscopic anatomy in knee surgery.* Baltimore: Williams & Wilkins, 1994.
24. Dorchak JD, et al. Arthroscopic treatment of symptomatic synovial plica of the knee: long-term followup. *Am J Sports Med* 1991;19:503–507.
25. O'Dwyer KJ, Peace PK. The plica syndrome. *Injury* 1988;19:350–352.
26. Arnoczky S, Warren SP. Microvasculature of the human meniscus. *Am J Sports Med* 1982;10:90–95.
27. Woo SL, Arnoczky SP, et al. Anatomy, biology, and biomechanics of tendon, ligament, and meniscus. In: Simon S, ed. *Orthopaedic basic science.* Rosemont, IL: American Academy of Orthopaedic Surgeons, 1994:45–88.
28. Fukubayashi T, Kurasawa H. The contact area and pressure distribution pattern of the knee: a study of normal and osteoarthritic knee joints. *Acta Orthop Scand* 1980;51:871–880.
29. Nordin M, Frankel VH. *Basic biomechanics of the musculoskeletal system,* 2nd ed. Philadelphia: Lea & Febiger, 1989.
30. Miller M, Palmer C. Arthroscopic meniscal repair. In: Hamer C, Vince KG, Fu FH, eds. *Techniques in knee surgery.* Philadelphia: Lippincott Williams & Wilkins, 2001.
31. Levy IM, Warren RF. The effect medial meniscectomy on anterior-posterior motion of the knee. *J Bone Joint Surg Am* 1982;64:883–885.
32. Smith FB. Tibial collateral strain due to occult derangements of the medial meniscus. *J Bone Joint Surg Am* 1954;36:88.
33. Johnson WO, Fu FH. Tibial meniscal dynamics using 3D reconstruction of MR images. In: *Proceedings of the orthopaedic research society.* Chicago, IL: 1990.
34. Pinar H, et al. Dislocating anterior horn of the medial meniscus. *Arthroscopy* 1998;14:246–249.

35. Berlet GC. The anterior horn of the medial meniscus: an anatomic study of its insertion. *Am J Sports Med* 1998;26:540–543.

36. Amin KB, Cosgarea AJ, Kaeding CC. The value of intercondylar notch visualization of the posteromedial and posterolateral compartments during knee arthroscopy. *Arthroscopy* 1999;15:813–817.

37. Williams P, Warwick R, Dyson M, et al., eds. *Gray's anatomy*, 37th ed. Edinburgh: Churchill Livingstone, 1989.

38. Nelson EW, LaPrade RF. The anterior intermeniscal ligament of the knee: an anatomic study. *Am J Sports Med* 2000;28:74–76.

39. Arnoczky SP. In: Feagin J, ed. *Anatomy of the cruciate ligaments*. New York: Churchill Livingstone, 1988:179–195.

40. Arnoczky S. *Blood supply to the anterior cruciate ligament and supporting structures.* Orthop Clin North Am 1985.16:15–28.

41. Schultz R, Miller DC, Kerr CS, et al. Mechanoreceptors in human cruciate ligaments. *J Bone Joint Surg Am* 1984;66:1072–1076.

42. Muller W. *The knee: form, function and ligament reconstruction.* New York: Springer-Verlag, 1983.

43. Girgis FG. Monajem A. The cruciate ligaments of the knee joint. *Clin Orthop* 1975;106:216–231.

44. Arnoczky SP, Buckwalter JA, et al. Anatomy of the anterior cruciate ligament. In: Jackson DW, Woo SL-Y, et al., eds. *The anterior cruciate ligament: current and future concepts.* New York: Raven Press, 1993:5–22.

45. Furman W, Marshall JL, Girgis FG. The anterior cruciate ligament: a functional analysis based on post-mortem studies. *J Bone Joint Surg Am* 1976;58:179–185.

46. Hovis W, Hawkins RJ. *Anatomy for ACL reconstruction.* Rosemont, IL: American Academy of Orthopaedic Surgeons, 1999.

47. Miller M, Cooper DE, Warner JP. *Review of sports medicine and arthroscopy.* Philadelphia: WB Saunders, 1995.

48. Morgan-Jones R, Cross MJ. *The intercruciate band of the human knee: an anatomical and histological study.* J Bone Joint Surg Br 1999;81:991–993.

49. Albright J, Carpenter JE, Graf BK, et al. Knee and soft tissue trauma. In: Beaty J, ed. *Orthopaedic knowledge update 6.* Rosemont, IL: American Academy of Orthopaedic Surgeons, 1999.

50. Kennedy J, et al. Nerve supply of the human knee and its functional importance. *Am J Sports Med* 1982;10:329–335.

51. Stoller D. *MRI, arthroscopy, and surgical anatomy of the joints.* Philadelphia: Lippincott Raven, 1999.

52. Brantigan O, Voshell AF. Ligaments of the knee joint: the relationship of the ligament of Humphry to the ligament of Wrisberg. *J Bone Joint Surg* 1946;28:66–67.

53. Heller L, Langman J. Menisco-femoral ligaments of the human knee. *J Bone Joint Surg Br* 1964;46:307–313.

54. Miller M, Bergfeld JA, Fowler PJ, et al. The posterior cruciate ligament injured knee: principles of evaluation and treatment. (Zuckerman J, ed.) *Instr Course Lect* 1999:199–207.

55. Matava M, Sethi NV, Totty WG. Proximity of the posterior cruciate ligament insertion to the popliteal artery as a function of the knee flexion angle. Implications for posterior cruciate ligament reconstruction. *Arthroscopy* 2000;16:796–804.

56. Cannon W. In: Johnson T, ed. *Arthroscopic meniscal repair.* Rosemont, IL: American Academy of Orthopaedic Surgeons, 1999.

57. Simonian PT, et al. Popliteomeniscal fasciculi and the unstable lateral meniscus: clinical correlation and magnetic resonance diagnosis. *Arthroscopy* 1997;13:590–6.

58. Fine K. Chondral fissures associated with the lateral meniscus. *Arthroscopy* 1995;11:292–295.

THE ANKLE

FERNANDO A. PENA GOMEZ
NED AMENDOLA

The first efforts at arthroscopic intervention, dating back to 1918, were made by Dr. K. Takagi at the University of Japan. Considering the technological limitations at that time, the knee joint was the focus of interest. Burman, in 1931, in New York, reported on arthroscopy of 100 knees, 25 shoulders, 20 hips, 15 elbows, 6 wrists, and 3 ankles (1). He stated that the ankle "is not suitable for arthroscopy." The congruency of the ankle joint and the diameter of the canula (4 mm) seemed to be the most limiting factors. Later, M. Watanabe, a protégé of Dr. K. Takagi, developed new arthroscopes and expanded arthroscopy to joints other than the knee. In 1977, Dr. Hiroshi Ikeuchi, a student of Dr. Watanabe, presented one of the first series on ankle arthroscopy with clear examples of intraarticular pathology (2). As described in Guhl's book (2), this presentation inspired Guhl and others to pursue further interest in this field of arthroscopy. More recently, several authors, among them Ewing, Ferkel, and Guhl, have popularized arthroscopy of the ankle joint (2–5). Although it is still an evolving area of arthroscopic surgery, ankle arthroscopy has demonstrated high rates of success and minimal complications with proper technique and indications.

Complications associated with ankle arthroscopy can be avoided or significantly decreased by a solid knowledge and familiarity with the anatomy of the ankle joint and the structures crossing along this joint. Feiwell and Frey (6), as well as Sitler et al. (5), described in detail the relationship of structures at risk with placement of standard ankle portals. These and other reports added to the improved visualization and access to the ankle joint, allowing an expansion in indications for ankle arthroscopy.

This chapter reviews the normal topographic anatomy, vital structures, and arthroscopic anatomy of the ankle joint.

F. Pena: Departmento Cirugía Ortópedica y Traumatología, Clinica Santa Elena, Madrid, Spain.
N. Amendola: Dept. of Orthopedics, University of Iowa Hospitals, Iowa City, Iowa.

TOPOGRAPHIC ANATOMY

The ankle joint consists of the distal tibia, the fibula, and the talus. The configuration of bony anatomy makes the ankle joint a very congruent joint with limited access if the soft tissue and bony structures are respected. Therefore, ankle arthroscopy represents a challenge to achieve full visualization and working access to the joint without creating any iatrogenic injury.

The medial malleolus extends approximately 1 cm distal to the joint line. The posterior tibialis tendon lies on the posterior half of the malleolus; posterior to it, the tibial nerve, the tibial artery, and the long flexor tendons are found and protected. Anterior to the medial malleolus lie the most distal and fine branches of the saphenous nerve, which are posterior and medial to the great saphenous vein. These branches may extend as far distal as the first metatarsophalangeal joint, where they anastomose with the most medial branches of the superficial peroneal nerve. Between the anterior tibialis tendon and the medial malleolus, the "soft spot" of the ankle joint is located. This represents a safe area in which to place an anteromedial portal; however, the portal should be placed as close as possible to the medial aspect of the anterior tibialis tendon, in order to avoid the saphenous nerve and vein as well as the medial malleolus (3) (Fig. 10.1).

Anteriorly, the thin subcutaneous tissue allows easy palpation of the anterior compartment structures. From medial to lateral, they are the anterior tibialis tendon, the extensor hallucis longus tendon, the anterior tibial artery and vein, the deep peroneal nerve, and the extensor digitorum longus tendon. Previous publications described the anterocentral portal, which provides a broad anterior visualization of the ankle joint (4,7,8). More recent reports (6,9) have pointed out the risk of injury to anterior structures with the use of this portal. In addition, adequate access through anteromedial and lateral portals has made the anterocentral portal unnecessary for full visualization (Fig. 10.2).

The superficial peroneal nerve may be found along the lateral half of the anterior aspect of the ankle (Fig. 10.3). Be-

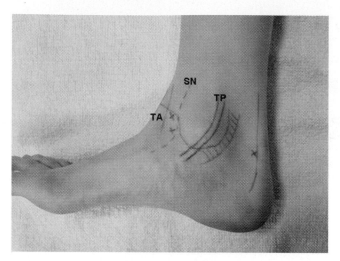

FIGURE 10.1 Medial aspect of the ankle with location of anteromedial, accessory medial, and posteromedial portals. EDL, extensor digitorum longus; Fi, fibula; NVB, neurovascular bundle; PerT, peroneal tendons; PITFL, posterior inferior tibiofibular ligament; SN, saphenous nerve; SPN, intermediate dorsal branch of peroneal nerve; SuN, sural nerve; TA, tibialis anterior tendon; Ta, talus; Ti, tibia; TP, tibialis posterior tendon.

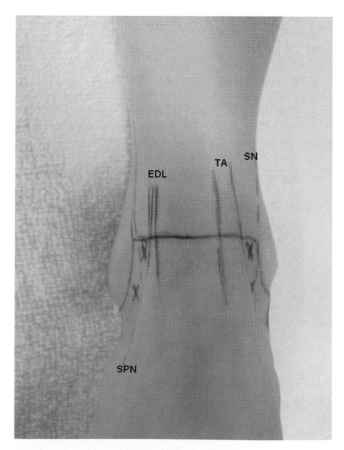

FIGURE 10.2 Anterior aspect of the ankle joint with location of the accessory medial, anteromedial, anterolateral, and accessory lateral portals. (Abbreviations as in Fig. 10.1.)

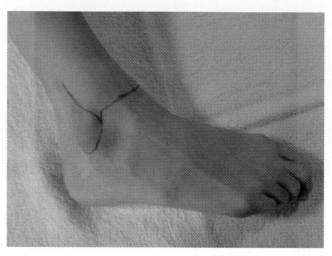

FIGURE 10.3 Lateral aspect of the foot and ankle with tenting of the intermediate dorsal cutaneous branch of the superficial peroneal nerve. (Abbreviations as in Fig. 10.1.)

cause injury to this nerve is the most common complication when using the anterolateral portal, it is important to discuss the anatomy in detail (2,4). Although multiple anatomic variations have been described, in 91% of specimens the nerve becomes subcutaneous approximately 10.5 cm proximal from the tip of the fibula (10). At this level it is most likely to be found along the anterior margin of the fibula. From that point, it branches into the medial terminal branch and the intermediate dorsal cutaneous branch. In 92% of specimens this division occurs at 6.5 cm proximal to the tip of the fibula (11). The medial terminal branch crosses the ankle joint line along the anterior middle third, adjacent to the extensor hallucis longus tendon. More distally, it trifurcates into three final branches to innervate the dorsal aspect of the medial half of the foot. The most lateral branch, the intermediate dorsal cutaneous branch, crosses the ankle joint subcutaneously at the level of the fourth and fifth extensor digitorum longus tendons, and from there it aims for the third intermetatarsal space (Fig. 10.4). This is the branch at risk when an anterolateral portal is created. More distally, it may have some anastomosis with the most dorsal branches of the sural nerve. The medial and the intermediate branches provide most of the dorsal skin sensation of the foot. The deep peroneal nerve innervates the dorsal aspect of the first web space.

The lateral malleolus extends more posteriorly and distally than its medial counterpart. The tip of the malleolus is, on average, 2 cm distal to the joint line and 1 cm posterior to the medial malleolus. Posterior to the fibula, the peroneal tendons curve inferiorly, and the sural nerve may be found more posteriorly. The sural nerve is located an average of 1 to 1.5 cm distal and 1.5 to 2 cm posterior to the tip of the fibula. It travels anteriorly and laterally to the lesser saphenous vein, which may be found in the immediate vicinity of the nerve. As mentioned previously, at the level of the

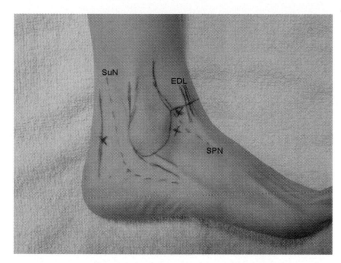

FIGURE 10.4 Lateral aspect of the ankle with location of the anterolateral, accessory lateral, and posterolateral portals. (Abbreviations as in Fig. 10.1.)

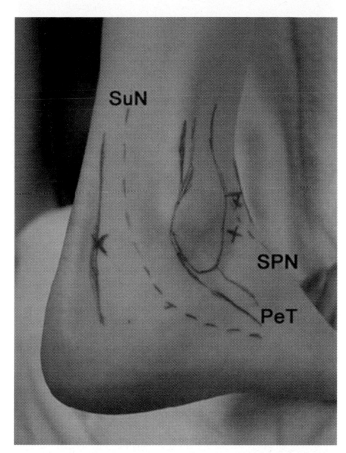

FIGURE 10.6 Posterior view of the lateral aspect of the ankle with location of the posterolateral, accessory lateral, and anterolateral portals. (Abbreviations as in Fig. 10.1.)

tuberosity of the fifth metatarsal it divides into its terminal medial and lateral branches to anastomose with the intermediate dorsal cutaneous branch of the superficial peroneal nerve (Fig. 10.4).

The posterior topographic anatomy of the ankle is better assessed with the patient in the prone position. At the level of the ankle joint, the Achilles tendon is slightly lateral to the midline. The joint line can be palpated and identified medial, lateral, and anterior to the tendon (Fig. 10.5). The superior border of the calcaneus is used as a reference, and dorsiflexion of the ankle joint helps in feeling the posterior process of the talus. Both medial and lateral portals are placed at the level of the tibiotalar joint (Fig. 10.6). The posterolateral portal is placed adjacent to the lateral border of the Achilles tendon, and the sural nerve remains anterior to

it by an average of 3.2 mm (5). On the medial side, the portal is again placed adjacent to the margin of the tendon, and the neurovascular bundle remains at a safe distance (on average, 9.7 mm) anterior to it (5) (Figs. 10.7 and 10.8).

We recommend identifying and delineating the structures described here with a marking pen before beginning the procedure, in order to have a better appreciation of their location and thus decrease the chances for injury. In addition, use of blunt dissection and a minimal number of reentries through the same portal decrease the risk of injury.

The technique and instrumentation required for ankle arthroscopy are discussed in Chapter 61.

INTRAARTICULAR ANATOMY

Ferkel (4) described a 21-point inspection for the intraarticular anatomy of the ankle. This method represents one of the many ways to explore the ankle joint. Regardless of the methodology used by the surgeon, we recommend, as with any joint arthroscopy, that a systematic procedure be used so as to avoid missing any portions or pathology of the ankle joint. The dome of the talus presents a convexity in the an-

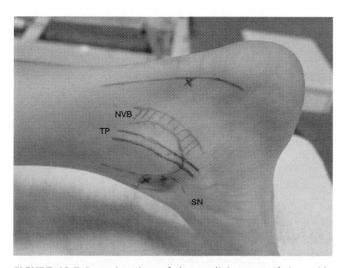

FIGURE 10.5 Posterior view of the medial aspect of the ankle with location of the posteromedial, accessory medial, and anteromedial portals. (Abbreviations as in Fig. 10.1.)

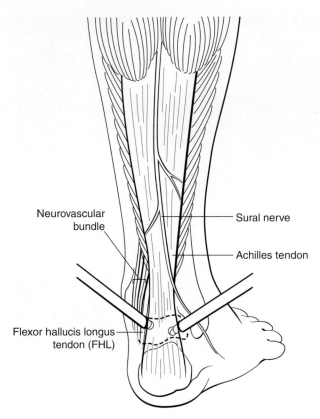

FIGURE 10.7 Diagram showing locations of the posterior portals and their relationship to neurologic structures. (Abbreviations as in Fig. 10.1.)

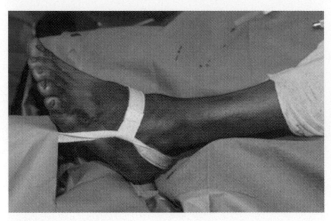

FIGURE 10.9 Noninvasive traction device used during ankle arthroscopy. (Abbreviations as in Fig. 10.1.)

scope and release of the distraction may take place, particularly to relax the capsule anteriorly. Dowdy and colleagues (12) concluded that noninvasive distraction of 30 lb for less than 60 minutes is a safe setup to avoid injury to the nerves crossing the ankle joint (Fig. 10.10).

Our preference is to begin with an anteromedial and anterolateral portal, with subsequent portals being created depending on the location of the pathology. As previously recommended by other authors (7,13), the medial and lateral portals provide better visualization of the medial and lateral structures, respectively. During surgery, the arthroscope is in general inserted opposite to the pathology, and the working instruments on the same side.

terior–posterior plane and a concavity in the medial–lateral plane. This particular morphology, as well as the inherent stability of the ankle joint, makes access to it more challenging than for some other joints.

The methodology and technique described in this chapter are performed with a 2.7-mm arthroscope and noninvasive ankle distraction (Fig. 10.9). Once the pathology has been identified and located, a change to the 4.0-mm arthro-

Anteromedial Portal

Through the anteromedial portal, the anterolateral part of the ankle joint is initially visualized. The junction of the anterior portion of the talus with the tibia superiorly and with the fibula laterally is inspected (Fig. 10.11). In this area, the intraarticular portion of the anterior inferior tibiofibular lig-

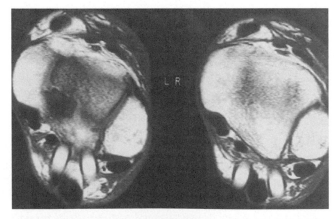

FIGURE 10.8 Magnetic resonance image of the location of the posterior portals in relation to the Achilles tendon and the neurovascular structures. (Abbreviations as in Fig. 10.1.)

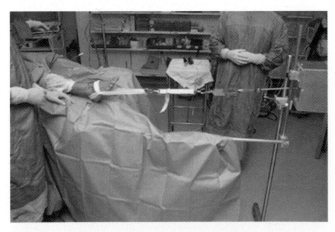

FIGURE 10.10 Setup for noninvasive traction during ankle arthroscopy. (Abbreviations as in Fig. 10.1.)

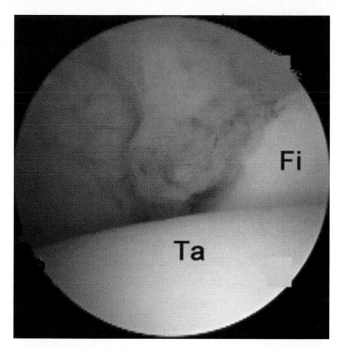

FIGURE 10.11 View of talofibular junction from anteromedial portal. (Abbreviations as in Fig. 10.1.)

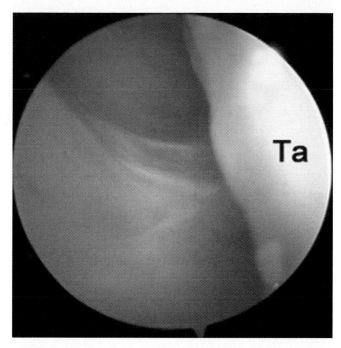

FIGURE 10.13 From anteromedial portal, insertion of anterior capsule into the talus. (Abbreviations as in Fig. 10.1.)

ament is seen (Fig, 10.12). These fibers run obliquely at 45 degrees from above the articular portion of the distal tibia. More anteriorly, the capsule inserts into the neck of the talus (Fig. 10.13). This area is difficult to assess if proper intraarticular pressure is not maintained, because the soft tissues collapse on themselves from lack of distention. More medi-

ally, the neck of the talus is inspected. Here can be visualized any anterior impingement between the neck of the talus and the anterior distal tibia. Some erosion of the dorsal aspect of the neck of the talus created by the anterior margin of the distal tibia may be noticed. Osteophytes may be present over the anterior aspect of the tibia, with the anteromedial portion the most common location. The capsule is reflected on intimate contact with the most superior portion of the osteophytes. This portion of the capsule must be peeled off before osteophyte removal.

Next, the surgeon may proceed posteriorly to assess the syndesmosis and the relationship between the tibia and fibula (Fig. 10.14). In posttraumatic cases, some impingement of soft tissues at the most superior aspect of the syndesmosis may be seen. Wolin et al. (14) described this as the meniscoid lesion of the ankle. Posterior to this level, the intraarticular portion of the posterior inferior tibiofibular ligament is also seen (Figs. 10.15 and 10.16). The most posterior aspect of the talus, the distal tibia, and the posterior capsule are visualized (Fig. 10.17). Continuing from lateral to medial, the medial half of the posterior aspect of the tibiotalar joint is also inspected and osteochondral injuries are ruled out (Fig. 10.18). Most of the posttraumatic osteochondral lesions are found between the middle and posterior thirds of the medial aspect of the dome of the talus (Fig. 10.19). The integrity of the medial wall of the body of the talus can be inspected, as can, more distally, the medial gutter (Fig. 10.20). Over the most distal portion of the gutter, the presence of loose bodies is ruled out and the status of the deepest fibers of the deltoid ligament is evaluated. Finally, moving anteriorly, the most

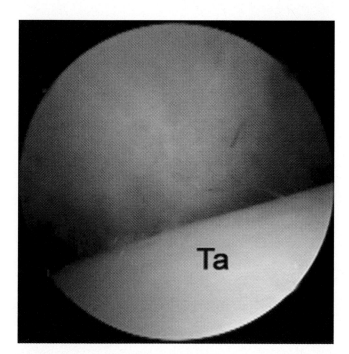

FIGURE 10.12 From anteromedial portal, view of lateral half of the talus. (Abbreviations as in Fig. 10.1.)

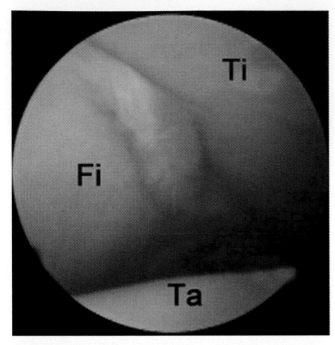

FIGURE 10.14 Intraarticular view of the syndesmosis from anteromedial portal. (Abbreviations as in Fig. 10.1.)

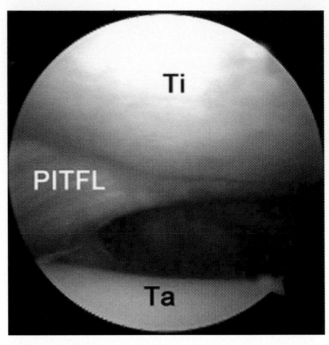

FIGURE 10.16 From anteromedial portal, posterior third of the lateral half of the ankle joint. (Abbreviations as in Fig. 10.1.)

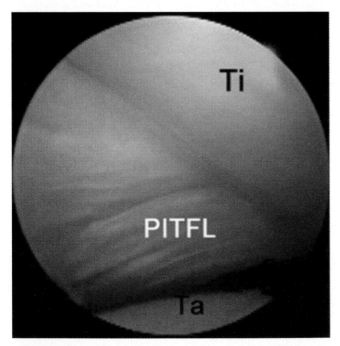

FIGURE 10.15 From anteromedial portal, view of posterior inferior tibiofibular ligament. (Abbreviations as in Fig. 10.1.)

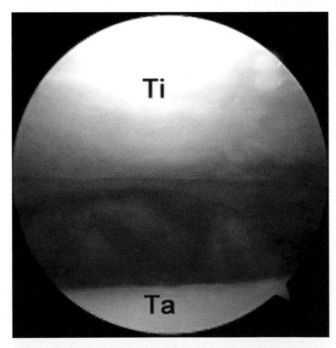

FIGURE 10.17 From anteromedial portal, posterior aspect of the ankle joint. (Abbreviations as in Fig. 10.1.)

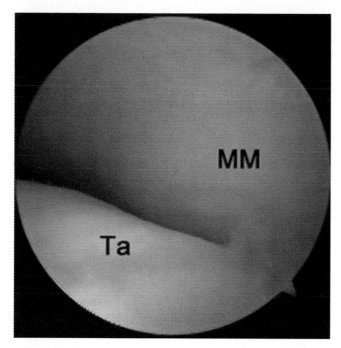

FIGURE 10.18 From anteromedial portal, medial half of the talus. (Abbreviations as in Fig. 10.1.)

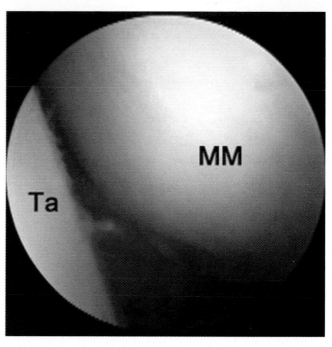

FIGURE 10.20 From anteromedial portal, most anterior aspect of medial gutter. (Abbreviations as in Fig. 10.1.)

anterior aspect of the medial malleolus may be seen. On some occasions, an anterior spur is seen in intimate relationship with the anteromedial aspect of the capsule (Fig. 10.21). As described for the anterior impingement, some kissing lesions between the talus and the medial malleolus may be seen during forced ankle dorsiflexion.

Anterolateral Portal

With the arthroscope in the anterolateral portal, the first area of inspection is the medial aspect of the tibiotalar joint. From here, similarly to the method from the anteromedial portal, the joint is inspected anteriorly, along with the most

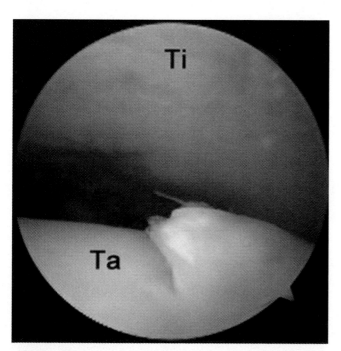

FIGURE 10.19 From anteromedial portal, view of anterior aspect of medial talus with chondral flap. (Abbreviations as in Fig. 10.1.)

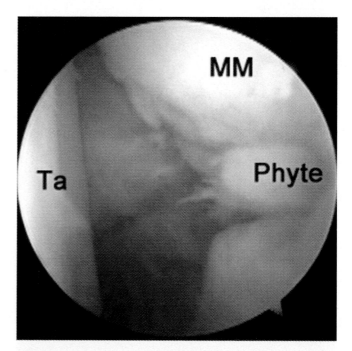

FIGURE 10.21 From anteromedial portal, most distal portion of the medial gutter with a tibial osteophyte. (Abbreviations as in Fig. 10.1.)

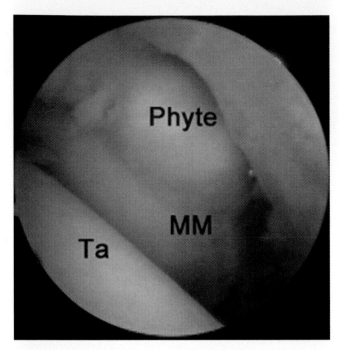

FIGURE 10.22 From anterolateral portal, medial gutter with tibial osteophyte. (Abbreviations as in Fig. 10.1.)

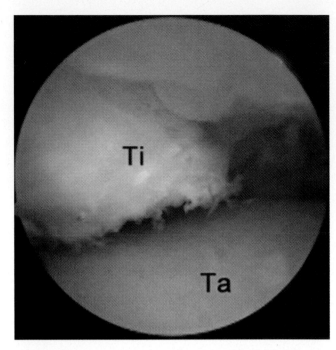

FIGURE 10.24 From anterolateral portal, medial half of the talus with tibial osteophytes. (Abbreviations as in Fig. 10.1.)

dorsal aspect of the talus and its capsular insertion. A better visualization of the anterior aspect of the medial malleolus can also be achieved. From this portal it is easier to identify the presence of spurs along the medial malleolus, as well as the amount that must be removed for adequate debridement, using the anterior cortex of the tibia as a reference point (Figs. 10. 22, 10.23, and 10.24).

As with the anteromedial portal, an inspection of the anteromedial aspect of the tibiotalar joint is carried out (Fig. 10.25). From there, evaluation of the posterior half of the articular surface of the ankle joint is possible (Fig. 10.26). Once the most posterior portion of the lateral aspect of the ankle is reached, the posterior inferior tibiofibular ligament can be identified. This ligament may be clearly visualized

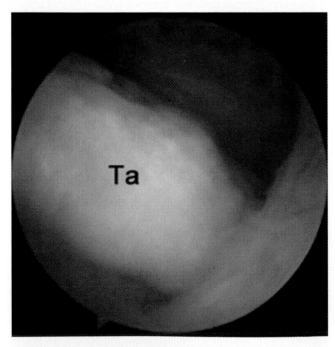

FIGURE 10.23 From anterolateral portal, medial aspect of the talus in dorsiflexion. (Abbreviations as in Fig. 10.1.)

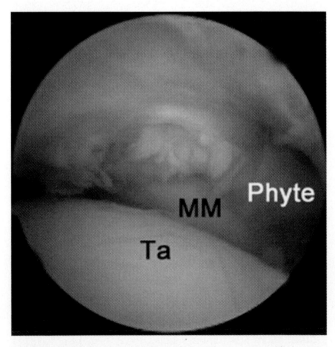

FIGURE 10.25 From anterolateral portal, posteromedial aspect of the talus. (Abbreviations as in Fig. 10.1.)

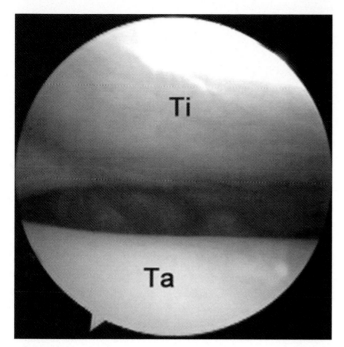

FIGURE 10.26 From anterolateral portal, posterior aspect of the ankle joint. (Abbreviations as in Fig. 10.1.)

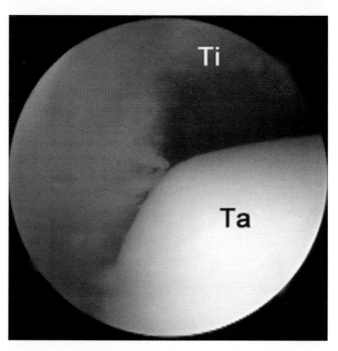

FIGURE 10.28 From anterolateral portal, lateral half of the talus. (Abbreviations as in Fig. 10.1.)

with distinct fibers running obliquely from anterior to posterior. A synovial fold may be seen which represents the intraarticular imprint of the transverse tibiofibular ligament (Fig. 10.27). Still moving anteriorly, the syndesmosis is visualized and, specifically, the most distal portion of the lateral gutter, where the presence of loose bodies or soft tissue impingement from previous trauma must be ruled out as a

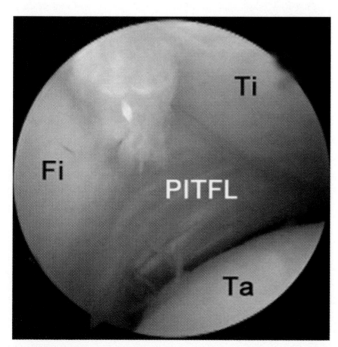

FIGURE 10.27 From anterolateral portal, posterior inferior tibiofibular ligament. (Abbreviations as in Fig. 10.1.)

source of pathology (Fig. 10.28). Finally, the most inferior fibers of the anterior inferior tibiofibular ligament are visualized as the inspection from this portal is concluded.

Accessory Anterior Portals

In certain cases, it is necessary to create accessory portals for better access to the most distal portion of the respective gutters (Fig. 10.29).

The accessory anteromedial portal provides exposure of the most distal fibers of the deltoid ligament. Its placement is approximately 1 cm anterior and distal to the medial malleolus, and still medial to the anterior tibialis tendon. As mentioned earlier, loose bodies embedded in the synovial tissue or ossicles from previous trauma may be found and removed from this portal (Fig. 10.30).

The accessory anterolateral portal allows better access with instruments to the lateral gutter. It is located at the level of the tip of the distal malleolus and 1 cm anterior to it. In addition, the anterior and posterior talofibular ligaments may be visualized from this portal, although their integrity should be evaluated from a dynamic perspective rather than during arthroscopy.

Posterolateral Portal

Via a posterolateral portal, the posterior aspect of the lateral gutter is examined and the structures previously mentioned should be visualized. This portion of the capsule does not allow a lot of mobility over this area, and it is fairly easy to be pushed away from the joint by the tight soft tissues. It usu-

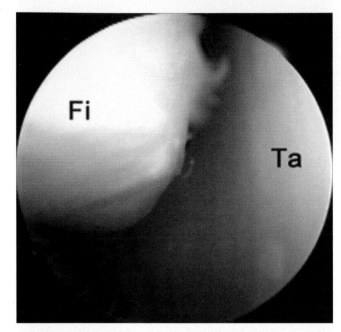

FIGURE 10.29 From anterolateral portal, most distal portion of the lateral gutter. (Abbreviations as in Fig. 10.1.)

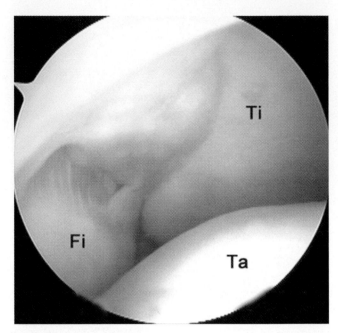

FIGURE 10.31 From posterolateral portal, posterior aspect of syndesmosis. (Abbreviations as in Fig. 10.1.)

ally is easier to enter the ankle joint below the transverse tibiofibular ligament (Fig. 10.31). These fibers are intraarticular but extrasynovial and represent the most inferior portion of the posterior inferior tibiofibular ligament. The remaining posterior lateral half of the articular surfaces for both talus and distal tibia may also be clearly visualized and treated from this approach (Fig. 10.32).

Posteromedial Portal

Several authors (6,9,15) have discouraged the use of a posteromedial portal because of an increased risk of injury to the calcaneal nerve, a branch of the tibial nerve. Sitler et al. (5) concluded that the tibial nerve and calcaneal nerve branches remain safe if this portal is approached with the patient in a prone position, and adjacent to the medial border

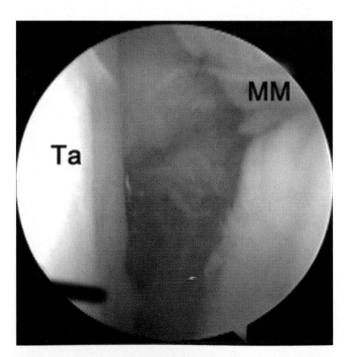

FIGURE 10.30 From accessory anteromedial portal, most distal portion of medial gutter. (Abbreviations as in Fig. 10.1.)

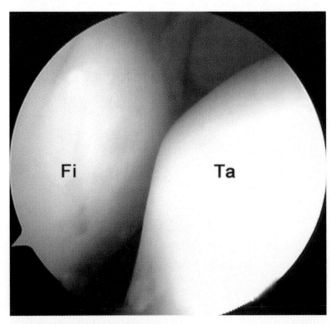

FIGURE 10.32 From posterolateral portal, posterior aspect of lateral gutter. (Abbreviations as in Fig. 10.1.)

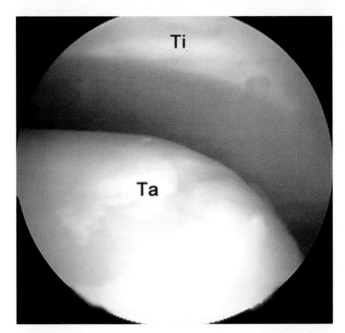

FIGURE 10.33 From posteromedial portal, flexor hallucis longus tendon at early portion of its excursion. (Abbreviations as in Fig. 10.1.)

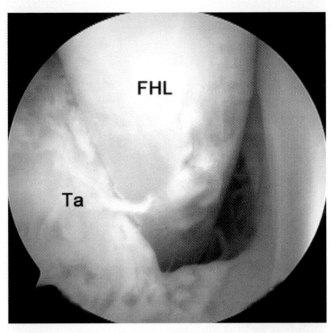

FIGURE 10.35 From posteromedial portal, flexor hallucis longus tendon at final portion of its excursion. (Abbreviations as in Fig. 10.1.)

of the Achilles tendon. We believe that a posteromedial portal may be safely used to address posterior pathology. Before getting into the ankle joint, a virtual space can be created between the posterior capsule anteriorly and the pre-Achilles bursa posteriorly. In this space, the tendon sheath for the flexor hallucis longus may be appreciated medially, as may the presence of an os trigonum (Figs. 10.33, 10.34, and

10.35). From this approach, this ossicle may be removed, although the posterior capsule must be violated during the resection, considering its intraarticular location. This portal allows evaluation of the most medial and posterior aspect of the talus and distal tibia (Fig. 10.36). Finally, the most posterior aspect of the medial gutter should be inspected to rule out the presence of loose bodies (Fig. 10.37).

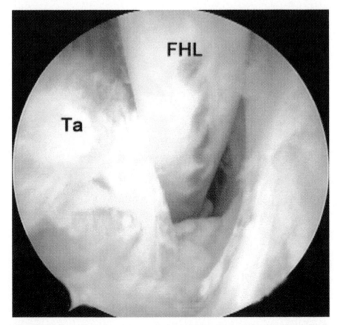

FIGURE 10.34 From posteromedial portal, flexor hallucis longus tendon at midportion of its excursion. (Abbreviations as in Fig. 10.1.)

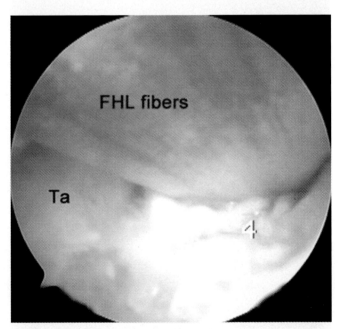

FIGURE 10.36 From posteromedial portal, posterior medial aspect of tibiotalar joint. (Abbreviations as in Fig. 10.1.)

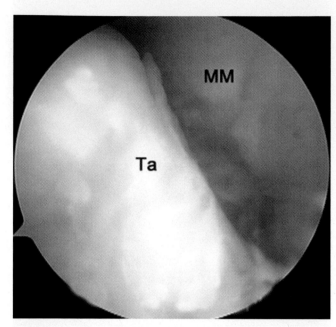

FIGURE 10.37 From posteromedial portal, posterior aspect of medial gutter. (Abbreviations as in Fig. 10.1.)

REFERENCES

1. Burman MS. Arthroscopy or the direct visualization of joints. *J Bone Joint Surg Am* 1931;13:669–695.
2. Guhl JF. *Ankle arthroscopy.* Thorofare, NJ: SLACK Inc., 1988: 1–6.
3. Ewing JW, Tasto JA, Tippett JW. Arthroscopic surgery of the ankle. *Instr Course Lect* 1995;44:325–340.
4. Ferkel RD. *Arthroscopic surgery: the foot and ankle.* Philadelphia: Lippincott-Raven, 1996:85–103.
5. Sitler DF, Amendola A, Bailey CS, et al. *Posterior ankle arthroscopy: an anatomic study.* Presented at the 68th American Academy of Orthopaedic Surgery, San Francisco, CA, 2001. *J Bone Joint Surg Am,* May 2000.
6. Feiwell LA, Frey C. Anatomic study of arthroscopic portal sites of the ankle. *Foot Ankle* 1993;14:142–147.
7. Drez D Jr, Guhl JF, Gollehon DL. Ankle arthroscopy: technique and indications. *Clin Sports Med* 1982;1:35–45.
8. Ferkel RD, Heath DD, Guhl JF. Neurological complications of ankle arthroscopy, *Arthroscopy* 1996;12:200–208.
9. Voto SJ, Ewing JW, Fleissner PR Jr, et al. Ankle arthroscopy: neurovascular and arthroscopic anatomy of standard and trans-Achilles tendon portal placement. *Arthroscopy* 1989;5:41–46.
10. Sarrafian SK. Anatomy of the foot and ankle: descriptive, topographic, functional. Philadelphia: Lippincott, 1993:356–374.
11. Horwitz MT. Normal anatomy and variations of the peripheral nerves of the leg and foot. *Arch Surg* 1938;36:626.
12. Dowdy PA, Watson BV, Amendola A, et al. Noninvasive ankle distraction: relationship between force, magnitude of distraction, and nerve conduction abnormalities. *Arthroscopy* 1996;12:64–69.
13. Carson WG, Andrews JR. Arthroscopy of the ankle. *Arthroscopy* 1987;6:503–512.
14. Wolin I, Glassman F, Sideman S. Internal derangement of talofibular components of the ankle. *Surg Gynecol Obstet* 1950; 91:193–200.
15. Stetson WB, Ferkel RD. Ankle arthroscopy: I. Technique and complications. *J Am Acad Orthop Surg* 1996;4:17–23.

THE ELBOW AND WRIST

TERRY L. WHIPPLE

ANATOMY OF THE ELBOW

The elbow joint consists of articulations among the distal humerus, the proximal ulna, and the proximal radius. Bony contours and ligaments restrict motion in the medial and lateral directions and limit motion in flexion, extension, rotation, distraction, and compression in the long axis of the arm. The tip of the olecranon, the medial epicondyle, and the lateral epicondyle are all palpable and help to form bony landmarks for surgical considerations. The flexion crease in the antecubital fossa overlies the distal humerus about 1 cm proximal to the joint space.

Bone Contours

The articular surface of the distal humerus is divided into separate and discrete surfaces. The trochlea is shaped somewhat like a spool and articulates with the proximal ulna. The olecranon fossa of the ulna rotates around the trochlea through elbow flexion and extension. The capitellum of the distal humerus lies lateral to the trochlea, and when viewed from the lateral side of the humerus it has an articular surface covering about 160 degrees of the anterior and distal humerus (1). The capitellum articulates with the head or proximal end of the radius and accommodates flexion and extension of the elbow as well as rotation of the forearm through 175 degrees of pronation and supination.

There is an anterior depression in the distal humerus proximal to the trochlea, called the coronoid fossa, into which the coronoid process of the proximal ulna inserts during elbow flexion (Fig. 11.1). Immediately opposite the coronoid fossa posteriorly is a similar depression in the distal humerus, known as the olecranon fossa, which accommodates the olecranon process of the proximal ulna in elbow extension. The coronoid and olecranon fossae are separated by a thin membrane of bone. On either side of the fossae radially and ulnarly are strong bony columns called the lateral and medial supracondylar columns, which provide strength to the distal ulna. The medial column is smaller than the lateral column; the lateral column is flat posteriorly and slightly concave anteriorly (Fig. 11.2).

The proximal radius, when viewed anteriorly, appears somewhat like a golf tee, with a slightly concave proximal end that articulates with the capitellum of the humerus. About 2 cm distal to the head of the radius on the medial side is a bony tuberosity where the strong biceps tendon attaches.

The proximal ulna, when viewed anteriorly, has a concavity on its lateral side against which the edge of the head of the radius articulates through pronation and supination (Fig. 11.3).

Elbow Ligaments

The medial and lateral collateral ligaments restrict lateral or valgus and medial or varus movement of the elbow, respectively. The medial collateral ligament consists of three separate bundles, which, when viewed from the medial side with the elbow flexed 90 degrees, form the limbs of an equilateral triangle (Fig. 11.4). The anterior bundle of the medial collateral ligament arises from the medial apophysis of the medial humeral epicondyle and inserts on the medial ridge of the proximal ulna between the flexor and extensor muscle compartments. The transverse bundle of the medial collateral ligament provides little valgus stability to the ulnohumeral joint, because it originates from the ulna on the medial margin of the olecranon process and inserts on the ulna just posterior to the insertion of the anterior bundle of the medial collateral ligament. Slightly deeper than the anterior and transverse bundles lies the posterior bundle of the medial collateral ligament, which originates from the medial humeral epicondyle and inserts on the ulna olecranon process just deep to the origin of the transverse bundle.

The lateral collateral ligament originates from the lateral epicondyle of the humerus and terminates diffusely in the annular ligament (2). The annular ligament encircles the

T. L. **Whipple:** Department of Orthopaedic Surgery, Medical College of Virginia; Director, Orthopaedics and Rehabilitation, American Self, Richmond, Virginia.

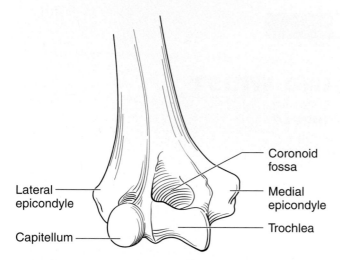

FIGURE 11.1 Anterior anatomy of the distal right humerus.

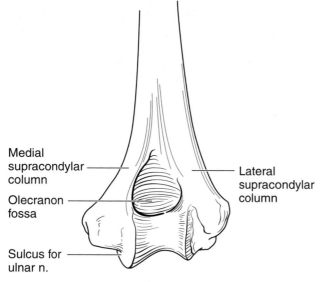

FIGURE 11.2 Posterior anatomy of the distal right humerus.

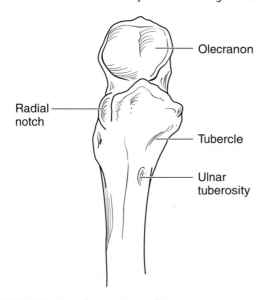

FIGURE 11.3 Anterior anatomy of the proximal right ulna.

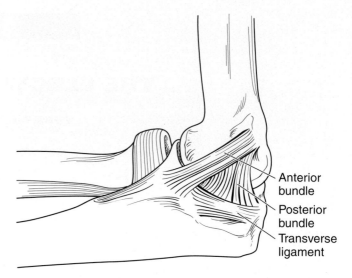

FIGURE 11.4 Medial collateral ligament of the elbow.

head and neck of the radius, originating and inserting on the lateral surface of the proximal ulna just distal to the concave facet for the radial head. A third ligament on the radial side of the elbow joint arises from the lateral humeral epicondyle and inserts on the ulna superficial to the annular ligament. This third ligament is called the lateral ulnar collateral ligament (Fig. 11.5).

Joint Capsule

The distal end of the humerus and the proximal ends of the radius and ulna articulate within a common space bounded

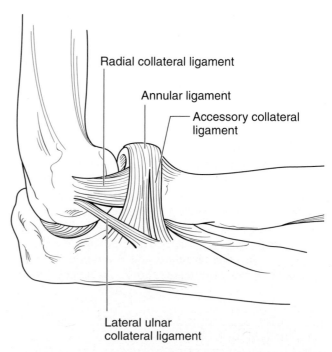

FIGURE 11.5 Lateral collateral ligament complex of the elbow.

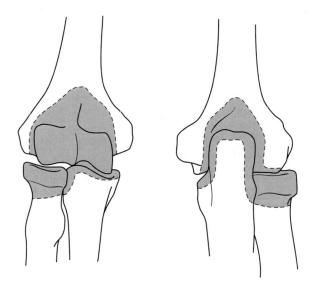

FIGURE 11.6 Attachments of the elbow capsule. **A**: Anterior. **B**: Posterior.

the flexor digitorum superficialis and the flexor digitorum profundus muscles.

Before bifurcation, the brachialis artery gives off the medial and radial collateral arteries. The radial collateral artery penetrates the lateral intermuscular septum from posterior to anterior and accompanies the radial nerve into the antecubital space. The medial collateral artery, also known as the ulnar collateral artery, penetrates the medial intramuscular septum from anterior to posterior and accompanies the ulnar nerve around the medial epicondyle and ulnar groove posteriorly. Both the radial and medial collateral arteries anastomose with the radial and ulnar recurrent arteries (3).

The ulnar artery anteriorly then gives off a common interosseous branch that subsequently bifurcates between the proximal radius and proximal ulna; the two divisions continue distally as the anterior and posterior interosseous arteries, accompanying similarly named branches of the medial and radial nerves (Fig. 11.7).

by the elbow joint capsule. The capsule is fibrous and inelastic in some regions, especially posteromedially. It is thin, flexible, and somewhat elastic in other areas to accommodate joint fluid and fibrofatty tissue movement anteriorly and posteriorly during joint motion. All of the ligament attachments lie outside the joint capsule, including the annular ligament that encircles the radial head. The joint capsule attaches to the distal humerus anteriorly along the medial and lateral columns and above the coronoid fossa. It attaches to the radius distal to the radial head and to the ulna distal to the coronoid process. Posteriorly, the elbow joint capsule attaches to the posterior surfaces of the medial and lateral columns, adjacent to the olecranon fossa of the humerus, and to the proximal ulna along the margins of insertion of the triceps tendon, leaving the entire bony olecranon process inside the intraarticular space posteriorly (Fig. 11.6).

Vascular Bundles

The superficial basilic vein anteromedially and the cephalic vein anterolaterally are the major venus conduits crossing the elbow. They lie between the skin and the muscle compartments and have numerous variable feeding channels and intercommunications in the antecubital fossa.

The deeper and more important arteries crossing the elbow require more explicit description for the arthroscopist. The brachial artery courses distally through the arm between the biceps and brachialis muscles. At the level of the radial head, the brachial artery bifurcates into the radial and ulnar arteries. The radial artery continues distally between the pronator teres muscle and the brachioradialis muscle. The ulnar artery continues distally in the forearm between

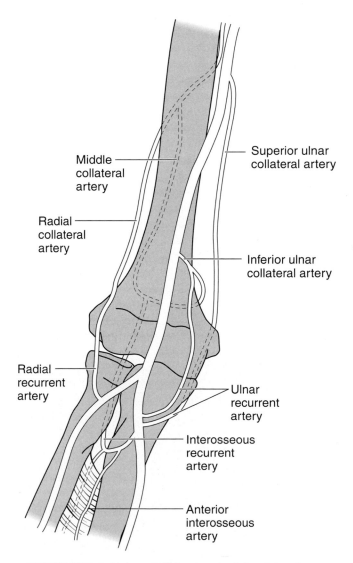

FIGURE 11.7 Anterior arterial network of the right elbow.

Nerves

It is imperative that arthroscopic surgeons know the precise locations of major motor and sensory nerve branches to avoid iatrogenic injury to these structures intraoperatively.

Three major mixed motor and sensory nerves cross the elbow: the radial, the median, and the ulnar nerves. The radial nerve consists principally of contributions from the C-6, C-7, and C-8 nerve roots continuing from the posterior cord of the brachial plexus. After penetrating the lateral intermuscular septum together with the radial collateral artery in the arm above the elbow, the radial nerve continues deep to the brachioradialis and brachialis muscles, superficial to the lateral metaphysis of the humerus (Fig. 11.8). Then, anteriorly, the radial nerve divides into superficial and deep branches (4). The superficial branch provides sensory innervation to the radial aspect of the forearm; the deep branch passes around the neck of the radius deep to the supinator muscle, which it innervates, and then continues as the posterior interosseous nerve to supply the extensor muscles on the dorsum of the forearm.

The median nerve includes fascicles from the C-5 through C-8 and T-1 nerve roots. It crosses from the lateral to the medial side of the brachial artery in the distal arm to enter the antecubital space. There it lies medial to the biceps tendon, passing beneath the bicipital aponeurosis, and gives ulnar motor branches to the pronator teres and flexor muscles of the forearm (5) (Fig. 11.8). Anteriorly, the median nerve is separated from the anterior elbow joint capsule by the interposed biceps tendon, the brachioradialis muscle, and the pronator teres muscle.

The ulnar nerve arises from the C-8 and T-1 nerve roots via the medial cord of the brachial plexus. The ulnar nerve lies posterior to the intermuscular septum above the elbow and passes around the medial epicondyle of the distal humerus, resting just superficial to the medial collateral ligament. Its first motor branch in the forearm supplies the flexor carpi ulnaris muscle, and then the ulnar heads of the flexor digitorum profundus muscle.

Sensory branches of the ulnar nerve arise in the distal forearm. The main trunk of the nerve is vulnerable to elbow arthroscopic procedures posterolaterally.

Arthroscopic Landmarks

Arthroscopic portals for the elbow joint are described elsewhere in this text (Chapters 43 and 44). From an anatomic rather than a surgical consideration, medial portals to the elbow should always be placed anterior to the intermuscular septum to avoid injury to the ulnar nerve (6). Both medial and lateral portals should always be established with the elbow in approximately 90 degrees of flexion and in the coronal plane, to avoid injury to the brachial artery and the median and radial nerves. Preliminary distention of the elbow joint with an isotonic irrigating solution displaces the anterior joint capsule and overlying structures approximately 10 to 15 mm from the joint, providing further protection.

The olecranon fossa of the elbow joint is covered by the triceps tendon. The joint may be safely insulated or penetrated through the triceps tendon in the olecranon fossa without risk to the neurovascular structures.

ANATOMY OF THE WRIST

The wrist is a complex joint that provides motion in three planes to position the hand on the end of the forearm. In addition to flexion, extension, and radial and ulnar deviation, the wrist functions in concert with the elbow to allow pronation and supination of the forearm and the hand. Al-

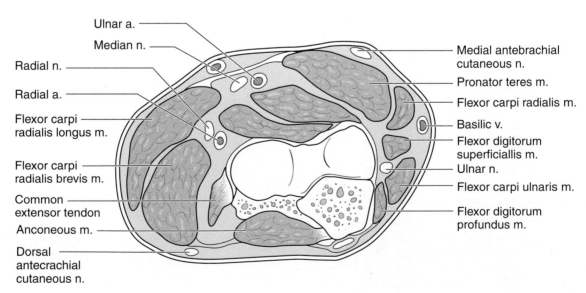

FIGURE 11.8 Cross-sectional anatomy of the elbow joint.

though most pronation and supination is a function of the elbow anatomy, there is a minor degree of pronation that occurs at the wrist together with extension and ulnar deviation, and a minor degree of supination at the wrist that occurs together with flexion and radial deviation.

Bones and Ligament

There are 15 bones that articulate at the wrist through some 27 facet surfaces (7).

The distal radius has a flat palmar surface and a generally convex dorsal surface. The medial side of the distal radius is concave with a facet that accommodates the head of the ulna through pronation and supination.

On its distal end, the radius has two articular facets covered with hyaline cartilage that articulate with the scaphoid and lunate bones, respectively.

The distal end of the ulna is rather blunt and articulates only with the radius around most of its circumference. The remainder of the circumference comprises the ulnar styloid process, which extends variably a couple of millimeters more distal.

Eight of the bones of the wrist, known collectively as the carpus, consist of proximal and distal rows of four bones each (Fig. 11.9). In the proximal carpal row, the scaphoid and lunate articulate with the two facets on the end of the radius. The triquetrum also articulates with the lunate and overlies

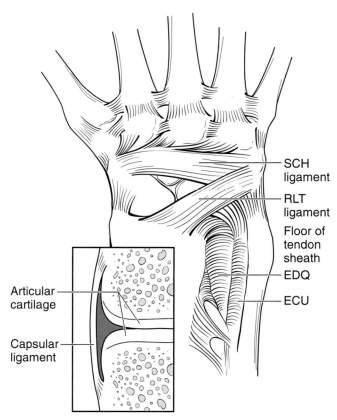

FIGURE 11.10 Dorsal extrinsic ligaments of the wrist. ECU, extensor carpi ulnaris tendon; EDQ, extensor digiti quinti tendon; RLT, radiolunotriquetral ligament; Sch, scaphocapitate–hamate ligament.

the distal end of the ulna but is separated from it by an interposed triangular fibrocartilage disk. Ulnar and volar to the triquetrum is the fourth bone of the proximal carpal row, the pisiform, which articulates only with the triquetrum and serves as the insertion for the flexor carpi ulnaris tendon.

The distal row of four carpal bones are the trapezium and the trapezoid, which articulate with the distal pole of the scaphoid proximally and the base of the first and second metacarpals distally. The capitate is the largest bone of the distal carpal row; it nestles proximally into the concave surface of the lunate. Distally, it articulates with the bases of the third and fourth metacarpals. Medial to the capitate is the hamate, which articulates proximally with the pisiform and, variably, with the distal medial corner of the lunate, and distally with the fourth and fifth metacarpals.

The carpal bones are held together by a system of dense dorsal (Fig. 11.10) and volar (Fig. 11.11) extrinsic ligaments and by a second system of thinner intrinsic ligaments (Fig. 11.9) that attach to adjacent bones in the proximal and distal carpal rows. Together, the extrinsic and intrinsic ligaments maintain the shape, integrity, and stability of the carpus.

As noted, the five metacarpals articulate with the distal carpal row and form the rays of the hand, extending to each of the five digits. The joints between the metacarpals and

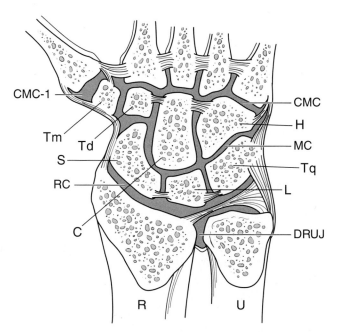

FIGURE 11.9 Graphic representation of wrist joint, and carpal anatomy. Dark areas represent separate joint compartments: the distal radioulnar joint (DRUJ), radiocarpal space (RC), and midcarpal space (MC) may communicate with the carpometacarpal (CMC) space. Note the intrinsic ligaments located between the bones of the proximal carpal row and those of the distal carpal row. C, capitate; H, hamate; L, lunate; P, pisiform; R, radius; S, scaphoid; Td, trapezoid; Tm, trapezium; Tq, triquetrum; U, ulna.

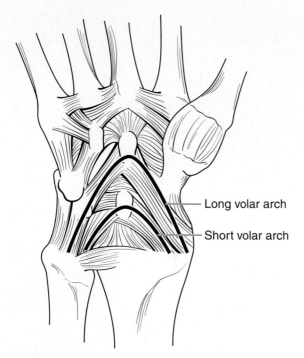

FIGURE 11.11 Volar extrinsic ligaments of the wrist. Note proximal and distal carpal arches.

the distal row of carpal bones are somewhat saddle-shaped, providing for movement in flexion, extension, and radial and ulnar deviation.

The triangular fibrocartilage complex interposed between the distal ulna and the triquetrum is composed of a central wafer of cartilage and a peripheral system of ligaments (8). Viewed from a distal point, the triangular fibrocartilage attaches to the convex medial edge of the radius and to the base of the ulnar styloid (Fig. 11.12). The volar and dorsal margins of this disk constitute strong ligaments that contribute largely to the stability of the distal radioulnar joint. These ligaments respectively blend with the volar

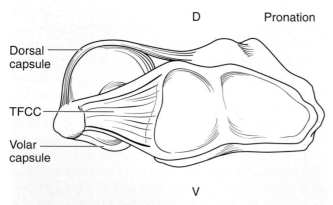

FIGURE 11.12 Graphic representation of the articular surface of the distal radius and triangular fibrocartilage complex (TFCC). Note the thickened dorsal and volar margins of the TFCC, which stabilize the distal radioulnar joint.

and the dorsal ulnocarpal ligaments extending from the ulna to the carpal bones.

There are three articular spaces in the wrist (Fig. 11.9). The triangular fibrocartilage complex separates the distal radioulnar joint from the radiocarpal space. The intrinsic ligaments of the proximal carpal row separate the radiocarpal space from the midcarpal space.

Capsule

The volar and dorsal capsules of the wrist joint are composed of discrete ligaments and looser condensations of fibrous tissue between the ligaments. Together they connect the carpus to the radius and ulna and limit distractibility of the wrist.

Dorsally, the principal ligament structures originate from the dorsal margin of the radius. Two principal bands course distally and ulnarward to insert on the dorsal rim of the scaphoid and lunate bones and into the dorsal rim of the lunate and triquetrum bones, respectively (Fig. 11.10).

The volar joint capsule is composed of an arch of ligament condensations inserting distally on the volar surface of the body of the capitate. The radial bundle extends proximally across the waist of the scaphoid as it arises from the volar margin of the radius and the radial styloid process. The ulnar arm courses proximally with insertions on the triquetrum and continues to its origin on the volar edge of the ulna as the ulnotriquetral ligament (Fig. 11.11).

Viewed arthroscopically, the volar radiocarpal ligaments can be identified standing in relief from the volar capsule. From the radial or lateral side of the wrist they can be seen as the radioscaphocapitate ligament, the radiolunotriquetral ligament, the ulnolunate ligament, and the ulnotriquetral ligament.

The membranous intrinsic ligaments extend from the dorsal capsule to the volar capsule in the coronal plane. Viewed arthroscopically in the radial carpal space, the intrinsic ligaments of the proximate carpal row are seen as concave continuations of the otherwise convex articular surfaces between the radius and the lunate, and between the lunate and the triquetrum.

In the midcarpal space, none of the intrinsic ligaments is visible (Fig. 11.9). There are open cleavages proximally between the scaphoid and lunate and between the lunate and triquetrum. Distally, there is an open cleavage plane between the trapezium and trapezoid, between the trapezoid and capitate, and between the capitate and hamate. The intrinsic ligaments in the distal carpal row are located at the middle and distal levels of these respective carpal bones.

Veins

The volar and distal superficial venous complexes are extremely variable in location and configuration. From an arthroscopic surgical perspective, they should be avoided by spreading the subcutaneous tissue with the tip of a hemostat when establishing a portal. The veins are so redundant that, even if one is inadvertently injured, there will be no significant consequence to the circulation.

Arteries

There are two major arteries that cross the wrist and should be protected from injury during arthroscopic surgical procedures. The radial artery crosses the volar surface of the radial styloid lateral to the flexor carpi radialis tendon. It then courses distally and dorsally beneath the abductor pollicis and the extensor pollicis brevis tendons, comprising the first extensor compartment, to enter the anatomic snuff box in the space between the first and second extensor compartments. The artery then continues distally and dorsally, crossing the base of the first metacarpal as the princeps pollicis artery. Because the artery lies in the volar aspect of the anatomic snuff box, identifying the snuff box by palpation and limiting arthroscopic portals to the dorsal aspect of the snuff box help protect the radial artery from surgical injury.

The ulnar artery crosses the volar aspect of the distal ulna lateral to the flexor carpi ulnaris tendon and alongside the ulnar nerve. All arthroscopic portals should be kept ulnar and dorsal to the flexor carpi ulnaris tendon to avoid surgical injury to the ulnar artery and ulnar nerve.

Nerves

The two mixed motor and sensory nerves that cross the wrist are the ulnar and median nerves. Both are fairly superficial structures on the volar surface of the wrist and should be in no jeopardy from arthroscopic procedures. The ulnar nerve courses parallel to the ulnar artery volar and medial to the flexor carpi ulnaris tendon. The median nerve courses medial to the palmaris longus tendon and is separated from the volar capsule of the wrist by the pronator quadratus muscle, the flexor digitorum profundus, and the flexor digitorum superficialis tendons.

The radial nerve contains no motor fibers at the level of the wrist. Its three sensory branches originate variably 1 to 5 cm proximal to the tip of the radial styloid, supplying sensation to the dorsal radial aspect of the hand and the dorsal aspect of the thumb, index, and long fingers. Because the origins of these three cutaneous branches are variable, they should be protected by spreading the subcutaneous tissue underlying portals with the tip of a hemostat, as described for protection of the veins.

Tendons

For arthroscopic considerations, knowledge of the anatomy of the extensor tendons at the wrist is imperative. Because all

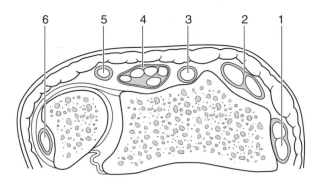

FIGURE 11.13 Graphic representation of the extensor tendon compartments.

arthroscopic portals are placed dorsal to the flexor carpi radialis and the flexor carpi ulnaris tendons, flexor tendons are of little concern.

The extensor tendons travel alone or in groups separated into six compartments, from lateral or radial to medial or ulnar (Fig. 11.13). The first extensor compartment defines the volar margin of the anatomic snuff box. It contains the abductor pollicis longus and the extensor pollicis brevis tendons.

The second extensor compartment contains the extensor carpi radialis longus and brevis tendons.

The third extensor compartment contains the extensor pollicis longus tendon alone.

The fourth compartment contains the extensor indicis proprius tendon and the extensor digitorum communis tendons. The contents of the fourth extensor compartment may be seen arthroscopically when the wall of a dorsal ganglion is resected to deflate the cyst.

The fifth extensor compartment contains the extensor digiti quinti tendon.

The extensor carpi ulnaris tendon traverses the sixth extensor compartment.

Arthroscopic portals to the radiocarpal space have been identified by a convention using the numbers of the extensor compartments between which the portals lie (9). The 3–4 portal is the principal arthroscopic portal to the radiocarpal space. Accessory portals include the 4–5 portal, the 1–2 portal, and the 6R and 6U portals, to the radial and ulnar sides of the extensor carpi ulnaris tendon, respectively.

Distraction

The articular spaces of the wrist are relatively small and confined. They cannot be adequately expanded by fluid distention as can the knee, shoulder, and elbow. Rather, the articular surfaces must be distracted from one another mechanically by applying soft finger traps to the index and long fingers through a mechanical distraction apparatus

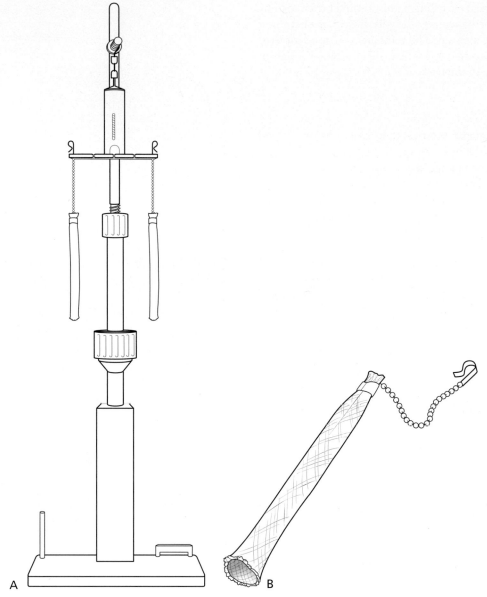

FIGURE 11.14 A and **B**: Wrist arthroscopy traction tower and nylon finger trap. (Courtesy of Linvatec, Largo, FL.)

(Fig. 11.14). Mechanical distraction approximately equal to the weight of the upper extremity (8 to 10 lb) will distract the radiocarpal spaces 3 to 4 mm, allowing sufficient room to use small-diameter surgical instruments.

Topographic Landmarks

On most wrists, certain structures can be identified by palpation and marked with indelible ink before the surgical examination is initiated. This is not always possible after fluid extravasation from the joint has caused dorsal synovial and subcutaneous swelling and obscured the landmarks.

After palpation, the bony contours can be sketched to resemble a posteroanterior radiograph of the wrist, identifying the distal radius and distal ulna contours and the base of the second and third metacarpals.

Then the tendons for the extensor pollicis longus, the extensor digitorum communis to the index and little fingers, and the extensor carpi ulnaris can be marked. The midcarpal space is located halfway between the distal edge of the radius and the base of the second and third metacarpals.

Use of sterile indelible ink preserves the landmarks for reference despite spillage of irrigation fluid and palpation with surgical gloves.

REFERENCES

1. Kapandji IA. *The physiology of joints. Vol. I: upper limb,* 2nd ed. Baltimore: Williams & Wilkins, 1970.
2. Basmajian JV. The unsung virtues of ligaments. Surg Clin North Am 1974;54:1259–1267.
3. Morrey BF, ed. *The elbow, and its disorders.* Philadelphia: WB Saunders, 1985.
4. Langman J, Woerdeman NW. *Atlas of medical anatomy.* Philadelphia: WB Saunders, 1976.
5. Anson BJ, McVay CB. Surgical anatomy, 5th ed., vol 2. Philadelphia: WB Saunders, 1971.
6. Eycleshymer AC, Schoemaker DM. A cross section anatomy. New York: D Appleton, 1930.
7. Whipple TL. *Arthroscopic surgery: the wrist.* Philadelphia: Lippincott, 1992.
8. Whipple TL, Geissler WB. Arthroscopic management of wrist triangular fibrocartilage complex injuries in the athlete. *Orthopaedics* 1993;16:1061–1067.
9. Whipple TL, Mirotta JJ, Powell JH III. Techniques of wrist arthroscopy. *Arthroscopy* 1986;2:244–252.

Operative Arthroscopy, third edition. Edited by John B. McGinty, Stephen S. Burkhart, Robert W. Jackson, Donald H. Johnson, and John C. Richmond. Lippincott Williams & Wilkins © 2003.

THE KNEE

12

ARTHROSCOPY OF THE KNEE: BASIC SETUP AND TECHNIQUE

W. HOWARD WU
JOHN C. RICHMOND

BASIC TECHNIQUE OF KNEE ARTHROSCOPY

Advances in instrumentation and technique during the twentieth century, particularly in the last two decades, have facilitated the surging interest in both diagnostic and therapeutic knee arthroscopy. Currently, knee arthroscopy is a well-accepted surgical technique and is among the most commonly performed procedures in orthopaedic surgery. This chapter describes the basic technique of knee arthroscopy, with the knowledge that there is no single "best" technique. The approach follows the tenet that must be adhered to for all arthroscopic techniques: they must demonstrate and allow treatment of intraarticular structures thoroughly, reliably, and without unnecessary trauma to the joint.

ANESTHESIA

The choice of general, regional, or local anesthesia depends on the patient, the anesthesia staff, and the operating surgeon. A brief overview is presented here, and detailed descriptions of the techniques are covered in a separate chapter.

General Anesthesia

New developments and anesthetic agents have made general anesthesia easier and safer. Use of general anesthesia in day-surgery cases such as knee arthroscopy has become commonplace as the incidence of side effects such as nausea and prolonged sedation has decreased. The procedure is reliable and allows complete relaxation of the patient. A tourniquet may be inflated, the leg fully manipulated, and any unforeseen incisions made without altering the anesthetic technique. It is especially useful in very young or very anxious patients. Disadvantages of general anesthesia are that more anesthetic agents are necessary, along with their side effects, and the small but finite risk inherent for anyone undergoing general anesthesia.

Regional Anesthesia

The preferred regional anesthetic technique in knee arthroscopy is single-injection spinal anesthesia. This method allows for an awake patient (if desired); a tourniquet can be applied and inflated, and the leg can be fully manipulated. With a skilled anesthesia team, it is usually a safe and effective choice. Disadvantages of this technique include the possibility of a difficult spinal puncture and spinal headache, although with the use of newer, smaller spinal needles, the incidence of this problem has fallen to approximately 1% for orthopaedic patients in general (1).

Local Anesthesia with Monitored Anesthesia Care

Knee arthroscopy under local anesthesia is best performed with monitoring and sedation when needed by the anesthesia department. This technique requires an experienced surgeon and an anesthesia team that is ready to convert to an alternative form of anesthesia in the event of patient discomfort. This method also limits use of a tourniquet, and forceful manipulation of the extremity may not be well tolerated by the patient. In addition, extraarticular pathologies are difficult to address, should they become evident during the procedure. Despite the obvious limitations, local anesthesia with monitored anesthesia care (MAC) is widely used for many routine arthroscopic knee procedures. Patients welcome the fact that only local anesthetic agents are required, and they generally recover with ease. The technique is also very useful in the setting of outpatient surgery centers.

W. H. Wu and J. C. Richmond: New England Medical Center, Tufts University School of Medicine, Boston, Massachusetts.

We find the technique to work best when the initial intraarticular injection is performed at least 15 minutes before instrumentation of the joint. We do this with sterile technique in the preoperative area under light sedation. Fifty to 60 mL of 1/4% bupivacaine with epinephrine is injected intraarticularly, which fixes to the synovium in the time before lavage of the joint through the arthroscope. This usually provides both adequate anesthesia of the synovium and constriction of the synovial blood vessels, so that a tourniquet is not needed. The portal sites can then be injected in the operating room. We prefer to use 1% lidocaine with epinephrine for both rapid onset and hemostatic properties.

PERIOPERATIVE ENVIRONMENT

Arthroscopy of the knee is typically performed in a general hospital surgical suite, an outpatient ambulatory surgical facility, or an office operatorium. In any setting, an established protocol to ensure the proper environment to perform the arthroscopy is essential. A surgical room with adequate space is required because of the large and bulky arthroscopic equipment. Nursing and ancillary staff should be properly trained, because a large array of specialized instruments are needed for arthroscopic surgery. The following are suggested guidelines for the proper setup for arthroscopic surgery of the knee. Although this is not the only method of performing knee arthroscopy, we have found that following this protocol carefully has led to a standard routine that is successful time after time.

Table Setup

A standard operative table with functional adjustment controls should be used. The patient is placed with his or her feet just reaching the end of the table. An unusually short or tall patient may need adjustments on the operative table. A leg holder or a lateral post is an extremely valuable piece of equipment that allows for adequate manipulation of the knee. A leg holder should be placed high on the thigh and snug, although not so overly tight as to cause a venous tourniquet. It should also be well padded to lessen the risks of pressure injury during the manipulation portion of the procedure.

Tourniquet

Use of a tourniquet is based on surgeon preference. We prefer to set up the tourniquet beforehand in every case, but we reserve routine inflation for those situations in which bleeding is typically problematic, such as total synovectomy. If unexpected bleeding is encountered during a routine procedure, then inflation of the tourniquet may be employed if increasing inflow pressure fails to maintain adequate visibil-

ity. Several points should be made regarding the use of tourniquets:

1. A pressure of 300 mm Hg appears to be safe in the lower extremity.
2. A wide tourniquet should be used with padding, to avoid direct damage in the zone of compression beneath the tourniquet.
3. Use of a tourniquet may induce quadriceps inhibition, complicating rehabilitation. It was found that 71% of patients undergoing routine meniscectomy with the use of a tourniquet still had electromyocardiographic (EMG) abnormalities after 6 weeks (2). Further increase in tourniquet time appears to cause increasing quadriceps inhibition, particularly with times exceeding 60 minutes (3,4).
4. The need for a tourniquet is less with high-pressure irrigation systems

Prophylactic Antibiotics

Single-dose prophylactic antibiotics are generally recommended for patients undergoing routine knee arthroscopy. Although the reported infection rate after knee arthroscopy is small (0.01% to 0.23%), full attention should be paid to stringent sterile techniques (5). In routine cases, it is preferable to administer the antibiotics 20 to 30 minutes before incision, often in the preoperative "holding area" (6). If a tourniquet is to be used, adequate time must be allowed for antibiotic circulation before inflation of the cuff.

The choice of an appropriate antibiotic depends on the intended organism, the coverage spectrum, and the patient's biologic constraints and tolerance. In most cases, broad-spectrum coverage, including staphyloccocal and streptococcal species, is recommended (7).

Surgeon Setup

The surgical team should scrub as they would for any other operative procedure. Impervious operating gowns and waterproof boots or shoe covers are preferred. The patient's extremity should be prepared with the same routine that is employed for open surgical procedures. Commercially prepared and specially designed arthroscopic draping material is preferred, because it has a reinforced, waterproof surface with fluid pouch. A surgical assistant is often needed to facilitate the operation, especially if more than two portals and frequent manipulations of the leg are required. Given the complex nature of arthroscopic instrumentation, it is prudent to review and request all required instruments before the start of the case.

Instrumentation

The nature of arthroscopic surgery necessitates a large array of instruments. These include the video system complete with arthroscope, camera, monitor, light source, and printer. A motorized shaving system and a cauterizing system are required. A large variety of arthroscopic hand instruments are commercially available. Finally, an irrigation-pump setup is indispensable. The surgeon should be familiar with the proper use of these instruments.

DIAGNOSTIC ARTHROSCOPY

All arthroscopic procedures of the knee should begin with a formalized diagnostic examination. Careful inspection of the entire joint in a systematic manner decreases the possibility of missed pathology. It may also bring to light any previously unsuspected lesion.

Standard Portals

Most routine knee arthroscopies can be performed with two portals: anterolateral and anteromedial (Fig. 12.1). In certain irrigation systems, a third portal (superomedial or superolateral) may be required for fluid flow. The incision for the anterolateral portal is made just off the lateral border of the patellar tendon at the level approximately 1 cm superior to the joint line. The most frequent use of the anterolateral portal is for placement of the arthroscope. It should be introduced into the joint with the use of a blunt obturator locked in the sheath and directed toward the intercondylar notch with the knee flexed to approximately 45 degrees. The obturator is then replaced with the 30-degree arthroscope to begin the diagnostic arthroscopy. The anteromedial portal is located just medial to the patellar tendon at the

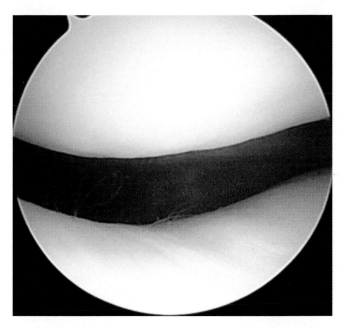

FIGURE 12.2 Patellofemoral joint. The patella is seen on top, and the trochlea on the bottom of the image.

level approximately 5 mm superior to the joint line. This portal is typically known as the "working portal," and it is most frequently used for placement of arthroscopic instruments. Care must be taken to avoid cutting the meniscus when creating these portals.

Patellofemoral Compartment

The patellofemoral compartment is readily in view when the arthroscope is placed beneath the patella while the knee is in extension (Fig. 12.2). The undersurface of the patella and its facets, as well as the femoral trochlear surface, are carefully inspected for defects by directing the arthroscope medially and laterally. A probe or blunt obturator inserted through the anteromedial portal can be used to palpate the articular surface. The superior portion of the patella may be better seen by manual compression of the patella from the skin surface to bring it into view. The suprapatella pouch should be viewed to assess for any loose bodies or signs of synovitis. There may be bands of adhesions in this compartment, particularly with a history of previous surgery. Assessment of patella mechanics may be made from the standard anterolateral portal, but it is probably better to use one of the superior portals if there is a question concerning patellofemoral alignment.

Lateral Gutter

The lateral gutter can be entered starting from the suprapatella pouch by sliding the arthroscope past the flare of the lateral femoral condyle with the knee in extension. Applying valgus stress to the joint to relax the iliotibial band allows

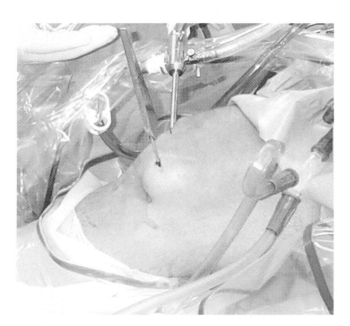

FIGURE 12.1 Standard setup for diagnostic and surgical arthroscopy of the knee. The arthroscope is in the anterolateral portal, with the probe in the anteromedial portal.

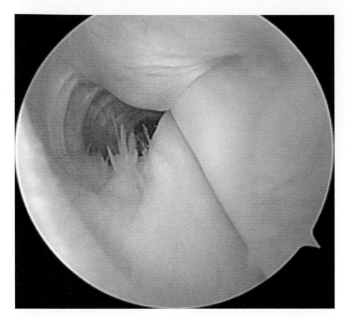

FIGURE 12.3 Posterolateral gutter and popliteal hiatus: a portion of the lateral meniscus can be seen beneath the lateral femoral condyle.

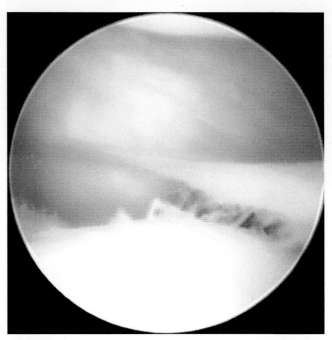

FIGURE 12.4 The mediopatella plica is commonly found and is asymptomatic in most people.

more space to maneuver. With the 30-degree arthroscope directed posteriorly, the posterolateral corner of the joint may be examined. The popliteal tendon should be identified between the lateral wall of the knee and the lateral meniscus (Fig. 12.3). If the incision is placed correctly, the arthroscope can be passed down the popliteal hiatus in front of the tendon, so that the tip lies just below the lateral meniscus. A defect may be seen in the meniscosynovial junction which is a normal variant. Care must be taken to look for loose bodies that may have settled in the lateral gutter or popliteal hiatus.

Medial Gutter

After completion of the inspection of the lateral gutter, the arthroscope is passed back to the patellofemoral compartment and moved medially over the flare of the medial femoral condyle to the medial gutter. Again, loose bodies should be sought. There frequently exists a shelf of redundant synovial fold extending medially from the superomedial portion of the patellofemoral joint in front of the medial femoral condyle (Fig. 12.4). Occasionally this plica is inflamed and requires resection.

Medial Compartment

The medial compartment may be entered from the medial gutter by following the medial edge of the medial femoral condyle down to the meniscosynovial junction and into the compartment. Valgus stress and slight knee flexion allow adequate visualization. The entire medial meniscus must be carefully inspected. The anterior horn is seen immediately

below the arthroscope, and the body of the meniscus is seen with its intimate relation to the medial capsule. With rotation of the 30-degree arthroscope so that it is directed posteriorly, the posterior horn of the medial meniscus should come into view (Fig. 12.5). The examination of the meniscus requires a probe for palpation. Care must be taken to reach all portions of the meniscus, especially the posterior horn, because visualization may be somewhat limited, particularly in "tight" knees. Careful palpation may reveal an

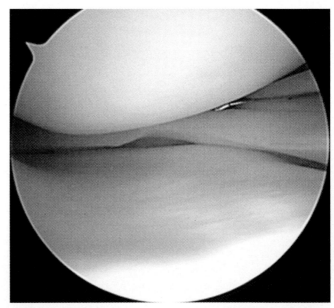

FIGURE 12.5 Medial compartment. The medial meniscus (with probing hook) is seen between the medial femoral condyle and medial tibial plateau.

otherwise obscured meniscal tear. Systematic inspection and palpation of the articular surfaces is also performed. The tibial surface should be carefully examined, including areas beneath the medial meniscus. The entire medial femoral condylar surface is then fully inspected for defects by flexing and extending the knee.

Intercondylar Notch

The intercondylar notch is the next compartment examined after the medial compartment. It contains the anterior cruciate ligament (ACL), the posterior cruciate ligament (PCL), the ligamentum mucosum (infrapatellar fold), and the entry to the posteromedial and posterolateral compartments. Care should be taken to limit any fluid flow into the fat pad overlying the intercondylar notch, which would block adequate view of the notch. The ACL is carefully examined from its origin on the lateral femoral condyle to its tibial insertion (Fig. 12.6). The proximal portion of the PCL is visible and should be carefully inspected as well. The overlying ligamentum mucosum may occasionally obstruct the view of the ACL or restrict movement of the arthroscope across the intercondylar notch. In this case, simply withdraw the arthroscope slightly while maintaining the tip in the joint, then swing the tip of the arthroscope over the ligamentum in order to redirect it to the lateral side of the ligamentum.

Lateral Compartment

To facilitate entry into the lateral compartment from the intercondylar notch, the arthroscopic probe is first parked just

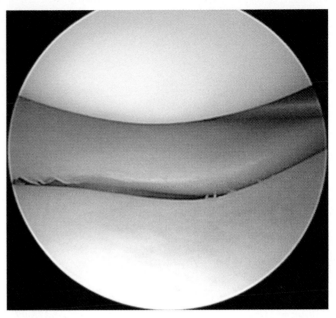

FIGURE 12.7 Lateral compartment. The lateral meniscus is seen between the lateral femoral condyle and lateral tibial plateau. The probing hook is visible to the right.

lateral to the ACL, at the junction of the lateral compartment. Next, the knee is placed into a figure-of-four configuration while the tip of the arthroscope is maintained in the intercondylar notch. With adequate varus stress applied and the lateral compartment open, the arthroscope is passed laterally into the compartment. With direction of the 30-degree arthroscope posteriorly, the posterior horn of the lateral meniscus is easily seen (Fig. 12.7). The popliteal hiatus with the popliteal tendon passing through it can usually be visualized. The arthroscope is then rotated to fully view the body and anterior horn of the lateral meniscus. At this point, the probe can easily be moved laterally and is used to palpate the meniscus and to carefully inspect for inconspicuous tears. As in the medial compartment, the lateral tibial and femoral articular surfaces must be systematically inspected as well.

Posterior Compartments

The posteromedial compartment should be entered if there is any suspicion of pathology. This includes symptoms arising from the medial compartment, loose bodies, and nonspecific mechanical symptoms. A peripheral posterior horn medial meniscus tear at the meniscosynovial junction can also be visualized posteromedially. The posteromedial compartment can be entered from the anterolateral portal in most patients by flexing the knee to approximately 90 degrees. This is most easily accomplished by elevating the operating table and simply letting the knee dangle off the side. The arthroscope is positioned in the space between the ACL and the medial femoral condyle and is then pushed gently and steadily past the ACL and into the posteromedial com-

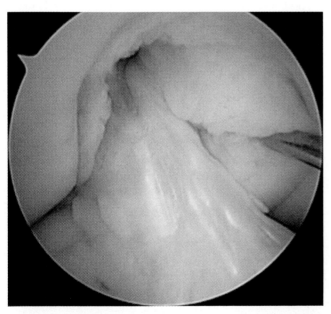

FIGURE 12.6 Intercondylar notch. Anterior cruciate ligament is seen in the center of the field. With retraction of the synovial fold by the probing hook, the proximal portion of the posterior cruciate ligament can be seen.

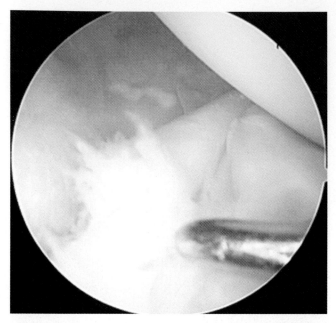

FIGURE 12.8 Posteromedial compartment. Shown to the right is the posterior portion of the medial femoral condyle. A tear of the posterior horn of the medial meniscus is seen.

partment (Fig. 12.8). This may not be possible in patients with extensive degenerative spurring. The rotation of the arthroscope should be directed downward to minimize iatrogenic injury during this maneuver. Once it is in the posteromedial compartment, movement of the arthroscope is generally limited to rotation. Visible structures include the posterior aspect of the medial femoral condyle, a portion of the posterior horn of the medial meniscus, and the posterior capsule. A 70-degree arthroscope may be exchanged to view further medially or distally, in particular the distal aspect of the PCL, although this is not routinely required.

The posterolateral compartment can similarly be entered through the space between the ACL and lateral femoral condyle while a gentle varus strain is applied. The posterior aspect of the lateral meniscus, lateral femoral condyle, and posterolateral capsule can all be inspected in this manner.

OTHER APPROACHES

Several other approaches are less frequently used in knee arthroscopy. They are described in the following paragraphs.

Posteromedial Portal

This portal is generally used for operative rather than diagnostic arthroscopy (8). The correct site of entry is identified by first entering the posteromedial compartment with the arthroscope, then transilluminating the overlying skin. A spinal needle in inserted posterior to the medial femoral condyle and into the posteromedial compartment. After satisfactory needle placement is verified, the needle is with-

drawn and a no. 11 scalpel blade is used to create the portal along the needle tract. Operating instruments or, if necessary, a cannula with a blunt trocar can be passed through this portal. The saphenous nerve is at risk with this approach.

Posterolateral Portal

This approach is not commonly used. The portal is made in a similar manner to a posteromedial portal. With the arthroscope in the posterolateral compartment and the skin of the knee transilluminated, a spinal needle, followed by a no. 11 blade, may be used. This portal must enter the skin well above the biceps tendon to avoid the peroneal nerve (9).

Central (Transpatella Tendon) Portal

This approach has the disadvantage of going through the patella tendon and the fat pad, which may result in tendon scarring. It should be placed proximally in the tendon and made sharply with the scalpel blade parallel to the tendon fibers to avoid tendon injury. This portal has the advantage of facilitating passage of the arthroscope into the posterior compartments (10,11). Although it can be used for routine diagnostic and most surgical procedures, we rarely use it, because of the risk to the patella tendon. Sometimes, when a small difference in entry point may be significant, such as in placing a screw or osteochondral graft into the articular surface, a more distal transpatella portal is needed. This should be located with a needle before the portal is established.

Suprapatella Portals

A suprapatella portal can be made medially or, more commonly, laterally. It is made above and lateral (or medial) to the patella, to enter the synovial cavity. It is useful for viewing the patellofemoral articulation as well as the fat fad and the anterior aspect of the knee joint. In certain irrigation systems, a suprapatellar portal is used for fluid flow. It bears reminding that the soft tissue in this area often does not provide a tight seal, and fluid extravasation is a common problem.

DRESSING AND POSTOPERATIVE CARE

At the conclusion of the procedure and after suction removal of excess irrigation fluid, a long-acting local anesthetic such as bupivacaine with epinephrine may be injected into the joint, unless otherwise contraindicated. This facilitates adequate pain control for the patient (12). Wound closure may be accomplished by a single buried absorbable suture or a simple nonabsorbable suture. Some surgeons choose to close only with a Steri-Strip or to leave the portal sites unclosed. A sterile dressing and a light but absorbent pad are applied, followed by a compressive wrap. Cryotherapy devices may also be of benefit to reduce postoperative pain and swelling (13,14). Before discharge, patients are instructed in the basic techniques of using crutches and exercises, according to the weight-bearing protocol dictated by the procedure performed. Finally, in routine cases, we have the patient remove the dressings and perform usual hygienic care to the knee in 48 hours.

REFERENCES

1. Puolakka R, Haasio J, Pitkanen MT, et al. Technical aspects and postoperative sequelae of spinal and epidural anesthesia: a prospective study of 3230 orthopedic patients. *Reg Anesth Pain Med* 2000;25:488–497.
2. Dobner JJ, Nitz AJ. Postmeniscectomy tourniquet palsy and functional sequelae. *Am J Sports Med* 1982;10:211–214.
3. Saunders KC, Louis DL, Weingarden SI, et al. Effect of tourniquet time on postoperative quadriceps function. *Clin Orthop* 1979;9:194–199.
4. Thorblad J, Ekstrand J, Hamberg P, et al. Muscle rehabilitation after arthroscopic meniscectomy with or without tourniquet control: a preliminary randomized study. *Am J Sports Med* 1985;13:133–135.
5. Keiser CH. A review of the complications of knee surgery. *Arthroscopy* 1992;8:79–83.
6. Boyd RJ, Burke JF, Colton T. A double-blind clinical trial of prophylactic antibiotics in hip fractures. *J Bone Joint Surg Am* 1973;55:1251–1258.
7. McEniry DW, Gorbach SL. Cephalosporins in surgery: prophylaxis and therapy. *Drugs* 1987;34:216–239.
8. Gold DL, Schaner DJ, Sapega AA. The posteromedial portal in knee arthroscopy: an analysis of diagnostic and surgical utility. *Arthroscopy* 1995;11.139–145.
9. Bennett WF, Sisto D. Arthroscopic lateral portals revisited: a cadaveric study of safe zones. *Am J Orthop* 1995;24:546–551.
10. Lindberg U, Hamberg P, Lysholm J, et al. Arthroscopic examination of the patellofemoral joint using a central, one portal technique. *Orthop Clin North Am* 1986;17:263–268.
11. Eriksson E, Sebik A. A comparison between the transpatellar tendon and the lateral approach to the knee joint during knee arthroscopy: a cadaver study. *Am J Sports Med* 1980;8:102–105.
12. Abbott PJ, Shiffrin J. Anesthesia and postoperative pain management for knee surgery. In: Fu F, ed. *Knee surgery.* New York: Lippincott Williams & Wilkins, 1994.
13. Whitelaw GP, DeMuth KA, Demos HA, et al. The use of the Cryo/Cuff versus ice and elastic wrap in the postoperative care of knee arthroscopy patients. *Am J Knee Surg* 1995;8:28–30.
14. Lessard LA, Scudds RA, Amendola A, et al. The efficacy of cryotherapy following arthroscopic knee surgery. *J Orthop Sports Phys Ther* 1997;26:14–22.

13

ARTHROSCOPIC MENISCECTOMY

PATRICK E. GREIS
ROBERT T. BURKS

Meniscus injury may cause pain and dysfunction of the knee joint requiring surgical intervention (1). Treatment options include arthroscopic meniscectomy and arthroscopic and/or open repair. Although the meniscus plays an important role in normal knee joint function, and retention of meniscus tissue is desirable, there are many circumstances in which repair of damaged tissue is not feasible and partial resection is necessary. When these circumstances arise, arthroscopic partial meniscectomy can provide relief of pain, eliminate mechanical symptoms caused by unstable meniscus fragments, and restore joint function to a more normal state. It is for this reason that arthroscopic meniscectomy has become one of the most common surgical procedures performed in many hospitals and outpatient surgical centers (2). Small et al. (3) reported that in a series of more than 10,000 arthroscopic procedures evaluated in one study of 21 surgeons, arthroscopic partial meniscectomy accounted for 35% of the total operations, and 41% of those performed on the knee joint (3).

The growth in the use of the arthroscope for the treatment of meniscus pathology was initiated by Japanese surgeons in the 1960s (4,5). In the mid-1970s, Dr. Richard L. O'Connor pioneered work that led to a marked increase in the use of the arthroscope as an operating tool in the treatment of knee pathology. During this same period, improvements in lens systems and fiber optics allowed for technical advances that made arthroscopy more practical. The clinical benefits of these techniques were quickly realized and included better visualization of the knee joint, improved diagnostic ability, decreased morbidity of surgical procedures, and improved clinical outcomes with regard to knee joint function and return to activity (6–10). For these reasons, arthroscopic treatment of meniscus pathology has replaced open techniques of treatment in most instances.

This chapter reviews pertinent information on arthroscopic meniscectomy, including surgical techniques and indications for this procedure. As technology continues to improve, new treatments for meniscus tears will surely evolve, including treatments such as gene therapy and meniscus replacement scaffolds. However, until these techniques become further advanced, arthroscopic partial meniscectomy will remain a mainstay for the treatment of meniscus tears in many circumstances.

PATHOLOGY

Meniscus tears have been demonstrated to occur with a mean annual incidence of 60 to 70 cases per 100,000 people (11,12). The male-to-female ratio has been shown to be between 2.5:1 and 4:1, probably because of the increased participation by boys and men in activities of sport. With increasing participation in sports by women, the incidence of meniscus tears in the younger female age group is sure to increase.

Studies evaluating the circumstances surrounding meniscus tears have demonstrated that more than one third of those tears that require treatment occur in association with traumatic rupture of the anterior cruciate ligament (ACL) (13). The peak incidence of meniscus tears in patients with traumatic ACL rupture was reported to be 21 to 30 years of age for men and 11 to 20 years of age for women. Degenerative tears not associated with ligamentous injury were shown to occur commonly in men during their fourth, fifth, and sixth decades of life.

In patients with an acute ACL rupture, studies have demonstrated that the lateral meniscus is more commonly torn, whereas in patients with chronic ACL-deficient knees, the medial meniscus is more commonly injured (14). These findings correlate with knowledge gained from magnetic resonance imaging (MRI) studies after an ACL ligament tear. The posterolateral tibia and anterolateral femoral condyle have a characteristic bone bruise pattern which indicates that a transient subluxation of the lateral plateau has occurred. It is during this event that injury to the lateral meniscus most likely occurs.

In the chronic ACL-deficient knee, the medial meniscus is more commonly torn, probably because of the sheer forces

P. E. Greis and R. T. Burks: University of Utah, Department of Orthopedics, Salt Lake City, Utah.

that are transmitted to the medial meniscus as it acts as a secondary restraint to anterior translation (15). Shoemaker and Markolf (16) showed that the posterior horn of the medial meniscus is the most important structure resisting anterior translation in the ACL-deficient knee (Fig. 13.1). Allen et al. (17) demonstrated that the resultant force in the medial meniscus is increased by 52% in full extension, and by 197% in 60 degrees of flexion under 134N anterior load in the ACL-deficient knee. With repetitive translation events, vertical tears within the medial meniscus are often seen, most commonly starting on the inferior surface of the posterior horn. Complete vertical tears may extend from the posterior horn anteriorly, and in certain circumstances may become displaced, creating a bucket-handle type of tear.

Meniscus tears may be classified according to the mechanism of injury or the tear pattern (18). Although both methods are useful, each classification scheme provides different information. With the first scheme, one can classify meniscus tears into two broad types: group I, tears that result from excessive force acting on what was a normal structure, and group II, tears that result from normal forces acting on an abnormal or weakened structure. In this classification scheme, meniscus tears that occur during a traumatic ACL rupture or a tibial plateau fracture fall into group I (i.e., excessive force acting on a previously normal structure). Tears that occur without a specific inciting event or with trivial trauma (e.g., squatting, bending, routine twisting) are in group II.

This distinction is important in that it may have a significant impact on treatment prognosis if meniscus salvage is being considered. In patients with group I tears, efforts at meniscus salvage could be considered even if the meniscus tear *pattern* would be less favorable for repair. Given the fact

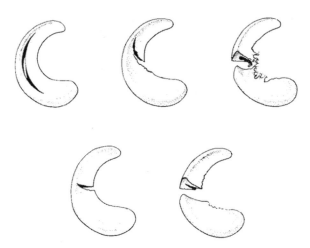

FIGURE 13.2 Classification of meniscus tears. A, vertical longitudinal; B, oblique; C, degenerative; D, transverse (radial); E, horizontal. (From Ciccotti MG, Shields CL Jr, El Attrache NS. Meniscectomy. In: Fu FH, Harner CD, Vince KG, eds. *Knee surgery,* vol 1. Philadelphia: Williams & Wilkins, 1994:591–613, with permission.)

that the involved meniscus was normal before injury, repair in this setting which "pushes the envelope" may be reasonable because of the beneficial effects that the meniscus has on joint function. With group II tears, efforts to salvage a meniscus with a repair are likely to be less successful because of the decreased intrinsic healing capacity of a weakened or degenerative structure. In these cases, partial meniscectomy may be the most appropriate treatment, even if the tear *pattern* might indicate that repair is technically possible, but with a low chance of long-term success.

The other classification scheme, which is more commonly used to describe meniscus tears, is based on tear configuration. With this classification, tear patterns commonly described include vertical longitudinal, oblique, complex (including degenerative), transverse (radial), and horizontal (Fig. 13.2). Metcalf (18) found that 80% of tears were of the vertical or oblique variety. Most of the tears that required treatment in his experience were in the medial meniscus (69%), with the lateral meniscus being involved to 24% of the time. Bilateral tears occurred in 7% of the cases, and most of the tears occurred in the posterior one half of the meniscus. With increasing age, degenerative complex tears were more commonly seen.

Of the various types, vertical longitudinal tears occur most commonly in younger individuals. As previously noted, they are commonly associated with ACL injury, and the medial meniscus is the most common site of injury.

Oblique tears tend to occur at the junction of the posterior and middle thirds of the meniscus. Mechanical symptoms of catching and pain from tension on the meniscus capsular junction may occur, because the torn edges catch between the tibia and femur. Tear propagation may also occur in this fashion.

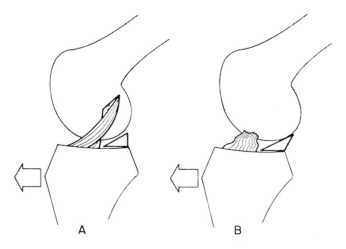

FIGURE 13.1 The posterior horn of the medial meniscus has been shown to be an important secondary restraint to anterior translation of the tibia. (From Levy IM, Torzilli PA, Warren RF. The effect of medial meniscectomy on anterior posterior motion of the knee. *J Bone Joint Surg Am* 1982;64:883–888, with permission.)

Horizontal cleavage tears begin as intrasubstance degeneration within the meniscus and then extend to the free margin of the meniscus. Extension toward the meniscus capsular junction is common, and cyst formation may cause localized swelling and pain as the tear extends along the line of the horizontally aligned middle perforating collagen bundles. Meniscus cysts are reported to represent 1% to 10% of meniscus pathology (19). They occur most commonly in the lateral meniscus. Histologic examination reveals that these cysts are often in direct continuity with the meniscus and are filled with a gel-like material that is biochemically similar to synovial fluid (20). They may cause pain due to direct pressure on the surrounding structures, and they are often palpable at or near the joint line.

Complex or degenerative tears are most commonly seen in older patients and may be associated with chondral degeneration. They are considered part of degenerative joint disease and osteoarthritis. Because of their complex pattern, free fragments can cause mechanical symptoms; however, pain associated with these types of tears is often part of a generalized inflammation that may occur with osteoarthritis. Histologically, degenerative tears exhibit myxoid degeneration, hyaline acellular degeneration, and dystrophic calcification (21). Work by Ferrer-Roca and ViLalta (21) characterized these changes along with the macroscopic findings commonly seen with degenerative meniscal pathology.

CLINICAL EVALUATION

History

The clinical evaluation of a patient with a suspected meniscus tear includes all aspects of a careful history and physical examination needed for any patient with knee pain, along with specialized tests for meniscus pathology. When taking the history, the onset of symptoms and the mechanism of injury are important factors in making the diagnosis. In isolation, meniscus tears often occur from a twisting injury or a hyperflexion event. Acute pain after injury, associated with swelling, loss of motion, and mechanical symptoms of catching, may be a clue to the diagnosis. However, in the degenerative setting, there may be an insidious onset of pain and/or swelling without a major inciting event. This is more common in older patients and may be associated with chondral injury and degeneration. In the setting of other major injury to the knee, such as an ACL tear or fracture, a high index of suspicion is required; meniscus injury is common in these settings but is more difficult to diagnose clinically because of the presence of ligament damage.

Physical Examination

Examination of the knee includes inspection, palpation, and special tests to evaluate for ligament integrity and possible signs of meniscus pathology. Inspection to assess for swelling is made, because many patients with meniscus tears have a joint effusion. Joint line swelling that is localized may be observed and may indicate a meniscus cyst. This is often more pronounced with knee flexion. Assessing range of motion to determine whether a mechanical block to flexion or extension exists is required. Palpation to assess tenderness and to feel for masses about the knee is also performed. After these generalized tests, ligament stability testing should be performed, and then specialized tests are added to aid in the diagnosis of meniscus tear. These specialized tests include joint line palpation, the flexion McMurray test (Fig. 13.3), the Apley grind test, and others. Studies examining the usefulness of these clinical tests have documented that none is perfect in the detection and diagnosis of meniscal pathology (22,23). Evans et al. (23) evaluated the flexion McMurray test to determine its reliability and accuracy. In their study, a medially based "thud" with rotation and flexion was the only McMurray sign to correlate well with meniscus tears. This finding, when present, was 98% specific for a meniscus tear; however, because it was not present in many patients with meniscus pathology, its sensitivity was only 15%. Weinstable et al. (22) found that the most useful clinical sign for a meniscus tear was joint line tenderness. This had a 74% sensitivity and a 50% positive predictive value.

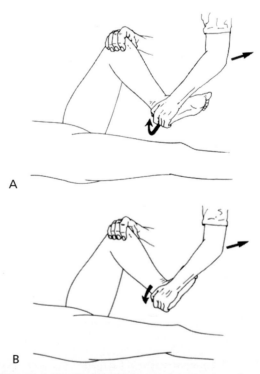

FIGURE 13.3 The flexion McMurray test may reproduce the mechanical symptoms of meniscal tear. (From McGee DJ. In: *Orthopaedic physical assessment.* Philadelphia: WB Saunders, 1992: 372–447, with permission.)

In the setting of ACL injury, the diagnosis of meniscus tear based on clinical grounds can be difficult. Shelbourne et al. (24) evaluated the finding of joint line tenderness in the setting of ACL injury and found that the accuracy was 54.9% for medial meniscus tears and 53.2% for lateral meniscus tears. They believed that variables such as associated collateral ligament damage, bone bruising, and swelling cause this physical finding to be unpredictable in the diagnosis of meniscus pathology in the setting of ACL injury.

Although clinical tests taken in isolation may have a poor reliability, and in the setting of ACL injury meniscus tear diagnosis is difficult, the clinical evaluation remains a powerful tool in the diagnosis of isolated meniscus tear. Terry et al. (25), using a complete history, physical examination, and plain radiographs, were able to accurately diagnosis meniscus pathology in the majority of patients with isolated tears. Using arthroscopic confirmation as the means of definitive diagnosis, they found that their clinical evaluation had a 95% sensitivity and 72% specificity for medial meniscal tears, and an 88% sensitivity and 92% specificity for lateral meniscus tears.

Diagnostic Studies

In addition to the history and physical examination, radiologic studies such as plain radiographs, arthrography, and MRI have been advocated as being helpful in the diagnosis of meniscus pathology (Fig. 13.4). As part of a routine orthopaedic examination, plain radiographs should be obtained to evaluate bone architecture and joint spaces. A stan-

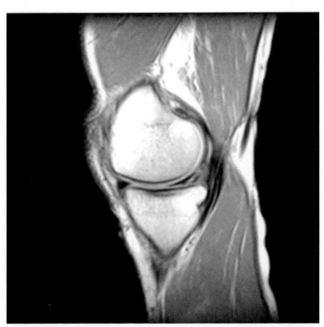

FIGURE 13.4 Magnetic resonance imaging scan of grade III change within the medial meniscus, consistent with meniscus tear.

dard series, which includes a 45-degree posteroanterior flexion weight-bearing view of both knees, a lateral view, and a Merchant's view of the patella, should be obtained. Rosenburg et al. (26) showed that the 45-degree posteroanterior weight-bearing view is more sensitive for detection of early joint space narrowing than is the standard anterior–posterior view in full extension. This is true because of the fact that osteoarthritis most commonly affects the posterior aspect of the femoral condyles early in the disease process. Unweighted x-ray studies are not as helpful. Patients with joint space narrowing are likely to have chondrosis, along with degenerative meniscal pathology, as the source of their pain.

Arthrography

Although it is mentioned for historical purposes, this imaging technique is infrequently used. MRI has replaced it as a more accurate, less invasive technique of imaging the meniscus.

Magnetic Resonance Imaging

Early studies using this technique were conducted with magnets of low field strength. During the early period of evaluation, accuracy for detecting meniscus tears was commonly reported to be 80% to 90%. This has improved as technology has allowed for the use of magnets with higher field strength and radiologists and orthopaedists have gained experience in reading scans. Accuracy is now believed to be in the middle to high 90s (27).

MRI technology continues to improve as software and hardware advancements are made. The advantages of MRI imaging in a patient with a suspected meniscus tear are its noninvasive nature, the absence of ionizing radiation, the ability to evaluate the meniscus in multiple planes, and the ability to fully evaluate the other bone, cartilage, and soft tissue structures within the joint. The limitations include the cost of the study and the potential for misinterpretation of the scan images due to technical shortcomings of the equipment or error on the part of the individual interpreting the scan.

On the MRI scan, the normal meniscus is usually a structure of uniformly low signal. Areas of increased signal that connect with the free edge of the meniscus are consistent with meniscus tearing. Areas of increased signal within the meniscus substance are found in young children, and also in adults with increasing age. These intrasubstance changes are a source of potential overreading of scans, which was a common error in early studies evaluating this technology.

Although MRI is a powerful tool in the diagnosis of meniscus tears, one should be careful to couple this information with the overall clinical picture. Positive findings from meniscus tears are common as patients age and in those with degenerative joint disease. Also, asymptomatic tears have been documented in younger age groups. In a study by LaPrade et al.(28), asymptomatic patients between 18 and 39 years of age with normal physical examinations had positive MRI scans in 5.6% of the cases. Boden et al. (28a) showed that 13% (8 of 63) of the MRI scans of asymptomatic subjects younger than 45 years of age were read as positive, and 36% (4 of 11) were positive in subjects older than 45 years of age.

Muellner et al.(27) demonstrated almost equal accuracy (94.5% versus 95.5%), sensitivity (96.6% versus 98%), and specificity (87% versus 85.5%) when MRI results were compared with clinical evaluation data in athletes with suspected meniscus pathology. In their study, the MRI scans infrequently changed the treatment plan or added to the clinical examination findings in making the diagnosis of meniscus tear.

INDICATIONS

The indications for arthroscopic meniscectomy include a consideration of two major questions: (a) Is there indication for surgical intervention? and (b) If surgical intervention is warranted, can and should meniscus repair be performed? In patients who have a meniscus tear and require surgical intervention, the answer to the second question often dictates whether a partial meniscectomy is performed. Because of the known deleterious effects of meniscectomy (29–38), efforts to enhance and expand the indications for meniscus repair have been made. The benefits of repair, when successful, include maintenance of a structure that plays a role in joint stability (15), load sharing (29–32), and shock absorption (39). These benefits, however, are not realized if the repair fails or if the repaired tissue is of poor quality or configuration and fails to function as an intact meniscus. Additionally, because repair techniques have traditionally resulted in greater perioperative morbidity, and because the rehabilitation period after repair necessitates a slower return to full activity, meniscus repair is often undertaken only if a reasonable expectation of success and benefit to the patient can be predicted.

Before setting up criteria for repair versus resection, criteria for operative intervention in patients with a suspected meniscus tear should be delineated (18). The surgical indications for arthroscopic treatment of meniscus pathology include (a) symptoms of meniscus injury that affect activities of daily living, work, and/or sports; (b) positive physical findings of joint line tenderness, joint effusion, limitation of motion, and provocative signs such as pain with squatting, a positive flexion McMurray test, or a positive Apley grind test; (c) failure to respond to nonsurgical treatment, including activity modification, medication, and a rehabilitation program; (d) absence of other causes of knee pain identified on plain radiographs or other imaging studies; and (e) presence of an unstable meniscus tear identified at the time of ligament reconstruction.

In many clinical situations not all of these criteria are present, but they should be considered before proceeding with operative treatment of meniscal pathology. In the setting of an ACL injury, the treatment of meniscus pathology is most often performed at the same time as ligament reconstruction. For this reason, surgical timing is often dictated by issues such as swelling, range of motion, quadriceps function, and other associated ligamentous injury. In rare instances, a displaced meniscus necessitates acute intervention, and surgeon preference may dictate whether concurrent ACL reconstruction is performed.

When deciding whether to repair or resect a torn meniscus, it is useful to consider the recommended criteria for meniscus repair (40). The criteria for repair include (a) a complete vertical longitudinal tear longer than 1 cm; (b) a tear within the outer one third of the meniscus (i.e., within 3 to 4 mm of the capsular rim); (c) a tear that can be displaced and is, therefore, unstable; (d) a tear in which the tissue to be repaired remains of good quality; and (e) a tear in which ligament stabilization is performed or the knee is ligamentously stable.

If these criteria are met, many would suggest that meniscus repair should be performed. If these criteria are not met and the tear requires treatment, partial meniscectomy may be required. In some situations, a tear is encountered and formal repair or resection is not required. Incomplete vertical longitudinal tears within the vascular zone that are not unstable, often less than 1 cm in length, and less than 50% of the depth of the thickness of the meniscus, as well as short complete vertical longitudinal tears smaller than 1 cm, may not require formal repair. These tears have been shown to remain asymptomatic in many situations, and they may even heal spontaneously after ligament stabilization. They may be left alone, or the technique of simple rasping and/or trephination may be used to enhance their healing potential.

Because many tears do not fall into the reparable or spontaneously healing categories, the need for partial meniscectomy remains. With the removal of unstable fragments, the clinical symptoms of locking and catching, along with the associated pain that these fragments cause, can be eliminated. In treating tears that are not suitable for repair, resection techniques should strive to remove the torn tissue and preserve stable, functioning meniscus tissue whenever possible, in an effort to minimize the deleterious effects of meniscectomy.

SURGICAL TECHNIQUE

The setup for arthroscopic meniscectomy is relatively standard, and most arthroscopic meniscus surgery can be performed on an outpatient basis. Anesthesia can be general, regional, or local, although general and regional anesthesia tend to provide better limb muscle relaxation, allowing for improved joint exposure and less risk of chondral injury.

Tourniquet use is not necessary in most cases and has been shown to have potential adverse effects that include electromyographic evidence of quadriceps muscle injury and a potential for increased risk of thrombophlebitis (41). Pump systems can now maintain a constant pressure and flow, which further obviates the need for tourniquet use. Fluid extravasation can occur with these systems, however, and one must maintain a degree of vigilance, especially with acute knee injuries in which capsular disruption may have occurred. Gravity flow into the knee for arthroscopy is safe, efficient, and inexpensive; however, it may result in suboptimal flow that does not allow for good visualization without the use of a tourniquet.

After anesthesia has been induced, the patient is usually supine on the operating room table. A leg holder or a lateral post may be used to provide a fulcrum around which pressure can be applied to gain access to the medial and lateral joints. When the patient is fully supine on a table, the figure-of-four position can be used to gain access to the lateral joint by resting the foot on the table with the knee in the flexed position. The leg holder or lateral post provides a fulcrum for valgus stress that opens the medial compartment (42).

Surgical instrumentation should include both a 30-degree and a 70-degree operating arthroscope. A 70-degree arthroscope is helpful for examining the posterior compartments of the knee and for visualizing very far anterior tears. Additionally, instrumentation such as manual resector forceps and a motorized shaver should be available. These are common instruments for all meniscectomy work. Because one may find a situation in which repair is preferable to resection, one should plan ahead and have instrumentation available for meniscal repair should that be the most appropriate treatment.

It is important during an arthroscopic examination of the knee to develop a standardized, systematic approach. Knowledge of a variety of portals should be available, although the basic anteromedial and anterolateral operating portals are used in most cases.

The technique of partial meniscectomy was well described by Dr. Robert Metcalf (18), who previously detailed the technical aspects of the surgery in earlier editions of this text. Over the years, improvements in technology and equipment have made many of the technical difficulties of this procedure much easier. Advances in fiberoptics and imaging have improved the field of view, and modern-day pump systems allow for surgery to proceed much of the time with a bloodless field without the use of a tourniquet. Advances in cutting instruments and shaver blades have made the mechanics of meniscus tissue removal much easier: with the sharp, aggressive instruments now available, rapid tissue removal is possible with little difficulty. The instruments and shavers now come in smaller sizes, which also makes surgery easier. The principles, however, remain the same and are outlined here.

Principles

Although the exact steps required for each type of tear are unique to the tear configuration, the principles of meniscectomy are, for the most part, the same. These were delineated by Metcalf et al. (18) (Fig. 13.5).

1. *Remove the mobile fragments*: Excise the torn portions of the meniscus that are unstable and move into the center portion of the joint. These fragments may catch within the joint, causing continued symptoms.
2. *Do not leave any sudden changes in rim contour*: Sharp edges of the meniscus may cause catching or folding of the meniscus with joint motion. Although one does not have to excise tissue to obtain the same rim width throughout, sudden changes in contour must be avoided. Trimming and tapering of the corners of a tear eliminates mechanical symptoms and allows preservation of meniscal tissue.
3. *Do not try to obtain a perfectly smooth rim*: Repeat arthroscopy has shown that by 6 to 9 months small irregularities in meniscus contour will smooth out. Although careful contouring is required, some biologic remodeling also occurs, and it is not necessary to spend an excessive amount of time making the meniscus perfectly smooth.
4. *Use the probe often*: By constantly evaluating the tear and the amount of meniscus resected, one can avoid an ex-

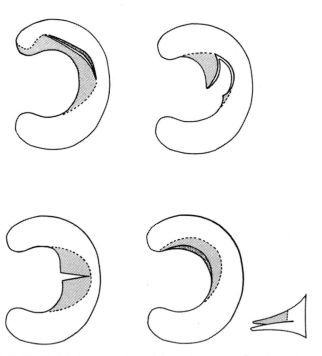

FIGURE 13.5 Principles of partial meniscectomy for the various types of meniscal tears—balancing meniscal resection. **A**: With a vertical longitudinal tear. **B**: With a flap tear. **C**: With a radial tear. **D**: With a horizontal cleavage tear. (From Newman AP, Daniels AU, Burks RT. Principles and decision making in meniscal surgery. *Arthroscopy* 1993;9:33–51, with permission.)

cessive resection. Mobility of remaining tissue should be assessed to avoid leaving behind unstable fragments.

5. *Protect the meniscus capsular junction*: If the meniscus is completely transected, the biomechanical effect is probably similar to that of a total meniscectomy, in that all hoop stresses within the meniscus are lost. Preserving a rim of tissue at the meniscus capsular junction lessens the effects of meniscus loss.

6. *Alternate between handheld and motorized instruments*: A more precise resection is possible with the handheld instruments, but aggressive shavers make quick work of unstable fragments. Medium-sized shavers often are a good compromise to allow mobility within the joint without damage to chondral surfaces.

7. *If unsure, leave more meniscus rim than less*: As mentioned previously, complete transection of the meniscus rim destroys the hoop stresses within the remaining meniscus. If a rim can be maintained, this problem will be avoided. At times, small, intact rim areas left behind can stabilize the meniscus, providing a more normal joint-loading environment. Occasionally, a second arthroscopy may be needed if tissue left behind continues to cause mechanical symptoms. However, this is believed to be preferable to an overly aggressive resection of tissue during the primary meniscectomy.

By following these principles, most types of tears encountered can be appropriately treated, leading to an improvement in knee function and a decrease in pain. In order to provide more detail with regard to specific treatment, sev-

eral types of tear configurations are used here to provide examples of the steps in arthroscopic meniscectomy.

Vertical Longitudinal Tears

The vertical longitudinal tear is commonly seen with chronic ACL injuries. When displaced, this tear configuration is commonly referred to as a "bucket-handle tear." If such a tear is more than 4 mm from the meniscus capsular junction, or if the inner portion of the meniscus is of poor quality and not suitable for repair, arthroscopic resection is appropriate, but in certain cases repair could still be considered.

Techniques for resection are well described with the use of a systematic approach, facilitating efficient removal of the torn fragment (43,44) (Fig. 13.6). In many instances, displaced tears can first be reduced to provide better visualization. This often allows the posterior horn to be seen well. When dealing with a bucket-handle medial meniscus tear, the arthroscope is placed in the lateral portal and manual basket forceps through the medial portal. With the use of the basket forceps, the posterior horn attachment of the torn meniscus can be partially transected. If a few fibers of the torn piece are left attached to the posterior horn, the fragment will stay in position, making the rest of the resection easier. The arthroscope is then placed in the medial portal, and the basket forceps are brought across the joint from the lateral portal. In this way, an appropriate cutting angle is achieved to transect the anterior attachment of the torn me-

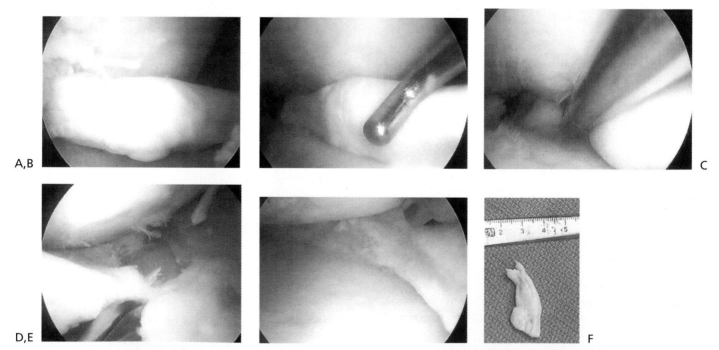

FIGURE 13.6 A chronic medial meniscus tear (**A**), can be reduced with the help of a probe (**B**). Posterior horn transection (**C**) is followed by anterior horn transection (**D**). The stable rim (**E**) and the removed fragment (**F**) are shown.

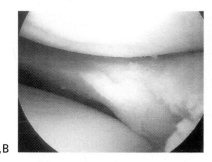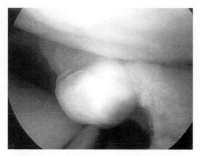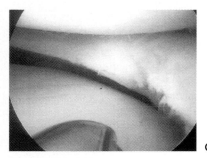

A,B   C

FIGURE 13.7 An oblique tear may fold under the meniscus rim and at first glance be undetectable (**A**). Probing can deliver the piece (**B**), and resection leaves a stable rim (**C**).

dial meniscus. When the anterior attachment is free, a grasper is used to hold the torn fragment, and it is pulled out of the lateral portal. Twisting of the grasper in a circular motion several times helps detach the small remaining portion of the posterior horn fragment. By this technique, the torn fragment is removed without leaving significant remnants behind, attached to either the anterior or posterior horn. If a small amount of meniscus tissue remains either anteriorly or posteriorly, it can easily be removed with the motorized shaver. An aggressive cutting blade facilitates tissue removal.

If the vertical longitudinal tear is confined to the posterior horn of the meniscus, tissue removal is usually performed in a piecemeal fashion. A wide "duck-billed" manual cutter is helpful and should be brought in through the ipsilateral portal to achieve the initial resection. Fragments are removed with the shaver, using suction. After the posterior portion of the meniscus has been removed, the more anterior part of the tear should be contoured to prevent an abrupt transition from the normal anterior meniscus. This is best accomplished by switching the arthroscope to the ipsilateral portal and using a manual cutter through the contralateral portal to form a transition from the anterior portion of the meniscus. Loose edges can be smoothed with the motorized shaver.

Radial Tears

Radial tears greater than 3 to 4 mm in depth can catch in the joint and should be treated with partial resection. Removal of meniscus tissue anterior and posterior to the radial component is best achieved with the use of a manual instrument brought in from either the ipsilateral or contralateral portal, depending on the tear site. Radial tears in the midportion of the meniscus (a common location) are usually best approached by bringing the basket or duck-billed forceps in from the contralateral portal. Tissue anterior and posterior to the radial tear is removed so that a smooth transition to the depth of the tear is achieved without abrupt changes in meniscus contour.

Oblique Tears

Oblique tears usually require resection in that at least a portion of the tear extends into the avascular zone of the menis-

cus. Removal of the torn fragment is accomplished with either manual or motorized instruments, and the remaining meniscus is contoured in a fashion similar to that for a radial tear. Oblique tears that extend deeply into the vascular zone may require a combination of partial resection and repair. If the injury is acute and resection will require removal of tissue all the way to the meniscus capsular junction, one should consider removing and contouring the inner one third of the meniscus tear and then using repair techniques to salvage the remaining tissue.

Oblique tears commonly displace if they are large, and the free fragment may slide underneath the normal meniscus (Fig. 13.7). At first glance with the arthroscope, these tears may be missed. Careful probing of the meniscus reveals the unstable portions, and they can be delivered into the joint. Once delivered, they can be resected using either basket forceps or a motorized shaver.

Additionally, large fragments may displace into the back of the knee, rotating on their posterior horn attachments. This is commonly seen in bucket-handle tears, in which the midportion of a vertical longitudinal tear becomes transected, leaving two mobile oblique fragments. These fragments may displace in and out of the joint and need to be resected. They are best identified by routinely placing a 70-degree arthroscope in the posterior compartment of the knee through the notch. Both the posteromedial and posterolateral corners can be examined in this way, and this technique should be used to avoid missing displaced mobile fragments. It helps to have a mental image as to how much meniscus is damaged. If the piece removed does not seem adequate to fill the defect, then diligence is needed to find what is missing.

Horizontal Tears

Horizontal tears are frequently encountered and most often involve the posterior and middle portions of the meniscus. The usual cleavage plane is fairly central, leaving two distinct leaves of tissue. Often the superior and inferior surfaces of the meniscus are relatively well preserved, and the cleavage plane extends a variable distance into the meniscus. If both leaves are intact, these horizontal tears may be treated with partial resection of the inner margin of the meniscus back to the end of the horizontal cleavage. At times, these cleavage planes extend deep into the meniscus and complete resection would necessitate a near-total meniscectomy. In such situations, partial resection of both the superior and inferior leaves is performed, with removal of any unstable fragments. If the two remaining leaves are of good quality, a small cleavage between them may be left.

At other times, either the inferior or the superior leaf has a more complex tear and is unstable. In these circumstances, resection of the unstable fragments leaves only one leaf remaining. If this tissue is of good quality, it may be left in place to provide a continuous meniscus rim. At times, however, the more intact leaf is structurally weak or damaged, with a vertical component of tearing seen more peripherally. This may be observed by careful probing of the intact side of the meniscus, noting a dimpling effect when probe pressure is applied. In these cases, the meniscus resection requires both removal of unstable fragments of the more involved leaf and partial resection of the more intact leaf to prevent recurrent tearing.

Complex and Degenerative Tears

Complex tears are most often seen in older individuals as a consequence of degenerative change within the joint and the meniscus (Fig. 13.8). However, they can also be seen in young individuals after significant traumatic events. In the younger age groups, consideration of salvage of complex tears should be made: The meniscus tissue is often of good quality, and the healing potential is high in the setting of sig-

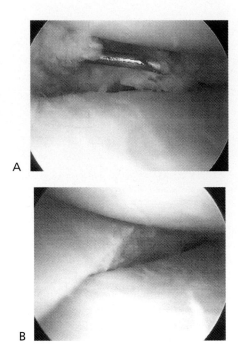

FIGURE 13.9 A spinal needle (**A**) may help manipulate fragments to allow a smooth resection (**B**).

nificant trauma such as major ligamentous injury or fracture. In the case of an older patient with a more degenerative complex tear, however, meniscectomy should be performed along with debridement of any loose chondral fragments seen at the time of surgery. As part of an overall degenerative process within the knee, these tears have little potential to heal and should be resected to eliminate mechanical irritation of the joint and joint capsule. The basic principles of resection should be followed to achieve a stable meniscus rim and preserve functioning tissue while removing all unstable fragments. However, because the knee is more degenerated and the patient is older, the value of meniscal retention is diminished, and a more aggressive approach to resection can be adopted. The motorized shaver is often very efficient in these cases, because the torn tissue is often soft and is easily cut and removed with the motorized shaver blades. In some instances, tear fragments are difficult to reach and manipulation with a percutaneously placed spinal needle may facilitate resection (Fig. 13.9).

Meniscus Cysts

Meniscus cysts have been reported to represent 1% to 10% of meniscus pathology and are commonly found with lateral meniscus tears (19). The patient presents with pain and swelling along the joint line. These cysts are often palpable and can be diagnosed by clinical examination (Fig. 13.10). MRI scans can confirm their presence and demonstrate the underlying meniscus tearing as the primary pathology (Fig. 13.11). Arthroscopic examination of the joint commonly confirms the presence of a tear (Fig. 13.12A), and resection

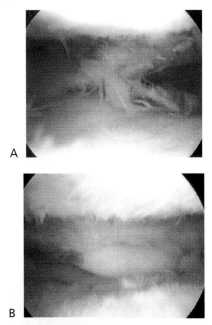

FIGURE 13.8 A degenerative tear (**A**) associated with significant chondrosis. After debridement (**B**), the articular surfaces show chondral degeneration.

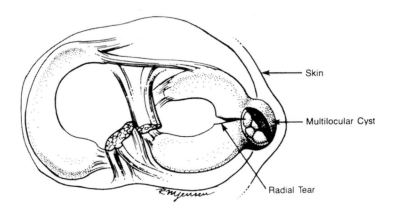

FIGURE 13.10 Cyst of the lateral meniscus. (From Cicotti MG, Shields CL Jr, El Attrache NS. Meniscectomy. In: Fu FH, Harner CD, Vince KG, eds. *Knee surgery,* vol 1. Philadelphia: Williams & Wilkins, 1994:591–613, with permission.)

of the torn tissue should be performed according to the tear pattern. Work can be done through the remaining horizontal tear after primary resection. The cyst is entered, and the clear, yellow fluid of the cyst can be seen to flow back into the joint (Fig. 13.12B,C). Further probing of the cyst is performed to ensure decompression, and then a rasp or mechanical shaver can be used to roughen the lining of the cyst so as to prevent recurrence. A spinal needle can be used from an outside-in approach to further puncture or decompress the cyst. With decompression and meniscectomy, cyst recurrence is unlikely; therefore, open excision is usually unnecessary. The outcome of arthroscopic meniscus cyst treatment has been reported to be 90% to 100% good results without recurrence (45,46).

Discoid Meniscus

Discoid meniscus may occur laterally or medially, with the great majority being lateral (Fig. 13.13A). When encountered as an incidental finding, they should be left alone. However, if either complete or partial variants are encountered that are inherently unstable and cause symptoms or that have torn fragments causing mechanical symptoms, partial resection must be considered (47,48). The goal of treatment is to contour the meniscus into a more normal C-

shaped structure. (49–51). This is performed by careful removal of the more central tissue with manual instruments (Fig. 13.13B,C). Care is taken to evaluate the size and shape of the remaining tissue as the resection proceeds and to assess posterior horn stability. Wrisberg varieties of discoid meniscus may require additional treatment with repair to

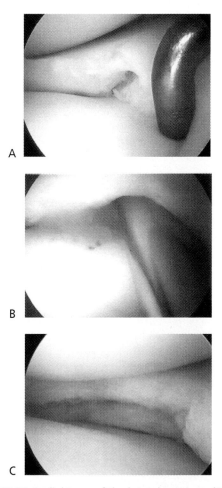

FIGURE 13.12 Radial tears of the lateral meniscus (**A**) can be associated with meniscus cysts. Probing (**B**) may decompress the cyst and release yellow cyst fluid. Resection of torn edges decompresses the cyst and alleviates symptoms (**C**).

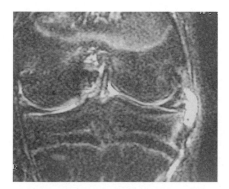

FIGURE 13.11 Magnetic resonance imaging scan of a lateral meniscus cyst associated with an underlying meniscus tear.

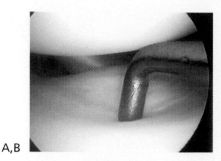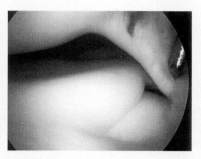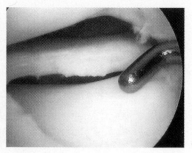

A,B

C

FIGURE 13.13 A discoid meniscus (**A**) may cause symptoms owing to free edges (**B**). Partial resection (**C**) leaves a more normally shaped meniscus.

the posterior capsule. Some discoid menisci are much thicker than a normal meniscus, and intrasubstance degeneration may be present. What appears to be a nice **C** shape is very thick at the inner edge and can cause symptoms. Recurrent tearing can occur, and subtotal or total meniscectomy may be necessary. Young patients who require total meniscectomy should be monitored closely, and meniscus transplantation should be considered if symptoms of pain and swelling occur.

REHABILITATION

Rehabilitation after partial meniscectomy can be aggressive, with the goal being a fast return to normal activities. At the completion of surgery, an intraarticular anesthetic is injected (0.25% or 0.5% Marcaine with Epinephrine) to achieve early pain relief and to decrease the need for postoperative narcotics (52,53). A light compressive dressing is applied, and ice or a cold delivery system is applied to the knee. Crutches may be used for 1 or 2 days, but immediate weight bearing and range of motion are allowed. The goal is for the patient to be walking without assistive devices as soon as possible. Stationary bicycle riding is begun on the second or third postoperative day, and strengthening exercises are initiated after the swelling has subsided and the patient is relatively free of pain with ambulation. Formal physical therapy, emphasizing closed-chain exercises, has been shown to be beneficial in achieving a faster return to full activity (54). However, many patients do not desire or require this. Full activities, including sports, can be resumed at 10 to 14 days, provided that the swelling is gone, the patient is pain free, and the knee has a nearly normal range of motion. In patients with degenerative chondral changes, return of function and pain resolution may be slower, requiring 6 to 8 weeks.

RESULTS

With the advent of arthroscopic meniscectomy, the era of open total meniscectomy has ceased. With the use of the

arthroscope, meniscus-preserving techniques are available that have obviated the need for open complete resection. Several authors have published results on the outcome after partial arthroscopic meniscectomy (42,55–58). The earliest literature compared this technique with the previous gold standard, which was the open total meniscectomy. Northmore-Ball et al. (59) reported a significant difference in results: With arthroscopic partial meniscectomy, 90% of the patients had good or excellent results, whereas patients undergoing open total meniscectomy had only 68% good or excellent results. Numerous other studies have demonstrated similar findings.

Arthroscopic treatment of meniscus tears by partial meniscectomy has resulted in excellent short-term results with major advantages over both partial and total open meniscectomy. These advantages include outpatient treatment, shorter recovery time, reduction in pain, reduction in the overall morbidity rate and in the rate of complications, and reduction in patient care costs. Although many of the early arthroscopic partial meniscectomy papers reported only short-term follow-up, many demonstrated 80% to 90% satisfactory clinical results after 2 to 3 years. Given the excellent short-term results of partial meniscectomy, one is left to question whether the long-term results will remain favorable. Certainly the results of open total meniscectomy were favorable with short follow-up, but they deteriorated significantly over time. In an effort to determine the long-term effects of partial meniscectomy on function, several authors have published studies of long-term follow-up on partial meniscectomy.

A number of long-term studies have raised the question of whether partial meniscectomy is, in fact, a benign procedure. Fauno and Nielsen (60) showed that osteoarthritic radiographic changes had occurred in 53% of operated knees undergoing partial meniscectomy, compared with 27% of the contralateral knees, at 8-year follow-up. A study by Rangger et al. (61) demonstrated that at 4-year follow-up degenerative radiographic changes were present in knees that had undergone partial meniscectomy. Thirty percent of the medial compartments that had undergone partial medial meniscectomy had radiographic changes consistent with osteoarthritis, and 24% of the lateral compartments that had undergone a lateral meniscectomy had degenerative changes. However, the authors noted that these poor radiographic findings did not correlate with subjective postoperative results. They found that 85% to 91% of the patients had good or excellent clinical outcomes based on subjective and objective criteria. Schimmer et al. (62) reported on patients after both 4 and 12 years of follow-up. Although 91.7% had good or excellent results at 4 years, by 12 years this was true of only 78.1% of the patients. The factor with the greatest impact on long-term outcome in their study was whether associated articular cartilage damage was seen at the time of meniscectomy. Only 62% of patients with articular cartilage damage at the time of meniscectomy had a good or excellent result at final follow-up, compared with 94.8% of patients who had no articular cartilage damage seen at the time of meniscectomy. Other studies of meniscectomy in patients older than 40 years of age have confirmed that articular cartilage damage seen at the time of meniscectomy can play a major role in outcome. Those patients with more changes were found to have poorer long-term outcomes.

Burks et al. (18,63) published a 15-year follow-up study of patients operated on by Dr. Robert W. Metcalf. Between June 1976 and August 1978, 282 arthroscopic meniscectomies were performed; 87% of these patients were contacted. A total of 102 patients were excluded from the study for a variety of reasons, such as subsequent surgery on the opposite (control) knee, age (older than 60 years), and ACL procedures performed at the time of arthroscopy. Patients were evaluated with a physical examination, a questionnaire, a Lysholm score for subjective satisfaction, and a Tegner functional activity score. They also had standing radiographs, which were objectively graded.

The average length of follow-up was 14.7 years, and 83% of the patients were men. The average age at meniscectomy was 35.8 years. There were 80% medial and 17% lateral meniscectomies, with 3% of patients having both menisci torn. Twenty percent of the men and 35% of the women had an associated ACL deficiency at the time of meniscectomy. There were no significant differences on the basis of age in any of the parameters tested. The men had better results than the women did, with a difference that was statistically significant for Lysholm scores and radiographic changes. In the evaluation of ACL-deficient knees, there was no significant difference between men and women. The Lysholm scores of medial and lateral meniscectomies were similar, although the lateral joint space was more narrow after lateral meniscectomy than the medial joint space was after medial meniscectomy. This variation was not statistically significant.

All parameters were worse for patients with ACL deficiency at the time of arthroscopic meniscectomy, and the differences were statistically significant. With the opportunity to monitor patients who had meniscectomies on an ACL-deficient knee without ACL reconstruction, the observation was made that these patients probably did better than those patients reported in previous series of open meniscectomies. However, the results were inferior to those of patients who had meniscectomies in stable knees. As would be expected, radiographs of ACL-deficient knees showed more joint space narrowing and other degenerative changes than those of stable knees. Patients with stable knees and normal preoperative radiographs who had simple partial medial meniscectomies were evaluated, and they had Lysholm scores of 95, and radiographic grade differences of only 0.25 when comparing one side with the other.

Extremity alignment and its effect on the results of meniscectomy were evaluated. A tibial–femoral angle greater than 4 degrees was considered to be a valgus knee, and one less than or equal to 4 degree was considered a varus knee. There was a statistically significant increase in radiographic grade changes in extremities that showed a varus alignment, compared with valgus knees, after medial meniscectomy. The medial joint space narrowing was also significantly greater in varus knees. The patient sampling was not great enough to draw conclusions about lateral meniscectomy and valgus knees. The authors' conclusions concerning arthroscopic partial meniscectomy from this follow-up study were as follows:

1. Results were almost universally good in stable knees at 15-year follow-up.
2. Age was not a factor in the results in this series.
3. ACL-deficient knees with meniscectomy had poorer results than stable knees with meniscectomy.
4. Results of medial and lateral meniscectomy showed no statistically significant difference.
5. Knees with alignment of less than 4 degrees showed poorer radiographic and Lysholm scores, compared with knees with alignment greater than 4 degrees, after medial meniscectomy. This was also true for alignment of less than 0 degrees compared with greater than 0 degrees.
6. Men had superior results than women if both had intact ACLs, but this difference was eliminated if both were ACL deficient.

COMPLICATIONS

The complications of arthroscopic meniscectomy include those complications common to all surgical procedures. However, there are also specific complications related to this procedure that bear mentioning. One of the most common complications after arthroscopic meniscectomy is continued pain. This is largely caused by other preexisting problems within the joint that are coexistent with meniscal tearing. In patients with significant chondral damage, results have been shown by numerous authors to be statistically worse than in patients with normal articular cartilage (62). For the patient undergoing partial meniscectomy who has significant degenerative changes, one must realize that complete relief of pain is unlikely and that continued symptoms of locking and catching may persist based on articular cartilage incongruity and not on catching of meniscus fragments.

Another complication of arthroscopic meniscectomy is hemarthrosis. Rarely, aggressive resection of meniscal tissue to the meniscus capsular junction can cause significant bleeding. This complication can cause severe pain and loss of motion in the knee joint. It may necessitate joint aspiration or even repeat arthroscopy if a tense hemarthrosis develops. Taking care to preserve the meniscus rim if possible, and to avoid aggressive meniscus capsular cutting, will help prevent hemarthrosis. Additionally, performing the procedure without a tourniquet will alert the physician to significant sources of bleeding that are encountered during the course of the procedure. Using an arthroscopic bovie or similar device, intraarticular bleeding can be stopped before completion of the procedure.

Infection after arthroscopic meniscectomy is extremely rare and is approximately equal to that reported for all other routine arthroscopic procedures. Other problems such as nerve injury, which can be encountered after meniscus repair, are infrequent. Most can be avoided with attention to detail, although occasional saphenous nerve injuries from the anterior portals can occur.

In unusual circumstances such as meniscus cyst or discoid meniscus, the complication rate may increase owing to recurrent problems such as cyst reaccumulation or recurrent tearing of abnormal tissue found in discoid menisci. Nevertheless, arthroscopic treatment in these situations is successful in more than 90% of the cases (45,46). Reflex sympathetic dystrophy and arthrofibrosis can occur after simple arthroscopy but are more related to patella procedures.

In general, arthroscopic meniscectomy is an extremely safe and effective procedure. Complications are few and, with attention to detail, a successful outcome can be obtained in more than 95% of the cases.

SUMMARY

Arthroscopic meniscectomy is a mainstay for the treatment of many types of meniscus pathology. Tear patterns that are not amenable to repair should be treated with arthroscopic partial meniscectomy to alleviate symptoms of pain, catching, and swelling of the joint. With careful attention to detail, arthroscopic partial meniscectomy has a success rate of more than 95% in the short term. Long-term studies have proven the efficacy of the procedure in patients whose articular surfaces were normal. In patients with significant degenerative changes, particularly nonalignment, the results of arthroscopic meniscectomy are less favorable, and recurrence of pain and swelling is a common problem resulting from associated chondral injury. As techniques develop that enhance repair and reconstruction efforts, arthroscopic meniscectomy may become a less frequently used procedure. However, at the present time, it remains an important tool for the treatment of many types of meniscus lesions.

REFERENCES

1. Smillie IS. Observations on the regeneration of the semilunar cartilage in man. *Br J Surg* 1943;31:398.
2. Renstrom P, Johnson RJ. Anatomy and biomechanics of the menisci. *Clin Sports Med* 1990;9:523–538.
3. Small NC. Complications in arthroscopic surgery performed by experienced arthroscopists. *Arthroscopy* 1988;4:215–221.
4. Ikeuchi H. The early days of arthroscopic surgery in Japan. *Arthroscopy* 1988;4:222–225.
5. O'Connor RL. The history of partial meniscectomy. In: Shahriaree J, ed. *Arthroscopic surgery*. Philadelphia: JB Lippincott, 1984:93–97.
6. Lysholm J, Gillquist J. Arthroscopic meniscectomy in athletes. *Am J Sports Med* 1983;11:436–438.
7. Hershman EB, Nisonson B. Arthroscopic meniscectomy: a follow-up report. *Am J Sports Med* 1983;11:253–257.
8. Zarris B, Boyle J, Harris BA. Knee rehabilitation following arthroscopic meniscectomy. *Clin Orthop* 1985;198:36–42.
9. Hamberg P, Gillquist J. Knee function after arthroscopic meniscectomy: a prospective study. *Acta Othop Scand* 1984;55:172.
10. Northmore-Ball MD, Dandy DJ, Jackson RW. Arthroscopic, open partial, and total meniscectomy. A comparative study. *J Bone Joint Surg Br* 1983;65:400–404.
11. Hede A, Jensen DB, Blyme P, et al. Epidemiology of meniscal lesions in the knee: 1,215 open operations in Copenhagen, 1982–1984. *Acta Orthop Scand* 1990;60:435–437.
12. Neilsen AB, Yde J. Epidemiology of acute knee injuries: a prospective hospital investigation. *J Trauma* 1991;31:1644–1648.
13. Peohling GG, Ruch DA, Chabon SJ. The landscape of meniscal injuries. *Clin Sports Med* 1990;9:539–549.
14. Duncan JB, Hunter R, Purnell M, et al. Meniscal injuries associated with acute anterior cruciate ligament tears in alpine skiers. *Am J Sports Med* 1995;23:170–172.
15. Levy IM, Torzilli PA, Warren RF. The effect of medial meniscectomy on anterior-posterior motion of the knee. *J Bone Joint Surg Am* 1982;64:883–888.
16. Shoemaker SC, Markolf KL. The role of the meniscus in the anterior-posterior stability of the loaded anterior cruciate-deficient knee. *J Bone Joint Surg Am* 1986;68:71–79.
17. Allen CR, Wong EK, Livesay GA, et al. Importance of the medial meniscus in the anterior cruciate ligament-deficient knee. *J Orthop Res* 2000;18:109–115.
18. Metcalf RW, Burks RT, Metcalf MS, et al. Arthroscopic meniscectomy. In: McGinty JB, Caspari RB, Jackson RW, et al., eds. *Operative arthroscopy*, 2nd ed. Philadelphia: Lippincott-Raven, 1996:263–297.
19. Lantz B, Singer KM. Meniscal cysts. *Clin Sports Med* 1990;9:707–725.
20. Ferrer-Roca O, ViLalta C. Lesions of the meniscus: part II. Horizontal cleavages and lateral cysts. *Clin Orthop* 1980;146:301–307.
21. Ferrer-Roca O, ViLalta C. Lesions of the meniscus: part I. Macroscopy and histologic findings. *Clin Orthop* 1980;146:289–300.
22. Weinstable R, Muellner T, Vecsei V, et al. Economic considerations for the diagnosis and therapy of meniscal lesions: can magnetic resonance imaging help reduce the expense. *World J Surg* 1997;21:363–368.
23. Evans PJ, Bell GD, Frank C. Prospective evaluation of the McMurray test. *Am J Sports Med* 1993;21:604–608.

24. Shelbourne KD, Martini DJ, McCarroll JR, et al. Correlation of joint line tenderness and meniscal lesions in patients with acute anterior cruciate ligament tears. *Am J Sports Med* 1995;23: 166–169.

25. Terry GC, Tagaert BE, Young MJ. Reliability of the clinical assessment in predicting the cause of internal derangements of the knee. *Arthroscopy* 1995;11:568–576.

26. Rosenberg TD, Paulos LE, Parker RD, et al. The forty-five-degree posteroanterior flexion weight-bearing radiographs of the knee. *J Bone Joint Surg Am* 1988;70:1479–1483.

27. Meullner T, Weinstable R, Schabus R, et al. The diagnosis of meniscal tears in athletes: a comparison of clinical and magnetic resonance imaging investigations. *Am J Sports Med* 1997;25: 7–12.

28. LaPrade RF, Burnett QM, Veenstra MA, et al. The prevalence of abnormal magnetic resonance imaging findings in asymptomatic knees. *Am J Sports Med* 1994;22:739–745.

28a. Boden SD, Davis DO, Dina TS, et al. A prospective and blinded investigation of magnetic resonance imaging of the knee. Abnormal findings in asymptomatic subjects. *Clin Orthop* 1992;(282): 177–185.

29. Ahmed AM, Burk DL. In vitro measurement of static pressure distribution in synovial joints: I. Tibial surface of the knee. *J Biomech Eng* 1983;105:216–225.

30. Radin EL, DeLamotte F, Maquest P. Role of the menisci in the distribution of stress in the knee. *Clin Orthop* 1984;185: 290–294.

31. Kettlekamp DB, Jacorb AW. Tibiofemoral contact area-determination and implications. *J Bone Joint Surg Am* 1972;54:349–356.

32. Fukubayaski T, Kurosawa H. The contact area and pressure distribution pattern of the knee: a study of normal and osteoarthrotic knee joints. *Acta Orthop Scand* 1980;51:871–879.

33. Johnson RJ, Kettlecamp DB, Clark W. Factors affecting the late results after meniscectomy. *J Bone Joint Surg Am* 1974;56:719.

34. Trapper EM, Hoover NW. Late results after meniscectomy. *J Bone Joint Surg Am* 1969;51:517–526.

35. Huckell J. Is meniscectomy a benign procedure? A long-term follow-up study. *Can J Surg* 1965;8:254–260.

36. Fairbank TJ. Knee joint changes after meniscectomy. *J Bone Joint Surg Br* 1948;30:664–670.

37. Allen PR, Denham RA, Swan AV. Late degenerative changes after meniscectomy. *J Bone Joint Surg Br* 1984;66:666–671.

38. Cox JS, Nye CE, Schaefer WW, et al. The degenerative effects of partial and total resection of the medial meniscus in dogs' knees. *Clin Orthop* 1975;109:178.

39. Voloshin AS, Wosk J. Shock absorption of meniscectomized and painful knees: a comparative in-vivo study. *J Biomed Eng* 1983;5:349–356.

40. Shelbourne KD, Patel DV, Adsit WS, et al. Rehabilitation after meniscal repair. *Clin Sports Med* 1996;15:595–612.

41. Saunders KC, Louis DL, Weingarden SI, et al. Effect of tourniquet time on postoperative quadriceps for function. *Clin Orthop* 1979;143:194–199.

42. Ciccotti MG, Shields CL, El Attrache NS. Meniscectomy. In: Fu F, Harner CD, Vince KG, ed. *Knee surgery* vol 1. Philadelphia: Williams & Wilkins, 1994:591–613.

43. Sprague NF. The bucket-handle meniscal tear: a technique using two incisions. *Orthop Clin North Am* 1982;13:337–348.

44. Dandy DJ. The bucket-handle meniscal tear: a technique detaching the posterior segment first. *Orthop Clin North Am* 1982;13: 369–385.

45. Glasgow MMS, Allen PW, Blakeway C. Arthroscopic treatment of cuts of the lateral meniscus. *J Bone Joint Surg Br* 1993;75: 299–302.

46. Ryu RKN, Jina AJ. Arthroscopic treatment of meniscal cysts. *Arthroscopy* 1993;9:591–595.

47. Comba D, Quaglia F, Magliano G. Massive discoid medial meniscus: a case report. *Acta Orthop Scand* 1985;56:340–341.

48. Herman G, Berson BL. Discoid medial meniscus: two cases of tears presenting as locked knee due to athletic trauma. *Am J Sports Med* 1984;12:74–76.

49. Vandermeer RD, Cunningham FK. Arthroscopic treatment of the discoid lateral meniscus: results of long-term follow-up. *Arthroscopy* 1989;5:101–109.

50. Ikeuchi H. Arthroscopic treatment of the discoid lateral meniscus: technique and long-term results. *Clin Orthop* 1982;167: 19–28.

51. Albertsson M, Gillquist J. Discoid lateral menisci: a report of 29 cases. *Arthroscopy* 1988;4:211–214.

52. Kneading C, Hill J, Katz J, et al. Bupivacaine use after knee arthroscopy: pharmacokinetics and pain control study. *Arthroscopy* 1990;6:33–39.

53. Henderson R, Campion E, DeMasi RA, et al. Post arthroscopy analgesis with bupivacaine. *Am J Sports Med* 1990;18:614–617.

54. Moffet H, Richards CL, Malouin F, et al. Early and intensive physiotherapy accelerates recovery postarthroscopic meniscectomy: results of a randomized controlled study. *Arch Phys Med Rehabil* 1994;75:415–426.

55. Newman AP, Daniels AU, Burks RT. Principles and decision making in meniscal surgery. *Arthroscopy* 1993;9:33–51.

56. Arnoczky SP, Warren RF. Microvasculature of the human meniscus. *Am J Sports Med* 1982;10:90–95.

57. Eggli S, Wegmuller H, Kosina J, et al. Long-term results of arthroscopic meniscal repair: an analysis of isolated tears. *Am J Sports Med* 1995;23:715–721.

58. Shrive N. The weight-bearing role of menisci of the knee. *J Bone Joint Surg Br* 1974;62:223–226.

59. Northmore-Ball MD, Dandy DJ, Jackson RW. Arthroscopic, open partial, and total meniscectomy. *J Bone Joint Surg Br* 1983;65:400–404.

60. Fauno P, Nielsen AB. Arthroscopic partial meniscectomy: a long-term follow-up. *Arthroscopy* 1992;8:345–349.

61. Rangger C, Klestil T, Gloetzer W, et al. Osteoarthritis after arthroscopic partial meniscectomy. *Am J Sports Med* 1995;23: 240–245.

62. Schimmer RC, Brulhart KB, Duff C, et al. Arthroscopic partial meniscectomy: a 12-year follow-up and two-step evaluation of the long-term course. *Arthroscopy* 1998;14:136–142.

63. Burks RT, Metcalf MH, Metcalf RW. Fifteen-year follow-up of arthroscopic partial meniscectomy. *Arthroscopy* 1997;13:673–679.

ARTHROSCOPIC MENISCAL REPAIR

W. DILWORTH CANNON, JR.

Thomas Annandale (1) was the first surgeon to perform an open meniscectomy in 1866, but his real claim to fame came on November 16, 1883, when he sutured back the anterior horn of the medial meniscus of a miner. This first open meniscal repair was considered a success when, 10 weeks later, the patient returned to work with a completely functioning knee. However, at that time there was little appreciation of this feat, because the body of the medical community believed, as Sutton (2) did, that the menisci were only "functionless remains of leg muscle origins." This tenet would remain prevalent for another 53 years. It was not until Don King's classic articles (3,4) in 1936 that the true function of the meniscus began to be understood. A patient with severe unicompartmental gonarthrosis of the knee stimulated his interest. This man had had a meniscectomy performed some 20 years previously, and King believed that there was a relationship between the meniscectomy and the subsequent arthritis. Through canine experiments, King was able to establish two important facts about the role of the menisci in the knee: (a) not only does meniscectomy cause degenerative changes in the knee, but these changes are directly related to the amount of meniscus removed, and (b) meniscal tears heal in the avascular portion of the menisci if the tears extend into the well-vascularized meniscosynovial junction. It was not until decades later that surgeons began to appreciate the significance of his work.

In 1969, Hiroshi Ikeuchi (5) performed the first arthroscopic meniscal repair in Tokyo. In the 1970s, DeHaven and others (6–10) began to perform open meniscal repair through a posterior arthrotomy. However, with the open technique, access to the mobile meniscal fragment can be difficult, limiting this type of repair to rim widths no greater than 2.5 to 3.0 mm (Fig. 14.1). After Henning performed the first arthroscopic meniscal repair in North America in 1980, surgeons began to take notice of this technique (11,12) (Fig. 14.2). Its widespread acceptance was slow, no doubt due to the inherent difficulty in performing it. Subsequently, other similar techniques were introduced (13–19).

The three types of meniscus repair are the inside-out, the outside-in, and the increasingly popular all-inside technique. The inside-out technique can be further subdivided into the double-barrel cannula and single needle passage techniques. Because collagen bundles are oriented predominantly circumferentially on the periphery of the meniscus, there is an advantage in being able to direct the individual throws of the mattress suture in superior and inferior directions so that the suture is oriented vertically on the periphery, thus securing more meniscal tissue for better fixation (Fig. 14.3). Horizontal sutures delivered through a double-barrel system may be more prone to pullout, or they may not provide adequate meniscal coaptation. However, a double-barrel cannula can be used like a single-barrel system if it is rotated between needle throws to create vertically oriented sutures. Barrett et al. (20) and Eggli et al. (21) reported better healing rates with the use of nonabsorbable sutures, compared with absorbable sutures. Asik et al. (22), Kohn and Siebert (23), and Rimmer et al. (24) concluded from their studies that vertically oriented sutures were stronger than horizontally placed sutures. Both Asik's group and Kohn and Siebert found that the weakest technique was knot-end sutures.

No matter what meniscal repair technique is used, abrasion of the tear site and perimeniscal synovium should be carried out. Such preparation is best done through a posterior incision and the anterior arthroscopic portals, using 2- and 3-mm rasps and burrs. A small powered shaver unit may also be used. I first suggested using abrasion for meniscus tear site preparation in 1983 (12), after which Richie et al. (25) and Okuda et al. (26) showed in animal studies that abrasion improved the rate of meniscus healing. In a goat study, trephination as an adjunct to suturing was demonstrated by Zhang et al. (27) to yield superior results compared with suturing alone. Trephination of incomplete meniscal tears produced good or excellent results in 90% of patients treated by trephination alone by Fox et al. (28). Shelbourne and Rask (29) showed that stable medial meniscal tears treated with abrasion and trephination alone had a 94% success rate. However, Talley and Grana (30) observed a higher failure rate for abraded stable medial meniscus tears compared with a similar treatment of stable lateral meniscus tears.

W. D. Cannon, Jr.: Department of Orthopaedic Surgery, University of California Medical School, San Francisco, California.

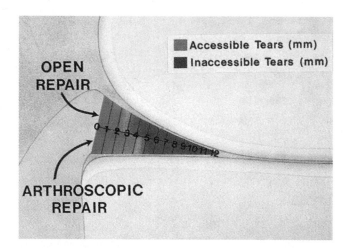

FIGURE 14.1 Arthroscopic versus open repair. The upper half of the meniscus shows the accessibility of the meniscus to open repair, the green area demonstrating that the surgeon cannot gain access to tears that have rim widths greater than 2.5 to 3.0 mm. In contrast, arthroscopic techniques can repair meniscal tears with rim widths greater than 4.0 mm. (Drawing courtesy of Jeanne Koelling.)

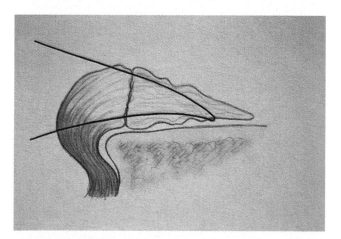

FIGURE 14.2 The Henning meniscal repair set consists of two rasps, a needle holder, a joint distractor, and a variety of cannulas.

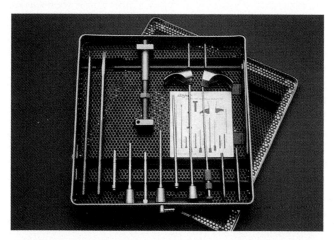

FIGURE 14.3 Using two separate needle passes, the surgeon can create a divergent suture containing enough meniscal tissue to provide excellent coaptation at the tear site. (Drawing courtesy of Jeanne Koelling.)

INDICATIONS

When making the decision whether to repair, partially excise, or leave alone a meniscus tear, there are many factors to consider, among them tear type, associated anterior cruciate ligament (ACL) tear, patient age, chronicity of the tear, medial versus lateral meniscus, and the presence of secondary tears. The ideal tear for repair is a vertical longitudinal tear within the peripheral 3 mm, placing it in the "red–red" zone, and associated with an ACL reconstruction. It is well documented that meniscus repair done in conjunction with an ACL reconstruction yields a significantly higher success rate (31–35). Tears with rim widths of 4 to 5 mm should still be considered for repair, especially if repair is undertaken in conjunction with an ACL reconstruction. Asahina et al. (36) found a higher failure rate in patients who were locking preoperatively. Complex radial split oblique tears of the posterior horn origin of the lateral meniscus should be considered for repair because of the rich blood supply in this area of the meniscus. This tear pattern is very common with acute tears of the ACL. Radial split tears of the middle third of the lateral meniscus have a low healing rate and may be better off left alone. Short tears (less than 1 cm) can be left alone, as can incomplete tears that do not result in an unstable meniscus fragment (Fig. 14.4). Fitzgibbons and Shelbourne (37) did not repair stable posterior horn tears of the lateral meniscus in knees undergoing ACL reconstruction. They encountered no symptomatic failures in 189 lateral meniscal tears with follow-up averaging 2.6 years after ACL reconstruction. A stable meniscal tear can be defined as one in which the meniscal fragment cannot be subluxed into the joint more than 3 mm. As mentioned earlier, Shelbourne and Rask (29) showed that stable medial meniscal tears treated with abrasion and trephination alone had a 94% success rate.

MODIFIED HENNING TECHNIQUE

Medial Meniscal Repair

A tourniquet is placed around the proximal thigh but is not used unless absolutely necessary. If ACL reconstruction is to be carried out at the same time, tourniquet use may be necessary, but ACL reconstruction still can easily be done without the use of a tourniquet. A well-padded leg holder is placed distal to the tourniquet, and if meniscal repair is planned, the thigh should be elevated approximately 45 degrees in the leg holder to gain access to the posteromedial corner of the knee (Fig. 14.5). It is important to pad the leg holder well and to place it on the thigh distal to the tourniquet, to prevent any pressure posteriorly on the sciatic nerve. Elevation of the thigh may not be necessary if the surgeon prefers to sit and flex the end of the table, but the thigh must extend far enough beyond the edge of the table break to provide access to the posterior corners of the knee. The leg may

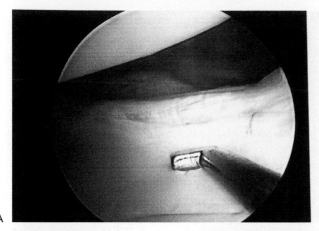

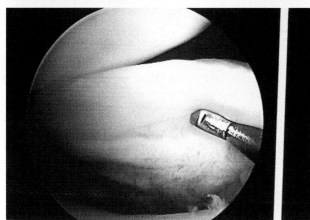

FIGURE 14.4 A: This incomplete tear of the superior surface of the posterior horn of the lateral meniscus in the right knee should be left alone. **B:** The inferior surface of the same meniscus does not show a tear.

be kept in this position without redraping if concomitant ACL reconstruction is done. After diagnostic arthroscopy has established the need for medial meniscal repair, a 6-cm longitudinal incision is made just posterior to the posterior border of the medial collateral ligament. The incision should be done with the knee flexed so that the pes anserinus and the sartorial branch of the saphenous nerve will lie posterior to the joint line, but care must be taken throughout the procedure to avoid excessive retraction or entrapping of the nerve with sutures. Dissection is carried down to the posterior capsule, deep to the semimembranosus, and half-way across the medial head of the gastrocnemius. If the direct head of the semimembranosus is too tight, it may be necessary to release several millimeters of its attachment. If suturing of the midcentral portion of the meniscus is contemplated, subcutaneous tissue should be dissected off the medial collateral ligament anterior to the posteromedial incision. A popliteal retractor is then inserted behind the posterior capsule. From the anterolateral portal, the arthroscope is run medial to the posterior cruciate ligament to inspect the posteromedial compartment of the joint.

Henning (11) used a joint distractor for repairs of the medial meniscus only. He inserted two 3/16-inch Steinmann pins, one just proximal to the adductor tubercle and the second in the anteromedial flair of the tibia, and then distracted the joint. If this did not allow adequate visualization of the posterior horn of the medial meniscus, Henning suggested making multiple transverse stab incisions in the medial collateral ligament in order to gain an additional 2 to 4 mm of joint opening. I rarely use the joint distractor, but I have used it to reduce displaced bucket-handle tears of the medial meniscus that otherwise were not reducible at surgery.

Since 1983, when I suggested that rasping of the perimeniscal synovium and tear site might improve neovascularization and hence healing, rasping has been done on all chronic and most acute repairs. Digital palpation, followed by insertion of a spinal needle through the synovium in the posteromedial incision, determines the optimal site for insertion of a 2- or 3-mm rasp. The ideal site should be close to the plane of the superior surface of the posterior horn of the meniscus. Perimeniscal synovial abrasion is then carried out under direct vision over the superior portion of the peripheral rim of the meniscus and in the tear site (Fig. 14.6). Both sides of the tear site should be freshened, especially if the tear is older than 8 weeks. Henning (11) showed statistically significantly improved results with rasping of the bucket-handle side of the tear. This debrides detritus that has a propensity to build up on the handle side of the tear site. The inferior surface of a posterior horn tear as well as the superior and inferior surfaces of a midcentral tear, are best rasped with a bur-type rasp (Bowen & Co., Rockville, MD) or an edge-cutting rasp introduced anteromedially. It is important to devote time to adequate abrasion of the synovium under the inferior portion of the meniscus.

Suturing is carried out with the use of 2-0 nonabsorbable Ethibond suture [Ethicon, Somerville, NJ [special order

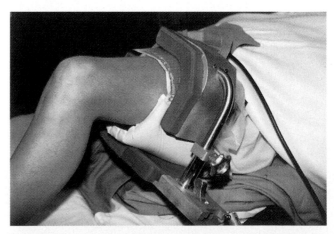

FIGURE 14.5 A thigh holder placed distal to the tourniquet and well padded posteriorly flexes the thigh up 45 degrees, providing excellent access to the posteromedial and posterolateral corners of the knee.

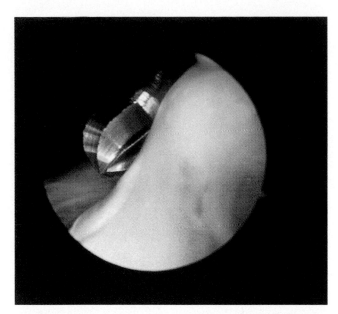

FIGURE 14.6 A 2-mm bur-type rasp has been introduced through the posteromedial incision while viewing through the intercondylar notch in this right knee. Abrasion of the tear site can be performed through this approach.

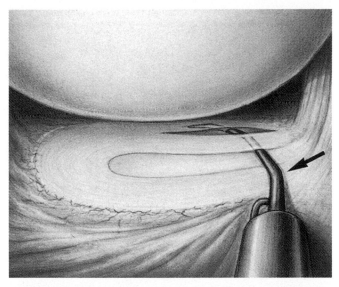

FIGURE 14.7 The first suture, placed close to the posterior horn of either medial or lateral meniscus, can be difficult to retrieve posteriorly. Therefore, a third bend in the needle is made by levering the cannula and needle holder into the intercondylar notch. The additional bend in the needle allows the surgeon to guide the needle into the popliteal retractor with greater ease. (Drawing courtesy of Jeanne Koelling.)

D-6702]) with double-armed taper-ended Keith needles. A 10- to 15-degree bend is made 4 mm from the needle tip, and a second 10- to 15-degree bend is made approximately 10 mm from the first bend in the same direction. The needle is then press fit–loaded into the needle holder (Stryker Corporation, Kalamazoo, MI). Suture placement for the posterior horn of the medial meniscus is carried out from the anteromedial portal. A short cannula is placed through the anteromedial portal close to the medial edge of the patellar tendon. Suturing is begun close to the posterior horn origin of the tear, and the first suture preferably should be placed on the inferior surface of the meniscus. Once the needle has been inserted approximately 3 to 4 mm from the tear site and up to the second bend in the needle, a third bend should be created in the needle by pushing the cannula and needle holder into the intercondylar notch (Fig. 14.7). The extra bend in the needle allows easier needle retrieval from the posteromedial incision. This first suture throw should be directed from the inferior surface upward through the meniscus so as to include as much meniscal tissue in a vertical orientation as possible. The surgeon may then carefully palpate the posterior capsule to determine whether the exit site of the needle will allow it to be contained by the popliteal retractor. Once this determination has been made, the needle may be advanced and grasped posteriorly with the needle holder. The needle should never be advanced while palpating posteriorly. After the needle is released anteriorly, it is pulled out through the posteromedial incision. The second throw of the first suture penetrates beyond the tear site near the meniscosynovial junction, thus creating a vertically oriented suture (Fig. 14.8). In an alternate suturing technique,

the second throw of the suture is made approximately 3 to 4 mm from the first throw, thus creating a horizontal mattress suture. The needles should be passed in divergent directions so as to include as much meniscal tissue in a vertical orientation as possible (Fig. 14.9). However, a horizontal suture is not as strong as a vertically oriented suture.

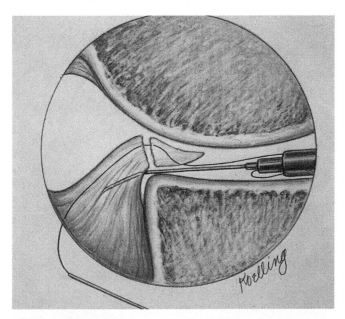

FIGURE 14.8 This diagram demonstrating the Henning technique shows excellent suture placement in the posterior horn with vertically divergent passes of the two needles. Note that one pass of the suture is close to the superior surface of the meniscus, and the second pass is underneath the inferior rim and penetrates through the meniscosynovial junction. (Drawing courtesy of Jeanne Koelling.)

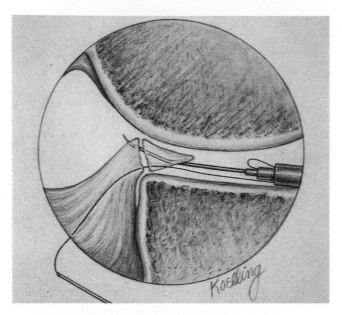

FIGURE 14.9 An alternative suturing technique employs the use of horizontally oriented mattress sutures. Note that the needle passes are divergent, securing more meniscal tissue. (Drawing courtesy of Jeanne Koelling.)

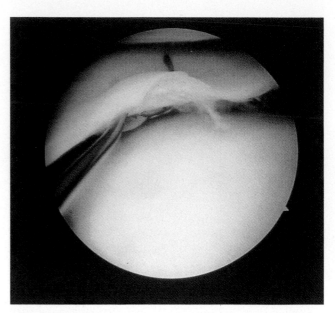

FIGURE 14.11 In the same patient as in Fig. 14.10, a suture is placed through the inferior surface of the medial meniscus via an ipsilateral portal.

Starting at the posterior horn origin, suture placement is alternated between the inferior and superior surfaces of the meniscus, with sutures spaced approximately 3 mm apart (Figs. 14.10 and 14.11). If the tear extends into the middle third of the medial meniscus, the arthroscope should be switched to the anteromedial portal, with suturing carried out through the anterolateral portal (Fig. 14.12). The most

anterior sutures may be directed out through a 1-cm incision placed between the posteromedial and the anteromedial incisions. Sutures placed in this fashion will avoid shear forces that may result from sutures directed obliquely out through the posteromedial incision. If difficulty is encountered in adequately visualizing or directing sutures through the posterior horn fragment, a probe inserted through an ac-

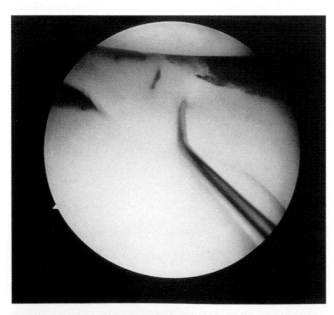

FIGURE 14.10 The needle is shown penetrating the superior surface of the medial meniscus in this right knee.

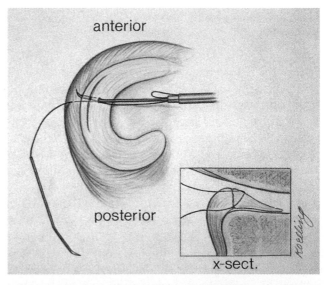

FIGURE 14.12 This diagram shows the technique for repair of the middle third of the medial meniscus. The arthroscope has been moved to the anteromedial portal, and suturing is carried out through the anterolateral portal. Note again the divergent needle placement, creating excellent coaptation of the meniscus. (Drawing courtesy of Jeanne Koelling.)

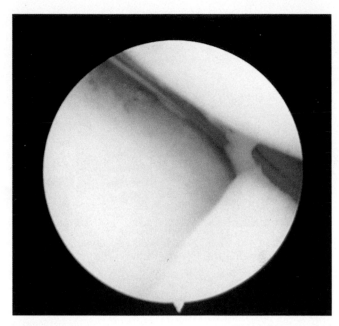

FIGURE 14.13 Arthroscopic view demonstrating another way of obtaining better suture placement for tears of the posterior horn and middle third of the medial meniscus. Notice that a nerve hook has been introduced through an accessory anteromedial portal (right side of photograph) and is lifting the meniscus up as the Keith needle is brought in through the anterolateral portal (left side of photograph). With this technique, more meniscal tissue can be skewered by the needle.

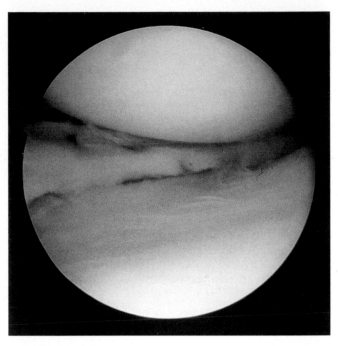

FIGURE 14.15 The displaced bucket-handle tear shown in Fig. 14.14 was repaired with eight sutures.

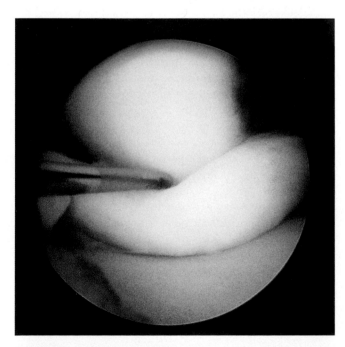

FIGURE 14.14 Most displaced bucket-handle tears such as this one can be successfully repaired.

cessory anteromedial portal may be used to bring the meniscal fragment anterior, or to tilt it so that suture placement can be optimized (Fig. 14.13). This is especially helpful when placing sutures through the inferior surface of the midcentral portion of the medial meniscus. Displaced bucket-handle tears also can be successfully repaired (Figs. 14.14 and 14.15).

If ACL reconstruction is to be performed, the sutures are not tied until the end of the reconstruction. The sutures can be kept tight in the meantime by threading them through 7-cm pieces of intravenous extension tubing and cross-clamping the tubing. Arnoczky (44) showed that meniscal healing in the avascular zone of canine menisci occurred when fibrin clot was inserted into punched-out defects in the meniscus, and all isolated meniscal repairs should have fibrin clot introduced into the tear site before the sutures are tied. Approximately 50 to 75 mL of venous blood is placed in a plastic container on the operative field, and the blood is stirred with one or two 10- or 20-mL glass syringe barrels for approximately 5 to 10 minutes until the clot adheres to the glass barrels (Fig. 14.16). It is then removed and blotted with moistened gauze. The same suture that is used for the meniscus repair (2-0 Ethibond) is placed and secured at each end of the tubulated clot, leaving one free needle at each end (Fig. 14.17). After introduction of a 6- or 7-mm cannula, the two free needles are bent in the same manner as for meniscal repair and loaded into the Henning needle holders. They are then passed through the cannula and under the inferior surface of the meniscus, through the meniscosyn-

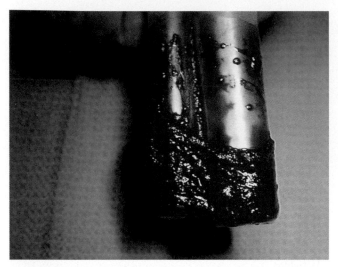

FIGURE 14.16 The appearance of the fibrin clot adhering to two glass syringe barrels after stirring 50 to 75 mL of venous blood for approximately 5 minutes.

ovial junction at the most posterior and anterior poles of the tear, and retrieved posteriorly. Tension is placed on these two sutures to align the clot in a linear direction. By pulling the two sutures together, the clot is fed into the opening of the cannula. Further advancement of the clot through the cannula is done by pulling on the two sutures while pushing the clot through the cannula with a blunt obturator. After the clot has been tucked into the tear site, all sutures are tied, trapping the fibrin clot in the tear site (Fig. 14.18). The single strands of the clot sutures are tied to adjacent meniscal repair sutures.

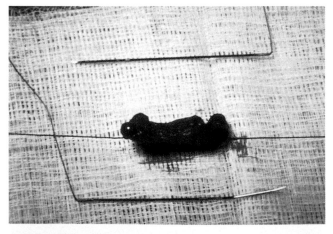

FIGURE 14.17 A 2-0 Ethibond suture has been placed through either end of the fibrin clot, facilitating its stable placement under the inferior surface of the meniscus at the tear site. (From Cannon WD, Vittori JM. Meniscal repair. In: Aichroth PM, Cannon WD, eds. *Knee surgery current practice.* London: Martin Dunitz, 1992, with permission.)

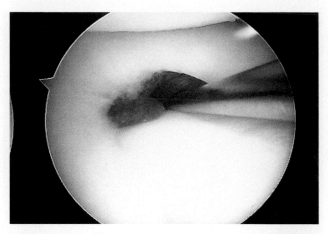

FIGURE 14.18 The fibrin clot has been placed under the meniscus at the repair site. Then the meniscus repair sutures are tied.

Lateral Meniscal Repair

The technique of lateral meniscal repair is similar to that of repair of the medial meniscus. A 6-cm vertical incision is made at the posterolateral corner of the knee. A longitudinal incision is made in the deep fascia along the posterior margin of the iliotibial band, and the biceps is retracted posteriorly with the knee flexed 90 degrees. The lateral head of the gastrocnemius is dissected off the posterior capsule to a point at which a nerve hook passed from the anteromedial portal over the top of the posterior horn origin of the lateral meniscus can be palpated through the posterolateral incision. With the knee flexed 90 degrees, the peroneal nerve will lie posterior to the biceps except in the proximal portion of the incision, where it crosses over behind the biceps to lie closer to the posterior surface of the lateral head of the gastrocnemius. The peroneal nerve does not have to be dissected out and identified. Abrasion of both tear surfaces is carried out as described for the medial side. Suture placement is done exclusively from the anteromedial portal. There should not be too much concern if a suture passes through the popliteus tendon, although it is preferable to avoid this situation.

Radial split tears of the posterior horn can be approximated by passing one suture through the posterior leaf, close to the inner margin of the meniscus, and the second suture through the anterior leaf of the tear. Because adequate healing has been difficult to achieve for radial split tears in the middle third of the lateral meniscus, I prefer to leave most of them alone. More complex tear types, including oblique flap tears, broken bucket-handle tears, and missing meniscal segments, have been repaired by Henning (21a) using fascial sheath fashioned from the fascia of the vastus lateralis and sutured superiorly and inferiorly over the tear site. Fibrin clot is then injected into the sheath. This difficult technique should not be attempted until the surgeon is comfortable with the use of standard meniscal repair techniques.

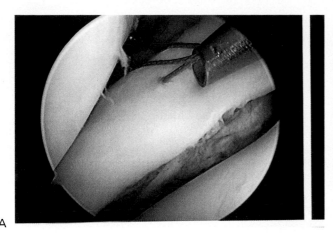

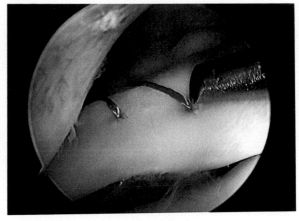

A

B

FIGURE 14.19 A: Arthroscopic view demonstrating an alternative method of meniscal repair. With the use of zone-specific curved cannulas, a pair of long needles are passed through the meniscus in individual throws. **B**: The suture is pulled tight.

ALTERNATIVE MENISCAL REPAIR TECHNIQUES

Zone-Specific Technique

Rosenberg (17) developed a zone-specific curved cannula system (Linvatec, Largo, FL) for meniscal repair. Long needles with swedged-on 2-0 Ethibond or 2-0 polydioxanone (PDS) sutures are passed through zone-specific cannulas placed against the superior or inferior surface of the torn meniscal fragment and advanced in 1-cm increments until identified and retrieved through a posterior incision (Fig. 14.19). Rosenberg has not found it a disadvantage to tie the sutures over the gastrocnemius heads, although I would be concerned that the amount of soft tissue interposition in the suture could result in a greater chance of suture loosening. Recently, Rosenberg designed a similar system using smaller cannulas and thinner needles, thus minimizing trauma to the meniscus.

I frequently use an alternative single-lumen malleable cannula technique (Fig. 14.20) (Arthrex, Naples, FL). It uses a nitinol needle threaded with off-the-shelf 2-0 nonabsorbable suture. It is a disposable, low-cost set of instruments.

Double-Barrel Techniques

Clancy and Graf (13) developed a popular double-barrel curved cannula system using a pair of long needles linked by 2-0 PDS (Ethicon) suture (Fig. 14.21). This technique is faster than the Henning technique, but it does have a disadvantage in that it is not possible to individually direct each throw of the suture as easily as with a single cannula technique, which enables the surgeon to obtain better coaptation of the meniscal fragments.

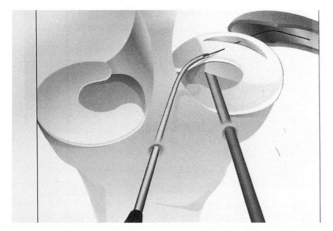

FIGURE 14.20 A nitinol needle is passed through a malleable cannula and penetrates the posterior horn of the medial meniscus. The popliteal deflector protects the neurovascular structures. (Drawing courtesy of Arthrex, Inc.)

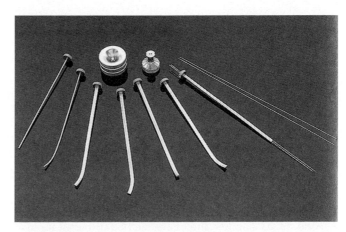

FIGURE 14.21 Graf and Clancy's double-barrel meniscal repair system. (Courtesy of Acufex Microsurgical, Norwood, MA.)

Outside-In Technique

Warren (16) developed an outside-to-inside technique using 18-gauge spinal needles to skewer the meniscal rim and fragment. Monofilament absorbable no. 0 PDS suture is then passed through the needle into the joint and retrieved through an anterior portal. Three to four knots are tied on the suture end, which is then pulled back into the joint against the superior or inferior surface of the meniscal fragment. The external ends of adjacent sutures are then tied together subcutaneously. In an alternative method, the two suture ends are brought out the anteromedial portal and tied together. The knot is then pulled back into the joint. The knot can be pulled through the meniscus tissue. If difficulty is encountered, then a small dilator knot can be tied on one of the two sutures; when the small knot is pulled through the meniscus, it creates a larger opening for the larger knot to pass through. Needle placement may be helped by counterpressure on the meniscus fragment and rim with a probe. Both needles of one suture should be placed across the tear site before the sutures are passed, to avoid the second needle's cutting the previously placed suture. For repair of the lateral meniscus, straight 18-gauge spinal needles should be kept anterior to the popliteus tendon. Curved needles (Smith and Nephew, Acufex, Mansfield, MA) provide better access to the posterior horn tears, obviating the need for a posterior incision and decreasing the risk of neurovascular injury (38). If delayed healing is expected, then nonabsorbable suture should be used. Morgan and Casscells (18) reported excellent results with this technique (Fig. 14.22).

Johnson (14) developed a similar technique using straight and curved spinal needles, with a wire loop to retrieve the end of the suture in the joint.

All-Inside Technique

Morgan (39) reported an all-inside technique for repair of the posterior horns using short curved needles placed through a large cannula posteromedially or posterolaterally and tying knots through the cannula.

REHABILITATION

If ACL reconstruction has been done along with meniscal repair, then early motion is emphasized to prevent an unacceptable incidence of stiffness and flexion contractures. My patients commence full passive extension and active flexion on the day after surgery. Partial weight-bearing is begun at 4 weeks, and patients are off their crutches by 6 weeks. Other surgeons (18,31) believe that early full weight bearing has no adverse effect on meniscal healing. Barber (40) compared two groups of patients; one group were braced and kept without weight bearing for 6 weeks, and the second group were allowed full motion without a brace and unrestricted return to pivoting sports once they had no effusion, full extension, and at least 120 degrees of flexion. In the unrestricted group of 58 repairs, the failure rate was 19%, compared with only 10% in the restricted group of 40 repairs. Mariani et al. (41) had a low failure rate in patients undergoing ACL reconstruction and concomitant meniscus repair who followed an aggressive rehabilitation program.

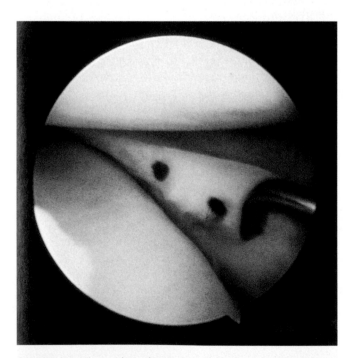

FIGURE 14.22 Another alternative method of meniscal repair uses knotted sutures passed from outside-in. (Courtesy of Craig D. Morgan, MD.)

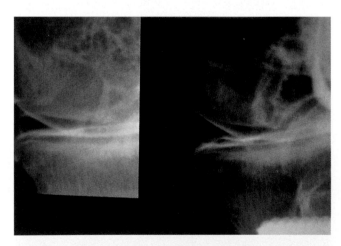

FIGURE 14.23 An arthrogram rather than a magnetic resonance imaging scan is the preferred method to assess the degree of meniscal healing for repairs of all medial menisci. *Left:* Preoperative vertical longitudinal tear of the posterior horn of the medial meniscus of a right knee. *Right:* Arthrogram at 6 months after meniscal repair, showing no evidence of residual cleft at the site of repair.

Some authors recommend that patients not flex their knees greater than 90 degrees for 4 weeks, believing that further flexion may stress the repair site.

In the 1980s and early 1990s, Henning and I felt that it was in the patient's best interest to know whether meniscal repair resulted in anatomic healing of the meniscus. Hence, 6 or more months after repair, an arthrogram (more accurate than a magnetic resonance imaging [MRI] scan) was done for medial meniscal repairs (Fig. 14.23) and arthroscopy under local anesthesia for lateral meniscal repairs. If a residual cleft at the repair site was less than 10% of the thickness of the meniscus, then it was considered healed. If a cleft was found that was less than 50% of the thickness of the meniscus, then the repair was considered partially healed. If the cleft was greater than 50% of the thickness, even if present only in one small region of the repair, then the repair was deemed to have failed (Fig. 14.24). Patients in the last category were advised to refrain from rigorous athletic activities.

The rehabilitative regimen for isolated meniscal repairs does not differ from that for meniscal repair carried out with ACL reconstruction. Straight-ahead running can be started at 5 months, and light sports begun at 6 months. Contact sports such as football and basketball are discouraged until 9 months. Again, some surgeons advocate early return to vigorous sports activity once the patient has regained strength and full range of motion.

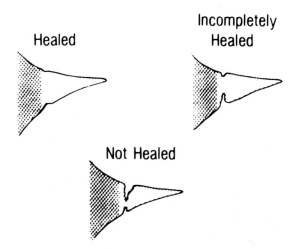

FIGURE 14.24 Six months after repair, the degree of healing can be determined by arthrography for the medial side and arthroscopy for the lateral side. A meniscus is classified as "healed" **(top left)** if it is healed over the full length of the tear with a residual cleft less than 10% of the thickness of the meniscus. A tear that is healed over its full length with a residual cleft that is less than 50% of its vertical height is classified as "incompletely healed" **(top right)**. A residual cleft of greater than 50% of the thickness of the meniscus at any point over the length of the tear is classified as "failed" **(bottom)**. (Drawing courtesy of Jeanne Koelling.)

RESULTS

From 1982 to 1997, I carried out 301 arthroscopic meniscal repairs. The average age of the patients was 27 years. Of the meniscal repairs performed, 59% were medial and 41% lateral; 78% were associated with an ACL reconstruction, and 22% were isolated repairs done in ACL-intact knees. Sixty-seven percent of the repairs were done in patients longer than 2 months after the time of injury. The average time between injury and surgery was 19 months. The Henning technique, either alone or in combination with another technique, was used in 91% of patients.

Of the 172 patients who had an anatomic assessment of the state of healing of their meniscal repairs, a follow-up arthrogram was done in 26% and second-look arthroscopy in 74%. This high number of arthroscopies can be accounted for by a number of patients who had both medial and lateral meniscal repairs and a number of patients with ACL reconstruction who had arthroscopic debridement for soft tissue impingement or arthroscopy at the time of hardware removal.

Because patients with incompletely healed meniscal repairs seemed to do as well as patients in the healed category, satisfactory results included both the healed and incompletely healed categories. Overall, based on *anatomic* assessment, 70% of meniscal repairs had a satisfactory outcome and 30% failed (Fig. 14.25). From purely a *clinical* assessment (absence of joint line pain or tenderness, clicking, locking, or swelling), 88% had a satisfactory outcome and 12% failed (Fig. 14.26).

The most important difference in this study was found in the healing rates of meniscal tears in knees with intact ACLs versus tears that were repaired in conjunction with ACL reconstruction (Fig. 14.25). Satisfactory anatomic healing in isolated meniscal repairs was only 53%, whereas in meniscal repairs associated with ACL reconstruction, there was a 75% rate of satisfactory healing ($p < .007$).

The width of the meniscal rim affected healing rates in both groups (Fig. 14.27). For rim widths up to 2 mm, healed and incompletely healed groups totaled 80%, whereas with rim widths of 4 to 5 mm, the avascular zone of the meniscus, this figure dropped to 44%.

There was also a relationship between tear length and healing (Fig. 14.28). Tear lengths less than 2 cm resulted in satisfactory healing in 81%, compared with 52% for tears 4 cm or longer.

Patients with older tears fared less well than those with acute tears (Fig. 14.29). Menisci that were repaired within 8 weeks after injury had a 77% incidence of satisfactory healing, but tears that were repaired more than 8 weeks after injury had a 67% healing rate. Lateral meniscal tears did better than those on the medial side, with 77% satisfactory healing in the former group but only 66% in the latter (Fig. 14.30).

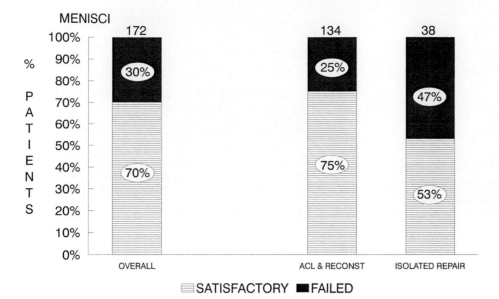

FIGURE 14.25 Meniscal repair results assessed anatomically. Overall results are shown on the left side bar. The right two bars show a comparison of isolated repairs versus anterior cruciate ligament (ACL) reconstructions with meniscal repairs. The rate of successful outcomes for meniscal repairs associated with ACL reconstructions was 75%, in sharp contrast to 53% in the isolated repair group. Note that a satisfactory outcome represents the sum of the healed and incompletely healed categories.

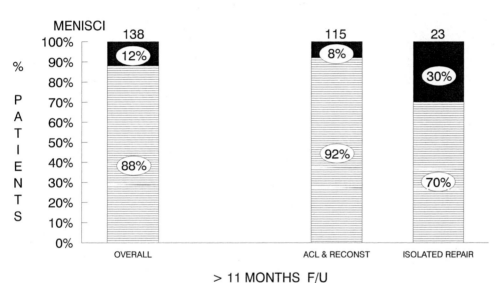

FIGURE 14.26 Meniscal repair results assessed clinically. In contrast to the results shown in Fig. 14.25, successful outcomes of meniscal repairs associated with anterior cruciate ligament reconstructions were 92%, versus 70% in the isolated repair group.

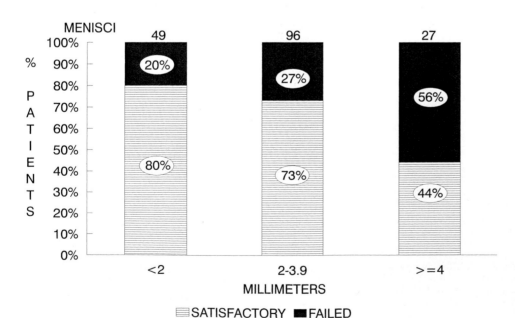

FIGURE 14.27 Rim width versus healing. As meniscal rim width increases, the incidence of repair failure increases.

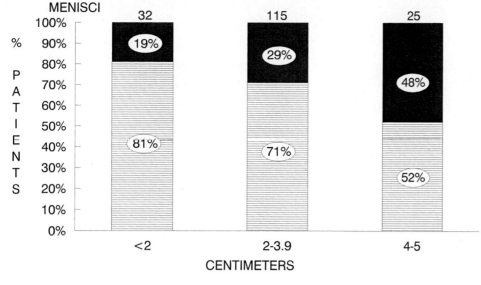

FIGURE 14.28 Length of tear versus healing. The incidence of meniscal healing is inversely correlated with tear length.

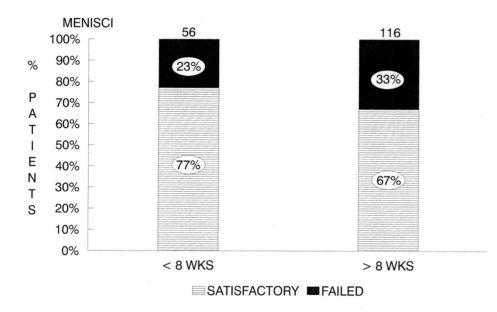

FIGURE 14.29 Time from injury versus healing. Menisci that were repaired within 8 weeks after injury had a 77% satisfactory outcome, whereas older tears had only a 67% satisfactory healing rate.

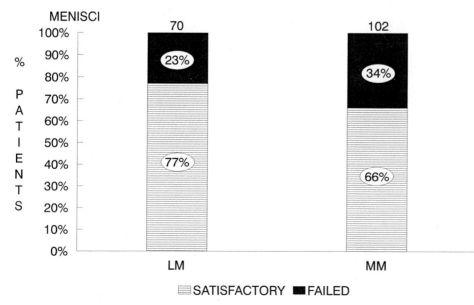

FIGURE 14.30 Side of repair versus healing. Lateral meniscal repairs had a 77% satisfactory healing rate, whereas medial meniscal repairs were only 66% successful.

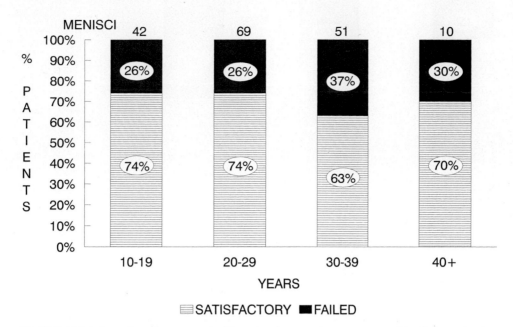

FIGURE 14.31 Age of patient versus healing. Age is not a deterrent to performing meniscal repair. The high failure rate in patients younger than 18 years of age may be related to poor postoperative compliance and a large number of isolated meniscal repairs.

The depth of peripheral vascular penetration of the meniscus decreases after birth until adolescence. In this group of patients, healing rates were not better among the younger patients (Fig. 14.31). Among those between 10 and 19 years of age, satisfactory healing was 74%, compared with 70% in patients 40 years of age and older.

Among patients who had a history of locking, only 59% had a satisfactory result (Fig. 14.32). In contrast, among pa-

tients with no history of locking, 79% had a satisfactory outcome (*p* = .007).

The use of fibrin clot for isolated meniscal repairs in ACL-stable knees improved the healing rate (Fig. 14.33), but because of the small number of repairs, the results were not statistically significant (*p* = .10). Nevertheless, fibrin clot insertion is still strongly recommended for use in isolated meniscal repair.

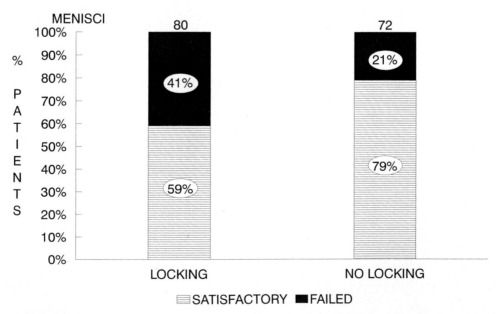

FIGURE 14.32 Among patients with a history of locking, only 59% had a satisfactory result. In contrast, among patients with no history of locking, 79% had a satisfactory outcome (*p* = .007).

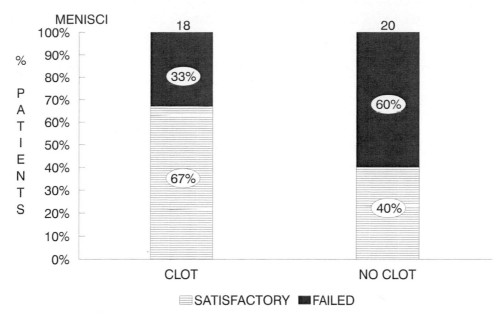

FIGURE 14.33 The use of fibrin clot for isolated meniscal repairs in anterior cruciate ligament–stable knees improved the healing rate.

COMPLICATIONS

No patient had any significant loss of range of motion that could be attributed to meniscal repair. There were no infections in the group. There were two cases of thrombophlebitis. There were no vascular injuries. One patient had partial peroneal nerve palsy during the repair of a displaced bucket-handle tear of a lateral meniscus with an associated proximal fibular fracture. The most anterior suture passed through 25% of the peroneal nerve, resulting in a partial foot

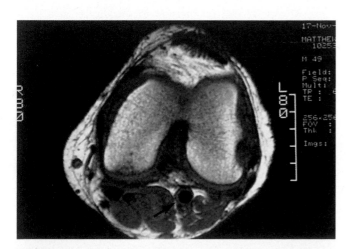

FIGURE 14.34 This magnetic resonance imaging scan demonstrates the intimate association of the popliteal artery and the posterior horn of the lateral meniscus. Without the insertion of a popliteal retractor in back of the posterior horn of the lateral meniscus, the artery can be easily injured. Black arrow indicates popliteal artery.

drop. Seven days later the suture was removed, and the patient went on to a full recovery. A small amount of articular cartilage scuffing may be inherent to the procedure but should be kept to a minimum. Not only may it occur during the movement of instruments through the anterior portals, but also the back ends of the Keith needles may scuff the cartilage as they are pulled out through the posterior incisions.

Small (42) reported a lower incidence of complications after meniscal repair (1.29%) compared with meniscectomy (1.69%), but this may reflect more importantly the experience of the 21 arthroscopists selected for this prospective study. In general, one would anticipate a higher incidence of serious neurovascular complications arising from meniscal repair compared with simple meniscectomy. Note the location of the popliteal artery (Fig. 14.34) lying immediately behind the posterior horn of the lateral meniscus. Unless one is using an all-inside technique with biodegradable devices, this location emphasizes the necessity of making a posterolateral incision and placing a popliteal retractor in back of the posterior horn to facilitate safe needle retrieval.

DISCUSSION

In 1984, I noted a significantly higher incidence of healing in meniscal repairs associated with ACL reconstruction compared with isolated meniscal repairs in ACL-stable knees (43). Subsequently, both Henning and I reported only 50% to 60% satisfactory healing in patients undergoing isolated meniscal repair (before the use of fibrin clot), in contrast to a success rate ranging from 75% to more than 90% among those patients undergoing combined meniscal repair and ACL stabilization (32). Other authors have reported a similar difference between these two groups of patients (31,34). This significant difference possibly can be explained by the following observations. First, the repair site, after ACL stabilization, is protected from the biomechanical forces accompanying anterior tibial subluxation that caused the meniscus tear. Second, ACL surgery results in more intraarticular trauma to the joint and hence more bleeding and fibrin clot formation, which provides an important adjunct to the healing process (44). Moreover, Thomas Tiling (45), from Cologne, Germany, performed biopsies from each side of the tear site in a group of 28 meniscal tears that were less than 12 days old. These biopsies were subjected to histologic and electron microscopic analysis. Biopsies from meniscal tears in ACL-stable knees revealed degenerative changes in 100% of the knees, but no degenerative changes were found in the biopsies of meniscal tears in patients with acute ACL tears.

I consider Tiling's findings as the most important explanation of my results. Also, in the case of isolated meniscal tears, there may be as yet unidentifiable joint configuration and biomechanical abnormalities that may have predisposed the meniscus to tearing, and these same factors may predispose a repaired meniscus to retear. This may account for the increased failure rate seen in the young adolescent group of isolated meniscal repairs. A case in point from my own practice is a 13-year-old girl who presented with bilateral displaced bucket-handle tears of her medial menisci that occurred during two episodes of squatting to pick up objects from the floor. Although one meniscus was repaired, it retore, and a second repair also failed. I used to think that meniscal tears associated with ACL tears were generally more peripheral and, hence, in a more vascular zone, but an analysis of rim widths in the ACL-associated versus the isolated meniscal repairs revealed no difference between the two groups.

The majority of meniscal repairs in one's practice will most likely be associated with torn ACLs. In Henning's series, 92% of meniscal tears were associated with ACL tears, as were 78% in my patient population, 50% in Lanny Johnson's patients, and 49% in Morgan's practice. Most surgeons (12,46,47) believe that, when a patient presents with both a reparable meniscal tear and a torn ACL, meniscal repair and ACL stabilization should be carried out at the same time. Some authors (48,49) have reported good results in a small number of patients whose meniscal repairs were carried out in the presence of ACL-deficient knees. In a long-term follow-up study, DeHaven et al. (50) found a 38% failure rate (6/16) in patients with open meniscal repair and chronic untreated ACL tears.

Henning (51) reported a fourfold reduction in arthritic changes among patients undergoing combined meniscal repair and ACL reconstruction, compared with partial or total meniscectomy and ACL reconstruction. Sommerlath (52) reported a statistically reduced incidence of degenerative arthritis among patients undergoing meniscal repair, compared with a similar group undergoing partial meniscectomy.

Whether there should be an upper age limit for meniscal repair is debatable. Certainly most reparable meniscal tears, such as vertical longitudinal tears, occur in the second and third decades of life, after which tear patterns tend to be more complex and oblique flap tears more prevalent. If a meniscal tear is associated with a torn ACL in an older person, the decision to repair rests with the decision to perform an ACL reconstruction. Among my patients, however, there was no dropoff of successful results with increasing age. In Henning's series, failures increased to 19% in patients older than 30 years of age, in contrast to 10% in patients younger than 30. In older patients, the frequency of mucoid degeneration within the meniscus might make repair tenuous (Fig. 14.35). Complex flap tears of the posterior horn of the lateral meniscus are frequently associated with ACL tears, and an effort should be made to repair them because of the good blood supply in this region, where small blood vessels frequently can be seen traversing to the inner edge of the meniscus. A case in point was a 45-year-old man who twisted his right knee, sustaining an ACL tear combined with a tear of his lateral meniscus. Repair of the lateral meniscus and ACL reconstruction were carried out (Fig. 14.36).

When one is performing inside-out arthroscopic meniscal repair using sutures, a posterior incision should be used to enable safe retrieval of needles. This should be done before the first needle is placed through the meniscus. On the medial side, the sartorial branch of the saphenous nerve passes close to the posteromedial corner of the knee and should be retracted away along with the pes anserinus, which lies posteriorly. On the lateral side, I am aware of several peroneal nerve injuries that most likely occurred because of the absence of a posterolateral incision for needle retrieval. The

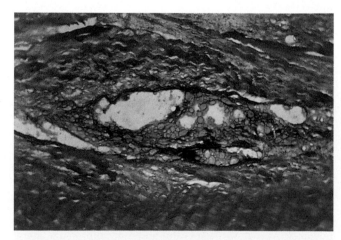

FIGURE 14.35 In older menisci, there is a greater incidence of mucoid degeneration, shown as blue on this colloidal iron stain.

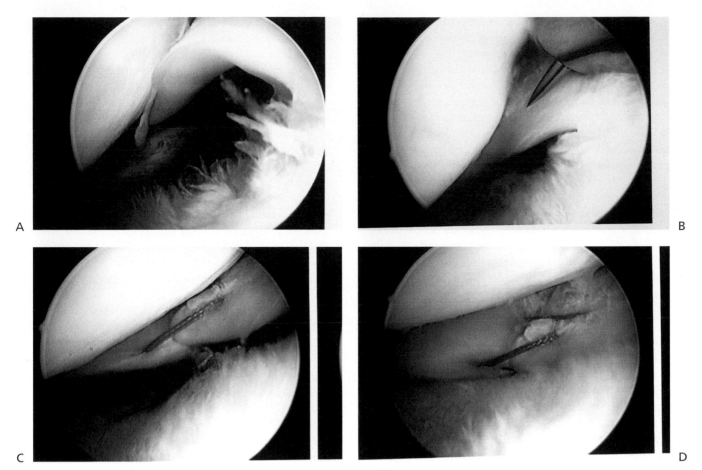

FIGURE 14.36 A: There is a radial oblique displaced flap tear at the posterior horn origin of this right lateral meniscus, a common tear pattern associated with a tear of the anterior cruciate ligament. **B**: With the Henning technique, the first needle pass close to the posterior horn origin reduces the displaced flap. **C**: The first suture, acting similar to a pursestring suture, on both sides of the flap, reduces the torn fragment. **D**: Final view of the repair after a second pursestring suture was placed.

knee should also be kept flexed close to 90 degrees to relax the nerve and move it away from the posterior horn origin of the lateral meniscus. If a tear in this region is to be adequately repaired, then placement of a popliteal retractor in back of the posterior horn is necessary to prevent risk of damage to the popliteal artery. However, I believe that lateral meniscal repair is inadequate if the surgeon does not place sutures in the posterior horn posterior to the popliteus tendon, and I have had failures of lateral meniscal repair in ACL-reconstructed patients. However, Fitzgibbons and Shelbourne (37) reported no known failures in a large series of lateral meniscal repairs with ACL reconstruction done without placing any sutures in the posterior horn of lateral meniscus tears that were reasonably stable.

The principle advantage of a single-needle technique over a double-barrel repair technique is that the former can produce a vertically oriented suture containing more meniscal tissue. Hence, there should be less likelihood of suture pullout and better meniscal tear coaptation, as well as more flexibility in repair technique. Asik et al. (22) and Rimmer et al. (24) found that a vertically oriented suture secures more of the circumferentially oriented collagen bundles than a horizontally placed suture does, and hence provides greater resistance against pullout. Asik's group also found that the weakest technique was knot-end sutures.

Whether one should use absorbable or nonabsorbable suture is also controversial. I believe that absorbable suture does not maintain adequate strength long enough for maturation of the fibrovascular tissue at the repair site to occur. Arnoczky (personal communication) has estimated that it takes 12 to 18 months for a repaired meniscus to regain normal biomechanical strength. Roddecker (53) found that the repaired meniscus only had 33% normal strength at 2 months, and 62% at 6 months after surgery. It would also appear that a meniscus sewn to the capsule by nonabsorbable suture placed by either open or arthroscopic technique behaves biomechanically in a manner similar to a normal meniscus (54). Barrett et al. (20), in a clinical study, showed that permanent suture was better than absorbable suture and that it provided for longer and more stable fixation, permitting more complete maturation and remodeling of the meniscus. Eggli et al. (21) also reported better healing rates with the use of nonabsorbable sutures.

It is difficult to compare different authors' results with meniscal repair when different criteria for healing are used. One should not merely assume that a meniscus is healed in the absence of clinical symptoms. Surgeons who evaluate the results of meniscus repair based on anatomic assessment invariably report poorer satisfactory results compared with surgeons who base their evaluation on clinical criteria. Davis (55) reported that 36% of asymptomatic people older than 45 years of age had grade III tears on MRI. Knowing the precise state of healing of the meniscus helps in intelligently informing a patient to what extent he or she can return to vigorous activities. For example, in an asymptomatic failed repair, the patient should be told to avoid highly competitive contact sports because of the risk of extending the region of nonhealing and creating a symptomatic meniscal tear. Assessment by MRI may be misleading, unless enhanced by gadolinium. Van Trommel et al. (56) reported the use of a noncontrast MRI technique in the evaluation of meniscal repair, which was more accurate than conventional MRI. The presence of type II and III signals in the repaired meniscus may indicate that most meniscal repairs do not heal perfectly, but on the other hand may be a stage of repair represented by a fibrovascular seam at the repair site, giving the false impression of a failure.

Through the precise anatomic assessment of results done in Henning's and my patients, we learned that failure of the meniscus to heal is not necessarily accompanied by symptoms of pain or catching. Two thirds of these anatomic failures had no accompanying symptoms of failure. The patients were advised to refrain from contact sports and to avoid extreme flexion of their knee. In contrast, Morgan et al. (47) reported no failures of meniscal repair among 62 asymptomatic patients with stable or reconstructed ACLs who underwent second-look arthroscopy, using criteria for healing similar to Henning's. Before the use of fibrin clot, according to Henning, the success rate of re-repair of the meniscus was only 10%, but substantially higher healing rates are now possible with the use of clot. Henning has routinely inserted fibrin clot, which has been shown to contain platelet-derived growth factor, fibronectin, and fibroblast growth factor, into the tear site during meniscal repair since early 1986. Because meniscal repair is so much more successful when it is done in conjunction with ACL reconstruction, I prefer to use clot only in cases of isolated meniscal repair. An exception is the use of clot for complex chronic tears associated with ACL reconstructions. Henning (57) reported preliminary results using clot in isolated meniscal repairs and found that the incidence of satisfactory healing rose from 59% to 92%; however, this difference was not statistically significant owing to the small number of patients. Clot insertion into the tear site has been the main technical problem with its use. Although prototype clot introducers are now becoming commercially available and should lessen this problem, sewing the clot into the tear site works well.

The type and location of the tear also influence results. In my own hands, repairs of single longitudinal nondisplaced tears have done better than those of displaced bucket-handle tears. Henning made an interesting unpublished observation that when both sides of vertical longitudinal tears were rasped, the results were statistically significantly better. He found an 18% failure rate when only the rim side of the tear was rasped, but the rate was only 3% when both sides were rasped.

Rosenberg (46) achieved a 92% incidence of clinically good or excellent results in meniscal repairs with rim widths less than 3 mm and recommended that meniscal repair be confined to tears in the peripheral one third of the meniscus. However, Henning (57) reported significant healing rates in tears with rim widths of 4 to 6 mm and also in complex tears of the meniscus. Johnson et al. (58) reported the findings of a long-term outcome study of Charles Henning's patients and found a clinical success rate of 76% (38/50) in isolated arthroscopic meniscal repairs, with an average follow-up of 10 years 9 months. Noyes and Barber-Westin (34), in a study of arthroscopic meniscal repair of tears extending into the avascular zone in patients 40 years of age and older, reported that only 12% of patients rating their overall knee condition as fair/poor. In a previous study, Rubman et al. (59) recommended repair of meniscal tears extending into the avascular region for selected patients, including those in their 20s and 30s and highly competitive athletes. Buseck and Noyes (60), in an evaluation of meniscal repairs after ACL reconstruction, found that the only factor that had a statistically significant impact on the rate of healing was rim width.

Factors that may dissuade some surgeons from attempting to repair more complex meniscal tears are surgical inexperience or a lack of surgical skill. With the advent of newer biodegradable all-inside devices, the technique of meniscal repair has become faster and easier, and more surgeons are resorting to repair. However, if surgeons choose to excise a reparable meniscus, they are denying patients the chance of a better long-term result.

CONCLUSIONS

Meniscal tears with 3 mm or less rim size can be repaired with a high success rate. In vertical longitudinal tears with greater rim width (i.e., "white–white" tears), it is still reasonable to perform meniscal repair despite a lower success rate. An attempt to repair meniscal tears that initially appear irreparable should be made if the tear is associated with a torn ACL, where the success rate is greater than 75%. More caution should be used with isolated repairs, but better results can be obtained in those cases with the use of fibrin clot. Increasing tear length correlates with an increasing failure rate. Lateral meniscal repairs do better than medial repairs. Posteromedial or posterolateral incisions and use of a popliteal retractor should be part of every inside-out repair procedure that employs sutures, in order to protect the popliteal neurovascular structures.

Meniscal repair technique using sutures has been emphasized in this chapter, but there are other good alternative techniques that can be used. In Chapter 15, Dr. Don Johnson reviews meniscus repair with the use of biodegradable devices. However, I believe that meniscal tears repaired with sutures represent the gold standard. With the advent of these quick and easier techniques using biodegradable devices, it is possible that there will be a higher failure rate compared with suturing alone. It is my personal recommendation that these new devices be used as a hybrid technique, employing them for tears at the posterior horn origin and suturing the remainder of the tear, especially long tears.

REFERENCES

1. Annandale T. An operation for displaced semilunar cartilage. *Br Med J* 1885;779.
2. Sutton JB. *Ligaments, their nature and morphology,* 2nd ed. London: HK Lewis, 1897.
3. King D. The healing of semilunar cartilages. *J Bone Joint Surg* 1936;18:333–342.
4. King D. The function of semilunar cartilages. *J Bone Joint Surg* 1936;18:1069–1076.
5. Ikeuchi H. Surgery under arthroscopic control. Proceedings of the Societe Internationale d'Arthroscopie, 1975. *Rheumatology* 1976;[Special Issue]:57–62.
6. DeHaven KE, Hales W. Peripheral meniscus repair: an alternative to meniscectomy. *Orthop Transact* 1981;5:399–400.
7. Price CT, Allen WC. Ligament repair in the knee with preservation of the meniscus. *J Bone Joint Surg* 1978;60:61–65.
8. Wirth CR. Meniscus repair. *Clin Orthop* 1981;157:153–160.
9. Cassidy RE, Schaffer AJ. Repair of peripheral meniscus tears: a preliminary report. *Am J Sports Med* 1981;9:209–214.
10. Hamberg P, Gillquist J, Lysholm J. Suture of new and old peripheral meniscus tears. *J Bone Joint Surg Am* 1983;65:193–197.
11. Henning CE. Arthroscopic repair of meniscus tears. *Orthopedics* 1983;6:1130–1132.
12. Scott GA, Jolly BL, Henning CE. Combined posterior incision and arthroscopic intra-articular repair of the meniscus. *J Bone Joint Surg Am* 1986;68:847–861.
13. Clancy WG Jr, Graf BK. Arthroscopic meniscal repair. *Orthopedics* 1983;6:1125–1128.
14. Johnson LL. *Meniscus mender II.* Technical bulletin. Okemos, MI: Instrument Makar, Inc.
15. Barber FA, Stone RG. Meniscal repair: an arthroscopic technique. *J Bone Joint Surg Br* 1985;67:39–41.
16. Warren RF. Arthroscopic meniscus repair. *Arthroscopy* 1985;1:170–172.
17. Rosenberg T, Scott S, Paulos L. Arthroscopic surgery: repair of peripheral detachment of the meniscus. *Contemp Orthop* 1985;10:43–50.
18. Morgan CD, Casscells SW. Arthroscopic meniscal repair: a safe approach to the posterior horns. *Arthroscopy* 1986;2:3–12.
19. Cannon WD, Vittori JM. Meniscal repair. In: Aichroth PM, Cannon WD, eds. *Knee surgery current practice.* London: Martin Dunitz, 1992.
20. Barrett GR, Richardson K, Ruff CG, et al. The effect of suture type on meniscus repair. a clinical analysis. *Am J Knee Surg* 1997;10:2–9.
21. Eggli S, Wegmuller H, Kosina J, et al. Long-term results of arthroscopic meniscal repair: an analysis of isolated tears. *Am J Sports Med* 1995;23:715–720.
21a. Henning CE, Yearout KM, Vequist SW, et al. Use of the fascia sheath coverage and exogenous fibrin clot in the treatment of complex meniscal tears. *Am J Sports Med* 1991;19:626–631.
22. Asik M, Sener N, Akpinar S, et al. Strength of different meniscus suturing techniques. *Knee Surg Sports Traumatol Arthrosc* 1997; 5:80–83.
23. Kohn D, Siebert W. Meniscus suture techniques: a comparative biomechanical cadaver study. *Arthroscopy* 1989;5:324–327.
24. Rimmer MG, Nawana NS, Keene GC, et al. Failure strengths of different meniscal suturing techniques. *Arthroscopy* 1995;11: 146–150.
25. Richie JR, Miller MD, Bents RT, et al. Meniscal repair in the goat model: the use of healing adjuncts on central tears and the role of magnetic resonance arthrography in repair evaluation. *Am J Sports Med*;26:278–284.
26. Okuda K, Ochi M, Shu N, et al. Meniscal rasping for repair of meniscal tear in the avascular zone. *Arthroscopy* 1999;15:281–286.
27. Zhang Z, Arnold JA, Williams T, et al. Repair is by trephination and suturing of longitudinal injuries in the avascular area of the meniscus in goats. *Am J Sports Med* 1995;23:35–41.
28. Fox JM, Rintz KG, Ferkel RD. Trephination of incomplete meniscal tears. *Arthroscopy* 1993;9:451–455.
29. Shelbourne KD, Rask BP. The sequelae of salvaged nondegenerative peripheral vertical medial meniscus tears with anterior cruciate ligament reconstruction. *Arthroscopy* 2001;17:270–274.
30. Talley MC, Grana WA. Treatment of partial meniscal tears identified during anterior cruciate ligament reconstruction with limited synovial abrasion. *Arthroscopy* 2000;16:6–10.
31. Barber FA, Click SD. Meniscus repair rehabilitation with concurrent anterior cruciate reconstruction. *Arthroscopy* 1997;13: 433–437.
32. Cannon WD, Vittori JM. The incidence of healing in arthroscopic meniscal repairs in anterior cruciate ligament-reconstructed knees versus stable knees. *Am J Sports Med* 1992;20: 176–181.
33. Jensen NC, Riis J, Robertsen K, et al. Arthroscopic repair of the ruptured meniscus: 1 to 6.3 years follow-up. *Arthroscopy* 1994;10: 211–214.
34. Noyes FR, Barber-Westin SD. Arthroscopic repair of meniscus tears extending into the avascular zone with or without anterior cruciate ligament reconstruction in patients 40 years of age and older. *Arthroscopy* 2000;16:822–829.
35. Warren RF. Meniscectomy and repair in the anterior cruciate ligament-deficient patient. *Clin Orthop* 1999;252:55–63.
36. Asahina S, Muneta T, Yamamoto H. Arthroscopic meniscal repair in conjunction with anterior cruciate ligament reconstruction: factors affecting the healing rate. *Arthroscopy* 1986;12: 541–545.
37. Fitzgibbons RE, Shelbourne KD. Aggressive nontreatment of lateral meniscal tears in anterior cruciate ligament reconstruction. *Am J Sports Med* 1995;23:156–159.
38. Rodeo SA. Technique of outside in repair. In: Cannon WD, ed. *Arthroscopic meniscal repair.* AAOS monograph. Rosemont, IL: American Academy of Orthopaedic Surgeons, 1999:35–37.
39. Morgan CD. The "all-inside" meniscus repair. *Arthroscopy* 1991; 7:181–186.
40. Barber FA. Accelerated rehabilitation for meniscal repairs. *Arthroscopy* 1994;10:206–210.

41. Mariani PP, Santori N, Adriani E, et al. Accelerated rehabilitation after arthroscopic meniscal repair: a clinical and magnetic resonance imaging evaluation. *Arthroscopy* 1986;12:680–686.

42. Small NC. Complications in arthroscopic surgery performed by experienced arthroscopists. *Arthroscopy* 1988;4:215–221.

43. Cannon WD. *Arthroscopic meniscal repair as related to ligamentous instability.* Presented at American College of Surgeons meeting, October 24, 1984, San Francisco, CA.

44. Arnoczky SP, Warren RF, Spivak JM. Meniscal repair using an exogenous fibrin clot - an experimental study in dogs. *J Bone Joint Surg Am* 1988;70:1209–1220.

45. Tiling T. Personal communication.

46. Rosenberg TD, Scott SM, Coward DB, et al. Arthroscopic meniscal repair evaluated with repeat arthroscopy. *Arthroscopy* 1986;2:14–20.

47. Morgan CD, Wojtys EM, Casscells CD, et al. Arthroscopic meniscus repair evaluated by second-look arthroscopy. *Am J Sports Med* 1991;19:632–638.

48. Hanks GA, Gause TM, Sebastianelli WJ, et al. Repair of peripheral meniscal tears: open versus arthroscopic technique. *Am J Sports Med* 1991;7:72–77.

49. Sommerlath K. The prognosis of repaired and intact menisci in unstable knees: a comparative study. *Arthroscopy* 1988;4:93–95.

50. DeHaven KE, Black KP, Griffiths HS. Meniscus repair. *Orthop Trans* 1987;2:469.

51. Lynch MA, Henning CE, Glick KR Jr. Knee joint surface changes: long-term follow-up meniscus tear treatment in stable anterior cruciate ligament reconstruction. *Clin Orthop* 1983;172: 148–153.

52. Sommerlath KG. Results of meniscal repair and partial meniscectomy in stable knees. *Int Orthop (SICOT)* 1991;15: 347–350.

53. Roeddecker K, Muennich U, Nagelschmidt M. Meniscal healing: a biomechanical study. *J Surg Res* 1994;56:20–27.

54. Baratz ME, Fu FH, Mengato R. Meniscal tears: the effect of meniscectomy and of repair on intraarticular contact areas and stress in the human knee. A preliminary report. *Am J Sports Med* 1986;14:270–275.

55. Boden SD, Davis DO, Dina TS, et al. A prospective and blinded investigation of magnetic resonance imaging of the knee. *Clin Orthop* 1992;282:177–184.

56. van Trommel MF, Potter HG, Ernberg LA, et al. The use of noncontrast magnetic resonance imaging in evaluating meniscal repair: comparison with conventional arthrography. *Arthroscopy* 1998;14:2–8.

57. Henning CE, Lynch MA, Yearout KM, et al. Arthroscopic meniscal repair using an exogenous fibrin clot. *Clin Orthop* 1990;252:64–72.

58. Johnson MJ, Lucas GL, Dusek JH, et al. Isolated arthroscopic meniscal repair: a long-term outcome study (more than 10 years). *Am J Sports Med* 1999;27:44–49.

59. Rubman MH, Noyes FR, Barber-Westin SD. Arthroscopic repair of meniscal tears that extend into the avascular zone:. a review of 198 single and complex tears. *Am J Sports Med* 1998;26:87–95.

60. Buseck MS, Noyes FR. Arthroscopic evaluation of meniscal repairs after anterior cruciate ligament reconstruction and immediate motion. *Am J Sports Med* 1991;19:489–494.

MENISCUS REPAIR WITH IMPLANTABLE DEVICES

DONALD H. JOHNSON

BIOABSORBABLE DEVICES

The original meniscal arrow (Fig. 15.1) was introduced in 1993 as an alternative to traditional suturing techniques for meniscal repair (1). It was released for clinical use in North America in 1996. Since then, several competitive products have been introduced to deal with the problems encountered with the original arrow. The principal advantage of these devices is that the difficult-to-repair posterior horn segment may be easily and quickly repaired with an all-inside technique. This also potentially shortens the operating time, because no posterior incision is required to retrieve and tie the sutures.

These devices may be evaluated on the basis of their material properties, load to failure, mechanism of failure, and clinical results.

Material Properties: The Polymers

The bioabsorbable implants are made from polyglycolic acid (PGA), polylevolactic acid (PLLA), racemic polylactic acid (PDLLA), and polydiaxonone (PDS). All these devices degrade into carbon dioxide and water. PLLA is more crystalline and takes longer to degrade than PDLLA does. The degradation occurs most rapidly near the center of the implant and progresses outward, producing a mantle of polymer on the outside. In bone, PGA has been associated with a more lytic reaction around the device. The device may be reinforced with fiber to increase the strength. The device fragments during the resorption but does not become a soft, jelly-like mass.

Not all of these devices are created equal. The original arrow was made with self-reinforced PLLA. The barbs are made by cutting the PLLA, which potentially can produce a stress riser (Fig. 15.1). The arrow was shown to have the same pullout strength as the horizontal loop suture (2,3). In an early presentation of second-look arthroscopies from Albrect-Olsen et al. (1), the arrows had been absorbed by 6 months, and 26 of 30 patients had healed completely. The BioStinger is also made from PLLA (Fig. 15.2). The Mitek anchor is made from both PDS and nonabsorbable Prolene. Arthrotek has used Lactosorb (a poly-L-lactide copolymer) in a staple configuration that is resorbed in 9 to 15 months. The SD Sorb Meniscus Staple is made of a copolymer of PGA/PLLA (18%/82%). The Dart is also made of a copolymer of 70% PLLA and 30% PDLA.

Load to Failure and Mechanism of Failure

Barber and Herbert (4) performed a pullout study of the various fixators on fresh porcine menisci. A peripheral tear was produced in the meniscus and repaired by a variety of techniques. The inner rim was pulled by a materials testing machine at 5 mm/min until failure. The load to failure and the mechanism of failure were noted. The types of repairs performed were as follows:

- Repair using single and double vertical suture of 2-0 Mersilene
- Repair using single and double horizontal 2-0 Mersilene suture
- Bionix arrow hand and crossbow
- BioStinger (Linvatec)
- T-fix (Smith and Nephew)
- SDsorb Meniscal Staple (Surgical Dynamics)
- Clearfix Screw (Innovasive Devices)
- Mitek Meniscal repair system
- Biomet staple
- Arthrex dart (two devices)

The data from Barber and Herbert's study are presented in Table 15.1.

Clinical Results

Kurzweil (5), at the Arthroscopy Association of North America 1999 fall course in San Diego, discussed his results and commented on his failures of repairs with the use of the bioabsorbable arrow. The 5 failures in the 40 patients all occurred in the first 10 patients. He believed that

D. Johnson: Sports Medicine Clinic, Carleton University, and University of Ottawa, Canada.

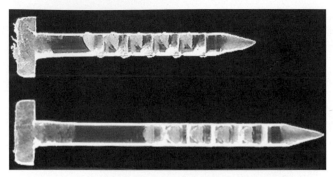

FIGURE 15.1 The Bionix meniscal arrow made from self reinforced polylevolactic acid (PLLA). The photograph shows how the meniscal arrow is cut to produce the barbs, which may lead to stress risers.

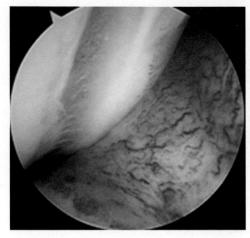

FIGURE 15.3 A longitudinal groove in the articular surface of the femur caused by the prominent head of the fixator. (Photo courtesy of Alan Barber.)

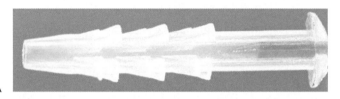

A

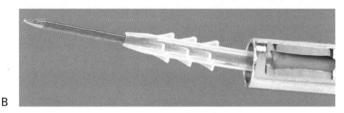

B

FIGURE 15.2 A and **B**: The BioStinger (Linvatec, Largo, FL) is a cannulated polylevolactic acid (PLLA) device produced from a mold. The cannulation makes placement of the device more accurate and facilitates reduction of the tear.

this result was related to the early learning curve. He found that two failures were caused by flexion injuries in the first 3 to 5 weeks. Three were caused by large peripheral bucket tears that were displaced at the time of diagnosis. Based on his experience, he suggested that there should be no accelerated rehabilitation, as has been used after traditional meniscal repair, and no flexion or squatting for 4 months (6). He suggested that the repair techniques of suture and arrows be combined for large displaced bucket tears. Also the knee should be cycled after the repair to make sure that the bucket tear does not redislocate into the notch. Furthermore, bioabsorbable devices should be avoided in red–red tears, in the popliteal tendon region, in small tight knees, and in large displaced bucket-handle tears.

Reported results with meniscal arrows, including second-look arthroscopies, from Albrecht-Olsen's group were

TABLE 15.1 COMPARISON OF LOAD TO FAILURE AND MECHANISM OF FAILURE OF MENISCAL REPAIR

Technique	Mean Load to Failure	Mechanism of Failure
Single vertical Mersilene suture	81 N	Break at knot
Double vertical Mersilene suture	113 N	Break at knot
Horizontal Mersilene suture	61 N	Break at knot
Bionix arrow (hand or gun)	33 N	Pull through inner rim
BioStinger	57 N	Pull through inner rim
SD Sorb Staple	31 N	Pull through outer rim
T-fix	50 N	Various
Clear fix	32 N	Various
Mitek	30 N	Pull through inner rim
Biomet staple	27 N	Staple breakage
Arthrex dart	61 N	Pull through inner rim

From Barber FA, Herbert MA. Meniscal repair devices. *Arthroscopy* 2000;16:613–618, with permission.

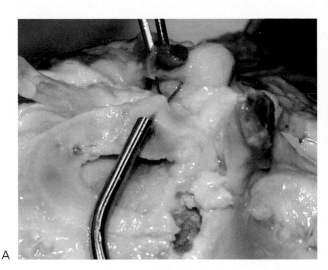

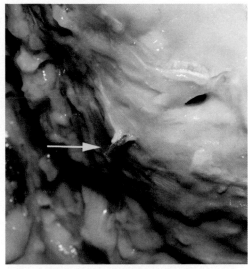

A

B

FIGURE 15.4 A: Cadaver specimen demonstrating a cannula with the wire penetrating posterior through the posterior horn of the lateral meniscus and into the popliteal artery. **B**: Cadaver specimen demonstrating a fixator that is protruding into the soft tissue of the medial aspect of the knee.

comparable to the results with traditional suturing techniques (1,7). Hurel et al. (8) presented clinical data demonstrating a success rate (88%) that was similar to that of suture repair.

As often occurs with the introduction of a new device or technique, complications that are specific to these devices have been reported. Although it is likely that each of these devices will have unique problems, the meniscal arrows, owing to their longer time on the market, were the first to have unique complications reported. Most alarming is the potential for damage to the articular surface (Fig. 15.3). In the October 2000 issue of the *Journal of Arthroscopy,* there were three separate case reports of similar damage to the articular surface of the femur caused by fixators (9–11). Migration and cystic hematoma formation have also been noted (12–14). A significant additional risk is penetration of the cannulated wire or arrow posteriorly, with injury to the neurovascular structures or other soft tissues (Figs. 15.4). If the procedure is perceived as simple, there may be overextension of the indications and complications that result from their inappropriate use.

PREFERRED TECHNIQUE

Because of its high holding power and potential to be countersunk into the meniscus, the BioStinger is my preferred implant for meniscal repair. The steps in its use are outlined in detail in this chapter. Each of the available implants has a learning curve associated with its use, as well as potential specific complications. Any surgeon using a meniscal repair implant should be familiar not only with the general principles of meniscal repair but also with technique and potential pitfalls associated with that device.

Preparing and Repairing the Meniscus

The tear should be initially probed to determine whether it is suitable for repair. The edges of the tear should be debrided of fibrous tissue with a rasp or a small shaver, as with traditional arthroscopic or open techniques (15–19). A technique of stimulation of the meniscal synovial border with electrocautery was described by Pavlovich (20,21). The principle is to lightly "burn" the synovium to produce a healing response (Fig. 15.5). Trephination may also improve healing rates in tears that are more central (22).

The sutures and bioabsorbable devices must be placed accurately to reduce the tear and hold it until it is healed. The common approach to large bucket-handle tears is to use sutures in the middle segment to reduce and hold the bucket tear and then to use the bioabsorbable devices in the difficult-to-repair posterior horn region. This has been termed a "hy-

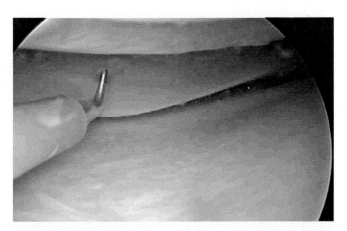

FIGURE 15.5 A monopolar electrode is used to stimulate the synovium at the tear.

brid" repair. Many of the implants have varied lengths. It is crucial to select the appropriate length to gain satisfactory fixation while not penetrating excessively into the periarticular soft tissues. The selection of a specific implant should be based on the experience of the surgeon. The technique for my preferred system is outlined in the following sections.

Technique of Meniscal Repair Using the BioStinger

The appropriate length of BioStinger is selected, usually 13 mm, and loaded on the cannulated wire of the delivery unit. The insertion tool is introduced into the joint through the appropriate portal, typically ipsilateral to the tear for use in the posterior horn, or from the contralateral side for use in the middle third of the meniscus. The cannula is placed against the meniscus, and then 2 mm of wire is delivered into the torn fragment. The fragment is then reduced to the peripheral rim (Figs. 15.6).

The delivery of the meniscus fixator is done with a manual gun. This device has three actions. The first pull advances the wire 2 mm into the meniscus. This can then be used to manipulate the meniscus into a reduced position. After the torn fragment is reduced, the cannulated wire is advanced into the rim by a second pull on the gun. The third pull on the trigger advances the fixator along the guide

wire (Figs. 15.7A,B). The BioStinger can be felt to ratchet into the meniscus.

To prevent bending of the cannulated wire, firm pressure must be exerted on the cannula to keep it against the meniscus. The cannula is backed up 5 mm, and the head of the BioStinger is inspected to be sure that it is countersunk under the surface of the meniscus (Fig. 15.7C). The head of the BioStinger must be countersunk to prevent gouging of the articular surface of the femur (Fig. 15.8). The low-profile head of the Linvatec BioStinger, the headless Innovasive screw, and the headless meniscal dart of Arthrex were designed to address this problem of the prominent head of the arrow.

The advantages of the BioStinger can be summarized as follows:

- Low-profile head
- Molded PLLA construction
- Four rows of prongs
- Cannulated insertion similar to inside-out suture repair
- Same load to failure as the horizontal suture
- Fast and easy to perform

The BioStinger's disadvantages are as follows:

- Expensive
- Damage to articular surface resulting from prominent head

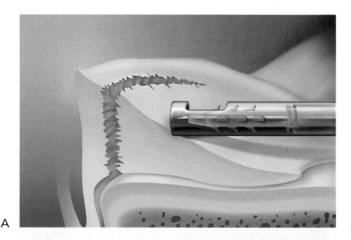

A

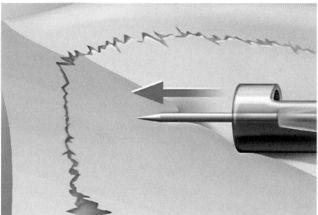

B

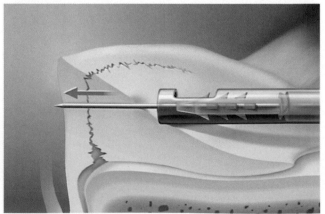

C

FIGURE 15.6 A: The cannula is placed against the meniscus 4 to 6 mm from the tear. **B**: Two millimeters of cannulated wire is delivered into the torn fragment. **C**: The fragment is then reduced to the peripheral rim and the wire is advanced into the periphery.

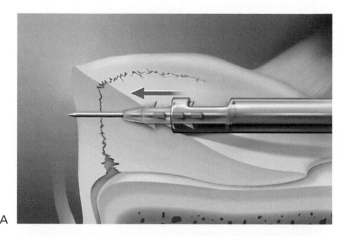

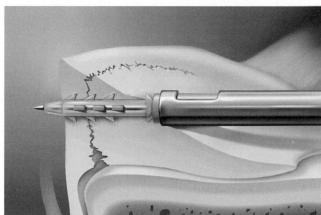

A

B

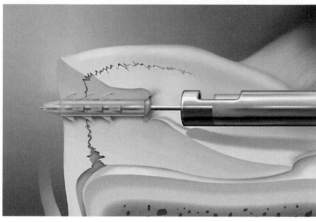

C

FIGURE 15.7 A through **C**: The BioStinger is inserted into the meniscus by the third pull of the trigger on the gun. The BioStinger can be felt to ratchet into the meniscus. The cannula is backed up 5 mm, and the head of the BioStinger is inspected to be sure that it is countersunk under the surface of the meniscus.

- Damage to neurovascular structures caused by overpenetration with the BioStinger
- Learning curve for insertion at the correct angle and position in the meniscus
- Difficult to use with a tight knee
- Prolonged time for resorption of the PLLA material

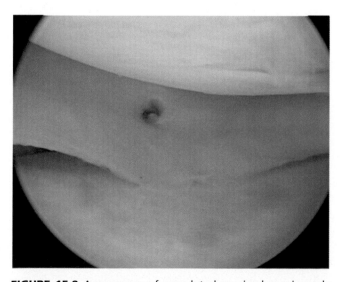

FIGURE 15.8 Appearance of completed meniscal repair made with the use of a BioStinger that has been countersunk.

Relative Contraindications for the Use of Meniscal Fixators

There are several contraindications for the use of meniscal fixators:

- Peripheral tear at the meniscal synovial junction. The fixator must have at least 3 mm of tissue to grasp.
- Lateral meniscal tear at the popliteus junction. This is an open space around the tendon that requires sutures to approximate the tissue.
- Chronic displaced bucket-handle tear. Such a tear may be repaired with a hybrid technique of sutures and fixators.
- Small, tight knee in young patient. It is difficult to insert the cannula under the condyle and into the correct position on the meniscus. The long needles of the sutures can be bent and directed into the correct position.

SUMMARY

Meniscus repair in a suitable patient with an appropriate tear is efficacious. Bioabsorbable devices should be used judiciously and, in large tears, in combination with sutures. At the present time, it is not known how much fixation is required to allow a torn meniscus to heal; consequently, any of the devices may work. The stimulation of the synovium with subsequent bleeding and production of a fibrin clot may be all that is necessary to promote healing of the meniscal tear (23). The final outcome of the procedure is judged by the clinical result.

My current approach is to use nonabsorbable sutures from inside-out, with a separate incision to retrieve the sutures and tie them over the capsule. I use the bioabsorbable fixators in the posterior region, which is difficult to access. If the tear is small (2 cm), I may use the fixators alone.

Above all, do no harm. Remember that it's not the arrow, but the Indian!

REFERENCES

1. Albrecht-Olsen PM, Kristensen G, Tormala P. Meniscus bucket handle fixation with an absorbable Biofix tack: development of a new technique. *Knee Surg Sports Traumatol Arthrosc* 1993;1: 104–106.
2. Albrecht-Olsen PM, Lind T, Kristensen G, et al. Failure strength of a new meniscus arrow repair technique: biomechanical comparison with horizontal suture. *Arthroscopy* 1997;13:183–187.
3. Dervin GF, Downing KJW, Keene GCR, et al. Failure strength of suture versus biodegradable arrow for meniscus repair: an in vitro study. *Arthroscopy* 1997;3:296–300.
4. Barber FA, Herbert MA. Meniscal repair devices. *Arthroscopy* 2000;16:613–618.
5. Kurzweil P. Personal communication, 1999.
6. Barber FA, Click CD. Meniscus repair rehabilitation with concurrent anterior cruciate ligament reconstruction. *Arthroscopy* 1997;13:433–437.
7. Albrecht-Olsen P, Kristensen G, Burgaard P, et al. The arrow versus horizontal suture in arthroscopic meniscus repair: a prospective randomized study with arthroscopic evaluation. *Knee Surg Sports Traumatol Arthrosc* 1999;7:268–273.
8. Hurel C, Mertens F, Verdonk R. Biofix resorbable meniscus arrow for meniscal ruptures: results of a 1-year follow-up. *Knee Surg Sports Traumatol Arthrosc* 2000;8:46–52.
9. Anderson K, Marx RG, Hannafin J, et al. Chondral injury following meniscal repair with a biodegradable implant. *Arthroscopy* 2000;16:749–753.
10. Ross G, Grabill J, McDevitt E. Chondral injury after meniscal repair with bioabsorbable arrows. *Arthroscopy* 2000;16:754–756.
11. Seil R, Rupp S, Dienst M, et al. Chondral lesions after arthroscopic meniscus repair using meniscus arrows. *Arthroscopy* 2000;16:E17.
12. Hechtman KS, Uribe JW. Cystic hematoma formation following use of a biodegradable arrow for meniscal repair. *Arthroscopy* 1999;15:207–210.
13. Ganko A, Engebretsen L. Subcutaneous migration of meniscal arrows after failed meniscus repair: a report of two cases. *Am J Sports Med* 2000;28;252–253.
14. Iannotti S, Goldberg MJ, Richmond JC. Subcutaneous migration of bioabsorbable meniscal arrows. *Am J Knee Surg* 2001;14: 122–124.
15. Morgan CD. The "all inside" meniscal repair. *Arthroscopy* 1991; 7:120–125.
16. DeHaven KE. Decision making factors in the treatment of meniscal lesions. *Clin Orthop* 1990;252:49–54.
17. Johnson LL. Meniscus repair: the outside-in technique. In: Jackson DW, ed. *Reconstructive knee surgery.* New York: Raven Press, 1995.
18. Money MF, Rosenberg TD. Meniscus repair: the inside-out technique. In: Jackson DW, ed. *Reconstructive knee surgery.* New York: Raven Press, 1995.
19. Rodeo S, Warren K. Meniscal repair using the outside to inside technique. *Clin Sports Med* 1996;15:469–481.
20. Pavlovich RI. Hi-frequency electrical cautery stimulation in the treatment of displaced meniscal tears. *Arthroscopy* 1998;14; 566–571.
21. Pavlovich R, Strobel M, Vazquez-Vela G, et al. Basic science on hi-frequency currents in arthroscopic knee surgery. *Am J Knee Surg* 1999;12:176–179.
22. Zhongnan A, Arnold JA. Trephination and suturing of avascular meniscal tears: a clinical study of the trephination procedure. *Arthroscopy* 1996;12:726–731.
23. Port J, Jackson DW, Lee TQ, et al. Meniscal repair supplemented with exogenous fibrin clot and autogenous cultured marrow cells in the goat model. *Am J Sports Med* 1996;24:547–555.

MENISCUS REPLACEMENT: ALLOGRAFTS AND COLLAGEN SCAFFOLDING

CHRISTOPHER K. JONES
WALTER R. SHELTON

The meniscus is vital to normal knee function, and knees that undergo total or partial loss of the meniscus are at risk for development of degenerative arthritis (1). Recent research has been focused on replacement and regeneration of menisci. Meniscus allografts heal and appear to function in a load-sharing manner. Collagen scaffolds may regenerate a meniscus-like structure using the patient's own tissue without the potential for disease transmission or immunologic incompatibility.

FUNCTIONS OF THE MENISCUS

The meniscus serves vital functions that are crucial to normal functioning of the knee, primarily load dissemination and shock absorption. The lateral meniscus carries 70% of the load of the lateral compartment, while load is shared equally between the articular cartilage and meniscus in the medial compartment (2,3). Meniscectomy can decrease contact between the femoral condyle and tibia plateau by more than 50% while doubling peak contact pressures (4–8). This mechanical alteration leads to stress concentrations surpassing failure levels of articular cartilage, resulting in shearing and fissuring and a degenerative joint.

The meniscus also has a secondary role in knee stability. Whereas meniscectomy in a stable knee does not produce instability, in the anterior cruciate ligament (ACL)–deficient knee medial meniscectomy results in a 10% increase in anterior translation, and concomitant lateral meniscectomy causes an additional 10% increase (8,9).

Additional functions of the menisci include joint lubrication, enhancing articular cartilage nutrition, and a role in proprioception. Every effort should be made to repair a torn meniscus if possible, but after total meniscectomy restoration of stress distribution can be achieved only by allograft or meniscus regeneration.

The ideal patient for consideration for meniscus replacement or regeneration should be young (less than 45 years of age), with well preserved articular cartilage and pain in the knee corresponding to the missing meniscus. Most knees are asymptomatic for several years after total meniscectomy and consideration of major knee surgery in a patient who has no pain is debatable. On the other hand, waiting to do a meniscus allograft until the knee has articular erosions to bone or severe blunting of the femoral condyle will result in failure of the meniscus allograft due to abrasive wear.

MENISCUS ALLOGRAFTS
Procurement and Processing

Early investigators, along with the evolving science of transplantation immunology, led to the development of modern tissue banks that provide a supply of high-quality allogeneic tissue for orthopaedic reconstructions. Procurement guidelines developed by the American Association of Tissue Banks ensure the quality and sterility of the allograft tissue (10). Potential donors must pass a detailed medical, social, and sexual history questionnaire completed by the next of kin or life partner. Any history of exposure to communicable diseases, reports of unprotected sexual contacts, drug use, neurologic diseases, autoimmune diseases, collagen disorders, or metabolic diseases will disqualify the individual as a donor.

A detailed physical examination, aerobic and anaerobic blood and tissue cultures, and blood tests to detect antibodies to the human immunodeficiency virus (HIV) types 1 and 2, hepatitis B surface antigen, hepatitis C antibodies, syphilis antibodies, and human T-cell lymphotropic virus antibodies are performed. A window of vulnerability between infection with a virus and production of detectable antibodies by the

C. K. Jones and W. R Shelton: Mississippi Sports Medicine and Orthopedic Center, Jackson, Mississippi.

donor exists. In the case of HIV, this window may be as short as 19 days but can last as long as 6 months.

Tissue harvest for musculoskeletal grafts takes place within a few hours after death of the donor, usually after other organ procurement teams have completed their tasks. Harvesting can be aseptic or clean. With an aseptic harvest, sterility of the graft is maintained throughout harvest and processing; a clean harvest requires secondary sterilization. After harvest, grafts are cooled and rapidly transported to the tissue bank.

Sterilization

All allografts should come with the highest possible assurance that they are free of pathogens. Unfortunately, most of the methods by which surgical materials are sterilized are unsuitable for use on human tissue. Heat and high doses of γ-radiation (greater than 3.0 mrad) are effective but weaken the collagen structure (11). The most common method of ensuring graft sterility is to adhere to sterile techniques during harvest, transport, and processing. The meniscus is soaked in antibiotic solution at 4°C for at least 1 hour, and multiple cultures are obtained during processing. Low-dose γ-radiation (2.0 to 3.0 mrad) may be used as an adjunct.

Despite measures to maintain graft sterility and extensive testing of the donor tissue, the potential for HIV or hepatitis transmission contamination remains because of the window of vulnerability. Buck et al. (12) calculated the risk of HIV transmission in properly screened and tested donors to be 1 in 1,600,000. One reported instance in which HIV was transferred from an allograft to a donor (13) occurred in 1985 to three recipients. The three grafts had been cleaned and frozen. Current screening methods, unavailable then, would probably have detected the presence of HIV. Patients receiving freeze-dried graft from the infected donor did not convert to HIV-positive status, suggesting that freeze-drying may kill the HIV virus.

Storage

Meniscus allografts may be stored by deep freezing or cryopreservation, or they may be implanted from a fresh cadaver. Many of the original grafts were implanted fresh in order to maintain graft cell viability (14). Screening considerations and timing of the surgery make fresh grafts more difficult to use.

Cryopreservation is a special process of controlled-rate freezing with extraction of cellular water that preserves up to 80% of cells in the graft. They can be stored for up to 10 years and are readily available in multiple sizes. Having viable meniscal cells at the time of transplantation has been thought to be advantageous, but several animal and clinical studies have failed to show an advantage for the use of cryopreserved grafts (15–21) compared with fresh-frozen grafts. Freeze-drying alters the collagen structure of the graft and is not acceptable for meniscus allografts.

Immunology

Antigens present on the donor cells in bone and cartilage do invoke a typical immune reaction, the severity depending on cell volume. Chondrocytes and fibrochondrocytes are deeply embedded in a matrix, which may account for the fact that a clinically significant immune reaction is not typically seen in the host. Careful analysis of synovial fluid and synovial biopsies have shown a slight increase in immunomarkers, but a clinically significant reaction does not appear to occur (22). No rejection of an allograft meniscus has been reported.

Animal Models

Early results of animal studies contributed to our understanding of allograft meniscal transplantation. Canham and Stanish (23) found that allograft menisci had healed to the surrounding capsule in dogs. Milachowski et al. (24) successfully transplanted into sheep medial menisci that were preserved either by deep freezing or by lyophilization and γ-irradiation. Zukor et al. (25), Arnocsky et al. (16), and Mikic et al. (20) all demonstrated cellular repopulation of meniscus allografts in animal models. Grafts were somewhat hypocellular at 6 to 8 months after transplantation, especially in the thicker areas of the posterior horns.

Jackson et al. (18) investigated the ability of transplanted menisci to function mechanically and biochemically in goats. Grafts demonstrated peripheral healing, revascularization, increased cellularity, and an almost normal gross appearance at 6 months, but showed increased water content and decreased proteoglycan content on biochemical examination. The articular cartilage in allograft knees tended to show more degeneration than controls.

Paletta et al. (26) and Alhalki et al. (27) examined the intraarticular contact area and pressures in the intact knee, after lateral meniscectomy, after implantation of size-matched meniscal allograft fixed with bone plugs, and after release of the anterior and posterior horns. Replacement of the menisci with allografts improved the contact area and pressures, but they did not return to normal. Anchoring of both horns of the menisci to bone is crucial in attaining the best mechanical function (28,29).

Results regarding whether meniscus allografts prevent articular cartilage degeneration have been varied. Edwards et al. (30) found no radiologic difference in sheep knees at 21 months after meniscectomy, allograft, or no operation. Other studies (31–33), however, showed a beneficial effect of implantation of an allograft meniscus compared with meniscectomy.

Clinical Studies

Milachowski et al. (24) implanted the first isolated human meniscal allograft in 1984. His series of 222 allografts, done in conjunction with ACL reconstruction, used fresh-frozen and freeze-dried grafts. At second-look arthroscopy, the freeze-dried grafts exhibited more shrinkage and synovial reaction than the fresh frozen grafts did. Garrett and Stevenson (14) first reported their results in six patients (four with medial and two with lateral tears) who underwent fresh meniscal allograft transplantation. Follow-up averaged 30 months, with no complaints of locking or catching episodes and only one patient with mild swelling. Four patients underwent second-look arthroscopy, and all menisci were completely healed and showed no shrinkage. In a later study, Garrett (15) presented 43 meniscal allografts with at least 2 years of follow-up. Seven patients had an isolated meniscal transplantation, and 24 had concomitant ACL reconstructions; 13 had osteotomies, and 11 had osteochondral allografts. Twenty-eight patients had second-look arthroscopy performed at 2 months to 2 years. Eight menisci exhibited fragmentation and failure of peripheral healing and were deemed failures. Twenty-seven cryopreserved grafts and 16 fresh grafts had no difference in outcome. The presence of significant arthritis was the factor found to be most associated with failure.

Noyes (34) reported on 96 fresh-frozen, irradiated allografts with a minimum of 2 years of follow-up. Twenty-nine failed and were removed. Of the 67 surviving menisci, only 9 (13%) were classified as healed and 30 (45%) as partially healed. There was a statistically significant relationship between overall healing rate and the arthrosis rating on MRI. Noyes recommended that allograft meniscal transplantation be reserved for symptomatic knees in young patients who have articular cartilage damage but no advanced deterioration.

Van Arkel and DeBoer (35) reported on 23 cryopreserved allografts at an average follow-up of 36 months. All knees had at least grade II articular cartilage changes, but only one had grade IV of the lateral compartment. Overall, 20 of the 23 patients had a satisfactory outcome with improvement in Knee Assessment Scoring System (KASS), modified Lysholm, and Tegner scores. Twelve patients underwent second-look arthroscopy. Five menisci were partially detached, and four healed with resuturing.

Goble et al. (36) reported on 19 cryopreserved meniscal allografts in 18 patients with a minimum of 2 years' follow-up. Seventeen patients reported a significant decrease in pain and improvement in function on a subjective evaluation. Second-look arthroscopy on 13 patients (14 grafts) showed that 10 had healed and were functioning normally. Four grafts demonstrated noticeable degenerative wear or peripheral detachment at the posterior horn. Only one required total excision.

More recently, Cameron and Saha (37) reported their experience with 67 fresh-frozen, irradiated meniscal allografts in 63 patients. Only 21 patients had the meniscal allograft as an isolated procedure. Forty-two had complex knee problems requiring combined procedures. At a minimum follow-up of 3 years, 86% of the patients had a good or excellent result based on a modified Lysholm score. Of those patients with isolated meniscal transplant, 90% had good or excellent results. The greatest gains in score occurred in the categories of pain and swelling.

Carter (38) reported on 46 patients with follow-up longer than 2 years. Thirty-nine of the grafts were medial, and seven were lateral. Eleven were isolated transplants, and 35 patients had concomitant procedures. Forty-five had decreased pain. Thirty-eight patients had repeat arthroscopy at 3 to 48 months after surgery. Four grafts showed shrinkage. Progression of arthritis by radiography was present in two patients. MRI did not reliably predict integrity of the graft. There were four failures (8.6%) in this group. Two menisci had advanced arthrosis, a third failed because of a technical error in placement, and a fourth failed because of patient noncompliance.

Stollsteimer et al. (39) analyzed the results of 23 nonirradiated, cryopreserved meniscal allografts in 22 of their patients at 1 to 5 years of follow-up. The primary indication for the procedure was disabling knee pain in the compartment where the meniscus had previously been removed. Twelve menisci were lateral and 11 were medial. Medial grafts were implanted with bone plugs, and a "keyhole" technique was used laterally. Reduction in pain was the most consistent improvement. Average loss of joint space was 0.882 mm (range, 0 to 3 mm) on radiograph. MRIs were obtained on both knees of patients to assess graft position and size. The allograft size ranged from 31% to 100% of the normal contralateral meniscus, with an average of 62%. Patients with Outerbridge scores of 2 or less in any area had significantly improved Lysholm and Tegner scores.

Rodeo et al. (22) took both synovial biopsies and two biopsy specimens measuring 3×4 mm from 28 meniscal allografts in 25 patients during routine second-look arthroscopy. Specimens were examined histologically and by immunohistochemical analysis. Repopulation with host cells was noted, but the central core was hypocellular. A low-level immune response directed against the allografts was also found, but it did not appear to affect the clinical outcome.

Preoperative Planning

Malalignment or instability should be corrected before or concomitantly with a meniscal replacement. The combination of a ligament reconstruction or corrective osteotomy with meniscal transplantation has been reported with good results (14,15,24,35–38,40,41).

The presence and degree of articular cartilage damage should be assessed. Joint incongruity, flattening of the femoral condyle, and grade IV articular cartilage changes all lead to a high failure rate (38). Best results are obtained in knees with little or no arthritic damage.

Proper graft sizing is crucial to the success of a meniscal allograft. Garrett and Stevenson (14). achieved a size match within 5% with plain x-ray. Carpenter et al. (42) performed a cadaveric study evaluating plain radiographs, computed tomograph (CT) scans, and MRI scans in determining the size of a meniscus. MRI consistently underestimated the size of the meniscus, whereas plain radiographs and CT scanning were more accurate. Pollard et al. (43) used bony landmarks and plain radiographs to perform meniscal sizing. Meniscal width was determined by measuring from the peak of the tibial plateau to the periphery of the tibial metaphysis on the anteroposterior radiograph. Meniscal length was determined as a percentage of the sagittal length of the tibial plateau (medial, 80%; lateral, 70%). The size of the meniscus can be determined to within 8% error. Shaffer et al. (44). found that MRI was only slightly more accurate than conventional radiography.

Patients must have reasonable expectations and understand that long-term results are unknown. No evidence proves that a meniscal allograft will prevent arthritis in the long term. The most reliable benefit is relief from pain.

SURGICAL TECHNIQUE

Meniscal transplantation can be performed arthroscopically, by an arthroscopic-assisted technique, or via an open approach. The choice of technique depends on surgeon preference, which meniscus (medial or lateral) is to be transplanted, and concomitant procedures. The first allografts were open, with collateral ligament release, but today the procedure can be performed arthroscopically or with a limited incision, reducing surgical morbidity.

A meniscus allograft functions best when the horns are anchored with bone (26–29). Medial menisci are implanted with separate bone plugs for each horn, whereas lateral menisci are implanted with a bone bridge, because of the close proximity of the anterior and posterior horns.

Medial Meniscus Replacement

After the allograft is thawed, residual capsular and ligament tissue is removed from its periphery. The anterior bone anchor is cut perpendicular to the accompanying tibial plateau and sized to a snug 9-mm size. The posterior bone plug is cut 45 degrees to the tibial plateau and undersized slightly to a 9-mm size. Both bone plugs should be 8 to 10 mm in length. A small drill hole is placed through the center of each bone anchor, and two no. 1 nonabsorbable sutures are inserted up the drill hole from below, across the meniscal horn, and back down the drill hole. After the allograft meniscus is prepared, the anterior aspect of each bone plug is marked to facilitate proper rotation. The graft is placed into the thawing solution and put on the back table.

Diagnostic arthroscopy is performed to completely assess the knee joint. If a concomitant ACL reconstruction is to be performed, the notchplasty and tunnels are drilled first. The remaining meniscus is debrided, leaving a thin rim of vascular meniscal bed. Anterior and posterior horn attachments serve as a guide for drilling the meniscal tunnels (45,46).

The 9-mm posterior meniscal tunnel is made by reaming over a guide pin placed into the posterior horn attachment of the old meniscus, from the lateral tibial metaphysis 3 cm distal to the tibial tubercle at a 45-degree angle. The rim of the posterior tunnel is debrided of remaining soft tissue, which otherwise might interfere with seating of the graft. The anterior medial portal is then enlarged to a 5-cm arthrotomy. The anterior horn attachment is identified. A guide pin is inserted perpendicular to the tibial plateau. A 9-mm socket, 10 mm deep, is made with a reamer. The ACL guide is used to make a small drill hole from the bottom of the socket outside to the medial cortex.

A longitudinal 3- to 5-cm incision is made posterior to the medial collateral ligament, beginning just above the joint line and extending distally. The posterior capsule is exposed, with careful protection of the saphenous nerve. Inside-out sutures will be passed through this capsule and delivered out the incision. A tissue protector is used to protect the neurovascular structures.

A single limb of double-armed 2-0 nonabsorbable suture on long needles is passed through the arthrotomy and out the posterior capsule approximately 1 cm from the posterior horn attachment. A mattress suture is placed in the meniscal allograft 1 cm from the posterior horn. The other limb of this suture is passed through the arthrotomy and out the posterior capsule adjacent to the other limb. A nasal speculum can be used to prevent the sutures from getting entangled in soft tissue anteriorly. A second suture is placed 1 cm from the first, by the same technique. These sutures will be used to pull the graft into the joint. The posterior bone anchor sutures cannot be used because the oblique pull will cause them to cut through the articular surface adjacent to the posterior tunnel. The posterior bone anchor sutures are then passed through the anterior arthrotomy and down the posterior tunnel. At this point it is important to ensure that no sutures have pierced any anterior soft tissues and that no sutures are twisted.

The posterior bone plug is introduced into the joint through the arthrotomy and, with the aid of a grasper, is teased either through the notch or around the periphery of the joint underneath the collateral ligament. The posterior horn capsular sutures are used to pull the meniscus into place. If difficulty is encountered during graft passage, the collateral ligament can be released to provide more room.

Once the meniscus is in its proper location, the anterior mark on the posterior bone plug is aligned and the plug is seated into the tunnel. The peripheral posterior horn sutures are then tied, securing the meniscus in place. Additional inside-out sutures are placed until adequate fixation of the meniscus is achieved. The anterior bone plug is seated with proper rotation, and the anterior and posterior anchor su-

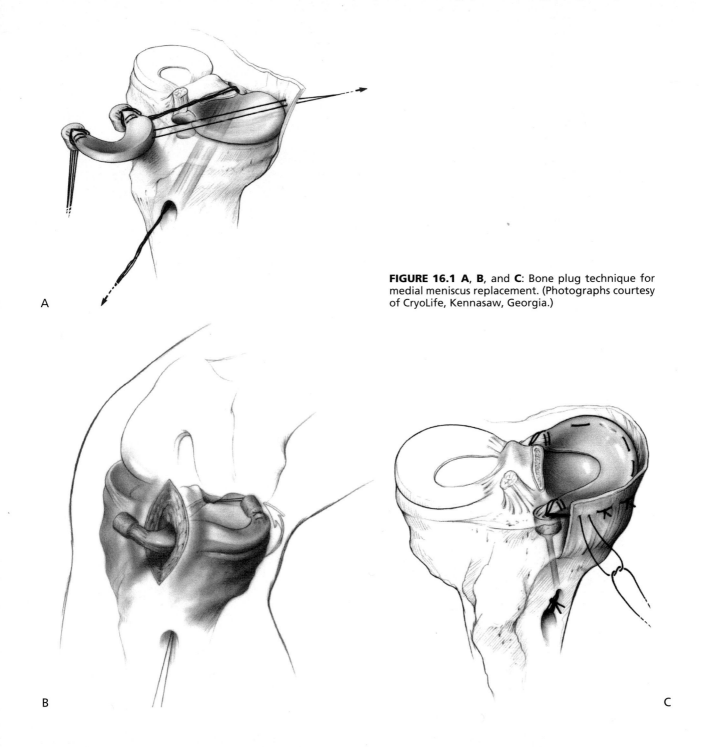

A

B

C

FIGURE 16.1 A, **B**, and **C**: Bone plug technique for medial meniscus replacement. (Photographs courtesy of CryoLife, Kennasaw, Georgia.)

tures are tied to each other over the anterior tibia. Inspection of the meniscus while taking the knee through a full range of motion should reveal any misplaced sutures or suture failures. The arthrotomy is closed in layers (Fig. 16.1).

Lateral Meniscus Replacement

The lateral meniscus is best replaced with a trough or keyhole technique (Fig. 16.2), which uses a bone bridge to maintain the connection between the anterior and posterior horns. The ACL tibial footprint's location on the medial side of the notch provides a space for placement of the trough without damage to the articular cartilage or ligaments. The close proximity of the lateral meniscus horns (11 to 13 mm, compared with 30 mm on the medial meniscus) facilitates this procedure. A 5-cm arthrotomy on the lateral border of the patella tendon will facilitate trough placement. The anterior and posterior horn attachments of the lateral meniscus are located and marked. The tibial eminence can be shaved down to facilitate visualization.

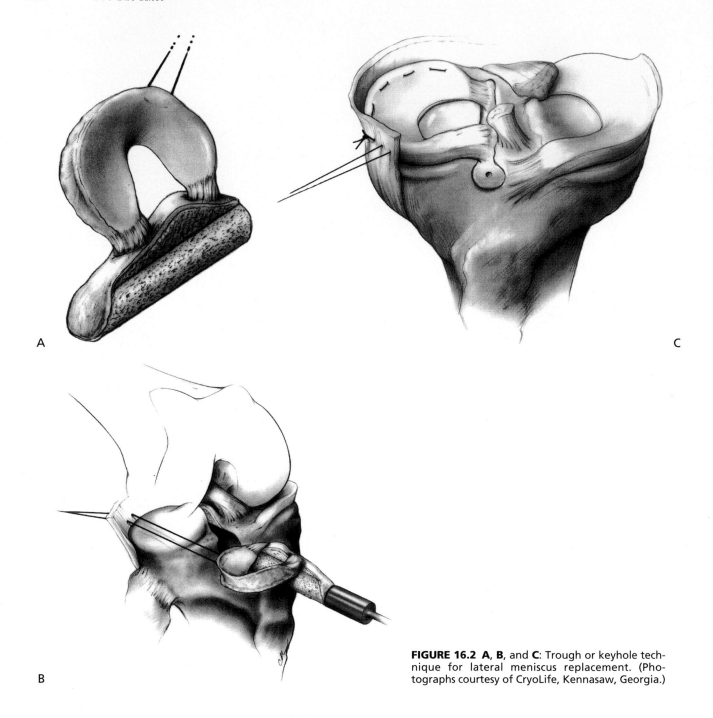

A

B

C

FIGURE 16.2 A, **B**, and **C**: Trough or keyhole technique for lateral meniscus replacement. (Photographs courtesy of CryoLife, Kennasaw, Georgia.)

Instrumentation is available from CryoLife, Inc. (Kennasaw, GA) and Arthrex, Inc. (Naples, FL) to make the trough and prepare the graft. With the use of a calibrated probe, the distance from the posterior aspect of the posterior horn attachment to the anterior tibia is measured. This distance represent the anterior-to-posterior trough length. An arthroscopic bur is used to create a shallow trough along the length of the trough. The desired trough width is determined, and the appropriate allograft starter and finishing chisels are selected. The starter chisel deepens the trough by several millimeters, and the finishing chisel completes the cut. The posterior tibial wall is left intact to protect neurovascular structures and to act as a buttress stop for the graft. The tibial trough sizing guide is used to confirm the length and depth of the trough.

With a small saw and bur, the lateral meniscal allograft is prepared with a bone bridge that corresponds to the size of the trough. The depth of the allograft bone from the site of the horn attachments is measured, and this depth should precisely match that of the trough. The mensical allograft sizing block is used to confirm that the size of the bone bridge is correct.

The posterolateral capsule of the knee is exposed, and a tissue protector is used to protect neurovascular structures. As with the medial meniscus technique, two sutures are placed in the posterior horn and the posterior capsule for use in pulling the graft into place. The graft is pulled into place with these two sutures, and the bone bridge is slid into the trough. The graft is then sutured using an inside-out technique. The bone plug is usually stable with press-fit fixation; however, if additional fixation is necessary, an absorbable pin or screw is sufficient.

MENISCAL REGENERATION

Meniscal regeneration may ultimately solve the problems of disease transmission, graft availability, graft sizing, and immune responses that are concerns with meniscal allografts. Scaffolds fabricated of purified type I collagen from bovine Achilles tendons have been used to support and promote the regeneration of a meniscus (47–54). The scaffolds are freeze-dried and inserted by suturing into the meniscus rim, using an open or arthroscopic-assisted technique similar to the one used with meniscus allografts.

Initial *in vitro* (47–50). and animal studies (51,52,54). resulted in a regenerated structure that was grossly and histologically similar to normal meniscus. Clinical trials were conducted in nine patients who had previously undergone total medial meniscectomy (51–54). Clinical and MRI evaluations were performed at 6, 12, 24, and 52 weeks, and evaluation for an immune response to the implant and relook arthroscopy were performed at 36 months; eight of the nine patients rated their knee as normal or near-normal and had returned to a higher level of activity. Second-look arthroscopy revealed regenerated tissue that grossly resembled meniscal tissue. Histologically, new matrix tissue was present that appeared chondroid, and there was no evidence of an immune response. A second study group of eight patients had similar results clinically, histologically, and grossly (53).

CONCLUSION

Although clinical and animal studies show that a meniscal allograft can heal, remain viable, and function, results are short term. The fact that loss of a meniscus leads to degenerative arthritis is proven, making replacement of a meniscus with an allograft both logical and promising. Caution must still be urged, because no long-term studies yet exist to prove that a meniscus allograft can prevent the progression of degenerative arthritis. Decrease in pain and increase in function have been consistently reported by most investigators.

Shrinkage of the graft, immunologic and disease transmission concerns, surgical difficulty, and reimbursement issues also remain considerations that must be addressed before a meniscus allograft is recommended.

Regeneration of the meniscus with a collagen scaffold remains experimental. Follow-up studies by multiple investigators will be needed before this procedure can become accepted.

REFERENCES

1. Rockborn P, Gillquist J. Long term results after arthroscopic meniscectomy: the role of preexisting cartilage fibrillation in a 13 year follow-up of 60 patients. *Int J Sports Med* 1996;17:608–613.
2. Walker PS, Erkman MJ. The role of the meniscus I force transmission across the knee. *Clin Orthop* 1975;109:184–192.
3. Seedhom BB, Wright V. Functions of the menisci. *J Bone Joint Surg Br* 1974;56:381.
4. Radin EL, Delamotte F, Maquet PG. Role of the meniscus in distribution of stress of the knee. *Clin Orthop* 1984;185:290–293.
5. Kurosawa H, Fukubayashi T, Nakajima H. Load-bearing mode of the knee joint: physical behaviour of the knee joint with or without menisci. *Clin Orthop* 1980;149:283–290.
6. Baratz ME, Fu FH, Mengato R. Meniscal tears: the effect of meniscectomy and repair on intra-articular contact areas and stress in the human knee. A preliminary report. *Am J Sports Med* 1986;14:270–275.
7. Fukubayashi T, Kurosawa H. The contact area and pressure distribution pattern of the knee: a study of normal and osteoarthrotic knee joints. *Acta Orthop Scand* 1993;51:871–979.
8. Shoemaker SC, Markolf KL. The role to the meniscus in the anterior-posterior stability of the loaded anterior cruciate-deficient knee. *J Bone Joint Surg Am* 1986;68:71–79.
9. Levy IM, Torzilli PA, Warren RF. The effect of medial meniscectomy on anterior-posterior motion of the knee. *J Bone Joint Surg Am* 1982;64:883–888.
10. American Association of Tissue Banks. *Standards for tissue banking.* McLean, VA: American Association of Tissue Banks, 1996.
11. Pelker RR, Friedlaender GE. Biomechanical aspects of bone autografts and allografts. *Orthop Clin North Am* 1987;18:235–239.
12. Buck BE, Malinin TI, Brown MD. Bone transplantation and human immunodeficiency virus: an estimate of risk of acquired immunodeficiency syndrome (AIDS). *Clin Orthop* 1989;240:129–136.
13. Simonds RJ, Holmberg SD, Hurwitz RL, et al. Transmission of human immunodeficiency virus type 1 from a seronegative organ and tissue donor. *N Engl J Med* 1992;326:726–732.
14. Garrett JC, Stevenson RN. Meniscal transplantation in the human knee: a preliminary report. *Arthroscopy* 1991;7:57–62.
15. Garret JC. Meniscal transplantation: a review of 43 cases with 2 to 7 year follow-up. *Sports Med Arthrosc Rev* 1993;1:164–167.
16. Arnoczky SP, Warren RF, McDevitt CA. Meniscal replacement using a cryopreserved allograft. *Clin Orthop* 1990;252:121–128.
17. Arnoczky SP, DeCarlo EF, O'Brien SJ, et al. Cellular repopulation of deep-frozen autografts: an experimental study in dogs. *Arthroscopy* 1992;8:428–436.
18. Jackson DW, McDevitt CA, Simon TM, et al. Meniscal transplantation using fresh and cryopreserved allografts: an experimental study in goats. *Am J Sports Med* 1992;20:644–656.
19. Fabbriciani C, Lucania L, Milano G, et al. Meniscal allografts: cryopreservation versus deep frozen technique. An experimental study in goats. *Am J Sports Med* 1992;5:124–134.
20. Mikic ZD, Brankov MZ, Tubic MV, et al. Transplantation of fresh-frozen menisci: an experimental study in dogs. *Arthroscopy* 1997;13:579–583.

21. Zukor DJ, Cameron JC, Brooks PJ, et al. The fate of human meniscal allografts. In: Ewing JW, ed. *Articular cartilage and knee joint function: basic science and arthroscopy.* New York: Raven Press, 1990:147–152.

22. Rodeo SA, Senevitatne A, Suzuki K, et al. Histological analysis of human meniscal allografts: a preliminary report. *J Bone Joint Surg Am* 2000;82:1071–1082.

23. Canham W, Stanish W. A study of the biological behavior of the meniscus as a transplant in the medial compartment of a dog's knee. *Am J Sports Med* 1986;14:376–379.

24. Milachowski KA, Weismeier K, Wirth CJ. Homologous meniscus transplantation: experimental and clinical results. *Int Orthop* 1989;13:1–11.

25. Zukor DJ, Rubins IM, Daigle MR, et al. Allotransplantation of frozen irradiated menisci in rabbits. *J Bone Joint Surg Br* 1991; 73:45.

26. Paletta GA, Manning T, Snell E, et al. The effect of allograft meniscal replacement of intraarticular contact area and pressures in the human knee: a biomechanical study. *Am J Sports Med* 1997;25:692–698.

27. Alhalki MM, Hull ML, Howell SM. Contact mechanics of the medial tibial plateau after implantation of a medial meniscal allograft: a human cadaveric study. *Am J Sports Med* 2000;28: 370–376.

28. Bylski-Austrow DI, Meade T, Majumed J, et al. Irradiated meniscal allografts: mechanical histological studies in the goat. *Trans Orthop Res Soc* 1992;3:175.

29. Chen MI, Branch TP, Hutton WC. Is it important to secure the horns during lateral meniscal transplantation: a cadaveric study. *Arthroscopy* 1996;12:174–181.

30. Edwards DJ, Whittle SL, Nissen MJ, et al. Radiographic changes in the knee after meniscal transplantation: an experimental study in a sheep model. *Am J Sports Med* 1996;24:222–226.

31. Cummins JF, Mansour JN, Howe Z, et al. Meniscal transplantation and degenerative articular change: an experimental study in the rabbit. *Arthroscopy* 1997;13:485–491.

32. Aagaard H, Jorgensen U, Bojsen-Moller F. Reduced degenerative articular cartilage changes after meniscal allograft transplantation in sheep. *Knee Surg Sports Traumatol Arthrosc* 1999;7:184–191.

33. Szomor ZL, Martin TE, Bonar F, et al. The protective effects of meniscal transplantation on cartilage: an experimental study in sheep. *J Bone Joint Surg Am* 2000;82:80–88.

34. Noyes FR. *Irradiated meniscus allografts in the human knee: a two to five year follow-up study.* Presented at the Orthopaedic Society for Sports Medicine Specialty Day, Orlando, Florida, February 19, 1995.

35. Van Arkel ER, DeBoer HH. Human meniscal transplantation: preliminary results at two to five year follow-up. *J Bone Joint Surg Br* 1995;77:589–595.

36. Goble EM, Kane SM, Wilcox TR, et al. Meniscal allografts. In: McGinty JB, Caspari RB, eds. *Operative arthroscopy,* 2nd ed. Philadelphia: Lippincott-Raven, 1996:317–331.

37. Cameron JC, Saha S. Meniscal allograft transplantation for uni-

compartmental arthritis of the knee. *Clin Orthop* 1997;337: 164–171.

38. Carter TR. Meniscal allograft transplantation. *Sports Med Arthrosc Rev* 1999;7:51–62.

39. Stollsteimer GT, Shelton WR, Dukes A, et al. Meniscal allograft transplantation: a 1 to 5 year follow-up of 22 patients. *Arthroscopy* 2000;16:343–347.

40. Yoldas EA, Irrgang J, Fu FH, et al. Arthroscopically assisted meniscal transplantation using non-irradiated fresh-frozen menisci. Presented at the Meniscus and Cartilage Transplantation Study Group, New Orleans, Louisiana, 1998.

41. Goble EM, Nelson KJ. Meniscal allograft transplantation. Presented at the *Meniscus and Cartilage Transplantation Study Group.* New Orleans, LA 1998.

42. Carpenter JE, Wojtys EM, Houston LJ, et al. Preoperative sizing of meniscal allografts. *Arthroscopy* 1993;9:344.

43. Pollard ME, Kang Q, Berg EE. Radiographic sizing for meniscal transplantation. *Arthroscopy* 1995;11:684–687.

44. Shaffer B, Kennedy S, Klimkiewicz J, et al. Preoperative sizing of meniscal allografts in meniscus transplantation. *Am J Sports Med* 2000;28:524–533.

45. Johnson DL, Swenson TM, Livesay GA, et al. Insertion-site anatomy of the human menisci: gross, arthroscopic, and topographical anatomy as a basis for meniscal transplantation. *Arthroscopy* 1995;11:386–394.

46. Berlet GC, Fowler PJ. The anterior horn of the medial meniscus: an anatomic study of its insertion. *Am J Sports Med* 1998;26: 540–543.

47. Stone KR, Rodkey WG, Webber RJ, et al. Future directions: collagen based prosthesis for meniscal regeneration. *Clin Orthop* 1990;252:129–135.

48. Stone KR, Rodkey WG, Webber RJ, et al. Meniscal regeneration with copolymeric collagen scaffolds: in vitro and in vivo studies evaluated clinically, histologically, biochemically. *Am J Sports Med* 1992;20:104–111.

49. Stone KR, Rodkey WG, Webber RJ, et al. Development of a prosthetic meniscal replacement. In: Mow VC, Arnoczky SP, Jackson DJ, eds. *Knee meniscus: basic and clinical foundations.* New York: Raven Press; 1992:165–173.

50. Li S-T, Yuen D, Li PC, et al. Collagen as a biomaterial: an application in knee meniscal fibrocartilage. *Meniscal Research Society Symposium Proceedings* 1994;331:25–32.

51. Stone KR, Steadman JR, Rodkey WG, et al. Regeneration of meniscal cartilage with use of a collagen scaffold: analysis of preliminary data. *J Bone Joint Surg Am* 1997;79:1770–1777.

52. Stone KR, Rodkey WG, McKinney LA, et al. Autogenous replacement of the meniscus cartilage: analysis of results and mechanisms of failure. *Arthroscopy* 1995;11:395–400.

53. Rodkey WG, Steadman JR, Li S-T. A clinical study of collagen meniscus implants to restore the injured meniscus. *Clin Orthop* 1999;367S:281–292.

54. Stone KR. Current and future directions for meniscus repair and replacement. *Clin Orthop* 1999;367S:272–280.

PATELLOFEMORAL DISORDERS:
DIAGNOSIS AND TREATMENT

DAVID J. NOVAK
JAMES M. FOX

At the Southern California Orthopedic Institute, patient visits resulting from problems referable to the patellofemoral joint are very common. In the practice of the senior author, which is confined to arthroscopic surgery of the knee, approximately 15% of new patients present with isolated patellofemoral pathology. Another 25% of patients have patellofemoral symptoms secondary to other diagnoses, such as anterior cruciate ligament (ACL) instability or meniscal tears. In most cases patellofemoral pathology can be treated conservatively, and surgery is rarely necessary (1–3). The causes of anterior knee pain are numerous. Chondromalacia, or softening of the articular cartilage, is one cause of anterior knee pain; however it can also be seen in the asymptomatic knee. Therefore, the term chondromalacia should not be used interchangeably with anterior knee pain. Chondromalacia can be caused by numerous factors, including abnormal tilt, subluxation, malalignment, and imbalance of the muscle tendon units. Malalignment and tracking problems, patellar tilt, patellar or quadriceps tendinosis, pathologic plica, fat pad impingement, and saphenous neuropathy can all cause symptoms related to the patellofemoral joint. Patellar instability can lead to subluxation or frank dislocation.

A careful patient history and thorough examination are paramount to the understanding and diagnosis of patellofemoral pathology. Radiographic and special studies, such as computed tomography (CT), dynamic magnetic resonance imaging (MRI), and radionuclide scans, can serve to support a suspected diagnosis. The arthroscope affords the surgeon not only a method of inspection and confirmation of a suspected diagnosis, but also a minimally invasive way to treat the problem. The arthroscope can also aid in examination and treatment when more extensive open surgery is necessary. An example is use the arthroscope to confirm a suspected case of tilt and subluxation. An arthroscopic lateral release could be performed first, followed by a mini-open proximal reefing. The arthroscope could then be reinserted to evaluate the appropriate tensioning of the sutures for the reefing, allowing for precise adjustments intraoperatively.

ANATOMY

The patella has five anatomic facets, although two main facets—the medial and the lateral—are clinically important. The central longitudinal ridge divides these two facets. The contact area of the patella moves proximally as the knee flexion angle increases and the joint reaction force also increases.

The shape of the patella can contribute to its stability. Wiberg (4) initially described patella types I through III (Fig. 17.1). In the type I patella, the medial and lateral facets are of equal proportions. Types II and III have a progressively smaller medial facet; a more dominant lateral facet is probably associated with patellar instability. This assumes that the final patellar shape is determined by the stresses imposed on it. For example, a lateralized gliding of the patella would result in a more prominent lateral facet (4). The shape of the trochlea can also influence patellar stability. Aglietti et al. (5) noted that the lateral condylar height in normal controls was almost twice that in patients with patellar subluxation, on average 9 mm versus 4.7 mm.

Medial Side

Warren and Marshall (6) delineated the anatomy of the medial side of the knee (Fig. 17.2). A three-layer system was described. The most important structure, the medial patellofemoral ligament (MPFL), is located within layer II, deep to the vastus medialis. Other authors have pointed out the importance of the ligament, including Feller et al. (7), who noted it to be a distinct structure in 20 cadavers dissected. The MPFL extends between the superomedial corner of the patella and the epicondyle of the femur. The

D. J. Novak and J. M. Fox: Southern California Orthopedic Institute, Van Nuys, California.

WIBERG

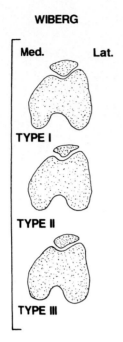

FIGURE 17.1 Wiberg patella types I, II, and III. (From Fox J, DelPizzo W, eds. *The patellofemoral joint.* New York: McGraw-Hill, 1993, with permission.)

MPFL is a static stabilizer of the patella. The MPFL has been shown to be the main static stabilizer, acting as a checkrein to lateral translation of the patellofemoral joint, while the quadriceps muscle acts as the main dynamic stabilizer. Much attention has been focused on the vastus medialis. The vastus medialis, specifically the oblique fibers (vastus medialis obliquus, or VMO), which are oriented at about 50 to 70 degrees relative to the long axis of the quadriceps tendon, are more efficient at resisting lateral translation (8). The patellomeniscal ligament and associated retinacular fibers were also found to be important, contributing another 22% of the total restraining force. The ligamentous structures may also contribute proprioceptive information to the surrounding musculature.

The MPFL may become avulsed from the femur at the time of lateral patellar dislocation. In addition, Koskinen and Kujala (9) showed that the medial vastus insertion is more proximal in patients who have sustained a dislocation than in normal controls.

Lateral Side

There is a superficial as well as a deep component to the lateral retinaculum (Fig. 17.3). The deep component inserts directly into the patella and is the primary restraint to patella translation on the lateral side of the joint. The deep transverse band attaches the iliotibial band to the patella. The sta-

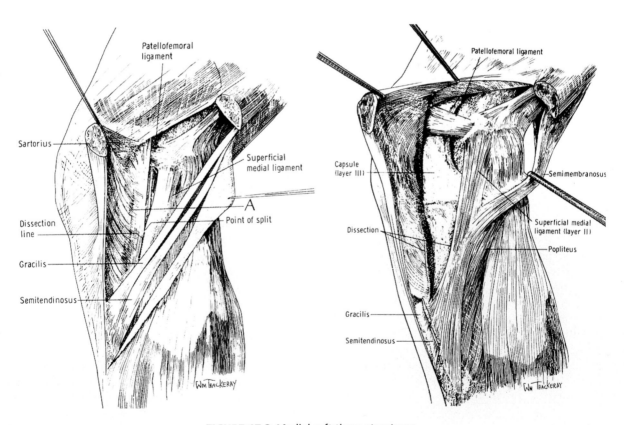

FIGURE 17.2 Medial soft tissue structures.

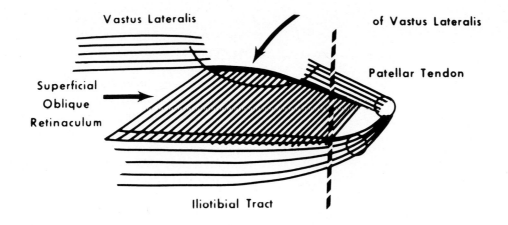

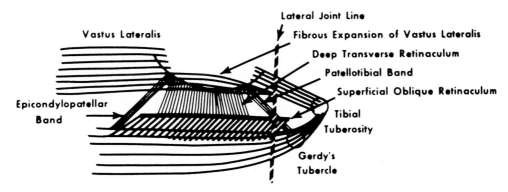

FIGURE 17.3 Lateral soft tissue structures.

bilizing effect of the lateral retinaculum is most notable at full knee extension, when the patella and trochlear articular surfaces are not in contact (10). As the iliotibial band moves posteriorly with knee flexion, the lateral pull of the patella is increased. If these forces act against weakened medial stabilizers, patellar tilt or subluxation may occur (11).

It is well known that some patients have an inherently tight lateral retinaculum. In patients with chronic patellofemoral malalignment and a tight lateral retinaculum, Fulkerson et al. (12) demonstrated a histologic pattern of small nerve injury (Fig. 17.4). This pattern of neuromatous degeneration may represent a source of pain in these patients. Sanchis-Alfonso et al. (13) also noted changes in the size and quantity of nerves in the lateral retinaculum. They examined the lateral retinacula of symptomatic patients by obtaining a biopsy of those patients undergoing a lateral release or a proximal realignment. In one group of 13 patients with isolated patellofemoral malalignment recalcitrant to nonoperative treatment, they noted increased neural growth factor production, indicating a proliferation of nociceptive axons in a perivascular location. In an earlier study (14), the same authors noted an increase in the proportion of innervated tissue in symptomatic patients, based on the total neural area as well as the size of the individual nerves.

The iliotibial tract, an extension of the tensor fascia lata muscle, extends from the muscle to Gerdy's tubercle. As the iliotibial band repetitively rubs over the lateral epicondyle with flexion and extension of the knee, pain can result.

BIOMECHANICS

The primary function of the patella is to improve the efficiency of the quadriceps by increasing the lever arm of the extensor mechanism. The patella increases the mechanical strength of the extensor mechanism by approximately 50% (15).

As the knee is flexed, the distal articular cartilage of the patella begins to articulate with the cartilage of the trochlear groove (Fig. 17.5). Initial patellofemoral contact occurs at approximately 10 to 15 degrees of knee flexion at the distal pole of the patella. In the case of patella alta, the initial contact does not occur until about 20 to 30 degrees of flexion (16,17). As flexion nears 90 degrees, the most proximal aspect of the patella is articulating with the trochlea. Depending on the location of an articular cartilage lesion, pain may be experienced at a particular degree of flexion.

CT images have aided the understanding of patellofemoral tracking at various angles of knee flexion (18). In

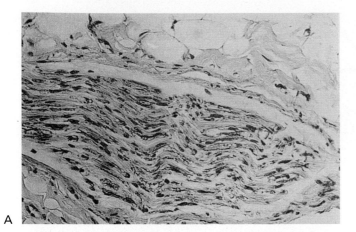

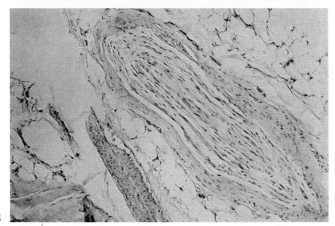

FIGURE 17.4 Nerve histology. **A**: Normal nerve with abundant myelin, considerable cellularity, and a normal, thin perineurium. **B**: Biopsy of the retinaculum of a patient with prolonged patellofemoral pain and malalignment. Note the gross demyelination and thickening of the perineurium. (From Fulkerson JP, Tennant R, Jaivin JS, et al. Histologic evidence of retinacular nerve injury associated with patellofemoral malalignment. *Clin Orthop* 1985;197:196–205, with permission.)

full extension, the patella normally sits slightly lateral to the trochlea and is lowered by the quadriceps into the center of the trochlea. The patella should sit centered by 15 to 20 degrees of knee flexion, without any evidence of tilt. The patella should then remain centered for the duration of knee flexion. Abnormal translation or subluxation, as well as rotation or tilt, can then be identified at various degrees of flexion.

HISTORY

As with any orthopaedic problem, a careful history will provide many clues to help determine the patient's problem. Acute traumatic injuries are less common than long-standing problems associated with malalignment.

Traumatic injuries, such as a fall onto the flexed knee, usually cause blunt force injury to the chondral surfaces of the patella, and in many cases to the femur, depending on the degree of flexion at the time of injury. In the case of an initial traumatic dislocation, the patient may describe a history of an external rotation-type injury of the femur on the tibia combined with valgus and knee flexion, after which the patella was noted to be laterally displaced on the outside of the knee. The patient may have manipulated the patella back into position by the time he or she is examined. Of course, this classic history has multiple variants.

In contrast, chronic patellofemoral malalignment is suggested by the insidious onset of progressive pain, recurrent instability, or bilaterality of symptoms. Nonspecific symptoms such as pain, crepitus, giving way, occasional locking, and swelling are common, but they may also be indicative of other, nonpatellofemoral pathology. Pain is the most common nonspecific complaint. Pain is usually a dull-type ache associated with an increase with flexed knee activities, especially stair climbing, squatting, or prolonged sitting. Obesity plays a distinct role in the worsening of patellofemoral arthrosis.

A recent study attempted to prospectively identify risk factors for the development of anterior knee pain in an athletic population (19). A total of 282 male and female students were evaluated for anthropometric variables, motor performance, general joint laxity, lower leg alignment characteristics, muscle length and strength, static and dynamic patellofemoral characteristics, and psychological parameters. Over a 2-year period, 24 of the 282 university athletes developed anterior knee pain. Significant correlation with the development of patellofemoral pain was noted for four factors: a shortened quadriceps muscle, an altered VMO muscle reflex response time, a decreased explosive strength, and a hypermobile patella.

Important factors that must be considered in the patient history include the following: the history of onset and progression of either instability or pain, whether there was a history of trauma or a documented dislocation, the characteristic of the pain, and whether there is any sensation of instability. In addition, problems with other joints should be sought, and generalized hyperlaxity should be determined, along with a comprehensive assessment of any prior treatments.

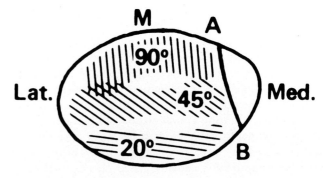

FIGURE 17.5 Contact area at increasing angles of flexion.

PHYSICAL EXAMINATION

The physical examination may focus on pathology referable to the knee once other causes, such as referred pain from the hip or lumbar spine, have been ruled out. One should also consider systemic causes, such as rheumatoid arthritis, as well as reflex sympathetic dystrophy. Careful examination also helps to identify other causes of knee pain, including meniscal pathology and cruciate pathology.

Gait should be carefully examined. Excessive tibio-femoral valgus, thrust, and excessive foot pronation may be noted. Excessive femoral anteversion, external tibial torsion, patella alta or baja, and abnormal medial or lateral rotation of the patella may also be observed (Fig. 17.6). Proximal and lateral rotation of the patella results in the so-called "grasshopper eyes" appearance. This may be noted with the patient seated and the knees flexed to 90 degrees (20). "Squinting patella" is caused by femoral anteversion and patellar malalignment.

The muscles around the knee can be examined and their girth measured, particularly the quadriceps and the vastus medialis, with any atrophy noted. The Q or quadriceps angle is measured with the patient supine. The Q angle is determined by a line drawn from the anterior superior iliac spine to the patella and from the patella center to the tibial tubercle (Fig. 17.7).

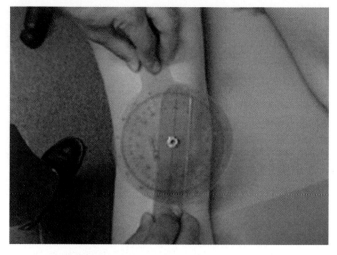

FIGURE 17.7 Measurement of quadriceps angle.

Aglietti et al. (5) studied 150 normal knees and found the average Q angle to be 11 degrees in men and 17 degrees in women. For this reason, a Q angle greater than 20 degrees is considered to be abnormal. Factors that may contribute to an abnormal Q angle include increased femoral anteversion, increased tibial external torsion, and lateralization of the tibial tubercle. The Q angle can also be examined with the knee in 90 degrees of flexion, as advocated by Fulkerson (23).

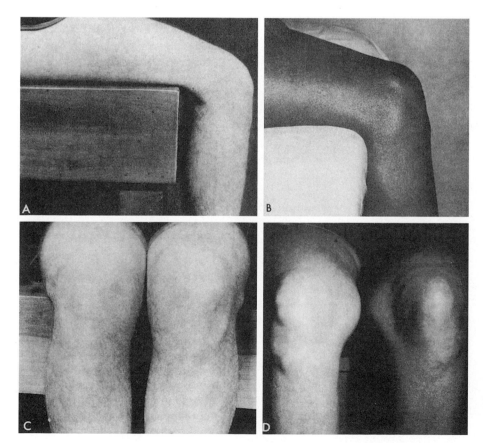

FIGURE 17.6 A: Normal knee from the side. **B**: Patella alta. **C**: Normal knee from the front. **D**: "Grasshopper eyes" patella. (From Hughston J, Walsh W, Puddu G: *Patellar subluxation and dislocation.* Philadelphia: WB Saunders, 1984, with permission.)

Examination in 90 degrees of flexion ensures that the patella is seated within the trochlear notch, which may actually reveal an increased abnormal Q angle. Fulkerson (23) established a normal range for this method of measurement, from −4 degrees to +6 degrees. Values greater than 8 degrees were considered pathologic.

With the patient seated, the patellofemoral motion can be observed as the patient actively moves the knee through a range of motion. The J-sign may be noted as the patella moves excessively in a lateral direction with a sudden jump as the knee is moved from a flexed position to complete extension. This may indicate an imbalance between medial and lateral forces (21).

The knee is examined for signs of effusion. The peripatellar soft tissues should then be examined carefully. The lateral retinaculum should be carefully palpated, as well as the quadriceps insertion to the patella, the patellar tendon, and the MPFL. The quadriceps and patellar tendon, and especially the peripatellar retinaculum, may exhibit signs of tenderness. The iliotibial band should be examined for tenderness as the knee is flexed and extended. The hamstrings should also be evaluated for relative tightness in the supine position. In the prone position, excessive tightness of the extensor mechanism can also be noted. In normal circumstances, the patient should be able to flex both knees symmetrically so that both heels are at or near the buttocks.

Crepitation can be noted simultaneously by placing a gentle posteriorly directed force over the patella while the knee is actively moved through a complete range of motion. By having the patient extend the tibia against resistance, crepitation is enhanced and the patient's typical pain is often duplicated (Fig. 17.8). The more proximal the articular lesion on the patella, the later in knee flexion pain may be reproduced.

The patellar lift-off test should be performed to evaluate for a tight lateral retinaculum (Fig. 17. 9). The patient

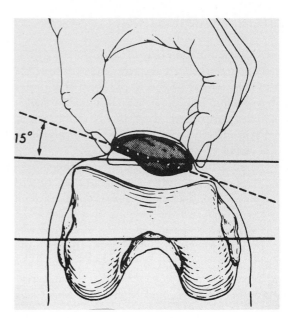

FIGURE 17.9 Patellar tilt test. (From Fox JM, DelPizzo W, eds. *The patellofemoral joint.* New York: McGraw-Hill, 1993, with permission.)

should be in the supine position, and the medial patella should be stabilized by the fingers of both hands while the thumbs are used to elevate the lateral patella. If the patella cannot be elevated to at least neutral, and usually slightly past neutral, then a tight lateral retinaculum exists and patellar tilt is probably present. Kolowich et al. (22) tested 100 patients with normal patella and noted a range of 0 to 20 degrees of excess tilt past neutral. They concluded that an inability to tilt to at least 0 degrees was abnormal, and noted further that this finding was correlated with a successful outcome after lateral retinacular release. Medial and lateral patella glide should also be carefully examined. Lateral patella glide assesses the integrity of the medial capsule, the medial retinaculum, and the VMO. The distance that the patella can be translated laterally can thus be assessed. This is somewhat similar to an apprehension test, although the patient must be thoroughly relaxed in order to perform this test. Medial patellar translation likewise assesses the lateral structures. Kolowich et al. (22) assessed medial and lateral glide at 30 degrees of knee flexion. A lateral glide of 3 quadrants suggests incompetent medial restraints, while a medial glide of 1 quadrant or less often indicates a tight lateral restraint. A medial glide of 3 quadrants suggests a hypermobile patella (23).

RADIOGRAPHIC STUDIES

At our institution, standard radiographs for evaluations of the knee include a lateral radiograph with bilateral weight-bearing anteroposterior (AP) and bilateral tangential (mod-

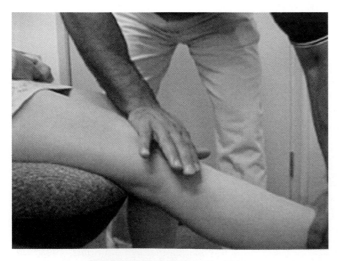

FIGURE 17.8 Patellar grind test.

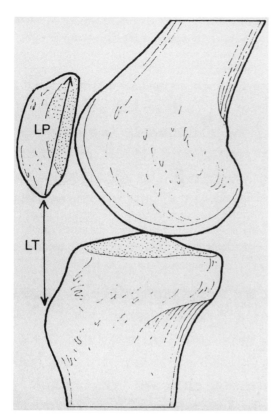

FIGURE 17.10 Insall–Salvati ratio. (From Insall J, Salvati E. Patella position in the normal knee joint. *Radiology* 1971;101:101–104, with permission.)

ified Merchant's) posteroanterior (PA) views. The lateral view may be used to assess for patella alta or baja. As an estimation, if the distance of the patellar tendon is more than 1.2 times the length of the patella, then patella alta may exist. The normal ratio of patellar bone length (LP) to patellar tendon length (LT) is 1% ± 20%, regardless of the angle of knee flexion (24) (Fig. 17.10).

The lateral view taken in 30 degrees of flexion can also be used to evaluate for patella alta or baja by using Blumensaat's line (25). The inferior pole of the patella should be approximately at the level of this line, which represents the roof of the intercondylar notch.

The bilateral AP view is useful for evaluating limb alignment as well as joint space narrowing, loose bodies, fractures, tumors, and patellar abnormalities including bipartite or tripartite patella. The 45-degree flexion PA view can accentuate tibiofemoral narrowing that otherwise would go undetected. The axial view should also be obtained to evaluate for patellar tilt or subluxation. Merchant described a method for obtaining this view at 45 degrees of knee flexion with the beam projected caudad at 30 degrees (26). At the Southern California Orthopedic Institute, a modified Merchant's view is used, with the knee placed in 30 degrees of flexion and both knees placed on one cassette for side-by-side comparison (Fig. 17.11).

Reference lines are then drawn tangential to the lateral facet, with a second line drawn across the condyles of the trochlea anteriorly, in a fashion similar to that described by Laurin et al. (27). The angle formed by these lines should open laterally. If the angle opens medially or the lines are parallel, the patella is probably tilted. This conclusion was reached by noting that 97% of normal subjects had diverging angles, whereas all patients with patellar tilt had parallel or converging angles. It is best to use the same method each time so that the results are reproducible.

Merchant's congruence angle may be used to interpret mediolateral subluxation (28) (Fig. 17.12). On the axial view, the central ridge of the patella should lie at or medial to the trochlear angle; if the ridge is lateral to the bisector, the patella is displaced laterally. In Merchant's original study of 100 normal patients, the average value of the congruence angle was −6 degrees, meaning again that the central ridge of the patella should be medial to the sulcus angle,

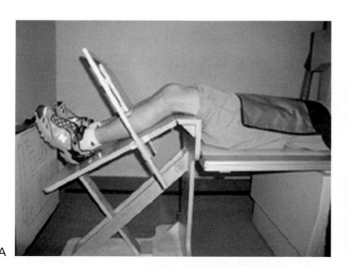

A

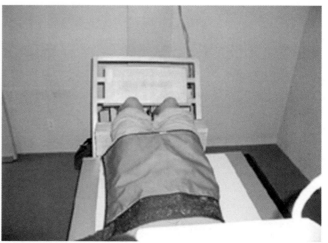

B

FIGURE 17.11 A and **B**: Technique for obtaining modified the Merchant's view.

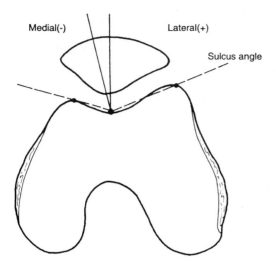

Medial(-)   Lateral(+)

Sulcus angle

FIGURE 17.12 Merchant's sulcus angle and congruence angle. (From Merchant A, Mercer R, Jacobson R, et al. Roentgenographic analysis of patellofemoral congruence. *J Bone Joint Surg Am* 1974;56:1391–1396, with permission.)

with a standard deviation of 11 degrees. A congruence angle of 16 degrees was considered abnormal. Aglietti, however, believed that this range was too wide. He studied 150 asymptomatic subjects and noted a mean congruence angle of −8 degrees with a standard deviation of 6 degrees (5).

CT has been shown to be useful in the evaluation of more difficult cases and for patients with more subtle degrees of tilt (29–31). CT views are precise midpatellar transverse images taken at varying degrees of knee flexion, usually 0, 15, 30, and 45 degrees of knee flexion, while the posterior femoral condyles are used as a reference line. The patient's normal standing alignment should be reproduced. The CT images are evaluated for patellar tilt angle and congruence angle.

MRI can also be used to evaluate patellar tracking in much the same fashion as CT. MRI is thought to be advantageous compared with CT because no ionizing radiation is administered to the patient (32). Transverse images are generated in the same pattern of knee flexion, namely 0, 15, 30, and 45 degrees (Fig. 17.13). The advantage of the MRI is that the surgeon can evaluate for chondral and other intraarticular pathology using one test. Nakanishi et al. noted good correlation between MRI and arthroscopic findings for moderate to advanced cartilage injury (33,34). Shellock et al. also found MRI to be useful in evaluation of the patellofemoral joint after lateral retinacular release if the patient continued to complain of anterior knee pain (35). In their study, medial subluxation was demonstrated in 74% of 43 knees with persistent symptoms after lateral retinacular

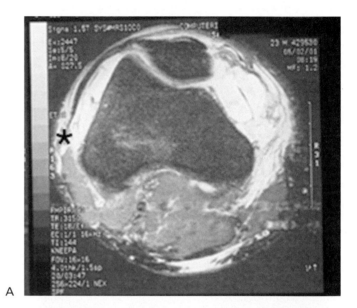

A

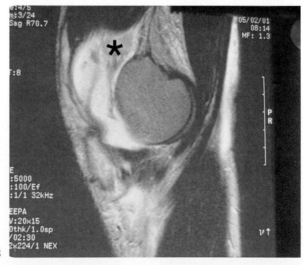

B

FIGURE 17.14 Magnetic resonance images showing medial patellofemoral ligament rupture. **A:** Axial view; asterisk indicates site of rupture. **B:** Sagittal view; asterisk indicates triangle of avulsion of the vastus medialis from the adductor magnus tendon.

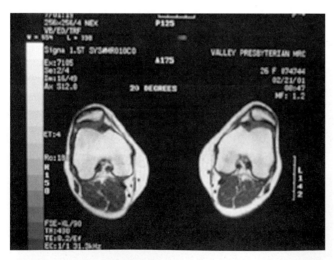

FIGURE 17.13 Magnetic resonance imaging tracking study with lateral subluxation and tilt.

release; 98% demonstrated malalignment. Forty-three percent had medial subluxation of the contralateral, unoperated knee. The authors concluded that some of the patients may have had medial subluxation before release, and that this might have been documented with preoperative MRI. The same authors also compared passive positioning with active motion MRI for the evaluation of tracking. They noted no difference in the qualitative assessment of patellofemoral pathology; however, the active movement techniques were less time-consuming and allowed for the evaluation of activated muscle and soft tissue structures (36).

MRI may also be useful in the situation of acute patellar dislocation (Fig. 17.14). MRI may be used in this situation to determine whether there is coexistent meniscal or cruciate ligament pathology, acute dislocation with incongruent reduction, or acute dislocation with point tenderness on the adductor tubercle. In the last situation, the patient may have sustained avulsion of the MPFL (37). In the Sallay study (37), 87% of patients with acute patellar dislocation had avulsion of the MPFL on MRI, and 94% of the patients had this diagnosis confirmed at the time of surgery.

Finally, bone scanning may be used to document increased tracer uptake, signaling increased metabolic activity in areas of chronic or acute trauma. Dye and Boll (38) noted that a bone scan may localize arthrosis to the patellofemoral joint and may further localize the arthrosis to the medial or lateral side. Bone scanning may also be useful to identify accessory bipartite fragments in the patient with bipartite patella who is symptomatic (39).

CLASSIFICATION OF PATELLOFEMORAL DISORDERS

Classification systems have been proposed by Merchant, Insall, Fulkerson, and others; the reader is directed to their published work for a full description (18,40,41). We have

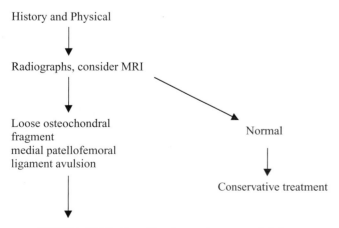

FIGURE 17.15 Algorithm for acute traumatic injury.

found a simple algorithm to be most helpful in the treatment of patients with patellofemoral disorders. The algorithm incorporates anatomic findings as well as history and mechanism of injury, and it also takes into account whether the injury was acute or chronic (Figs. 17.15 and 17.16).

NONOPERATIVE TREATMENT

Nonoperative treatment should be used first in all chronic conditions of the patellofemoral joint and is successful in 75% to 80% of cases. A recent study evaluated the long-term outcome of conservative therapy (42). The authors started with 49 patients in a prospective, randomized, double blind study of unilateral chronic patellofemoral pain. The patients were treated with quadriceps muscle exercises either alone or in combination with intraarticular injection of glycosaminoglycan or placebo. The patients were examined after 6 months to assess short-term results. At that time, complete subjective, functional, and clinical recovery had occurred in almost three fourths of the patients, and no clinically significant differences among the three groups were detected. The authors then reexamined 45 of the original 49 patients at 7 years. Again almost three fourths of the patients had full subjective and functional recovery, although objective evaluation revealed that the number of patients with no symptoms on patellar compression and apprehension tests had decreased over time, and the number with crepitation had increased. The authors concluded that the overall outcome was good in approximately two thirds of patients (42).

The physician must establish a good working relationship with the patient. The patient must understand that patellofemoral problems can be successfully treated, usually without surgery, but that nonoperative treatment may be prolonged and will require significant commitment on the part of the patient. Furthermore, the patient should be fully educated that variances in their anatomy may be contributing to their problem, such as weak quadriceps or tight hamstrings, and that targeting these problem areas with directed physical therapy is often beneficial. However, they should be cautioned that there is usually no quick and easy treatment for their problem.

Brief periods of rest and modification of activities can be beneficial. Short-term use of antiinflammatory medication can also help control inflammation. Increasing the strength of the quadriceps muscle is the focus of a rehabilitation program; the vastus medialis is specifically targeted (Fig. 17.17). Biomechanical analysis has shown that patellofemoral contact pressures are lowest between 0 and 30 degrees of knee flexion, and for this reason short-arc extensions in this range are recommended. Biofeedback may be used during quadriceps exercises to let the patient know when the VMO is contracting (Fig. 17.18). Performing these exercises in a closed-chain fashion further decreases contact pres-

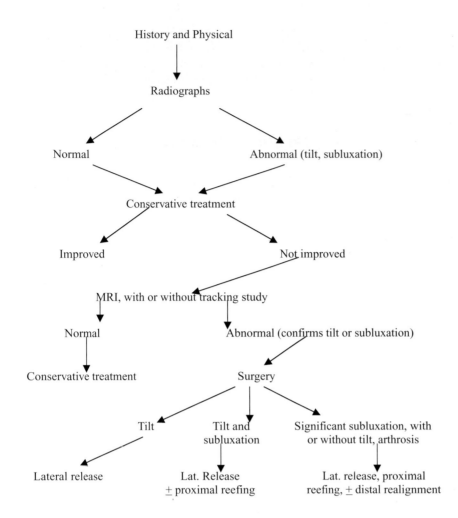

History and Physical

↓

Radiographs

Normal   Abnormal (tilt, subluxation)

Conservative treatment

Improved   Not improved

MRI, with or without tracking study

Normal   Abnormal (confirms tilt or subluxation)

Conservative treatment   Surgery

Tilt   Tilt and subluxation   Significant subluxation, with or without tilt, arthrosis

Lateral release   Lat. Release ± proximal reefing   Lat. release, proximal reefing, ± distal realignment

FIGURE 17.16 Algorithm for a chronic problem.

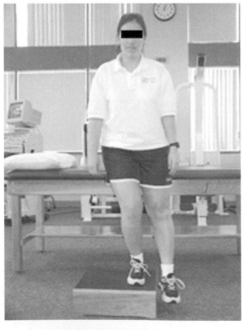

FIGURE 17.17 Stepdowns.

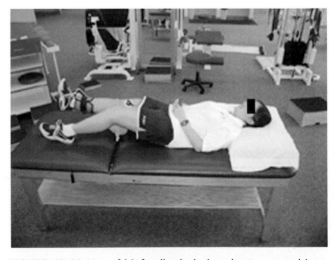

FIGURE 17.18 Use of biofeedback during short-arc quadriceps exercises.

sures. Isometric exercises are also more beneficial than isokinetic exercises. Isokinetic, eccentric, and high torque exercises only cause higher articular cartilage pressures and should be avoided. Strength gains can be measured at the start of physical therapy, and quadriceps strength increases can be monitored as therapy progresses.

Therapy should also stress stretching of the lateral retinaculum and of the iliotibial band if they are tight. The lateral retinaculum may be stretched and mobilized using passive manual displacement of the patella and deep massage of the lateral retinaculum. Emphasis should also be placed on stretching of the hamstrings as they are often tight. Bracing may also be used (Fig. 17.19). Bracing probably has little effect on kinematic knee function, although in one evaluation 75% of patients believed that the main benefit of the brace was improved patellar stability, and most had some degree of pain relief (43). With a specific guided rehabilitation program, most patients should notice improvement and be able to transfer to a home program for maintenance therapy after a 10- to 12-week formal, supervised physical therapy program.

McConnell taping has been evaluated and noted to be beneficial, although possibly not to the degree that its initial authors had noted. Taping can be used to control tilting or subluxation so as to reduce anterior knee pain. Gilleard and McConnell noted a change in activation of the VMO and the vastus lateralis (44). They studied 14 patients with patellar pain and noted earlier activation of the VMO when the patella was taped. However, they also stated that further research was necessary to determine whether and how this change is beneficial. Kowall et al. (45) conducted a retrospective review of patellar taping for the treatment of patellofemoral pain and concluded that the benefit of patellar taping may not be as great as previously found. Furthermore, in a recent study, 16 female patients with anterior knee pain were evaluated with CT both before and after McConnell patellar taping, and no significant effect on patellofemoral lateralization or tilt was noted, although the authors agreed that taping did decrease pain in many cases (46). Patients with excessive pronation may benefit from orthotics.

SURGICAL TREATMENT

Because this is an arthroscopy textbook, the arthroscopic treatment of patellofemoral disorders will be discussed, although specific malalignment patterns are best treated with open surgery. Still, even in the case of a planned open procedure, the arthroscopic evaluation of the cartilaginous surfaces to determine evidence of arthrosis plays an important role in treatment. At the Southern California Orthopedic Institute, the full evaluation of the patellofemoral joint commences with standard knee arthroscopy. The examination should be done in a systematic manner each time to avoid missing pathology.

The patient is placed in the supine position and prepared and draped in a standard fashion. A lateral leg post is placed at the midthigh level and adjusted for valgus stress and medial compartment viewing. A standard inferolateral portal is made for viewing with the arthroscope. An inferomedial portal is then made for placement of a cannula for fluid outflow. Standard systematic diagnostic arthroscopy is performed with careful palpation of the menisci and cartilage surfaces in each compartment, as well as evaluation and palpation of the cruciate ligaments. The patellofemoral joint is then evaluated for arthrosis, and mechanical debridement with a shaver is performed to remove fibrillated cartilage and stabilize defects (Fig. 17.20). The arthroscope may need to be changed to the inferomedial portal, with instruments introduced through the lateral portal, for the best access to cartilage lesions. We do not recommend the use of monopo-

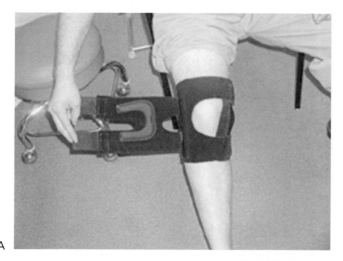 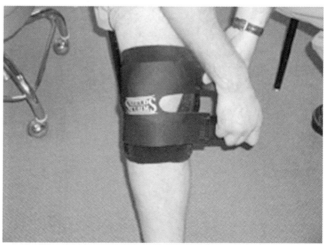

A   B

FIGURE 17.19 A and **B**: Patellofemoral brace.

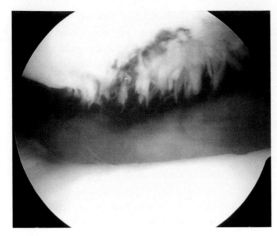

FIGURE 17.20 Arthroscopic view from the inferolateral portal. Note grade III chondromalacia of the lateral facet.

lar or bipolar radiofrequency to stabilize or debride articular lesions at the present time, because the long-term implications of this treatment on normal cartilage cells are unknown.

Using a needle for localization, a superlateral portal is then created. This portal is placed approximately 3 cm proximal to the superior pole of the patella (Fig. 17.21). The arthroscope is changed to the superolateral portal to look "down" on the patellofemoral articulation (Fig. 17.22). With passive flexion of the knee, the lateral facet aligns at a mean flexion angle of 20 degrees, the central ridge at 35 degrees, and the medial facet at 50 degrees (47). When evaluating patellar maltracking arthroscopically, malalignment is defined by failure of the midpatellar ridge to seat within the intercondylar groove by 45 degrees of knee flexion. This differs from the radiographic data previously described by Fulkerson and Merchant. Some of the discrepancy can be explained by arthroscopic fluid distension, tourniquet inflation if one is used, or surgical paralysis of the quadriceps (48). Johnson et al. noted a significant difference in patellar tracking when examining 11 normal volunteers arthroscopically under local anesthesia. The patella was noted to center at 20 degrees during active knee flexion and at 45 degrees during passive knee flexion (49). The patella is normally superior and slightly lateral to the intercondylar groove in full extension. The surgeon should routinely view patellar tracking in normal individuals to become comfortable with the normal expected appearance. Patellar tracking is first evaluated, and then, if lateral patellar tilt is confirmed, a lateral retinacular release is performed arthroscopically.

TECHNIQUE: ARTHROSCOPIC LATERAL RELEASE

The technique for arthroscopic lateral retinacular release is as follows. An electrosurgical cutting hook is placed through the nonconductive cannula in the inferolateral portal. Alternatively, a monopolar or bipolar radiofrequency device may be used, although this is not the preferred instrument at our institution. The release is performed starting at the inferolateral portal and working proximally (Fig. 17.23). The arthroscope is usually placed in the inferomedial portal for best viewing. If necessary, the electrosurgery can be introduced through the superolateral portal. The vastus lateralis muscle should be avoided proximally. The release should be performed 5 mm to 1 cm from the edge of the patella. The deep and then the superficial retinaculum are divided, and the release is complete when subcutaneous tissue is identified (Fig. 17.24). The skin is vulnerable to thermal injury, and the depth of the cutting tip should be closely visualized. After completion of the procedure, the surgeon should again evaluate passive patellar tilt-up. The patella should be able to be inverted passively at least 60 degrees (Fig. 17.25). All bleeding points should be meticulously cauterized, and the pump pressure should be lowered to check for additional bleeding. Wounds are closed with Steri-Strips, and a sterile dressing is applied. The dressings are held in place with a standard full-length compressive stocking to minimize distal swelling. A cold compressive device is used if possible to aid in control of postoperative swelling.

In general, in the correct patient population, lateral reticular release has been found to be beneficial, with a relatively low complication rate of less than 10% (50). The overall complication rate in this series of 446 procedures from surgeons at multiple centers was 7.2%, with hemarthrosis being the most common complication. The author found that the most significant risk for complication was the use of a drain for 24 hours or longer and performing the release with a scissors while viewing arthroscopically. The technique we describe is safe and minimizes the risk of hemarthrosis because bleeding vessels are cauterized directly.

Postoperatively, weight bearing is encouraged immediately. Quadriceps setting, range of motion, and straight leg

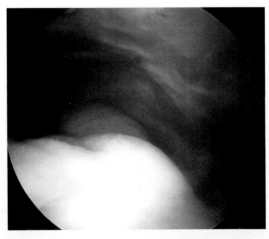

FIGURE 17.21 Arthroscopic view. Needle localization for the superolateral portal.

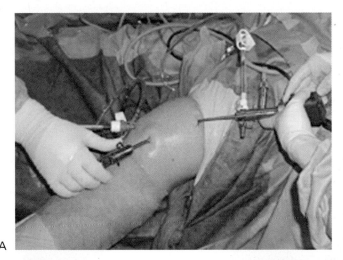

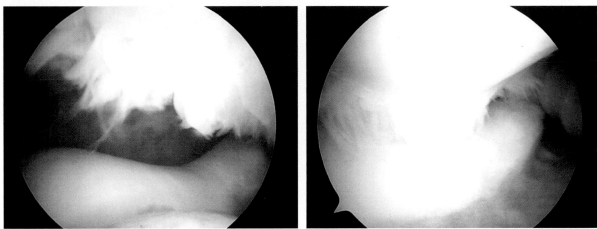

FIGURE 17.22 A: Arthroscope in the superolateral portal. **B**: Corresponding arthroscopic view at full extension **(left)** and at 30 degrees of flexion **(right)**.

A

B

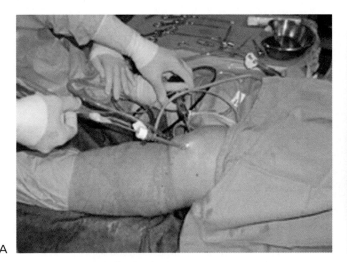

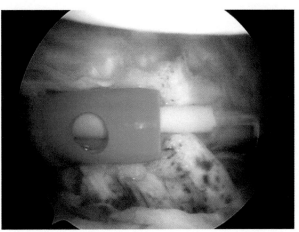

A

B

FIGURE 17.23 A: Arthroscope in inferomedial portal with electrosurgery in inferolateral portal. **B**: Corresponding arthroscopic view. Note the proximal division of the retinaculum on the right.

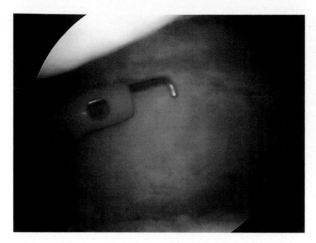

FIGURE 17.24 Arthroscopic view after lateral release. Note the distance between the superior border (tip of probe) and the inferior border (bottom of photograph) of the divided retinaculum.

raising are started on postoperative day 1. Most patients need crutches for less than 1 week. Formal physical therapy is usually continued for a period of 4 to 6 weeks, followed by a home program. Physical therapy includes progressive quad strengthening exercises, followed by resistance exercises.

After arthroscopic lateral release, patellofemoral tracking should again be evaluated as the knee is placed through a range of motion. If subluxation exists but the Q angle is within normal limits or mildly increased, a proximal realignment on the medial side should be considered.

A complete description of various realignment techniques is beyond the scope of this chapter; however, both open and arthroscopic procedures have been described. The arthroscopic realignment as described by Henry and Pflum (51) involves placing multiple no. 2 polydioxanone (PDS) sutures percutaneously and through the medial retinaculum to plicate the tissues and then tying these sutures with the use of a knot pusher (51). We use a mini-open medial capsular reefing procedure (Fig. 17.26). A 3- to 4-cm incision is made over the medial retinaculum adjacent to the patella, leaving the synovium intact. The medial retinaculum is then divided and advanced and reefed onto the superomedial aspect of the patella. Patellar position, rotation, and tracking are evaluated with the arthroscope in the superolateral portal as each suture is placed. Tension is held on the sutures as the knee is placed through a range of motion to allow for adjustment. The no. 1 Vicryl sutures are then tied. A range-of-motion brace set from 0 to 60 degrees is used postoperatively.

If the tracking is still abnormal, or if preoperatively the patient has a highly abnormal Q angle with significant subluxation, a tibial tubercle osteotomy is performed. We use an oblique tibial tubercle osteotomy as initially described by Bandi (52). We prefer to osteotomize the patellar tendon insertion with a 2 × 3 cm piece of the tubercle and transfer this anteromedially (Fig. 17.27). The degree of obliquity

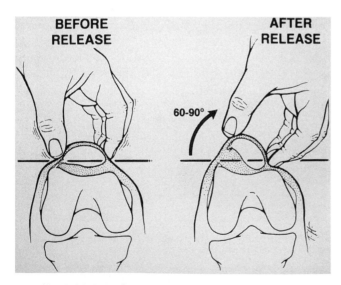

FIGURE 17.25 Postrelease evaluation. (From Fox JM, DelPizzo W, eds. *The patellofemoral joint.* New York: McGraw-Hill, 1993, with permission.)

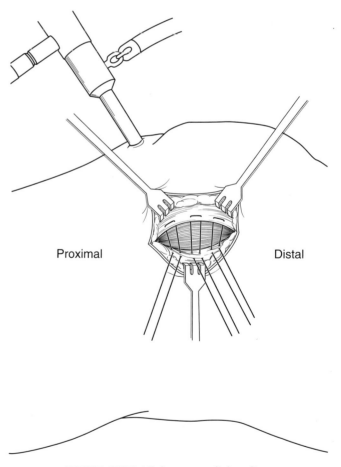

FIGURE 17.26 Mini-open medial reefing.

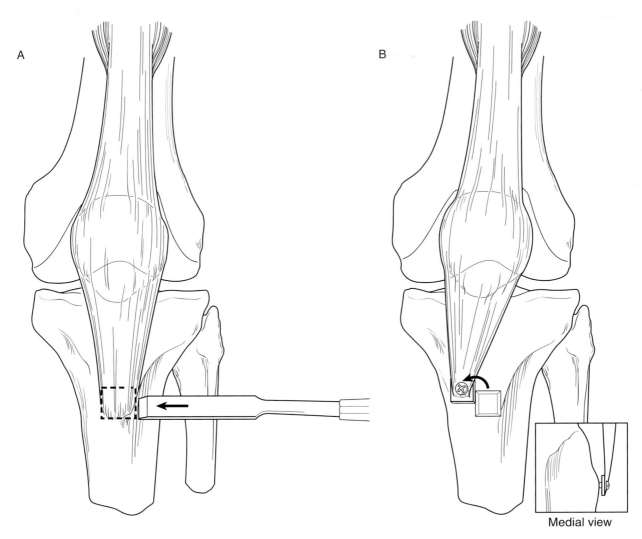

FIGURE 17.27 Tibial tubercle osteotomy.

and the exact position in which the transferred tubercle is placed determine the medialization and anteriorization. If significant patellofemoral arthrosis is encountered, we increase the amount of anterior displacement; if the primary problem is lateral subluxation with an abnormal Q angle, the amount of medialization is more important. Tracking can again be assessed, using provisional k-wire fixation if necessary, before final fixation with a cancellous screw. A range-of-motion brace set from 0 to 60 degrees is used postoperatively.

Arthroscopic Treatment of Other Patellofemoral Pathologies: Chondromalacia

As stated previously, softening or wear of the articular cartilage of the knee is a common finding in asymptomatic patients. The four-level grading system for chondromalacia described by Outerbridge is well known: Grade I indicates swelling and softening, and the grades progress through fissuring and fragmentation to grade IV, which designates complete erosion of the articular surface and exposed subchondral bone (53). Grade II or III chondrosis should be mechanically debrided to remove a possible source of loose bodies and possibly stabilize articular defects. An attempt should be made to leave as much normal cartilage undisturbed possible. As stated previously, we prefer a mechanical form of debridement such as a motorized shaver (Fig. 17.28).

We do not advocate the use of monopolar or bipolar radiofrequency at this time. If bare subchondral bone is exposed, microfracture technique may be used to provide vascular channels in the hope of generating fibrocartilage to fill the defect. Furakawa et al. (54) studied the composition of this repair tissue in rabbits and noted reversal in the normal ratio of type I and type II cartilage. They noted an abnormally large amount of type I collagen, whereas in normal cartilage type II tissue makes up 90% to 95%. This repara-

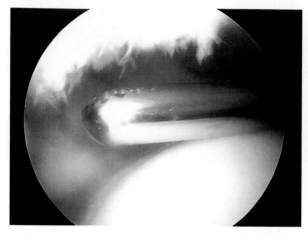

FIGURE 17.28 Arthroscopic view showing mechanical debridement with a motorized shaver.

tive tissue has an imperfect structure, and the integrity of the repair tissue is not maintained, resulting in likely fibrillation and breakdown of the repair cartilage.

If chondral changes are associated with patellofemoral malalignment, then the source of the changes—the malalignment—must be addressed. As previously stated, if only patellar tilt is present, it can often be adequately treated by lateral retinacular release. If subluxation is present, with an abnormal congruence angle, then a proximal or distal open realignment procedure may be needed.

CONCLUSION

The patellofemoral joint is a common source of pathology, either as a primary problem or as a significant secondary problem that may eventually become the most troubling to the patient. As with any orthopedic problem, a careful history and thorough examination are important. Radiographs, CT, and MRI studies all may be used to aid in diagnosis. Patellofemoral arthroscopy is very beneficial to confirm an initial diagnosis and to treat pathology. Arthroscopic examination should be performed in a routine manner so as to avoid inadvertently missing critical findings. Arthroscopic lateral release is very beneficial in treating patellar tilt. If significant subluxation is also present, the arthroscope can be used in conjunction with a planned open procedure, such as a proximal reefing or distal realignment, to assess correction intraoperatively. The surgeon should not forget that the mainstay of treatment for patellofemoral disorders in all cases initially, and in the majority of cases definitively, is patient education combined with appropriate physical therapy.

REFERENCES

1. Karlsson J, Thomee R, Sward L. Eleven year follow-up of patellofemoral pain syndrome. *Clin J Sports Med* 1996;6:22–26.

2. Whitelaw G, Rullo D, Markowitz H, et al. A conservative approach to anterior knee pain. *Clin Orthop* 1989;246:234–237.

3. DeHaven K, Dolan W, Mayor P. Chondromalacia patellae in athletes: clinical presentation and conservative management. *Am J Sports Med* 1979;77:5–11.

4. Wiberg G: Roentgenographic and anatomic studies on the patellofemoral joint with special reference to chondromalacia patella. *Acta Orthop Scand* 1941;12:319–410.

5. Aglietti P, Insall JN, Cerulli G. Patellar pain and incongruence I: measurements of incongruence. *Clin Orthop* 1983;176:217–224.

6. Warren LF, Marshall JL. The supporting structures and layers on the medial side of the knee: an anatomical analysis. *J Bone Joint Surg Am* 1979;61:56–62.

7. Feller JA, Feagin JA Jr, Garrettt WE Jr. The medial patellofemoral ligament revisited: an anatomical study. *Knee Surg Sports Traumatol Arthrosc* 1993;1:184–186.

8. Conlan T, Garth WP Jr, Lemons JE. Evaluation of the medial soft tissue restraints of the extensor mechanism of the knee. *J Bone Joint Surg Am* 1993;75:682–693.

9. Koskinen SK, Kujala UM. Patellofemoral relationships and distal insertion of the vastus medialis muscle: a magnetic resonance imaging study in nonsymptomatic subjects and in patients with patellar dislocation. *Arthroscopy* 1992;8:465–468.

10. Heegaard J, Leyvraz PE, Van Kampen A, et al. Influence of soft structures on patellar three dimensional tracking. *Clin Orthop* 1994;299:235–243.

11. Fulkerson J, Gossling H. Anatomy of the knee joint lateral retinaculum. *Clin Orthop* 1980;153:183.

12. Fulkerson JP, Tennant R, Jaivin JS, et al. Histologic evidence of retinacular nerve injury associated with patellofemoral malalignment. *Clin Orthop* 1985;197:196–205.

13. Sanchis-Alfonso V, Rosello-Sastre E. Immunohistochemical analysis for neural markers of the lateral retinaculum in patients with isolated symptomatic patellofemoral malalignment: a neuroanatomic basis for anterior knee pain in the active young patient. *Am J Sports Med* 2000;28:725–731.

14. Sanchis-Alfonso V, Rosello-Sastre E, Monteagudo-Castro C, et al. Quantitative analysis of nerve changes in the lateral retinaculum in patients with isolated symptomatic patellofemoral malalignment: a preliminary study. *Am J Sports Med* 1998;26:703–709.

15. Sutton F, Thompson C, Lipke J, et al. The effect of patellectomy and knee function. *J Bone Joint Surg Am* 1976;58:537–540.

16. Goodfellow J, Hungerford D, Zindel M. Patellofemoral joint mechanics and pathology: functional anatomy of the patellofemoral joint. *J Bone Joint Surg Br* 1976;58:287–290.

17. Hungerford G, Barry M. Biomechanics of the patellofemoral joint. *Clin Orthop* 1979;149:9–15.

18. Fulkerson J, Shea K. Disorders of patellofemoral alignment. *J Bone Joint Surg Am* 1990;72:1424–1429.

19. Witvrouw E, Lysens R, Bellemans J, et al. Intrinsic risk factors for the development of anterior knee pain in an athletic population: a two year prospective study. *Am J Sports Med* 2000;28:480–489.

20. Hughston J, Walsh W, Puddu G. *Patellar subluxation and dislocation.* Philadelphia: WB Saunders, 1984.

21. Greenfield M, Scott W. Arthroscopic evaluation and treatment of the patellofemoral joint. *Orthop Clin North Am* 1992;23:587–600.

22. Kolowich PA, Paulos LE, Rosenberg TD, et al. Lateral release of the patella: indications and contraindications. *Am J Sports Med* 1990;18:359–365.

23. Fulkerson JP, Kalenak A, Rosenberg TD, et al. Patellofemoral pain. *Instr Course Lect* 1992;41:57–71.

24. Insall J, Salvati E. Patella position in the normal knee joint. *Radiology* 1971;101:101–104.

25. Blumensaat C. Die Lageabweichungen und Verrenkungen der Kniescheibe. *Ergeb Chir Ortho* 1938;31:149.

26. Merchant A, Mercer, R, Jacobson R, et al. Roentgenographic analysis of patellofemoral congruence. *J Bone Joint Surg Am* 1974;56:1391–1396.

27. Laurin C, Dussault R, Levesque H. The tangential x-ray investigation of the patellofemoral joint. *Clin Orthop* 1979;144: 16–26.

28. Merchant AC. Patellofemoral disorders: biomechanics, diagnosis, and nonoperative treatment. In: McGinty JB, ed. *Operative arthroscopy*. New York: Raven Press, 1990:273.

29. Martinez S, Korobkin M, Fonder FB, et al. Diagnosis of patellofemoral malalignment by computed tomography. *J Comput Assist Tomogr* 1983;7:1050–1053.

30. Schutzer S, Ramsby G, Fulkerson J. The evaluation of patellofemoral pain using computerized tomography: a preliminary study. *Clin Orthop* 1986;204:286–293.

31. Fulkerson J, Schutzer S, Ramsby G, et al. Computerized tomography of the patellofemoral joint before and after lateral release or realignment. *Arthroscopy* 1987;3:19–24.

32. Shellock F, Mink J, Fox J. Patellofemoral joint, kinematic MR imaging to assess tracking abnormalities. *Radiology* 1988;168: 551–553.

33. Van Leersum MD, Schweitzer ME, Gannon F, et al. Thickness of patellofemoral articular cartilage as measured on MR imaging: sequence comparison of accuracy, reproducibility, and interobserver variation. *Skeletal Radiol* 1995;24:431–435.

34. Nakanishi K, Inoue M, Harada K, et al. Subluxation of the patella: evaluation of patellar articular cartilage with MR imaging. *Br J Radiol* 1992;65:662–667.

35. Shellock F, Mink J, Deutsch A, et al. Evaluation of patients with persistent symptoms after lateral retinacular release by kinematic magnetic resonance imaging of the patellofemoral joint. *Arthroscopy* 1990;6:226–234.

36. Shellock F, Mink J, Deutsch A, et al. Kinematic MR imaging of the patellofemoral joint: comparison of passive positioning and active movement techniques. *Radiology* 1992;184:574–577.

37. Sallay PI, Poggi J, Speer KP, et al. Acute dislocation of the patella: a correlative pathoanatomic study. *Am J Sports Med* 1996;24: 52–60.

38. Dye S, Boll D. Radionuclide imaging of the patellofemoral joint in young adults with anterior knee pain. *Orthop Clin North Am* 1986;17:249–261.

39. Iossifidis A, Brueton RN, Nunan TO. Bone scintigraphy in painful bipartite patella. *Eur J Nucl Med* 1995;22:1212–1213.

40. Merchant A. Classification of patellofemoral disorders. *Arthroscopy* 1988;4:235–240.

41. Insall J. Patellar pain. *J Bone Joint Surg Am* 1982;64:147–152.

42. Kannus P, Natri A, Paakkala T, et al. An outcome study of chronic patellofemoral pain syndrome: seven-year follow-up of patients in a randomized, controlled trial. *J Bone Joint Surg Am* 1999;81:355–363.

43. Greenwald MS, Bagley AM, France EP, et al. A biomechanical and clinical evaluation of a patellofemoral knee brace. *Clin Orthop* 1996;324:187–195.

44. Gilleard W, McConnell J, Parsons D. The effect of patellar taping on the onset of vastus medialis obliquus and vastus lateralis muscle activity in persons with patellofemoral pain. *Phys Ther* 1998;78:25–32.

45. Kowall MH, Kolk G, Nuber GW, et al. Patellar taping in the treatment of patellofemoral pain: a retrospective study. *Am J Sports Med* 1996;24:61–66.

46. Gigante A, Pasquinelli FM, Paladini P, et al. The effects of patellar taping on patellofemoral incongruence: a computed tomography study. *Am J Sports Med* 2001;29:88–92.

47. Sojbjerg J, Lauritzen J, Hvid I, et al. Arthroscopic determination of patellofemoral alignment. *Clin Orthop* 1987;215:243–247.

48. Grana W, Hinkley B, Hollingsworth S. Arthroscopic evaluation and treatment of patellar malalignment. *Clin Orthop* 1984;186: 122–128.

49. Johnson L. Arthroscopic evaluation of the patellofemoral articulation. In: Fox JM, DelPizzo W, eds. *The patellofemoral joint*. New York: McGraw-Hill, 1993:335–350.

50. Small NC. An analysis of complications in lateral retinacular release procedures. *Arthroscopy* 1989;5:282–286.

51. Henry JE, Pflum FA. Arthroscopic proximal patella realignment and stabilization. *Arthroscopy* 1995;11:424–425.

52. Bandi W. Chondromalacia patellae und femoro-patellare arthrose. *Helv Chir Acta* 1972;39[Suppl 1]:1–70.

53. Outerbridge RE, Dunlop J. The problem of chondromalacia patellae. *Clin Orthop* 1975;110:177–196.

54. Furukawa T, Eyre DR, Koide S, et al. Biochemical studies on repair cartilage resurfacing experimental defects in the rabbit knee. *J Bone Joint Surg Am* 1980;62:79–89.

18

ARTICULAR CARTILAGE: BASICS OF DIAGNOSIS AND TREATMENT

CHARLES A. BUSH-JOSEPH
MICHAEL D. GORDON

Articular cartilage injuries in the knee are commonly seen at arthroscopy, and the appropriate management of these lesions continues to be debated. Curl et al., in a review of 31,516 knee arthroscopies, found a 63% incidence of chondral lesions (1). Although the lesions were found throughout all three compartments of the knee, the most frequent locations were the patella and medial femoral condyle. In patients undergoing anterior cruciate ligament (ACL) reconstruction, Bach et al. reported chondromalacia of the patella in 31% and medial femoral condyle changes in 33% of patients studied (2,3). Fortunately, most articular cartilage injuries seen at arthroscopy are incidental and are associated with meniscal or ligamentous injuries. These are typically small or partial-thickness lesions that may remain asymptomatic.

The arthroscopic surgeon faces the common dilemma of deciding which lesions warrant observation and which require treatment. The decision to treat straightforward cartilage lesions is based on the biologic nature of the cartilage lesion as well as on patient-related factors of age, activity demands, and rehabilitation potential.

STRUCTURE AND FUNCTION OF ARTICULAR CARTILAGE

The principal functions of articular cartilage are to distribute loads evenly across the ends of bones and to provide a smooth, near-frictionless gliding surface. The basic architecture is composed of chondrocytes, collagen, extracellular matrix proteoglycans, noncollagenous proteins, and water. Chondrocytes make up 1% to 10% of the volume and are derived from undifferentiated mesenchymal marrow stem

C. A. Bush-Joseph: Department of Orthopaedic Surgery, Rush Presbyterian St. Luke's Medical Center, Chicago, Illinois 60612.

M. D. Gordon: Department of Orthopaedic Surgery, Rush Presbyterian St. Luke's Medical Center, Chicago, Illinois 60612.

cells (8). These cells synthesize and maintain the balance of the other components in articular cartilage.

Collagens, predominantly type II, are 60% of the dry weight of cartilage and provide the form and tensile stiffness of this tissue (9). Proteoglycans, comprising 2% to 35% of the dry weight, provide the compressive strength of articular cartilage (10). Proteoglycans are composed of a central structural protein with chains of highly charged glycosaminoglycans. The polarity of these molecules traps water within the matrix of the cartilage. Water is 75% to 80% of the wet weight of articular cartilage.

Articular cartilage is highly structured and is organized into four distinct histologic zones (Fig. 18.1). The superficial zone is the thinnest, and the collagen fibrils are oriented parallel to the joint surface. The transitional zone has a higher concentration of proteoglycans and a lower amount of water and collagen. In the middle, or radial, zone, the chondrocytes are arranged in columns, and there is the highest concentration of proteoglycans. The *tidemark* is located at the base of this zone, and the collagen fibrils extend through this landmark. The calcified cartilage zone is the deepest and is a thin layer of calcified cartilage that separates the radial zone from the underlying subchondral bone.

Articular cartilage lacks blood vessels, lymphatic vessels, and nerves. It receives its nutrition primarily by diffusion from the synovial fluid. The avascular status of articular cartilage is what causes its very limited response to injury, one that is far different from the way other tissues react to damage (13). Reparative cells may originate from synovial tissue, bone marrow, or other vascular elements (11). The matrix acts as a diffusion barrier as well as plays a key role in signal transduction throughout the chondral surface (9,12). This highly restricted location limits the potential for spontaneous repair unless the tidemark is violated and the lesion extends into the subchondral bone. When this occurs, such as in an osteochondral fracture, a vascular proliferative response initiated in the subchondral bone takes place.

Numerous studies have documented the poor response of partial-thickness articular cartilage injuries. These are

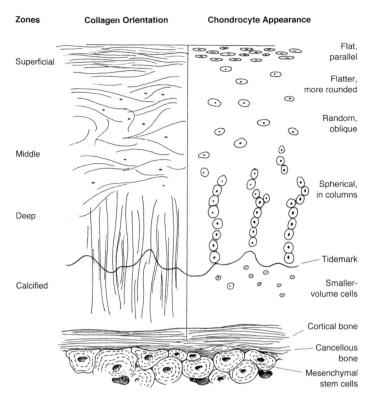

FIGURE 18.1 Modified Outerbridge classification of articular cartilage lesions. (From Browne JE, Branch TP. Surgical alternatives for treatment of articular cartilage lesions. *J Am Acad Orthop Surg* 2000;8:180–189, with permission.)

use. The system described by Outerbridge in 1961 is the simplest and most commonly cited working tool for describing chondral lesions (10). This grading system is based on the gross appearance of the defects, with grade I being softening or blistering of the surface. A grade II lesion is characterized by fissures or clefts measuring less than 1 cm in diameter. Grade III is characterized by deep fissures extending to subchondral bone measuring more than 1 cm, whereas grade IV is when subchondral bone is exposed (21) (Fig. 18.2). The Outerbridge grade, combined with the size, shape, and location of the damaged surface, provides an excellent method to communicate about chondral injuries. A "modified" Outerbridge scale, frequently used in the literature, does not depend on the size of the lesion, but rather is based solely on the depth of the fissuring or fibrillation (Fig. 18.3).

marked by a short-lived metabolic and enzymatic rush that is ultimately ineffectual (14). A region of necrosis is present in the immediate area around the lesion, with a limited increase in cellular activity. Studies have demonstrated no progression of healing over time, and these lesions remain stable, without significant progression (14–18).

When lesions extend deep through the tidemark, one sees in-growth of capillaries from the vascular bed and the formation of a fibrin clot, which soon leads to vascular fibroblastic repair tissue. Shapiro et al. showed that the source of the repair cells is from the undifferentiated mesenchymal cells of the marrow (19). Nehrer et al. evaluated specimens from failed cartilage repair procedures and demonstrated a variable healing response (20). The procedures that involved mechanically violating the tidemark, such as abrasion arthroplasty, were associated with fibrous tissue formation that underwent rapid degeneration. These investigators found that only 2% of the cross-sectional area had the appearance of healthy articular cartilage.

CLASSIFICATION OF ARTICULAR CARTILAGE LESIONS

Multiple grading systems of articular cartilage lesions have been devised over the years, but few have led to sustained

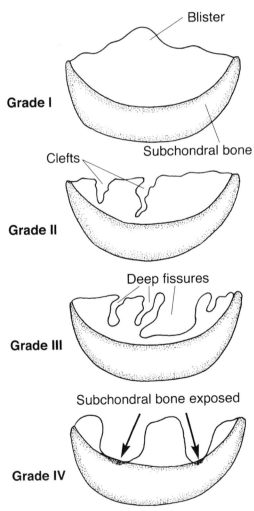

FIGURE 18.2 Basic structure of articular cartilage. (From Browne JE, Branch TP. Surgical alternatives for treatment of articular cartilage lesions. *J Am Acad Orthop Surg* 2000;8:180–189, with permission.)

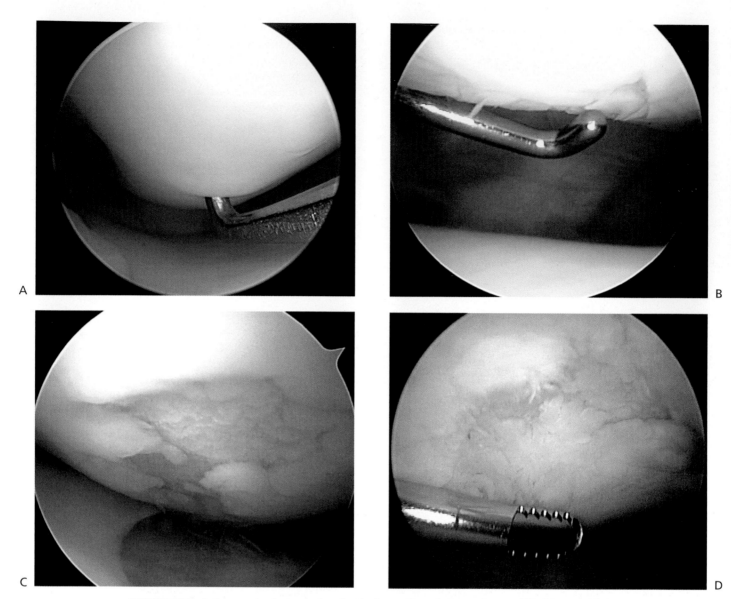

FIGURE 18.3 Arthroscopic photographs of articular cartilage lesions using modified Outerbridge classification. **A**: Grade I softening. **B**: Grade II partial-thickness fissuring. **C**: Grade III full-thickness fissuring and fibrillation. **D**: Grade IV articular changes with exposed bone centrally surrounded by diffuse grade III articular cartilage.

HISTORY AND PHYSICAL EXAMINATION

Articular cartilage injuries may occur as an isolated injury, they may be associated with meniscal or ligamentous injuries, or they may develop as a result of degenerative or inflammatory arthrosis. Patients with a traumatic onset often give a history of patellar dislocation or subluxation, a twisting injury, or a direct blow to the knee. Patients may report sudden pain and often describe a "snap" within the knee. Others have vague complaints of aching with chronic or intermittent swelling. Pain is the most common symptom and may or may not be associated with an effusion or locking resulting from the presence of loose bodies within the knee

joint (22–25). Pain related to activity can be suggestive of the location of the lesion (i.e., pain with jumping or the extension phase of kicking suggests patellar or trochlear disease; pain with the flexion phase of kicking suggests posterior condylar lesions) (26).

The key to early diagnosis is suspicion, based on the history and mechanism of injury. Johnson-Nurse and Dandy found that 95% of patients reported having pain, 76% swelling, and 18% locking. In addition, 51 of their 76 patients noted acute trauma instigating their condition. These investigators also reported that one-third of their cases "escaped early diagnosis" (23).

The physical examination in patients with articular injuries is often dictated by the severity of the associated injuries. Small lesions may cause no localized findings other than tenderness in the affected area. The presence of joint crepitation from exposed subchondral bone suggests a larger lesion. Hemarthrosis and the presence of fat globules are highly suggestive of osteochondral injury, particularly in the setting of an acute patellar dislocation (22). Noyes et al. reported that 20% of patients with traumatic hemarthrosis with minimal to no instability had chondral fractures (27). Butler and Andrews found that 11% of their patients with acute hemarthrosis had an osteochondral fracture at arthroscopy (28). Patients with chronic articular injuries often have localized tenderness in the involved area and may develop activity-related joint swelling.

Joint osteophytes, limb malalignment, and contractures are ominous findings of more advanced joint arthrosis in which the treatment of articular cartilage lesions remains unpredictable. Synovial thickening and polyarticular involvement suggest inflammatory arthrosis, in which case articular cartilage lesions rarely warrant treatment as an isolated entity.

RADIOGRAPHIC AND DIAGNOSTIC TESTS

Because of the variable and broad presentation of articular cartilage injuries, many attempts have been made to develop a simple test to diagnosis these lesions. Weight-bearing radiographs of the knee have not consistently revealed defects in either prospective or retrospective studies (22), but they are necessary to identify global joint space loss and the presence of limb malalignment. Weight-bearing posteroanterior flexion views are useful in diagnosing compartment narrowing (primarily on the flexion surface of the femur) or the presence of osteochondritis dissecans lesions. Skyline and merchant radiographs have been more sensitive in identifying osteochondral defects involving the patellofemoral articulation. Ultrasound has also been evaluated as a method to evaluate for articular cartilage injuries, but its current use remains investigational (29).

The ability to visualize articular cartilage with magnetic resonance imaging (MRI) has advanced with the development of new sequences, receiver coils, and gradient technology (30). The two most widely used imaging techniques are the T1-weighted fat-suppressed three-dimensional spoiled gradient-echo technique and the T2-weighted fast spin-echo technique. Accuracy is highest in the patellofemoral joint with both techniques because the cartilage is thickest there (Fig. 18.4). Disler et al. found that the fat-suppressed three-dimensional spoiled gradient-echo sequence provides 91% accuracy, with a sensitivity of 86% and a specificity of 97%. The T2-weighted fast spin-echo techniques, both without and with fat suppression, also have a high accuracy

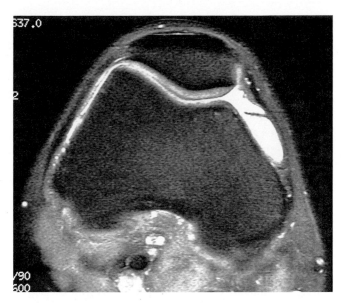

FIGURE 18.4 Magnetic resonance imaging photograph of normal patellofemoral joint articular cartilage.

of 92%, with a sensitivity of 87% and a specificity of 92% (31) (Fig. 18.5). In contrast to these good results, Munk et al. found very poor correlation between arthroscopic and MRI findings, with a sensitivity and positive predictive value of 0% (32). Multiple other techniques have been described, with variable results (31–37). Adding intraarticular contrast to the MRI does not appear to improve the accuracy of the technique (38).

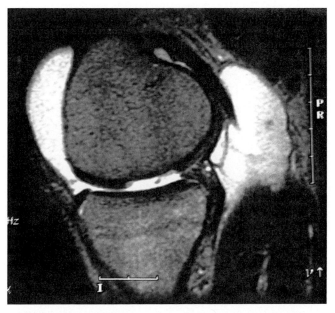

FIGURE 18.5 Magnetic resonance imaging of a full-thickness articular cartilage defect of the medial femoral condyle.

TREATMENT

The treatment of articular cartilage lesions has a long history of simple and increasingly complex procedures, with variable results. The uncertainty of the natural history of chondral injuries makes it especially difficult to determine the ideal method of management. Several authors believe that many lesions are nonprogressive, and the joints will return to an asymptomatic state once the transient synovitis resolves or the associated injuries are treated (4,13–15, 39–41). The dilemma is determining which lesions will follow this nonprogressive course and which will gradually degenerate over time. Messner and Maletius reported that 22 of 28 patients with isolated chondral lesions (smaller than 1 cm in diameter) who were followed-up over a 14-year period had good or excellent clinical results without treatment (7). When the history, physical examination, and radiographs are suggestive of degenerative joint disease, arthroscopic treatment remains an adjunct to alleviate mechanical symptoms resulting from loose bodies, meniscal tears, or unstable chondral flaps.

All treatment regimens, except joint lavage and debridement, are based on interventions to increase the cellular access to the injury site. This can be accomplished by increasing the vascular flow, by recruiting local cells, or by transplanting cells to the affected region. The end result is one of two pathways: a *repair* or a *restorative* response.

Lavage and Debridement

Lavage and mechanical debridement comprise the simplest operative approach and have been described extensively in the treatment of knees with significant degenerative joint disease. Chondral flaps or fibrillation can cause mechanical symptoms as well as lead to reactive synovitis and joint effusion (42). Conservative shaving of these lesions does not stimulate repair; however, multiple authors have demonstrated relief with simple debridement back to stable margins (43–51). In addition, other authors have demonstrated temporary relief of symptoms with lavage alone (52,53). In one study considering chondral injuries in collegiate soccer players, Levy et al. noted 100% good or excellent results at 1-year follow-up after simple debridement (26). In summary, lavage and debridement can predictably provide *temporary* relief of the symptoms of chondral injuries; however, the duration of the benefit is extremely variable. Care must be taken to avoid overzealous chondral debridement that exposes large surface areas and leads to increased contact stresses in neighboring tissue.

Lasers and Radiofrequency Energy

Lasers have long been used for tissue ablation and cauterization. Evidence also indicates that laser light can trigger a cellular healing response (54). Multiple studies have been performed to evaluate whether the different types of lasers can affect chondral injuries in a positive way. Most of these studies have been extremely limited in number of specimens and length of follow-up. They suggest that there is probably no benefit over simple mechanical debridement, and lasers may even increase the risk of complications of necrosis and cartilage slough (55,56). An *ex vivo* study of laser-induced cartilage injury that used confocal microscopy demonstrated that standard histologic analysis greatly underestimated the degree of acute tissue damage (57). Given the potential increased risk, as well as the expense, it appears that lasers have a limited role in the treatment of chondral injuries. Lasers, with proper caution, remain an effective tool for simple tissue debridement and hemostasis control.

Monopolar and bipolar *radiofrequency energy* has been evaluated in the treatment of partial-thickness defects of articular cartilage. Initially, this technology was noted to "smooth" and "stabilize" the chondral surface, and these findings led to further study. Despite early enthusiasm for the contouring potential of radiofrequency energy, gross and histologic studies using highly sensitive confocal laser microscopy to evaluate cell viability are now clearly showing that thermal chondroplasty results in immediate chondrocyte death and overall decrease in proteoglycan levels (58–60). Lu et al. demonstrated that bipolar radiofrequency energy devices penetrate 78% to 92% deeper than the monopolar system and reach the subchondral bone (59) (Fig. 18.6). Until further studies have been completed and technical advances have been made to limit the depth of penetration of this technology, radiofrequency energy has a limited role in the treatment of articular cartilage injuries other than as an effective means of tissue debridement.

Marrow Stimulation Techniques

The avascularity of the articular cartilage has been a major target of the treatments for injuries to the joint surface. Techniques focusing on marrow stimulation were first described in open surgery and have since been tailored to arthroscopy (61,62). Penetration of the subchondral bone provides vascular access to the lesion and, theoretically, access to the pluripotent marrow cells. The repair tissue that forms is predominantly fibrous and generally deteriorates over time (12,13,15,48).

In 1959, Pridie first described the concept of drilling through eburnated bone to stimulate reparative fibrocartilage (61). Johnson popularized *abrasion arthroplasty,* a treatment in which a bur is used to resect the bone to a depth of 1 to 2 mm (63). Despite Johnson's enthusiasm, other authors have not had comparable results and actually have reported a greater than 20% incidence of clinical worsening (47,50,64). These procedures are largely discussed out of historical interest and have been replaced by other treatment methods.

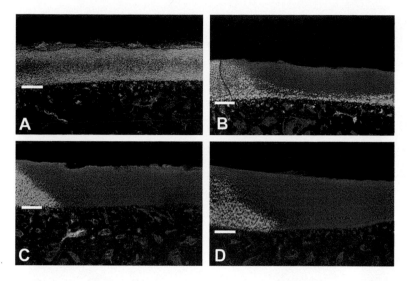

FIGURE 18.6 Confocal microscopic image demonstrating radiofrequency energy–treated cartilage surface *(top of each image)* and subchondral bone *(bottom of each image)* using a paintbrush pattern in bovine articular cartilage. The *green dots* indicate viable chondrocytes, and the *red dots* indicate dead chondrocytes. **A**: Control. **B**: Oratec monopolar radiofrequency energy treatment caused immediate chondrocyte death that did not extend to the subchondral bone. Mitek (**C**) and Arthrocare (**D**) bipolar radiofrequency energy treatments caused immediate cell death that extended to the subchondral bone. The *white bars* demonstrate the boundary between the cartilage and subchondral bone. (From Lu Y, Edwards RB III, Cole BJ, et al. Thermal chondroplasty with radiofrequency energy: an *in vitro* comparison of bipolar and monopolar radiofrequency devices. *Am J Sports Med* 2001;29:42–49, with permission.)

Microfracture is a technique in which multiple holes are made using awls into the subchondral bone 3 to 5 mm apart. This technique produces a vascular response while maintaining the structural integrity of the underlying subchondral plate. Unstable chondral flaps are removed, and the calcified cartilage layer is lightly debrided without damaging the underlying subchondral bone (Fig. 18.7). Using awls theoretically has the advantage of not creating heat necrosis associated with power drilling techniques. Steadman et al. found that 75% of their patients had an improvement in their pain at a follow-up of 3 to 5 years (65). The greatest improvement occurred in the first postoperative year, and then the results tended to plateau over the next 4 to 5 years (66). These surgeons described an involved postoperative protocol that included continuous passive motion (CPM) and protected weight bearing for 6 to 8 weeks. Steadman et al. described that the regenerated tissue appeared to be a hybrid of hyaline cartilage and fibrocartilage, whereas numerous animal and human studies have shown that the tissue is predominantly fibrocartilage (65). Despite the relative clinical success of this method, the durability of the fibrocartilage tissue remains in doubt. The authors have experienced greatest success with microfracture techniques when they are used in combination with ligament reconstruction in unstable knees or in combination with unloading procedures for patients with mechanical malalignment (65).

Periosteal and Perichondral Grafts

Periosteal or perichondral grafts were described in the past as cellular donors. Homminga et al. in 1990 used costal perichondrium to fill 30 articular cartilage defects in 25 patients (68). These investigators noted the presence of hyaline repair tissue at follow-up arthroscopy and biopsy. Calcific radiodensity in the grafts occurred by 2 years in more than two-thirds of the patients. In his series, Farnworth

noted that these calcific densities represented enchondral ossification within the graft that ultimately led to graft failure in seven of his ten patients (22).

Periosteum is derived from perichondrium embryologically and has been shown to have chondrogenic potential from the cambium layer producing a hyaline-like cartilage (69,70–76). Many laboratory studies have been performed on these grafts; however, few good clinical studies exist. Lorentzon treated 26 patellar defects with tibia-based periosteal grafts in conjunction with debridement, microfracture, and postoperative CPM (77). Lorentzon found 16 excellent and nine good results at 3½ years and recommended the treatment for patients with disabling patellofemoral pain. Potential ossification of this tissue through time has led to very limited application of this technique.

Cell and Tissue Transplantation

Autologous chondrocyte implantation was first reported in 1994 by Brittberg et al. Autologous chondrocytes were harvested during arthroscopy and were grown in culture before being reimplanted under periosteal flaps into chondral defects (78). The subchondral bone was not violated, thereby limiting the fibrovascular response. These investigators found hyaline-like tissue in 11 of 16 lesions at second-look arthroscopy. At follow-up of 2 to 9 years, 92% of isolated femoral condyle lesions, 65% of patellar lesions, and 89% with osteochondritis dissecans had good or excellent results (79). These investigators suggest that the indications for this technique are for the repair of symptomatic, cartilaginous defects of the femoral condyle and trochlea in younger patients with good alignment and stability. Newman raised questions about the initial studies and whether the good results were caused specifically by the chondrocyte transplantation, the natural history of partial-thickness chondral injuries, or the debridement performed as part of the procedure (13). Minas

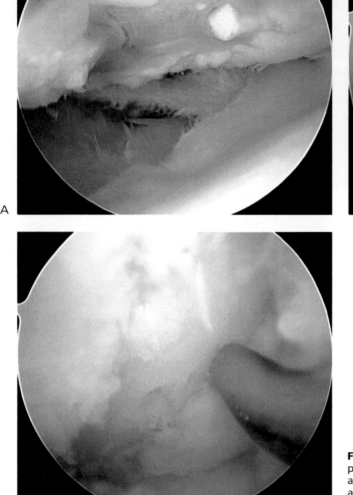

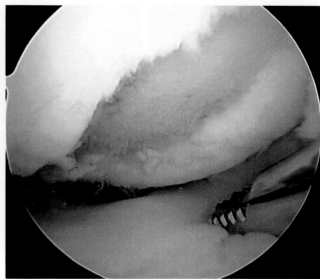

FIGURE 18.7 Microfracture of the medial femoral condyle in a patient with a chondral fracture with acute anterior cruciate ligament injury. **A**: Condyle lesion. **B**: Debridement of the margins and calcified cartilage layer. **C**: Microfracture of the base using angled awls.

reported a 37% complication rate in his series of 70 patients (80) (Fig. 18.8). Details of this technique, as well as potential indications, are covered in Chapter 19.

Osteochondral autografts are osteochondral plugs that are harvested from a nonarticulating portion of the joint and are transferred to a defect in a weight-bearing region. Hangody et al. compared mosaicplasty with abrasion arthroplasty, microfracture, and subchondral drilling of articular lesions from 1 to 9 cm^2. These investigators concluded that the results of procedures that penetrated the subchondral bone deteriorated over time, with improvements ranging from 48% to 62%, whereas osteochondral autografts results remained at 86% to 90% at 5 years (81). The limited supply of donor tissue and the difference in the surface contour of the donor plug to the recipient site are concerns that restrict the use of this procedure. In addition, when multiple plugs are used, the space between the grafts is filled in with fibrocartilage. Finally, CPM in the postoperative period and firm

fixation of the plugs have also been found to be beneficial (82) (Fig. 18.9).

Osteochondral allografts have been extensively studied and have had mixed results, depending on the way in which they are preserved or prepared and the time in which they are reimplanted (83,84). The potential advantages of allografts are the ability to fill a larger defect, the lack of donor site morbidity, and the increased congruency of the graft with the surrounding and opposing joint surfaces. The central problem in the preparation of these grafts is that to ensure the greatest survival of the chondrocytes, the grafts must be implanted very soon after harvest, possibly within 24 hours, and they cannot be frozen. Although this approach preserves the articular surface, the underlying bone is not rid of its cellular elements, and thus antigenic exposure and the risk of viral transmission are increased (85,86). When these grafts fail, it is usually because of collapse of the subchondral bone. Zukor et al. reported a success rate in 92 knees with osteo-

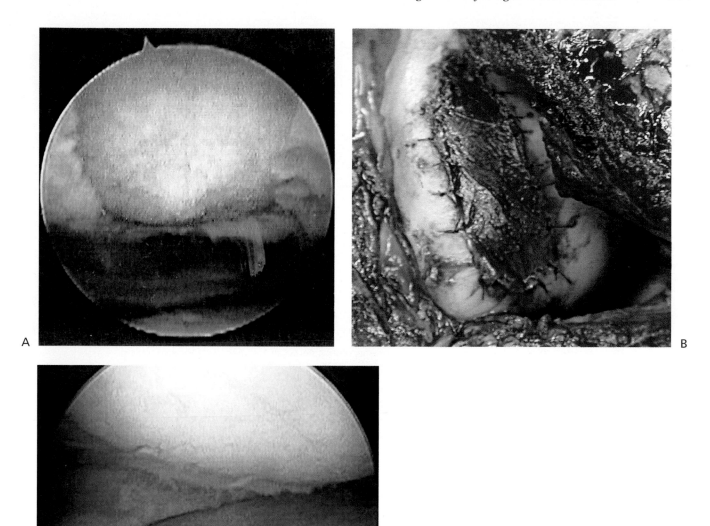

FIGURE 18.8 Clinical photographs of a full-thickness chondral defect of a medial femoral condyle (**A**), after autologous chondrocyte transplantation with periosteal grafting (**B**), and during an arthroscopic second-look procedure 18 months postoperatively (**C**).

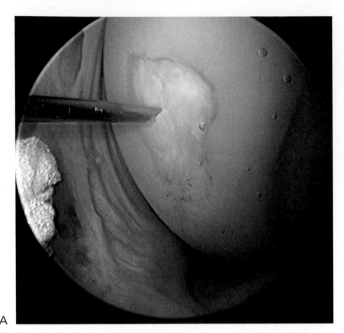
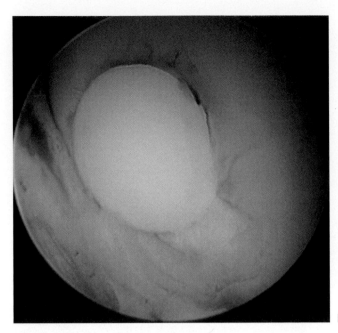

A   B

FIGURE 18.9 A: Clinical photograph of a symptomatic defect of the medial femoral condyle despite microfracture treatment of the defect 12 months earlier. **B**: Appearance of a single osteochondral autologous plug in the defect.

chondral allografts of 75% at 5 years, 64% at 10 years, and 63% at 14 years (85). Gross reported the success rate in 123 knees to be 95% at 5 years, 71% at 10 years, and 66% at 20 years (86).

REHABILITATION

Preoperative education of the patients on the nature and goals of rehabilitation can prevent postoperative fear and apprehension that may lead to delayed recovery. General principles after arthroscopic surgery include early range of motion, joint swelling control, and muscle activation. Weight-bearing status is determined by the specifics of the procedure performed. The use of ice in the early postoperative period can be helpful to control joint swelling and to allow improved motion. Analgesics and antiinflammatory medications are encouraged for pain relief. An early emphasis on quadriceps activation and on recovery of full extension of the knee encourages a faster return to ambulation. Patients with poor muscle activation often require a supervised physical therapy program for 1 to 3 months.

Patients undergoing an extensive procedure involving multiple osteochondral plugs or multiple microfracture holes may develop hemarthrosis requiring joint aspiration. Prolonged joint swelling can lead to quadriceps inhibition and the development of joint fibrosis. Compressive wraps and support hose may be helpful. Isometric exercises and the use of stationary bicycles are helpful to control edema, to regain motion, and to reestablish a more normal gait pattern. Strengthening exercises (with the use of weights) are avoided

until near-normal range of motion is recovered. Closed-chain exercises avoid shear forces over the joint surfaces and are generally much safer than open-chain exercises in these patients.

Recovery time varies with the complexity of the procedure. Patients who undergo simple lavage and debridement generally recover within 6 to 8 weeks. Patients who undergo a more extensive debridement, marrow stimulation techniques, or chondrocyte transplant procedures often require 3 to 6 months before improvement is noted.

FUTURE AND ADJUNCTIVE TREATMENTS

CPM and its beneficial effects on the healing response of articular cartilage are concepts that have been championed since 1970 by Salter. His basic science research demonstrated that CPM has a significant stimulating effect on the healing of articular tissues, and CPM can contribute to regeneration of articular cartilage through neochondrogenesis both with and without periosteal grafts (87). Multiple trials have been published incorporating CPM in the standard postoperative regimen, including microfracture, autologous chondrocyte transplantation, and mosaicplasty.

Current research includes considering harnessing bone morphogenetic proteins to try to stimulate chondrogenesis. Sellers et al. reported the 1-year results of implanting a collagen sponge impregnated with recombinant human bone morphogenetic protein-2 (rhBMP-2) into rabbit knee full-thickness chondral defects (88,89). These researchers found that the addition of rhBMP-2 resulted in improved histologic appearance and composition of the extracellular matrix that was sustained throughout the year of the project. Another area of research is the evaluation of the role of implantable synthetic scaffolding that is placed within the chondral defect.

REFERENCES

1. Curl WW, Krome J, Gordon ES, et al. cartilage injuries: a review of 31,516 knee arthroscopies. *Arthoscopy* 1997;13:456–460.
2. Bach BR Jr, Levy ME, Bojchuk J, et al. Single-incision endoscopic anterior cruciate ligament reconstruction using patellar tendon autograft: minimum two-year follow-up evaluation. *Am J Sports Med* 1998;26:30–40.
3. Bach BR Jr, Tradonsky S, Bojchuk J, et al. Arthroscopically assisted anterior cruciate ligament reconstruction using patellar tendon autograft: five-to nine-year follow-up evaluation. *Am J Sports Med* 1998;26:20–29.
4. Campbell CJ. The healing of cartilage defects. *Clin Orthop* 1969;64:45–63.
5. Coletti JM Jr, Akeson WH, Woo SL-Y. A comparison of the physical behavior of normal articular cartilage and the arthroplasty surface. *J Bone Joint Surg Am* 1972;54:147–160.
6. Furukawa T, Eyre DR, Koide S, et al. Biochemical studies on repair cartilage resurfacing experimental defects in the rabbit knee. *J Bone Joint Surg Am* 1980;62:79–89.
7. Messner K, Maletius W. The long-term prognosis for severe damage to weight-bearing cartilage in the knee. *Acta Orthop Scand* 1996;67:165–168.
8. McDevitt CA, Marcelino J. Composition of articular cartilage. *Sports Med Arthrosc Rev* 1994;2:1–12.
9. Buckwalter JA, Mankin HJ. Articular cartilage: part I. Tissue design and chondrocyte–matrix interactions. *J Bone Joint Surg Am* 1997;79:600–611.
10. Browne JE, Branch TP. Surgical alternatives for treatment of articular cartilage lesions. *J Am Acad Orthop Surg* 2000;8:180–189.
11. Hunziker EB, Rosenberg LC. Repair of partial-thickness defects in articular cartilage: cell recruitment from the synovial membrane. *J Bone J Surg Am* 1996;78:721–733.
12. Buckwalter JA, Mankin HJ. Articular cartilage: part II. Degeneration and osteoarthrosis, repair, regeneration, and transplantation. *J Bone Joint Surg Am* 1997;79:612–632.
13. Newman AP. Articular cartilage repair. *Am J Sports Med* 1998;26:309–324.
14. Mankin HJ. The response of articular cartilage to mechanical injury. *J Bone Joint Surg Am* 1982;64:460–466.
15. Buckwalter JA, Rosenberg L, Coutts R, et al. Articular cartilage: injury and repair. :In Woo SL-Y, Buckwalter JA, eds. *Injury and repair of the musculoskeletal soft tissues*. Park Ridge, IL: American Academy of Orthopaedic Surgeons, 1988:465–482.
16. Meachim G. The effect of scarification on articular cartilage in the rabbit. *J Bone Joint Surg Br* 1963;45:150–161.
17. Meachim G, Roberts C. Repair of the joint surface from subarticular tissue in the rabbit knee. *J Anat* 1971;109:317–327.
18. Thompson RC. An experimental study of surface injury to articular cartilage and enzyme responses within the joint. *Clin Orthop* 1975;107:239–248.
19. Shapiro F, Koide S, Flimcher MJ. Cell origin and differentiation in the repair of full-thickness defects of articular cartilage. *J Bone Joint Surg Am* 1993;75:532–553.
20. Nehrer S, Spector M, Minas T. Histologic analysis of tissue after failed cartilage repair procedures. *Clin Orthop* 1999;365:149–162.
21. Outerbridge RE. The etiology of chondromalacia patellae. *J Bone Joint Surg Br* 1961;43:752–757.
22. Farnworth L. Osteochondral defects of the knee. *Orthopedics* 2000;23:146–157.
23. Johnson-Nurse C, Dandy DJ. Fracture separation of articular cartilage in the adult knee. *J Bone Joint Surg Br* 1985;67:42–43.
24. Matthewson MH, Dandy DJ. Osteochondral fractures of the lateral femoral condyle: a result of indirect violence to the knee. *J Bone Joint Surg Br* 1978;60:199–202.
25. Vellet AD, Marks PH, Fowler PJ, et al. Occult posttraumatic osteochondral lesions of the knee: prevalence, classification, and short-term sequelae evaluated with MR imaging. *Radiology* 1991;178:271–276.
26. Levy AS, Lohnes J, Sculley S, et al. Chondral delamination of the knee in soccer players. *Am J Sports Med* 1996;24:634–639.
27. Noyes FR, Bassett RW, Grood ES, et al. Arthroscopy in acute traumatic hemarthrosis of the knee. *J Bone Joint Surg Am* 1980;62:687–695.
28. Butler JC, Andrews JR. The role of arthroscopic surgery in the evaluation of acute traumatic hemarthrosis. *Clin Orthop* 1988;228:150–152.
29. Disler DG, Raymond E, May DA, et al. Articular cartilage defects: in vitro evaluation of accuracy and interobserver reliability for detection and grading with US. *Radiology* 2000;215:846–851.
30. McCauley TR, Disler DG. MR imaging of articular cartilage. *Radiology* 1998;209:629–640.
31. Disler DG, McCauley TR, Kelman CG, et al. Fat-suppressed three-dimensional spoiled gradient-echo MR imaging of hyaline cartilage defects in the knee: comparison with standard MR imaging and arthroscopy. *AJR Am J Roentgenol* 1996;167:127–132.
32. Munk B, Madsen F, Lundorf E, et al. Clinical magnetic resonance imaging and arthroscopic findings in knees: a comparative prospective study of meniscus anterior cruciate ligament and cartilage lesions. *Arthroscopy* 1998;14:171–175.
33. Ochi M, Sumen Y, Kanda T, et al. The diagnostic value and limitation of magnetic resonance imaging on chondral lesions in the knee joint. *Arthroscopy* 1994;10:176–183.
34. Heron CW. Review article: MRI of the knee. *Br J Radiol* 1993;66:292–302.
35. Potter HG, Linklater JM, Allen AA, et al. Magnetic resonance imaging of articular cartilage in the knee: an evaluation with use of fast-spin echo imaging. *J Bone Joint Surg Am* 1998;80:1276–1284.
36. Mori R, Ochi M, Sakai Y, et al. Clinical significance of magnetic resonance imaging (MRI) for focal chondral lesions. *Magn Reson Imaging* 1999;17:1135–1140.
37. Gold GE, Thedens DR, Pauly JM, et al. MR imaging of articular cartilage of the knee: new methods using ultrashort TE's. *AJR Am J Roentgenol* 1998;170:1223–1226.
38. McCauley TR, Disler DG. Magnetic resonance imaging of articular cartilage of the knee. *J Am Acad Orthop Surg* 2001;9:2–8.
39. Fuller JA, Ghadially FN. Ultrastructural observations on surgically produced partial-thickness defects in articular cartilage. *Clin Orthop* 1972;86:193–205.
40. Ghadially FN, Thomas I, Oryschak AF, et al. Long term results of superficial defects in articular cartilage: a scanning electron-microscope study. *J Pathol* 1977;121:213–217.
41. Mankin HJ, Boyle CJ. The acute effects of lacerative injury on DNA and protein synthesis in articular cartilage. In: Bassett CAL, ed. *Cartilage degradation and repair*. Washington, DC: National Research Council/National Academy of Sciences/National Academy of Engineering 1967:185–199.
42. Evans CH, Mazzocchi RA, Nelson DD, et al. Experimental arthritis induced by intraarticular injection of allogenic cartilaginous particles into rabbit knees. *Arthritis Rheum* 1984;27:200–207.

43. Kim HKW, Moran ME, Salter RB. The potential for regeneration of articular cartilage in defects created by chondral shaving and subchondral abrasion: an experimental investigation in rabbits. *J Bone Joint Surg Am* 1991;73:1301–1315.

44. Mitchell N, Shepard N. Effect of patellar shaving in the rabbit. *J Orthop Res* 1987;5:388–392.

45. Baumgaertner MR, Cannon WD Jr, Vittori JM, et al. Arthroscopic debridement of the arthritic knee. *Clin Orthop* 1990;253:197–202.

46. Bert JM. Role of abrasion arthroplasty and debridement in the management of osteoarthritis of the knee. *Rheum Dis Clin North Am* 1993;19:725–739.

47. Bert JM, Maschka K. The arthroscopic treatment of unicompartmental gonarthrosis: a five-year follow-up study of abrasion arthroplasty plus arthroscopic debridement and arthroscopic debridement alone. *Arthroscopy* 1989;5:25–32.

48. Buckwalter JA, Lohmander S. Operative treatment of osteoarthritis: current practice and future development. *J Bone Joint Surg Am* 1994;76:1405–1418.

49. Jackson RW, Silver R, Marans R. Arthroscopic treatment of degenerative joint disease. *Arthroscopy* 1986;2:114.

50. Rand JA. Role of arthroscopy in osteoarthritis of the knee. *Arthroscopy* 1991;7:358–363.

51. Hubbard MJS. Articular debridement versus washout for degeneration of the medial femoral condyle: a five-year study. *J Bone Joint Surg Br* 1996;78:217–219.

52. Gibson JNA, White MD, Chapman VM, et al. Arthroscopic lavage and debridement for osteoarthritis of the knee. *J Bone Joint Surg Br* 1992;74:534–537.

53. Livesley PJ, Doherty M, Needoff M, et al. Arthroscopic lavage of osteoarthritic knees. *J Bone Joint Surg Br* 1991;73:922–926.

54. Hansson TL. Infrared laser in the treatment of craniomandibular disorders: arthrogenous pain. *J Prosthet Dent* 1989;61:614–616.

55. Vangness CT Jr, Ghaderi B. Lasers in orthopedic surgery: a literature review of lasers and articular cartilage. *Orthopedics* 1993;16:593–598.

56. Thal R, Danziger MB, Kelly A. Delayed articular cartilage slough: two cases resulting from holmium:YAG laser damage to normal articular cartilage and a review of the literature. *Arthroscopy* 1996;12:92–94.

57. Mainil-Varlet P, Monin D, Weiler C, et al. Quantification of laser-induced cartilage injury by confocal microscopy in an *ex vivo* model. *J Bone Joint Surg Am* 2001;83:566–571.

58. Lu Y, Edwards RB III, Kalscheur VL, et al. Effect of bipolar radiofrequency energy on human articular cartilage: comparison of confocal laser microscopy and light microscopy. *Arthroscopy* 2001;17:117–123.

59. Lu Y, Edwards RB III, Cole BJ, et al. Thermal chondroplasty with radiofrequency energy: *in vitro* comparison of bipolar and monopolar radiofrequency devices. *Am J Sports Med* 2001;29:42–49.

60. Lu Y, Hayashi K, Hecht P, et al. The effect of monopolar radiofrequency energy on partial-thickness defects of articular cartilage. *Arthroscopy* 2000;16:527–536.

61. Pridie KH. A method of resurfacing osteoarthritic knee joints. *J Bone Joint Surg Br* 1959;41:618–619 (abst).

62. Ficat RP, Ficat C, Gedeon P, et al. Spongialization: a new treatment for diseased patellae. *Clin Orthop* 1979;144:74–83.

63. Johnson LL. Arthroscopic abrasion arthroplasty historical and pathologic perspective: present status. *Arthroscopy* 1986;2:54.

64. Friedman MJ, Berasi CC, Fox JM, et al. Preliminary results with abrasion arthroplasty in the osteoarthritic knee. *Clin Orthop* 1984;182:200–205.

65. Steadman JR, Rodkey WG, Singleton SB, et al. Microfracture technique for full thickness chondral defects: technique and clinical results. *Oper Tech Orthop* 1997;7:300–307.

66. Blevins FT, Steadman JR, Rodrigo JJ, et al. Treatment of articular cartilage defects in athletes: an analysis of functional outcome and lesion appearance. *Orthopedics* 1998;21:761–768.

67. Mitchell N, Shepard N. The resurfacing of adult rabbit articular cartilage by multiple perforations through the subchondral bone. *J Bone Joint Surg Am* 1976;58:230–233.

68. Homminga GN, Bulstra SK, Bouwmeester PS, et al. Perichondral grafting for cartilage lesions of the knee. *J Bone Joint Surg Br* 1990;72:1003–1007.

69. Kon M. Cartilage formation from perichondrium in a weight-bearing joint: an experimental study. *Eur Surg Res* 1981;3:387–396.

70. Poussa M, Rubak J, Ritsila V. Differentiation of the osteochondrogenic cells of the periosteum in chondrogenic cells of the periosteum in chondrotropic environment. *Acta Orthop Scand* 1981;52:235–239.

71. O'Driscoll SW, Salter RB. The induction of neochondrogenesis in free intra-articular periosteal autografts under the influence of continuous passive motion: an experimental investigation in the rabbit. *J Bone Joint Surg Am* 1984;661248–1257.

72. Poussa M, Ritsila V. The osteogenic capacity of free perosteal and osteoperiosteal grafts: a comparative study in growing rabbits. *Acta Orthop Scand* 1979;50:491–499.

73. Rubak JM. Reconstruction of articular cartilage defects with free periosteal grafts: an experimental study. *Acta Orthop Scand* 1982;53:175–180.

74. Rubak JM, Poussa M, Ritsila V. Chondrogenesis in repair of articular cartilage defects by free periosteal grafts in rabbits. *Acta Orthop Scand* 1982;53:181–186.

75. Rubak JM, Poussa M, Ritsila V. Effects of joint motion on the repair of articular cartilage with free periosteal grafts. *Acta Orthop Scand* 1982;53:187–191.

76. O'Driscoll SW, Keeley FW, Salter RB. The chondrogenic potential of frcc autogenous periosteal grafts for biological resurfacing of major full-thickness defects in joint surfaces under the influence of continuous passive motion. *J Bone Joint Surg Am* 1986;68:1017–1035.

77. Lorentzon R. Treatment of cartilage defects of the patella with periosteum transplantation. In: *Proceedings of the 2nd Freiburg International Symposium on Cartilage Repair*. Freiburg, Switzerland: 1997.

78. Brittberg M, Lindahl A, Nilsson A, et al. Treatment of deep cartilage defects in the knee with autologous chondrocyte transplantation. *N Engl J Med* 1994;331:889–895.

79. Peterson L, Minas T, Britberg M, et al. Two-to-9-year outcome after autologous chondrocyte transplantation of the knee. *Clin Orthop* 2000;374:212–234.

80. Minas T. The role of cartilage repair techniques, including chondrocyte transplantation, in focal chondral knee damage. *AAOS Instr Course Lect* 1999;48:629–643.

81. Hangody L, Kish G, Karpati Z, et al. Mosaicplasty for the treatment of articular cartilage defects: application in clinical practice. *Orthopedics* 1998;21:751–756.

82. Jackson DW, Scheer MJ, Simon TM. Cartilage substitutes: overview of basic science and treatment options. *J Am Acad Orthop Surg* 2001;9:37–52.

83. Shelton WR, Treacy SH, Dukes AD, et al. Use of allografts in knee reconstruction: part I. Basic science aspects and current status. *J Am Acad Orthop Surg* 1998;6:165–168.

84. Shelton WR, Treacy SH, Dukes AD, et al. Use of allografts in knee reconstruction: part II. Surgical considerations. *J Am Acad Orthop Surg* 1998;6:169–175.

85. Zukor DJ, Paitich B, Oakeshott RD, et al. Reconstruction of post-traumatic articular surface defects using fresh small-fragment osteochondral allografts. In: Aebi M, Regazzoni P, eds. *Bone transplantation*. Berlin: Springer, 1989:293–305.

86. Gross AE. Fresh osteochondral allografts for post-traumatic knee defects: surgical technique. *Oper Tech Orthop* 1997;7:334–339.
87. Salter RB. The biologic concept of continuous passive motion of synovial joints: the first 18 years of basic research and its clinical application. *Clin Orthop* 1989;242:12–25.
88. Sellers RS, Peluso D, Morris EA. The effect of recombinant human bone morphogenetic protein-2 (rhBMP-2) on the healing of full-thickness defects of articular cartilage. *J Bone Joint Surg Am* 1997;79:1452–1463.
89. Sellers RS, Zhang R, Glasson SS, et al. Repair of articular cartilage defects one year after treatment with recombinant human bone morphogenetic protein-2 (rhBMP-2). *J Bone Joint Surg Am* 2000;82:151–160.

TREATMENT OF COMPLEX ARTICULAR SURFACE INJURIES

SCOTT D. GILLOGLY
TIMOTHY S. HAMBY

Articular cartilage is one of the most complex tissues of the body, composed of a unique structure with complex biomechanical functions (17,31,58). It is a resilient load-bearing tissue, providing joint surfaces with the low friction, lubrication, and wear characteristics required for repetitive gliding motion. It is also responsible for absorbing mechanical shock and for distributing this load on the subchondral bone. Damage to the articular cartilage of the knee often leaves patients with a painful, swollen knee (18). Unlike most biologic tissues in the body, articular cartilage does not have the regenerative capacity to repair itself, thus leaving the patient and the orthopaedic surgeon with a practical problem and no good solution. These cartilage defects variably progress to the degenerative changes seen in osteoarthritis (3,13,39,44). Adequate treatment of articular damage has long been sought. For more than 2 centuries, surgeons have understood that articular cartilage lesions do not heal (46). Despite a plethora of procedures and techniques developed to encourage some degree of healing, articular cartilage lesions remain a practical problem, often leading to functional disability and osteoarthritis. These lesions are associated with unpredictable symptoms and a pathophysiologic response to injury (57).

Healthy articular cartilage is a viscoelastic material that functions to reduce stress on subchondral bone and to minimize friction (20,21). It is composed of matrix, chondrocytes, and water, overlying the subchondral bone. More than 50% of the dry weight of articular cartilage consists of collagen, and, of this, more than 90% is considered type II collagen (18,58). Articular cartilage collagens provide the tissue's tensile and shear properties, as well as immobilize the proteoglycans within the extracellular matrix. As with most human tissue injuries, injuries that result in full-thickness chondral defects initiate a healing response producing type I collagen (19,56,59). However, articular cartilage receives its nutrition through its bathing synovial fluid, and it lacks a true blood supply (72). Additionally, cartilage lacks undifferentiated cells within it that can migrate to the injury site, proliferate, and participate in the repair response. Thus, the fibrous repair cartilage (composed of type I collagen) is not fully repaired to form the original hyaline cartilage, composed of predominantly type II collagen. This fibrous cartilage has decreased resilience and stiffness, and it frequently breaks down, thus allowing progression to degenerative changes (57,68). Today, these chondral lesions remain significant public health issues.

Chondral lesions in young adult knees are frequent injuries encountered by orthopaedic surgeons (44,51,90). A retrospective review of 31,516 knee arthroscopies reviewed the prevalence of chondral injuries (26). There were 41% Outerbridge grade III chondral injuries and 19.2% Outerbridge grade IV chondral injuries. It was estimated that 3% to 4% were isolated grade IV chondral lesions larger than 2 cm². These larger lesions in young, healthy persons tend to have significant associated morbidity and often limit their employment opportunities, participation in sports, and activities of daily living (28,51). These lesions are also at a higher risk to progress to osteoarthritis (60,73). The challenge remains to find a repair method that allows these patients to resume active, productive lifestyles (61).

Goals of articular cartilage repair are to restore the biomechanical properties of normal articular cartilage, improve the patient's symptoms, return the patient to preinjury functional level, and prevent the progression of focal chondral injuries to end-stage osteoarthritis (23). Historically, treatment of chondral lesions primarily consisted of lavage (45,53) and debridement (6,34), as well as techniques to penetrate the subchondral bone, including abrasion (7,8,49,50,80), drilling (48), and microfracture (9,35,89). These techniques are predicated on stimulation and aggregation of undifferentiated mesenchymal stem cells to the site of injury (64). During the 1990s, the evolution of cartilage repair was dramatically changed. New techniques became

S. D. Gillogly: Atlanta Sports Medicine & Orthopaedic Center, Atlanta, Georgia 30327.

T. S. Hamby: Atlanta Sports Medicine & Orthopaedic Center, Atlanta, Georgia 30327.

available for treatment of full-thickness chondral defects of the knee. Tissue transfer with osteochondral autografts (10,42) and allografts (24,32,55,93), as well as cellular repair with autologous chondrocyte implantation (ACI) (15,37,62), opened new avenues for treatment of chondral defects. Whereas treatment techniques of marrow stimulation and osteochondral transfer are covered in Chapter 18, this chapter focuses on the treatment of larger, full-thickness chondral defects, often with coexisting knee disorders, by using ACI.

Although the interest in cartilage injuries and repair techniques over the 1990s led to a better understanding of the scope of the clinical problem, classification of cartilage injuries, and encouraging clinical results with newer treatment techniques, we have many unanswered issues, particularly with the natural history across the range of chondral injuries. There is a wide diversity of patients and chondral injuries; thus, all injuries do not merit the same treatment. Treatment needs to be tailored to the individual patient and the characteristics of the chondral lesion, and deciding on the best treatment must address the degree of knee disease and the patient's expectations. Consideration must be given to the size and location of the lesions, the number of defects, prior surgical treatments, and the patient's age, body mass, activity demands, and any comorbid conditions, both in the knee and systemically. Clinical algorithms have focused on the size of the lesion as well as level on the demands of the patient (16,23,64). Lesions larger than 2 cm^2 are considered more difficult to treat by other available techniques and are covered in this chapter using ACI as the treatment technique. It is essential that treatment of the chondral lesions match the needs of the patient (23).

In 1994, Brittberg et al. published their initial experience with autologous cultured chondrocytes used to treat large chondral lesions (15). The long-term results have shown good clinical outcomes in larger lesions in which traditional techniques failed (76,79). Animal models and clinical experience have shown that ACI can produce a hyaline-like repair tissue (5,14,39,75,82), which is responsible for its long-term durability.

The clinical results with ACI have been reported from numerous centers worldwide (4,22,36,65,74,82). Peterson et al. reported a retrospective analysis of their first 100 patients, ranging in follow-up between 2 and 9 years (79). These investigators had a 92% success rate in the isolated femoral condyle lesions, a 89% success rate with osteochondral defects, a 65% success rate with patellar chondral defects, and a 67% success rate in patients with multiple chondral lesions. One-third of the multiple lesions involved bipolar lesions. Additionally, they reported a 96% durability factor with the first 31 patients treated who were evaluated at 2 years and then again at an average of 7.5 years (76).

The Cartilage Registry Report (2), an international multicenter observational assessment of patients treated with ACI, released data on 5-year clinical experience involving more than 800 surgeons. Patient assessment revealed a 78% improvement for all defects treated, with an 81% improvement in isolated femoral condyle defects. Clinician evaluations showed a 79% improvement for all lesions and an 85% improvement in femoral condyle lesions. The most common adverse events reported with ACI were intraarticular adhesions (2.0%), detachment or delamination (1.4%), hypertrophic tissue (1.3%), and catching or popping (1.0%). The overall adverse event rate and safety profile were less than 7%. There was a 1.5% cumulative index of treatment failures at 5 years. Peterson et al. reported a 7% failure rate with the first 100 patients treated in Sweden (79).

Minas et al. (70) reported on 235 patients treated with ACI; these investigators showed an 87% improvement in a 6-year experience treating patients with complex or salvage cases. Our series, involving the first 112 patients treated with ACI, had a 91% good to excellent success rate. We showed that patients were able to return to, and to maintain, a high level of activity over a 5-year period after treatment (36).

ACI has been demonstrated to be a safe and effective treatment for large and complex full-thickness chondral injuries, if it is performed in properly selected patients. However, many challenges are frequently encountered during the procedure, as well as in patient selection. To ensure the best opportunity for a successful outcome, the orthopaedic surgeon needs to be conscious of these challenges.

INDICATIONS FOR AUTOLOGOUS CHONDROCYTE IMPLANTATION

ACI is indicated for symptomatic, large (>2 cm^2) full-thickness chondral lesions located on the femoral condyles and trochlear groove, including osteochondritis dissecans in patients from adolescence to their 50s in age (61) (Fig. 19.1A). Patients must be able to comply with the rehabilitation protocol. ACI is not indicated as a treatment option for osteoarthritis, such as in the presence of bipolar bone-on-bone lesions. If a lesion is present on the reciprocal surface, greater than grade III chondromalacia, the opposing surface will not be suitable for this technique (Fig. 19.1B).

Perhaps equally important as the presence of a predominantly focal chondral defect is the status of the remainder of the knee. The presence of coexisting disease, such as ongoing ligamentous instability, bony malalignment, bone deficiency, patellar malalignment, or complete meniscal deficiency, will prevent an environment conducive for cartilage restoration. Therefore, the prerequisites for a successful outcome include appropriate bony alignment, ligamentous stability, adequate motion and muscle strength, and compliance. Ideally, some meniscal function should also be present in the involved compartment. It is essential that in addition to a comprehensive physical examination, weight-bearing

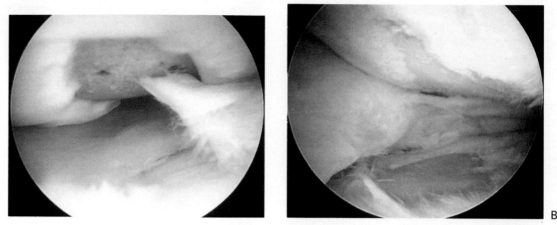

FIGURE 19.1 A: Full-thickness chondral defect of the femoral condyle with good surrounding articular cartilage appropriate for autologous chondrocyte implantation. **B**: Bipolar defects of both femoral condyle and tibial plateau with scant surrounding degenerative cartilage and absent peripheral meniscus.

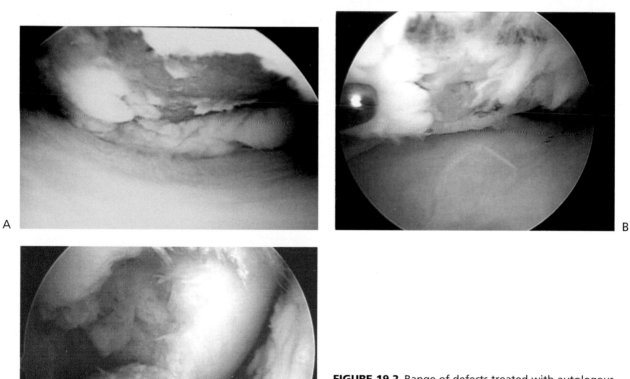

FIGURE 19.2 Range of defects treated with autologous chondrocyte implantation. **A**: Large traumatic defect associated with an anterior cruciate ligament tear. **B**: Traumatic 7 cm² defect with irregular borders in an otherwise normal healthy compartment. **C**: Osteochondritis dissecans defect with a greater than 8-mm deep bone loss that will require bone graft before autologous chondrocyte implantation.

anteroposterior, 45-degree, and patellar alignment radiographs be obtained (83). If there is any question about malalignment, full-length standing alignment radiographs should be obtained. Radiographs and magnetic resonance imaging (MRI) scans are also used as the first indicator of the status of the underlying subchondral bone (38,47, 81,83). Any bony loss of more than 7 to 8 mm in depth requires bone grafting before cell implantation. Deficiencies in any of these prerequisites need to be addressed before or concomitant with ACI. It has become more apparent with further experience in treating large chondral injuries that failure to recognize or treat these coexisting factors leads to poorer outcomes or treatment failure.

The final decision to determine the suitability of a chondral lesion for ACI comes at the time of arthroscopic assessment. The size, location, and depth of the defect, the status of the surrounding articular cartilage and underlying bone, and the status of the opposing chondral surfaces are all evaluated. Arthroscopic assessment also affords an opportunity for examination with the patient under anesthesia to confirm ligament stability and allows for evaluation of the menisci. The ideal chondral lesion for repair with ACI is one that has full-thickness involvement with exposed subchondral bone and is well shouldered on all sides by normal-appearing articular cartilage in an otherwise healthy knee. In general, the defects treated by this technique are larger than 2 cm^2 (67), and in our series, the average size of the defects was larger than 5.8 cm^2. Furthermore, the ideal defect is more the exception rather than the rule because many defects occur in the presence of other knee disorders and have some degree of border uncontainment (Fig. 19.2).

AUTOLOGOUS CHRONDROCYTE IMPLANTATION SURGICAL TECHNIQUE

The surgical technique for ACI has been well defined and published in numerous articles (15,22,37,69). The essential steps include an initial chondral biopsy for autologous chondrocyte cell culture, followed by a separate implantation procedure consisting of arthrotomy, defect preparation, periosteal procurement, fixation of the periosteal tissue, securing of a watertight seal with fibrin glue, implantation of the chondrocytes, and wound closure (Fig. 19.3).

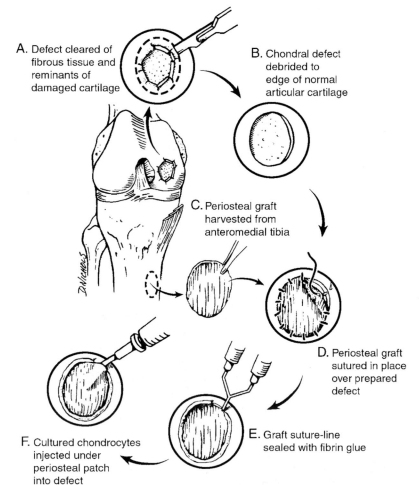

A. Defect cleared of fibrous tissue and reminants of damaged cartilage

B. Chondral defect debrided to edge of normal articular cartilage

C. Periosteal graft harvested from anteromedial tibia

D. Periosteal graft sutured in place over prepared defect

E. Graft suture-line sealed with fibrin glue

F. Cultured chondrocytes injected under periosteal patch into defect

FIGURE 19.3 Autologous chondrocyte implantation technique.

Chondral Biopsy for Chondrocyte Culture

Once the patient and the defect have been determined to be suitable for the ACI technique and the prerequisites have been addressed or can be addressed, a chondral biopsy is obtained for chondrocyte cell culture. The biopsy tissue is obtained from the superior edge of the medial or lateral femoral condyles in an area that is nonarticulating with the tibia and has limited contact with the patella. It can also be obtained from the lateral intercondylar notch in the same location as notchplasty is performed during anterior cruciate ligament (ACL) reconstruction. An arthroscopic gouge or ring curette is used to obtain several small slivers of full-thickness chondral tissue totaling the approximate volume of a pencil eraser. The chondral tissue is then placed in the biopsy medium and shipping vial while still using sterile technique. The specimen is then forwarded for chondrocyte cell culture. Although the cells could be available for implantation as early as 3 weeks from that point, the process can be temporarily suspended for later ACI when the surgeon and patient deem it appropriate.

Surgical Approach

A medial or lateral parapatellar arthrotomy is typically used to expose the corresponding chondral lesion. As with any surgical procedure, good exposure is essential to adequate performance of the intended technique and essential for a favorable outcome. The surgeon must be able to visualize the defect well enough to debride all damaged cartilage adequately. Additionally, the surgeon should have access comfortably to secure a periosteal patch to the defect's healthy cartilage margins with 6.0 absorbable suture. Inadequate exposure can lead to incompetent securing of the periosteal patch to the defect. A watertight seal of the periosteal graft must be obtained with the surrounding healthy cartilage margins; otherwise, the cultured chondrocytes risk leaking from under the graft, with resulting graft failure. For multiple, complex, or hard-to-reach chondral defects, a midline incision, with a medial parapatellar arthrotomy and eversion of the patella, is recommended. The end result should not be compromised for the sake of an ill-advised concern to keep the approach small. In some cases, particularly in patients with multiple defects or for trochlea or patellar defects when bony patellar realignment such as an anteromedialization of the tibial tubercle (Fulkerson procedure) (29) is contemplated in conjunction with the ACI procedure, the tubercle osteotomy can be incorporated into the exposure by turning the tubercle proximally, thus greatly enhancing exposure.

Debriding the Defect

After adequate exposure of the defect has been achieved, all damaged and undermined cartilage and fibrocartilage must be debrided from the defect. The ultimate goal of ACI is to acquire a durable, hyaline-like cartilage that integrates with the host bone and surrounding healthy cartilage. Failure to debride the tidemark or calcified zone of cartilage (deepest cartilage layers overlying subchondral bone) can inhibit the repair tissue's ability to integrate with host bone. This has been demonstrated in canine models, in which the calcified cartilage left on the subchondral plate resulted in failure of integration of cartilage with bone (11).

Chondral defects often have surrounding fissures in the cartilage extending from the lesion. Additionally, areas of damaged, thinned, or undermined cartilage are frequently present around a chondral defect (59). These areas of cartilage surrounding chondral defects also represent unhealthy, injured cartilage (Fig. 19.4A). Periosteal graft securing must be obtained to healthy cartilage margins. If these damaged areas are not excised, the repair tissue's ability to integrate with the host cartilage will be compromised (82). Furthermore, securing the periosteal graft to a margin of soft, damaged cartilage compromises the integrity of the patch graft

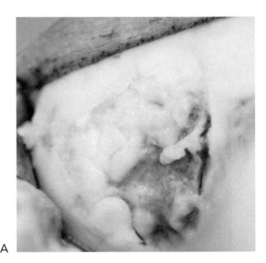

A

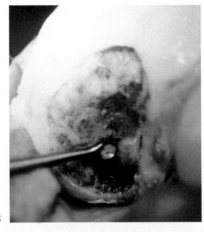

B

FIGURE 19.4 A: Extensive damaged cartilage and fibrocartilage surrounding an osteochondritis dissecans defect. **B**: The defect after debridement to a stable peripheral border of healthier-appearing articular cartilage.

and potentially allows it to pull loose during the early motion phase of rehabilitation. These regions of damaged cartilage surrounding the chondral defect should be excised with a no. 15 blade scalpel to healthy, undamaged cartilage, to remove any damaged cartilage down to the subchondral bone (Fig. 19.4B).

Internal intraarticular osteophytes in the subchondral bone are sometimes encountered and may be a consequence of penetration of the subchondral bone either from injury or prior surgical procedures (73) (Fig. 19.5A and B). These in-

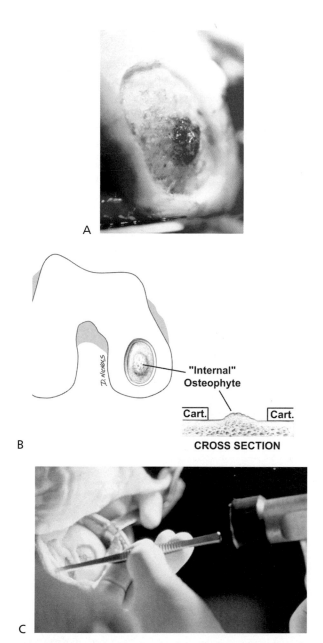

FIGURE 19.5 A: Note the internal osteophyte extruding from defect that would create a stress riser on the periosteum. **B**: Cross-sectional schematic showing the intralesional or internal osteophyte. **C**: Using a bone tamp, the osteophyte can be compressed down to the level of the surrounding subchondral bone without creating any significant bleeding.

ternal osteophytes may be more likely seen in patients who have had prior penetrating subchondral bone procedures performed for the chondral defect, including drilling, abrasion, or microfracture. These osteophytes can also occur in more chronic lesions. These bony prominences leave a stress riser, which may interfere with periosteal attachment, or they may damage the patch when the knee is put through its range of motion. These osteophytes should be gently tapped back into the subchondral bone to the level of the subchondral plate with a smooth, noncorrugated bone tamp (73) (Fig. 19.5C). Trying to curette or excise these osteophytes results in bleeding, which can be difficult to control, and it is necessary to obtain a dry defect field before implanting the cultured chondrocytes. Additionally, fibrous plugs remaining from a previous procedure (drilling or microfracture) may be encountered. These should also be debrided to the level of the subchondral bone. However, the fibrous tissue should not be removed from the drill holes, because this will also result in loss of hemostasis.

During debridement, the surgeon should avoid any violation of the subchondral bone that increases bleeding and the potential introduction of stem cells and fibroblasts that could compromise the quality of the repair tissue (69). If bleeding occurs, hemostasis needs to be obtained. There are three practical means of controlling oozing blood from the subchondral surface. Epinephrine- and thrombin-impregnated neuro-patty sponges can be used. These neuropatties should be placed in the bed of the defect, and slight compression should be applied. Secondly, fibrin glue can be injected into the bleeding defect, and pressure with the surgeon's finger can be applied. Holding for 30 seconds often controls the bleeding. A third means of obtaining hemostasis is using electrocautery with a needle point bovy. By placing the bovy on a low setting, between 5 and 8 W, bleeding can often be controlled at the punctate point of penetration. However, this should be the last resort for obtaining hemostasis, because the possible effect of localized necrosis from the cautery on the bone or the repair process is unknown.

After debridement, there should be a dry defect with subchondral bone at the base and more normal surrounding articular cartilage at the periphery. When this effect is achieved, the defect is measured to determine the size of the periosteal graft. This can be done by measuring the longest anteroposterior and mediolateral dimension and then adding 1 to 2 mm to each measurement to obtain the size of the periosteal graft. Another method that works well for clearly circumscribed defects is to make a template from the sterile paper that comes with surgical gloves. Once the template is cut out, it can be used to trace the defect size and configuration on the periosteal harvest site, with about 1 mm added to its border. The purpose of adding 1 to 2 mm in size when cutting the periosteal graft is to account for the shrinkage factor that occurs when periosteum is harvested.

Periosteal Harvesting

The recommended periosteal graft harvest site is the proximal medial tibia, just distal to the pes anserinus and the medial collateral ligament insertion (79). The periosteum is thicker on the posterior cortex of the tibia, compared with the anterior ridge. The underlying fat and fascia layers that cover the periosteum must be removed from the harvest site, and this is much easier to do before the graft is harvested. One of the most common mistakes made in harvesting the periosteal graft is leaving the thin fascia layer on the periosteum (12). Before removing the periosteal graft, the periosteum should appear as a white, glistening tissue. If it still appears to have a yellowish tinge, the fascia is probably still overlying the periosteum. Sharp dissection with scissors is recommended to remove this thin outer layer. A wet sponge also assists in removing redundant tissue over the periosteum.

Increased age, inactivity, obesity, and smoking may lead to atrophy of the periosteum (71,73). Periosteal atrophy has also been seen in female patients who are more than 40 years old. If the proximal tibia periosteal tissue is extremely thin and fragile, this tissue should not be used. An alternate site, which is infrequently necessary for harvesting the periosteum, is proximal to the articular surface of the medial and lateral femoral condyles. This distal femoral periosteum is a thicker tissue than that found on the tibia, so it is easier to handle. Harvesting this distal femoral periosteum requires a synovial incision and a subsynovial dissection to the periosteum. A T-incision is recommended, pulling back the synovial lining and thus exposing the periosteum. This structure is frequently covered with small blood vessels, which can be carefully cauterized after the synovial incision, but before the removal of the periosteum. After a femoral periosteal graft has been harvested, the synovium should be repaired in its original location with sutures to discourage additional bleeding into the joint (73). The final periosteal graft should be a clean, thin flap that leaves adequate space for cultured chondrocyte expansion. This graft can usually be acquired from the proximal medial tibia, with the femoral condyles serving as a backup source only if necessary.

Periosteal Suturing

Periosteal fit and the technique of fixation are extremely important to the outcome. The periosteum is attached with 6-0 Vicryl suture using a simple interrupted suture technique. The corners of the periosteal graft should be anchored to host cartilage first, to ensure the fit and tension of the graft. The tension of the periosteum should fit like skin over a drum. It should have a manhole-cover appearance with the periosteum up to, but not extending over, the cartilage rim. Any redundant periosteum is trimmed with sharp fine scissors, to keep appropriate tension on the graft.

The amount of tension on the flap should be taut with no excessive tissue. The knots should be tied on the side of the periosteum, not on the surface of the cartilage; thus avoiding any frictional force that could cause loosening of the knots. A short 1- to 2-mm tail should be left when cutting the suture. If the sutures are cut at the base of the knot, the knot may loosen. Various needle choices are available for the fine sutures, and they offer a wide range of applicability in different situations. A smaller needle with a shorter radius of curvature works best around thick normal cartilage, whereas a thin curve of greater radius allows a longer pass through thinner cartilage (Fig. 19.6).

When the graft is fully secure with only a small opening left to accommodate an angiocatheter, the repair is checked for a watertight seal. This is accomplished with a small syringe filled with saline and an angiocatheter (Fig. 19.7). The saline is slowly injected under the periosteal patch while one watches for any leakage around the peripheral suture line. Any obvious areas of leakage are carefully reinforced with an additional suture or two, as needed. When the saline overflows only at the injection site, the repair is watertight and ready to be sealed with fibrin glue. Commercial preparations of fibrin glue are available in most operating rooms.

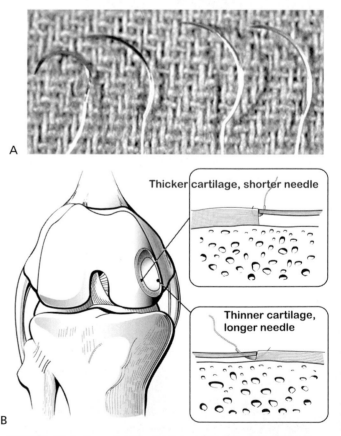

FIGURE 19.6 A: variously sized needles (P1, P2, PC1) allow greater flexibility in suturing the periosteum to the articular cartilage. **B**: The larger radius of curvature needle allows one to secure the suture in more tissue when the surrounding cartilage is thinned.

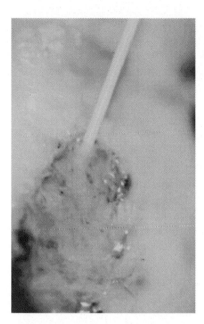

FIGURE 19.7 When securing the periosteal graft, a small opening is left for insertion of a plastic angiocatheter initially to inject saline to check for a watertight seal along the suture line and then finally to inject the cells into the defect.

With appropriate warming and mixing, these preparations provide a consistent flow of a rapidly setting sealant to further ensure a watertight interface between the chondral edges and the periosteum. The repair is then ready for the autologous cells.

Implanting Autologous Chondrocytes

The autologous chondrocytes are shipped sterile to arrive the morning of the procedure. While in the shipping container packaged with dry ice, they remain viable for at least 36 hours, thus offering at least a short window of flexibility. Each vial of cells contains between 10 and 12 million autologous chondrocytes and provides more than adequate cells for a defect up to 10 cm^2. Although the cells are sterile within the vial, the outer vial is not sterile. The surgeon should wear an extra glove to hold the nonsterile vial while aspirating the cells to a tuberculin syringe. The needle of the angiocatheter is used to penetrate the rubber stopper, and then the syringe is attached to the angiocatheter for cell aspiration. The cells, which settle during shipping, are mixed by aspirating and injecting back into the vial several times. The total volume is typically between 0.25 and 0.35 cc. When all the cells are in the syringe, the hub of the catheter and the syringe are grasped by the surgeon's sterile hand and are withdrawn from the vial. The extra, now nonsterile glove is removed. The cells are then injected under the periosteal patch into the defect. The catheter is passed distally across the defect and is slowly withdrawn as the cells are injected. The small opening left for the injection site is then closed

with one or two additional 6-0 Vicryl sutures and is sealed with fibrin glue as well.

After completion of the implantation, the retractors are removed, and the knee is brought to full extension, thus ensuring no contact with any opposing surface during the maneuver. Any further wound hemostasis or irrigation is then done to ensure that there is no inadvertent contact, such as with a suction tip, with the graft. Any concomitant procedures should be completed before the cells are implanted. The patient's knee should not be placed through a range of motion after the cells are implanted. The wound is then closed routinely. A drain is not routinely used because of the potential for contact with the graft or the suction effect of the drain. The postoperative course and rehabilitation are covered later in this chapter.

CHALLENGES ENCOUNTERED DURING AUTOLOGOUS CHRONDROCYTE IMPLANTATION

The previous discussions of surgical technique generally deal with the ideal straightforward lesion, which is isolated and well contained by healthy chondral margins to suture the periosteal graft, has no coexisting knee disease, and has no subchondral bone loss. Unfortunately, this ideal situation does not always exist. Patients often have some degree of uncontainment of cartilage borders. Additionally, what appears to be a well-contained isolated defect on initial arthroscopic evaluation can become a difficult challenge at implantation, for many reasons. For example, the lesion may be difficult to reach, as in a posterior condylar lesion, or the lesion may be difficult to reconstruct the normal articular contours, as in an isolated central patellar defect that involves the longitudinal ridge between the facets. The surgeon must be aware of these situations that can be encountered intraoperatively, so they can be handled in an appropriate fashion. Furthermore, coexisting knee disease is frequently present. Chondral defects often result from some other soft tissue or mechanical failure of the knee, including, but not limited to, ligamentous insufficiency or bony malalignment (39,88). Another situation requiring alteration in technique is subchondral bone loss greater than 7 to 8 mm in depth. The surgeon must also be aware of these frequent coexisting conditions, so they can be evaluated preoperatively to allow for staging or other alterations in technique. The following sections of this chapter focus on the treatment of difficult chondral lesions and of lesions in a knee with coexisting disease.

Uncontained Lesions

The periosteal graft should ideally be sutured to healthy, well-defined host cartilage margins. Often, initial arthroscopic examination shows that the defect appears to be contained by healthy cartilage; however, at implantation, it is found that some of surrounding cartilage is, in fact, damaged and must be debrided. This situation can leave the patient with some areas of the defect that do not have a healthy cartilage border, as a result of its extension to the peripheral borders of the femoral condyles or intercondylar notch. Ideally, the surgeon knows from initial arthroscopic evaluation that the chondral lesion extends beyond the cartilage margin and is uncontained. Regardless, the surgeon must be ready to handle uncontained lesions, which are not as straightforward as an isolated, well-contained chondral defect.

A chondral defect that extends into the intercondylar notch is an example of an uncontained chondral defect. This type of lesion is obviously on the weight-bearing portion of the articular cartilage and thus can cause significant symptoms. This presents a challenge in that there is no host cartilage border for suturing the graft at the intercondylar border of the defect. The intercondylar synovium can serve as a margin to which the periosteal graft can be secured. To ensure good fixation, the interrupted sutures should be placed slightly closer together than the standard 3 to 4 mm. Additionally, a running stitch may be added to help to secure the graft and to make it more stable and tight. This prevents spilling of cultured chondrocytes and minimizes any type of mechanical friction that may occur. Furthermore, periosteal graft hypertrophy is minimized by this technique.

A longer needle may be useful to obtain a larger bite into the soft tissue, to make the graft more secure. If the soft tissue margin has been stripped away from the bone, however, then another method if fixation will be needed.

The peripheral borders of the femoral condyles are another location where uncontained defects can occur (Fig. 19.8). There may be variable soft tissue at the border to secure the periosteum. Another option may be to place multiple peripheral drill holes 3 to 5 mm apart with a Keith needle. A P1 cutting edge needle can be flattened out and passed through the drill holes. To ensure the tightest attachment of the periosteal graft to the bone, all sutures should be passed through the graft and bone before they are tied down and secured.

A further option for securing the periosteum to the bone is using mini-Mitek suture anchors (Fig. 19.9). The microanchor is the best option, because it is the smallest anchor available. Before each anchor is placed, the nonabsorbable suture should be removed and replaced with absorbable 5-0 or 6-0 Vicryl suture. Each anchor is put in place spaced 3 to 5 mm apart. A small free needle is used on each suture to pass through the periosteum. Again, all the sutures should be passed before they are tied down. This allows adjustment of the periosteal tension. This technique results in watertight securing of the graft to bone and is applicable anywhere necessary.

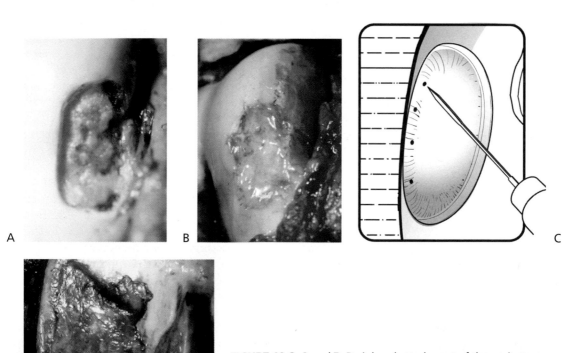

A   B   C

D

FIGURE 19.8 A and **B**: Peripheral attachment of the periosteum can use the bordering soft tissue, as in this case along the edge of the lateral femoral condyle, provided the soft tissue is naturally secure to the bone edge. **C** and **D**: Where there is no soft tissue firmly attached to bone to secure the periosteum, an alternative is to make small drill holes with a Keith needle to allow passing of the periosteal securing sutures directly through the bone edge.

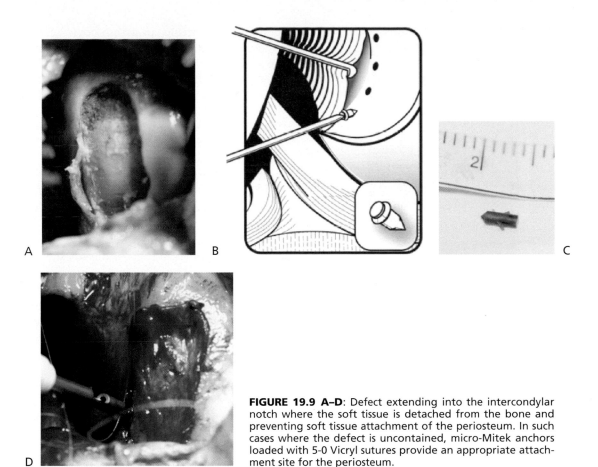

FIGURE 19.9 A–D: Defect extending into the intercondylar notch where the soft tissue is detached from the bone and preventing soft tissue attachment of the periosteum. In such cases where the defect is uncontained, micro-Mitek anchors loaded with 5-0 Vicryl sutures provide an appropriate attachment site for the periosteum.

Defects extending posteriorly, especially in the lateral compartment, can be difficult to reach with an anterior exposure. It is therefore challenging to secure the periosteum to the posterior chondral margin. These compartments can be maximally opened by hyperflexing the patient's knee as far as possible and externally or internally rotating the leg. Smaller needles with tighter curvatures allow for a quicker bite. Using a free needle may be beneficial in very tight compartments. After the needle tip is passed partially through the periosteal graft and host cartilage, the suture can then be passed through the eye of the needle. The needle should then be pulled through the graft and host cartilage and removed, thus leaving the suture passed through the graft and posterior cartilage margin. Another useful method is to pass the needle through the periosteum and chondral tissue and into the posterior meniscus. Then, the surgeon cuts the suture just above the needle and pulls the suture back into the knee. The needle can then be grasped with the needle holder and retrieved separately. The sutures can then be tightened and tied. Usually by maneuvering the patient's leg externally and internally, as well as using either of these techniques, most posteriorly extending lesions can be reached. If the posterior margin is lacking a cartilage rim to suture to, the a series of the microanchors into the bone, as described earlier, can be used to help secure the periosteum.

Bony Deficiency

As part of the evaluation for the suitability of this treatment, the surgeon must assess whether bone deficiency is associated with a chondral defect, such as an osteochondral fracture or osteochondritis dissecans. If bony deficiency exists, the depth of bone loss must be carefully considered. The best evaluation method appears to be a combination of MRI and arthroscopy. MRI allows assessment by the usual criterion of the viability of underlying bone and any possible depth of necrotic bone (27,47,81) (Fig. 19.10). During arthroscopic assessment, a probe can be used to gauge the depth of involvement. The probe can also be used to check the stability and viability of the exposed bone. If radiographs or MRI scans show suspicious bone, then the probe will usually find the fissure of nonviable bone and allow it to be removed. This approach will allow the true depth of involvement to be appreciated.

Shallow lesions, defined as up to 6 to 7 mm of bony involvement, do well with just implantation of the cultured cells, and bone grafting is not necessary. Shallow osteochondral lesions should have the sclerotic bottom of the defect gently debrided, with care taken not to elicit a bleeding response. The cartilage should be debrided back to healthy peripheral edges. The periosteum can then be secured over

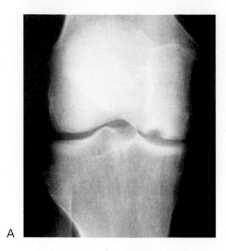

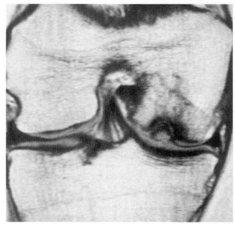

FIGURE 19.10 Radiograph (**A**) of a medial femoral condyle defect with underlying necrotic bone noted on magnetic resonance imaging (**B**). This defect was treated with staged arthroscopic bone grafting 6 months before the autologous chondrocyte implantation procedure.

the lesion, and then the cultured chondrocytes can be implanted under the periosteum.

Although Peterson (78) reported an 84% success rate in 32 patients with osteochondritis dissecans (with some lesions exceeding 10 mm of bony involvement), current recommendations now include bone grafting for defects with bone deficiency more than 8 mm in depth (67). Bone grafting, when consolidated, essentially creates a new subchondral bone plate and reconfigures the concavity of the lesion closer to its normal convexity. Additionally, it minimizes the depth of repair tissue that needs to be regenerated, thus hastening the overall healing process. Staged bone grafting is typically initiated at the time of arthroscopic evaluation and cartilage biopsy. In general, it takes 4 to 6 months or longer for the graft to heal and consolidate before cell implantation.

Bone grafting can be done as an open procedure or arthroscopically, depending on the size, location, number of lesions, and surgeon's preference (69). Although we initially used an open technique with a limited arthrotomy, it was

desirable to develop an arthroscopic technique, which would avoid an arthrotomy. With further experience, we now use an arthroscopic technique exclusively. Furthermore, we have now made greater use of allograft bone preparations, thereby obviating the need for iliac crest bone graft harvest. This has been especially practical in adolescent patients with osteochondritis dissecans lesions who require considerable bone graft volume to fill the bony defects. The arthroscopic technique can be performed as an outpatient procedure and is well tolerated by these patients. When a defect is determined to require bone grafting based on the foregoing assessment factors, the final consideration is arthroscopic evaluation. The surgeon should counsel the patient and family of this possibility preoperatively, thereby allowing the surgeon to proceed directly to bone grafting at this point.

The arthroscopic technique requires debridement of necrotic bone, placement of the graft, and securing of the graft with fibrin glue (Fig. 19.11). When one prepares the defect for bone grafting, the superficial surface dimensions should be less than the deep dimensions, thus creating an overhanging edge to help secure the bone graft. The debridement and shaping of the defect are accomplished with a motorized bur and handheld curettes. All necrotic bone fragments are removed. It is typically clear when the margin of healthy bone is reached, based on the color and appearance of healthy cancellous bone. This portion of the procedure is done with the usual arthroscopic distention medium. The bone graft source can be morselized autologous cancellous bone from the iliac crest or proximal tibia or allograft paste with interspersed cancellous bone, depending on the size of the deficiency and the surgeon's and patient's preferences. Some of the newer commercially available allograft mixtures have a paste-like quality particularly conducive for this arthroscopic technique. The allograft offers further advantages of off-the-shelf availability and avoids the donor site morbidity of harvesting a graft from the iliac crest.

When the defect is appropriately debrided to healthy bone, the irrigating fluid inflow is stopped, and the bone graft is inserted. We use an 8- or 9-mm metal canula and obturator that allows the bone graft to be inserted in one end of the canula, and the obturator then pushes the graft out the other end inserted under arthroscopic view into the base of the defect. The graft comes out much like squeezing toothpaste. With the obturator fully inserted, the canula-obturator becomes an impacter to shape and control the graft material. This sequence is repeated several times to bring the graft material up to, but not more than, the level of the subchondral bone. During this phase of the procedure, the tourniquet needs to be elevated if not already up. Any bone graft fragments that spill out of the defect can be removed with an arthroscopic grasper. Next, a layer of fibrin glue is placed over the bone graft up to the chondral surface to seal the graft. The double-barrel syringe, which comes with the fibrin glue preparation kit, also has a self-

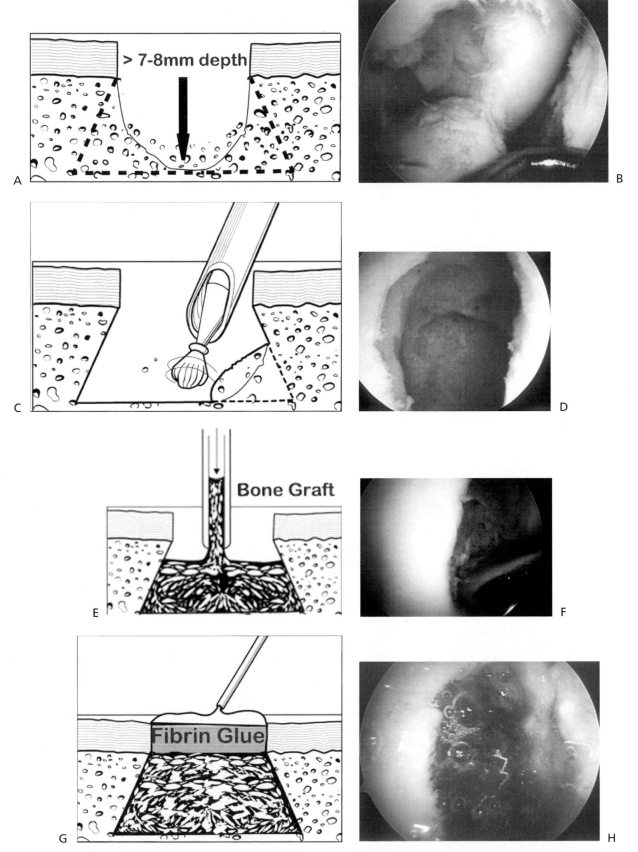

FIGURE 19.11 Arthroscopic bone grafting technique for defects greater than 7 to 8 mm in depth. After the bone graft heals, usually in 4 to 6 months, autologous chondrocyte implantation can be performed to repair the persistent chondral defect.

mixing delivery tube that easily reaches the defect through standard arthroscopic portals. When the fibrin glue is in place, the tourniquet can then be deflated to form a fibrin clot, which further helps to secure the bone graft. The instruments are then withdrawn and the knee is brought to full extension and closed routinely. Postoperatively, patients are allowed to advance their range of motion as tolerated and are permitted partial weight bearing on crutches for about 3 to 4 weeks. Patients tolerate this procedure very well, and symptoms are reduced, often dramatically.

Coexisting Knee Disorders

Autologous chondrocytes, like any method of cartilage repair, should not be expected to perform when placed in a compromised environment. Chondrocytes implanted into a knee that has ongoing ligamentous instability, maltracking, or biomechanical malalignment will ultimately fail because of the altered intraarticular environment that promotes excessive friction, shear stresses, and abnormal compressive loads across the injured chondral surface (63). It is absolutely essential that associated knee disorders including ligamentous instability, mechanical malalignment (both of the tibiofemoral joint as well as of the patellofemoral articulation), and meniscal attrition be corrected before or in conjunction with ACI. Failure to recognize coexistent pathologic conditions of the knee before chondrocyte implantation will markedly increase the chance of a poor outcome and an unhappy patient.

Corrective procedures may be done initially as a staged procedure or concomitant with ACI. In general, it is preferred to only perform one concomitant procedure at the time of ACI. If two or more reconstructive procedures are indicated, in addition to the ACI procedure, it is more appropriate to address these in a staged manner. The objective of using concomitant procedures is to facilitate the healing process of the repair tissue by unloading overloaded compartments, balancing soft tissues, and ensuring proper tracking. Peterson et al. stated that addressing these background factors is the single most important factor in improving the initial outcomes (77).

Ligamentous Insufficiency

Ligamentous insufficiency may jeopardize any newly regenerated repair tissue from excessive shear force. Even subtle giving way of the knee produces unacceptable forces across the maturing cells. ACL tears are the most common ligament injuries we have seen with full-thickness chondral defects (36). ACL reconstruction may be performed at the time of cell implantation, or in a prior staged procedure. If performed concomitantly, ACL reconstruction should precede the ACI and should be performed in the standard manner with whatever technique and graft best suits the situation. The arthroscopic ACL reconstruction is done before

proceeding with the arthrotomy for the ACI. When exposure may be a problem, such as very posteriorly on the condyles or any tibial defect, it is beneficial to wait for final fixation of the tibial side of the ACL graft until the ACI procedure is completed. However, this securing of the tibial side should be done with no significant manipulation of the knee. The obvious advantages of performing both procedures at the same time are that the patient has one surgery, one rehabilitation, and a lower cost. There is very little modification to ACL rehabilitation protocols needed because the ACI rehabilitation program is more limiting and is the overriding guidance postoperatively.

Biomechanical Alignment

Biomechanical alignment needs to be evaluated before chondrocyte implantation. This includes assessment of the tibiofemoral joint as well as the patellofemoral articulation. If physical examination or initial radiographs (weight-bearing anteroposterior, 45-degree, and axial views) indicate any malalignment, bilateral weight-bearing, full-length films from hip to ankle should be obtained. If the mechanical axis passes through the compartment in which the chondral lesion is located, an unloading osteotomy should be performed (Fig. 19.12). Numerous tibial or femoral osteotomies can be done to unload the knee (1,25,41,43,85,87), but the choice depends on the patient's specific angular deformity and characteristics. In addition to the standard closing wedge osteotomy of the proximal tibia with plate fixation, we have increasingly used medial opening wedge high tibial osteotomy either with plate fixation or external fixation with medial hemicallotasis. We tend to favor a closing wedge in patients who are smokers. The medial hemicallotasis technique is better suited for staged ACI procedures. If it is elected to perform the osteotomy concomitantly with chondrocyte implantation, the cartilage defect should be prepared first, followed by harvesting the periosteal graft. The osteotomy should then be performed through the same incision as for the periosteal graft harvest. The high tibial osteotomy should be completed with stable fixation before the periosteal patch is secured for the chondral defect. Continuous passive motion and early active range-of-motion exercises should be initiated 24 hours postoperatively. Once again, the protocol for the ACI is the overriding guidance and does not necessitate any change with an added high tibial osteotomy.

Patellofemoral Malalignment

If a patellar or trochlear chondral defect is present, patellofemoral maltracking should be suspected, particularly in chronic situations. Acute patellar subluxation or dislocation events producing chondral defects are more obvious. In chronic conditions, however, the underlying patellar malalignment or maltracking may be more subtle. In these

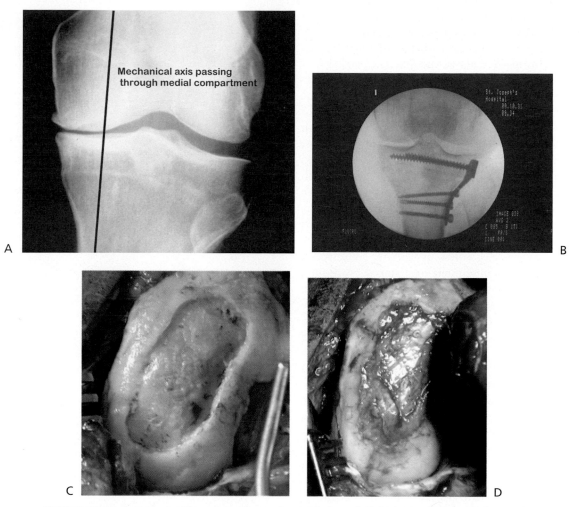

FIGURE 19.12 A: Patient with a medial femoral condyle large full-thickness chondral defect and malalignment with the mechanical axis passing through the medial compartment. **B**: Osteotomy is necessary to correct malalignment either with a medial opening high tibial osteotomy or, as in this case, a lateral closing wedge high tibial osteotomy. **C** and **D**: A medial femoral condyle defect after debridement and after securing the periosteum.

patients, a thorough history and physical examination is the first-line indicator raising suspicion of patellofemoral malalignment. Additional workup should include axial and lateral patella radiographs, and possible computed tomography or MRI scans, as discussed in Chapter 17 (30). Whereas no one method of evaluation fully defines the degree of dynamic patellar malalignment, arthroscopic assessment may become the final determinant in deciding on a concomitant realignment procedure for trochlea or patellar full-thickness chondral defects. This arthroscopic assessment can be done at the time of chondral biopsy. While visualizing the patellofemoral joint through the arthroscope, the surgeon should put the patient's knee through slow flexion and extension and should observe the patellofemoral tracking. Assessment should be through more than one portal, to substantiate the findings. Any abnormal patellar tracking not only is the likely source of the patellar or trochlear defects, but also would preclude a satisfactory environment for the maturation of the implanted chondrocytes into ideal repair

chondral tissue. In addition to concerns for the lateral maltracking of the patella, the concept of decreasing the patellofemoral contact forces also is desirable. Depending on the degree of lateral maltracking, the amount of medialization can be correspondingly adjusted. The anteromedialization of the tibial tubercle procedure as described by Fulkerson offers the options of adjusting the degree of medialization while still elevating the tubercle anteriorly (29). In some patients without lateral maltracking of the patella, anterior transfer alone may be sufficient to reduce the contact pressure on the patellofemoral joint. In most cases of patellar or trochlear defects, a distal patellar realignment procedure should be performed.

Although patellar realignment can be performed during the initial arthroscopy, we have found it almost always more prudent to combine the distal realignment procedure with the ACI for patellar or trochlea defects. Performing a tibial tubercle osteotomy at the time of implantation offers the distinct advantage of excellent exposure of the patellar or trochlear defects. The tubercle osteotomy and lateral release are combined with a medial parapatellar incision of the retinaculum from the tubercle proximally to the level of the vastus medialis. This method allows the tubercle, patellar tendon, and patella to be reflected proximally and affords wide access to the trochlea and patella (Fig. 19.13). Before the cells are implanted, the tubercle is placed in the various transferred positions while the patient's knee is put through a range of motion to determine which position is the most appropriate anteromedial transfer. The position is marked for later reference after completing the ACI. This approach alleviates the need to do much manipulation of the knee after the cells are implanted, rather just allowing the tubercle to be replaced in its predetermined position and secured with internal fixation and closure of the medial retinaculum without reefing. Regardless of whether the surgeon elects a concomitant realignment or a staged procedure, patellofemoral alignment, tracking, and load distribution need to be optimized at the time of ACI. This provides the cells an optimal environment for the maturation process.

Patellar defects can range from isolated facet defects to diffuse large central defects involving both facets and crossing the median ridge. Clinical experience has shown that single facet lesions tend to have better outcomes than lesions that cross the median ridge. Moreover, contained patellar lesions do better than uncontained lesions (76). Thus, when one debrides a patellar lesion, a cartilage rim should always be preserved whenever possible. For defects isolated to one facet, the same technique recommended for a condyle defect is preferred, thus leaving the periosteum flush and firm to the surface. However, for patellar chondral defects involving both facets, it is a greater challenge to recreate the normal contour of the patella when suturing the periosteum over a large centralized defect (Fig. 19.14). To accomplish this, the periosteum should be oversized in both the medial and lateral directions by 3 to 4 mm, as opposed to the standard 1 to 2 mm. The apex of the medium ridge should be sutured first (at the highest point). Then sutures should be placed in an alternating fashion medially and laterally, extending out

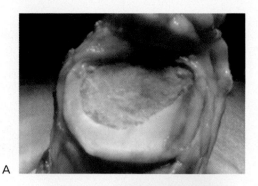

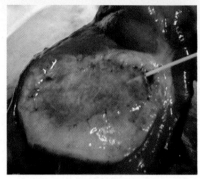

FIGURE 19.14 A: Large central patellar defect involving both medial and lateral facets. **B**: Periosteum secured to recreate the contour of the patella (note the angiocatheter during injection of the cells through a small unsecured edge of the periosteum). After injection, two additional sutures close the injection site.

peripherally, to create a tent-like structure. This technique helps to recreate the normal articular facet architecture of the patella (69).

Uncontained patellar lesions can be repaired in a fashion similar to that of condylar uncontained lesions. The periosteal graft can be sutured into soft tissue with interrupted knots and then reinforced with a running suture to make it as secure as possible. Longer needles can be used to provide a larger bite in soft tissue. As with condylar lesions, drill holes through the bone edges or microanchors can also be used to secure the periosteal graft. It is essential to reduce any high spots or areas of bunching of the periosteum to minimize concentrating friction or stress on the periosteal edges. Mechanical friction can be a catalyst for the complication of periosteal hypertrophy (73).

Trochlear lesions can also be challenging because of the concave anatomy of the trochlear groove, which can be difficult to reconstruct. However, the key to avoiding excessive tension and shear stresses across the graft is to recreate the normal contour of the sulcus. A large centralized trochlear lesion is best reconstituted by oversizing the periosteum by about 3 to 4 mm in the proximal to distal dimension. Suturing should begin at the central sulcus and should then progress medially and laterally. This helps to recreate the normal topography of the sulcus and thus avoids central wear and risk of delaminating the graft (Fig. 19.15). Trochlea defects are seldom uncontained unless they are

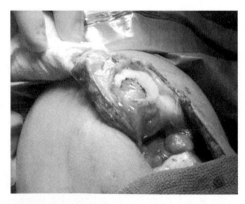

FIGURE 19.13 Tibial tubercle reflected proximally to give broad exposure for autologous chondrocyte implantation of a patellar defect combined with anteromedialization of the tibial tubercle.

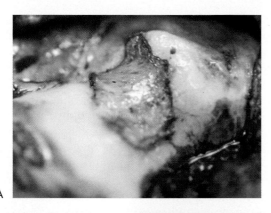

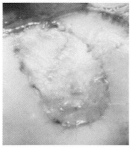 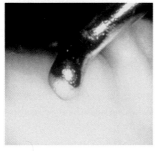

FIGURE 19.15 A: The double contour of the trochlea, medial to lateral and anterior to posterior, is recreated by the periosteum. **B** and **C**: A well-contained trochlear defect at autologous chondrocyte implantation and at second-look arthroscopy 6 months later.

very large. In such cases, the same principles are followed in attaching the periosteum.

Meniscal Deficiency

In addition to assessing the ligamentous stability and mechanical alignment of the knee, the quality and function of the meniscus should also be assessed before ACI (52). The meniscus plays an important role in knee function, and whenever possible it should be preserved or repaired (92). At what point a partial meniscectomy leads to a loss of meniscal function equivalent to a total meniscectomy is not easily determined. The posterior third of the menisci is more important than the anterior third in terms of function. Moreover, the peripheral fibers of the menisci providing hoop stress function are particularly essential (40). Even a relatively small-appearing radial tear that disrupts the periphery of the meniscus may greatly diminish its function. If a total meniscectomy has been performed in the same compartment as the chondral lesion, a meniscal allograft transplant should be considered (86,91). The advantages of a meniscal allograft with an ACI are that the meniscus helps to reduce concentrated forces in the involved compartment and it helps to protect the newly formed repair tissue. Once again, the decision to stage a meniscal transplant or to perform it concomitantly with ACI depends on surgeon and patient decision making. If there is any doubt, staging the two pro-

cedures may be more prudent. When one performs concomitant meniscal allograft and ACI, the meniscal transplant should be completed first, using the surgeon's standard technique. Any incisions used during the transplant should be easily extensile to expose for the ACI procedure. Finally, the meniscal graft should be placed and secured, followed by completion of the ACI. Clinical experience in this area is limited. Gersoff et al. reported on ten patients who had concomitant ACI and meniscal allografts. The follow-up was only between 12 and 26 months, but no differences were noted in the clinical results when they were compared with outcomes of isolated chondral lesions. Eight of ten patients preliminarily had successful outcomes (33).

Massive Chondral Lesions

Surgeons are frequently concerned about the potential for good outcomes in patients with very large chondral defects. As long as the knee is free of arthritic changes, or bipolar bone on bone lesions, and coexisting pathologic conditions of the knee are corrected, excellent outcomes comparable to those with smaller lesions can be expected. Larger (more than 6 cm^2) chondral lesions have been shown to have outcomes with ACI similar to those of smaller lesions (36). The only significant difference is the time necessary for healing, because the maturation of repair tissue clearly requires more time for a much larger defect. These massive defects are more likely to have a greater percentage of their periphery uncontained. It is therefore important to have adequate exposure for secure attachment of the periosteal graft with all the available previously described techniques. Attachment to the posterior margin of these very large condylar lesions can be extremely difficult, especially in the lateral compartment. The previously described techniques, however, provide good options for successfully establishing a watertight posterior seal.

If the grafted area extends over the entire circumference of the condyle, having two injection sites reduces the risk of damaging the patch when one tries to advance the catheter tip down to the apex of the lesion. One opening should be at the middle of the patch to fill the lower portion, and the other should be at the top, for subsequent filling of the upper half of the defect. These massive defects require two vials of cells each injected separately through the respective filling sites. As a general rule, one vial of cells representing 10 to 12 million autologous chondrocytes should be used for each 8 to 10 cm^2 of a defect. Postoperatively, an unloading brace should be considered for the first 6 months, to assist in preventing the overloading of the massive repair area.

Multiple Lesions

Another not infrequent presentation of chondral injury is that of multiple defects within the knee (Fig. 19.16). Again, in the nonarthritic knee, multiple cartilage defects respond to ACI as do isolated lesions (36). However, more periosteal

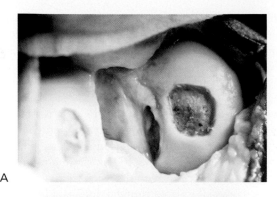

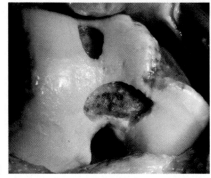

FIGURE 19.16 A: Multiple defects including both the medial and lateral femoral condyles. **B**: Multiple defects of the trochlea.

graft is obviously required for multiple lesions. All defects should be measured at the initial diagnostic arthroscopy, to establish an initial plan regarding how much surface area of periosteum will be required. Although the proximal tibia distal to the pes insertion is the optimal site, periosteum can also be obtained through the same arthrotomy incision from the distal femur (73). More than one donor site may be required for periosteal harvesting. When more than one donor site is used for periosteum, the surgeon should attempt to match the thickness of the periosteum to the depth of the healthy cartilage surrounding the defect. Thus, for example, the thicker periosteum should be used for trochlea or patella defects, whereas the thinner periosteum should be used on the femoral condyles. Thinner periosteum results in fewer complications and a better repair tissue (66). A final alternative is to plan preoperatively to use the contralateral proximal tibia. This may be particularly indicated in patients who have had prior surgical procedures involving the proximal tibia. For very large defects or if the periosteum becomes torn or damaged on one edge, two pieces of periosteum can be sutured together to increase the total size. A very small noncutting needle is used for this technique or for repairing any inadvertent hole in the periosteum.

MANAGEMENT OF COMPLICATIONS

Complications associated with ACI can be categorized as those occurring with the graft, those associated with the arthrotomy, or those associated with any concomitant procedures. The most common complication that occurs with the graft is periosteal overgrowth or hypertrophy (67). Periosteal overgrowth tends to develop between 5 and 9 months after implantation. Symptoms include catching, popping, or swelling, which may or may not be painful (73). Activities associated with these symptoms need to be analyzed carefully, and the patient's rehabilitation and exercise programs need to be altered accordingly. If symptoms still persist, arthroscopic evaluation will be indicated. If the periosteum appears hypertrophied or protrudes above the level of the surrounding chondral surface, it can be managed by removing the protruding redundant tissue to the level of the surrounding cartilage. This is best performed with an arthroscopic knife cutting tangential to the chondral surface (Fig. 19.17). A less aggressive arthroscopic shaver blade such as the Turbowhisker™ (Dyonics) can be used to remove any remaining fibrillated periosteum. Radiofrequency energy heat is contraindicated to debride the periosteal overgrowth because of its variable depth of penetration that potentially can produce cell death (54).

Periosteal graft failure can also occur as a result of periosteal graft delamination. Minas et al. described a classification system for graft delamination, depending on the amount of tissue that has delaminated (69). Marginal delamination is defined as less than 10 mm of graft loosening.

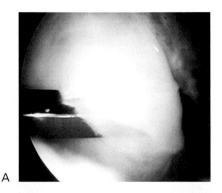

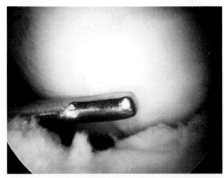

FIGURE 19.17 A: At second-look arthroscopy, periosteal hypertrophy is seen on this a medial femoral condyle defect. Note the arthroscopic banana knife cutting tangential to the articular surface to remove the periosteal overgrowth. **B**: After resection of the periosteal hypertrophy, note the smooth contour of the underlying repair.

This small of an area can be excised, thus exposing the subchondral bone, which can be microfractured or drilled to try to fill the gap with fibrocartilage. A partial delamination is defined as delamination of less than 50% of the graft, but more than 1 cm of tissue loss. Treatment of this class of delamination is a little more controversial. It can be treated by rcimplantation of chondrocytes, or it can be treated as a marginal delamination with debridement and microfracture or drilling. When more than 50% of the graft has loosened, or only a small rim of repair tissue is attached to a portion of host cartilage, it is considered a total graft delamination, and this should be treated with reimplantation of chondrocytes or other alternatives.

Of the causes of graft failure, overload of the maturing graft is typically involved. Unexpected or sudden trauma to the knee occurring during the first 6 months after chondrocyte implantation is the typical situation. This may occur when a patient slips or falls, thus placing a shear load across the graft. It may also result from noncompliance with the rehabilitation protocol during the critical postoperative period. Both these situations underscore the importance of a protected gradual rehabilitation course. Patients should wear a rehabilitation hinged brace at least during the first 6 weeks until they have good leg control and weight bearing. Patients should also understand the critical importance of the gradual rehabilitation protocols, not designed to hassle them but to optimize their results. These points frequently need to be reiterated to patients, especially as they start to feel more comfortable with the knee. These issue become less of a concern after about 6 months postoperatively. Although the implanted chondrocytes and graft have not fully matured and developed at 6 months, the graft is usually firm enough and is integrated with the host cartilage to withstand higher levels of force. A final cause of graft failure is progression of advanced osteoarthritis. This may occur as a result of the host cartilage's being chondrodysplastic, thus disabling the repair tissue's ability to integrate into the host cartilage. Additionally, the chondrodysplastic host cartilage will continue to progressively degenerate over time.

Arthrofibrosis, or adhesion formation, is a risk of any knee arthrotomy and occurs in approximately 2% of ACIs (69,73). There is an increased risk of this complication in patients undergoing concomitant procedures. Patients with multiple implants, female patients undergoing tibial tubercle osteotomy with manipulation of the fat pad, or patients with lateral closing wedge osteotomy appear to be more at risk, based on our experience. The key to avoiding stiffness is early motion. Continuous passive motion should be started in the immediate postoperative period (84). Patellar mobility and maintaining full extension are also critical components of early rehabilitation. During surgery, the articular cartilage and soft tissues should be kept moist with irrigation solution, to avoid any collateral tissue trauma. When arthrofibrosis does occur, it unfortunately can be a difficult problem to manage. Rather than immediate closed

manipulation, which could injure the graft, an aggressive motion program in therapy should be the first line of treatment. Use of various motion orthoses may also be helpful. If however, by 4 to 6 months postoperatively the patient is not progressing, then arthroscopic lysis of adhesions followed by gentle manipulation is appropriate. Typically, dense scar tissue is found anteriorly and about the suprapatellar pouch. In a methodical manner, the scar is released using a radiofrequency ablator probe and a large resector shaver blade. Care is taken to avoid any contact with the graft. Once the scar is resected and the patella is mobilized, visualization of the graft typically shows good healing and maturation. We have not found that arthrofibrosis affects the outcome of the graft or the ACI procedure. An aggressive postoperative motion and weight-bearing protocol is then followed. Normal or near-normal range of motion can almost always be regained.

REHABILITATION

Rehabilitation after ACI is a slow, gradual progression (37). The biologic nature of this repair tissue needs to be respected and cultivated (Fig. 19.18). This healing process relies on a balance between the appropriate amount of stimuli for the cells to be able to form a durable matrix and graft protection. There is a degree of individual variation with the rehabilitation process, just as there is with tissue healing. The program needs to be designed according to the patient's status and needs, along with such factors as the size and location of the lesion and any possible concomitant procedures that were performed. It is important that there be regular contact among the patient, physical therapist, and physician, especially during the first 3 months. An overly aggressive rehabilitation program could certainly jeopardize the repair tissue. The foundation principles for a successful ACI rehabilitation program are centered on mobility and motion exercises, protection of the graft, muscle strengthening, progressive weight bearing, and patient education. Motion helps with cellular orientation and helps to prevent a stiff joint. However, protection of the repair tissue from excessive forces is essential in the early phases. An overaggressive patient, for example, bearing weight on a freshly repaired condylar defect, puts too much stress on the graft, and this potentially leads to graft delamination and failure. Continuous passive motion and a touch–weight-bearing status of the repaired extremity should be the initial steps in rehabilitation. Isometric strengthening exercises to reestablish muscle tone are introduced early, followed by gradual progression to progressive resisted exercises and a return to greater degrees of functional activities.

Rehabilitation of patellofemoral ACI requires some special considerations to achieve early motion while protecting the forces across the graft. Patellofemoral contact pressure is maximized between 40 and 70 degrees of knee flexion and

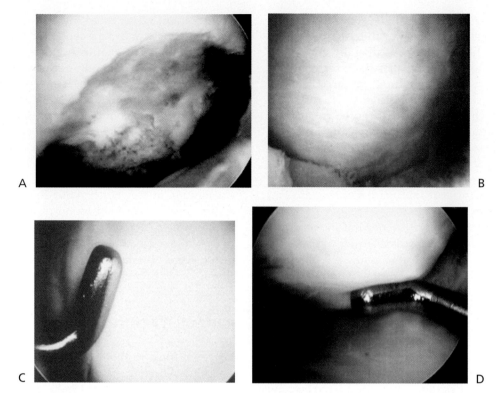

FIGURE 19.18 Maturation of the repair tissue over time. **A**: A lateral femoral condyle defect after failed osteochondral allograft and subsequent staged bone grafting. **B**: Five months after autologous chondrocyte implantation with complete fill of the defect: the surface is still undulated and soft. **C**: Same lesion at 1 year: now with a smooth surface, firmer, and integrated with surrounding articular cartilage. **D**: Defect at 3 years: asymptomatic, with a surface virtually indistinguishable from the remaining condyle.

should therefore be avoiding during active knee extension. Exercises to promote patella mobility should be initiated early, to avoid adhesions. Patients are not allowed to perform active knee extension during the first 12 weeks postoperatively. Passive motion, either with continuous passive motion or by using the well leg to extend the involved leg from flexion, is allowed and encouraged. The addition of active extension exercises is based on the size and location of the defect as observed intraoperatively. The surgeon should guide the patient and therapist in the rehabilitation process.

Finally, the surgeon must educate patients, so they have an understanding of the time-sensitive maturation process of ACI (69). Thus, they can set appropriate expectation levels for their progress.

PATIENT EDUCATION

Patient education by the surgeon cannot be overemphasized. The rehabilitation protocol must be followed, and patients must be informed that failure to do so may well compromise their results. The regenerated repair tissue has a time-sensitive maturation associated with it that needs to be carefully developed. If the graft is overloaded too early, it can be compromised. In speaking with patients, it is impor-

tant to explain to them about the distinct phases of the healing process (67). For the first 3 to 4 weeks, the cells are developing the tissue matrix and are filling the defect. At this point, the tissue is very soft and tenuous. Motion exercises are very important at this stage to help with cellular orientation and to prevent joint stiffness (69). At 3 months, the repair tissue has a wave-like gelatin texture that should be secure to the subchondral bone, but not fully bonded to the lateral borders. At this point, patients are allowed to participate in low-impact activities such as walking, cycling, and swimming. Patients need to be informed that if a specific activity is causing pain, this activity should be decreased or restricted. Patients need to be responsible and not overdo it. At 6 months, the repair tissue has a firm, putty-like substance and should be well fixed to the underlying bone and to the adjacent cartilage. Patients should really start to see significant improvements in pain relief at this point. However, patients need to be reminded that the repair tissue is not fully developed and matured yet. At 9 months, the repair tissue should be firm enough to tolerate aerobic classes, playing golf, and taking long hikes. By the twelfth to the fourteenth month, patients should generally be able to participate in high-impact sporting activities, involving lateral movements. By 24 months, activities are usually unrestricted, and patients are free of symptoms. In our clinical series, patients have actually shown continued clinical improvement as late as 3 and 4 years postoperatively.

CONCLUSION

Large full-thickness articular cartilage defects of the knee are a significant problem, often leading to significant morbidity in a young population. They often result in pain, swelling, and restriction of normal activities, and they not uncommonly progress to degenerative arthritis. Inherently, chondral defects have a poor capacity for intrinsic repair, despite a multitude of procedures developed to meet this challenge. ACI has shown good to excellent clinical outcomes across multiple centers even with patients in whom other previous procedures have failed. Although numerous challenges exist with this procedure, with experience and an understanding of potential difficulties, these challenges can be efficiently managed. Long-term outcomes support ACI as a valid treatment option for symptomatic patients with large chondral lesions who want to resume an active lifestyle.

REFERENCES

1. Aglietti P, Stringa G, Buzzi R, et al. Correction of valgus knee deformity with a supracondylar V osteotomy. *Clin Orthop* 1987; 217:214–220; 1987.
2. Anderson AF, Browne JE, Ergglet C, et al. *Cartilage repair registry,* vol 7. Cambridge, MA: Genzyme Biosurgery: a division of Genzyme Corp., 2001;1–7.
3. Angermann P, Riegels-Nielsen P, Pedersen H. Osteochondritis dissecans of the femoral condyle treated with periosteal transplantation: poor outcome in 14 patients followed for 6–9 years. *Acta Orthop Scand* 1998;69:595–597.
4. Bahuaud J, Maitrot RC, Bouvet R, et al. Autologous chondrocyte implantation for cartilage repair: presentation of 24 cases. *Chirurgie* 1998;123:568–571.
5. Barone LM. Cultured autologous chondrocyte implantation for cartilage repair. *Genzyme tissue repair.* Cambridge, MA: Genzyme Corp., 1996.
6. Baumgaertner MR, Cannon WD, Vittori JM, et al. Arthroscopic debridement of the arthritic knee. *Clin Orthop* 1990;253:197–202.
7. Bert JM. Abrasion arthroplasty. *Oper Tech Orthop* 1997;7:294–299.
8. Bert JM, Maschka K. The arthoscopic treatment of unicompartmental gonarthrosis: a five-year follow-up study of abrasion arthroplasty plus arthoscopic debridement and arthroscopic debridement alone. *Arthroscopy* 1989;5:25–32.
9. Blevins FT, Steadman JR, Rodrigo JJ, et al. Treatment of articular cartilage defects in athletes: an analysis of functional outcome and lesion appearance. *Orthopedics* 1998;21:761–768.
10. Bobic V. Osteochondral autologous graft transplantation in the treatment of focal articular cartilage lesions. *Semin Arthoplasty* 1999;10:21–29.
11. Breinan HA, Minas T, Hsu H, et al. Effect of cultured autologous chondrocytes on repair of chondral defects in a canine model. *J Bone Joint Surg Am* 1997;79:1439–1451.
12. Brittberg M. Autologous chondrocyte transplantation. *Clin Orthop* 1999;367[Suppl.]:S147–S155.
13. Brittberg M, Lindahl A, Homminga G, et al. A critical analysis of cartilage repair. *Acta Orthop Scand* 1997;68:186–191.
14. Brittberg M, Nilsson A, Lindahl A, et al. Rabbit articular cartilage defects treated with autologous cultured chondrocytes. *Clin Orthop* 1996;326:270–283.
15. Brittberg M, Lindahl A, Nilsson A, et al. Treatment of deep cartilage defects in the knee with autologous chondrocyte transplantation. *N Engl J Med* 1994;331:889–895.
16. Browne JE, Branch TP. Surgical alternatives for treatment of articular cartilage lesions. *J Am Acad Orthop Surg* 2000;8:180–189.
17. Buckwalter JA, Mankin HJ. Articular cartilage: part I. Tissue design and chondrocyte–matrix interactions. *J Bone Joint Surg Am* 1997;79:600–611.
18. Buckwalter JA, Mankin HJ. Articular cartilage: part II. Degeneration and osteoarthrosis, repair, regeneration and transplantation. *J Bone Joint Surg Am* 1997;79:612–632.
19. Buckwalter JA, Mankin HJ. Articular cartilage repair and transplantation. *Arthritis Rheum* 1998;41:1331–1342.
20. Buckwalter JA, Rosenberg LC, Hunziker EB. Articular cartilage: composition, structure, response to injury, and methods of facilitating repair. In: Ewing JW, ed. *Articular cartilage and knee joint function: basic science and arthroscopy.* New York: Raven Press, 1990:19–56.
21. Camosso ME, Marotti G. The mechanical behavior of articular cartilage under compressive stress. *J Bone Joint Surg Am* 1962;44: 699–709.
22. Cole BJ, D'Amato M. Autologous chondrocyte implantation. *Oper Tech Orthop* 2001;11:115–131.
23. Cole BJ, Farr J. Putting it all together. *Oper Tech Orthop* 2001; 11:151–154.
24. Convery FR, Akeson WH, Meyers MH. The operative technique of fresh osteochondral allografting of the knee. *Oper Tech Orthop* 1997;7:340–344.
25. Coventry MB. Osteotomy about the knee for degenerative and rheumatoid arthritis. *J Bone Joint Surg Am* 1973;55:23–48.
26. Curl WW, Krome J, Gordon ES, et al. Cartilage injuries: a review of 31,516 knee arthroscopies. *Arthroscopy* 1997;13:456–460.
27. Disler DG, McCauley TR. Clinical magnetic resonance imaging of articular cartilage. *Top Magn Reson Imaging* 1998;9:360–376.
28. Dzioba RB. The classification and treatment of acute articular cartilage lesions. *Arthroscopy* 1988;4:72–80.
29. Fulkerson JP. Anteromedialization of the tibial tuberosity for patellofemoral malalignment. *Clin Orthop* 1983;177:176–181.
30. Fulkerson JP. Patellofemoral pain disorders: evaluation and management. *J Am Acad Orthop Surg* 1994;2:124–132.
31. Furukawa T, Eyre DR, Koide S, et al. Biochemical studies on repair cartilage resurfacing experimental defects in the rabbit knee. *J Bone Joint Surg Am* 1980;62:79–89.
32. Garrett JC. Fresh osteochondral allografts for treatment of articular defects in osteochondritis dissecans of the lateral femoral condyle in adults. *Clin Orthop* 1994;303:33–37.
33. Gersoff W. Clinical experience with autologous chondrocyte implantation: a preliminary report. Presented at the Western Orthopaedic Society meeting, Steamboat Springs, CO, 2001.
34. Gibson JN, White MD, Chapman VM, et al. Arthroscopic lavage and debridement for osteoarthritis of the knee. *J Bone Joint Surg Br* 1992;74:534–537.
35. Gill TJ. The role of the microfracture technique in the treatment of full-thickness chondral injuries. *Oper Tech Sports Med* 2000;8:138–140.
36. Gillogly SD, Hamby TH. Clinical results of autologous chondrocyte implantation for large full-thickness chondral defects of the knee: five-year experience with 112 consecutive patients. Presented to the American Orthopaedic Society for Sports Medicine, Keystone, CO, 2001.
37. Gillogly SD, Voight M, Blackburn T. Treatment of articular car-

tilage defects of the knee with autologous chondrocyte implantation. *J Orthop Sports Phys Ther* 1998;28:241–251.

38. Graf BK, Cook DA, De Smet AA, et al. "Bone bruises" on magnetic resonance imaging evaluation of anterior cruciate ligament injuries. *Am J Sports Med* 1993;21:220–223.

39. Grande DA, Pitman MI, Peterson L, et al. The repair of experimentally produced defects in rabbit articular cartilage by autologous chondrocyte transplantation. *J Orthop Res* 1989;7:208–218.

40. Grood ES. Meniscal function. *Adv Orthop Surg* 1984;7:193–197.

41. Ha'Eri GB, Orth MC, Wiley AM. High tibial osteotomy combined with joint debridement: a long-term study of results. *Clin Orthop* 1980;151:153–159.

42. Hangody L, Kish G, Karpati Z, et al. Autogenous osteochondral graft tehcnique for replacing knee cartilage defects in dogs. *Orthop Int* 1997;5:175–181.

43. Hernigou P, Medevielle D, Debeyre J, et al. Proximal tibial osteotomy for osteoarthritis with varus deformity: a ten to thirteen-year follow-up study. *J Bone Joint Surg Am* 1987;69:332–354.

44. Homminga GN, Bulstra SK, Bouwmeester PM, et al. Perichondral grafting for cartilage lesions of the knee. *J Bone Joint Surg Br* 1990;72:1003–1007.

45. Hubbard MJ. Articular debridement versus washout for degeneration of the medial femoral condyle: a five-year study. *J Bone Joint Surg Br* 1996;78:217–219.

46. Hunter W. On the structure and diseases of articulating cartilages. *Philos Trans R Soc Lond B Biol Sci* 1743;42:514–521.

47. Imhof H, Sulzbacher I, Grampp S, et al. Subchondral bone and cartilage disease: a rediscovered functional unit. *Invest Radiol* 2000;35:581–588.

48. Insall J. The Pridie debridement operation for osteoarthritis of the knee. *Clin Orthop* 1974;181:61–67.

49. Johnson LL. Arthroscopic abrasion arthroplasty historical and pathologic perspective: present status. *Arthroscopy* 1986;2:54–69.

50. Johnson LL. Arthscopic abrasion arthoplasty. In: McGinty JB, Caspari RB, Jackson RW, et al., eds. *Operative arthroscopy.* New York: Raven Press, 1991:341–360.

51. Johnson-Nurse C, Dandy DJ. Fracture-separation of articular cartilage in the adult knee. *J Bone Joint Surg Br* 1985;67:42–43.

52. Lewandrowski K, Muller J, Schollmeier G. Concomitant meniscal and articular cartilage lesions in the femorotibial joint. *Am J Sports Med* 1997;25:486–494.

53. Lively PJ, Doherty M, Needoff M, et al. Arthroscopic lavage of osteoarthritic knees. *J Bone Joint Surg Br* 1991;73:922–926.

54. Lu Y, Edwards RB, Cole BJ, et al. Thermal chondroplasty with radiofrequency energy: an *in vitro* comparison of bipolar and monopolar radiofrequency devices. *Am J Sports Med* 2001;29:42–49.

55. Mahomed MN, Beaver RJ, Gross AE. Allograft bones and soft tissues: the long-term success of fresh, small fragment osteochondral allografts used for intraarticular post-traumatic defects in the knee joint. *Orthopedics* 1992;15:1191–1199.

56. Mandelbaum BR, Browne JE, Fu F, et al. Articular cartilage lesions of the knee. *Am J Sports Med* 1998;26:853–861.

57. Mankin HJ. The response of articular cartilage to mechanical injury. *J Bone Joint Surg Am* 1982;64:460–466.

58. Mankin HJ, Mow VC, Buckwalter JA, et al. Articular cartilage structure, composition, and function. In: Buckwalter JA, Einhorn TA, Simon SR, eds. *Orthopaedic basic science: biology and biomechanics of the musculoskeletal system.* Rosemont, IL: American Academy of Orthopaedic Surgeons, 2001:443–470.

59. Mankin HJ, Mow VC, Buckwalter JA. Articular cartilage repair and osteoarthritis. In: Buckwalter JA, Einhorn TA, Simon SR, eds. *Orthopaedic basic science: biology and biomechanics of the musculoskeletal system.* Rosemont, IL: American Academy of Orthopaedic Surgeons, 2001:471–488.

60. Messner K, Maletius W. The long-term prognosis for severe damage to weight-bearing cartilage in the knee: a 14-year clinical and radiographic follow-up in 28 young athletes. *Acta Orthop Scand* 1996;67:165–168.

61. Minas T. Treatment of chondral defects in the knee. *Orthopedics* 1997;3:69–74.

62. Minas T. Autologous cultured chondrocyte implantation in the repair of focal chondral lesions of the knee: clinical indications and operative technique. *J Sports Traumatol Rel Res* 1998;20:90–102.

63. Minas T. Nonarthoplasty management of knee arthritis in the young individual. *Curr Opin Orthop* 1998;9:46–52.

64. Minas T. The role of cartilage repair techniques, including chondrocyte transplantation, in focal chondral knee damage. *Instr Course Lect* 1999;48:629–643.

65. Minas T. Chondrocyte implantation in the repair of chondral lesions of the knee: economics and quality of life. *Am J Orthop* 1998;27:739–744.

66. Minas T. Techniques on the horizon, articular cartilage techniques, biologic joint preservation. Presented at the 20th Annual Meeting of the Arthroscopy Association of North America, Seattle, WA, 2001.

67. Minas T, Chiu R. Autologous chondrocyte implantation. *Am J Knee Surg* 2000;13:41–50.

68. Minas T, Nehrer S. Current concepts in the treatment of articular cartilage defects. *Orthopedics* 1997;20:525–538.

69. Minas T, Peterson L. Advanced techniques in autologous chondrocyte transplantation. *Clin Sports Med* 1999;18:13–44.

70. Minas T, Gross A, O'Driscoll S, et al. Surgical treatment for articular cartilage defects in the knee. Presented at the 68th Annual Meeting of the American Academy of Orthopaedic Surgeons, San Francisco, CA, 2001.

71. O'Driscoll SW. Articular cartilage regeneration using periosteum. *Clin Orthop* 1999;367[Suppl.]:S186–S203.

72. O'Driscoll SW. The healing and regeneration of articular cartilage. *J Bone Joint Surg Am* 1998;80:1795–1812.

73. Peterson L. Cartilage cell transplantation. In: Malek MM, ed. *Knee surgery: complications, pitfalls, and salvage.* New York: Springer, 2001:440–449.

74. Peterson L. Articular cartilage injuries treated with autologous chondrocyte transplantation in the human knee. *Acta Orthop Belg* 1996;62[Suppl.]:196–200.

75. Peterson L. Long-term clinical results of using autologous chondrocytes to treat full-thickness chondral defects. *J Sports Traumatol Rel Res* 1998;20:103–108.

76. Peterson L, Frolunda V, Lindahl A, et al. Durability of autologous chondrocyte transplantation of the knee. Presented at the 67th Annual Meeting of the American Academy of Orthopaedic Surgeons, Orlando, FL 2000.

77. Peterson L. Articular cartilage injury in the athlete: treatment options in 2001. Presented at the 68th Annual Meeting of the American Academy of Orthopaedic Surgeons, San Francisco, CA, 2001.

78. Peterson L. Durability of autologous chondrocyte transplantation of the knee. Presented at the MacArthur Cartilage Repair Workshop, New York, NY, 2000.

79. Peterson L, Minas T, Brittberg M, et al. Two- to 9-year outcome after autologous chondrocyte transplantation of the knee. *Clin Orthop* 2000;374:212–234.

80. Rand JA. Role of arthroscopy in osteoarthritis of the knee. *Arthroscopy* 1991;7:358–363.

81. Recht MP, Resnick D. Magnetic resonance imaging of articular cartilage: an overview. *Top Magn Reson Imaging* 1998;9:328–336.

82. Richardson JB, Caterson B, Evans EH, et al. Repair of human articular cartilage after implantation of autologous chondrocytes. *J Bone Joint Surg Br* 1999;81:1964–1968.

83. Rosenberg TD, Paulos LE, Parker RD, et al. The forty-five-degree posteroanterior flexion weight-bearing radiograph of the knee. *J Bone Joint Surg Am* 1988;70:1479–1483.

84. Salter RB, Simmonds DF, Malcolm BW, et al. The biological effect of continuous passive motion on the healing of full-thickness defects in articular cartilage: an experimental investigation in the rabbit. *J Bone Joint Surg Am* 1980;62:1232–1251.

85. Schwartsman V. Circular external fixation in high tibial osteotomy. *Instr Course Lect* 1995;44:469–474.

86. Shelton WR, Dukes AD. Meniscus replacement with bone anchors: a surgical technique. *Arthroscopy* 1994;10:324–327.

87. Slocum DB, Larson RL, James SL, et al. High tibial osteotomy. *Clin Orthop* 1974;104:239–243.

88. Spindler KP, Schils JP, Bergfeld JA, et al. Prospective study of osseous, articular and meniscal lesions in recent anterior cruciate ligament tears by magnetic resonance imaging and arthroscopy. *Am J Sports Med* 1993;21:551–557.

89. Steadman JR, Rodkey WG, Singleton SB, et al. Microfracture technique for full-thickness chondral defects: technique and clinical results. *Oper Tech Orthop* 1997;7:300–304.

90. Terry GC, Flandry F, Van Manen JW, et al. Isolated chondral fractures of the knee. *Clin Orthop* 1988;234:170–177.

91. Veltri DM, Warren RF, Wickiewicz TL, et al. Current status of allograft meniscal transplantation. *Clin Orthop* 1994;303:44–55.

92. Walker PS, Erkman MJ. The role of the menisci in force transmission across the knee. *Clin Orthop* 1975;109:184–192.

93. Zukor DJ, Gross AE. Osteochondral allograft reconstruction of the knee. *Am J Knee Surg* 1989;2:139–149.

DEGENERATIVE ARTHRITIS

ROBERT W. JACKSON

Degenerative arthritis, or osteoarthritis as it is sometimes called, may very well be the world's oldest and most chronic disease. Traces of degenerative arthritis have been found in the fossil remains of dinosaurs and prehistoric humans. Written accounts of osteoarthritis date back to ancient times, and its existence is borne out of examination of Egyptian mummies, which clearly show evidence of the disease. There are basically two classifications of degenerative arthritis: the primary type, which apparently develops spontaneously but may be associated with some minor or repetitive and subclinical level of traumatic insult to the joint with a possible genetic predisposition, and the secondary type, which results from a recognizable problem, usually traumatic. Degenerative arthritis is relatively rare before the age of 40 years, except in secondary cases. As aging occurs, an increasing proportion of the population develops degenerative arthritis in one or more joints. Statistics suggest that 80% of people more than 50 years old have arthritis, with spine, hip, and knees the most frequently affected joints (1).

Orthopaedic surgeons are therefore faced with increasing numbers of patients who have degenerative arthritis of the knee. The two main factors that contribute to the situation are the advancing general age of our population and the increasing and sustained activity seen at all ages, in terms of sports and recreational activities. In the past, treatment generally consisted of conservative measures and, in severe cases, referral to an orthopaedic surgeon, who would perform realignment, replacement, or ablation of the joint. However, with the advent of arthroscopy, a newer concept of treatment has evolved based on minimal intervention. With the aid of arthroscopic visualization of the joint, degenerative arthritis in its earliest stage can be identified by the softening and fragmenting of articular cartilage. This condition is frequently associated with degenerative changes in the menisci.

The effect of lavage or washing of degenerative joints in reducing symptoms was perhaps first noted by Bircher in

1921 (2), when he wrote an article on degenerative arthritis of the knee diagnosed by arthroscopic means. Burman et al., in 1934 (3), noted the beneficial effect of washing the knee joint, and they were first to describe "the lavage effect." Watanabe et al. (4) also reported on the beneficial effect of lavage alone in eliminating symptoms of osteoarthritis. In several publications, Jackson and others (5–10) speculated on the mechanism of this lavage phenomenon and also encouraged the use of minimally invasive techniques to remove symptomatic meniscal and articular cartilage fragments from osteoarthritic knees. Although this positive symptomatic effect is not yet not fully explained, arthroscopic lavage and debridement are now being extended to other joints, and similar beneficial effects are being noted. Other detractors, however, have commented on the unpredictability of the procedure and the recurrence of symptoms after varying periods of time (11,12).

SPECTRUM OF TREATMENT

When a patient presents with degenerative arthritis of the knee joint, treatment usually begins with conservative management. This customarily consists of relative rest, weight reduction, methods of cushioning heel-strike impact (e.g., soft rubber heels or insoles with energy-absorbing characteristics), a cane or other weight-relieving mechanisms, analgesics, nonsteroidal antiinflammatory medications, and the occasional intraarticular injection of steroids. Steroid usage has fewer and fewer proponents because the adverse effect of the steroid on already damaged articular cartilage seems to outweigh the potential beneficial effect of the steroid on the inflamed synovium of the joint. More recently, the effect of bracing to unload the affected compartment of the knee has shown promise as a temporizing measure. The injection of high-molecular-weight hyaluronic acid or "viscosupplementation" is also currently in use.

When nonoperative treatment fails to relieve symptoms or the initial degree of degenerative change is so severe at the time of presentation that conservative measures offer no hope of relief, operative treatment is generally contem-

R. W. Jackson: Department of Orthopaedic Surgery, Baylor University Medical Center, Dallas, Texas 75246.

plated. In the past, operative treatment usually consisted of open debridement of the joint or a realignment procedure through either the upper tibia or the lower femur. More recently, operative treatment has been centered around arthroplasty, either total or unicompartmental, and in the United States alone, surgeons perform more than 250,000 knee replacements each year.

We are now able to offer an additional category of treatment, consisting of minimally invasive arthroscopic surgery. Arthroscopic treatment combines lavage of the arthritic joint with debridement of articular cartilage surfaces and meniscal tears, in addition to the occasional partial synovectomy and the removal of osteophytes on which sensitive soft tissues are impinging. Pridie, as reported by Insall (13), noted that drilling through eburnated bone could result in a fibrocartilaginous resurfacing of the arthritic area. This observation resulted in efforts to achieve biologic regeneration of articular surfaces by marrow stimulating techniques. Additionally, cartilage transfer (mosaicplasty) and autologous chondrocyte harvest, culturing, and reimplantation have been developed (see Chapters 6 and 19).

PHILOSOPHY OF MANAGEMENT

The philosophy of management is that patients with degenerative joint disease have, by the time they report and seek treatment, often reached a point at which the damage to the articular cartilage is irreversible. Therefore, in these instances, a return to a state of youthful normality is not possible, and treatment is directed toward minimizing symptoms in the simplest way possible with the least complications. The patients are informed that arthroscopic lavage and debridement are not a cure, but merely comprise temporizing therapeutic method that can give significant relief of discomfort in most cases. Patients readily accept this concept, because they are usually reluctant to undergo major surgical procedures. Their hope is that by the time further treatment is necessary, additional knowledge and techniques for repair and regeneration will be available to give them a better chance at an excellent end result. Moreover, some patients believe that, if they can manage to function for a few more years, their activity level will be less in retirement or in later life, and perhaps major replacement surgery to the affected joint will not be necessary.

INSTRUMENTATION AND TECHNIQUES

The operative instruments are miniaturized cutting tools, such as punch forceps, knives, rongeurs, curettes, rotating suction shavers, and, more recently, laser or radiofrequency delivery tips, ranging in diameter from 3.8 to 5.2 mm (14).

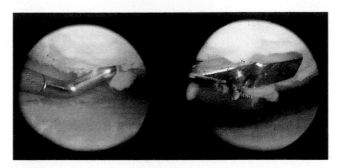

FIGURE 20.1 Loose or scaling fragments of articular cartilage, demonstrated by probing, can be removed with manual or powered instruments.

The basic principle of arthroscopic treatment is to remove any loose, scaling, or desquamating articular cartilage fragments from the articular surfaces and to excise any loose flaps or degenerative tears of meniscal cartilage (Figs. 20.1 and 20.2). Osteophytes that are rimming the edges of the articular surfaces and are believed to cause impingement against adjacent soft tissues can also be removed with a small rongeur, an osteotome, or an abrasion tool. Associated with the removal of degenerative tissue that has no reasonable opportunity for repair is the process of lavage, which washes the joint with copious amounts of irrigating solution. In many instances, both large and small fragments of fibrin or articular cartilage debris are noted to be washed out in the irrigating solution (Fig. 20.3).

Along with these visible fragments, it is assumed that enzymes and other microscopic debris fragments are also washed from the joint, and it is currently postulated that the removal of such enzymes is the reason behind the improvement in symptoms. Removing the larger scaling or desquamating articular and meniscal cartilage fragments not only eliminates the source of elements that are perpetuating the painful process (15), but also eliminates some of the mechanical problems of instability and crepitus.

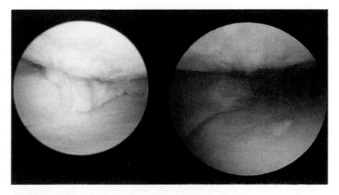

FIGURE 20.2 A torn meniscus associated with degenerative changes in the articular cartilage was removed under arthroscopic control. The immediate relief from discomfort was gratifying and lasted for more than 3 years.

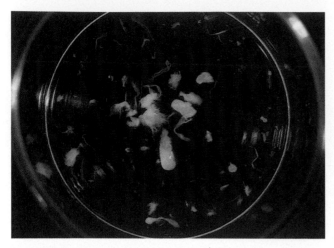

FIGURE 20.3 Washings from an arthritic knee joint, showing fibrous debris and other macroscopic articular cartilage fragments.

SELECTION OF SUITABLE PATIENTS

Bauer and Jackson described six types of symptomatic articular cartilage lesions that were seen arthroscopically (16). These investigators suggested that four types of chondral lesions were caused by singular exposures to direct trauma, and two types of degenerative lesions were probably the results of repetitive indirect or subclinical traumatic insults. In cases of traumatic lesions with loose flaps of articular cartilage (type III), the removal of the flaps completely relieved the patient's symptoms. Moreover, in cases of degenerative arthritis with diffuse fibrillation (type V) and some articular cartilage base still left covering the weight-bearing area of the joint, arthroscopic lavage appeared to be very beneficial. Patients in whom the articular cartilage had been worn away to expose subchondral bone (type VI) appeared to receive a less beneficial effect from the lavage and debridement process.

In an effort to recognize and define those patients who predictably would not do well and therefore to avoid unnecessary arthroscopic procedures, a retrospective study was carried out to correlate the clinical picture of signs, symptoms, and radiographic appearance with the known outcome of a large number of cases, with a minimum 2-year follow-up. From these data, four clinical stages, representing the increasing severity of degeneration, were described (17) (Table 20.1).

As a prospective guide to treatment, the following were postulated:

- Patients with *stage I* cases should primarily be treated by nonoperative measures, unless there are mechanical symptoms.
- Patients with *stage II* cases should be ideal for arthroscopic lavage and debridement.
- Patients with *stage III early stage IV* cases (i.e., loss of articular cartilage resulting in exposed bone on either the femur or tibia but not both sides) cases may also be considered suitable for arthroscopic treatment and moreover provide the opportunity to obtain biologic repair of the damaged surface of the joint with arthroscopic surgical techniques. Resurfacing techniques that can be performed arthroscopically include drilling, microfracture, abrasion arthroplasty and, more recently, autotransplantation with osteochondral plugs.
- Patients with *late stage IV* cases (erosion of articular cartilage on both femur and tibia, i.e., bone-on-bone contact) would probably *not* obtain any long-term benefit from an arthroscopic procedure and should be considered for a realignment or a replacement procedure, if the symptoms warrant such treatment (Fig 20.4).

PROSPECTIVE STUDY OF ARTHROSCOPIC TREATMENT OF OSTEOARTHRITIS

During a 2 1/2-year period from January 1, 1995 to June 30, 1997, 208 "new" patients were seen and diagnosed as having osteoarthritis of the knee. (Patients who had been diagnosed as having osteoarthritis and who had previously been treated by any surgical method were excluded.) All these patients were referred for consideration of some form of orthopaedic surgical treatment, because they had been

TABLE 20.1 STAGING SYSTEM FOR DEGREE OF DEGENERATION OF THE ARTICULAR SURFACE

Stage	Clinical Presentation	Radiographic Image	Arthroscopy Appearance	Arthroscopy Treatment
I	Minimal pain and swelling	Essentially normal with slight early changes	Softening	Nonoperative
II	Pain with activity, swelling, loss of range of motion	Joint space narrowing and early osteoarthritic changes	Fibrillation	Lavage and debridement
III	Pain with activity, swelling/warmth, loss of range of motion, slipping, catching	Joint space narrowing, osteophyte formation and angulation	Fragmentation	Lavage, debridement, and resurfacing if indicated
IV	Pain at rest, deformity, varus instability (lateral thrust)	Narrowing, osteophytes, joint destruction, bone-on-bone articulation	Eburnation	Realignment or replacement

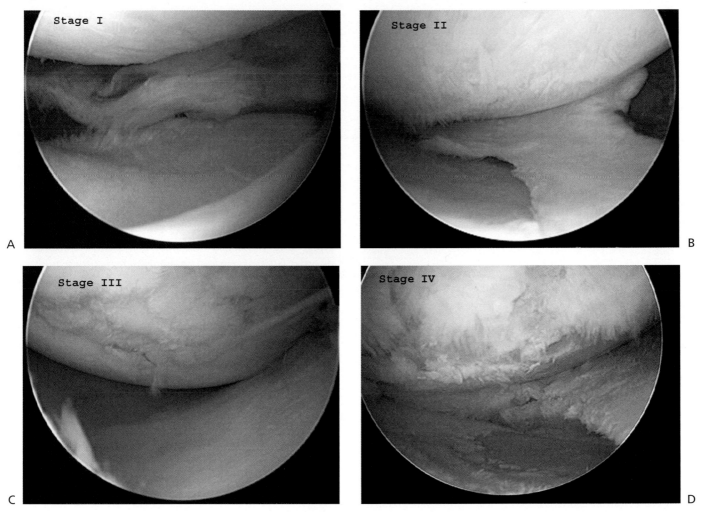

FIGURE 20.4 Arthroscopic pictures of different cases representing progressively severe degeneration of articular cartilage, sometimes in association with meniscal disease. **A**, Stage I; **B**, Stage II; **C**, Stage III; **D**; Stage IV.

unresponsive to physical therapy, analgesics, nonsteroidal antiinflammatory drugs, and other conservative measures instituted by primary care physicians. Only three patients were lost to follow-up. Follow-up was carried out 4 to 6 years after the primary, prospective treatment (18).

Of the 205 patients with adequate follow-up, seven were not considered surgical candidates and were continued on conservative treatment. None of these patients received surgical treatment in the 4- to 6-year span of the study. Seventy-seven patients were treated by primary replacement arthroplasty or osteotomy. One hundred twenty-one patients had arthroscopic surgery as their initial treatment, and a current outcome was obtained on all the 121 consecutive arthroscopic cases (Table 20.2).

The outcomes were subjectively placed into four categories of results:

1. Patients with *excellent* results had virtually no further symptoms.

TABLE 20.2 SYMPTOMATIC RESULTS: 4–6 YEARS AFTER ARTHROSCOPIC SURGERY OF 121 CONSECUTIVE CASES

Stage	Excellent/Good	Fair	Poor
I (8)	8 (100%)	0	0
II (32)	29 (90.6%)	0	3 (9.4%)
III (39)	19 (48.7%)	11 (28.2%)	9 (23.1%)
IV (42)	5 (11.9%)	22 (52.4%)	15 (35.7%)

2. Patients with *good* results had slight pain and swelling with higher level activities.

3. Patients with *fair* results had some discomfort with regular activities and often controlled pain and swelling with nonsteroidal antiinflammatory drugs.

4. Patients with *poor* results had night pain, they had received other surgical treatment, or the knee was constantly limiting their activities.

These 121 patients therefore provided a snapshot of the symptomatic results of conservative arthroscopic surgery, with a minimum 4-year follow-up and with prospective treatment based on staging of the severity of the osteoarthritis.

The term *arthroscopic surgery* can have many interpretations. In this series, it included lavage or irrigation of the knee, removal of loose bodies, trimming of meniscal fragments, and the conservative or minimal removal of separating or desquamating articular cartilage fragments (chondroplasty). Patients in whom other methods of treatment, such as abrasion arthroplasty, microfracture, or transplantation of osteochondral plugs and extensive synovectomy, were *not* included in this study.

RESULTS

Stage IV Cases

Of the 119 patients classified as having stage IV cases, 77 did not undergo arthroscopy, and their initial surgical treatment was replacement arthroplasty. The 42 patients with cases labeled stage IV and who underwent arthroscopy usually requested the procedure. Although the so-called "beneficial lavage effect" was experienced to some degree in 27 patients with stage IV lesions (23% of total), it was not predictable and not very dramatic. Only five patients (12%) of this group were considered to have good or excellent results at 4-year follow-up. Twenty-two patients (52%) were considered to have fair results, because they still had residual symptoms, but all stated that they were improved to some degree by the arthroscopic procedure. Fifteen patients (36%) had no significant relief, and 12 of these went on to replacement surgery in an average of 1.2 years. Three patients had a second arthroscopy; one was slightly improved, and the other two showed no improvement but elected no further treatment because of health problems. These findings confirmed my opinion that arthroscopy should probably not be done on stage IV lesions, unless it is to buy some time before definitive replacement or realignment surgery is performed.

Stage II and III Cases

A total of 71 patients (32 stage II and 39 stage III) comprised the moderately advanced arthritic group. Sometimes the prospective clinical assessment of stage II turned out to be a stage III at arthroscopy, and a stage III actually turned out to be an early stage IV. However, patients with stage II and stage III cases appear to benefit most from arthroscopic treatment. In this study, of the 71 patients in the stage II to stage III category, only six had a repeat arthroscopy, and three subsequently underwent replacement arthroplasty, resulting in 62 patients (87%) who were improved symp-

tomatically for 4 to 6 years by the initial arthroscopic surgery procedure.

Stage I Cases

The greatest benefit of arthroscopic surgery is seen in the earlier stages of the degenerative process. All eight of the patients who were considered to have stage I cases and who were treated by arthroscopy had complete relief of symptoms, at least as long as our follow-up period. Granted, these patients were primarily treated for other reasons, such as meniscal disease, but all of them demonstrated stage I degenerative changes at arthroscopy. This observation has potential significance in that, by performing arthroscopic lavage with the added capability of treating a mechanical disorder (such as removing a meniscal tear, a loose body, or a chondral flap), the danger of gastrointestinal bleeding and other adverse systemic effects from the prolonged use of nonsteroidal antiinflammatory medications is eliminated. There is, of course, the risk of surgery, but it was believed that, because the surgical procedure was performed on an outpatient basis with minimal anesthesia (and in many instances local anesthesia), this was an acceptable risk, and the procedure provided quick and lasting relief. The benefits of tidal irrigation or outpatient needle lavage, without arthroscopic examination of the joint, have been noted in the rheumatology literature (19,20).

COMPLICATIONS

The complications associated with arthroscopic treatment of degenerative arthritis include those of any arthroscopic procedure (21). Usually, the procedure is performed while the patient is under a general anesthetic, because the patient with an arthritic joint is relatively uncomfortable when the joint is stressed to obtain access to the posterior regions or with the inflation of the tourniquet. The complications of anesthesia and the minor morbidity associated with the operative procedure must also be considered. The risk of infection is possibly increased in older patients, who may not have a normally functioning immune system. If previous steroid injections have been given to the joint, there may also be a reduced resistance to bacterial invasion. Removal of deranged tissue can be carried out to a harmful degree, thus producing a more painful situation than that existing before the arthroscopic intervention. An aggressive abrasion, for example, may cause further malalignment in the weight-bearing area if excessive amounts of cortical bone are removed. Instances have been recorded in which arthrofibrosis, perhaps secondary to bleeding within the joint postoperatively or scar tissue enhanced by the removal of synovium, has led to decreased range of motion and increased pain. If laser energy is used to perform a chondroplasty, adverse photodynamic effects may be seen much later in the subchondral areas.

DISCUSSION

There are many ways to look at these data, but the overall message appears to be that arthroscopic surgery can give significant relief from the symptoms of osteoarthritis in its early stages, and for many patients, it provides symptomatic relief for a long time. The theory of why lavage works is centered largely on the removal of debris from the joint, which can cause synoviris. In addition, degradative enzymes and other factors, which may contribute to the pain syndrome, are washed out by this method.

Our prime consideration in all stages of treatment during this study (especially stages II and III) was merely to remove, in a very conservative manner, any loose, scaling, or desquamating articular cartilage fragments or any degenerative or loose meniscal fragments. This was occasionally associated with a minor degree of synovectomy when synovial fronds appeared to be impinging between the articulating joint surfaces. Care was taken to preserve as much articular cartilage as possible and not to remove it. Before this study, abrasion arthroplasty or multiple drilling was attempted in many instances. Although improvement in 80% to 85% of patients has been reported after abrasion arthroplasty (22), the lack of good short-term results, usually associated with increased morbidity, led to the discontinuance of this approach as a routine treatment modality in my practice. Authors who are critical of the abrasion arthroplasty technique point out that abrasion alone does not address the question of why the weight-bearing surface of the joint had been denuded of articular cartilage in the first place (23). Usually, this is a malalignment phenomenon or a chronic instability problem, and neither is addressed by purely debriding the exposed bone surface. Our goal therefore, during the time frame of this study, was to remove only the loose, fragmenting, or fibrillating articular surfaces, with minimal debridement whenever possible.

The advantages of arthroscopic treatment of degenerative arthritis are obviously the minimal morbidity and the low complication rates. Most of the procedures are done as same-day surgical or short-stay cases. Patients generally are most appreciative of the opportunity to have something done that could delay or postpone major surgery until a more optimal time in their life. Many middle-aged people prefer to wait until they retire before they undergo major surgery. Others choose to wait for improved technology before they undergo arthroplasty.

SUMMARY

Osteoarthritis or degenerative arthritis of the knee is a condition that presents itself to the treating physician at any stage in the spectrum, from early to severe destruction of the joint. A clinical staging system based on the severity of the degenerative process has been proposed to enable better comparison of treatment modalities and also to provide a guide to treatment. A prospective study has shown that arthroscopic surgery can give significant relief of symptoms for long periods of time, if treatment is appropriately initiated in the earlier stages of the degenerative process. Patients with more advanced stages of the condition may receive temporary relief from arthroscopic lavage or debridement, but any benefit is unpredictable and lasts only a few months. Current efforts at marrow stimulation and other autogenous techniques for biologic resurfacing of the arthritic knees will, one hopes, improve these statistics in the future.

It is recommended that the surgeon's armamentarium in the treatment of degenerative arthritis should involve interventional arthroscopy at an earlier stage rather than at a later stage in the disease process. It is also recommended that the arthroscopist should be very conservative in debridement and should remove only the loosened and scaling fragments that will not become reattached to the articular surface. In the presence of eburnated articular surfaces, realignment or replacement surgery would appear to be a more appropriate and reasonable way of treating the patient. In the future, it may be possible to repair damaged articular cartilage in a more effective way, through a biologically resurfaced joint, or even through the application of a synthetic surface to the articular weight-bearing areas. At this point in our knowledge, however, arthroscopic lavage and debridement comprise an acceptable treatment method for degenerative arthritis unresponsive to conservative measures.

Finally, when assessing the overall place of arthroscopy in the management of degenerative arthritis, we must consider not only its role in the treatment of the established disease process, but also its role in the prevention of degenerative arthritis (5). It is extremely difficult to provide objective data regarding prevention at this stage. However, it is believed that the early and accurate diagnosis of trauma, associated with minimal intervention techniques, such as meniscal repair, partial meniscectomy, and the early stabilization of ligamentous or capsular ruptures, can prevent or at least minimize the progressive degenerative changes that have been seen in the past associated with traumatic injury to the joint. Although it is speculative at present, it is entirely possible that the future major role of arthroscopy will primarily be the prevention of arthritis, and subsequent generations will see much less of this type of disease than present orthopaedic surgeons are encountering. In the meantime, however, there is no question that we now have an additional modality (lavage and debridement associated with arthroscopic treatment) to help treat the patient who is afflicted with a painful arthritic degenerative joint.

REFERENCES

1. Peyron JG, Altman RD. The epidemiology of osteoarthritis. In: Moskowitz RW, Howell DS, Goldberg VM, et al., eds. *Osteoarthritis: diagnosis and medical/surgical management,* 2nd ed. Philadelphia: WB Saunders, 1992:15–37.
2. Bircher E. Die Arthroendoskopie. *Zentralbl Chir* 1921;48:1460–1461.
3. Burman MS, Finkelstein H, Mayer L. Arthroscopy of the knee joint. *J Bone Joint Surg* 1934;16:255–268.
4. Watanabe M, Takeda S, Ikeuchi H. *Atlas of arthroscopy.* Tokyo: Igaku Shoin, 1957.
5. Jackson RW. The role of arthroscopy in the management of the arthritic knee. *Clin Orthop* 1974;101:28–35.
6. Dandy DJ. Arthroscopic debridement of the knee for osteoarthritis. *J Bone Joint Surg Br* 1991;73:877–878.
7. Ewing JW. Arthroscopic treatment of degenerative meniscal lesions and early degenerative arthritis of the knee. In: Ewing JW, ed. *Articular cartilage and knee joint function: basic science and arthroscopy.* New York: Raven Press, 1990:137–145.
8. Rand JA. The role of arthroscopy in osteoarthritis of the knee. *Arthroscopy* 1991;7:358:363.
9. Shahariaree H. Arthroscopic debridement. In: Shahriaree H, ed. *O'Conner's textbook of arthroscopic surgery,* 2nd ed. Philadelphia: JB Lippincott, 1992:433–436.
10. Livesley PJ, Doherty M, Needoff M, et al. Arthroscopic lavage of osteoarthritic knees. *J Bone Joint Surg Br* 1991;73:922–926.
11. Sharkey PF. The case against arthroscopic debridement. *J Arthroplasty* 1997;12:467–469.
12. Moseley JB, Wray NP, Kuykendall D, et al. Arthroscopic treatment of osteoarthritis of the knee—a randomized, double-blind, placebo-controlled trial: two year follow-up of 180 patients. Presented at the 68th Annual Meeting of the American Association of Orthopaedic Surgeons, San Francisco, CA, 2001.
13. Insall JN. Intra-articular surgery for degenerative arthritis of the knee: a report of the work of the late K.H. Pridie. *J Bone Joint Surg Br* 1967;49:211–228.
14. Gobel EM, Kane SM, Wilcox, TR, et al. Advanced arthroscopic instrumentation. In: McGinty JB, ed. *Operative arthroscopy,* 2nd ed. Philadelphia: Lippincott–Raven, 1996:7–12.
15. Jackson RW, Marans HJ, Silver RS. The arthroscopic treatment of degenerative arthritis of the knee. *J Bone Joint Surg Br* 1988;70: 332.
16. Bauer M. Jackson RW. Chondral lesions of the femoral condyles: a system of arthroscopic classification. *Arthroscopy* 1988;4:97–102.
17. Jackson RW. The role of arthroscopy in diagnosis and management of osteoarthritis. In: *Osteoarthritis: diagnosis and medical/surgical management,* 2nd ed. Philadelphia: WB Saunders, 1992:527–534.
18. Jackson RW, Dieterichs C. Results of arthroscopic lavage and debridement of osteoarthritic knees using the degree of degeneration as a guide to treatment: a prospective study. Submitted to *Arthroscopy* 2002.
19. Ike RW, Arnold WJ, Rothschild E, et al. Tidal irrigation versus conservative medical management in patients with osteoarthritis of the knee: a prospective, randomized study. *J Rheumatol* 1992;19:772–779.
20. Chang RW, Falconer J, Stulberg SD, et al. A randomized, controlled trial of arthroscopic surgery versus closed needle joint lavage for patients with osteoarthritis of the knee. *Arthritis Rheum* 1993;36:289.
21. Sprague NF III. *Complications in arthroscopy.* New York: Raven Press, 1989.
22. Johnson LL. *Diagnostic and surgical arthroscopy.* St. Louis: CV Mosby, 1981.
23. Bert JM, Maschka K. The arthroscopic treatment of unicompartmental gonarthrosis: a five-year follow-up study of abrasion arthroplasty plus arthroscopic debridement and arthroscopic debridement alone. *Arthroscopy* 1989;5:25–32.

ARTHROSCOPIC SYNOVECTOMY OF THE KNEE

DARRELL J. OGILVIE-HARRIS

Arthroscopic synovectomy is a technique by which the synovium can be resected from the knee joint. The advantages of arthroscopic synovectomy compared with traditional open synovectomy are significantly less joint stiffness and the ability to reach a greater portion of the synovium of the knee joint. The disadvantage of arthroscopic synovectomy is that the operation can be technically difficult to perform.

EQUIPMENT REQUIREMENTS

Arthroscopic synovectomy can be carried out with a standard arthroscope. Sometimes a 70-degree arthroscope is valuable for viewing posteriorly. Most of the time, however, the 30-degree arthroscope is adequate.

It is vital to have good flow. Arthroscopic synovectomy, therefore, does require a pressure pump. It should have separate volume and pressure controls. Without this type of pump system, the arthroscopic synovectomy is potentially hazardous because of obstruction of view. Usually, a low pressure setting is started initially, at, say, 35 mm Hg. This can be increased to 50 or 60 mm Hg if intraarticular bleeding occurs. It is essential that the field be kept clear at all times.

A power shaver with a synovial resector blade is necessary. Generally, a blade with a 5.5-mm diameter works best in the anterior compartment. This is supplemented by a 4.5-mm curved blade to reach into the smaller areas around the menisci and also in the posterior compartment. A variably curved blade is ideal because it allows the angle to be changed, particularly when working in the posterior compartments. This approach allows maximum access to the joint lining.

A tourniquet is essential. This controls the bleeding into the joint. Anything that obscures the adequate visualization

D. J. Ogilvie-Harris: Associate Professor, Deptartment of Surgery, Toronto Western Hospital, Toronto, Ontario, Canada.

of the synovium increases the risk of damage to structures around the joint.

The type of anesthetic used can either be general anesthetic or spinal. The operation is too technically difficult to perform using a local anesthetic, especially because of the requirement to have access to the posterior portals.

PREOPERATIVE PLANNING

It is essential to have established the diagnosis of the synovial disorder before performing synovial resection. In patients with rheumatoid arthritis or seronegative arthritis, this may depend on the clinical features, radiographic features, and appropriate blood work. When one suspects pigmented villonodular synovitis, it is in my view essential to have an established histologic diagnosis. This may have required previous diagnostic arthroscopy with synovial biopsy. If the patient has been referred for arthroscopic synovectomy, then the original histologic diagnosis must accompany the patient. Similar considerations apply in the case of synovial chondromatosis. Informed consent from the patient is essential. In discussing arthroscopic synovectomy, particular care must be taken to discuss the posterior portals and posterior aspect of the arthroscopic synovectomy. This does increase the risk to the neurovascular structures of the posterior aspect of the knee compared with anterior arthroscopy. In addition, the postoperative rehabilitation is longer that with normal arthroscopy, and there is a possibility of developing knee stiffness with the requirement for manipulation, although this complication is rare.

TECHNIQUE

Arthroscopic synovectomy is carried out in a systematic manner (1,23). Initially, the tourniquet is inflated. The arthroscope is introduced through a standard anterolateral portal. Diagnostic arthroscopy is carried out probing the appropriate structures such as the menisci, the articular cartilage, and the cruciate ligaments. The patient may have concurrent intraarticular disease such as a torn meniscus that needs treatment at the same time as the arthroscopic synovectomy.

Five basis steps are used to carry out the synovectomy:

Step 1: The arthroscope is place through the anterolateral portal (Fig. 21.1). A synovial resector is introduced into the lateral suprapatellar portal. Under direct vision, the synovium is removed from the suprapatellar pouch, much of the lateral gutter, the medial gutter, and the intercondylar notch, where it can be visualized.

Step 2: The arthroscope is kept in the anterolateral portal (Fig. 21.2). A synovial resector is moved to the anteromedial portal. The synovium is then resected from the medial gutter, from the intercondylar notch, and from around the medial meniscus. Sometimes it is necessary to switch to a small shaver to remove the synovium from around the meniscus. Care is taken in the intercondylar notch not to resect the portions of the anterior or posterior cruciate ligament.

Step 3: The arthroscope is then removed and is replaced into the anteromedial portal (Fig. 21.3). The shaver is placed into the anterolateral portal. It is then possible to resect the remaining portions of the synovium in the lateral gutter, the remaining synovium in the intercondylar notch, and the remaining synovium around the medial and lateral meniscus. Again, a 4.5-mm resector is sometimes necessary to clear the synovium away from underneath the meniscus.

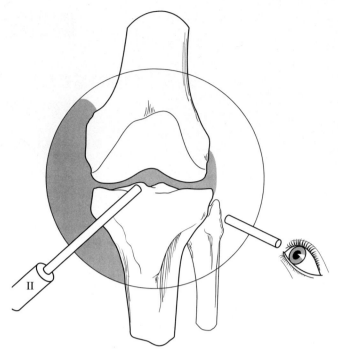

FIGURE 21.2 The second step involves keeping the arthroscope in the same portal and moving the shaver to the inferomedial portal. The synovium in the medial gutter and the intracondylar notch can be resected. The *shaded area* shows the synovium reached.

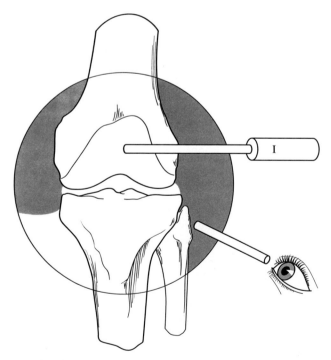

FIGURE 21.1 Initially a diagnostic arthroscopy is carried out. Then the first step consists of placing the arthroscope in the inferolateral portal with the shaver in the superolateral portal. The synovium in the suprapatellar pouch and both gutters can be resected. The shaded area shows the synovium reached.

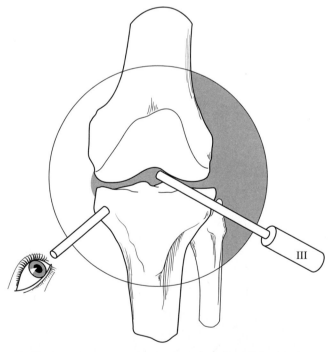

FIGURE 21.3 Then the third step consists of placing the arthroscope in the inferomedial portal with the shaver in the inferolateral portal. The synovium in the lateral gutter and the intercondylar notch can be resected. The *shaded area* shows the synovium reached.

Step 4: The arthroscope is kept in the anteromedial portal (Fig. 21.4). The shaver is introduced into the supramedial portal. This portal is made at the superomedial border of the patella, 1 cm above and 1 cm medial to the corner of the patella. Through this portal the remaining synovium in the suprapatellar pouch and the medial gutter and lateral gutter can be resected. In addition, any portion of the fat pad, which is hypertrophic, can be resected. There is usually abundant synovium around the fat pad itself, particularly in diseases such as rheumatoid arthritis.

Step 5: This step consists of visualizing and resecting the synovium from the posteromedial and posterolateral compartments (3) (Fig. 21.5). This is usually left until last. The reason for this sequence is that once the anterior synovium has been resected, it is easier to access the posterior joint. Moreover, if there is difficulty in accessing the posterior compartment such that synovectomy posteriorly is not possible, at least the anterior component of the surgical procedure will have been performed. It has been suggested that the posterior compartments be accessed first (4). However, I consider this strategy to be more risky.

To access the posterior component with the arthroscope, the knee must be flexed to 90 degrees. This approach opens up the intercondylar notch but also allows the neurovascular structures to move posteriorly. If a leg holder is used, it must be sufficiently proximal to allow the posterior neu-

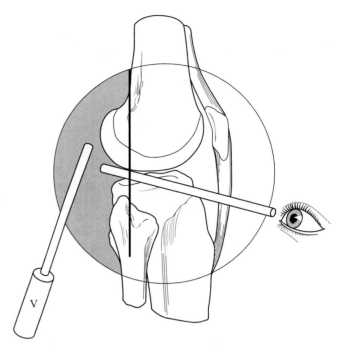

FIGURE 21.5 The posterior compartments undergo instrumentation after the anterior synovectomy is complete.

rovascular structures to fall back so they are not brought into the operative field.

To establish the posteromedial and posterolateral portals, the posterior compartments can be transilluminated with the light of the arthroscope. The operating room lights are dimmed. It is then possible to see the site of entry for the posteromedial and posterolateral portals.

To establish a posteromedial portal, the posteromedial corner of the joint is palpated (Figs. 21.6 and 21.7). A small-bore needle is introduced into the joint to establish the portal. This must be clearly visualized within the posterior compartment of the joint before establishing a larger portal.

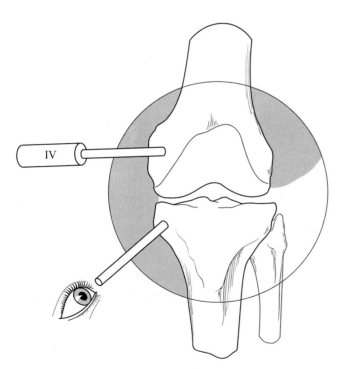

FIGURE 21.4 The fourth step consists of keeping the arthroscope in the inferomedial portal with the shaver in the superolateral portal. The synovium in the lateral gutter and suprapatellar pouch can be resected. The *shaded area* shows the synovium reached.

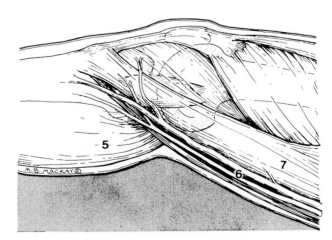

FIGURE 21.6 The structures at risk on the medial side of the knee in extension.

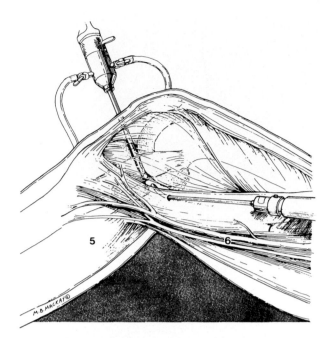

FIGURE 21.7 The structures at risk on the medial side of the knee in flexion. The neurovascular structure move into a relatively safe zone. A needle and the shaver can be introduced at the posteromedial joint line.

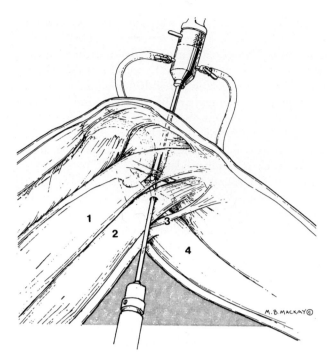

FIGURE 21.9 In flexion, the neurovascular structures move posteriorly. Care must be exercised to remain well anterior to the biceps tendon, to clear the common peroneal nerve.

Our anatomic studies indicate that when a knee is flexed to 90 degrees, the saphenous nerve and vein are about 1 cm posterior to the posteromedial corner of the joint. Putting a needle in at this site and aiming anteriorly safely clear the neurovascular structures.

Once the needle has been used to establish the portal clearly, a small incision is made in the skin. Blunt dissection is carried out using artery forceps. This technique lessens the chance to damage any of the superficial nerves in this area. A sharp obturator is then used to make a portal, and the shaver is introduced. In the posterior compartment, a 4.5-mm curved shaver is used.

To establish the posterolateral portal, the knee must be flexed to 90 degrees (Figs. 21.8 and 21.9). The posterolat-

eral compartment is transilluminated with the arthroscope. If the knee is in extension, the common peroneal nerve is at risk. At 90 degrees of flexion, the common peroneal nerve is well away, under the biceps tendon. The posterolateral portal therefore must always be established anterior to the biceps tendon, to leave 1 to 2 cm of clearance.

The posterolateral joint line is palpated. A thin-bore needle is put into the posterolateral joint and is aimed anteriorly. The needle must be clearly visualized within the posterolateral joint. A small incision is made in the posterolateral corner. The skin is opened using artery forceps. A sharp trocar is then introduced into the joint, followed by a shaver. A 4.5-mm shaver blade is used.

The posterior compartment can be visualized by putting the arthroscope directly through the intercondylar notch on the same side as the posterior compartment is visualized or by crossing the intercondylar notch. The posteromedial compartment can be visualized from the anteromedial portal (Fig. 21.10). The arthroscope is passed medial to the posterior cruciate ligament. It can also be accessed on the contralateral portal (i.e., the posterolateral portal) when one introduces the arthroscope medial to the anterior cruciate and medial to the posterior cruciate. In my experience, the ipsilateral portal technique and the contralateral portal technique are used equally.

In a similar manner, the posterolateral joint can be accessed from the anterolateral compartment, coming lateral to the posterior cruciate ligament (Fig. 21.11). The contralateral portal is the anteromedial portal and takes the arthroscope lateral to the anterior and posterior cruciate ligaments.

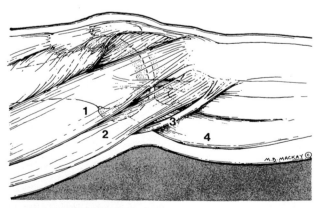

FIGURE 21.8 The structures at risk at the posterolateral side of the knee in extension.

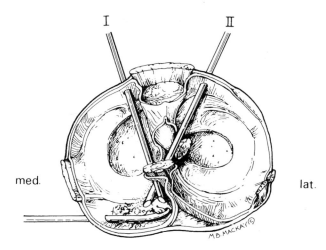

FIGURE 21.10 The ipsilateral and contralateral approaches to the medial posterior compartment of the knee through the intercondylar notch.

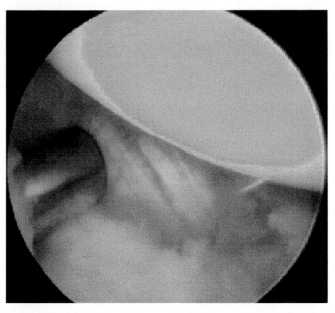

FIGURE 21.12 Rheumatoid synovium being resected. The small area of shiny normal tissue is seen below the margins of the synovium.

A special technique is used to resect the synovial from the posterior compartments. It is critical that the capsule is not violated because extraarticular structures can then be sucked into the joint. Careful control of the suction is therefore used to minimize damage to the capsule and then carefully to resect the synovium from the posterior joint. If there is any doubt whatsoever regarding the visualization of the tip of the shaver or the structure being resected, the operation is halted. If there is blockage of the view through bleeding or technical difficulties, it is safer to stop the operative procedure rather than to proceed without adequate visualization.

Synovial Resection

It can be difficult to know when sufficient synovium has been resected. Basically, the synovium needs to be removed until the shiny capsular surface below it is seen (Figs. 21.12 and 21.13). This means resecting the synovium and the subsynovial tissue. When the synovium is pigmented, the lines of distinction are easier to see. The surgeon must

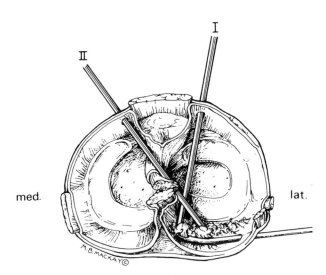

FIGURE 21.11 The ipsilateral and contralateral approaches to the medial posterior compartment of the knee through the intercondylar notch.

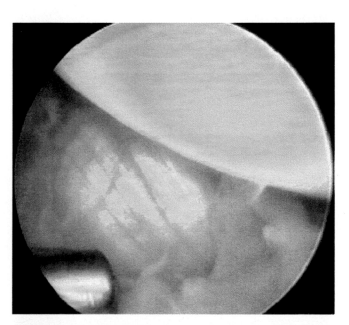

FIGURE 21.13 Rheumatoid synovium being resected. The area of synovial hypertrophy is progressively resected to expose more of the normal underlying tissues.

move the shaver progressively around the joint to remove all visible synovium using steps 1 to 5, as described earlier.

POSTOPERATIVE MANAGEMENT

A drain is left in the knee for at least a few hours postoperatively. If bleeding is significant, the drain may be left in overnight. If bleeding is minimal, the drain can be removed 1 to 2 hours after the surgical procedure.

Adequate pain management is necessary. Patients do experience a significant amount of pain after synovectomy. This can be relieved by femoral nerve blocks.

It has not been my practice to use continuous passive movement machines. However, this method is certainly an acceptable form of treatment. I start patients on an aggressive program of active range of movement and quadriceps muscle strengthening. It is important that patients have an actively supervised therapy program, starting immediately postoperatively, if they are to achieve optimal results with regard to knee flexion, extension, and return of quadriceps strength. Without an adequate postoperative treatment program, the risk of complications such as knee stiffness or reflex sympathetic dystrophy will probably increase.

RHEUMATOID ARTHRITIS

Indications

Patients must have an established diagnosis of rheumatoid arthritis (Fig. 21.14). Good medical management is necessary for at least 6 months before surgical synovectomy is considered. This medical management is usually supervised by a rheumatologist. If the patient has persistent swelling of

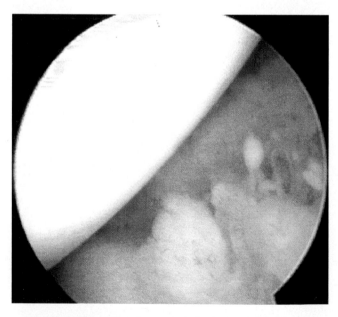

FIGURE 21.14 Villous hyperplasia in rheumatoid synovitis.

the knee joint for more than 6 months, despite good medical control, then arthroscopic synovectomy may help the patient.

It is important to have an established diagnosis of rheumatoid arthritis. It is also important to rule out other causes of unilateral joint swelling, particularly any form of septic arthritis.

Special Considerations

The patient's general medical condition needs to be carefully considered, including such aspects as neck instability and management of drugs such as prednisone or methotrexate. The patient should have minimal radiologic changes. The procedure is not indicated for patients with advanced rheumatologic changes with significant joint damage. Posterior synovial masses cannot be easily reached or removed—they may require open excision combined with arthroscopic anterior synovectomy (5).

Results

Published articles of our own results indicate that this operation is good for local control of the disease; 70% to 80% of patients will be relieved of their symptoms for 4 to 5 years (6,7). It is not known whether the procedure changes the natural history of the disease. The operation is, however, highly effective for localized control of synovitis in patients meeting the foregoing criteria.

SERONEGATIVE ARTHRITIS

Indications

The indications for arthroscopic synovectomy in patients with seronegative arthritis are not as clear as in rheumatoid arthritis (seropositive). Patients have various conditions such as psoriasis, Reiter's disease, or ankylosing spondylitis. The indications are persistent synovitis of one or both knees for more than 6 months despite adequate medical control. Patients should have minimal radiographic changes.

Special Considerations

These patients tend to become stiff postoperatively. It is essential therefore that they have a good postoperative rehabilitation program. This includes the use of a continuous passive movement machine.

Results

The results in seronegative arthritis are not as good as in patients with rheumatoid arthritis. Approximately 50% to 60% of patients will have significant benefit (8,9). Benefits include local relief of synovitis, pain, and limitations. The effect of the procedure on the long-term evolution of the disease is unknown (10).

SYNOVIAL CHONDROMATOSIS

Indications

There are two major forms of this condition (11,12). Some patients have only one or two loose bodies associated with minimal synovial reaction. This may well be a different condition than the diffuse form. In this situation, it may be sufficient to remove the one or two loose bodies and to perform a localized resection of the synovium.

The more common variety is diffuse synovial chondromatosis. These patients have many loose bodies, sometimes hundreds. These are small cartilaginous loose bodies and are associated with actively inflamed synovium.

Saleh and I published a series of cases in 1994 that indicated that the removal of loose bodies alone is not sufficient (13). In these patients, we had excellent results of removal of the loose bodies associated with arthroscopic synovectomy. This is the treatment of choice.

In some cases, previous diagnostic arthroscopy has been performed. Multiple loose bodies have been seen and removed. However, the patient has developed a recurrence. In this situation, arthroscopic synovectomy is necessary to control the disease.

Special Considerations

It is difficult to determine how much synovium is involved. Sometimes the area of synovial hyperplasia may be in the posterior compartment and sometimes in the anterior compartments (Fig. 21.15). Generally, I look for any area of abnormal synovium and resect it.

Sometimes it is impossible to know whether all the loose bodies have been removed. Having completed the synovectomy, I spend several minutes inspecting all aspects of the joint to see whether any further loose bodies remain. Copious irrigation is carried out after the synovectomy to try to ensure that all the loose bodies have been removed.

In the informed consent for this procedure, I warn patients that loose bodies may be missed. On occasion, it may be necessary to go back again later to remove further loose bodies. In this situation, the synovium again should be carefully examined to make sure that areas of synovial hyperplasia or metaplasia have not recurred.

Results

Generally, the results in the literature indicate about a 10% recurrence rate. However, this is usually associated with removal of the loose bodies alone. In our series, we had a significant recurrence rate in patients when the loose bodies alone were removed. However, after arthroscopic synovec-

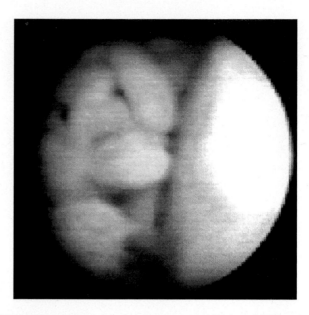

FIGURE 21.15 The posterior compartment in synovial chondromatosis. The localized metaplastic synovium is forming early loose bodies from the synovial lining. Synovectomy of this abnormal tissue is essential.

tomy, with removal of the loose bodies, the recurrence rate is extremely low.

PIGMENTED VILLONODULAR SYNOVITIS

Indications

It is important to have a biopsy-proven diagnosis of this condition before proceeding with a synovectomy. If the patient has been referred without a histologic diagnosis, the initial arthroscopy and biopsy may be necessary to establish clearly that this is the condition one is treating. This distinction is important because, if there is a recurrence, more radical treatments may be necessary, such as irradiation. Magnetic resonance imaging can be very helpful in establishing a diagnosis preoperatively (14).

Special Considerations

There are two forms of this condition: a localized form and a generalized form. In the localized form, patients often present with a history of locking (Fig. 21.16). A pedunculated mass is found attached to the synovium. Arthroscopically, it is dark reddish brown. The synovium at the point of attachment show similar changes.

The pedunculated mass can be resected either as a whole or in part. Localized synovectomy should be carried out, to remove all the synovium from the area of the attachment. This synovium should be removed until the shiny capsular fibers below it are seen.

The diffuse form of the condition is much more difficult to deal with and has a high recurrence rate. The synovium is

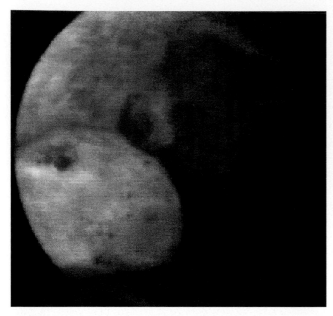

FIGURE 21.16 Typical *deep orange* discoloration in pigmented villonodular synovitis. This is a pedunculated nodule with localized extension. Local excision is indicated.

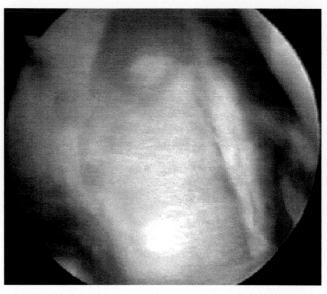

FIGURE 21.18 The synovium in pigmented villonodular synovitis must be resected down to normal tissue below it. The shaver has been used to remove the deeply pigmented abnormal synovium, and the shiny capsular layer can be seen showing through it.

diffusely involved with masses of villous hypertrophy, with deep orange pigmentation (Fig. 21.17). Complete synovectomy should be attempted. The more synovium that can be removed, the greater the chance is eradication of the disease. The resection lines between normal and abnormal tissue are seen more easily because of the pigment (Fig. 21.18). Great care should be taken to reach the healthy, undiseased tissue below it. Small shavers are needed around the menisci (Fig.

21.19). The procedure includes a complete anterior and posterior synovectomy, involving all the compartments. It is necessary to use shavers of different sizes to access fully all areas of the joint that can be visualized.

Postoperatively, these patients are followed-up with magnetic resonance scans every 6 months or so. Significant recurrence of the disease radiologically and clinically may necessitate a second or even third synovectomy. This increases

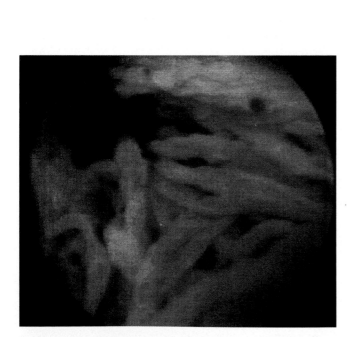

FIGURE 21.17 Diffuse pigmented villonodular synovitis. A complete anterior and posterior synovectomy is warranted.

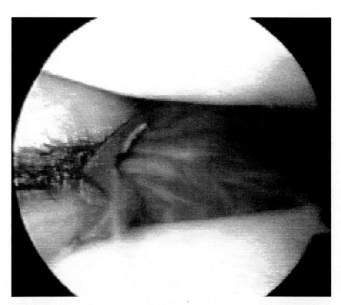

FIGURE 21.19 Small shavers will be necessary to remove the synovium above and below the meniscus. A 4.5-mm curved shaver is used to excise the synovium above the medial meniscus in this patient with pigmented villonodular synovitis.

the risk of potential harm to the patient because of scarring from the first synovectomy.

In the event that the disease becomes invasive locally and cannot be adequately controlled, other, more radical methods for control may be necessary. I currently use irradiation in this situation. It is wise to refer patients to specialized centers for this type of care.

In advanced pigmented villonodular synovitis, with destruction of the joint surfaces or significant erosion of the bone, arthroscopic synovectomy is not adequate. These patients usually require joint reconstruction.

Where there is a huge mass posteriorly, arthroscopic synovectomy may not be effective. This is particularly the case if the mass has broken through the posterior capsule, where the risk of damage to the neurovascular structures with the arthroscopic technique is significant. In this situation, anterior arthroscopic synovectomy, combined with posterior open excision of the posterior fossa extension, could be considered.

Results

Patients with the localized nodular form of pigmented villonodular synovitis should do very well with localized excision and localized synovectomy (15–18). There seems to be little chance of recurrence if this procedure is carried out effectively.

Patients with the diffuse form of pigmented villonodular synovitis do have a significant recurrence rate (19–21). In our series, the recurrence rate was 10%, but in some series, it is substantially higher. The keys to a lower recurrence rate are early establishment of the diagnosis and as complete a synovectomy as possible. Careful follow-up is necessary in view of the recurrence rate, with serial physical examinations and magnetic resonance scan evaluation. Recurrence should be treated early and effectively, to avoid joint destruction (22).

NONSPECIFIC SYNOVITIS

Indications

Patients who have monoarthropathy with no established cause for it are considered to have nonspecific synovitis. Initially, arthroscopy and biopsy are performed. The biopsy is examined for pathologic and histologic features as well as sent for cultures for infective organisms. If the pathology laboratory establishes that the condition is a nonspecific synovitis, then synovectomy will be indicated if medical management has failed.

Special Considerations

It is important to rule out other intraarticular disorders of a mechanical nature as causes of the synovitis.

Results

In our series, about two-thirds of patients had adequate control of the synovitis. Approximately half the patients had relief of their pain. Function was improved in approximately three-fourths of the patients with this diagnosis. These patients require ongoing follow-up and observation to determine whether they develop any of the more classic causes of arthritis at a later date.

POSTTRAUMATIC SYNOVITIS

Indications

By definition, these patients have persistent synovitis of the knee after trauma when significant intraarticular factors have been ruled out by appropriate investigations or diagnostic arthroscopy (23). When the swelling has been present for 6 months despite adequate control, synovectomy can be attempted.

Special Considerations

In many cases, psychological and emotional factors affect the patient's outcome.

Result

In our series, the main indication for the synovectomy was pain. Only approximately one-third of our patients benefited with substantial pain relief. We were able to eliminate the synovial reaction in two-thirds of the patients, as shown by the absence of synovitis or effusion postoperatively, but the pain persisted. Caution is therefore necessary in dealing with this group of patients.

HOFFA'S DISEASE: INFRAPATELLAR FAT PAD

Indications

In 1904, Hoffa first described this syndrome of impingement of the infrapatellar fat pad. In his original article, excision of the fat pad relieved the patient's symptoms (24).

Patients with this condition have a positive Hoffa sign. This test consists of applying pressure to the medial side of the fat pad with the knee flexed. On extension, the patient experiences pain, and the fat pad is trapped underneath the patellar tendon.

Before accepting this diagnosis, it is very important to rule out other significant disease. Other synovial diseases, such as rheumatoid arthritis and pigmented villonodular synovitis, also cause anterior knee pain and fat pad hypertrophy. A thorough history, physical examination, laboratory tests, radiographs, magnetic resonance scans, and bone scans may be necessary to rule out other significant disorders.

Special Considerations

At arthroscopy, it is important to rule out other significant causes of disease. For example, if the patient has significant chondromalacia of the patella, or meniscal or chondral disease, the diagnosis of Hoffa's syndrome really should not be entertained. Hypertrophy of the fat pad may be secondary to other joint inflammation.

If the fat shows significant signs of inflammation with fibrosis and extension up under the patella into the patellofemoral joint, or with villous change, resection should be performed. In this case, only an anterior portion of the synovectomy is carried out, with focus on the fat pad alone. Care must be taken not to violate the patellar tendon itself.

Results

In patients without any other chronic inflammatory synovial disease, results are good. In our series, nine of 11 patients had excellent results, one had a fair result, and one had a poor result. The patients with fair and poor results turned out to have significant other synovial diseases that became apparent later.

BAKER'S CYST

Indications

During routine knee arthroscopy of the posterior compartments, many patients are found to have a patent foramen into Baker's cyst or a semimembranous bursa (25). Generally, the bursa is only directly instrumented when it is associated with other significant intraarticular disease such as pigmented villonodular synovitis, synovial chondromatosis, or rheumatoid arthritis. The bursa is often inflamed and distended when there is other intraarticular disease such as a torn meniscus or osteoarthritis. In this situation, I regard the bursal inflammation as being secondary to the intraarticular disease (26). When the intraarticular disease is dealt with, the bursa either spontaneously heals or causes minimal symptoms (27).

Special Considerations

The bursa can be accessed by visualizing the posteromedial compartment, by using either an ipsilateral or contralateral approach. In the case of a significant synovial pathologic process, a posteromedial portal is established, and a shaver is introduced into the bursa. Great care must be taken not to violate the walls of the bursa because the neurovascular structures are in proximity.

Where Baker's cyst is associated with other significant articular disease, this is dealt with in the usual manner. This may involve such activities as excision of the meniscus or removal of chondral debris from the femoral condyles.

In the unusual situation of Baker's cyst without significant intraarticular disease, the opening of the cyst can be enlarged. The lining of the cyst is excised arthroscopically, and the mouth of the cyst is made as wide as possible without violating the capsule of the joint. In this way, free communication of fluid is allowed between the cyst and the knee joint itself and eliminates the buildup of pressure in this cyst resulting from the one-way valve system.

Results

The results depend on the pathologic features. If the pathologic process has been adequately dealt with, then the cyst will usually disappear or will cause minimal symptoms.

MISCELLANEOUS CONDITIONS OF THE SYNOVIUM

Some synovial conditions are rare. These conditions may be seen and treated under the guidelines outlined earlier. It is important to establish a pathologic diagnosis. Some of these entities are synovial hemangioma (28,29), hemophilic synovitis (30,31), or tumors (32).

PLICA SYNDROME

Plicae are normal synovial structures of the knee joint (33). They are remnants of the mesenchymal tissue that occupies the space between the distal femoral and proximal tibial epiphyses in the 8-week-old embryo. Incomplete resorption leaves synovial plicae in most knees. The superior and inferior plicae are the most common (50% to 65%), but they have extremely little clinical relevance. The lateral plica is rare (1% to 3%). The medial plica is found in 75% of knees. It can be markedly thickened in about 5% of cases (34). Arthrography, ultrasonography, computed tomography scan with arthrography, and magnetic resonance imaging can demonstrate the presence of plicae and can measure their size with good accuracy (35). Arthroscopy allows a very precise assessment of the plica, including dynamic examination. I look for medial impingement against the patellofemoral articular surfaces and local articular cartilage softening (chondromalacia) or damage. In 5% or so of cases, the medial plica becomes symptomatic. Circumstances such as a history of blunt trauma or, more often, overuse of the knee can cause symptoms. The plica causes symptoms such as pain, crepitus, snapping or popping, or effusion related to flexion of the knee joint. The clinical picture may mimic a torn medial meniscus or a maltracking patella. Clinical examination is extremely helpful when the snapping plica is palpated at the medial edge of the patella and reproduces the patient's symptoms. If the condition is chronic, these symptoms may be treated with nonsteroidal antiinflammatory drugs, physical therapy, electrophoresis, or local injection. Surgical treatment is indicated if conservative therapy fails. Arthroscopic complete resection of the plica usually cures the symptoms (36). Care should be taken not to resect the joint capsule aggressively or the patient may develop painful intraarticular scarring at this point. Histologic examination often confirms the chronic inflammatory response in the plica and damage to the femoral condyle.

PREPATELLAR BURSA: HOUSEMAID'S KNEE

Indications

Patients who have a persistent prepatellar bursa despite adequate conservative treatment are candidates for excision (37). This can be carried out very effectively arthroscopically. The patient should have had repeated aspirations and injections of cortisone. The patient should also be free of infection (38).

Special Considerations

The prepatellar bursa is entered 1 cm distal to its distal edge. The arthroscope is therefore introduced from below or distally. The arthroscope is initially introduced subcutaneously. It is then introduced into the bursa itself. If the bursa is not fully distended, it can be distended with a syringe and needle before the arthroscope is inserted, to improve access.

Once the arthroscope has been introduced into the bursa, inflation with low pressure is used. A curved 4.5-mm synovial resector is introduced, again from below the inferior edge of the bursa, to make a small subcutaneous tunnel of cm.

The bursa is then completely resected from inside outward. On the deep surface, one should see the shiny fibers of the patella. On the superficial surface, one should see the subcutaneous fat. Care must be taken not to penetrate the skin.

Postoperatively, a small-bore drain is placed into the space created for a short time. The knee is placed in extension with a pressure dressing.

Results

My results with resection of the prepatellar bursa have been excellent. More than 90% of patients have good long-term results. Some patients have residual hypersensitivity, with difficulty kneeling on the kneecap, particularly if they have a job such as a tile setter, which has this requirement. It is important to ensure the patient does not have other inflammatory conditions such as rheumatoid arthritis or the bursa and inflammation can return. Generally, this is a highly effective procedure with minimal morbidity.

COMPLICATIONS OF ARTHROSCOPIC SYNOVECTOMY

The complications of synovectomy are similar to those of arthroscopy in general. They can consist of minor irritation around the portals or more major complications such as joint infection, reflex sympathetic dystrophy, or persistent stiffness and pain.

Specific complications are associated with the posterior portals. Great care must be taken not to damage the neurovascular structures of the posterior aspect of the knee. In a clinical study that was conducted of 179 consecutive cases, we had five complications, all resulting from the posteromedial portal. Three patients had residual numbness down the medial aspect of the calf but not into the foot. The numbness took 6 months to 1 year to resolve, and only one case persisted. There were also cases of small neuromas at the posteromedial portal site. Care should be taken here especially to flex the knee to 90 degrees and to use subcutaneous dissection. Two patients had damage to the saphenous vein that was noted when the tourniquet was released. In each case, the vein was isolated and tied.

In our series of synovectomies, we noted reflex sympathetic dystrophy, which needs to be diagnosed early and treated aggressively. If the patient has persistent knee stiffness with a lack of 90 degrees of knee flexion at more than 6 weeks postoperatively, I consider manipulation with the patient under anesthesia or further arthroscopy with release of adhesions. In these cases, it is usually the suprapatellar pouch that becomes full of adhesions and can be released arthroscopically. After this type of procedure, the patient is given epidural morphine for analgesia and is placed on a continuous passive movement machine to regain flexibility.

There is a recurrent rate of synovitis after arthroscopic synovectomy. Although not really a complication, this should certainly be discussed with the patient preoperatively. Careful consideration needs to be given to the cause of the recurrence. For example, if the reason is inadequate disease control on a systemic basis, this needs to be addressed. If the reason is occurrence of the local disorder, consideration has to be given to other forms of treatment, including, if necessary, repeat synovectomy.

REFERENCES

1. Ogilvie-Harris DJ, Basinski A. Arthroscopic synovectomy of the knee for rheumatoid arthritis. *Arthroscopy* 1991;7:91–97.
2. Klein W, Jensen KU. Arthroscopic synovectomy of the knee joint: Indication, technique and follow up results. *Arthroscopy* 1988;4:63–71.

3. Ogilvie-Harris DJ, Biggs DJ, MacKay M, et al. Posterior portals for arthroscopic surgery of the knee. *Arthroscopy* 1994;10;608–612.

4. Kim JM. Direct posterior-posterior triangulation of the knee joint. *Arthroscopy* 1997;13:262–264.

5. Tanaka N. Yamamura M. Ishii S. Anterior arthroscopic synovectomy plus capsuloplasty with a pedicle graft for the treatment of rheumatoid popliteal cysts. *J Rheumatol* 1999;26:1481–1485.

6. Ogilvie-Harris DJ, Basinski A. Arthroscopic synovectomy for rheumatoid arthritis: a prospective study. *Arthroscopy* 1991;7:91–97.

7. Klug S, Wittmann G, Weseloh G. Arthroscopic synovectomy of the knee joint in early cases of rheumatoid arthritis: follow-up results of a multicenter study. *Arthroscopy* 2000;16:262–267.

8. Ogilvie-Harris DJ, Weisleder L. Arthroscopic synovectomy of the knee: is it useful? *Arthroscopy* 1995;11:91–95.

9. Dirienzo G, Osti L, Merlo F. Our experience in the treatment of rheumatoid knee by arthroscopic synovectomy. *Chir Organi Mov* 1997;82:275–278.

10. Ayral X, Bonvarlet JP, Simonnet J, et al. Arthroscopy-assisted synovectomy in the treatment of chronic synovitis of the knee. *Rev Rhum Engl Ed* 1997;64:215–226.

11. Colican MR, Dandy DJ. Arthroscopic management of synovial chondromatosis of the knee. *J Bone Joint Surg Am* 1989;71;498–500.

12. Dorfman H, DeBie B, Bonvarlet JP, et al. Arthroscopic treatment of synovial chondromatosis of the knee. *Arthroscopy* 1989;5, 48–51.

13. Ogilvie-Harris DJ, Saleh K. Diffuse synovial chondromatosis: a comparison of removal of the loose bodies with arthroscopic synovectomy. *Arthroscopy* 1994;10:166–170.

14. Bravo SM, Pugh DG. Pigmented villonodular synovitis. *Radiol Clin North Am* 1996;34:311–321.

15. Ogilvie-Harris DJ, McLean J, Zarnett ME. Pigmented villonodular synovectomy of the knee. *J Bone Joint Surg Am* 1992;74:119–123.

16. Zvijac JE, Lau AC, Hechtman KS, et al. Arthroscopic treatment of pigmented villonodular synovitis of the knee. *Arthroscopy* 1999;15:613–617.

17. Perka C, Labs K, Zippel H, et al. Localized pigmented villonodular synovitis of the knee joint: neoplasm or reactive granuloma? A review of 18 cases. *Rheumatology* 2000;39:172–178.

18. Lee BI, Yoo JE, Lee SH, et al. Localized pigmented villonodular synovitis of the knee: arthroscopic treatment. *Arthroscopy* 1998;14:764–768.

19. Rochwerger A, Groulier P, Curvale G, et al. Pigmented villonodular synovitis of the knee. Treatment results in 22 cases. *Rev Chir Orthop Reparatrice Appar Mot* 1998;84:600–606.

20. de Visser E, Veth RP, Pruszczynski M, et al. Diffuse and localised pigmented villonodular synovitis: evaluation of treatment of 38 patients. *Arch Orthop Trauma Surg* 1999;119:401–404.

21. Rydholm U. Pigmented villonodular synovitis. *Acta Orthop Scand* 1998;69:203–210.

22. Flandry FC, Hughston JC, Jacobson KE, et al. Surgical treatment of diffuse pigmented villonodular synovitis of the knee. *Clin Orthop* 1994;300;183–192.

23. Comin JA, Rodriguez-Merchan EC. Arthroscopic synovectomy in the management of painful localized post-traumatic synovitis of the knee joint. *Arthroscopy* 1997;13:606–608.

24. Ogilvie-Harris DJ, Giddens J. Hoffa's syndrome: arthroscopic resection of the fat pad. *Arthroscopy* 1994;10:186–187.

25. Johnson LL, van Dyk GE, Johnson CA, et al. The popliteal bursa (Baker's cyst): an arthroscopic perspective and the epidemiology. *Arthroscopy* 1997;13:66–72.

26. Sansone V, De Ponti A. Arthroscopic treatment of popliteal cyst and associated intra-articular knee disorders in adults. *Arthroscopy* 1999;15:368–72.

27. Burger C, Monig SP, Prokop A, et al. Baker's cyst—current surgical status: overview and personal results. *Chirurg* 1998;69:1224–1229.

28. Farkas C, Morocz I, Szappanos L, et al. The importance of arthroscopy in diagnosing synovial haemangioma of the knee joint. *Acta Chir Hung* 1998;37:17–22.

29. Price NJ, Cundy PJ. Synovial hemangioma of the knee. *J Pediatr Orthop* 1997;17:74–77.

30. Rodriguez-Merchan EC, Magallon M, Galindo E, et al. Hemophilic synovitis of the knee and the elbow. *Clin Orthop* 1997;343:47–53.

31. Eickhoff HH, Koch W, Raderschadt G, et al. Arthroscopy for chronic hemophilic synovitis of the knee. *Clin Orthop* 1997;343:58–62.

32. Tandogan RN, Aydogan U, Demirhan B, et al. Intra-articular metastatic melanoma of the right knee. *Arthroscopy* 1999;15:98–102.

33. Dupont JY. Synovial plicae of the knee. Controversies and review. *Clin Sports Med* 1997;16:87–122.

34. Kim SJ, Choe WS. Arthroscopic findings of the synovial plicae of the knee. *Arthroscopy* 1997;13:33–41.

35. Jee WH, Choe BY, Kim JM, et al. The plica syndrome: diagnostic value of MRI with arthroscopic correlation. *J Comput Assist Tomogr* 1998;22:814–818.

36. Bae DK, Nam GU, Sun SD, et al. The clinical significance of the complete type of suprapatellar membrane. *Arthroscopy* 1998;14:830–835.

37. Ogilvie-Harris DJ, Gilbart M. Endoscopic bursal resection: the olecranon bursa and prepatellar bursa. *Arthroscopy* 2000;16:249–253.

38. Kaalund S, Breddam M, Kristensen G. Endoscopic resection of the septic prepatellar bursa. *Arthroscopy* 1998;14:757–758.

Operative Arthroscopy, third edition. Edited by John B. McGinty, Stephen S. Burkhart, Robert W. Jackson, Donald H. Johnson, and John C. Richmond.
Lippincott Williams & Wilkins © 2003.

ARTHROFIBROSIS

JOHN C. RICHMOND

Arthrofibrosis is a restriction of motion of a joint that can result from injury or surgery. It is a particularly bothersome complication when it involves the knee, because even small losses of knee extension are poorly tolerated. Although restrictions of knee motion have resulted from minor injuries or diagnostic arthroscopy, they are more common after major ligament or fracture reconstruction (1–9). In general, both the incidence and the severity of postoperative arthrofibrosis are correlated with the extent of the surgical procedure, any presurgical limitations of motion, and the duration of postoperative immobilization. In the treatment of acute anterior cruciate ligament (ACL) tears, an inverse correlation exists between the time from injury to surgery and the frequency of arthrofibrosis.

The classification of arthrofibrosis of the knee is based on the motions that are limited, the extent of these limitations, and any entrapment of the patella. The typical classification scheme (Table 22.1) has four categories, as follows:

1. Loss of extension
2. Loss of flexion
3. Loss of both flexion and extension
4. Infrapatella contracture syndrome (IPCS), which has limitation of both flexion and extension, with entrapment of the patella

IPCS, as first described by Paulos et al., results from an abnormal fibrosclerotic response in the infrapatella fat pad and peripatella tissues (2). Progressive shortening of the patella tendon typically results in patella infera (8,9). This often leads to the rapid onset (within 6 months) of patellofemoral arthrosis as the result of a bent knee gait (2,4,6).

Localized areas of scar tissue may lead to restrictions of motion, if these areas occur in inopportune locations, such as anterior in the intercondylar notch or between the quadriceps mechanism and the anterior femur (Fig. 22.1). This condition probably should not be termed arthrofibrosis because it is quite different from the diffuse scarring that occurs in arthrofibrosis. The diagnosis and treatment of these localized lesions are also covered in this chapter.

HISTORICAL PERSPECTIVES

Restriction of knee motion after injury or surgery has long been a problem. The advent of arthroscopic surgery, with a resultant decrease in joint trauma, has helped to decrease the frequency and severity of motion limitation that may result from surgical intervention. In the 1940s, Thompson described an extensive open quadricepsplasty for the problem of arthrofibrosis (10,11). Nicoll, in the 1960s, recognized four potential sites of disease that could contribute to the problem (12). These included (a) fibrosis of the vastus intermedius in and just proximal to the suprapatella pouch, (b) intraarticular adhesions between the patella and the femur, (c) fibrosis of the vastus lateralis with adhesion to the femoral condyle, and (d) shortening of the rectus femoris. His recommended treatment was open serial release of each of these areas, until full motion was restored. These were extensive, often heroic, associated with significant morbidity. Sprague et al. were the first to recognize the potential of the arthroscope in the evaluation and treatment of arthrofibrosis (1). Since then, innumerable authors have contributed to our understanding, evaluation, and treatment of this problem. Most important has been identification of strategies for prevention.

PREVENTION TECHNIQUES

Elimination of arthrofibrosis is not yet attainable, but we should focus our efforts on reducing the frequency and severity of this complication. Although each specific condition and procedure will have its own optimal scheme to minimize the risk of arthrofibrosis, important generalities should be reviewed. Several specific areas can readily be identified and addressed: optimal surgical timing, inflammatory conditions, mechanical blocks to motion, and tailored rehabilitation programs.

J. C. **Richmond:** Department of Orthopaedic Surgery, Tufts University School of Medicine; New England Medical Center, Boston, Massachusetts.

TABLE 22.1 TYPES OF ARTHROFIBROSIS BASED ON MOTION LIMITATION AND PATELLA MOBILITY

Type	Extension Loss	Flexion Loss	Patella Mobility
1	>5 degrees	None	Normal
2	None	>25 degrees	Limited inferior glide
3	>10 degrees	>25 degrees	Limited in all planes
4	>10 degrees	>30 degrees	Patella infera

TIMING OF TREATMENT

The majority of information concerning the timing of surgery and arthrofibrosis is based on the treatment of ACL injuries (1–9). This likely developed because of the high frequency of this injury and the recommendation by numerous authors in the 1980s that the optimal period for ACL reconstruction was within the first few weeks after injury. In 1991, Shelbourne et al. and Mohtadi et al. identified early ACL reconstruction as a significant risk factor for postoperative arthrofibrosis (13,14). If surgical treatment is delayed until nearly full motion has been recovered, quadriceps control allows full active extension, and acute hemarthrosis has resolved, then the risk of postsurgical arthrofibrosis necessitating arthroscopy or manipulation will be substantially reduced (15). Hunter et al. showed that it is possible to achieve good results with ACL reconstruction with in the first 3 weeks after injury, if an aggressive rehabilitation protocol is used (16). This approach, however, results in 6% of patients' requiring additional surgical procedures to regain motion.

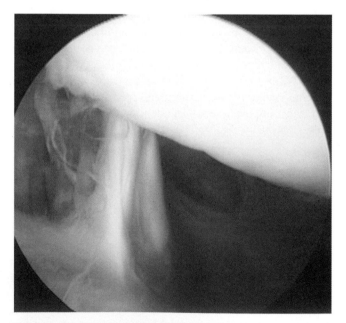

FIGURE 22.1 Isolated suprapatella adhesion, representing localized scarring, not arthrofibrosis.

Certain injuries, such as knee dislocations and intraarticular fractures, are best treated with early surgery. To delay surgical treatment in these cases, to improve motion, may significantly compromise long-term stability and function. In a series reported by Noyes and Barber-Westin, only 25% of patients who underwent late ACL and posterior cruciate ligament reconstruction after knee dislocation were able to return to sport activity without symptoms, whereas more than 70% of patients who had acute reconstructions were not limited in sport activity (17). Both the magnitude and the timing of the surgical treatment in these cases contribute to a potentially high rate of postoperative stiffness requiring manipulation or arthroscopy. Even with immediate protected mobilization after early surgical treatment of knee dislocations, the frequency of stiffness requiring mobilization was greater than 50% in two series (17,18).

MECHANICAL PROBLEMS

Mechanical causes include immobilization, malpositioned ligament grafts, and displaced tissues (19–22). ACL reconstruction remains the most frequent cause of arthrofibrosis in virtually all series reporting on the treatment of arthrofibrosis (1–9). Although biologically induced arthrofibrosis may occur after ACL reconstruction, particularly when the procedure is done early after injury, the condition more commonly occurs as a result of a mechanical issue (22–26). This is typically the result of suboptimal graft positioning or excessive tensioning of a nonanatomically positioned graft (Fig. 22.2). Common positioning errors include: (a) anterior placement of the femoral drill hole leading to a shortened intraarticular graft and (b) anterior placement of the tibial drill hole resulting in impingement on the roof of the notch. There is a definite interplay between the placement of ACL drill holes and the tensioning technique. Optimal tensioning technique is one that results in reproducibly stable knees, with full range of motion. Several authors have recommended techniques that rely on high tensioning forces applied with the knee in full extension and fixation with the knee at or near full extension (27,28). This approach ensures that the graft will not limit extension. Whichever tensioning technique is employed, it is critical that the knee comes to full extension intraoperatively, because anything less markedly increases the risk of extension

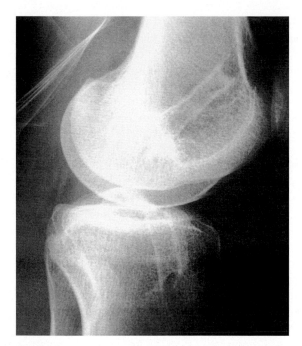

FIGURE 22.2 Lateral radiograph after anterior cruciate ligament reconstruction, demonstrating anterior placement of the femoral drill hole. This positioning often leads to motion limitation, as a result of shortened intraarticular graft length.

loss. Postoperative limitation of extension (either mechanical from technical error or by rehabilitation protocol) may result in the formation of a *cyclops lesion,* which is a proliferative nodule of fibrovascular scar that forms anterior to the ACL graft (29). This scar may be caused by organization of the hematoma anterior to the graft.

Immobilization has been eliminated from the postoperative rehabilitation protocols after ACL reconstruction, but it continues to be recommended after other surgical procedures. Immobilization after other surgical procedures also leads to an increased risk of arthrofibrosis when compared with early mobilization. This problem has been identified with numerous procedures including meniscal repair, patellar realignment, posterior cruciate ligament reconstruction, repair of tibial spine fractures, and multiligament reconstructions (17,18,21,30–32). Although immobilization for short periods may offer protection of various structures from excessive stress, one must be cognizant of the potential harm of immobilization when considering its use. The myriad deleterious effects of longer periods of immobilization include not only stiffness, but also loss of strength of ligaments and muscles, calcium loss from bone, and articular cartilage injury (33–35).

Continuous passive motion (CPM) has been recommended as a modality to reduce the risk of motion-limiting arthrofibrosis after surgery. The use of CPM after several different procedures has been studied. Although it has proven to be of significant value with some procedures, it is not universally beneficial. Total knee arthroplasty is the procedure in which CPM has demonstrated the most benefit; it

reduces the risk of arthrofibrosis requiring manipulation substantially (from 10% to 0% in one study) (36). The risk of arthrofibrosis after patella realignment is also reduced with the use of CPM (30). The risk of motion limitation after ACL reconstruction, however, has not been altered by the use of postoperative CPM (37–40).

Quadriceps weakness with a resulting extensor lag may also inadvertently result in a limitation of extension. There is a complex intermingling of this with the issues of timing of surgery after injury. Inability of the patient actively to extend the knee fully before the surgical procedure substantially increases the risk of extension loss postoperatively.

Hyaluronic acid films have proven of benefit in the reduction of intraabdominal adhesions after bowel surgery (41,42). Hyaluronic acid films or gels may, in the future, offer a mechanical means to reduce intraarticular adhesions by acting as a barrier to their formation after surgical procedures. In prior unpublished work, my colleagues and I used hyaluronic acid films in a rabbit knee model. There was a significant reduction in both the number and the density of adhesions when the film was used.

INFLAMMATORY CONDITIONS

Many authors have noted an inflammatory phase, as manifested by warmth and induration of the knee, in a large percentage of patients who develop significant arthrofibrosis (2,4–9). Pharmacologic methods for reducing inflammation postoperatively, although intuitively attractive, have not been studied as a potential means of limiting arthrofibrosis. Some data relating to antiinflammatory drugs are interesting and may be extrapolated to this issue. Routine perioperative use of nonsteroidal antiinflammatory drugs (NSAIDs) has resulted in a significant reduction in postoperative narcotic analgesic demands, as well as increased early motion (up to 3 weeks postoperatively) (43,44). This finding argues strongly for the routine postoperative use of NSAIDs in those patients with no known contraindications to the use of these agents. Oral corticosteroids have similarly reduced demand for postsurgical analgesics and have increased the rate of recovery from numerous arthroscopic procedures (45,46). Because most surgical procedures do carry a relatively low risk of arthrofibrosis, and several significant potential complications are related to the use of oral corticosteroids (e.g., osteonecrosis and gastrointestinal ulceration), the routine use of oral corticosteroids after knee surgery is not recommended. One can consider the use of oral corticosteroids after those procedures that may have an exceptionally high risk of postsurgical motion-limiting arthrofibrosis. A significantly increased risk of postoperative septic arthritis has been associated with the intraarticular use of corticosteroids at the time of surgery (47). Although intraarticular corticosteroids seem to be a means to reduce the risk of scar formation, this increased risk of sepsis precludes their routine use. An exception could be those procedures that carry a very high risk of motion-limiting arthrofibrosis.

Postoperative cryotherapy has the attraction of being a simple, inexpensive, and low-risk means to reduce postoperative inflammation, pain, and swelling. There have been several studies on the use of cryotherapy, and the results have been contradictory. Although its use may reduce swelling and pain in the immediate postoperative period, no evidence indicates a long-term reduction in the rates of arthrofibrosis (48–51).

Investigators have noted an increased risk of arthrofibrosis after ACL and medial collateral ligament (MCL) injury treated with early ACL reconstruction and MCL repair, when the MCL tear is proximal (52). Although this may be a purely mechanical issue, it may result from a localized inflammatory condition, because this is the typical location of the metaplastic formation of bone in the MCL in Pellegrini-Stieda syndrome.

REHABILITATION

As noted earlier, a major factor in reducing the risk of motion loss after injury or surgery is the rehabilitation protocol. This really begins preoperatively in many cases, because regaining full motion after injury and before surgical treatment diminishes the risk of motion problems postoperatively. If possible, full passive extension should be encouraged in the immediate postoperative period. This prevents the accumulation of a hematoma in the notch, which may lead to an extension-limiting cyclops lesion. This also reduces the tendency for the fat pad to scar to the notch (13–16).

Early recognition by the treating orthopaedic surgeon or physical therapist of patients who are not regaining flexibility at the expected rate after injury or surgical treatment is key to reducing the long-term morbidity of the condition. Greater than anticipated pain is often a precursor of motion issues and should alert the practitioner to this issue. The appropriate steps after identification of the problem are covered later in this chapter, in the discussion of treatment.

PATHOLOGY

Several common causes of arthrofibrosis have been identified. The most common causes are mechanical, including inappropriately positioned or tensioned ligament grafts, prolonged immobilization, and displaced tissues such as fracture fragments or meniscal tears (1–7,23–26). Periarticular inflammatory processes, including infection or inflammatory arthropathies, may lead to arthrofibrosis. Exciting work in the basic biology of normal scar formation and in the abnormal processes of arthrofibrosis has identified abnormal growth factor expression and inappropriate immune response as pathways that may define the common cause and new potential preventions and treatments for arthrofibrosis.

Normal healing includes a series of successive and interrelated processes that lead to the formation of a scar. These processes begin with the migration and proliferation of primitive and inflammatory cells. Neovascularization, extracellular matrix deposition, and stromal cell proliferation follow (53–56). Numerous different growth factors, which are produced locally by cells that migrate to the area of injury, regulate this process. The best-known of these growth factors include platelet-derived growth factors (PDGF-α and PDGF-β), transforming growth factors (TGF-α and TGF-β), and insulin-like growth factors (ILGF-I and ILGF-II). At the time of injury and active tissue repair, the expression of these growth factors is highest. Their expression normally declines as healing progresses and is absent in mature scar (54,57,58). TGF-β is the most thoroughly studied and has been implicated in numerous fibrotic conditions in other organs, including liver, kidney, and lung. Abnormal expression of some of these growth factors has been identified in several of the fibroproliferative disorders of the musculoskeletal system, such as fibrous dysplasia, palmar fibromatosis (Dupuytren's disease), aggressive fibromatosis, and arthrofibrosis (59–63). Adhesive capsulitis of the shoulder has shown a marked similarity to these conditions on immunohistochemistry (64). Failure of normal regulatory mechanisms for the various growth factors may contribute to these conditions. Preliminary *in vitro* studies have demonstrated that blocking of PDGF-α, TGF-β, and ILGF-I inhibits the proliferation in cell culture of the fibroblasts derived from arthrofibrosis of the knee (59,60).

Abnormal reaction to stretching has been noted in the clinical treatment of arthrofibrosis, with signs of increased local inflammation and reduced motion reported when aggressive manipulative stretching has been employed in the early phases of IPCS (2,6). Laboratory support for this finding comes from the comparison of Dupuytren's fibroblasts with normal fibroblasts under cyclic loading in tissue culture (65). With cyclic repetitive strain, there is a significant increase in the proliferation of these abnormal fibroblasts when compared with normal fibroblasts. This proliferation appears to be mediated by growth factors. Aggressive stretching of joints in the inflammatory phase of arthrofibrosis may accentuate the problem.

The common finding in arthrofibrosis is dense intraarticular and periarticular scar. This scar may obliterate the suprapatella pouch and intercondylar notch. Adhesions to the articular surface are common. Histologically, this tissue is dense fibrovascular tissue, which may demonstrate areas of chondroid or osteoid metaplasia (1–8).

CLINICAL EVALUATION

Any patient who fails to gain knee motion at the expected rate after injury or surgical treatment may be developing arthrofibrosis. Mechanical blocks to motion need to be identified early in the treatment of the motion-limited knee. After acute injury, failure to gain expected range of motion may result from a displaced bucket-handle meniscal tear (21). Magnetic resonance imaging should be used to identify potential soft tissue blocks to motion. Displaced articular fracture fragments are best assessed with plain radiographs or computed tomography scanning.

Malpositioned ACL grafts are still one of the most common causes of postoperative stiffness. Often routine radiographs are adequate to identify the misplaced bone tunnels (Fig. 22.2), although magnetic resonance imaging is occasionally helpful to visualize the graft impinging on the notch (Fig. 22.3). Identifying and treating a mechanical block motion can prevent the more serious consequences that can develop. The identification of a malpositioned ACL drill hole can be a difficult issue to confront, because the best treatment depends on early elimination of the mechanical block to motion. This may necessitate early surgical treatment, either to expand the notch when anterior placement of the tibial drill hole leads to impingement of the graft on the roof of the notch or to remove a graft that is too anterior on the femur. Delaying surgical correction by even a few months may be ill advised, because even a few months of a bent knee gait can result in significant patellofemoral arthrosis (4,6,8). It is better to remove a misplaced ACL graft early, to regain full motion, and then perform a revision ACL reconstruction in the correct location than it is to continue with a program of physical therapy and serial casting if this is destined to fail because of a technical error.

Pain is often a prominent component of arthrofibrosis. Complex regional pain syndromes should be included in differential diagnosis, and they can be difficult to differentiate from arthrofibrosis. Stiffness, with associated warmth and swelling, is typically the most prominent symptom of a developing arthrofibrosis. These symptoms should also alert the clinician to consider sympathetically mediated pain syndromes and to take the necessary steps, such as lumbar sympathetic blockade, to rule them out, when appropriate.

Although numerous patterns of arthrofibrosis have been identified, a simple scheme with four classes, based on motion limitation and patella mobility, is adequate for treatment planning (Table 22.1) (1–3,6,8,9,24,29,66,67). Based on this schema, we have developed a straightforward treatment algorithm for the management of arthrofibrosis (Fig. 22.4). Limitation of patella mobility, especially superior glide, can often be elicited in IPCS. Although this may occur secondary to a timing, mechanical, or rehabilitative issue, this is often the beginning of primary arthrofibrosis, which can be particularly bothersome to treat. Not infrequently, patients who develop IPCS are keloid formers. We have anecdotally noted this phenomenon to be more common in fair-skinned redheads.

TREATMENT

Using the classification scheme and treatment algorithm presented earlier will facilitate the management of arthrofibrosis. Early recognition of the peripatella inflammation that portends the development of IPCS allows prompt treatment. I believe that a short course of high-dose oral corticosteroids offers a good chance to treat this early inflammatory phase successfully and to reduce or prevent the major problems associated with a full-blown IPCS (6). Oral NSAIDs may also be of value, but my experience suggests that corticosteroids work better. Aggressive stretching in this early inflammatory phase seems to exacerbate the inflammation in many patients, and it is usually counterproductive. Perhaps the reason is the paradoxic increase in scar formation that can occur when abnormal fibroblasts are stretched, as noted earlier in the discussion of pathology (29). The best rehabilitation program at this juncture is gentle, nonforceful mobilization performed actively by the patient. This seems to allow some patients' conditions at least to stabilize, if not improve, early in the course of IPCS.

The treatment of arthrofibrosis depends both on the type and the time elapsed from the inciting event. Treatment of each type is discussed individually. In general, application of the treatment algorithm shown in Fig. 22.4 has simplified our decision-making process in these complex cases.

In type 1 arthrofibrosis, the involved knee lacks the full extension (including physiologic recurvatum) equal to the contralateral knee. This often results from the early lack of extension and resulting scar formation anterior in the notch or between the fat pad and the notch (24–29) (Fig. 22.5) Although this condition is most frequent after ACL surgery, it

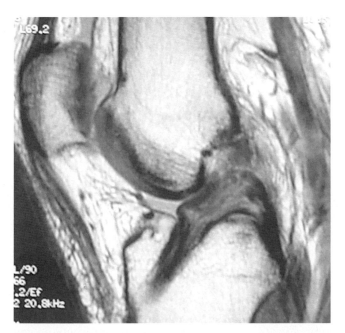

FIGURE 22.3 Magnetic resonance imaging scan demonstrating impingement of the anterior notch on the anterior cruciate ligament graft in extension.

Arthrofibrosis: Algorithm for Management

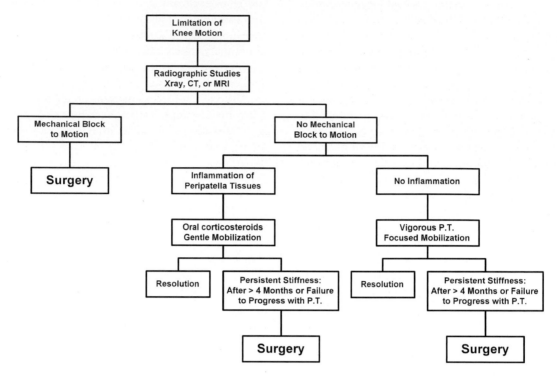

FIGURE 22.4 Algorithm for management of arthrofibrosis.

is not limited to ACL reconstructions. Imaging studies, as noted in the discussion of mechanical problems, should be performed to identify any mechanical cause that must be addressed surgically. When the condition is identified in the first several months after the index injury or surgery, mechanical stretching techniques are often of benefit. Among

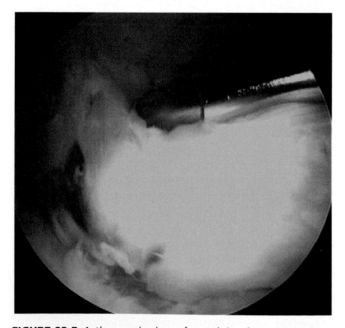

FIGURE 22.5 Arthroscopic view of a nodule of scar located anterior in the notch (cyclops lesion) after anterior cruciate ligament reconstruction.

the techniques that have been employed are dynamic extension braces, dropout casts, extension boards, and serial extension casts. My preference is the extension board because of it simplicity and ease of use. Serial extension casts are associated with a risk of articular cartilage injury and must be employed cautiously. Cartilage damage may occur both from immobilization and from the pressure on the joint surface from forced extension. If employed, serial extension casts should be changed at least every 48 hours, to minimize this risk. The longer the time elapsed from the index surgery or injury, the less likely these mechanical modalities are to be effective. My own experience is that after 4 months, the scar tissue that is limiting motion has matured to the point at which surgical removal is necessary. Although other authors have used manipulation with the patient under anesthesia as a technique, I favor arthroscopic debridement in any patient ho is more than 4 months from the index event (68). This is because adhesions to articular cartilage may be strong enough to avulse the joint surface cartilage after this point (33,34). In those cases that follow total knee arthroplasty, this is obviously not an issue.

Because flexion deformities of as little as 5 to 8 degrees often result in a limp or anterior knee pain, these may require surgical treatment. With flexion contractures of 10 degrees or more, most patients are symptomatic. Surgery is indicated for those patients who have pain or who limp and for those who have more than a 10-degree loss of extension. Most patients can be treated arthroscopically or with the combination of arthroscopic and limited open technique.

There is usually scarring anterior in the notch or between the infrapatella fat pad and the notch or proximal tibia. When a nodule of scar forms anterior to the graft after ACL reconstruction, this variant is termed *cyclops syndrome* (29) (Fig. 22.5). This nodule may cause mechanical symptoms. It has also been described after total knee arthroplasty (69). Complete resection of the nodule, as well as any of additional notch scarring, is necessary. If impingement on an ACL graft is found, then the notchplasty must be expanded. Any scarring in the fat pad should be removed. Rarely is the suprapatella pouch involved in type 1 arthrofibrosis. Any scarring identified in the pouch should be resected, because this may limit the proximal excursion of the quadriceps muscle and active extension postoperatively. If full extension is still limited after all intraarticular scar has been removed, then attention should be focused on the extrasynovial region between the patella tendon and the tibia. Scar can be resected from here either arthroscopically or through a small incision (6,24). Failure to do this may result in persistent lack of extension postoperatively, and it has been shown in cadaver experiments possibly to result in patella infera (70).

Immediate postoperative extension splinting or use of an extension board is recommended. Typically, regaining flexion does not present a problem, unless extension splinting is employed for a protracted period. CPM use is typically not required, and it may even be counterproductive, because full knee hyperextension is often not reached in CPM. Pain management, although less of an issue than after surgery in higher grades of arthrofibrosis, is important. Femoral nerve blocks, single or repetitive, can be important adjuncts in pain management.

In type 2 arthrofibrosis, only flexion is limited. This typically results from immobilization in extension and the associated suprapatella scarring. This can also be the result of extraarticular adhesions between the quadriceps and the femur. In type 2, the patella is only limited in inferior excursion and is not entrapped by scar. Early on, in the first few months after the index injury or surgery, physical therapy remains the mainstay of treatment. Aggressive manipulative physical therapy should be avoided, particularly as the interval from injury or surgery approaches 4 months and there is a risk of avulsion of articular cartilage by a mature adhesion to the joint surface (33,34). Early manipulation while the patient is under anesthesia has been used successfully, but it may not be necessary. My preference is to delay correction until the 4-month anniversary, unless there is a clear lack of progress after 4 to 6 weeks of supervised physical therapy, and then to perform arthroscopic lysis of adhesions followed by manipulation. The intraoperative findings usually include suprapatella pouch that contains multiple adhesions. Less often, the pouch has been obliterated with scar (Fig. 22.6A).

In the surgical treatment of this isolated lack of flexion, all visible scar should be removed, and meticulous hemostasis should be obtained (1,3,4). Traditionally, the motorized shaver is the instrument of choice, but newer radiofrequency devices offer the ease of resection and cauterization simultaneously. The dissection should be carried up under the distal quadriceps muscle to free it from the femoral shaft, to restore the normal volume to the suprapatella pouch (Fig. 22.6B). A blunt obturator or a 1/4-inch curved osteotome can be employed for this purpose (4). The entire procedure can often be done without the use of a tourniquet, and this improves both hemostasis and postoperative quadriceps

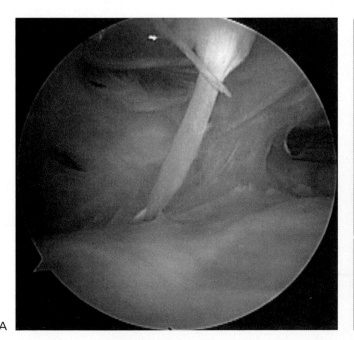
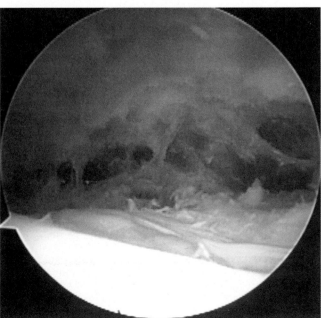

A
B

FIGURE 22.6 A: Marked obliteration of the suprapatella pouch by scar. **B:** Restoration of the suprapatella pouch by resection of the thick adhesive bands.

function. If a tourniquet is required, it should be deflated before manipulation to allow free quadriceps excursion.

Postoperative drainage of the joint and CPM are of benefit after arthrolysis in patients with type 2 arthrofibrosis (4,6). Although the drains can easily be placed into the gutters from a suprapatella portal, old incision sites should be avoided, because this may lead to delayed healing, persistent drainage, and an increased risk of infection. The maximum tolerated range of motion for the CPM should be selected both for flexion and extension in the immediate postoperative period. The drains may be removed early if the volume of drainage is limited (more than 75 mL/8 hours) or maintained for up to 48 hours if needed. Postoperative pain management is often an issue after arthrolysis in patients with any type of arthrofibrosis. The use of femoral nerve blocks or indwelling epidural catheters can be of marked benefit in the perioperative period.

Patella entrapment syndromes encompass types 3 and 4 arthrofibrosis and extend to IPCS (2,4,6,8,9,24). Surgical treatment is almost always required, but it should be delayed until complete resolution of the inflammatory stage. As previously noted, a short course of high-dose oral corticosteroids may be of significant benefit. Aggressive stretching and manipulation while the patient is under anesthesia are contraindicated, particularly when there is warmth and inflammation in the fat pad or peripatella region (6). IPCS can be recognized by the development of patella infera, in association with entrapment of the patella. Wide variability exists in the ratio of patella tendon length to patella length (range 0.75 to 1.46) among patients, but almost no variation between sides in the same patient. Flexed-knee lateral radiographs to compare involved with uninvolved patella tendon length are indicated to identify patella infera (8). More than 8 mm of shortening of the patella tendon will require specific attention to this tendon during surgical treatment. This is best accomplished with a DeLee-type tibial tubercle osteotomy (Fig. 22.7), which not only restores the patella toward its normal vertical position but also helps to decrease patellofemoral contact pressures by bringing the insertion of the patella tendon more anteriorly (71,72).

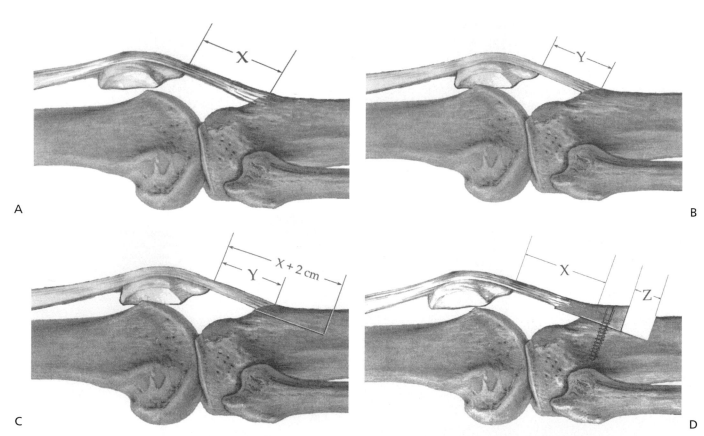

FIGURE 22.7 DeLee osteotomy designed to restore the patella to its normal location when there has been significant loss of length of the patella tendon. Measurements should be made from lateral radiographs of both knees at the same degree of flexion, to ensure that the patella tendons are taut. **A:** The length of the normal patella tendon (X) is measured from the noninvolved knee. **B:** The length of the shortened tendon (Y) on the involved knee. **C:** X + 2 cm is the overall length of the shortened tendon plus the osteotomy. **D:** Once the osteotomy is completed, the bone block is slid proximally the distance Z, where Z = X − Y. Fixation is with one or two screws, and the defect Z should be grafted. (From Malik MM, ed. *Knee surgery: complications, pitfalls, and salvage.* New York: Springer, 2001, with permission.)

Open, arthroscopic, and combined procedures have been employed and reported on in the treatment of types 3 and 4 arthrofibrosis (1–9,24). Results have been similar, and the selection depends on the comfort and skill of the individual surgeon. All intraarticular adhesions must be released. Lateral and medial retinacular releases are necessary, as is removal of all scar, often including the fat pad, that tethers the patella to the tibia. The bursa deep to the distal patella tendon must be completely freed. Notch impingement must be corrected. If a malpositioned ligament graft is identified, this must be removed, motion must be regained, and late reconstruction should be considered if instability develops. In our own series, this was usually not necessary, because more than 50% of patients who had an ACL graft resected remained clinically stable through more than 2 years of follow-up (4). This is in part the result of reduced activity levels, because most patients who develop true patella entrapment have long-term patellofemoral symptoms related to articular surface damage. Extraarticular bands from the patella to the femur have been described, but direct exposure of these bands may not be necessary, because the lateral and medial releases are usually adequate to lyse them.

Although the DeLee tibial tubercle slide osteotomy can be used to restore the patella to a near-normal location, patella femoral symptoms often remain a long-term issue, as the result of significant patella chondromalacia (Fig. 22.8) and the shortened patella tendon. In some patients who have been treated with only soft tissue releases, progressive shortening of the patella tendon in time has been reported, a finding suggesting an ongoing fibrotic process (9).

In the immediate postoperative period, intraarticular drains are important to reduce the potential for hemarthrosis. Early motion, including CPM, cryotherapy, and regional pain management techniques, such as femoral nerve block or an indwelling epidural catheter, should all be employed. Daily physical therapy for patella mobilization, joint motion, and recruitment of the quadriceps is indicated, often for the first few weeks (24). There is often a biphasic improvement in joint motion, with immediate postoperative motion decreasing over the next 7 to 10 days in the early inflammatory phase of healing. As the warmth and inflammation fade, motion can again regained. Oral corticosteroids, in a high-dose tapered course over 3 to 4 weeks, can be of significant benefit for patients with significant postrelease inflammation (6).

Because of the significant cortical defect created just distal to the tibial tubercle by the DeLee osteotomy, even when grafted, these patients require long-term protection with crutches and a hinged brace, often up to 12 weeks postoperatively. This area is also prone to stress reactions or stress fractures if the patient returns to running, even after complete healing.

RESULTS

The arthroscopic treatment of types 1 or 2 arthrofibrosis has proven effective in most cases. Normal or near-normal motion and function can be anticipated and maintained for the long term. When patella entrapment or IPCS is encountered, the long-term results are less satisfactory (1–9,24,29). In large part, this can be attributed to damage to the articular surfaces of the patellofemoral joint. Observations of progressive shortening of the patella tendon after treatment point to either an ongoing inflammatory process or persistent abnormal growth factor expression. Substantial motion gains in both flexion (approximately 30 degrees) and extension (approximately 15 degrees) can be achieved in those patients with patella entrapment but no patella infera. Functional recovery and return to athletics are determined, in large part, by the status of the patellofemoral articular surfaces. Whereas motion gains in those patients with IPCS are nearly as good as in patients with just patella entrapment, their function typically remains limited by articular surface damage and the long-term abnormal patellofemoral mechanics related to the shortened patella tendon. Late loss of patella tendon length with return to a mechanically suboptimal patella location is a concern.

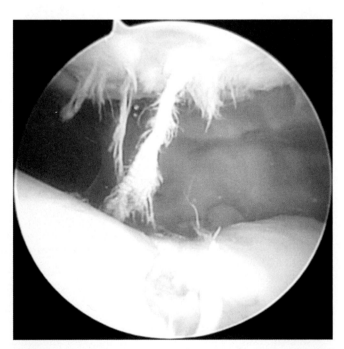

FIGURE 22.8 Significant chondromalacia of the patella and femoral trochlea groove resulting from arthrofibrosis with patella baja.

SUMMARY

Reducing the incidence and severity of arthrofibrosis through careful preoperative rehabilitation before ACL reconstruction, and progression to early full motion after surgery, have been major advances over the past decade. Extrapolation of these principles to other injuries and surgeries has also contributed to a decline in problems associated with limitations of motion. Physicians and therapists involved in treatment of the knee must be aware of the devastating long-term problems that can result from patella entrapment syndromes. Early recognition of developing motion issues should promote more rapid treatment and improved results.

When motion problems are identified, the type of arthrofibrosis should be categorized, and treatment should be instituted. If the patient's condition is in an inflammatory stage, mobilization should be gentle. Oral corticosteroids should be considered important adjuncts that can reduce inflammation before more aggressive manipulative or surgical therapy. Early (typically in the first 4 months) after the inciting injury or surgical procedure, nonoperative treatment is indicated. Surgical intervention should not be delayed, however, when there is failure to progress or a mechanical block to motion. Any surgical treatment, whether it be open, arthroscopic, or a combination, need be based on the following principles: (a) complete removal of all intraarticular scar; (b) release of any extraarticular adhesions; (c) elimination of any mechanical block to motion, including malpositioned grafts; and (d) restoration of patella mobility and position. Failure to achieve any of these will result in persistent limitations of motion and the potential for further articular cartilage injury. After surgical treatment of arthrofibrosis, rehabilitation protocols should stress early motion (particularly full passive extension, if it was limited preoperatively), rapid return of quadriceps function and excursion, and patella mobilization. CPM can be an important adjunct, if flexion was limited preoperatively. In the future, the use of hyaluronic acid films or gels or manipulation of the various growth factors may reduce the incidence of arthrofibrosis in high-risk situations.

REFERENCES

1. Sprague NJ III, O'Connor RL, Fox JM. Arthroscopic treatment of postoperative knee fibroarthritis. *Clin Orthop* 1982;166: 165–172.
2. Paulos LE, Rosenberg TD, Drawbert J, et al. Infrapatellar contracture syndrome: an unrecognized cause of knee stiffness with patella entrapment and patella infera. *Am J Sports Med* 1987; 15:331–341.
3. Parisien JS. The role of arthroscopy in the treatment of postoperative fibroarthrosis of the knee joint. *Clin Orthop* 1988;229: 185–192.
4. Richmond JC, Assal MA. Arthroscopic management of arthrofibrosis of the knee, including infrapatellar contraction syndrome. *Arthroscopy* 1991;7:144–147.
5. Cosgarea AJ, DeHaven KE, Lovelock JE. The surgical treatment of arthrofibrosis of the knee. *Am J Sports Med* 1994;22:184–191.
6. Paulos LE, Wnorowski DC, Greenwald AE. Infrapatellar contracture syndrome diagnosis, treatment, and long-term follow-up. *Am J Sports Med* 1994;22:440–449.
7. Klein W, Shah N, Gasse A. Arthroscopic management of postoperative arthrofibrosis of the knee joint: indication, technique, and results. *Arthroscopy* 1994;10:591–597.
8. Noyes FR, Wojtys EM, Marshall MT. The early diagnosis and treatment of developmental patella infera syndrome. *Clin Orthop* 1991;265:241–252.
9. Millett PJ, Riley RJ 3rd, Wickiewicz TL. Open debridement and soft tissue release as a salvage procedure for the severely arthrofibrotic knee. *Am J Sports Med* 1999;27:552–562.
10. Thompson TC. Quadricepsplasty to improve knee function. *J Bone Joint Surg* 1944;25:366–379.
11. Hesketh KT. Experiences with the Thompson quadricepsplasty. *J Bone Joint Surg Br* 1963;45:491–495.
12. Nicoll EA. Quadricepsplasty. *J Bone Joint Surg Br* 1963;45:483–490.
13. Shelbourne KD, Wilckens JH, Mollabashy A, et al. Arthrofibrosis in acute anterior cruciate ligament reconstruction: the effect of timing of reconstruction and rehabilitation. *Am J Sports Med* 1991;19:332–336.
14. Mohtadi NGH, Webster-Bogaert S, Fowler PJ. Limitation of motion following anterior cruciate ligament reconstruction: a case-control study. *Am J Sports Med* 1991;19:620–625.
15. Shelbourne KD, Foulk DA. Timing of surgery in acute anterior cruciate ligament tears on the return of quadriceps muscle strength after reconstruction using an autogenous patellar tendon graft. *Am J Sports Med* 1995;23:686–689.
16. Hunter RE, Mastrangelo J, Freeman JR, et al. The impact of surgical timing on postoperative motion and stability following anterior cruciate ligament reconstruction. *Arthroscopy* 1996;12: 667–674.
17. Noyes FR, Barber-Westin SD. Reconstruction of the anterior and posterior cruciate ligaments after knee dislocation. *Am J Sports Med* 1997;25:769–778.
18. Shapiro MS, Freedman EL. Allograft reconstruction of the anterior and posterior cruciate ligaments after traumatic knee dislocation. *Am J Sports Med* 1995;23:580–587.
19. Harner CD, Irrgang JJ, Paul J, et al. Loss of motion after anterior cruciate ligament reconstruction. *Am J Sports Med* 1992;20: 499–506.
20. Berg EE. Comminuted tibial eminence anterior cruciate ligament avulsion fractures: failure of arthroscopic treatment. *Arthroscopy* 1993;9:446–450.
21. Shelbourne KD, Johnson GE. Locked bucket-handle meniscal tears in knees with chronic anterior cruciate ligament deficiency. *Am J Sports Med* 1993;21:779–782.
22. Graf BK, Ott JW, Lange RH, et al. Risk factors for restricted motion after anterior cruciate reconstruction. *Orthopedics* 1994;17: 909–912.
23. Fisher SE, Shelbourne KD. Arthroscopic treatment of symptomatic extension block complicating anterior cruciate ligament reconstruction. *Am J Sports Med* 1993;21:558–564.
24. Shelbourne KD, Johnson GE. Outpatient surgical management of arthrofibrosis after anterior cruciate ligament surgery. *Am J Sports Med* 1994;22:192–197.
25. Lane JG, Daniel DM, Stone ML. Graft impingement after anterior cruciate ligament reconstruction: presentation as an active extension "thunk." *Am J Sports Med* 1994;22:415–417.
26. Reider B, Belniak RM, Preiskorn DO. Arthroscopic arthrolysis for flexion contracture following intra-articular reconstruction of the anterior cruciate ligament. *Arthroscopy* 1996;12:165–173.
27. Bach BR, Jones GT, Sweet FA, et al. Arthroscopy-assisted anterior cruciate ligament reconstruction using patellar tendon substitution: two- to four-year follow-up results. *Am J Sports Med* 1994;22:758–767.
28. Nabors ED, Richmond JC, Vannah WM, et al. Anterior cruciate

ligament graft tensioning in full extension. *Am J Sports Med* 1995;23:488–492.

29. Jackson DW, Schaefer RK. Cyclops syndrome: loss of extension following intra-articular cruciate ligament reconstruction. *Arthroscopy* 1990;6:171–178.

30. Fulkerson JP Becker GJ, Meaney JA, et al. Anteromedial tibial tubercle transfer without bone graft. *Am J Sports Med* 1990;18:490–497.

31. Austin KS, Sherman OH. Complications of arthroscopic meniscal repair. *Am J Sports Med* 1993;21:864–869.

32. Fanelli GC, Gianotti BF, Edson CJ. Current concepts review: the posterior cruciate ligament arthroscopic evaluation and treatment. *Arthroscopy* 1994;10:673–688.

33. Evans EB, Eggers GWN, Butler JK, et al. Experimental immobilization and remobilization of rat knee joints. *J Bone Joint Surg Am* 1960;42:737–758.

34. Enneking WF, Horowitz M. The intra-articular effects of immobilization on the human knee. *J Bone Joint Surg Am* 1972;54:973–985.

35. Frank CB. Ligament healing: current knowledge and clinical applications. *J Am Acad Orthop Surg* 1996;44:74–83.

36. Ververeli PA, Sutton DC, Hearn SL, et al. Continuous passive motion after total knee arthroplasty: analysis of costs and benefits. *Clin Orthop* 1995;321:208–215.

37. Richmond JC, Gladstone J, MacGillvray J. Continuous passive motion after arthroscopically assisted anterior cruciate ligament reconstruction: comparison of short- versus long-term use. *Arthroscopy* 1991;7:39–44.

38. Rosen MA, Jackson DW, Atwell EA. The efficacy of continuous passive motion in the rehabilitation of anterior cruciate ligament reconstruction. *Am J Sports Med* 1992;20:122–127.

39. Witherow GE, Bollen SR, Pinczewski LA. The use of continuous passive motion after arthroscopically assisted anterior cruciate ligament reconstruction: help or hindrance? Knee Surgery, Sports Traumatology, *Arthroscopy* 1993;1:68–70.

40. McCarthy MR, Yates CK, Anderson MA, et al. The effects of immediate continuous passive motion on pain during the inflammatory phase of soft tissue healing following anterior cruciate ligament reconstruction. *J Orthop Sports Phys Ther* 1993;17:96–101.

41. Becker JM, Dayton MT, Fazio VW, et al. Prevention of postoperative abdominal adhesions by a sodium hyaluronate-based bioresorbable membrane: a prospective, randomized, double-blind multicenter study. *J Am Coll Surg* 1996;183:297–306.

42. Burns JW, Colt MJ, Burgess LS, et al. Preclinical evaluation of Sperafilm bioresorbable membrane. *Eur J Surg Suppl* 1997;577:40–48.

43. Nelson WE, Henderson RC, Almekinders LC, et al. An evaluation of pre- and post-operative nonsteroidal anti-inflammatory drugs in patients undergoing knee arthroscopy: a prospective, randomized, double-blind study. *Am J Sports Med* 1993;21:510–516.

44. Rasmussen S. Thomsen S, Madsen SN, et al. The clinical effect of naproxen sodium after arthroscopy of the knee: a randomized, double-blind, prospective study. *Arthroscopy* 1993;9:375–380.

45. Vargas JH, Ross DG. Corticosteroids and anterior cruciate ligament repair. *Am J Sports Med* 1989;17:532–534.

46. Highgenboten, CL, Jackson AW, Meske NB. Arthroscopy of the knee: ten-day pain profiles and corticosteroids. *Am J Sports Med* 1993;21:503–506.

47. Armstrong RW, Bolding F, Joseph R. Septic arthritis following arthroscopy: clinical syndromes and analysis of risk factors. *Arthroscopy* 1992;8:213–223.

48. Cohn BT, Draeger RI, Jackson DW. The effects of cold therapy in the postoperative management of pain in patients undergoing anterior cruciate ligament reconstruction. *Am J Sports Med* 1989;17:344–349.

49. Daniel DM, Stone ML, Arendt DL. The effect of cold therapy on pain, swelling, and range of motion after anterior cruciate ligament reconstructive surgery. *Arthroscopy* 1994;10:530–533.

50. Edwards DJ, Rimmer M, Keene GCR. The use of cold therapy in the postoperative management of patients undergoing arthroscopic anterior cruciate ligament reconstruction. *Am J Sports Med* 1996;24:193–195.

51. Konrath GA, Lock T, Goitz HT, et al. The use of cold therapy after anterior cruciate ligament reconstruction: a prospective, randomized study and literature review. *Am J Sports Med* 1996;24:629–633.

52. Robins AJ, Newman AP, Burks RT. Postoperative return of motion in anterior cruciate ligament and medial collateral ligament injuries: effect of medial collateral ligament rupture location. *Am J Sports Med* 1993;21:20–25.

53. Grotendorst GR, Grotendorst CA, Gilman T. Production of growth factors (PDGF and TGF-β) at the site of tissue repair. *Prog Clin Biol Res* 1988;266:47–54.

54. Steefnos H, Lossing C, Hansson HA. Immunohistochemical demonstration of endogenous growth factors in wound healing. *Wounds* 1990;2:218–226.

55. Antoniades HN, Galanopoulos T, Neville-Golden J, et al. Injury induces *in vivo* expression of PDGF and PDGF-receptor mRNAs in skin epithelial cells and PDGF mRNA in connective tissue fibroblasts. *Proc Natl Acad Sci USA* 1991;88:565–569.

56. Antoniades HN, Galanopoulos T, Neville-Golden J, et al. Expression of growth factor and receptor mRNAs in skin epithelial cells following acute cutaneous injury. *Am J Pathol* 1993;142:1099–1110.

57. Ross R, Raines EW, Bowen-Pope DF. The biology of platelet-derived growth factor. *Cell* 1986;46:155–169.

58. Whitby DJ, Ferguson MWJ. Immunohistochemical localization of growth factors in fetal wound healing. *Dev Biol* 1991;147:207–215.

59. Richmond JC, Alman BA, Pojerski M. Growth factor expression in arthrofibrosis. *Arthroscopy* 1996;12:352–353.

60. von Deck MD, Richmond JC, Alman BA. Arthrofibrosis: a potential treatment based on growth factor manipulation. *Arthroscopy* 1997;13:393–394.

61. Alman BA, Goldberg MJ, Nabor SP, et al. Aggressive fibromatosis. *J Pediatr Orthop* 1992;12:1–10.

62. Alman BA, Nabor SP, Terek RM, et al. Platelet-derived growth factor in fibrous musculoskeletal disorders: a study of pathologic tissue sections and primary cell cultures. *J Orthop Res* 1995;13:66–77.

63. Terek RM, Jiranek WA, Goldberg MJ, et al. The expression of platelet-derived growth factor gene in Dupuytren contracture. *J Bone Joint Surg Am* 1995;77:1–9.

64. Bunker TD, Anthony PP. The pathology of frozen shoulder: a Dupuytren-like disease. *J Bone Joint Surg Br* 1995;77:677–683.

65. Alman BA, Greel DA, Ruby LK, et al. Regulation of proliferation and platelet-derived growth factor expression in palmar fibromatosis (Dupuytren contracture) by mechanical strain. *J Orthop Res* 1996;14:722–728.

66. Murakami S, Muneta T, Ezura Y, et al. Quantitative analysis of synovial fibrosis in the infrapatellar fat pad before and after anterior cruciate ligament reconstruction. *Am J Sports Med* 1997;25:29–34.

67. Mariani PM, Santori N, Rovere P, et al. Histological and structural study of the adhesive tissue in knee fibroarthrosis: a clinical-pathological correlation. *Arthroscopy* 1997;13:313–318.

68. Dodds JA, Keene JS, Graf BK, et al. Results of knee manipulations after anterior cruciate ligament reconstructions. *Am J Sports Med* 1991;19:283–287.

69. Carro LP, Suarez GG. Intercondylar notch fibrous nodule after total knee replacement: a case report. *Arthroscopy* 1999;15:103–105.

70. Ahmad CS, Kwak SD, Ateshian GA, et al. Effects of patellar tendon adhesion to the anterior tibia on knee mechanics. *Am J Sports Med* 1998;26:715–724.

71. Ferguson AB Jr, Brown TD, Fu FH, et al. Relief of patellofemoral contact stress by anterior displacement of the tibial tubercle. *J Bone Joint Surg Am* 1979;61:159–166.

72. Nakamura N, Ellis M, Seedhom BB. Advancement of the tibial tuberosity: a biomechanical study. *J Bone Joint Surg Br* 1985;67:255–260.

ARTHROSCOPIC TREATMENT OF ANTERIOR CRUCIATE LIGAMENT INJURIES

NICK A. EVANS
DOUGLAS W. JACKSON

FUNCTIONAL ANATOMY

The *anterior cruciate ligament* (ACL) is an intraarticular collagenous structure located in the center of the knee joint and covered with a synovial sheath. The ligament has an average length of 31 to 38 mm and an average width of 11 mm (1). Proximally, it is attached to the posterior aspect of the lateral femoral condyle's medial surface. The ligament passes anteriorly, medially, and distally within the joint to its attachment at the anteromedial region of the tibial plateau between the tibial eminences. The distal portion of the ligament fans out to create a larger tibial attachment, known as the *footprint*.

The ACL is a continuum of fibers that have no distinct bundle morphologic features. The microanatomy consists of multiple collagen fibers 20 μm wide, grouped into larger fascicles ranging from 20 to 400 μm in diameter (2). Despite the lack of anatomic delineation, the fiber arrangement has been "functionally" divided into two subdivisions or bundles: an anteromedial band and a posterolateral band. The fibers of the anteromedial band pass from the proximal part of the femoral attachment to the anteromedial aspect of the tibial footprint. The posterolateral band fibers attach distally to the femur and posterolaterally to the tibia. The posterolateral band is taut when the knee is extended, and the anteromedial band becomes taut when the knee is flexed. Because of its internal architecture and attachment sites on the femur and tibia, the ACL provides restraint to anterior translation and internal rotation of the tibia, varus and valgus angulation, and hyperextension of the knee.

As a knee joint stabilizer, the ACL is able to resist a tensile force of 2,000 N load. However, during normal daily function, the ligament sees loads of less than 20% of its failure capacity. The highest loads are provided by quadriceps-powered knee extension, moving from approximately 40 degrees to full extension.

INJURY

In the United States, the prevalence of ACL injury is about one in 3,000 (3), and approximately 250,000 new injuries occur each year (4). Current estimates indicate that 100,000 ACL reconstruction operations are performed annually in the United States (5). Many of these injuries occur during sporting activities that involve deceleration, twisting, cutting, and jumping movements. The ligament fails as a consequence of excessive valgus stress, forced external rotation of the femur on a fixed tibia with the knee in full extension, or forced hyperextension.

The spectrum of ACL injury ranges from a partial sprain (grade I or II) to complete disruption (grade III). Most diagnosed ACL injuries are complete disruptions (85%), and partial sprains occur less frequently (15%). ACL damage may occur in isolation (25% of cases) or in combination (75%) with injury to other structures in the knee joint, including meniscus, articular cartilage, collateral ligament, or joint capsule (6–8).

Because of its intraarticular location, the ACL has poor healing potential. Extraarticular ligaments heal by progressing through a series of inflammatory, proliferative, and remodeling phases, which result in the formation of organized scar tissue. This process is incited by the formation of a localized hematoma. In contrast, when the ACL is torn, its synovial envelope is damaged, and blood dissipates within the joint. Without the formation of a blood clot, the normal sequence of soft tissue repair will not initiate (9). The ruptured ACL does not form a bridging scar after complete disruption. Instead, a layer of synovial tissue forms over the damaged surface, and the ruptured ends retract (10).

N. A. Evans and D. W. Jackson: Southern California Center for Sports Medicine, Long Beach, California.

NATURAL HISTORY

The fate of different injuries to the ACL is variable. The prognosis for a partially torn ACL may be favorable, if the synovial envelope remains intact (8,9). Complete ACL ruptures have a less favorable outcome. The development of symptomatic knee instability after ACL injury occurs in an unpredictable fashion, ranging from 16% to almost 100% (11). Some patients are disabled for sport activities, whereas others appear to have minimal impairment. The functional outcome is difficult to predict, because symptomatic instability depends on the degree of joint laxity and on the athletic demands of the individual patient.

Repeated episodes of subluxation in the ACL-deficient knee can result in further intraarticular damage. Meniscus injury occurs in association with 50% of acute ACL tears, and this figure rises to 90% in ACL-deficient knees assessed 10 years or more after the initial injury. The incidence of articular cartilage lesions rises from 30% in acute ACL injuries to approximately 70% of knees with chronic ACL instability. Such intraarticular deterioration increases the subsequent risk of developing joint arthrosis. The progression to radiographically detectable osteoarthritis in ACL-deficient knees is variable, ranging from 15% to 65%, and it depends on the length of follow-up. The success of surgical ACL reconstruction in preventing the development of arthrosis has not been demonstrated (12,13).

PATIENT SELECTION

Without treatment, a complete ACL injury can result in progressively increasing symptomatic knee instability, which inflicts recurrent intraarticular damage and eventually causes osteoarthritis. The fundamental rationale for surgical reconstruction of the disrupted ACL is to prevent future meniscal tears and associated joint damage. Patient selection for surgical intervention is not straightforward, however, because not all patients with an injured ACL become symptomatic, and not all knees with chronic ACL deficiency progress to osteoarthrosis. Hence, not all such injuries warrant surgical reconstruction. However, certain characteristics indicate that a patient is at high risk of developing symptomatic knee instability after ACL injury (6). The high-risk features are as follows:

- Complete ACL disruption: grade III injury
- Greater than 5 mm side-to-side difference (KT-1000 measured displacement)
- Combined injury: meniscus or other ligament
- High-demand sport: level 1 (jumping, pivoting, cutting)
- Young age

Patients exhibiting high-risk features are candidates for surgical reconstruction. Other (low-risk) patients may be managed with a nonoperative treatment program of reha-bilitation and selective bracing. If, however, symptoms of instability and recurrent traumatic effusions persist despite rehabilitation and activity modification, surgical reconstruction may be appropriate at a later date.

PREOPERATIVE ASSESSMENT

The preoperative assessment of the patient with an injured ACL requires a thorough history and physical examination. The patient's age, occupation, and level of sporting activity are important to establish. Initially, the patient with an acutely injured knee presents with hemarthrosis and restricted range of motion. Later, the symptomatic patient complains of knee instability and disability for sports or occupation and usually presents after an episode of subluxation.

During physical examination of the injured knee, the range of motion is documented, and any effusion is evaluated. When testing for laxity, the anterior drawer test is more specific for anteromedial band rupture, whereas the Lachman and pivot shift tests are preferred to diagnose a disrupted posterolateral band. All three tests are likely to be positive when the ACL is completely torn.

Radiographs are useful to document degenerative disease, to assess lower extremity alignment, and to exclude bony fracture. Although not routinely necessary, a magnetic resonance scan confirms ACL disruption and reveals associated meniscus tears, bone contusions, and other ligament damage.

The informed and written consent obtained preoperatively should explain the procedure, risks, rehabilitation, and prognosis. We try to provide the patient with a clear understanding of ACL instability, the objectives of reconstruction in alleviating symptoms, and the expected outcome. On the day of the surgical procedure, the surgeon should confirm that the correct limb is identified and clearly marked.

SURGICAL TECHNIQUE

ACL reconstructive surgery is performed in a stepwise fashion as follows:

1. Knee evaluation with the patient under anesthesia and confirmation of ACL rupture
2. Graft harvesting and preparation
3. Arthroscopic documentation and treatment of intraarticular disease
4. Preparation of the intercondylar notch
5. Osseous tunnel placement
6. Graft implantation and fixation
7. Wound closure and postoperative assessment of stability
8. Postoperative rehabilitation

Ligamentous Evaluation with the Patient under Anesthesia

The patient is positioned supine on the operating table, and identification of the correct limb is confirmed before surgical preparation and draping. General, regional, or epidural anesthesia is administered, depending on the patient's choice. A tourniquet is applied to the proximal thigh, but it is inflated only to aid hemostasis should bleeding obscure arthroscopic visualization. We use a lateral thigh post to facilitate limb positioning and administer a cephalosporin (cefazolin, 1 g) for perioperative antibiotic prophylaxis.

Preoperatively, the injured knee and the contralateral knee are evaluated and compared, with the patient under anesthesia, by means of physical examination and a KT-1000 knee arthrometer. In the event of an equivocal pivot shift test or a side-to-side-difference of less than 5 mm with the KT-1000 arthrometer at maximal manual displacement, diagnostic arthroscopy should precede graft harvest. When complete rupture of the ACL is clinically obvious, we harvest the autograft before the arthroscopic portion of the surgical procedure. This approach allows graft preparation by an assistant while the surgeon simultaneously prepares the osseous tunnels and can reduce overall operating time.

Graft Harvest

Graft selection largely depends on the individual surgeon's and patient's preference. We prefer using the middle third of the patellar tendon with bone plugs at both ends (14), although we commonly use other sources of autograft or allograft. We inject the planned incision site with a mixture of 0.25% bupivacaine (Marcaine) and 1:200,000 epinephrine, which we believe helps to reduce bleeding and postoperative pain.

A vertical skin incision is made from the inferior pole of the patella downward over the patella tendon to a point 1 cm medial to the tibial tubercle (Fig. 23.1). This single incision accommodates graft harvest and arthroscopic portals, and the slight medial obliquity facilitates tibial tunnel preparation (Fig. 23.2). The graft can also be harvested through two small transverse incisions overlying the bony insertions of the patellar tendon. However, this approach does not allow direct visualization of the entire tendon, and additional incisions are required for the tibial tunnel and arthroscopic portals.

With the single-incision technique, the paratenon is incised vertically and is carefully dissected off the tendon to identify its medial and lateral borders. Flexing the patient's knee places the exposed tendon under tension and facilitates graft harvest. We use a double-handle scalpel with parallel blades to harvest the central third of the tendon (Fig. 23.3). The size of the graft is determined by the overall width of the tendon. Our preference is that the graft width should not exceed 40% of the overall patellar tendon width, and the

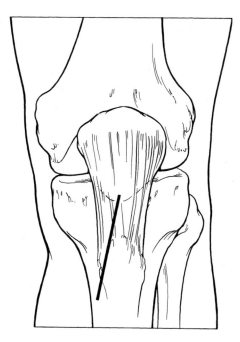

FIGURE 23.1 Our preferred incision for arthroscopically assisted anterior cruciate ligament reconstruction extends from the inferior pole of the patella to a point just medial to the tibial tubercle.

scalpel blades are set accordingly. When the tendon width is at least 25 mm, the blades are set 10 mm apart. In smaller patients, we harvest a 9-mm wide graft. Beginning at a bony attachment, the central third of the tendon is incised in the line of its fibers. Electrocautery is then used to delineate the bone–tendon junctions and to outline the margins of the bone plugs (Fig. 23.4). Care should be taken to avoid damage to either the graft or the remaining patella tendon.

The technique used to harvest the bone plugs should reproducibly obtain a plug that fits snugly into the osseous tunnels with minimal contouring to allow secure fixation. It should also minimize the risk of patella fracture at the site of harvest. We use a circular oscillating saw (Stryker) (Fig. 23.5), which provides cylindrical bone plugs of varying diameter (9, 10, or 11 mm). In most cases, a saw blade 10 mm in diameter is selected. This device affords the following advantages: (a) ease and rapidity of harvest, (b) reproducible cylindrical bone plug 1 mm smaller in diameter than the corresponding osseous tunnel, (c) decreased stress riser at the patella harvest site, and (d) ease of graft insertion because of uniform sizing. We harvest the tibial bone plug first, using a saw blade 10 mm in diameter. Once the bone plug has been harvested, the tendon graft is dissected from the underlying fat pad. With a towel clip, distal traction is applied to the tibial bone plug; this delivers the patella into the wound and avoids the need to extend the skin incision proximally. The circular saw with a 10-mm diameter blade is then used to harvest a 20- to 22-mm long patellar plug (Fig. 23.6). Other techniques for harvesting the bone plugs use a straight-blade oscillating saw, an osteotome, or semicircular

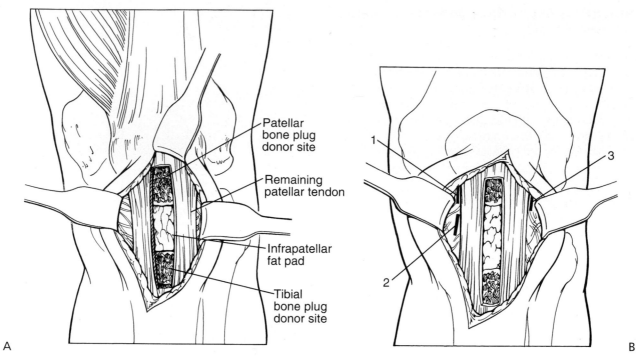

A

B

FIGURE 23.2 A: Exposure after graft harvest. **B:** Arthroscopic portals may be placed within the margins of the incision: 1, anteromedial portal; 2, accessory anteromedial portal; 3, anterolateral portal.

gouges. Whichever technique is used, it should provide a reproducible graft, avoid potential stress risers, minimize trauma to the underlying articular cartilage, and fit snugly into the osseous tunnel with minimal gaps.

Graft Preparation

Once harvested, the autograft is prepared for implantation at a side table by the surgeon or an assistant. If an autograft

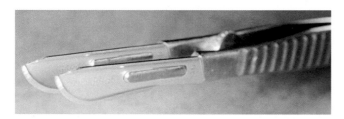

FIGURE 23.3 Adjustable double-handled scalpel used to harvest patella tendon graft.

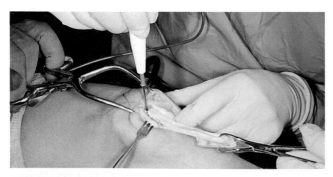

FIGURE 23.4 Electrocautery delineates the bone–tendon junction.

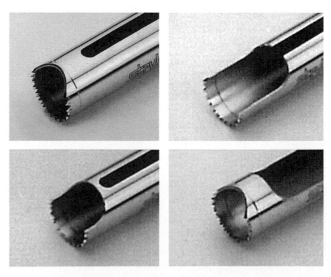

FIGURE 23.5 Circular oscillating saw blades.

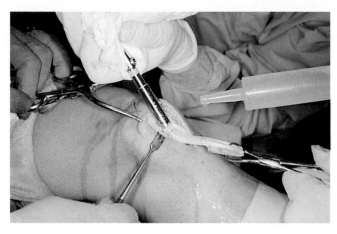

FIGURE 23.6 Distal traction on the tibial bone plug with a towel clip exposes the inferior pole of the patella for bone plug harvest.

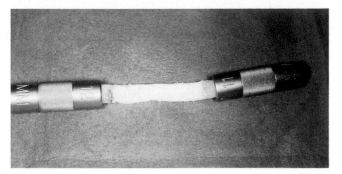

FIGURE 23.8 Passage through cylindrical sizers ensures that the graft will pass easily through the osseous tunnels.

is used, we prefer the assistant to start shaping the graft at the commencement of the arthroscopic evaluation. Instruments that aid graft preparation include the following:

1. A bone nibbler or rongeur
2. Dissecting scissors
3. Plug sizers 9, 10, 11, and 12 mm in diameter
4. A bone plug holder
5. A drill (with a ³⁄₃₂-inch bit) and a drill guide for placement of the passing sutures
6. A spring-loaded device to pretension the graft
7. A measuring device to determine the length of the bone plugs and overall graft length (Fig. 23.7)

The bone plugs are trimmed first. We prefer the bone plug harvested from the tibia to measure 25 mm in length and the bone plug harvested from the patella to measure 20 to 22 mm. Next, a simulation of bone plug passage through the osseous tunnels is performed using the cylindrical sizers.

The bone plugs are trimmed as necessary until they slide easily through the appropriate sizer (Fig. 23.8).

The smaller bone plug, typically from the patella, is placed in the femoral tunnel. Using a 3/32-inch drill bit, we place a single drill hole through the cortical surface of the bone plug (Fig. 23.9), through which we thread a 30-inch no. 2 nonabsorbable suture. The drill hole is sited fairly close to the tip of the bone plug (Fig. 23.10), to provide better directional control during graft passage into the femoral tunnel. Three evenly spaced drill holes are made in the tibial bone plug and are threaded with no. 5 polyester sutures. The holes are oriented perpendicular to each other, to minimize the chance of suture laceration during interference screw insertion.

We prefer to mount the graft in the spring-loaded graft holder under 8 pounds of tension while final trimming of fat and extraneous tissue is performed with curved Mayo scissors. The bone–tendon junction of the femoral plug is then marked with methylene blue using a sterile pen (Fig. 23.11). In addition, the center of the bone plug is marked longitudi-

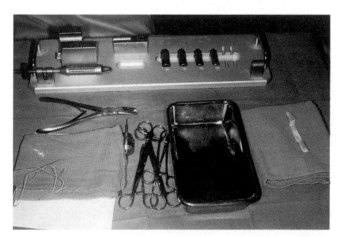

FIGURE 23.7 Our work station for preparation of the bone–patellar tendon–bone graft.

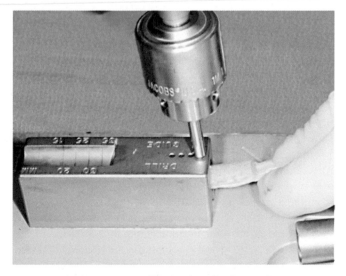

FIGURE 23.9 Drill hole placed in bone plug.

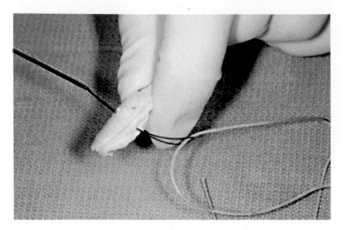

FIGURE 23.10 Bone plug threaded with suture.

nally, to facilitate bone plug rotation and positioning during passage into the femoral tunnel. When preparation of the graft is complete, it is covered with an antibiotic-soaked sponge until the surgeon is ready for graft implantation.

The total length of the typical bone–patellar tendon–bone graft is usually 90 to 105 mm after preparation. The required length of the tibial tunnel can be calculated by subtracting the length of the femoral tunnel and intraarticular length from the overall graft length. Thus, with a 25-mm femoral tunnel length and 30 mm for the intraarticular portion, a 100-mm graft requires a 45-mm tibial tunnel. However, because of the oblique distal opening of the tibial tunnel, we add an additional 5 mm so the bone plug will not protrude. Therefore, a 50-mm tunnel is drilled (Fig. 23.12).

An alternative means to reduce the potential for length mismatch between the graft and tunnel was recommended by Schaeffer, Gow, and Tibone (15). The recommendation involves harvesting additional bone from the tibia proximal to the tubercle. This additional length bone block can be inserted into the femoral tunnel, thus effectively recessing the entire graft further into the femur and reducing the potential for the graft to protrude from the tibia. This technique can effectively recess the graft up to 8 mm into the femoral tunnel. It does require insertion of the tibial bone block into the femur.

Alternative Autografts

A popular alternative graft is the semitendinosus–gracilis (hamstring) autograft (16). Graft harvest is performed through a 2- to 5-cm incision at the insertion of the pes anserinus tendons. The landmark for the superior edge of the pes anserinus is 1 cm medial and level with the tibial tubercle, approximately two fingerbreadths below the joint line. We prefer a slightly oblique incision parallel to the pes anserinus to reduce the risk of injury to the infrapatellar branches of the saphenous nerve. Once the subcutaneous tissue is reflected from the deep fascia, the tendons can be rolled under the finger at the posteromedial corner of the tibia. A fascia incision is made along the superior aspect of the pes tendons to the

edge of their anterior insertion. The cut is then directed perpendicular and is continued distally along the anterior border of the pes tendons. The pes attachment is then dissected from the periosteum, to create a triangular flap allowing the tendons to be seen from the inside outward. With the tendons exposed in this manner, scissors are used to incise along the cleft between the gracilis and semitendinosus. The gracilis is protected behind a retractor. The semitendinosus is carefully freed from its aponeurotic attachments to the medial gastrocnemius and is dissected off the sartorius expansion. The free end of the tendon is held with an Allis clamp or a whipstitch. Gentle traction and blunt finger dissection can be used to confirm the mobility of the tendon. A tendon stripper is then passed over the tendon and is advanced proximally with a twisting and pushing movement.

Great care is taken to keep the tendon stripper parallel to the tendon. If any fascial bands impede the passage of the tendon stripper, they should be carefully divided with scissors. The patient's knee is flexed at least 30 degrees during this maneuver, and placing the limb in a figure-4 position may aid exposure. The tendon can then be detached from its muscle belly in the thigh and delivered into the wound. The gracilis tendon is harvested in a similar manner, but, again, care must be taken to release the sartorius attachment in its expansion, to free the gracilis tendon completely. Harvest usually yields 25 to 30 cm of good-quality tendons with nearly equal lengths.

Graft preparation begins with removal of residual muscle tissue from the tendons. The semitendinosus will have residual muscle tissue present on only one side of the tendon, whereas the gracilis will have muscle present on two sides. The graft construct is fashioned by folding each tendon in half, to form a four-stranded graft. The folded end is whipstitched with a no. 5 nonabsorbable polyester suture for 30 to 40 mm to create the femoral end of the graft. The intraarticular segment is between 25 and 40 mm in length. The distal portion of the graft is whipstitched for 40 to 50 mm to incorporate the four strands together. The graft is passed through the cylindrical sizers to determine the tibial and femoral tunnel diameters needed.

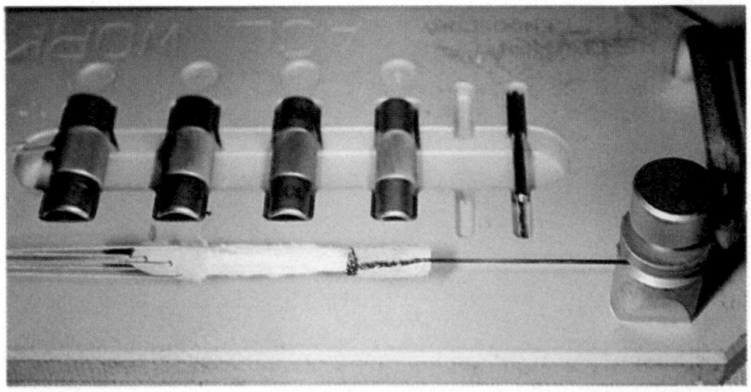

FIGURE 23.11 The bone–tendon junction is marked with a sterile pen for enhanced visualization during seating of the proximal bone plug.

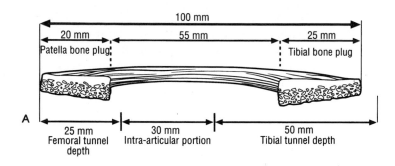

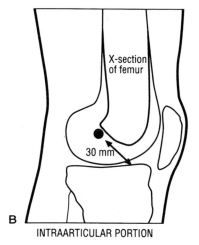

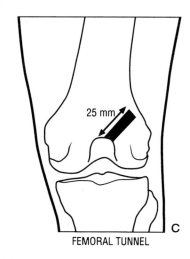

100 mm (total graft length)
- **30** mm (intraarticular portion)
- **25** mm (femoral tunnel length)
+ **5** mm (to prevent tibial plug protrusion)

50 mm (= TIBIAL TUNNEL LENGTH)

FIGURE 23.12 A: The length of the graft is used to determine the tibial tunnel length required. **B** and **C:** With a 100-mm graft, a 25-mm femoral tunnel depth plus 30 mm for the intraarticular portion of the graft leaves a 45-mm length of graft. However, because we drill the tunnel with an oblique opening, an extra 5 mm is needed to prevent protrusion of the tibial bone plug. Therefore, a 50-mm tibial tunnel is required.

Another alternative autograft is the central quadriceps tendon using a patella bone block at one end (17). This graft may also be used without a bone block. This graft is harvested through a 4-cm incision starting centrally at the upper pole of the patella and extending proximally. A graft 10 mm in width is carefully delineated, from the center of the upper pole of the patella. We prefer to use a double-handle scalpel to harvest a central quadriceps tendon graft 7 to 8 cm in length. A hemostat is used to separate the graft within the substance of the vastus intermedius, such that adequate thickness is harvested, but without entering the suprapatellar pouch. The graft is released proximally, and a 10-mm circular oscillating saw is used to create a 20- to 25-mm cylindrical bone plug form the upper pole of the patella. A single drill hole is placed in the bone plug, through which we thread a 30-inch no. 2 nonabsorbable suture. The tendinous end of the graft is whipstitched with a no. 5 polyester suture.

Documentation and Treatment of Intraarticular Disease

The intraarticular portion of the surgical procedure can be performed while the graft is prepared at a side table by an as-

sistant. The arthroscope is inserted into an anterolateral portal, created by retracting the skin flap to expose the lateral border of the patella tendon. An anteromedial portal is made in a similar way, and both portals can be placed within the margins of the existing skin incision (Fig. 23.13). Separate standard arthroscopic portals are required when using alternative grafts. ACL reconstruction requires high fluid

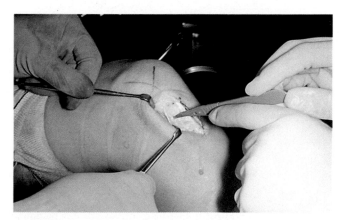

FIGURE 23.13 Arthroscopic portal created within the margins of skin incision used for graft harvest.

flows, which may be achieved through a separate cannula or by a pump through the arthroscope.

A thorough diagnostic arthroscopic examination is performed to confirm the torn ACL and to assess the status of the menisci and articular cartilage. Each intraarticular structure is probed using a hook, and sequential photographic images are taken for documentation purposes (Fig. 23.10).

We prefer to treat any associated intraarticular injuries before proceeding with the ligament reconstruction. Intraarticular visualization and suture placement are easier while the patient's knee is unstable and before notchplasty or osseous tunnel drilling can cause bleeding. Meniscal tears are repaired or resected, depending on their configuration. Articular cartilage damage is documented and treated if deemed appropriate, by chondroplasty or microfracture. If mosaicplasty is to be considered, we believe that it should be carefully discussed before the surgical procedure, to obtain the patient's consent.

Preparation of the Intercondylar Notch

Remnants of the torn ACL are debrided using a full-radius resector, and the tibial footprint should be clearly identified. The ligamentum mucosum is removed to enhance visualization. The infrapatellar fat pad is seldom resected, and the posterior cruciate ligament (PCL) is protected. Notchplasty begins with debridement of the soft tissue and periosteum from the lateral wall of the notch. We prefer an oscillating resector for soft tissue removal under direct visualization, to prevent localized gouging or production of ridges in the notch. The entire surface of the lateral wall that will involve the opening to the osseous tunnel is debrided. Bleeding encountered at this point may be controlled with electrocautery, inflation of the tourniquet, or both. Sufficient hydrostatic pressure by means of gravity inflow irrigation or infusion pump seems to minimize undesired intraarticular bleeding and the need for tourniquet. Once the notch has been adequately debrided of soft tissue, an assessment can be made regarding the need for additional bony notchplasty. We perform a notchplasty when there is difficulty in visualizing the lateral wall or when the presence of notch osteophytes will impinge and guillotine the ACL graft. A bony notchplasty is done more frequently in chronic than in acute ACL deficiency. The procedure is carried out using an arthroscopic bur or a full-radius resector (Fig. 23.14). If the notch requires significant widening, a ¼-inch curved osteotome may be introduced through the medial portal, and the large bone fragments may be removed with a grasper. Minimal articular cartilage removal is desirable. Regardless of the technique used, the posterior margin of the notch should be clearly identified, to avoid misinterpreting the so-called "resident's ridge" as the over-the-top position. This error in landmark selection may cause the femoral tunnel to be placed more anteriorly than desired.

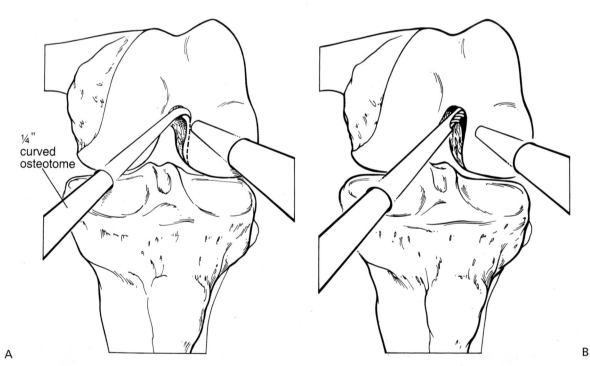

FIGURE 23.14 A: The extent of bony notchplasty may be demarcated with a 1/4-inch curved osteotome placed through the anteromedial portal. **B:** Fine tuning of the notchplasty may be completed using an arthroscopic bur or shaver.

Osseous Tunnel Placement and Preparation

The selection of ideal osseous tunnel sites is a crucial step in ACL reconstruction (18). The normal ACL is composed of a large number of fibers. Each fiber is a different length, has a different origin and insertion, and is under different tension during the range of motion of the knee (19). The graft replacing the ACL will have parallel fibers. Even with optimal selection of the placement of the osseous tunnels, the fibers of the graft will undergo length and tension changes with range of motion (20). Therefore, the ACL replacement will not duplicate the original ligament. However, placing the center of the osseous tunnels at the most isometric points maximizes the stability that can be obtained during motion.

The site for the femoral tunnel is selected once the notch has been prepared. It requires visualization of the over-the-top position, which is enhanced by flexing the patient's knee to 70 degrees or more. If interference screw fixation is desired, the femoral site selected should result in an osseous tunnel with a 1- to 2-mm thick posterior cortical wall. This provides a posterior buttress for the interference screw and thereby prevents posterior wall blow out, at the same time protecting the posterior neurovascular bundle.

To locate the desired center of the femoral tunnel, we prefer to use a placement guide that keys off the over-the-top position. A cannulated endoscopic femoral guide selects a tunnel site as far posteriorly as possible, without destroying the posterior cortex (Fig. 23.15). When a 10-mm tunnel is desired, the center of the osseous tunnel is located with a guide that centers the tunnel 7 mm anterior to the over-the-top position. This creates a tunnel 5 mm in radius, which leaves a 2-mm rim of posterior cortex. The guide is inserted through an accessory anteromedial portal placed more inferiorly, just above the joint line. The center of the selected femoral tunnel site is then marked with a guide wire. This point is verified visually and is checked with a nerve hook, to confirm the correct distance from the over-the-top position.

Selecting the properly positioned femoral tunnel site ensures maximum postoperative knee stability. The intraarticular site of the tibial tunnel has less effect on changes in graft length, but its position is important in preventing intercondylar notch impingement. The extraarticular opening of the tibial tunnel can be altered, depending on the tunnel length required to accommodate the graft. We locate the center of the intraarticular opening immediately posterior to the anatomic center of the ACL tibial footprint. Four consistent anatomic landmarks can be used to locate the tibial tunnel center (21): the anterior horn of the lateral meniscus, the medial tibial spine, the PCL, and the ACL stump. The site can be located in the anteroposterior plane by extending a line in continuation with the inner edge of the anterior horn of the lateral meniscus. This point is consistently located 6 to 7 mm anterior to the anterior border of the PCL. If an 11-mm diameter tunnel is desired, this places the center 7 mm anterior to the PCL and yields a tunnel with a 5.5-mm radius, with 1 to 2 mm of bone separating the posterior wall of the tunnel from the PCL. The mediolateral placement of the tunnel center should correspond to the depression medial to the medial tibial spine in the mediolateral center of the ACL stump (Fig. 23.16). This tunnel placement should allow the ACL graft, once in place, to touch the

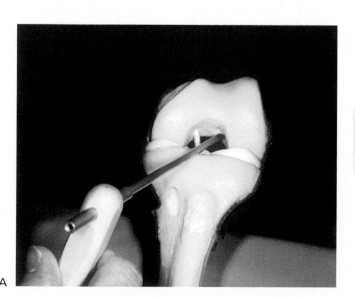
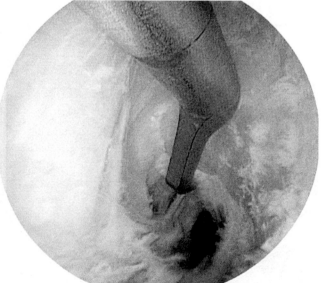

A   B

FIGURE 23.15 A: The anatomic model illustrates the over-the-top drill guide. **B:** The over-the-top drill guide allows reproducible selection of the femoral tunnel site by placing the drill tip a chosen distance anterior to the posterior notch.

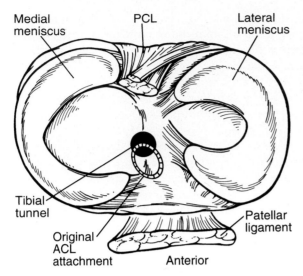

FIGURE 23.16 The center of the tibial tunnel is in line with the posterior edge of the anterior horn of the lateral meniscus, in the depression just lateral to the medial tibial spine.

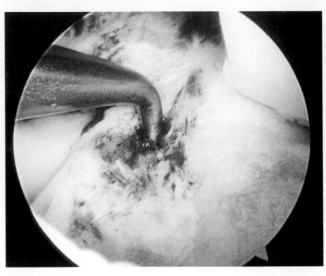

FIGURE 23.18. The tibial guide is placed into position through the anteromedial portal.

lateral aspect of the PCL but not be significantly deflected by it. Similarly, it should neither abrade nor impinge against the medial aspect of the lateral femoral condyle or the roof of the intercondylar notch when the knee is in full extension (22). Anterior graft placement results in impingement and subsequent graft failure (Fig. 23.17).

With the tunnel center chosen, the patient's knee is flexed 90 degrees, and the tip of the tibial drill guide is positioned through the anteromedial portal (Fig. 23.18). The angle of this guide is adjusted to create the desired tunnel length. The skin incision is retracted medially and distally while the drill sleeve is placed against the tibial cortex, medial to the tubercle, and a guide wire is drilled into place. Vi-

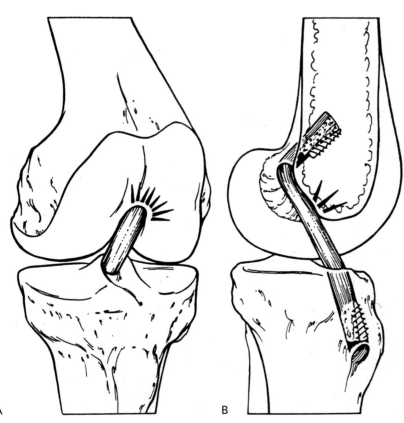

FIGURE 23.17 A: Graft impingement against the lateral femoral condyle. **B:** Graft impingement against the roof of the notch.

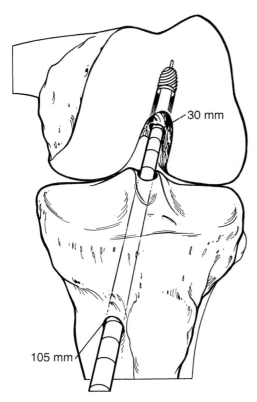

FIGURE 23.19 When the femoral tunnel depth has been reached, the length of the calibrated drill at the tibial tunnel mouth should show the length of the graft plus the extra 5 mm added to prevent plug protrusion.

sualization of the tip of the guide wire as it enters the joint allows any adjustments in pin location to be made at this time. The residual ACL stump may deceive the surgeon into believing the guide wire is positioned more posteriorly than it is when it actually enters the joint. Because of the angle with which the wire penetrates the plateau, the entry point is actually 2 to 3 mm anterior to where the tip is first visualized. Careful confirmation as the pin enters the joint or removal of an adequate amount of the ACL remnant helps to minimize this source of error.

We prefer to drill the tunnel with a cannulated core drill that cuts a dowel plug of bone from the tibia. This affords clean removal of the tibial ACL stump, and the bone plug can be used later to graft the patellar defect. The tibial tunnel is usually 10 or 11 mm in diameter, depending on the diameter of the harvested graft. As the drill is advanced, a curette or curved snap may be used to prevent proximal migration of the guide wire, as well as accidental plunging of the drill into the joint. The tibial tunnel is then plugged to preserve fluid distention while a shaver is used to remove any debris in the joint and to chamfer the tunnel edges. It is important to remove debris anterior to the tunnel edge, because residual tissue anteriorly can contribute to formation of a postoperative cyclops lesion (23). If the tibial tunnel ends up too anteriorly placed, a femoral drill bit or a bur

placed through the tibial tunnel can be used to move the entrance posteriorly.

Once the tibial tunnel is drilled and any debris is cleared from its intraarticular margin, the femoral tunnel can be prepared. With the patient's knee flexed 70 degrees, the guide wire is placed through the tibial tunnel and is advanced into the premarked position on the lateral wall of the femoral notch. An alternative technique for placing the femoral guide wire is to use a drill guide through the tibial tunnel that measures down from the over-the-top position. If applied properly, these guides can facilitate anatomic placement of the femoral graft in a reliable fashion (24). A calibrated cannulated drill is advanced manually over the wire until it engages the lateral wall of the intercondylar notch. Care should be taken to prevent damage to the PCL while the drill is being advanced. The drill bit diameter is chosen to accommodate the corresponding bone plug. The femoral tunnel is then reamed to the desired depth. We prefer to ream 5 mm longer than the patellar bone plug, and the depth is read directly off the calibrated drill using the arthroscope. When this depth has been reached, the measurement at the distal end of the tibial tunnel should be slightly longer than the total graft length (Fig. 23.19). If the overall graft length is longer than the total tunnel length, the surgeon may either shorten the bone plugs or deepen the femoral tunnel. The drill is then removed from the power driver, and the drill bit is removed by hand. A full-radius resector is then used to remove residual soft tissue debris that could impede graft passage. A suction device is passed up through the tibial tunnel and into the femoral tunnel to remove osseous debris. We make a small notch in the femoral tunnel at 2 o'clock (left knee) or 10 o'clock (right knee) for the future placement of the interference screw guide wire (Fig. 23.20). Confirmation of an intact 2 mm of posterior cortex is needed if interference fixation is to be used.

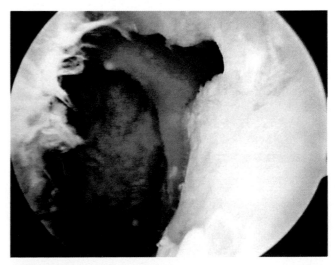

FIGURE 23.20 The femoral tunnel entrance is notched for guide wire insertion.

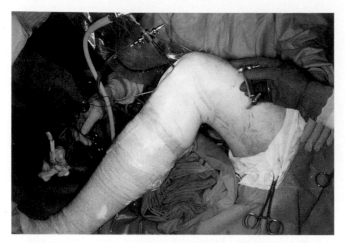

FIGURE 23.21 The knee is flexed to at least 90 degrees for passage of the Beath pin. The knee must remain flexed until suture passage, to prevent accidental bending or breakage of the pin.

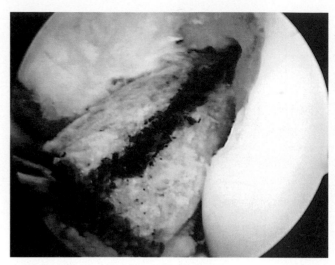

FIGURE 23.22 As the graft is passed into the femoral tunnel, the ink marking the bone–tendon junction confirms the correct rotation and depth of bone plug placement.

Next, a Beath pin is advanced through both tunnels with the patient's knee flexed between 90 and 110 degrees. The pin contains an eyelet that will be threaded with the graft's sutures for passage. It is drilled through the femoral tunnel to exit the thigh anterolaterally. To assist the pin's emergence through the skin, the flat edge of a metallic instrument may be placed just proximal to the exit point as the drill tents the skin. A drill puller may then be placed over the tip to stabilize the pin and to cover the sharp tip. Care must be taken to ensure that the knee remains flexed to the same degree to prevent bending or breaking the Beath pin during its passage (Fig. 23.21).

Graft Passage and Fixation

The graft is now ready for implantation, and it is transferred from the tension board to the operating table. The nylon suture attached to the patellar bone plug is threaded through the eyelet of the Beath pin. The drill puller is used to deliver the suture through the joint, to exit the skin over the anterolateral thigh. A hemostat is attached to the free ends of the suture to pull the graft into the tibial tunnel. Under arthroscopic visualization, the graft is passed into the femoral tunnel with cephalad traction on the proximal suture. The cancellous surface is placed anterolaterally so the collagen fibers of the new ligament are posterior in the femoral tunnel. A hemostat or nerve hook may be placed through the anteromedial portal to help guide the proximal plug past the PCL and to orient the graft properly in the femoral tunnel (Fig. 23.22). The graft is fully seated when the junction of the bone plug and ligament, marked earlier with a pen, is visualized at the tunnel mouth.

Our preferred method of securing the graft is cannulated interference screw fixation, although there are many alternative methods (25). The femoral interference screw is placed first. We prefer a bioabsorbable cannulated screw,

7 mm in diameter by 20 mm in length, with a buttress head and dull threads for the femoral fixation. A guide wire is inserted through the accessory anteromedial portal and is sited in the anterolateral notch, created earlier in the femoral tunnel (Fig. 23.23). This will position the screw against the cancellous side of the plug, away from the collagen. The guide wire is placed during graft passage and is advanced as the femoral plug is seated. We advance it no more than 10 mm

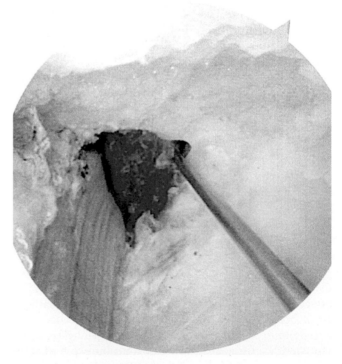

FIGURE 23.23 With the graft seated, a guide wire is sited in the premade notch, for screw placement.

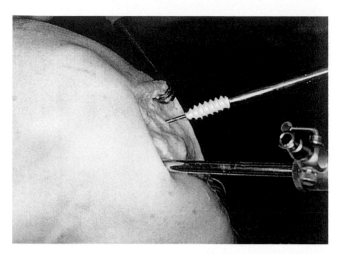

FIGURE 23.24 The cannulated interference screw is placed through the accessory anteromedial portal against the cancellous surface of the bone plug. Knee flexion to 110 degrees helps to prevent screw divergence.

so it can be removed easily once the screw has been placed. With the patient's knee flexed at 90 degrees, the screw is advanced over the wire (Fig. 23.24), under arthroscopic visualization to ensure that the threads do not damage the graft and that the screw does not rotate around the graft. The screw is seated flush with the marked bone–tendon junction (Fig. 23.25). The screw drive and guide wire are then removed from the joint.

If the semitendinosus–gracilis (hamstring) graft is used, our preferred method of fixation is a round-headed, soft-threaded, cannulated interference screw. The blunt threads protect the soft tissue graft during screw insertion. The round head reduces fiber stress as the graft exits the tunnel, and it also compresses the graft against the tunnel aperture to provide a secure fixation. We prefer aperture fixation, with the graft secured at or near the intraarticular graft margin, rather than suspensory fixation, in which the graft is secured at a more remote site (26). The use of an EndoPearl device (Linvatec, Largo, FL) may provide additional fixation strength and may eliminate construct slippage when hamstring tendon grafts are fixed with interference screws (27). We fix the bone plug of the central quadriceps tendon autograft using the same technique as that described for the patellar tendon.

The femoral fixation may be tested by applying distal traction to tibial bone plug sutures. We prefer to pull vigorously during the testing, because this is the best time to correct an inadequate proximal fixation. The knee is then cycled five to ten times through a full range of motion with the graft under tension. Observing the excursion of the bone plug within the tibial tunnel allows an estimation of the overall graft isometry. Although true isometry is not possible with a linear, cylindrical graft, we expect less than 2 mm of excursion of the tibial plug. Excursion of more than 2 mm suggests inadequate proximal fixation, graft damage, or

improperly placed tunnels. If there is no excursion, the tibial bone plug may have become trapped within the tibial tunnel.

During knee motion, the position at which the tibial plug is most distal in the tunnel is noted. This position is typically at approximately 30 degrees of flexion. To prevent capture of the knee, the tibial interference screw is placed with the bone plug in the position where the knee is in full extension. The graft is placed under approximately 10 pounds of longitudinal traction on the suture, to prevent proximal migration of the plug if the screw is advanced. Care must be taken not to overtension the graft. The distal plug is rotated 90 degrees externally, so the cancellous bone surface is posterior in the tibial tunnel. We use a 9 × 25 mm bioabsorbable interference screw without a buttress head, placed posterior to the tibial plug against the cancellous surface. The screw is inserted until the end is buried within the tunnel entrance. We prefer to use a round-head, soft-thread, cannulated screw to secure the graft in the tibial tunnel when we use hamstring or quadriceps tendon autograft.

After the graft has been fixed, it is evaluated arthroscopically to assess notch impingement and to confirm graft tensioning during Lachman's maneuver. The arthroscopic instruments are removed after the knee joint has been drained of fluid. The Lachman and pivot shift tests are performed, and if stability has been restored to the knee, the bone plug sutures are removed. If stability testing is not acceptable, the graft is retensioned. This is an infrequent experience, occurring less than 5% of the time.

Wound Closure

The bony defect in the patella is grafted using the core of bone obtained from the tibial tunnel. The retinacular tissue is closed over the defect to hold the graft in place. The patella tendon is loosely reapproximated to minimize any palpable

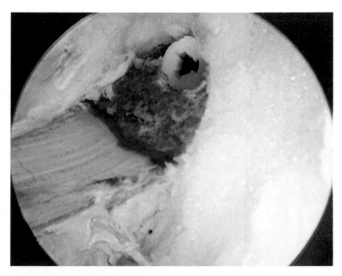

FIGURE 23.25 Completion of screw placement.

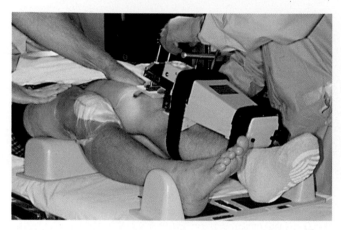

FIGURE 23.26 Postoperative arthrometry can be performed while one maintains the sterility of the wound by covering the wound with a sponge, followed by a Steridrape.

gaps, without shortening the tendon. The paratenon, subcutaneous tissue, and skin are closed in separate layers. To provide postoperative analgesia, the joint is injected with 25 mL of 0.25% bupivacaine with 1:200,000 epinephrine and 5 mg of morphine.

A sterile gauze and adhesive drape are used to cover the wound, and knee stability is assessed by KT-1000 arthrometry (Fig. 23.26), for comparison with the preoperative value and with the contralateral knee. A fresh sterile dressing is then applied to the wound and is held in place using a compressive antiembolism stocking. A cold therapy wrap and a knee immobilizer are applied. The patient is transported to the recovery room. We perform ACL reconstructions as an outpatient procedure, and patients are discharged home on the same day, with oral pain medication (hydrocodone). We find that selective femoral nerve blocks are helpful for postoperative pain relief. On a rare occasion, the patient may require an overnight stay to control pain or to treat persistent nausea and vomiting. The patient is instructed to use crutches, with weight bearing as tolerated on the operated limb. Intermittent ice application is recommended for 3 to 4 days. Patients are allowed to shower on the day after the surgical procedure, provided they keep the wound covered. The first postoperative office visit is arranged at 3 to 5 days. We perform an evaluation of the wound, change the dressing, and schedule the rehabilitation program.

Technical Pitfalls

Difficulties in Harvesting the Graft

In attempting to harvest the patellar tendon graft, the circular saw may start to advance too deeply and may lacerate the tendon. This can be avoided by gently redirecting the saw; however, sudden changes in direction can fracture the plug. Switching to a larger-diameter saw or using an osteotome to complete the harvest can minimize this problem.

Problems with the Femoral Screw Guide Wire

If the guide wire for the femoral screw is inserted too deeply, it may be difficult to extract, or it may break. Failure to place the guide wire directly between the bone plug and osseous tunnel wall may misdirect the screw and thus compromise interference fixation. Many of the newer screwdrivers have detachable handles that allow removal of the guide wire soon after the screw is engaged.

Blowout of the Posterior Wall of the Femoral Tunnel

It is important to check for blowout of the posterior wall of the femoral tunnel because it may preclude endoscopic femoral interference fixation. If blowout does occur, the procedure should be converted to the two-incision technique, with the interference screw inserted laterally. Alternately, Endo-button fixation could be considered. The risk of blowout during femoral drilling is minimized by flexing the patient's knee to 70 degrees or more.

Problems with the Tibial Interference Screw

Two problems with the tibial interference screw may result in graft laxity. First, the screw can push the tibial bone plug into the tunnel, with resulting loss of tension on the graft. This is best avoided by maintaining tension on the bone plug sutures and watching the position of the plug as the screw is inserted. Second, the soft medullary bone of the tibia may result in inadequate interference fixation. A feeling for good interference fixation develops with increased resistance with turns of the screwdriver. If the tibial fixation is believed to be inadequate, a larger-diameter interference screw may be used, or the sutures can be tied over a post or a bone bridge.

Graft Protrusion

If the tibial plug protrudes from the tibial tunnel, distal interference fixation may not be possible. This can be avoided by matching the length of the graft and osseous tunnels, as described earlier. Small discrepancies may sometimes still exist, requiring some adjustments. Shortening of the bone plugs by 2 to 3 mm or deepening the femoral tunnel by 3 to 5 mm can compensate for a small difference. If necessary, the graft sutures can be tied around a screw-and-washer fixation post.

REHABILITATION

We routinely perform ACL reconstruction in all age groups on an outpatient basis. A knee immobilizer is worn for 2 to 4 weeks during ambulation and sleep. Weight bearing is allowed as tolerated, and crutches are recommended until adequate muscular control of the knee and lower extremity is regained. Rehabilitation therapy is commenced within the first postoperative week. Emphasis is placed on regaining knee extension and muscle strengthening. Our goal is to achieve full knee motion, without effusion, by 2 months postoperatively. Patients who fail to achieve the desired goals by 2 months deserve special attention to determine why they have not made satisfactory progress. We have a close working relationship with physical therapists, and they alert us if any problems develop. Our standard rehabilitation protocol after ACL reconstruction is shown in Table 23.1. The patient's return to specific activities is guided by the surgeon and the therapist.

RESULTS

The long-term satisfactory results in terms of functional stability, symptom relief, and return to preinjury level of activity have been reported to be between 75% and 90% (28–31). Many factors influence the outcome of ACL reconstruction including the integrity of the secondary restraints, the preoperative knee laxity, the status of the articular and meniscal cartilages, graft selection, surgical technique, postoperative rehabilitation, and the motivation and expectation of the patient (32–34).

There is no universally accepted definition of an unsatisfactory outcome after ACL reconstruction. However, failure can be classified into one of the following categories: loss of motion, persistent pain, extensor mechanism dysfunction, or recurrent instability. The causes of failure include poor surgical technique, failure of graft incorporation, infection, arthrofibrosis, excessive or aggressive rehabilitation, postoperative trauma, and failure to treat a combined instability that involves damaged secondary restraints. Errors in surgical technique are probably the most common cause of graft failure. Technical errors include nonanatomic tunnel placement, graft impingement, improper graft tensioning, and inadequate graft fixation in the osseous tunnels (28).

COMPLICATIONS

As with any surgical treatment, there are inherent risks and potential complications. We can divide these risks into three major categories.

1. General complications of knee surgery
2. Specific complications of ACL reconstruction
3. Complications of graft procurement

The general complications of surgical procedures at the knee include hemarthrosis, hematoma, infection, thrombophlebitis or deep venous thrombosis, skin necrosis, nerve injury, vascular injury, tourniquet palsy, and reflex sympathetic dystrophy. When these complications occur, early recognition and treatment will minimize their long-term effects.

Failure of Anterior Cruciate Ligament Reconstruction

The specific complications relating to ACL reconstruction can be classified into one of the following categories:

1. Loss of motion
2. Recurrent instability
3. Patellofemoral dysfunction
4. Pain

Failure to regain full range of motion after ACL reconstruction can be related to surgical error in graft placement, arthrofibrosis, prolonged immobilization, or inadequate participation in a rehabilitation program. Early aggressive postoperative mobilization is helpful in preventing contractures. Most patients regain full range of motion within 6 to 8 weeks. If the range of motion plateaus postoperatively and does not respond to therapy, arthroscopic intervention and gentle manipulation may be indicated. We recommend considering operative intervention to our patients if full motion has not been regained by 3 months. The incidence of arthrofibrosis may be increased when reconstruction is performed immediately after injury. We prefer to delay reconstruction until after the acute postinjury inflammatory response has subsided and the knee has regained close to full range of motion. This may require a 1- to 3-week period in some patients. Postoperative loss of extension is a more difficult problem to treat than is loss of flexion. Even a 5- or 10-degree loss of extension can result in significant disability. The quadriceps muscles fatigue much more quickly if the patient's knee cannot lock during stance, and the condition causes the patient to ambulate with a relatively short leg gait. Flexion is usually easily regained with manipulation and arthroscopic lysis of adhesions.

Technical errors that affect the range of knee motion include anterior placement of the tibial tunnel, graft impingement, and improper tensioning of the graft. Accurate placement of the femoral tunnel is also important. If the femoral tunnel is sited too anteriorly, it may limit knee flexion, whereas if it is placed too far posteriorly, it can restrict knee extension. When the tibial tunnel is positioned too far anteriorly, the ACL graft may impinge against the intercondylar notch, thereby restricting knee extension. Over time, the notch has a guillotine effect on the graft and causes it to fail. An adequate notchplasty and careful selection of osseous tunnel sites will minimize the risk of impingement. A mechanical block to knee extension can also be the result of a *cyclops lesion,* an organized nodule of fibrous tissue located anterior to the tibial tunnel. Arthroscopic debridement of this lesion often restores knee extension. Overzealous tensioning of the graft in knee flexion is associated with a decreased range of motion. The knee flexion angle at the time of graft fixation is critical in preventing knee "capture." We prefer to fix the tibial bone plug with the knee in the last 10 degrees of extension to avoid overconstraining the joint.

Inadequate graft tensioning, conversely, produces a nonfunctioning graft that may lead to persistent instability.

TABLE 23.1 ANTERIOR CRUCIATE LIGAMENT RECONSTRUCTION REHABILITATION PROTOCOL[a]

Immobilization
  Knee immobilizer worn at night and when ambulating for 2–4 weeks
  Immobilizer discontinued by 4 weeks

Ambulation
  Two-crutch ambulation in the knee immobilizer allowed immediately with weight bearing as tolerated
  Crutches discontinued when quadriceps control is acquired and knee extension of 10 degrees or less is achieved

Range of motion
  Early range of motion (out of the knee immobilizer) encouraged
  Passive flexion to full extension with untreated leg assistance: immediate (as tolerated)
  Passive extension with weighted assistance: immediate (as tolerated)
  Patellar mobilization (as required)
  Stationary bicycle: begin at 3–4 weeks

Strength return[a]
Quadriceps
  Cocontraction with hams: immediate
  Leg raises: bent knee raise with cocontraction: weeks 2 to 6
  Knee dips with adduction squeeze: at 3 weeks
  Wall sits: 3 weeks
  Stairmaster: 4 weeks
  Set-up: 5 weeks
  Lunges: 8–10 weeks
  Step-down: 10–14 weeks

Hamstrings
  Ham sets/slides: first week
  Resisted ham curls: 2–3 weeks
  Resisted hip extension: 2–8 weeks
  Resisted hip flexion after 90 degrees knee flexion is achieved

Lower extremity conditioning
  Isometric abduction and adduction: 1–8 weeks
  Machine hip abduction and adduction: 3 weeks
  Calf strengthening after 90-degree knee flexion achieved
  Road bicycle if patient requests after 3 months

Functional exercises
  Weight shift: 1 week
  Weight shift on trampoline: 3 weeks
  One-leg bounce (supported): 4 weeks
  Walking and gait review: 4 weeks
  Slide board: 3 months

Return to activity[b]
  Jogging: 3–4 months
  Straight-line running: 4 months
  Directional changes/sport-specific adaptations: 4–6 months

[a] Emphasis is on closed-chain quadriceps exercises, which include use of Stairmaster, squat machines, leg press, and ski machines. Open-chain quadriceps isokinetic testing is not routinely performed. Effusions must be under control and the vastus medialis oblique functioning to progress quadriceps exercises.
[b] Return to sports and progression of the program requires timely return of motion (especially extension), quadriceps, and vastus medialis oblique control, and HOP test 85% of uninvolved limb.
From the Southern California Center for Sports Medicine, Long Beach, CA, with permission.

Initial graft fixation must be secure enough to prevent changes in graft tension before biologic fixation occurs in the tunnels. Interference screw fixation is usually replaced by bone-to-bone and aperture soft tissue healing by 6 weeks postoperatively. Aggressive rehabilitation protocols require stable fixation that permits immediate knee motion without compromising graft tension. Initial fixation strength depends on the type of graft, the gap or space between the graft and tunnel walls, the fixation device, and the bone quality at the fixation sites. We believe that documenting graft stability and knee motion at the conclusion of the surgical procedure is important. Graft failure can occur during the operation as a result of bone plug fracture, loss of fixation, or collagen avulsion. These perioperative complications are best recognized and remedied before the patient leaves the operating room.

Donor Site Morbidity

Harvesting the central third of the patella tendon for use as an autograft has been associated with donor site morbidity including patellar pain, patella fracture, and patellar tendon rupture. Reports of patellar pain range from 4% to 40% (35). The development of patella baja after complete closure of the tendon defect has been suggested as a possible reason for postharvest anterior knee pain. The incidence of patellar tendon rupture is low with or without closure of the tendon defect. Similarly, the incidence of patellar fracture at the time of surgery and during the first postoperative year is low, and bone grafting the donor site does not seem to affect outcome. Postoperative patellofemoral symptoms are minimized by early rehabilitation to regain range of motion and muscle strength. Overall, it appears that the functional deficit associated with patellar tendon harvest is relatively minor and, if present, usually resolves after 3 to 6 months. Patellofemoral dysfunction after ACL reconstruction may be the result of trauma at the time of ACL injury. It may also be contributed to by the nature of the reconstructive surgery itself, or the rehabilitation program, rather than directly caused by graft harvest (36–42).

One of the advantages of the hamstring tendon graft is the avoidance of interference with the knee extensor mechanism. Despite removing the tendon for the medial muscular stabilizers of the knee, the functional deficit after semitendinosus and gracilis tendon harvest seems to be minimal. It has been reported that hamstring strength is restored to around 95% of preoperative values, and there is evidence of a postharvest scar formation in the semitendinosus–gracilis region that resembles a "neotendon" (43,44).

Nerve injury may also occur during autograft harvest. One common problem is injury to one of the infrapatellar branches of the saphenous nerve. Although often considered a single branch, this plexus of sensory nerves crosses over the patellar tendon and is difficult to avoid. We warn patients that there may be a small area of numbness over the lateral aspect of the proximal tibia. We also warn them about the possibility that a neuroma may form, but we rarely encounter it postoperatively. Direct injury to the saphenous nerve is more likely related to hamstring tendon harvest, but the risk may be reduced with knee flexion during graft harvest to relax the nerve and blunt dissection to free the tendons before passage of the tendon stripper.

GRAFT SELECTION

The lack of any single graft that meets all the surgeon's desired criteria has led to the use of various grafts for ACL reconstruction, each with its own advantages and disadvantages (9,45). Because of the unfavorable results of synthetic ligament replacements, biologic tissue grafts (autografts or allografts) have remained the most widely used grafts. The use of autograft minimizes the risk of disease transmission, delayed incorporation, adverse inflammatory reactions, and potential antigenicity problems and reduces the cost of the procedure, whereas allograft avoids donor site morbidity, decreases surgical time, and may diminish postoperative pain during the first month (45).

The process of graft incorporation includes graft necrosis, revascularization, cellular repopulation, collagen deposition, and matrix remodeling (46). This "ligamentization" process is influenced by the graft source, host response, and the biomechanical loading of the graft during rehabilitation. The rate of graft incorporation also depends on the type of graft material and on the method of fixation. The biologic healing response should be respected during the design of rehabilitation programs and when making the decision about when the patient can resume normal activities.

Autografts

Autograft tissue from the same person is harvested from the patient at the time of surgical reconstruction. Using the patient's own tissue avoids the risks of disease transmission and immunogenic reaction and is currently the most popular graft choice. Sources of tissue include the patella tendon, hamstring tendons (semitendinosus–gracilis), and quadriceps tendon. The concern common to all autografts is that of donor site morbidity.

The most commonly used graft today is the patella tendon, and it is our graft of choice. The bone–patella tendon–bone complex has high ultimate strength (2,300 N) and stiffness 620 N/mm) that allow for a more predictable restoration of knee stability. Bone-to-bone interference screw fixation provides a solid fixation with rapid graft incorporation, and this facilitates an accelerated rehabilitation that consistently achieves satisfactory results. However, compared with other sources of autograft, donor site morbidity is reported to be more frequent. Complications after patella tendon harvesting include patellar fracture, tendon rupture, patella baja, anterior knee pain, and quadriceps weakness. The use of an alternative autograft may be favorable in the patient with extensor mechanism maltracking, patellofemoral osteoarthritis, or previous patella tendon harvest.

Attention has shifted more recently to the use of hamstring tendon graft with its relatively low donor site morbidity and smaller surgical incisions. The technique has involved double-, triple-, and quadruple-strand semitendinosus–gracilis tendon graft, which has an ultimate tensile strength as high as 4,000 N. The results with hamstring reconstruction are comparable to those obtained with patella tendon autograft (47,48). The disadvantages of this soft tissue graft include the lack of rigid bony fixation for early aggressive rehabilitation and return to full activity. Complications after hamstring harvesting include altered hamstring function, sartorius nerve injury, and tendon transection.

The quadriceps tendon graft has become an alternative replacement graft, especially for revision ACL surgery, and for use in reconstructing knees with multiple ligament injuries that require grafts. It has a comparable ultimate tensile strength to patella tendon, but its donor site morbidity is reported to be somewhat less.

Allografts

The types of allografts harvested from human donors to reconstruct the ACL include patellar tendon, Achilles tendon, quadriceps tendon, and tibialis anterior tendon. Allografts are particularly useful when reconstructing multiple ligament injuries in the same knee. The advantages of using allograft tissue include shorter surgical time, reduced surgical morbidity, smaller incisions, and the ability to shape and prepare the graft in a unique manner in comparison with what can be done with autografts. Disadvantages include increased financial cost, the risk of disease transmission, and slower incorporation of the graft (45,49).

Xenografts

Donor graft tissue from a different species is a potential source of collagen that can be preshaped and stored at a lower cost than allografts. The main disadvantage at this time is immune reactivity to the antigens associated with residual cell fragments, membranes, and matrix molecules. These problems may be reduced by future technologies in biocleansing. Xenograft sources include porcine small intestinal submucosa (SIS graft), demineralized bone, and bovine tendon and ligament.

Synthetic Ligaments

Prosthetic devices used for ACL replacement have a relatively high failure rate as a result of fatigue, abrasion, and particulate debris. In addition, chronic effusion, synovitis, and osteolysis have made many synthetic grafts undesirable. There are limited, if any, current indications for using prosthetic ligament substitutes based on their financial cost and long-term outcomes.

CONCLUSIONS

Arthroscopic management of ACL injuries has gradually evolved to its present state. Skilled surgeons have used their experience and knowledge to refine the instrumentation and techniques to allow widespread use. Previous problems with postoperative lack of full range of motion and graft impingement or failure have decreased in incidence as tunnel placement has become better defined. Improved fixation devices have allowed smaller incisions to be used regardless of graft type. These refinements have resulted in less operative morbidity, shorter hospitalization, and faster, more predictable postoperative rehabilitation.

Re-creation of the functions of the normal ACL remains an elusive goal. Current reconstructions have been able to provide a check-rein function to restore stability, but true isometry and proprioceptive feedback are still lacking. With further refinements, the goal of restoring patients to normal preinjury function may yet be attained.

REFERENCES

1. Odensteim M, Gillquist J. Functional anatomy of the anterior cruciate ligament and rationale for surgery. *J Bone Joint Surg Am* 1985;67:257–262.
2. Arnoczky SP, Matyas JR, Buckwalter JA, et al. Anatomy of the anterior cruciate ligament. In: Jackson DW, ed. *The anterior cruciate ligament: current and future concepts.* New York: Raven Press, 1993:5–22.
3. Miyasaka KC, Daniel DM, Stone ML. The incidence of knee ligament injuries in the general population. *Am J Knee Surg* 1991; 4:43–48.
4. Johnson DL, Warner JJP. Diagnosis for anterior cruciate ligament surgery. *Clin Sports Med* 1993;12:671–684.
5. Brown CH, Carson EW. Revision anterior cruciate ligament surgery. *Clin Sports Med* 1999;18:109–171.
6. Daniel DM. Selecting patients for ACL surgery. In: Jackson DW, ed. *The anterior cruciate ligament: current and future concepts.* New York: Raven Press, 1993:251–258.
7. Hirshman HP, Daniel DM, Miyasaka K. The fate of unoperated knee ligament injuries. In: Daniel D, Akerson W, O'Connor J, eds. *Knee ligaments: structure, function, injury and repair.* New York: Raven Press, 1990:481–503.
8. Jackson RW. The torn ACL: Natural history of untreated lesions and rationale for selective treatment. In: Feagin JA, ed. *The cruciate ligaments,* 2nd ed. New York: Churchill Livingstone, 1994: 485–493.
9. Fu FH, Bennett CH, Lattermann C, et al. Current trends in anterior cruciate ligament reconstruction: part I. Biology and biomechanics of reconstruction. *Am J Sports Med* 1999;27: 821–830.
10. Murray MM, Martin SD, Martin TL, et al. Histological changes in the human anterior cruciate ligament after rupture. *J Bone Joint Surg Am* 2000;82:1387–1397.

11. Frank CB, Jackson DW. The science of reconstruction of the anterior cruciate ligament. *J Bone Joint Surg Am* 1997;79:1556–1576.
12. Daniel DM, Stone ML, Dobson BE, et al. Fate of the ACL-injured patient: a prospective outcome study. *Am J Sports Med* 1994;22:632–644.
13. Casteleyn PP, Handelburg F. Non-operative management of anterior cruciate ligament injuries in the general population. *J Bone Joint Surg Br* 1996;78:446–451.
14. Jackson DW, Jennings LD. Arthroscopically assisted reconstruction of the anterior cruciate ligament using a patella tendon bone autograft. *Clin Sports Med* 1988;7:785–800.
15. Schaeffer B, Gow W, Tibone JE. Graft-tunnel mismatch in endoscopic anterior cruciate ligament reconstruction: a new technique of intraarticular measurement and modified graft harvesting. *Arthroscopy* 1993;9:643–646.
16. Brown CH, Steiner ME, Carson EW. The use of hamstring tendons for anterior cruciate ligament reconstruction: technique and results. *Clin Sports Med* 1993;12:723–756.
17. Fulkerson JP, Langeland R. An alternate cruciate reconstruction graft: the central quadriceps tendon. *Arthroscopy* 1995;11:252–254.
18. Fineburg MS, Zarins B, Sherman OH. Practical considerations in anterior cruciate ligament replacement surgery. *Arthroscopy* 2000;16:715–724.
19. Welsh R. Knee joint structures and functions. *Clin Orthop* 1980;147:7.
20. Graf B. Isometric placement of substitutes for the anterior cruciate ligament. In: Jackson D, Drez D, eds. *The anterior cruciate deficient knee.* St. Louis: CV Mosby, 1987:55–71.
21. Jackson D, Gasser S. Tibial tunnel placement in ACL reconstruction. *Arthroscopy* 1994;10:124–131.
22. Yaru N, Daniel D, Pennar D. The effects of tibial attachment site on graft impingement in an anterior cruciate ligament reconstruction. *Am J Sports Med* 1992;20:217–220.
23. Jackson D, Shaefer R. Cyclops syndrome: loss of extension following intraarticular anterior cruciate ligament reconstruction. *Arthroscopy* 1990;6:171–178.
24. Marans HJ, Hendrix MR, Patterson RS. A new femoral drill guide for arthroscopy sutured anterior cruciate ligament placement. *Arthroscopy* 1992;8:234–238.
25. Brand J, Weiler A, Caborn DNM, et al. Graft fixation in cruciate ligament reconstruction. *Am J Sports Med* 2000; 28: 761–774.
26. Allen AD, Sitler MR, Marchetto P, et al. Assessment of the endoscopic semitendinosus/gracilis autograft procedure with interference screw fixation for reconstruction of the anterior cruciate ligament. *Orthopedics* 2001;24:347–353.
27. Weiler A, Richter M, Schmidmaier G, et al. The EndoPearl device increases fixation strength and eliminates construct slippage of hamstring grafts with interference screw fixation. *Arthroscopy* 2001;17:353–359.
28. Harner CD, Giffin JR, Dunteman RC, et al. Evaluation and treatment of recurrent instability after anterior cruciate ligament reconstruction. *J Bone Joint Surg Am* 2000;82:1652–1664.
29. O'Neill DB. Arthroscopically assisted reconstruction of the anterior cruciate ligament: a prospective randomized analysis of three techniques. *J Bone Joint Surg Am* 1996;78:803–813.
30. Shelbourne KD, Gray T. Anterior cruciate ligament reconstruction with autologous patellar tendon graft followed by accelerated rehabilitation: a two to nine year follow-up. *Am J Sports Med* 1997;25:786–795.
31. Bach BR, Tradonsky S, Bojchuk J, et al. Arthroscopically assisted anterior cruciate ligament reconstruction using patellar tendon autograft: five to nine year follow-up evaluation. *Am J Sports Med* 1998;26:20–29.
32. Johnson DL, Harner CD, Mayday MG, et al. Revision anterior cruciate ligament surgery. In: Fu FH, Harner CD, Vince KG, eds. *Knee surgery,* vol 1. Baltimore: Williams & Wilkins, 1994: 877–895.
33. Shelbourne KD, Gray T. Results of anterior cruciate ligament reconstruction based on meniscus and articular cartilage status at the time of surgery. *Am J Sports Med* 2000;28:446–452.
34. Murrell GAC, Maddali S, Horovitz L, et al. The effects of time course after anterior cruciate ligament injury in correlation with meniscal and cartilage loss. *Am J Sports Med* 2001;29:9–14.
35. Fu FH, Bennett CH, Ma CB, et al. Current trends in anterior cruciate ligament reconstruction: part II. Operative procedures and clinical correlations. *Am J Sports Med* 2000;28:124–130.
36. Shelbourne KD, Nitz P. Accelerated rehabilitation after anterior cruciate ligament surgery. *Am J Sports Med* 1992;18:292–299.
37. Shelbourne KD, Trumper RV. Preventing anterior knee pain after anterior cruciate ligament reconstruction. *Am J Sports Med* 1997;25:41–47.
38. Jarvela T, Paakkala T, Kannus P, et al. The incidence of patellofemoral osteoarthritis and associated findings 7 years after anterior cruciate ligament reconstruction with bone-patella tendon-bone autograft. *Am J Sports Med* 2001;29:18–24.
39. Eilerman M, Thomas J, Marsalka D. The effect of harvesting the central one third of the patellar tendon on patellofemoral contact pressure. *Am J Sports Med* 1992;20:738–741.
40. Lephart S, Kocher M, Harner C, et al. Quadriceps strength and functional capacity after anterior cruciate ligament reconstruction: patellar tendon autograft versus allograft. *Am J Sports Med* 1993;21:738–743.
41. Rosenberg T, Franklin J, Baldwin G, et al. Extensor mechanism function after patellar tendon graft harvest for anterior cruciate ligament reconstruction. *Am J Sports Med* 1992;20:519–526.
42. Shino K, Nakagawa S, Inoue M, et al. Deterioration of patellofemoral articular surfaces after anterior cruciate ligament reconstruction. *Am J Sports Med* 1993;21:206–211.
43. Simonian PT, Harrison SD, Cooley VJ, et al. Assessment of morbidity of semitendinosus and gracilis tendon harvest for ACL reconstruction. *Am J Knee Surg* 1997;10:54–59.
44. Rispoli DM, Sanders TG, Miller MD, et al. Magnetic resonance imaging at different time periods following hamstring harvest for anterior cruciate ligament reconstruction. *Arthroscopy* 2001;17: 2–8.
45. Tifford CD, Simon TM, Jackson DW. Graft selection for ligamentous reconstruction. In: *The adult knee.* Philadelphia, Lippincott Williams & Wilkins, 2001.
46. Amiel D, Kleiner JB, Roux RD, et al. The phenomenon of "ligamentization": anterior cruciate ligament reconstruction with autologous patellar tendon. *J Orthop Res* 1986;4:162–172.
47. Corry IS, Webb JM, Clingeleffer AJ, et al. Arthroscopic reconstruction of the anterior cruciate ligament: a comparison of patellar tendon autograft and four-strand hamstring tendon autograft. *Am J Sports Med* 1999;27:444–454.
48. Yumes M, Richmond JC, Engels EA, et al. Patellar versus hamstring tendons in anterior cruciate ligament reconstruction: a meta-analysis. *Arthroscopy* 2001;17:248–257.
49. Peterson RK, Shelton WR, Bomboy AL. Allograft versus autograft patellar tendon anterior cruciate ligament reconstruction: a 5-year follow-up. *Arthroscopy* 2001;17:9–13.

24

ARTHROSCOPIC TREATMENT OF THE POSTERIOR CRUCIATE LIGAMENT

J. ROBERT GIFFIN
CHRISTOPHER D. HARNER

Treatment algorithms for the management of posterior cruciate ligament (PCL) injuries continue to evolve. Long-term studies of patients with chronic PCL deficiency have shown that while many maintain a high level of function in spite of persistent laxity, some are predisposed to developing increased knee instability and degenerative changes over time. Although our present understanding of the "true" natural history of PCL injuries remains somewhat unclear, recent laboratory investigations have improved our understanding of the effects of PCL injury on knee function as well as provided a more scientific basis for reconstruction.

As our understanding of the anatomy and biomechanics of the PCL has continued to improve, the surgical techniques used to address reconstruction have evolved accordingly. While biomechanical studies have provided a more scientific rationale for tunnel placement and the selection of grafts, no single reconstruction technique has emerged as the consistent approach accepted among all surgeons. Most surgical series reported to date have limited numbers of patients and relatively short follow-ups. Reconstructive options that are currently in practice include single-bundle or double-bundle transtibial techniques, tibial onlay technique, or a combination of these techniques. A myriad of auto- and allograft materials have been utilized. This trend will likely continue until better prospective outcome studies are published in the literature. Finally, inconsistent results following PCL reconstruction reported commonly in the past may be attributed to clinicians' failing to recognize and treat associated injuries. Fortunately, the synergistic relationship between the PCL and posterolateral structures (PLS) has become better understood in recent years.

J. R. Giffin: Department of Orthopaedic Surgery, Fowler Kennedy Sport Medicine Clinic, University of Western Ontario, London, Ontario.

C. D. Harner: Section for Sports Medicine, University of Pittsburgh, Pittsburgh, Pennsylvania.

PATHOLOGY

Posterior cruciate ligament injuries are more common than previously thought. Injuries to the PCL have been reported to comprise approximately 3% of all knee injuries in the general population and as high as 37% in the trauma patients with acute hemarthroses (1–3). Furthermore, the setting in which the injury occurred has diagnostic and therapeutic implications, as 95% of the PCL injuries in the trauma setting have associated ligamentous injuries as well (2). By contrast, athletes suffer mainly isolated PCL injuries (4,5), although the overall incidence in this population remains unknown.

PCL injuries can be classified according to severity, timing, and associated injuries (6). Each of these variables affects treatment and outcome. Severity corresponds to the degree of laxity in the PCL, being either a partial (grades I or II) or a complete tear (grade III). This is typically determined by the physical examination. Isolated injuries, in general, may be successfully treated with rehabilitation (4,5,7–9). Combined injuries, however, have a more guarded prognosis. Better results may be possible in this group with early surgical intervention rather than with conservative treatment (6,10).

The distinction between the acute and chronic PCL-injured knee is somewhat arbitrary, but it is important, particularly for associated ligament injuries. In the acute setting, typically defined as within 3 weeks from injury, early surgery facilitates primary repair of associated collateral ligaments, the posteromedial corner (PMC), and PLS injuries. Chronic injuries may become associated with significant scar formation that limits the success of a delayed primary repair, and typically commits the surgeon to waiting a full 3 months to allow completion of the healing response before surgical reconstruction can be implemented. Furthermore, chronic injuries may become associated with significant pericapsular stretching, resulting in increased instability or the development of arthrosis. In these cases, it may be difficult to determine the extent of the initial injury as well as devise an optimal treatment plan.

Distinguishing between the isolated and combined PCL injuries is critical, because the prognosis and treatment can be vastly different. Isolated injuries typically represent partial PCL disruptions. While grade III PCL tears can occur in isolation, most occur as part of a combined ligament injury pattern, typically involving the PLS (2,6,11). Many other combined PCL injury patterns are possible; however, the importance lies in the proper identification of this multiligament injured group.

CLINICAL EVALUATION

Evaluation of a patient with an injured knee begins with obtaining a detailed history; the physician should delineate the mechanism and severity of injury, as well as possible associated injuries. Unlike patients with isolated ACL tears, patients with acute, isolated PCL injuries do not typically relate a sense of instability. They may complain of knee pain, swelling, and stiffness, but this is usually only of mild severity. Chronic injuries involving the PCL can cause disability ranging from almost no functional limitations to severe limitations during activities of daily living (4,5,12–14). In general, patients with isolated injuries of the PCL tend to function at higher levels than patients with other associated ligamentous injuries (15).

After observation of the patient's stance and gait, a thorough knee examination is essential and should include evaluation of range of motion, palpation, ligamentous examination, and specialized testing. Assessment for meniscal damage or other ligamentous injury, aside from the PCL, should be routinely performed. Special care must be undertaken when evaluating the anterior cruciate ligament (ACL) in the setting of a PCL-insufficient knee. The noninvolved knee must be examined first to determine the normal relationship of the tibia to the femur, since, in the PCL-injured knee, the tibia will sublux posteriorly. Once this subluxation is manually corrected in the injured knee, standard anterior drawer and Lachman tests can be performed. Despite the increased awareness of PCL injuries, they are still frequently missed at the initial evaluation.

The most accurate clinical test to assess PCL integrity is the posterior drawer test (7,16). The patient is placed supine and the knee is flexed to 90 degrees while a posteriorly directed force is placed on the proximal tibia. The extent of translation is evaluated by noting the change in the distance of step-off between the medial tibial plateau and the medial femoral condyle. Equally important during this test is to assess the quality of the endpoint. Normally, the tibial plateau is positioned approximately 1 cm anterior to the femoral condyle, but this can vary, making examination of the contralateral knee essential. PCL injury can be graded with respect to the amount of laxity determined by this test. Grade I is classified as <5 mm of posterior tibial displacement as demonstrated by excessive posterior translation with main-

tenance of an anterior step-off. Grade II is classified as a 5- to 10-mm translation corresponding to the plateau being displaced flush to the level of, but not posterior to the femoral condyle. Both of these grades represent partial tears of the PCL. More than 10 mm of translation constitutes a grade III injury, with the plateau displaced posterior to the condyle, and is consistent with a complete tear of the PCL. The degree of sagittal translation should also be assessed with the knee flexed 30 degrees. A slight increase in translation at 30 degrees and not at 90 degrees of flexion may indicate a PLS injury; increased sagittal translation at both 30 and 90 degrees, with maximal translation at 90 degrees of knee flexion, is consistent with a PCL injury. The posterior sag test, performed with the hip and knee flexed to 90 degrees, may provide additional information in evaluating the PCL. With a complete PCL tear, the pull of gravity will displace the tibia posterior to the femur while the examiner supports the weight of the limb by the foot.

Proper evaluation of the PCL is not complete unless all the other ligamentous structures of the knee are evaluated, especially the PLS. This can be difficult with the tibia subluxed posteriorly as in a grade III PCL injury, and so manually reducing the tibia to neutral is essential (7,17). Testing for the PLS is best performed with the patient positioned prone while an external rotation force is applied to tibia at 30 and 90 degrees. The degree of external rotation is measured by comparing the medial border of the foot to the axis of the femur. Since wide variability of external rotation is possible at these positions, it is essential to compare the results to the contralateral side (15,18). More than a 10-degree difference is considered abnormal (18). The popliteus complex portion of the PLS is the primary restraint to external rotation at all degrees of knee flexion but its effect is maximal at 30 degrees. An increase of 10 degrees or more of external rotation at 30 degrees of knee flexion, but not at 90 degrees, is considered diagnostic of an isolated PLS injury (19). On the other hand, the PCL is the secondary restraint to external rotation when the knee is at 90 degrees of flexion (18,20,21). Increased external rotation at both flexion angles indicates that a combined injury may be present. The recognition of this posterolateral instability component is imperative, since it may significantly affect treatment.

Varus and valgus stress tests are important in assessing the integrity of the LCL portion of the PLS as well as the medial collateral ligament (MCL). These should be performed with the knee both in full extension and in 30 degrees of flexion. Isolated PCL injury does not significantly affect varus or valgus stability. Increased varus opening at 30 degrees of knee flexion indicates an injury to the LCL and possibly the popliteus complex. An additional slight increased opening also at full extension is consistent with injuries to both of these structures. If there is a large degree of varus opening at full extension, a combined injury of the PLS, PCL, and/or the ACL may be present (18,20–24). Increased valgus laxity at 30 degrees indicates injury to the

MCL, while increased valgus laxity in full extension indicates additional injury to the posteromedial corner.

The evaluation of gait and limb alignment is particularly important for patients with chronic PCL injuries. In this situation, the stabilizers of the posterior and possibly the lateral knee may not be functioning optimally (17,25). This may lead to a combination of excessive posterior translation, posterolateral rotation, and varus thrust in the stance phase of gait (25). Varus malalignment may also accentuate this dynamic instability pattern. If unrecognized during the evaluation, these factors may aversely affect the result of PCL reconstruction.

Imaging

Standard anteroposterior (AP) and lateral radiographs are an essential part of the diagnostic evaluation. The films must also be carefully scrutinized for both tibial subluxation and associated bone injuries particularly involving the PCL (Fig. 24.1). These can be very subtle findings, but when recognized and repaired acutely, have resulted in a good outcome (26,27). Stress and contralateral views, although not routine, may be helpful in some situations (28,29). Finally, in the setting of a chronic injury, flexion weight-bearing and full-length lower extremity films are also necessary to determine the presence of arthritis or malalignment, which can affect management decisions.

Magnetic resonance imaging (MRI) has become the diagnostic study of choice in evaluating the knee with a presumed PCL injury. This study is 96% to 100% sensitive in detecting tears of the PCL and can also determine the pre-

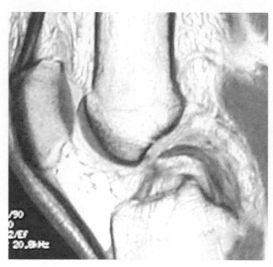

FIGURE 24.2 Magnetic resonance imaging (MRI) showing "peel-off" of the femoral attachment of the PCL, with hemorrhage throughout the rest of the ligament.

cise location of the tear, with implications for treatment (30–32). For example, the femoral "peel-off" injury is particularly amenable to primary repair (33,34) (Fig. 24.2). The MRI can be used to assess the menisci, articular surfaces, and other ligaments of the knee, which also have relevance to treatment and prognosis. The addition of a coronal oblique technique aligned along the axis of the popliteus tendon may prove to be of further assistance in evaluating this region (35).

A bone scan may prove helpful in the evaluation and management of the chronic PCL injured knee. Patients with long-standing PCL injuries are predisposed to early medial and patellofemoral compartment chondrosis (8,16,36). In the setting of an isolated PCL-deficient knee with medial and/or patellofemoral compartment pain and normal radiographs, a bone scan to assess these compartments may be helpful. If there is increased uptake, then surgical intervention may be beneficial (10). If there is no increased uptake, then a continued nonoperative approach has been our treatment of choice.

TREATMENT OPTIONS

Despite recent advances in PCL research, controversy still exists with respect to the definite indications for surgical intervention for the PCL-injured knee. The treatment protocol depends on many factors. Selecting the best option must take both patient and injury factors into consideration. While the location, timing, severity, and extent of associated injuries are important prognostic factors, the patient's age, occupation, health, and expectations play an equally important role in the decision-making process. While investiga-

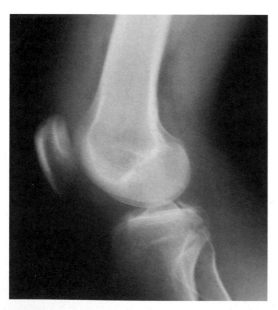

FIGURE 24.1 Lateral radiograph revealing a relatively subtle bony avulsion of the tibial insertion of the posterior cruciate ligament (PCL).

tors have been unable to consistently identify prognostic factors to help predict which patients will develop long-term disability, indications for surgical management are becoming better defined.

The general consensus at present is that most acute, isolated partial PCL injuries (grades I and II) do not require surgical intervention (4–10,13,14). The likely benign course of these injuries is related to the remaining integrity both of the secondary restraints and of various portions of the PCL (6). Furthermore, these partial tears have been shown to have a strong propensity to heal (37). Our current treatment schema for acute, presumed isolated PCL injuries is presented in Table 24.1. Chronic residual posterior laxity may occur if these injuries are not treated appropriately, causing the ligament to heal in an elongated position (38). Therefore, the initial treatment of partial PCL injuries should consist of protected weight bearing, the use of a knee immobilizer or brace with drop-lock hinges, and a quadriceps and triceps surae rehabilitation program to counteract posterior tibial subluxation. Closed kinetic chain quadriceps and gastroc-soleus strengthening are favored through an arc from 0 to 60 degrees of flexion to limit the stresses on the healing PCL.

The nonoperative course for isolated, complete tears of the PCL (grade III) has not been as predictable in the acute setting. This is likely due to inadequate healing of unrecognized associated capsular injuries. Because of the significant risk of an associated PLS injury, most authors would recommend 2 to 4 weeks of immobilization in full extension. This minimizes the posterior displacing effect of both gravity and the hamstrings on the tibia and allows the PLS injury, if present, to heal with less stress (6). Following the period of immobilization, a similar rehabilitation protocol is followed. Unfortunately, many of these injuries do not heal, and over time these patients may develop symptoms secondary to increased shear stresses to the articular cartilage, especially in the medial and patellofemoral compartments (5,8,10,16,39,40). Thus surgery has been recommended for these patients, especially if they continue to be symptomatic

despite maximizing physical therapy, as current surgical techniques can potentially improve stability and diminish pain.

Grade III PCL injuries, when combined with other major ligament disruptions, have not done well with nonoperative management. This has led to current treatment regimens that encourage early PCL reconstruction with appropriate repair and/or reconstruction of the associated injuries (Table 24.1). While the complexity of the PLS and the less than optimal results when PLS reconstruction is delayed necessitate early repair of PLS injuries, the MCL may be more forgiving. Similar to current ACL/MCL treatment regimes, which suggest protection in a brace to allow MCL healing, prior to delayed ACL reconstruction, acute PCL/MCL injuries may be considered for delayed PCL reconstruction. The knee is immobilized near full extension, with radiographic confirmation that there is no posterior tibial subluxation (a true lateral radiograph must confirm this) for 2 to 4 weeks, prior to mobilization and rehabilitation in preparation for PCL reconstruction (41).

The literature suggests that patients with persistent symptoms after adequate therapy for an isolated grade III PCL injury likely have an occult, concomitant ligamentous injury, particularly involving the PLS (3,6,15,42). These combined injuries have a more guarded prognosis and should be treated surgically (6,10,15). Depending on the severity, this particular combination can lead to significant disability (43). Therefore, we would recommend a PLS reconstruction in conjunction with the PCL reconstruction. When a coexistent PLS injury is overlooked, surgical treatment of the PCL may have a higher risk of failure (44).

In the chronic situation, symptoms from PCL laxity are typically pain and swelling, indicative of articular surface injury, or instability due to combined laxities. Our treatment schema for chronic PCL insufficiency is presented in Table 24.2. Careful attention to alignment is crucial, particularly when there is PCL and PLS laxity in the varus knee. Osteotomy to correct the malalignment is necessary, or the soft tissue reconstruction will fail.

TABLE 24.1 ACUTE POSTERIOR CRUCIATE LIGAMENT (PCL) INJURY

	Isolated		Combined
Grade I	4 to 6 weeks of limited activity, quadriceps strengthening, and proprioceptive training	PCL and LCL or PLS	PCL reconstruction with repair/augmentation capsular structures within 2 to 3 weeks
Grade II	4 to 6 weeks of limited activity, quadriceps strengthening, and proprioceptive training	PCL and MCL	PCL reconstruction with repair/augmentation capsular structures within 2 to 3 weeks. Possible brace, then PCL reconstruction (see text)
Grade III	Brace in extension × 4 weeks, then rehab as above. Surgery if "peel-off" or young athlete	PCL and ACL, med./lat. corner, disloc. knee	PCL reconstruction with repair/augmentation capsular structures within 2 to 3 weeks

ACL, anterior cruciate ligament; MCL, medial collateral ligament; PLS, posterolateral structure.

TABLE 24.2 CHRONIC PCL LAXITY

	Isolated		Combined
Grade I	Quadriceps rehab Activity modification	PCL and LCL or PLS	PCL reconstruction with reconstruction of capsular structures
Grade II	Quadriceps rehab Activity modification	PCL and MCL	PCL reconstruction with reconstruction of capsular structures
Grade III	Quadriceps rehab Activity modification Surgery if symptomatic or positive bone scan	PCL and ACL, med./lat. corner	PCL/ACL reconstruction with reconstruction of capsular structures

SURGICAL TECHNIQUE

Current PCL reconstructive techniques continue to evolve but should adhere to basic principles:

1. All associated pathology must be identified and treated.
2. The risk of neurovascular injury must be minimized.
3. An adequately strong graft should be placed anatomically, appropriately tensioned, and rigidly fixed.
4. Prepare for prolonged rehabilitation and delayed return to athletics.

To ensure optimal surgical outcome, the surgeon must be familiar with and capable of performing the repair or reconstruction options for the PCL as well as those of the collateral and capsular structures. Our surgical approach depends on which structures are injured. This is typically determined by the information obtained from the preoperative examination, imaging studies. and, most importantly, the examination under anesthesia. This is valuable not only for confirming the PCL injury but also for assessing the other potentially injured structures. These cases should be performed in a semi-elective setting with a skilled operating room staff. In addition, because of the proximity of the vessels to the tibial PCL graft placement, a vascular surgeon should be readily available.

Operating Room Setup

The patient is positioned supine on the operating table and an examination under anesthesia is performed. The setup should permit the operative knee to be taken through a full range of motion. It is important to completely define all ligamentous injuries and range of motion. Special attention is focused on the collateral ligaments in combined injury patterns, as injuries to these structures will generally determine the placement of surgical incisions. We use the contralateral knee for comparison. A well-padded tourniquet is applied to the upper thigh, but it is usually not inflated. A Foley catheter may be placed if significant capsular surgery with a prolonged operative time is anticipated, and a Doppler ultrasound is used to confirm the distal pulses at the start and finish of the procedure.

Role of Arthroscopy

To decrease the amount of surgical dissection, arthroscopic techniques are utilized as much as possible using standard arthroscopy portals. Arthroscopy is utilized to confirm the extent of the injury and, furthermore, to assist with the repair or reconstructive procedure whenever possible. However, it is not always possible (*or safe*) to use arthroscopy in the acute or subacute setting because of capsular disruption. Sufficient capsular healing needs to have occurred (~2 weeks) in order to maintain joint distention and avoid developing an iatrogenic compartment syndrome. In these cases, the procedure is usually begun using gravity flow or a fluid pump (low-pressure setting), and the thigh and calf must be palpated prior to as well as intermittently throughout the procedure to monitor for fluid extravasation. If extravasation is noted, the arthroscopic procedure is discontinued and the remainder of the procedure is performed using an open technique. The arthroscope, however, can still be extremely valuable, improving visualization and magnification in a "dry" field as various portions of the procedure are performed through mini-arthrotomies.

Arthroscopic examination is carried out through anteromedial and anterolateral portals using a 30-degree arthroscope. The typical findings in a PCL-deficient knee are a soft and/or scarred PCL with a lax, but otherwise normal-appearing ACL, due to the posterior tibial subluxation (Fig. 24.3). Drawing the tibia forward will restore normal tension to the ACL.

Repair vs. Reconstruction

The decision to repair or reconstruct a torn ligament depends on a number of factors. MRI is particularly helpful in determining which structures are repairable and which must be reconstructed. In general, repairs are not as strong as reconstructions, and modification of the postoperative protocols must reflect this difference.

Unfortunately, as with ACL injuries, primary repair of midsubstance PCL tears has not been consistently successful (45). The exception is cases of PCL bony or ligament insertion avulsions, where repair of these injuries typically results

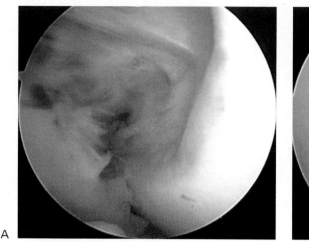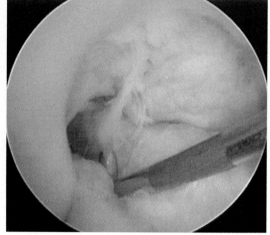

FIGURE 24.3 A: Arthroscopic view demonstrates a scarred, ghost-like PCL in this right knee. **B:** The anterior cruciate ligament (ACL) in the same knee is lax to probing, but normal in appearance, confirming the PCL laxity.

in a favorable outcome (25,45–47). Several surgical approaches can be utilized depending on other associated ligament and meniscal injuries that may require treatment and include the posteromedial, posterolateral, and posterior approach to the knee as well as all arthroscopic techniques (46–48). In addition, various fixation methods have been described and depend on the size of the bony fragment. For large avulsion fragments, AO screws can be used, whereas smaller fragments can be stabilized with Kirschner wires or tension band wiring, or by suture repair through drill holes.

Techniques of Reconstruction

Several different methods have been developed for PCL repair or reconstruction, emphasizing the fact that no current technique has met with reproducibly excellent results. Most surgeons now agree that restoration of normal anatomy yields the best potential for consistent results after PCL reconstruction (6,23,49). Numerous variables exist, including graft choice, type of fixation, tunnel placement, as well as inlay versus tibial tunnel techniques. The two most commonly employed reconstructive techniques of today are the transtibial tunnel and the tibial inlay techniques. Both are reviewed here. While Harner et al. (50) have shown that a double-bundle construct has the best chance of reproducing the biomechanics of the PCL *in vitro*, clinical studies have not confirmed improved results of this technique over single-bundle reconstructions *in vivo*.

Graft Choices and Fixation Methods

A variety of tissues have been used for knee reconstructions (51). Autologous tissues typically used today include patellar, hamstring, or quadriceps tendon. Achilles tendon, patellar tendon, and tibialis anterior tendon are the most commonly used allograft tissues. Several studies have documented by arthroscopy and histologic methods that the transplanted allograft tendons revascularize, undergo cellular repopulation and reach maturity just as autograft tissue does, although this process may take longer with the allograft tissue (52–54).

Mixed results have been reported using the various types of grafts. However, this difference may be strictly dependent on the technique utilized and not necessarily related to the graft type. We continue to favor Achilles tendon allograft because of its high tensile strength, shorter operating time, ease of passage, and lack of donor-site morbidity in an already compromised knee. Additional benefits include its exceptional size and length and bony attachment at one end, making it quite versatile when compared to other graft options.

Multiple methods of fixation also exist, including metal and bio-interference screws, buttons, cortical screws and soft tissue washers, or staples (55). No single technique is universally accepted. We prefer to use a screw and soft tissue washer when securing soft tissue to bone in most instances, as this has been shown to be the most stable fixation (56). The treating surgeon should be familiar with several of these options so that the final choice can depend on the surgical situation.

Tunnel Placement and Graft Tensioning

Biomechanical studies support reconstruction of the anterolateral bundle when performing single-bundle technique (6,57–59) (Fig. 24.4). Anterior placement of the femoral tunnel in the anatomic footprint has been shown to restore normal knee laxity better than isometric graft placement (57,60). Variations in tibial tunnel placement affect graft behavior to a lesser degree than variations in femoral tunnel placement (61,62). Furthermore, the position in which the

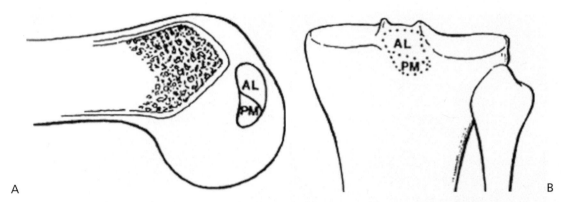

A   B

FIGURE 24.4 A: Femoral attachment sites of the main components, anterolateral bundle (AL) and posteromedial bundle (PM), are indicated schematically. **B:** Tibial insertion sites of the main components, AL and PM, are indicated schematically.

nonisometric graft is tensioned and fixed has a significant effect on knee mechanics (63). The surgeon should tension the anterolateral bundle at 90 degrees of knee flexion under an applied anterior drawer, since tensioning in full extension may lead to graft failure or overconstraint of the knee and eventual loss of flexion (57,63).

Single-Bundle Reconstruction

The single-bundle technique was developed to reconstruct the anterolateral bundle because of its larger size and greater biomechanical properties when compared with the posteromedial bundle (6,7,64,65). In an attempt to place the graft in the anatomic position of the native anterolateral bundle, single tibial and femoral tunnels are utilized. Several studies have attempted to determine the optimum femoral tunnel position for reconstructing the anterolateral PCL bundle (58,59,62,66–68). We believe that reproduction of the normal anatomy is the ideal location with anterior placement of the tunnel in the anatomic anterolateral bundle footprint of the femur (Fig. 24.4). Good results have been reported using this technique along with tensioning of the graft in 90 degrees of knee flexion with an anterior drawer force (57,63).

Similarly, studies have been conducted to determine the optimal tibial tunnel placement for PCL reconstruction (58,59,61,69,70). While transtibial drilling techniques from the anteromedial tibia creates the so-called killer curve, this has not been a problem in our experience. Nonetheless, techniques have been developed to limit this graft angulation using a posterolateral tibial tunnel (71) as well as the tibial inlay technique (see below).

Authors' Preferred Surgical Technique (Single Bundle)

At our institution, we use a single-bundle reconstruction using Achilles tendon allograft in acute PCL injuries. An examination under anesthesia confirms an isolated PCL defi-

ciency with no evidence of posterolateral or posteromedial insufficiency. We then proceed with arthroscopy, addressing any associated meniscal pathology. The injured PCL is debrided, leaving a remnant of the tibial and femoral attachments, and preserving the meniscofemoral ligaments whenever possible (Fig. 24.5). We utilized an accessory posteromedial arthroscopic portal and a 70-degree arthroscope for improved visualization (72). Curved 90 degrees, over-the-back instruments are made by a number of commercial companies, and facilitate the exposure of the PCL tibial footprint.

The tibia is exposed anteromedially through a 3-cm incision that begins at the same level as the proximal tibial tubercle. Passage of the guide pin requires a PCL drill guide that has a shield to reduce the chance of penetration by the guide pin into the popliteal space. The use of image intensification when passing the guide pin facilitates this step, or an acceptable alternative is to obtain a lateral radiograph after passage of the pin, to ascertain appropriate placement, low-

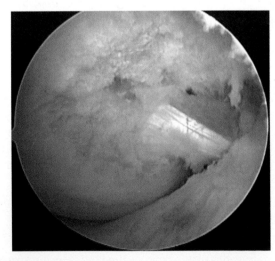

FIGURE 24.5 Arthroscopic view of the left knee femoral PCL attachment demonstrates a well-preserved meniscofemoral ligament of Wrisberg.

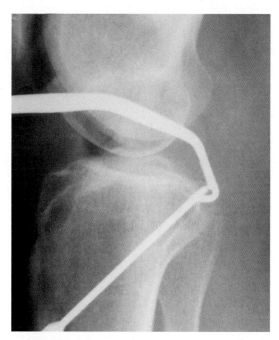

FIGURE 24.6 Intraoperative lateral radiograph demonstrates the tibial guide pin in an appropriate position. The shield of the guide does offer some protection of the popliteal contents, but this step still requires extreme care.

in the PCL tibial footprint (Fig. 24.6). Fanelli (41) has described a posterior medial "safety incision," which allows the surgeon to place a finger between the popliteal vessels and the site of penetration of the tibial posterior cortex by the guide pin and drill. This is another strategy that can be used to protect the popliteal structures (Fig. 24.7). Once the correct location of the tibial guide pin has been confirmed, drilling the tibial tunnel is done under direct arthroscopic visualization with the knee flexed to 90 degrees and a curette placed over the guide pin to prevent its proximal migration into the popliteal space. Drilling the tibial tunnel is begun with power and completed by hand to minimize the penetration of the drill-bit as the hole is completed. The C-arm may be utilized at the surgeon's preference. The tibial tunnel is drilled carefully to a 10-mm diameter, followed by an 11-mm tunnel dilator. A rasp must be used to circumscribe the superior edge of the drill hole into the joint to reduce abrasion on the graft.

A guide pin is then placed in the footprint of the anterolateral bundle of the PCL on the femur through the anterolateral arthroscopy portal at the 1 o'clock position in a right knee, 6 mm off of the articular margin. Visualization is via the arthroscope in the anteromedial portal. This pin should angle away from the articular surface to reduce the risk of avascular necrosis (AVN) of the femoral condyle from disruption of the blood supply. The femoral tunnel is then hand drilled to an 11-mm diameter with a depth of 30 mm. We then drill a 3.2-mm hole in the end of the tunnel out of the anteromedial femur. The Achilles tendon allograft has

previously been prepared on the back table to fit an 11-mm tunnel and whipstitched with No. 5 braided nonabsorbable suture. An 18-gauge wire loop is placed up through the tibial tunnel, into the knee, and pulled out of the anterolateral arthroscopic portal to be used to retrieve the tendon through the tibial tunnel. A Beath pin is then placed from the anterolateral arthroscopic portal through the femoral tunnel and out of the anteromedial thigh and skin. The bone plug suture is placed through the Beath needle and pulled into the femoral tunnel with the cancellous side facing posteriorly. Using a nitinol guide pin, a 7- × 20-mm metal interference screw is placed, securing the Achilles tendon bone plug in the femoral tunnel. The soft tissue end of the Achilles tendon allograft is then pulled into the knee through the anterolateral arthroscopic portal and down the tibial tunnel using the 18-gauge wire loop.

The graft is tensioned and the knee brought through several cycles of flexion and extension. The knee is flexed to 90 degrees, and an anterior drawer is applied to the knee. With 15 to 20 pounds of tension applied to the graft, a screw and soft tissue washer are used to fix the Achilles tendon allograft to the anteromedial tibia. We often supplement our tibial tunnel fixation with a bioabsorbable interference screw. If collateral ligament surgery is necessary, it should be performed prior to final fixation of the tibial end of the graft, to minimize the possibility of loosening the graft during the manipulation necessary for the extraarticular surgery. Final tensioning of the PCL graft is done after cycling the knee. The knee is then examined to assess stability. The graft is checked arthroscopically (Fig. 24.8). Pulses are then rechecked and the knee is closed in a standard fashion. We

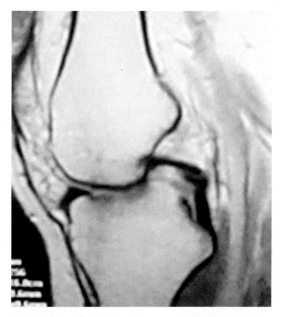

FIGURE 24.7 MRI scan illustrates that the popliteal vessels are less than a centimeter away from the point where the tibial guide pin penetrates the posterior cortex.

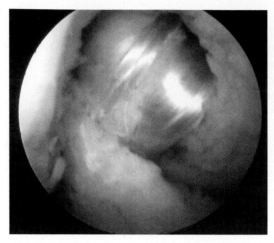

FIGURE 24.8 Arthroscopic view of a completed single-bundle PCL reconstruction in this right knee using an Achilles allograft.

brace the knee in full extension for 4 weeks to allow our reconstruction to heal before beginning gradual progressive motion and resistive exercises.

Double-Bundle Reconstruction

Double-bundle reconstruction techniques have been introduced in an attempt to reproduce more accurately the complex functional anatomy of the PCL (73–75). It has been hypothesized that double-bundle PCL reconstruction would more closely restore normal knee biomechanics throughout its full range of motion, and this has been shown in several biomechanical cadaver studies (50,73–76). While traditional single-bundle reconstruction restores knee biomechanics at mid- to high knee flexion angles, there still tends to be residual laxity when the knee is near full extension (50). Biomechanical studies have shown the addition of the posteromedial bundle reduced posterior tibial translation in knee flexion, as well as extension, suggesting that this bundle serves an important role throughout knee flexion (50,75,77). Although technically challenging, double-bundle reconstruction has become our preferred surgical technique in chronic PCL deficiency because of its improved restoration of normal knee mechanics. Additional clinical studies are necessary, however, to determine the long-term outcomes of this newer reconstructive technique.

Authors' Preferred Surgical Technique (Double-Bundle)

At our institution, we use a double-bundle reconstruction for chronic PCL injuries. Our technique is similar to the single-bundle reconstruction with the addition of a posteromedial bundle reconstruction using a semitendinosus autograft. This is harvested in a standard fashion through our anteromedial tibial incision, doubled over, whipstitched with No. 2 braided nonabsorbable suture, and fashioned to fit

usually a 6- or 7-mm tunnel. We use the same tibial tunnel as with our single-bundle reconstruction. For the posteromedial femoral tunnel, a guide pin is placed through the anterolateral arthroscopic portal in the footprint of the posteromedial bundle. This is at the 2:30 clock position in a right knee, 3 to 4 mm off of the articular margin (depending on tunnel size) and at least 4 to 5 mm away from the anterolateral (AL) tunnel. It is important to direct the guide pin divergent from the AL tunnel to prevent collapse. This will ensure that there is an adequate bone bridge between the two tunnels (Fig. 24.9).

We then drill the posteromedial tunnel to a 6- or 7-mm diameter and a 30-mm depth. A 3.2-mm drill hole is then placed through the end of our tunnel and a Beath pin is placed through this drill hole out of the anteromedial femoral cortex and skin. A skin incision is then made, and the Beath pin is followed to its exit from the outer femoral cortex. The doubled over end of the semitendinosus graft is pulled up into the femoral tunnel, and the sutures are tied on the outer femoral cortex with a button. An alternative fixation technique utilizes a soft tissue bio-interference screw placed arthroscopically, obviating the need for a separate incision. Using the same technique as for the anterolateral bundle, the semitendinosus graft is pulled into the tibial tunnel. The anterolateral component Achilles graft is tensioned and fixed first, using the method noted above for the single bundle graft. For the tibial fixation of the posteromedial bundle graft, the knee is brought to 15 degrees of flexion with an applied anterior drawer. The semitendinosus graft is then fixed to the tibia with a separate screw and soft tissue washer. We often supplement our tibial tunnel fixation with a bioabsorbable interference screw. As with the single-bundle technique, collateral ligament surgery should be performed prior to tibial fixation of both components of the graft. Pulses are then rechecked and the knee is closed in

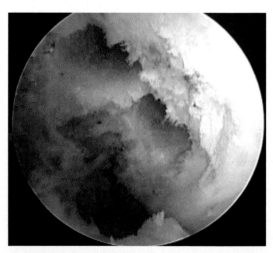

FIGURE 24.9 Arthroscopic view of the femoral tunnels for a double-bundle technique illustrates an adequate bone bridge to allow interference fixation.

a standard fashion. We brace the knee in full extension for 4 weeks to allow our reconstruction to heal before beginning gradual progressive motion and resistive exercises.

Tibial Inlay

This technique was initially described by Berg (78) to circumvent the issues of bone plug passage through the long tibial tunnel and potential abrasion at the posterior tibial exit point, or "killer turn." It also facilitates protection of the popliteal neurovascular structures. Utilization of the posterior approach to the tibial insertion of the PCL as described by Burks and Schaffer (79) simplifies the posterior exposure. The technique has been utilized most commonly with patella tendon autograft, but recently Bergfeld and Graham (80) have described its use with a double-bundle Achilles allograft. Early results with this technique are promising (78,81,82).

Positioning with the tibial inlay technique is challenging. It is simplest with the patient in the lateral decubitus position, with the operative leg up. A tourniquet is applied to

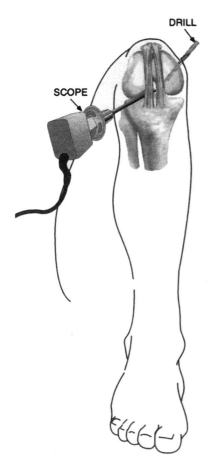

FIGURE 24.10 Position of the leg for arthroscopic examination and patella tendon graft harvest in the tibial inlay technique. (From Miller MD. Posterior cruciate ligament reconstruction: tibial inlay technique. *Sports Med Arthrosc Rev* 1999;7(4), with permission.)

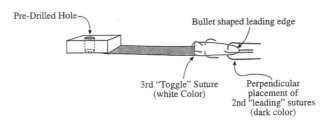

FIGURE 24.11 Preparation of a patella tendon graft for the tibial inlay technique. (From Miller MD. Posterior cruciate ligament reconstruction: tibial inlay technique. *Sports Med Arthrosc Rev* 1999;7(4), with permission.)

the upper thigh, but is rarely needed. With the hip abducted, flexed, and externally rotated, the arthroscopic portion of the procedure, as well as harvesting of the patella tendon autograft, if desired, are accomplished (Fig. 24.10). The patella tendon autograft is prepared by predrilling the larger bone block with a 4.5-mm drill, to allow lag fixation with a bicortical screw and washer. The graft is prepared with the smaller bone block bullet shaped, to facilitate retrieval into the femoral drill hole (Fig. 24.11). Three drill holes for retrieval sutures are placed in this block. An Achilles allograft can be prepared similarly for placement of the bone block posteriorly, with the tendon in the femur (80). Standard arthroscopy is then performed, and the PCL remnant is resected. The femoral guide pin is passed either from outside in, with a commercial drill guide, or from inside out, as described above in the transtibial tunnel technique. Placement of the guide pin is to replicate the anterolateral component of the PCL. The femoral tunnel is then drilled and circled (Fig. 24.10). A twisted wire (18 or 20 gauge) is placed through the tunnel, positioned at the PCL tibial attachment, and held in place with bone plug.

The patient is now repositioned with the foot on a padded Mayo stand, and the PCL tibial insertion is exposed through a "hockey-stick" incision (Fig. 24.12). The interval between the semimembranosis and the medial head of the gastrocnemius is developed, and the gastrocnemius is retracted laterally to expose the posterior capsule of the knee. The medial gastrocnemius muscle belly protects the popliteal neurovascular structures. Smooth Steinmann pins can be drilled into the posterior tibial cortex to act as retractors. Partial release of the medial head of the gastrocnemius may be necessary for exposure in some cases. The PCL sulcus is palpated on the back of the tibia, and the popliteus muscle fibers are elevated to expose the PCL insertion. Osteotomes, curettes, and burs are used to create the inlay site with a depth that will have the cortical surface of the bone block flush with the tibia (Fig. 24.13).

The block may be provisionally fixed to the posterior tibia with a staple that is intentionally left proud for removal, if necessary. The bulleted bone block is then retrieved into the femoral tunnel through the joint using the prepositioned wire. In some cases this is facilitated by ini-

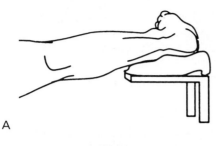

A

LATERAL

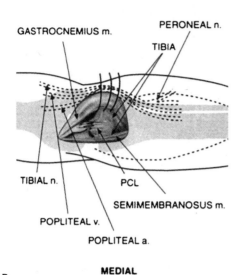

GASTROCNEMIUS m.   PERONEAL n.
TIBIA

TIBIAL n.   PCL

SEMIMEMBRANOSUS m.

POPLITEAL v.

POPLITEAL a.

B   **MEDIAL**

FIGURE 24.12 A,B: Positioning for the popliteal exposure for the inlay technique. (From Miller MD. Posterior cruciate ligament reconstruction: tibial inlay technique. *Sports Med Arthrosc Rev* 1999;7(4), with permission.)

tially pulling the bone block into the notch through the anteromedial arthroscopy portal, and then pulling the block into the femoral tunnel. The additional suture in the bone block may be used through the portal to toggle the bone block into alignment with the femoral tunnel. It is intended to fix the bone block in the femoral tunnel such that the block is at the aperture to the joint. If the bone block is re-

cessed too far up the femoral tunnel, then the tibial attachment site is advanced distally. The tibial side is fixed with a cortical lag screw and supplemented with the staple. The femoral side is then fixed with an interference screw placed posterior to the bone block from outside in (Fig. 24.13). The graft is tensioned at 80 to 90 degrees with an anterior drawer applied to the tibia and 15 to 20 pounds of tension on the graft. Pulses are then rechecked and the knee is closed in a standard fashion. We brace the knee in full extension for 4 weeks to allow our reconstruction to heal before beginning gradual progressive motion and resistive exercises.

Combined Injuries

The combined PCL-PLS injury is one of the most complicated knee injury patterns that an orthopaedic surgeon may have to manage. When both the PCL and PLS are ruptured, substantial posterior translation, external rotation, and varus opening may all be present at differing angles of knee flexion (15). This combination creates a complex surgical dilemma that usually necessitates the surgeon having more than one surgical plan (23). Many techniques of reconstruction have been recommended, including arcuate ligament advancement, biceps tenodesis, and popliteofibular ligament reconstruction with allograft or autograft tissue. However, no consensus exists as to the best procedure (23,83–88). This combined injury must be appropriately identified since posterior and posterolateral instability will invariably persist if the injury is managed nonsurgically as an isolated PCL injury (1,2,27,50,63,84,89). Chronic cases of posterolateral instability demonstrate tissue redundancy and excessive scarring posterior to the LCL, making identification of the particular structures of the popliteus complex difficult. Therefore, the timing of surgical treatment of the injured PLS is critical, with acute repairs consistently giving more favorable results than reconstruction of chronic injuries (3,15,18,35).

Chronic PCL injuries involving the PLS are even more surgically challenging. If an injury to the PLS is ignored or goes unrecognized, repair or reconstruction of other ligaments will have a significant risk of failure due to chronic

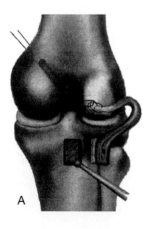

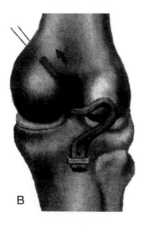

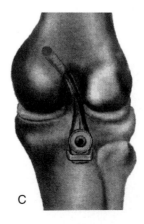

A   B   C

FIGURE 24.13 A–C: Composite illustration of passage and fixation of the tibial inlay graft. (From Miller MD. Posterior cruciate ligament reconstruction: tibial inlay technique. *Sports Med Arthrosc Rev* 1999;7(4), with permission.)

repetitive stretching of the reconstruction (15,18,35). Surgical treatment of PLS injuries in the chronic injury setting is centered on reconstruction rather that repair of deficient structures. We recommend anatomic reconstruction of the popliteofibular ligament and, if necessary, the LCL. If varus malalignment or a lateral thrust exists, a proximal tibial osteotomy may be necessary to correct the alignment. Although the osteotomy may be performed in conjunction with the PLS reconstruction, we favor staging the operation since the osteotomy alone may alleviate the patient's symptoms, thereby avoiding further surgical intervention (18).

Authors' Preferred Surgical Technique (PLS)

The PCL is reconstructed first using the double-bundle technique. Then attention is focused on the reconstruction of the PLS prior to tensioning and tibial fixation of the PCL grafts. Our approach for a combined PCL-PLS reconstruction begins with a lateral "hockey-stick" incision that parallels the posterior edge of the iliotibial band. The iliotibial band is then split, thereby exposing the deep structures of the LCL anteriorly and the lateral head of the gastrocnemius

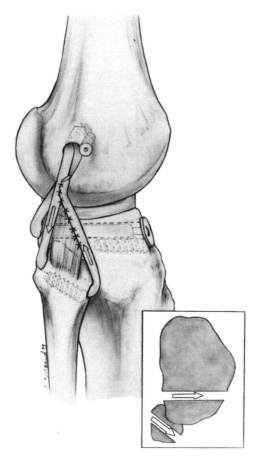

FIGURE 24.14 Use of a split Achilles allograft to reconstruct the PLS. (From Ferrari JD, Bach BR Jr. Posterolateral instability of the knee: diagnosis and treatment of acute and chronic instability. *Sports Med Arthrosc Rev* 1999;7(4), with permission.)

muscle and underlying popliteus complex more posteriorly. The injured structures must then be properly identified. If the LCL is part of the injury pattern, we reconstruct it according to the following steps. An oblique tunnel that is oriented similarly to the course of the lateral collateral ligament is created in the proximal fibula (Fig. 24.14). A proximal, blind femoral tunnel is then created at the anatomic insertion site of the popliteus tendon along the epicondylar axis of the femur. The popliteus tendon portion requires an anterior to posterior drill hole in the lateral tibia (Fig. 24.14). An Achilles tendon allograft is then passed under the LCL into the proximal and distal tunnels. After preparing the posterolateral aspect of the knee, the PCL graft is secured into the tibia. The knee is then placed in 30 degrees of flexion where final posterolateral stabilization is performed. Fixation at the fibular tunnel is achieved with soft tissue or conventional interference screws and fixation at the femoral side is performed with either a soft tissue interference screw, a button tied over the medial cortex through a separate skin incision, or a combination of these fixation methods. Fixation of the tibial arm of the PLS graft is with a bioabsorbable screw supplemented by tying over a button. As the graft is tensioned and secured, the knee is maintained in 20 to 30 degrees of flexion with neutral to slight internal rotation of the foot.

REHABILITATION

Immediately after the operation, the injured limb is placed in a well-padded hinged knee brace locked in extension. This should be performed with care to avoid any posterior translation of the tibia while it is applied. Immobilization in extension enables the knee joint to remain reduced and minimizes the effects of gravity and hamstring forces that create posterior tibial sag, thus allowing the collateral ligament repair and/or reconstruction a chance to heal (6). The rehabilitation protocol is, in general, slower than that for isolated ACL reconstruction. Reconstructions of PCL-PLS combined injuries are progressed even more slowly. In particular, crutches are continued for 3 months to allow the lateral soft tissue repair or reconstruction to heal without undue tension. This program is broken down into four phases: (a) 0 to 4 weeks, (b) 1 to 3 months, (c) 3 to 9 months, and (d) 9 to 12 months. Supervised physical therapy takes place for approximately 3 to 5 months after surgery.

Phase 1

The hinged knee brace is maintained in extension for the first postoperative month. During this time the patient is allowed to bear full weight to tolerance on the limb with the brace locked. Crutches should be used for assistance during the first 6 to 8 weeks. Quadriceps exercises form the mainstay of rehabilitation and are begun in the form of quadriceps sets and straight leg raises starting the first postoperative day. Active hamstring exercises are avoided because of the potential for the muscles to sublux the tibia posteriorly and stress the repair.

Phase 2

This phase begins 4 weeks after surgery and lasts 8 weeks. The goals are to allow the healing of the soft tissue reconstruction to bone, which takes 6 to 8 weeks, and the return of normal motion and gait. The brace is unlocked between 4 and 6 weeks after surgery for controlled gait training and range of motion (ROM) exercises. These exercises are performed with the assistance of a physical therapist who applies an anterior drawer to the proximal tibia as the patient flexes the knee or with the patient in a prone position. This is important to prevent posterior tibial sag. The brace is then unlocked for all activities during the 6- to 8-week period. Crutches and the brace are removed at 8 weeks if the patient exhibits good quadriceps strength and control, full knee extension, knee flexion of 90 to 100 degrees and a normal gait pattern. If the PLS was also reconstructed, the brace and crutches are continued until 3 months after surgery. At this point, the patient begins wall slides (0–45 degrees) and ambulation in a swimming pool. At 8 weeks, a stationary bike is added with the heel forward on the pedal and the seat slightly higher than normal. Balance and proprioception exercises are also begun.

Phase 3

Phase 3 extends from 3 to 9 months after surgery. The patient is expected to achieve full pain-free ROM, normal gait, good quadriceps strength and should have no patellofemoral complaints. Obtaining the last 10 to 15 degrees of flexion may take up to 5 months. Exercises are advanced to jogging in the pool and walking on the treadmill. Closed-chain kinetic exercises are also begun during this time period.

Phase 4

This period extends from approximately 9 to 12 months after surgery. The goal during this time period is the gradual return to work and athletic participation as well as the maintenance of strength and endurance. This may involve sports-specific training, work hardening, or job restructuring as needed. Education is essential to provide the patient with a clear understanding of the possible limitations.

COMPLICATIONS

Failure to recognize and appropriately treat associated ligament injuries are the most frequent problems encountered in PCL surgery. These problems may contribute to the lack of reproducibly excellent results often noted by authors following PCL surgery. Careful examination both prior to surgery and in the operating room, with attention to both MRI and arthroscopic findings, will improve identification of all injured structures. Successful results depend on repair and/or reconstruction of all torn structures (84–87).

Injury to the popliteal artery and vein or the tibial nerve are potentially devastating complications. Injury can occur at the time of guide pin passage, or while reaming. Specially designed PCL tibial guides, with protective aiming arms, are helpful, but caution must be exercised, since twisting the guide may cause the pin to miss the spoon. Jackson et al. recognized that "winding-up" of these structures may occur with a large drill bit, even if the guide pin is visualized. Drilling through the posterior cortex of the tibial tunnel by hand is an important safety measure for the transtibial tunnel technique (90,91). The posteromedial safety incision, described by Fanelli (41), is another strategy that will reduce this risk. The tibial inlay technique, by eliminating the transtibial tunnel, is another way to limit the risk of neurovascular injury.

Avascular necrosis of the medial femoral condyle following PCL reconstruction is infrequent (90). It probably results from a femoral drill hole that passes too close to the articular surface. Femoral guide pin passage should take this into account, and aim away from this surface.

SUMMARY

Isolated and combined posterior cruciate ligament injuries remain a challenging problem to orthopaedic surgeons. Variations in patient outcomes following PCL reconstruction in the past may be attributed to clinicians' failing to restore posterior stability as well as recognize and treat associated injuries. Fortunately, the synergistic relationship between the PCL and PLS has become better understood in recent years.

Although basic science investigations have provided a more scientific rationale for the selection of grafts and tunnel placement, no single reconstruction technique has emerged as the consistent approach accepted among all surgeons. A debate that will likely continue until better long-term prospective studies are published in the literature.

REFERENCES

1. Fanelli GC. Posterior cruciate ligament injuries in trauma patients. *Arthroscopy* 1993;9:291–294.
2. Fanelli GC, Edson CJ. Posterior cruciate ligament injuries in trauma patients: Part II. *Arthroscopy* 1995;11:526–529.
3. Miller MD, Bergfeld JA, Fowler PJ, et al. The posterior cruciate ligament injured knee: principles of evaluation and treatment. In:

Zuckerman JD, ed. *Instructional course lectures, Vol. 48.* Rosemont, IL: American Academy of Orthopaedic Surgeons, 1999: 199–207.

4. Fowler PJ, Messiah SS. Isolated posterior cruciate ligament injuries in athletes. *Am J Sports Med* 1987;15:553–557.

5. Parolie JM, Bergfeld JA. Long-term results of nonoperative treatment of isolated posterior cruciate ligament injuries in the athlete. *Am J Sports Med* 1986;14:35–38.

6. Harner CD, Höher J. Current Concepts: evaluation and treatment of posterior cruciate ligament injuries. *Am J Sports Med* 1998;26:471–482.

7. Covey DC, Sapega AA. Current concepts review: injuries to the posterior cruciate ligament. *J Bone Joint Surg* 1993;75A:1376–1386.

8. Keller PM, Shelbourne KD, McCarroll JR, et al. Nonoperatively treated isolated posterior cruciate ligament injuries. *Am J Sports Med* 1993;21:132–136.

9. Shelbourne KD, Davis TJ, Patel DV. The natural history of acute, isolated, nonoperatively treated posterior cruciate ligament injuries: a prospective study. *Am J Sports Med* 1999;27:276–283.

10. Torg JS, Barton TM, Pavlov H, et al. Natural history of the posterior cruciate ligament-deficient knee. *Clin Orthop* 1989;246:208–216.

11. Fanelli GC, Giannotti BF, Edson CJ. Current concepts review: the posterior cruciate ligament arthroscopic evaluation and treatment. *Arthroscopy* 1994;10:673–688.

12. Cain TE, Schwab GH. Performance of an athlete with straight posterior knee stability. *Am J Sports Med* 1981;9:203–208.

13. Cross MJ, Powell JF. Long-term followup of posterior cruciate ligament rupture: a study of 116 cases. *Am J Sports Med* 1984;12:292–297.

14. Dandy DJ, Pusey RJ. The long-term results of unrepaired tears of the posterior cruciate ligament. *J Bone Joint Surg* 1982;64B:92–94.

15. Cooper DE, Warren RF, Warner JJP. The posterior cruciate ligament and posterolateral structures of the knee: anatomy, function and patterns of injury. In: Tullos HS, ed. *Instructional course lectures,* vol 40. Park Ridge, IL: American Academy Orthopaedic Surgeons, 1991:249–270.

16. Clancy WG, Jr, Shelbourne KD, Zoellner GB, et al. Treatment of knee joint instability secondary to rupture of the posterior cruciate ligament. Report of a new procedure. *J Bone Joint Surg* 1983;65A:310–322.

17. Noyes FR, Barber-Westin SD. Treatment of complex injuries involving the posterior cruciate and posterolateral ligaments of the knee. *Am J Knee Surg* 1996;9:200–214.

18. Veltri DM, Warren RF. Posterolateral instability of the knee. In: Jackson DW, ed. *Instructional course lectures,* vol 44. Rosemont, IL: American Academy of Orthopaedic Surgeons, 1995:441–453.

19. Albright JP, Brown AW. Management of chronic posterolateral rotatory instability of the knee: surgical technique for the posterolateral sling procedure. In: Zuckerman JD, ed. *Instructional course lectures,* vol 48. Rosemont, IL: American Academy Orthopaedic Surgeons, 1999:369–378.

20. Gollehon DL, Torzilli PA, Warren RF. The role of the posterolateral and cruciate ligaments in the stability of the human knee. A biomechanical study. *J Bone Joint Surg* 1987;69A:233–242.

21. Grood ES, Stowers SF, Noyes FR. Limits of movement in the human knee. Effect of sectioning the posterior cruciate ligament and posterolateral structures. *J Bone Joint Surg* 1988;70A:88–97.

22. Veltri DM, Deng X-H, Torzilli PA, et al. The role of the cruciate and posterolateral ligaments in stability of the knee. A biomechanical study. *Am J Sports Med* 1995;23:436–443.

23. Cooper DE. Treatment of combined posterior cruciate ligament and posterolateral injuries of the knee. *Oper Tech Sports Med* 1999;7:135–142.

24. Veltri D, Deng X-H, Torzilli PA, et al. The role of the popliteofibular ligament in the stability of the human knee. A biomechanical study. *Am J Sports Med* 1996;24:19–27.

25. Noyes FR, Barber-Westin SD. Surgical restoration to treat chronic deficiency of the posterolateral complex and cruciate ligaments of the knee joint. *Am J Sports Med* 1996;24:415–426.

26. Meyers MH. Isolated avulsion of the tibial attachment of the posterior cruciate ligament of the knee. *J Bone Joint Surg* 1975;57A:669–672.

27. Müller W. *The knee: form, function and ligament reconstruction.* Berlin: Springer-Verlag, 1983.

28. Hewett TE, Noyes FR, Lee MD. Diagnosis of complete and partial posterior cruciate ligament ruptures: stress radiography compared with KT-1000 arthrometer and posterior drawer testing. *Am J Sports Med* 1997;25:648–655.

29. Shino K, Mitsuoka T, Horibe S, et al. The gravity sag view: a simple radiographic technique to show posterior laxity of the knee. *Arthroscopy* 2000;16:670–672.

30. Grover JS, Bassett LW Gross ML, et al. Posterior cruciate ligament: MR imaging. *Radiology* 1990;174:527–530.

31. Polly DW, Callaghan JJ, Sikes RA, et al. The accuracy of selective magnetic resonance imaging compared with the findings of arthroscopy of the knee. *J Bone Joint Surg* 1988;70A:192–198.

32. Turner DA, Prodromos CC, Petasnick JP, et al. Acute injuries of the ligaments of the knee: magnetic resonance evaluation. *Radiology* 1985;154:717–722.

33. Barrett G, Savoie F. Operative management of acute PCL injuries with associated long term results. *Orthopaedics* 1991;14:687–692.

34. Pouranas J, Symeonides P. The results of surgical repairs of acute tears of the posterior cruciate ligament. *Clin Orthop* 1991;267:103–107.

35. LaPrade RF. The medial collateral ligament complex and the posterolateral aspect of the knee. In: Arendt EA, ed. *Orthopaedic knowledge update: sports medicine 2.* Rosemont, IL: American Academy of Orthopaedic Surgeons, 1999:317–326.

36. Dejour H, Walch G, Peyrot J, et al. The natural history of rupture of the posterior cruciate ligament. *Fr J Orthop Surg* 1988;2:112–120.

37. Shelbourne KD, Jennings RW, Vahey TN. Magnetic resonance imaging of posterior cruciate ligament injuries: assessment of healing. *Am J Knee Surg* 1999;12:209–213.

38. Tewes DP, Fritts HM, Fields RD, et al. Chronically injured posterior cruciate ligament: magnetic resonance imaging. *Clin Orthop* 1997;335:224–232.

39. Boynton MD, Tietjens BR. Long-term followup of the untreated isolated posterior cruciate ligament-deficient knee. *Am J Sports Med* 1996;24:306–310

40. Lipscomb AB, Anderson AF, Norwig ED, et al. Isolated posterior cruciate ligament reconstruction: long-term results. *Am J Sports Med* 1993;21:490–496.

41. Fanelli GC. Arthroscopically assisted posterior cruciate ligament reconstruction: transtibial tunnel technique. In: Fanelli GC, ed. *Posterior cruciate ligament injuries, a practical guide to management.* New York: Springer, 2001:141–156.

42. Veltri DM, Warren RF. Posterolateral instability of the knee. *J Bone Joint Surg* 1994;76A:460–472.

43. Saddler SC, Noyes FR, Grood ES, et al. Posterior cruciate ligament anatomy and length-tension behavior of PCL surface fibers. *Am J Knee Surg* 1996;9:194–199.

44. Harner CD, Vogrin TM, Höher J, et al. Biomechanical analysis of a posterior cruciate ligament reconstruction: deficiency of the

posterolateral structures as a cause of graft failure. *Am J Sports Med* 2000;28:32–39.

45. Bianchi M. Acute tears of the posterior cruciate ligament: clinical study and results of operative treatment in 27 cases. *Am J Sports Med* 1983;11:308–314.

46. Kim SJ, Shin SJ, Choi NH, et al. Arthroscopically assisted treatment of avulsion fractures of the posterior cruciate ligament from the tibia. *J Bone Joint Surg* 2001;83A:698–708.

47. Deehan DJ, Pinczewski LA. Technical note: arthroscopic reattachment of an avulsion fracture of the tibial insertion of the posterior cruciate ligament. *Arthroscopy* 2001;17:422–425.

48. Espejo-Baena A, Lopez-Arevalo R, Urbano V, et al. Case report: arthroscopic repair of the posterior cruciate ligament: two techniques. *Arthroscopy* 2000;16:656–660.

49. Noyes FR, Stowers SF, Grood ES, et al. Posterior subluxations of the medial and lateral tibiofemoral compartments. An in vivo ligament sectioning study in cadaveric knees. *Am J Sports Med* 1993;21:407–414.

50. Harner CD, Janaushek MA, Kanamori A, et al. Biomechanical analysis of a double-bundle posterior cruciate ligament reconstruction. *Am J Sports Med* 2000;28:144–151.

51. Noyes FR, Butler DL, Grood ES, et al. Biomechanical analysis of human ligament grafts used in knee-ligament repairs and reconstructions. *J Bone Joint Surg* 1984;66A:344–352.

52. Jackson DW, Corsetti J, Simon TM. Biologic incorporation of allograft anterior cruciate ligament replacements. *Clin Orthop* 1996;324:126–133.

53. Nikolaou PK, Seaber AV, Glisson RR, et al. Anterior cruciate ligament allograft transplantation: long-term function, histology, revascularization, and operative technique. *Am J Sports Med* 1986;14:348–360.

54. Shino K, Inoue M, Horibe S, et al. Maturation of allograft tendons transplanted into the knee: an arthroscopic and histological study. *J Bone Joint Surg* 1988;70B:556–560.

55. Brand J, Weiler A, Caborn DNM, et al. Current concepts: graft fixation in cruciate ligament reconstruction. *Am J Sports Med* 2000;28:761–774.

56. Robertson DB, Daniel DM, Biden E. Soft tissue fixation to bone. *Am J Sports Med* 1986;14:398–403.

57. Burns WC II, Draganich LF, Pyevich M, et al. The effect of femoral tunnel position and graft tensioning technique on posterior laxity of the knee. *Am J Sports Med* 1995;23:424–430.

58. Covey DC, Sapega AA, Sherman GM. Testing for isometry during reconstruction of the posterior cruciate ligament: anatomic and biomechanical considerations. *Am J Sports Med* 1996;24:740–746.

59. Galloway MT, Grood ES, Mehalik JN, et al. Posterior cruciate ligament reconstruction: An in vitro study of femoral and tibial graft placement. *Am J Sports Med* 1996;24:437–445.

60. Pearsall AW, Pyevich M, Draganich LF, et al. In vitro study of knee stability after posterior cruciate ligament reconstruction. *Clin Orthop* 1996;327:264–271.

61. Bach BR Jr, Daluga DJ, Mikosz R, et al. Force displacement characteristics of the posterior cruciate ligament. *Am J Sports Med* 1992;20:67–72.

62. Grood ES, Hefzy MS, Lindenfeld TN. Factors affecting the region of most isometric femoral attachments: part I—the posterior cruciate ligament. *Am J Sports Med* 1989;17:197–207.

63. Harner CD, Janaushek MA, Ma CB, et al. The effect of knee flexion angle and application of an anterior tibial load at the time of graft fixation on the biomechanics of a posterior cruciate ligament-reconstructed knee. *Am J Sports Med* 2000;28:460–465.

64. Girgis FG, Marshall JL, Al Monajem ARS. The cruciate ligaments of the knee joint: anatomical, functional and experimental analysis. *Clin Orthop* 1975;106:216–231.

65. Race A, Amis AA. The mechanical properties of the two bundles of the human posterior cruciate ligament. *J Biomech* 1994;27:13–24.

66. Markolf KL, Slauterbeck JR, Armstrong KL, et al. A biomechanical study of replacement of the posterior cruciate ligament with a graft: part I—Isometry, pre-tension of the graft, and anterior-posterior laxity. *J Bone Joint Surg* 1997;79A:375–380.

67. Ogata K, McCarthy JA. Measurements of length and tension patterns during reconstruction of the posterior cruciate ligament. *Am J Sports Med* 1992;20:351–355.

68. Ortiz GJ, Schmotzer H, Bernbeck J, et al. Isometry of the posterior cruciate ligament: Effects of functional load and muscle force application. *Am J Sports Med* 1998;26:663–668.

69. Racanelli JA, Drez D. Posterior cruciate ligament tibial attachment anatomy and radiographic landmarks for tibial tunnel placement in PCL reconstruction. *Arthroscopy* 1994;10:546–549.

70. Sidles JA, Larson RV, Garbini JL, et al. Ligament length relationships in the moving knee. *J Orthop Res* 1988;6:593–610.

71. Ohkoshi Y, Nagasaki S, Yamamoto K, et al. A new endoscopic posterior cruciate ligament reconstruction: minimization of graft angulation. *Arthroscopy* 2001;17:258–263.

72. Lysholm J, Gillquist J. Arthroscopic examination of the posterior cruciate ligament. *J Bone Joint Surg* 1981;63A:363–366.

73. Petrie RS, Harner CD. Double bundle posterior cruciate ligament reconstruction technique: University of Pittsburgh approach. *Oper Tech Sports Med* 1999;7:118–126.

74. Clancy WC, Bisson LJ. Double-bundle technique for reconstruction of the posterior cruciate ligament. *Oper Tech Sports Med* 1999;7:110–117.

75. Race A, Amis AA. PCL reconstruction: in vitro biomechanical comparison of "isometric" versus single and double-bundled "anatomic" grafts. *J Bone Joint Surg* 1998;80B:173–179.

76. Mannor DA, Shearn JT, Grood ES, et al. Two-bundle posterior cruciate ligament reconstruction: an in vitro analysis of graft placement and tension. *Am J Sports Med* 2000;28:833–845.

77. Fox RJ, Harner CD, Sakane M, et al. Determination of the in situ forces in the human posterior cruciate ligament using robotic technology: a cadaveric study. *Am J Sports Med* 1998;26:395–401.

78. Berg EE. Posterior cruciate ligament tibial inlay reconstruction. *Arthroscopy* 1995;11:69–76.

79. Burks RT, Schaffer JJ. A simplified approach to the tibial attachment of the posterior cruciate ligament. *Clin Orthop* 1990;254:216–219.

80. Bergfeld JA, Graham SM. Tibial inlay procedure for PCL reconstruction: one tunnel and two tunnel. *Oper Tech Sports Med* 2001;8:69–75.

81. Miller MD, Olszewski AD. Posterior cruciate ligament injuries: New treatment options. *Am J Knee Surg* 1995;8:351–355.

82. Jung YB, Tae SK, Yum JK. Reconstruction of the posterior cruciate ligament with modified inlay technique. *Arthroscopy* 1998;14(suppl):S19(abst).

83. Clancy WG. Repair and reconstruction of the posterior cruciate ligament. In: Chapman M, ed. *Operative orthopaedics*. Philadelphia: 1981:1651–1655.

84. Fanelli GC, Giannotti BF, Edson CJ. Arthroscopically assisted combined posterior cruciate ligament/posterolateral complex reconstruction. *Arthroscopy* 1996;12:521–529.

85. Fleming RE, Blatz DJ, McCarroll JR. Posterior problems in the knee: Posterior cruciate insufficiency and posterolateral rotatory insufficiency. *Am J Sports Med* 1981;9:107–113.

86. Hughston JC, Jacobson KE. Chronic posterolateral rotatory instability of the knee. *J Bone Joint Surg* 1985;67A:351–359.

87. Noyes FR, Barber-Westin SD. Surgical reconstruction of severe chronic posterolateral complex injuries of the knee using allograft tissues. *Am J Sports Med* 1995;23:2–12.

88. Watanabe Y, Moriya H, Takahashi K, et al. Functional anatomy of the posterolateral structures of the knee. *Arthroscopy* 1993;9: 57–62.

89. Staubli HU, Birrer S. The popliteus tendon and its fascicles at the popliteal hiatus: gross anatomy and functional arthroscopic evaluation with and without anterior cruciate ligament deficiency. *Arthroscopy* 1990;6:209–220.

90. Fanelli GC, Monahan TJ. Complications in posterior cruciate ligament surgery. In: Fanelli GC, ed. *Posterior cruciate ligament injuries, a practical guide to management.* New York: Springer, 2001:291–302.

91. Jackson DW, Proctor CS, Simon TM. Arthroscopic assisted PCL reconstruction: a technical note on potential neurovascular injury related to drill bit configuration. *Arthroscopy* 1993;9:224–227.

25

ARTHROSCOPIC TREATMENT OF FRACTURES ABOUT THE KNEE

ROBERT E. HUNTER
ROBERT C. SCHENCK, JR.

FRACTURES OF THE PROXIMAL TIBIA

Proximal tibia fractures represent a complex spectrum of injuries involving the tibial knee joint surface; they can occur secondary to a variety of causes, including motor vehicle trauma, falls from a height, and collisions in sports. The classic history is a fall or impact causing valgus and compression across the knee joint whereby the femoral condyle or condyles impact the articular surface, creating a fracture. Other mechanisms occur secondary to a direct blow (e.g., "bumper fracture"), and these fracture types are frequently more complex (in both fracture pattern and soft tissue injury) than those created by the femoral condyles (36).

Classification

In our experience, the use of a classification in the management of proximal tibial fractures is crucial. Although not all fractures can be classified, and certainly interobserver discrepancies occur, the application of the Schatzker classification system has been extremely useful in our hands. Furthermore, the concept of fracture-dislocations, as popularized by Tillman Moore in the early 1980s, is very useful alongside the Schatzker system in directing management and predicting outcome in cases of fractures about the proximal tibia. Although the Hohl classification has been used in the past, in our experience it is not as universally applicable as the Schatzker classification system (12,14,17,20,21,36) (Fig. 25.1A). The Schatzker system, as originally described, classifies fractures into six types, described as a Schatzker I through VI (39). An important and ingenious concept of the Schatzker system is energy of injury. As one progresses through the Schatzker classification system, the higher numbers portend higher levels of energy of injury. This is an ex-

tremely important point in management of the soft tissues about the knee as well as specific components of the system (e.g., the Shatzker IV fracture, discussed later).

The classification system is as follows. Schatzker I fracture type is a minimally displaced split of the lateral tibial plateau that can usually be treated with percutaneous screw fixation or with arthroscopic methods of reduction and simultaneous percutaneous fixation. As noted later, a displaced split fracture may occasionally have an associated incarcerated lateral meniscus, necessitating management of both the fracture and soft tissue interposition.

A Schatzker II fracture is the historically common, "split-depressed" fracture. This routinely requires elevation of the depressed segment, which can be performed with arthroscopically assisted indirect methods or, depending on fragment position (i.e., in the case of a completely rotated fragment), with open reduction internal fixation using a classic AO technique (38). In the split-depressed fracture (Schatzker II), the articular surface is depressed and sometimes rotated, with bone impaction present. Depending on the degree of split and the position of the depressed fracture, the pattern must be individualized for either an arthroscopic approach with percutaneous screw fixation or an open approach with reduction of the articular surface and biologic bone restoration with screw and side plate fixation.

Schatzker III is a depression-type fracture of the lateral tibial plateau. It usually requires fracture elevation, either arthroscopically assisted or open, and can frequently be internally fixed with percutaneous screw fixation.

The Schatzker IV through VI types are higher-energy injuries and should be handled with a careful eye to the soft tissues, because final fracture management significantly depends on the adequacy of the soft tissue envelope. The Schatzker IV fracture is a medial condyle fracture of the proximal tibia and is often erroneously viewed as a benign fracture. Although the surgeon is tempted to treat this fracture with a few percutaneous screws from medial to lateral, the risk of late varus collapse is significant, especially in the situation of a high-energy fracture. For that reason, this frac-

R. E. Hunter: Aspen Foundation for Sports Medicine, Education, and Research, Aspen, Colorado.

R. C. Schenck, Jr.: Department of Orthopaedics and Rehabilitation, University of New Mexico School of Medicine, Albuquerque, New Mexico.

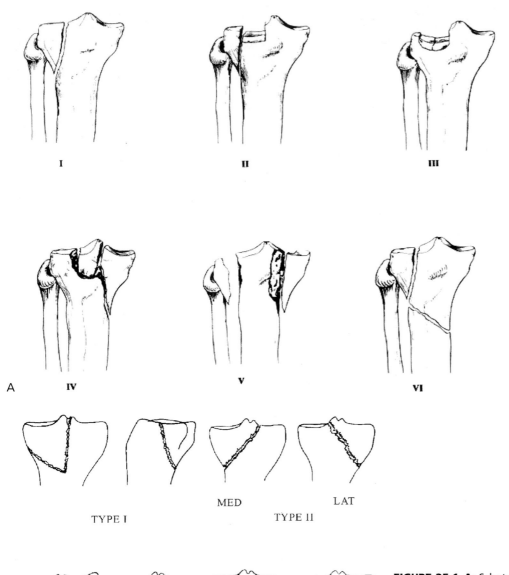

I

II

III

A   IV

V

VI

TYPE I

MED   LAT

TYPE II

B   TYPE III

MED   LAT

TYPE IV

TYPE V

FIGURE 25.1 A: Schatzker classification (types I through VI) of proximal tibial fractures. (From Schatzker J, McBroom R, Bruce D. The tibial plateau fracture: the Toronto experience 1968–1975. *Clin Orthop* 1979; 138:94–98, Figs. 1 through 6, with permission). **B:** Moore's classification of fracture-dislocations. (From Moore TM. Fracture-dislocation of the knee. *Clin Orthop* 1981; 156:129, Fig. 1, with permission.)

ture type must be handled with care. For the majority of displaced medial tibial condylar fractures, a medial approach with open reduction and internal fixation is recommended, with the plate placed in a posteromedial position.

The Schatzker V fracture is a bicondylar fracture in which the proximal tibia is still in continuity (usually a portion of the eminence) with the tibial shaft (but with fractures of both condyles). These fractures require care of the soft tissues and can be treated with screw or plate fixation only if the soft tissues are in good condition (evidence of normal skin lines, minimal swelling). The archaic approach of a "dead bone sandwich," with medial and lateral plating accompanied by required incisions, is a high-risk operation and should rarely be performed. The decision usually lies between unilateral plating and hybrid external fixation (17,36).

The Schatzker VI fracture (described as metaphyseal diaphyseal dissociation) is a high-energy injury and requires treatment of the articular pieces as well as reestablishment of continuity between the condyles and the tibial shaft. Use of percutaneous cannulated fixation in combination with hybrid external fixation is frequently required (36,38,39).

Lastly, in treatment of the proximal tibia fracture, it is important to understand and identify the injury classified as a fracture-dislocation (13,20,33,34). This simply implies a fracture of the articular proximal tibia with an associated ligamentous injury (cruciate and/or collateral ligament). In such injuries the fracture is often obvious, but the ligamentous injury cannot be overlooked and frequently requires repair or reattachment. The system described by Moore is specifically designed for classification of fracture-dislocations, in which both ligamentous injury and plateau fracture occur concomitantly (17,33) (Fig. 25.1B). Frequently one sees a combination of the depressed lateral plateau fracture with a completely torn medial collateral ligament (MCL) (13,33). This injury pattern requires treatment with fracture reduction and fixation and repair of the MCL. In contrast to the nonoperative management seen with collateral ligaments in association with the torn anterior cruciate ligament (ACL), fracture-dislocations involving the plateau and opposite collateral ligament require operative stabilization of both (36).

Fracture displacement is a commonly discussed topic, with varying opinions on what is acceptable for a good outcome in the long term (15,36). Contact pressure measurements have been studied in the cadaver; stress aberrations were seen with displacement greater than 2.5 mm (8). However, there is controversy over the exact degree that is acceptable clinically. Although many orthopaedic surgeons discuss an "anatomic" reduction, the clinical result after minimally displaced fractures is usually quite good. Several studies have shown good clinical results with displacement up to 5 mm. In the young patient with no evidence of arthritis, a guideline of 2.5 mm as an acceptable degree of displacement is useful. However, in patients older than 50 years of age, 5 mm of displacement can be well tolerated in the situation of knee stability in full extension, as noted later. In one study displacement of 10 mm was associated with a poor result, and this does imply an upper limit of articular displacement that can be tolerated clinically (26,38).

Although the classification of fractures by displacement is well known, a less known but equally important concept is that based on knee stability. Rasmussen (37), in a series of proximal tibia fractures treated by both open and closed methods, described his technique of examination under anesthesia (EUA) to determine the need for operative intervention. With the knee placed in full extension, less than 10 degrees of varus or valgus "instability" was an indication for closed treatment. These results were verified on longer follow-up of the same patients by Lansinger et al. (28). Fracture displacement of up to 5 mm was found to be tolerated well at long-term follow-up. Although fracture displacement may seem the most important factor in determining the treatment plan, knee stability is a clinical finding of at least equal importance in the management of proximal tibial fractures (9,12). Stability is evaluated by applying a varus and then a valgus force to the knee in full extension and comparing the resulting movement with that on the contralateral, normal side. Because most fractures are of the lateral tibial plateau,

one usually is evaluating for valgus stability. Lastly, the description of degrees of instability, in our opinion, is often difficult and is an estimate at best. Nonetheless, the presence of normal varus and valgus stability with the knee positioned in full extension indicates an ideal situation for nonoperative management. Using fracture type, displacement, and knee stability, in the context of the overall state of the soft tissue envelope, the surgeon can determine the appropriate surgical approach (14,20,21,28,33,36,37).

Diagnosis and Treatment

Clinically, patients with fractures of the proximal tibia present with acute pain that is exacerbated with any effort at weight bearing and, at times, noticeable deformity. Physical examination demonstrates a tense effusion in almost all cases. Of all of the possible causes for intraarticular bleeding, fractures precipitate the most aggressive bleeding and result in a painful and tense effusion. Palpation reveals joint line tenderness, principally on the tibial side in the area of the fracture. In addition, the examiner should look for medial pain and swelling and palpate for collateral ligament tenderness, especially in the area of the MCL, when evaluating a lateral plateau fracture (13). Range of motion (ROM) is usually restricted secondary to the effusion and protective muscle spasm. Stability examination is very important but can be difficult in the acute setting. It frequently must be delayed until an EUA can be performed, owing to patient intolerance to examination in the acute setting and evaluation in the emergency room (36).

Radiographic Evaluation

Standard radiographic assessment should include anteroposterior and lateral radiographs of the knee. If there is a suspicion of a fracture or if further clarification is sought, oblique views can be helpful. Several studies have shown underestimation of fracture displacement on plain radiographs. In a cadaveric study, Kearns et al. (25) found that anteroposterior and lateral radiographs revealed 3-mm defects 50% of the time and 5-mm defects 85% of the time but underestimated the displacement by an average of 2.5 mm. When oblique views were added to the study, 3-mm defects were revealed 80% of the time and 5-mm defects 90% of the time. Therefore, radiographs are a very important initial study for plateau fractures but tend to underestimate fracture displacement and can completely miss subtle fractures that appear entirely normal (Fig. 25.2).

Computed tomography (CT) scans have traditionally been used to help to identify fracture patterns about the proximal tibia (14). Classically, any study of bone integrity requires the use of CT scanning. However, in proximal tibial fractures, the occurrence of associated soft tissue injuries make magnetic resonance imaging (MRI) an attractive alternative to CT scanning. In a study comparing CT with

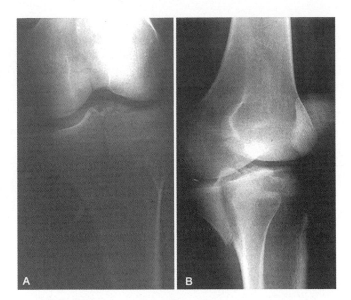

FIGURE 25.2 A: Anteroposterior radiograph of the proximal tibia without obvious evidence of fracture. **B:** Oblique radiographic view of the same patient in (A), with clear visual evidence of a posterior third medial condyle fracture of the proximal tibia. (From Perry CR, Hunter R, Ostrum R, et al. Fractures of the proximal tibia. *Instr Course Lect* 1999;48:497–513, with permission.)

MRI in the evaluation of tibial plateau fractures, Kode et al. (26) found a significant number of additional soft tissue findings with MRI and concluded that MRI was the preferred technology. Hunter et al. reviewed the role of MRI in preoperative assessment of plateau fractures (23), finding that MRI changed the fracture classification in 29% of knees and also changed surgical planning in one of three patients. In addition to the benefits demonstrated in identifying bony pathology, soft tissue injury was identified in a large percentage of the cases reviewed, including an incidence of 45% for lateral meniscus tear, 9% for medial meniscus tears, and 19% for MCL tears. Lastly, the ability to view MRI scans in sagittal, coronal, and transverse planes without additional reconstructive techniques, makes MRI a more user-friendly modality than CT. Certainly, the greater clinical availability of CT, especially for the patient with multiple traumatic injuries, can affect the decision between CT and MRI. All things being equal, however, it is our clinical preference to use MRI in the evaluation of proximal tibia fractures (3,7,23,26) (Fig. 25.3).

Indications

A number of authors have addressed the arthroscopic management of plateau fractures and have demonstrated quite clearly the feasibility of using arthroscopy in selected cases (6,9,10,11,18,19,22,29,30,35,42). Fowble et al. (18) compared arthroscopic reduction and percutaneous fixation with traditional techniques of open reduction with internal fixation (ORIF) in 23 selected cases of split or split depres-

sion fractures. They obtained anatomic reduction in 100% of the arthroscopically treated group, compared with 55% in the ORIF group. The hospital stay in the arthroscopic group was half as long as that of the ORIF group, and restoration of ROM was more easily obtained with arthroscopic techniques. Nonetheless, the indications for arthroscopic treatment of fractures of the proximal tibia are not well defined in the literature. In one series by Bennett and Browner (5), the effectiveness of the arthroscope in evaluating fractures of the proximal tibia was demonstrated. They recommended that arthroscopy be used in the evaluation of all nondisplaced fractures and in conjunction with all fractures percutaneously fixed. We agree with the usefulness of arthroscopy in the management of proximal tibial fractures but find that MRI evaluation can frequently replace the arthroscope in minimally or nondisplaced fractures. Surgical goals, whether the fracture is addressed arthroscopically or with open techniques, remain the same: anatomic reduction, rigid internal fixation, and soft tissue repair as necessary to achieve early return to ROM (16). The arthroscopic option is best suited for the lateral split and lateral depression fractures (Schatzker types I and III, respectively), as well as many split depression fractures (Schatzker type II). The arthroscopic option can be used in some nondisplaced or minimally displaced low-energy medial plateau fractures (Schatzker type IV), and occasional for a minimally displaced or nondisplaced low-energy bicondylar fracture (Schatzker type V). However, the application of arthroscopic techniques must be used with care in fracture patterns IV, V, and VI, which are more commonly seen in higher-energy injuries. Lastly, the simple fracture-dislocation pattern, involving a lateral plateau fracture and a concomitant MCL injury, can also be approached with the arthroscope for fracture fixation, but with open repair of the MCL (36).

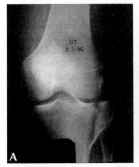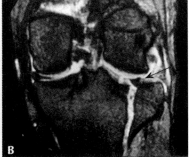

FIGURE 25.3 A: Minimally displaced Schatzker I fracture of the proximal tibia. (From Perry CR, Hunter R, Ostrum R, et al. Fractures of the proximal tibia. *Instr Course Lect* 1999;48:497–513, with permission.) **B:** Magnetic resonance imaging scan demonstrating a displaced lateral meniscus tear into the fracture, which at the time of surgery was reduced arthroscopically with repair of the meniscus and percutaneous cannulated screw fixation of the lateral plateau. (From Perry CR, Hunter R, Ostrum R, et al. Fractures of the proximal tibia. *Instr Course Lect* 1999;48:497–513, with permission.)

The advantages of the arthroscopic treatment are a thorough joint evaluation and lavage; complete visualization of the fracture, especially posteriorly; and minimization of incisions and avoidance of a large knee joint arthrotomy. Theoretically, this results in minimization of soft tissue dissection but must be used in conjunction with percutaneous screw fixation. Meniscal detachment is avoided, as is the need for collateral ligament repair. The disadvantages of arthroscopic treatment include the fact that it is technically demanding and can be used only with selected fractures. Furthermore, equipment setup and the need for both arthroscopy (with fluid flow) and fluoroscopy, frequently simultaneously, require coordination of operating room (OR) nursing staff and technicians and radiology technicians. Furthermore, there is a stated risk of compartment syndrome with arthroscopic intervention, and the surgeon must identify fluid extravasation and be prepared to abandon an arthroscopic approach for an open procedure in the presence of gross soft tissue swelling about the knee, especially posterior or in the area of the anterior compartment (4). Lastly, the use of arthroscopy has not been justified in higher-energy and complex fracture patterns for which hybrid external fixation is used, compared with fluoroscopic control and mini-open joint inspection arthrotomy (36).

Surgical Technique

Before embarking on an arthroscopic approach to tibial plateau fractures, it is important to do a thorough preoperative evaluation in order to determine the appropriate treatment strategy. The preoperative workup includes a complete history and physical examination, anteroposterior and lateral knee radiographs, and an ancillary study as indicated—CT or MRI. Fractures that are most effectively treated arthroscopically are Schatzker I, II, and III and occasional Schatzker IV or V. Certainly, high-quality plain radiographs are invaluable in determining the appropriate treatment. MRI or CT can be particularly helpful in identifying those fractures that can be treated nonsurgically. These studies also assist in identifying the appropriate reduction maneuvers that are necessary for closed treatment. If surgical treatment is necessary, MRI or CT assists in optimal screw placement. Joint depression fractures that are most amenable to an arthroscopic approach are those that are pushed down symmetrically, rather than with a large anteriorly displaced fragment. Ease of reduction by indirect (arthroscopic) methods can frequently be reliably judged from preoperative MRI.

Technique and Setup

The technical exercise of arthroscopic-assisted fixation of the proximal tibial fracture can be straightforward with proper setup and synchronous use of arthroscopic and fluoroscopic imaging. The patient is initially carefully evaluated with an EUA, and if gross valgus instability is present a visual inspection under fluoroscopic control should be performed to differentiate between fracture depression and MCL injury (or to establish the presence of both). A standard clinical EUA of both cruciates and collaterals should be

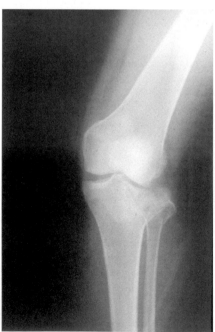
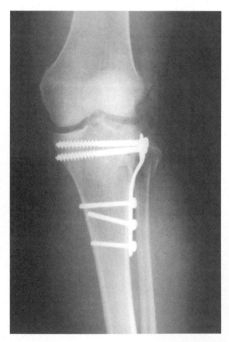
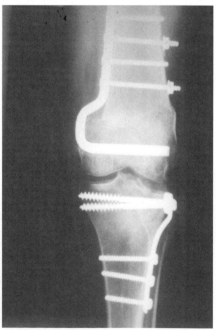

A, B   C

FIGURE 25.4 A: Lateral split fracture on anteroposterior radiograph. **B:** Lateral split fracture in (A) after open reduction with internal fixation and no medial collateral ligament repair. **C:** Late collapse of lateral plateau "fracture-dislocation."

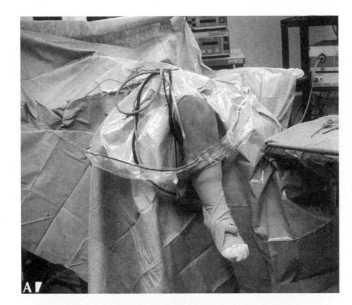

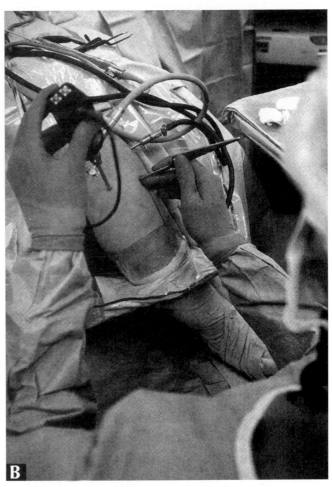

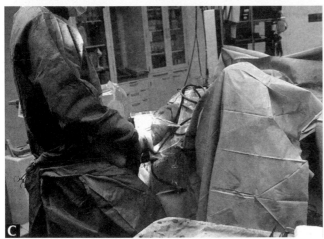

FIGURE 25.5 A: The injured extremity is placed in a leg holder with the operating room table end "dropped" or "broken," allowing complete access to the leg. **B:** The foot is placed across the surgeon's lap to provide varus stress for access and visualization of the lateral compartment. **C:** After arthroscopic fixation, the knee is extended and percutaneous cannulated screws are placed with fluoroscopic guidance to hold the reduction. (From Perry CP, Hunter R, Ostrum R, et al. Fractures of the proximal tibia. *Instr Course Lect* 1999;48:497–513, with permission.)

performed. Associated ligament injuries must be recognized and frequently must be addressed at the time of fracture fixation to prevent deformity or late collapse (Fig. 25.4). Patient setup for arthroscopic fixation requires patient positioning for both simultaneous arthroscopic and fluoroscopic control. Use of a leg holder on the upper thigh (padded tourniquet) and a contralateral lithotomy leg holder, with the end of the table "broken," allows for both ease of arthroscopic visualization and intermittent fluoroscopy (Fig. 25.5).

The arthroscope is introduced through the standard infralateral parapatellar portal with gravity or "low flow" pump inflow. A separate superolateral outflow portal frequently allows for hematoma evacuation, but suction shaving is often needed in addition to fluid lavage. A probe is in-

serted through the anteromedial portal, and a routine examination of the knee joint is performed. It is not common to find medial-sided articular cartilage or meniscal pathology given the valgus load in creating the majority of plateau fractures, but one should visualize the medial meniscus as well as the articular surfaces in the medial compartment. An examination of the intercondylar notch allows one to identify ACL pathology and the occasional posterior cruciate ligament injury, but again, this should be recognized or at a minimum suspected after MRI and intraoperative, careful EUA. During arthroscopy, varus pressure is applied to the knee to open the lateral joint, and the plateau fracture can be visualized; fat pad debridement is routinely performed to aid in fracture visualization. The arthroscope is then switched to the anteromedial portal, and the anterolateral

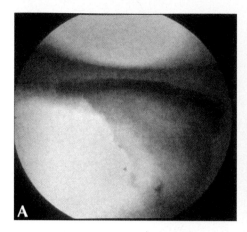
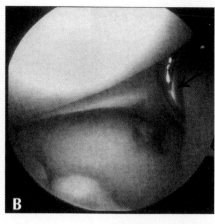

FIGURE 25.6 A: Visualization of the lateral plateau after debridement of the anterior fat pad. **B:** An ancillary lateral portal can be used to retract the lateral meniscus for complete visualization of the fracture extension. (From Perry CP, Hunter R, Ostrum R, et al. Fractures of the proximal tibia. *Instr Course Lect* 1999;48:497–513, with permission.)

portal becomes the working site. If the plateau fracture is predominately anterior, an accessory lateral portal can be very helpful. This portal is made approximately 2 cm lateral to the patellar tendon (anterolateral portal) and along the lateral joint line. Through this portal, and using an arthroscopic probe, one can retract the lateral meniscus for better visualization of the compartment (Fig. 25.6).

A tibial guide is used to find the center of the depressed area of the plateau, although most commercially available ACL tibial guides are somewhat difficult to use owing to the depth of the hook. Preferably, the guide should be modified to have a simple flat surface, in order to accomplish accurate positioning of the pin in the lateral articular fracture frag-

ment. Furthermore, the pin should enter the lateral tibial flare away from fracture lines in preparation for creation of a cortical window. Once positioned, a guide wire is inserted percutaneously through the anterolateral tibial cortex and passed into the knee joint under direct visualization. Ideally, the pin enters the joint slightly posterior in the fracture fragment and midway between the medial and lateral extents of the depressed segment (Fig. 25.7). A small skin incision is made around the percutaneous pin to allow a 9-mm cannulated drill to be inserted "percutaneously." The tibial cortex is carefully drilled, avoiding penetration past the cortical rim and avoiding the articular surface. An angled, cannulated tamp is introduced through the tibial hole and is used to

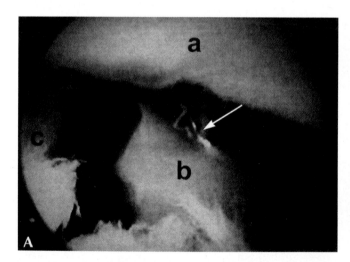
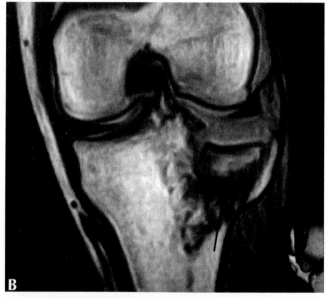

FIGURE 25.7 A: The guide wire *(arrow)* is ideally placed in the fractured articular segment in the posterior third, midway between the medial and lateral extent of the fracture fragment. a, lateral femoral condyle; b, displaced lateral tibial plateau fracture; c, intact portion of the lateral tibial condyle. **B:** The entry point *(arrow)* of the drill guide is crucial. It must enter the anterolateral cortex of the tibia low enough that the reamed cortical window is below the depressed articular fragment, in order to avoid damage to the articular segment and allow for elevation of the fragment. (From Perry CP, Hunter R, Ostrum R, et al. Fractures of the proximal tibia. *Instr Course Lect* 1999;48:497–513, with permission.)

carefully tap and elevate the depressed fragment while simultaneously visualizing the lateral compartment arthroscopically. First, the central aspect of the depression is first elevated, and then, by rotation of the angled tamp, the edges at the 3-, 6-, and 9-o'clock positions are effectively elevated to ensure anatomic reduction. The inferior surface of the lateral meniscus serves as a reduction guide, because on complete reduction of the articular surface, the lateral meniscus will lie normally against the hyaline surface (36) (Fig. 25.8).

After the fracture has been anatomically reduced, fluoroscopy is used to demonstrate alignment of the plateau, confirming anatomic reduction. It is very important to align the fluoroscope so that it is completely tangential to the articular surfaces, to preclude false perception of anatomic fracture alignment. After the reduction has been deemed adequate, bone graft is placed through the drill hole in the anterolateral tibia, completely filling the void created by the elevation of the fragment and the tamp itself. Although a variety of materials are available, either allograft or other osteoinductive bone graft substitutes work well (40). Avoiding an iliac crest harvest and its associated complications is becoming more clinically applicable with good patient acceptance. Although autogenous graft is still the gold standard, the added morbidity (8% major, 20% minor complications in one series) to provide cells and osteoinductive growth factors must be weighed by the treating surgeon (1,40).

Using fluoroscopy, guide wires are passed from lateral to medial approximately 1 cm below the articular surface, exiting the medial metaphysis. Then, 7.0- or 7.3-mm Synthes (Paoli, PA) cannulated screws are used to internally fix the fracture and simultaneously reduce any remaining plastic deformation of the lateral metaphyseal cortex. At a mini-

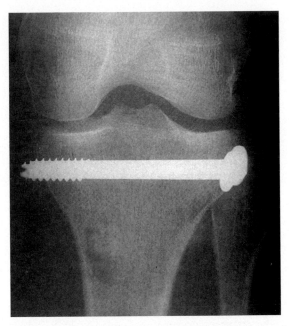

FIGURE 25.9 Once the fracture is reduced, the joint line and lateral tibial condyle are located under fluoroscopic guidance, and percutaneous cannulated 7.0- or 7.3-mm screws are inserted (7.3 mm in this patient). A washer is an excellent hardware adjunct for fracture compression and prevention of screw head penetration past the lateral tibial cortex. (From Perry CP, Hunter R, Ostrum R, et al. Fractures of the proximal tibia. *Instr Course Lect* 1999;48:497–513, with permission.)

mum, two screws are employed for simple split or split depression fractures (Fig. 25.9). If such fixation is not considered adequate, then conversion to an open approach with buttress side plate fixation may be necessary. Lastly, evidence of a complete contralateral ligamentous injury, as seen with fracture-dislocations, should be addressed at the time of fracture fixation (Fig. 25.10).

We prefer intraoperative plain radiographs (not just hard copies of the fluoroscopic images) at the conclusion of the procedure, because the detail is much greater than with fluoroscopy, especially in the evaluation of fractures about the proximal tibia. It is our preference to obtain this added information in the OR, so that changes can be made in the reduction or internal fixation if necessary.

Postoperatively, knees are placed in a hinged brace that allows full ROM as pain and swelling allow. Crutch walking is initiated on the day after surgery, employing a non–weight-bearing strategy for the first 6 to 10 weeks after fixation and depending on fracture stability and surgeon preference. In most circumstances, partial weight bearing is allowed after 6 to 8 weeks, and approximately 10% to 15% of the body weight is added per week over the remaining 4 to 6 weeks, with full weight bearing by 12 weeks after surgery. The addition of a concomitant ligament (MCL) repair requires aggressive ROM exercises to avoid arthrofibrosis, but strict prohibition of weight bearing is required to avoid late collapse (36).

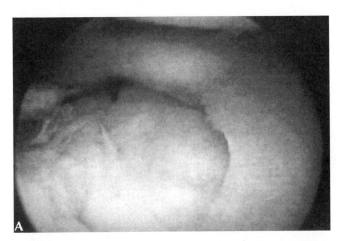

FIGURE 25.8 After complete reduction, the tibial plateau should contact the undersurface of the lateral meniscus throughout its periphery, with the edges of the fractured surface level with the adjoining intact surface medially. (From Perry CP, Hunter R, Ostrum R, et al. Fractures of the proximal tibia. *Instr Course Lect* 1999;48:497–513, with permission.)

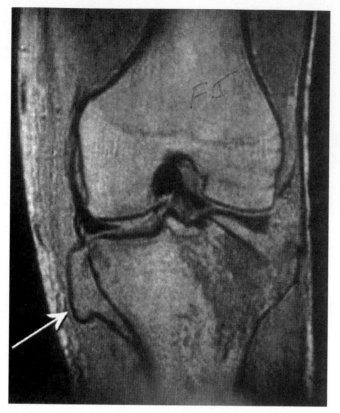

FIGURE 25.10 Magnetic resonance image of a fracture-dislocation of the proximal tibia with a depressed lateral plateau segment and a complete medial collateral ligament (MCL) injury. Fracture elevation and internal fixation were used in combination with MCL reattachment distally. (From Perry CP, Hunter R, Ostrum R, et al. Fractures of the proximal tibia. *Instr Course Lect* 1999;48:497–513, with permission.)

TIBIAL SPINE AVULSIONS

Tibial spine avulsion fractures represent an avulsion of the tibial eminence most commonly involving the ACL insertion. It has been described as "the childhood equivalent of the ACL rupture" and is frequently seen in an arthroscopic practice. Although the injury represents a ligamentous avulsion of the ACL insertion, there can be overlap between split-type tibial plateau fractures and this injury, placing it into the category of a fracture-dislocation requiring fracture and ligamentous fixation. In the following discussion, the eminence fracture is treated as an isolated entity, with the caution that it can occur in combination with other fractures about the proximal tibia.

Although it was first described in 1875, the early literature described this diagnosis as one exclusive to knees with open growth plates (i.e., a childhood injury) (32). However, this injury was later demonstrated to occur in the adult population, accounting for up to 40% of all the eminence injuries seen in one series. The mechanism of injury is similar to that of an ACL rupture with valgus external rotation, deceleration injury, and hyperflexion and internal rotation as seen in skiing (i.e., phantom foot phenomenon). These in-

juries are also frequently seen as a result of motor vehicular accidents in both the adult and pediatric populations. It is important for the surgeon to remember that some degree of ligamentous substance injury can occur in combination with an avulsion pattern (41).

Myers and McKeever (32) provided the most widely used classification system for eminence fractures. The system classifies tibial spine avulsions into three types. Type I is a nondisplaced or minimally displaced spine avulsion (32). Type II is an avulsion in which the fracture is rotated with the posterior aspect of the avulsion still in place. Type III represents a completely displaced fracture fragment (Fig. 25.11). There are some shortcomings to the system. The radiograph classifies the fracture based on its final position and does not represent maximum displacement at the time of injury; therefore, it probably underrepresents the amount of instability associated with the fracture. It is likely that some fractures classified as type II were type III at the time of injury. The classification system describes only the bony position and does not provide any information about soft tissue injury about the ligament substance or knee joint itself. Some injuries classified as type I injuries with minimal displacement have been shown to have an entrapped meniscus or intermeniscal ligament blocking complete reduction.

Treatment recommendations have varied, but the classic recommendation calls for extension casting for type I injuries, extension casting or possibly ORIF for type II injuries, and ORIF for type III lesions. With current commonplace use of arthroscopy, the ability to evaluate visually the reduction of the tibial spine fracture, as well as the presence of articular or midsubstance cruciate injury, makes arthroscopic applications appealing for even the nondisplaced tibial spine fractures. Also, the ability to internally fix such fractures, creating a scenario for early ROM, is another

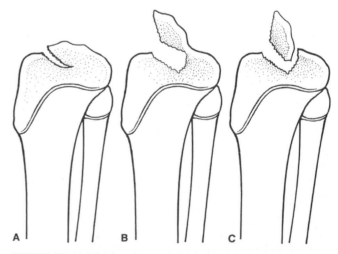

FIGURE 25.11 Tibial eminence (tibial spine avulsion) fractures of the proximal tibia as described by Meyers and McKeever. (From Meyers MH, McKeever FM. Fracture of the intercondylar eminence of the tibia. *J Bone Joint Surg Am* 1959;41:4209–4222, with permission.)

argument for the arthroscopic approach. If closed reduction is used, we recommend MRI afterward to evaluate any concomitant joint injury and the adequacy of tibial spine avulsion fracture reduction.

McLennan (31) presented a study reviewing management of type III fractures that compared closed reduction and casting (group I), arthroscopic reduction and casting (group II), and arthroscopic reduction with internal fixation (group III) (31). Lysholm scores were higher in groups II and III than in group I. Both Tegner and International Knee Documentation Committee (IKDC) scores were highest in group III, intermediate in group II, and lowest in group I. When the knees were reexamined postoperatively (arthroscopically), only group III showed the fragment to be reduced, with groups I and II having greater than 3 mm of fracture fragment offset. McLennan concluded that the arthroscopic approach produced more predictable results and was the treatment of choice for type III fractures. This recommendation was extended to include type II fractures by other authors. Certainly indications for tibial spine avulsion fractures are evolving. Preoperative MRI is very useful in identifying fracture extent and the presence of involvement of the posterior cruciate ligament. If the tibial spine is comminuted, caution should be exercised, because rigid fixation may not be possible. Failure to achieve rigid fixation may lead the surgeon to immobilize the knee postoperatively, causing significant problems with mobility.

Surgical Technique

The knee is placed in a leg holder off the side of the operating table. The nonoperative leg is supported on foam. A radiolucent table should be used if fluoroscopic control is desired. An alternative method can be used, as noted previously with fractures of the proximal tibia, but fluoroscopic is not as crucial in this scenario. In any case, plain radiographs are taken at the end of the procedure so that reduction and fixation are satisfactorily verified before the patient leaves the OR. Reduction of tibial spine fractures can be difficult, and it is better to have the plain films in the OR so that changes in reduction or fixation can be made if necessary.

The arthroscope is placed through an anterolateral portal, and the probe and operating instruments through an anteromedial portal. Variations on outflow, either superomedial or superolateral, depend on surgeon preference and experience. We first evacuate the hematoma with the use of a motorized suction shaver. Usually it is not necessary to employ a tourniquet, because the pump provides adequate joint distension. The fragment or fragments are identified and debrided of all soft tissue around the margin to allow for good visualization of both the bony bed and the fragment (Fig. 25.12). The fat pad is debrided as necessary to obtain complete visualization of the anterior aspect of the joint. The knee is carefully inspected for any entrapped meniscus or intermeniscal ligament. Any interposed soft tissue is re-

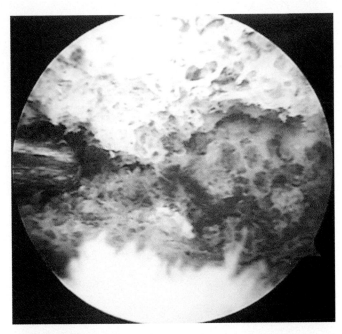

FIGURE 25.12 The synovial resector is used to debride all clot and loose bone from between the avulsed fragment and the tibial bed. (From Hunter RE. Arthroscopic management of intraarticular tibial fractures. In: *Master techniques in orthopaedic surgery,* 2nd ed [in press], with permission.)

tracted, and the avulsion fracture is reduced with "firm but gentle" (27) pressure with an arthroscopic probe. The presence of fracture extension into the plateau or plastic deformation can make reduction difficult, and occasionally a mini-open technique just medial to the patellar tendon is required to obtain adequate fracture reduction.

One of two fixation techniques is employed: cannulated screws (retrograde or antegrade) or nonabsorbable suture (tied over a bony bridge). We prefer suture fixation in patients with open growth plates. Nonetheless, when cannulated screws are used, the fracture fragment is reduced into its bony bed and held with a probe through the anteromedial portal. A guide wire is drilled percutaneously through a midmedial portal into the fragment and with care to engage only the posterior cortex of the tibia (Fig. 25.13). Fluoroscopic control is used to be certain that the guide wire does not overpenetrate the posterior cortex. Once reduction is verified and the guide wire is checked for appropriate screw length selection, a 4.0-mm cannulated screw (Synthes) is passed through the spine and to the posterior cortex of the tibia (Figure 25.14). We use real-time fluoroscopy as the screw is advanced to prevent injury to the neurovascular structures by an advancing guide wire posteriorly. Typically, one screw completely stabilizes the fracture, but a second screw can be added depending on fracture fragment size and stability after initial screw placement.

Screw fixation is an excellent technique in those cases in which the bony fragment is large enough to accommodate the screw and in those patients in whom the growth plate is almost closed or completely fused. In children with open

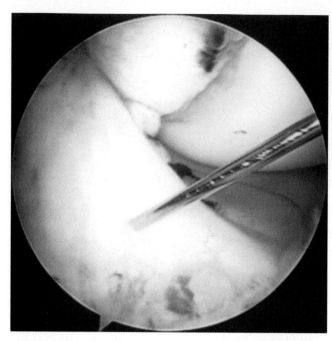

FIGURE 25.13 Percutaneous fixation of the spine avulsion through a midmedial patellar portal. (From Hunter RE. Arthroscopic management of intraarticular tibial fractures. In: *Master techniques in orthopaedic surgery,* 2nd ed [in press], with permission.)

growth plates and in situations in which the fragment is not large enough to accommodate a screw, or if the surgeon desires to avoid intraarticular metallic fixation, suture fixation becomes an excellent surgical option. The knee is positioned in a similar fashion, fracture reduction is performed, and a 0.045 K-wire is inserted through a midmedial portal into the fragment directed posteriorly for temporary fixation. An ACL guide is used to pass a $5/_{64}$ inch pin retrograde from the subcutaneous tibial border at the level of the tibial tubercle (midway between the posteromedial tibial edge and the tibial tubercle laterally), entering the joint at the medial aspect of the avulsed fragment. A small incision is made in the area of the guide pin to expose the cortical surface. The guide wire is removed and replaced with a Hewson suture passer (Fig. 25.15) (Smith and Nephew Endoscopy, Andover, MA). Through the anteromedial portal, a no. 5 Ethibond suture (Ethicon, Somerville, NJ) is passed into the joint, then through the loop in the suture passer, and is pulled distally, exiting the anteromedial tibial cortex (Fig. 25.16). Using the ACL guide, a second guide wire is started 5 mm from the first pin site and drilled into the lateral aspect of the spine avulsion. The wire is removed and replaced with the Hewson suture passer (Fig. 25.17). The opposite end of the no. 5 Ethibond is passed through the loop and then pulled through the joint and out the anteromedial tibial cortex, creating a loop of no. 5 Ethibond suture that passes from the medial to the lateral aspect of the spine avulsion, exiting the

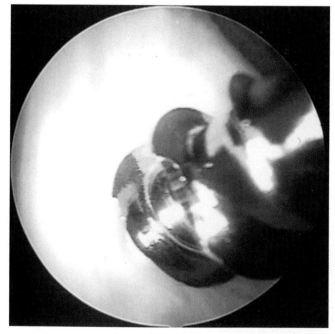

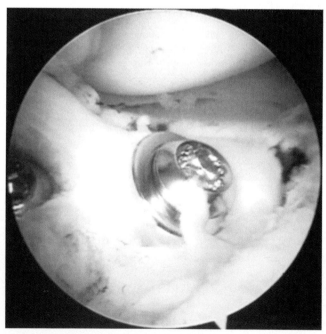

A

B

FIGURE 25.14 A: A 4.0-mm cannulated screw is passed through a midmedial puncture wound into the spine avulsion. (From Hunter RE. Arthroscopic management of intraarticular tibial fractures. In: *Master techniques in orthopaedic surgery,* 2nd ed [in press], with permission). **B:** Arthroscopic image of a spine avulsion after percutaneous fixation with two cannulated screws. A washer has been used in this case but generally is not necessary. (From Hunter RE. Arthroscopic management of intraarticular tibial fractures. In: *Master techniques in orthopaedic surgery,* 2nd ed [in press], with permission.)

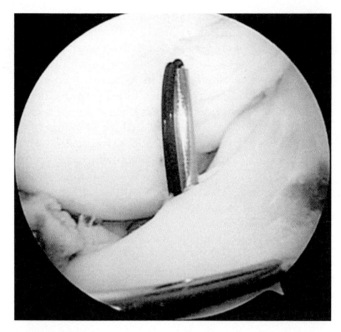

FIGURE 25.15 Hewson suture passer has been placed through the tibial hole entering the joint on the medial aspect of the spine avulsion. (Reprinted with permission from Hunter, RE. *Arthroscopic Management of Intraarticular Tibial Fractures, Master Techniques in Orthopaedic Surgery*, second edition, *in press*).

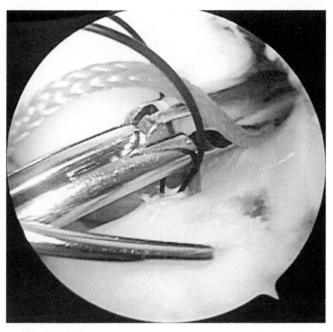

FIGURE 25.16 A no. 5 Ethibond is passed through the antero-medial portal, through the Hewson suture passer, and pulled out the anteromedial cortex. (Reprinted with permission from Hunter, RE. *Arthroscopic Management of Intraarticular Tibial Fractures, Master Techniques in Orthopaedic Surgery*, second edition, *in press*).

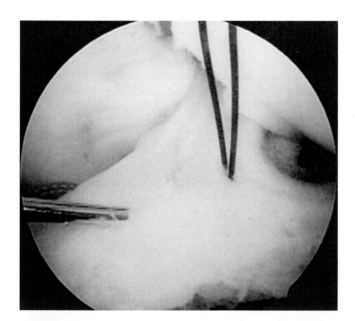

FIGURE 25.17 A second guide wire has been drilled and replaced with a second Hewson suture passer. This will receive the opposite end of the no. 5 Ethibond suture. (Reprinted with permission from Hunter, RE *Arthroscopic Management of Intraarticular Tibial Fractures, Master Techniques in Orthopaedic Surgery*, second edition, *in press*).

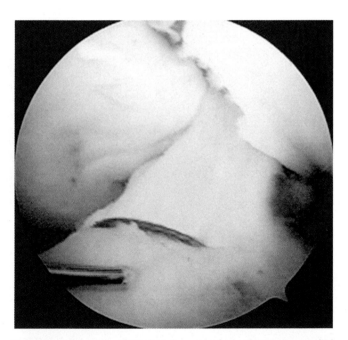

FIGURE 25.18 A no. 5 Ethibond crosses from the anteromedial to the anterolateral aspect of the spine avulsion with temporary fixation maintained with the guide wire. (Reprinted with permission from Hunter, RE. *Arthroscopic Management of Intraarticular Tibial Fractures, Master Techniques in Orthopaedic Surgery*, second edition, in press).

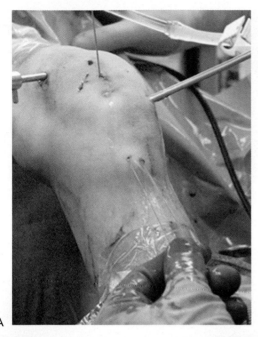

A

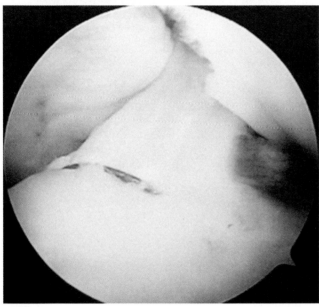

B

FIGURE 25.19 Final arthroscopic imaging demonstrating tension in the no. 5 Ethibond suture and anatomic reduction of the spine avulsion. **A:** Outside view of a left knee showing both limbs of the no. 5 Ethibond exiting the anteromedial tibia. (Reprinted with permission from Hunter, RE. *Arthroscopic Management of Intraarticular Tibial Fractures, Master Techniques in Orthopaedic Surgery*, second edition, *in press*.)

tibial metaphysis (Fig. 25.18). The suture ends are tied over a bony bridge with a minimum of four throws (preferably six), ensuring arthroscopic reduction and tension of the tibial spine avulsion fracture (Fig. 25.19).

Postoperative ROM is dictated by fracture stabilization and surgeon experience. Short-term use of an extension brace for ambulation, with twice-daily passive ROM out of the brace from 0 to 90 degrees, is used for the first 2 to 3

weeks. Straight leg raising and quadriceps isometrics are employed to try to maintain quadriceps tone. Thereafter, ROM limits are removed and closed-chain quadriceps exercises are begun.

An arthroscopic approach to these fractures can be successful in the vast majority of cases. Either screw fixation or suture fixation can effectively reduce and hold the fracture in place. Because screw fixation is perhaps more rigid, it is the treatment of choice when the fracture is large enough to accommodate a screw and in knees in which the growth plate is closed. Suture fixation becomes an excellent alternative in the growing child and in situations in which there is comminution or the fragment is too small to accommodate screw fixation. Indications for surgery are evidence of fracture displacement on radiography or evidence of clinical laxity on examination. If the fracture is reduced, held firmly, and allowed to heal, the return to a preinjury level of participation is quite predictable.

REFERENCES

1. Arrington ED, Smith WJ, Chambers HG, et al. Complications of iliac crest bone graft harvesting. *Clin Orthop Rel Res* 1996;329: 300–309.
2. Apley A. Fractures of the lateral tibial condyle treated by skeletal traction and early mobilization. *J Bone Joint Surg Br* 1956;38: 699–708.
3. Barrow BA, Fajman WA, Parker LM, et al. Tibial plateau fractures: evaluation with MR imaging. *RadioGraphics* 1994;14: 564–559.
4. Belanger M, Fadale P. Compartment syndrome of the leg after arthroscopic examination of a tibial plateau fracture: case report and review of the literature. *Arthroscopy* 1997;13:646–651.
5. Bennett WF, Browner B. Tibial plateau fractures: a study of associate soft tissue injuries. *J Orthop Trauma* 1994;8:183–188.
6. Bobic V, O'Dwyer KJ. Tibial plateau fractures: the arthroscopic option. *Knee Surg Sports Traumatol Arthrosc* 1993;1:239–242.
7. Brophy DP, O'Malley M, et al. MR imaging of tibial plateau fractures. *Clin Radiol* 1996;51:873–878.
8. Brown TD, Anderson DD, Nepola JV, et al. Contact stress aberrations following imprecise reduction of simple tibial plateau fractures. *J Orthop Res* 1988;6:851–862.
9. Buchko GM, Johnson DH. Arthroscopy assisted operative management of tibial plateau fractures. *Clin Orthop* 1996;332:29–6.
10. Carro LP. Arthroscopic management of tibial plateau fractures: special techniques [Technical note]. *Arthroscopy* 1997;13:265–267.
11. Caspari RB, Hutton PM.J, Whipple TL, et al. The role of arthroscopy in the management of tibial plateau fractures. *Arthroscopy* 1985;1:76–82.
12. Daniel E, Rice T. Valgus-varus stability in the hinged cast used for controlled mobilization of the knee. *J Bone Joint Surg Am* 1979;61:135–136.
13. Delamarter RB, Hohl M, Hopp E Jr. Ligament injuries associated with tibial plateau fractures. *Clin Orthop* 1990;250:226–233.
14. Dias J, Stirling A, Finlay D, et al. Computerized axial tomography for tibial plateau fractures. *J Bone Joint Surg Br* 1987; 69:84–88.

15. Duwelius PJ, Connolly JF. Closed reduction of tibial plateau fractures: a comparison of functional and roentgenographic end results. *Clin Orthop* 1988;230:116–126.
16. Enneking W, Horowitz M. The intra-articular effects of immobilization on the human knee. *J Bone Joint Surg Am* 1972;54:973–985.
17. Fernandez D. Anterior approach to the knee with osteotomy of the tibial tubercle for bicondylar tibial fractures. *J Bone Joint Surg Am* 1988;70:1208–1219.
18. Fowble CD, Zimmer JW, et al. The role of arthroscopy in the assessment and treatment of tibial plateau fractures. *Arthroscopy* 1993;9:584–590.
19. Guanche CA, Markman AW. Arthroscopic management of tibial plateau fractures. *Arthroscopy* 1993;9:467–471.
20. Hohl M. Fractures of the knee: part I. Fractures of the proximal tibia and fibula. In: Rockwood CA, Green DP, eds. *Fractures.* pp. 1725-1761. Philadelphia: JB Lippincott, 1991:1725 1761.
21. Hohl M. Tibial condylar fractures. *J Bone Joint Surg Am* 1971;49:1455–1467.
22. Holzach P, Matter P, et al. Arthroscopically assisted treatment of lateral tibial plateau fractures in skiers: use of a cannulated reduction system. *J Orthop Trauma* 1994;8:273–281.
23. Hunter RL. Personal communication, 2001.
24. Kaar TK, Schenck RC Jr, Wirth MA, et al. Complications of metallic suture anchors in shoulder surgery: a report of 8 cases. *J Arthrosc* 2001;17:31–37.
25. Kearns RJ, Mendelow M, Soltes G, et al. Radiographic view and quality in the assessment of the tibial plateau fracture: are we missing something? *J Orthop Trauma* 1989;3:167 (abst).
26. Kode L, Lieberman JM, Motta AO, et al. Evaluation of tibial plateau fractures: efficacy of MR imaging compared with CT. *AJR Am J Roentgenol* 1994;163:141–147.
27. Krackow, KA. Personal communication, 1986.
28. Lansinger O. Tibial condylar fractures: a twenty-year follow-up. *J Bone Joint Surg Am* 1986;68:13–19.
29. Lobenhoffer P, Schulze M, et al. Closed reduction/percutaneous fixation of tibial plateau fractures: arthroscopic versus fluoroscopic control of reduction. *J Orthop Trauma* 1999;13:426–431.
30. Mazoue CG, Guanche CA, et al. Arthroscopic management of tibial plateau fractures: an unselected series. *Am J Orthop* 1999;28:508–515.
31. McLennan JG. Lessons learned after second-look arthroscopy in type III fractures of the tibial spine. *J Pediatr Orthop* 1995;15:59–62.
32. Meyers MH, McKeever FM. Fracture of the intercondylar eminence of the tibia. *J Bone Joint Surg Am* 1959;41:209–222.
33. Moore T. Fracture-dislocation of the knee. *Clin Orthop* 1981;156:128–140.
34. Moore T, Harvey P. Roentgenographic measurement of tibial plateau depression due to fracture. *J Bone Joint Surg Am* 1974;56:155–160.
35. Muezzinoglu US, Guner G, et al. Arthroscopically assisted tibial plateau fracture management: a modified method. *Arthroscopy* 1995;11:506–509.
36. Perry CP, Hunter R, Ostrum R, et al. Fractures of the proximal tibia. *Instr Course Lect* 1999;48:497–513.
37. Rasmussen PS. Tibial condylar fractures. *J Bone Joint Surg Am* 1973;55:1331–1350.
38. Rüed TP, Murphy WM. *AO principles of fracture management.* New York: AO Publishing, Thieme, 2000:864.
39. Schatzker J, McBroom R, Bruce D. The tibial plateau fracture: the Toronto experience. *Clin Orthop* 1979;138:94–140.
40. Schenck RC. Strategic strategies: contemporary tissue engineering. *Medscape* 2001.
41. Schenck RC, Kovach IS, Agarwal A, et al. Cruciate injury patterns in knee hyperextension: a cadaveric model. *J Arthrosc* 1999;15:489–495.
42. Scheerlinck T, Ng CS, et al. Medium-term results of percutaneous, arthroscopically-assisted osteosynthesis of fractures of the tibial plateau. *J Bone Joint Surg Br* 19998;80:959–964.

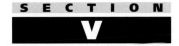

SECTION
V

THE SHOULDER

HISTORY, PHYSICAL EXAMINATION, AND DIAGNOSTIC MODALITIES

NEIL S. ROTH
LOUIS U. BIGLIANI

Arthroscopy of the shoulder has provided an enormous opportunity to understand the anatomy and physiology of the shoulder joint (1). While shoulder arthroscopy is an effective surgical tool for both the diagnosis and management of many pathologic conditions, it does not replace a thorough history and physical examination (2).

Successful shoulder arthroscopy relies on proper patient selection by establishing the correct preoperative diagnosis, and can be utilized to treat both intraarticular as well as extraarticular shoulder pathology. Preoperatively, conditions that have symptoms similar to those of shoulder pathology, such as cervical radiculopathy, tumors, infection, and systemic rheumatologic disorders, must be carefully discerned (3).

This chapter discusses the relevant history, physical examination, and diagnostic modalities necessary for a thorough preoperative assessment essential for evaluating a patient for shoulder arthroscopy.

HISTORY

Shoulder problems affect a broad age range of patients with varying activity levels. A systematic, reproducible approach to each patient will ensure comprehensive information gathering and proper diagnosis. Initially, the patient's age, hand dominance, occupation, athletic activities, medical history, and family history are recorded (Table 26.1).

While a patient's age is not necessarily diagnostic, full-thickness rotator cuff tears are found almost exclusively in patients older than 40 years of age (4). Rarely do patients younger than 30 have primary rotator cuff pathology; they usually have "impingement" pain due to underlying shoulder instability (5).

Hand dominance is important in treatment recommendations, as the dominant arm of an athlete in a sport involving overhead arm movements will provide a different therapeutic challenge than the nondominant shoulder of a sedentary individual. The majority of rotator cuff tears affect the dominant shoulder (6).

Understanding the daily demands and level of disability that patients have with regard to their occupation as well as their intensity and level of competition in athletic activities is essential. Certain activities have a predilection for specific pathology, such as distal clavicle osteolysis in a weight lifter (7) or anterior shoulder instability with repetitive overhead arm activity seen in a baseball pitcher, tennis player, or swimmer (8).

A complete general medical history should be obtained with special attention to any systemic or rheumatologic disorders. Diabetes mellitus and metastatic cancer are often associated with adhesive capsulitis. Additionally, a family history of generalized ligamentous laxity will assist in treating a patient with multidirectional shoulder instability.

The patient's chief shoulder complaint usually consists of some element of pain, instability, weakness, or loss of motion. The pattern of these symptoms is important to document, most notably the duration, severity, provocation, and location. The mechanism of shoulder injuries can be due to a traumatic event, but is often atraumatic in nature due to repetitive microtrauma. Night pain and pain at rest are common in patients with mechanical shoulder pathology and are usually due to impingement or glenohumeral arthritis; however, infection and tumor must be ruled out.

Pain with overhead arm activity is common in patients with rotator cuff tears as well as in overhead arm activity athletes with underlying instability. The pattern of pain and exacerbating activities has to be well documented. A classification scheme has been developed for the treatment of overhead arm athletes, which describes shoulder pain along an impingement-instability spectrum (9). A frequent complaint of overhead arm athletes with underlying instability may be early fatigue, loss of velocity, or lengthier warmup periods.

N. S. Roth and L. U. Bigliani: Shoulder Service, New York Orthopaedic Hospital, Columbia-Presbyterian Medical Center, New York, New York.

TABLE 26.1 HISTORY

Patient
  Age
  Hand dominance
  Occupation
  Athletics
    Sports
    Level of competition
    Relation to shoulder problem (e.g., weight lifting and oste-
      olysis of the distal clavicle)
  Medical history (e.g., diabetes, cancer)
  Family history (e.g., arthritis, ligamentous laxity)

Shoulder disorder
  Chief complaint
    Pain
    Weakness
    Stiffness
    Instability
  Symptom pattern
    Duration
    Provocation
    Severity
    Location
  Injury
    Traumatic
    Atraumatic
    Repetitive microtrauma
    Preexisting condition?
  Level of disability
    Athletics
    Occupation
    Daily tasks

Related symptoms
  Cervical pain
  Neurologic
    Cervical radiculopathy
    Brachial plexus
    Peripheral nerve
  Chest (e.g., cardiac, lung, herpes zoster)

Patients with rotator cuff tears can have episodic symptoms of bursitis and tendonitis prior to an acute extension of a rotator cuff tear, usually with seemingly trivial trauma. However, presentation of patients with rotator cuff tears may be variable, as patients with full-thickness tears may have no symptoms, while patients with partial-thickness tears may exhibit marked weakness and loss of motion. More severe rotator cuff injuries may occur, especially when associated with a shoulder dislocation in an older patient.

Impingement shoulder pain is usually felt deeply and down the front of the upper arm, but usually not extending beyond the elbow. Anterior shoulder pain does not correlate well with any one pathologic process nor does biceps tendonitis, which occurs in both impingement, instability, and as an isolated entity. Posterior shoulder pain occurs with glenohumeral joint arthritis, but can also occur with anterior shoulder instability in overhead arm athletes. If pain in the posterior aspect of the shoulder or trapezius radiates down past the elbow into the hands, this is more consistent with a cervical radiculopathy (10). Severe episodic pain and inflammation may be suggestive of calcific tendonitis.

The etiology of shoulder instability is usually easier to identify than when shoulder pain is the presenting symptom. While most shoulder problems are due to overuse, in a traumatic event the position of the arm at the time of injury is critical to the history. A patient with an abducted, externally rotated arm will typically have anterior instability, while a dislocation with the hand below shoulder level implies posterior instability (11). If a patient is suspected of having underlying instability, information pertaining to the direction, trauma, volition, and degree of instability must be obtained. The mechanism of any injury and exacerbating activities should be documented. If a shoulder dislocation occurs, the degree of instability can be dictated by whether a closed reduction was required or if a spontaneous reduction occurred.

Weakness of the affected shoulder is a frequent complaint, but splinting from pain often contributes to this lack of strength. Patients with large rotator cuff tears often report weakness or fatigue with overhead arm use, but can also have surprisingly good motion and function. Patients will complain of "crackling" in their shoulders with motion, which can be due to a variety of disorders, including full-thickness tears producing crepitus when the greater tuberosity comes into contact with the undersurface of the acromion, glenohumeral osteoarthritis, or acromioclavicular arthritis.

Rowe described the "dead arm syndrome" in a young patient who complains of weakness, numbness, or tingling with a specific activity. These complaints are often due to underlying shoulder instability and can be due to labral pathology, capsular laxity, or rotator cuff overuse (12). Loss of motion is difficult to assess in patients with shoulder pain due to splinting, and should be assessed during the physical examination.

Symptoms from related areas must be considered and distinguished from intrinsic mechanical shoulder problems. A thorough history must be taken to rule out sources of referred pain such as the neck, chest, heart, upper back, and arm, while recognizing that these disorders may coexist. Numbness or tingling below the elbow and into the hand may be indicative of cervical disease or peripheral nerve entrapment. Brachial plexopathy can occur with shoulder instability, especially when an inferior component exists, or with an acromioclavicular dislocation or trapezius palsy (13).

PHYSICAL EXAMINATION

Physical examination of the shoulder should proceed in an organized reproducible manner (Table 26.2). The physical exam of the shoulder includes five basic parts: inspection,

TABLE 26.2 EXAMINATION

Cervical spine
  Rotation
  Flexion/extension
  Pain with motion
  Provocative testing—Spurling's test
  Sensory, motor, deep tendon reflexes

Inspection
  Muscle atrophy/hypertrophy
  Bone prominences
  Deformity (e.g., biceps long head rupture)
  Generalized ligamentous laxity (e.g., thumb, elbow)

Palpation
  Sternoclavicular joint
  Acromioclavicular joint
  Rotator cuff/tuberosities (e.g., calcium deposits)
  Biceps tendon/bicipital groove
  Glenohumeral joint line
  Trapezius muscle spasm

Range of motion
  Motion quality—rhythm, synchrony, scapulothoracic
  Range of motion
    Elevation—active, passive
    External rotation—at neutral and 90 degrees of abduction
    Internal rotation

Strength
  Supraspinatus
  External rotation
  Internal rotation—"lift-off" test, abdominal compression
  Scapular stabilizers

Provocative tests
  Impingement
    Neer
    Hawkins
    Arc of pain
    Impingement test
    Acromioclavicular (AC) joint—horizontal adduction, selective injection
  Instability—anterior
    Apprehension sign
    Relocation test
    Load and shift test
    Drawer sign
  Instability—posterior
    Posterior stress test
    Drawer sign
  Instability—inferior
    Sulcus test—neutral and 90 degrees abducted
  Labral tests
  Biceps
    Speed's test
    Yergason's test

palpation, range of motion, strength testing, and provocative tests.

The shoulder is often the site for referred pain, commonly from the cervical spine. Therefore, a thorough examination of the cervical spine must be performed for any potential coexisting or referred pathology. The cervical spine is brought through a range of motion, including flexion, ex-

tension, and lateral rotation. Pain and crepitation with motion should be noted. The Spurling test, which is effective in distinguishing cervical spine radiculopathy from intrinsic shoulder pathology, is performed with gentle cervical extension, and rotation toward the affected shoulder with axial compression; it is positive if it produces posterior shoulder pain and radiculopathy. Bilateral deep tendon reflexes as well as a thorough dermatomal sensory and motor evaluation shoulder be performed.

Inspection

Patients should be examined with both shoulders exposed, allowing access anteriorly as well as posteriorly. Women are placed in gowns so that they are "strapless" and men disrobe above the waist. Thorough inspection of the shoulder should note any muscular atrophy, hypertrophy, asymmetry, or deformity as well as bony prominences. Examination may reveal a prominent scapular spine due to spinati atrophy, which is often indicative of a long-standing rotator cuff tear, but may also be present with suprascapular nerve entrapment. The shoulder is evaluated for any deformity of the biceps muscle, as the long head of the biceps tendon is often ruptured in patients with rotator cuff disease. Additionally, bony prominences and contour of the shoulder are noted, as a patient with an anterior shoulder dislocation loses normal contour with squaring and anterior fullness.

Palpation

Palpation around the shoulder joint should be done systematically so that each muscle, joint, and bony prominence is evaluated. The sternoclavicular joint; the clavicle; the acromioclavicular joint (AC); the anterior, lateral, and posterior acromion; the anterior and posterior joint lines; and the biceps tendon should each be tested for discrete tenderness. Localized tenderness over the AC joint is often overlooked as a source of symptoms and may be implicated in rotator cuff pathology or degenerative joint disease. Palpation of the greater tuberosity, assisted by extension of the shoulder slightly (14), is often positive with rotator cuff pathology, but may be due to calcific tendonitis and should be correlated with rotational radiographs of the humerus (Fig. 26.1). Tenderness in the bicipital groove may be present with involvement of the biceps tendon, and can be implicated in both rotator cuff pathology and glenohumeral instability. Anterior and posterior joint line tenderness may be present with glenohumeral instability, while posterior joint line tenderness is commonly noted in patients with glenohumeral arthritis.

Range of Motion/Strength Testing

Range of motion and strength testing can be performed simultaneously and should be compared to the asymptomatic

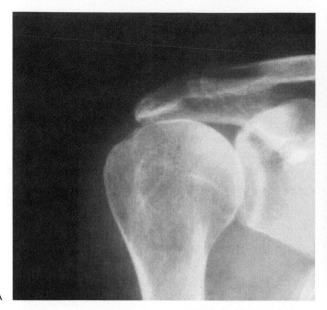

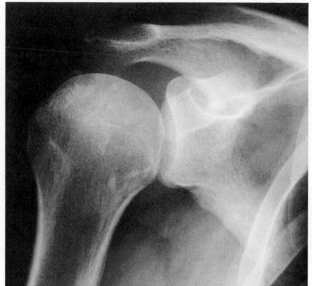

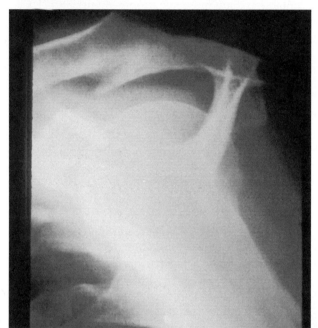

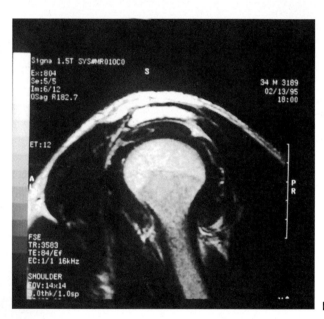

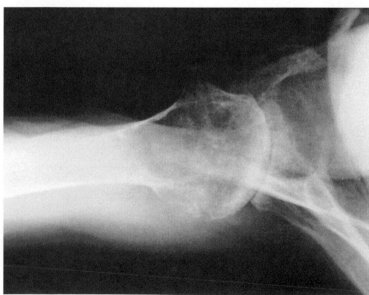

FIGURE 26.1 As a part of a comprehensive examination, all patients should have plain radiographs that include anteroposterior (AP) views in neutral and in external and internal rotation, a lateral in the scapular plane, and an axillary view. **A:** With advanced rotator cuff disease, AP radiographs may show degenerative changes of the anterior acromion and greater tuberosity, as well as a decreased acromiohumeral interval. **B:** Rotational AP views may demonstrate evidence of calcific tendonitis, as seen here, or the presence of a Hill-Sachs defect. **C:** Acromial morphology is best visualized through a "supraspinatus outlet" view. A hooked, type III acromion (38) is associated with a majority of rotator cuff tears. **D:** Sagittal oblique views on magnetic resonance imaging (MRI) are useful in demonstrating acromial morphology and allows visualization of outlet pathology. **E:** Axillary views are useful in demonstrating fractures associated with instability as well as glenoid reactive changes, as seen here.

side (15). General motion of the shoulder is observed for glenohumeral rhythm, scapulothoracic motion, and overall synchrony of motion. The current recommendation of the American Shoulder and Elbow Surgeons is to measure four functionally necessary arcs of motion both actively and passively: total elevation, external rotation at neutral abduction, external rotation at 90 degrees abduction, and internal rotation (Fig. 26.2). A patient with limited motion in a single or multiple planes must be carefully examined to differentiate among some of the possible etiologies such as a rotator cuff tear, adhesive capsulitis, or calcific tendonitis (Fig. 26.1B). Manual strength testing may be difficult to assess quantitatively because of coexistent pain (16). Crepitation with motion from the glenohumeral joint, subacromial space, or scapulothoracic joint should be noted.

Total elevation, including both glenohumeral and scapulothoracic motion, is more reproducibly measured than attempting to isolate glenohumeral motion, and is more functionally relevant. Passive elevation is more accurately measured in the supine position, while active elevation is measured erect. Motor testing of the supraspinatus is tested with the arm in 90 degrees of forward elevation and 20 degrees of internal rotation with the elbows extended (17).

External rotation is tested with the arm at the side and the patient supine (Fig. 26.2), to eliminate trunk rotation, as well as with the arm at 90 degrees of abduction. Motor testing in external rotation is done with the elbow flexed and the arm at the side to avoid deltoid contribution, and weakness in this position is a common finding with a tear involving the infraspinatus tendon. Weakness in external rotation at neutral may indicate a long-standing rotator cuff tear (18), and with concomitant weakness in shoulder abduction shows a statistically significant correlation with the size of the tear (6).

Motor testing of the shoulder in external rotation above 45 degrees of abduction tests primarily for the teres minor. Patients with large or massive tears involving the infraspinatus will often be unable to maintain their arm in external rotation at neutral as well as in the abducted arm, producing the "signe de clairon" (19). The external rotation lag sign is designed to test the integrity of the supraspinatus and infraspinatus tendons and is performed by passively flexing the elbow to 90 degrees, and the shoulder to 20 degrees of elevation and near maximal external rotation. The patient is asked to maintain this position while the physician releases the wrist; the test is positive if a lag, or angular drop, occurs (20). The drop sign is designed to assess infraspinatus function and is performed with the patient seated with his back to the physician, who holds the affected arm at 90 degrees of elevation and maximal external rotation with the elbow at 90 degrees of flexion. The patient is asked to maintain this position while the physician supports the elbow and releases the wrist; the test is positive if a lag occurs.

Internal rotation is measured according to the highest vertebral level an upright patient can reach with his thumb. Patients with subscapularis tears have an increase in passive external rotation and weakness of internal rotation. The competence of the subscapularis muscle can be tested utilizing the "lift-off" test, which has been shown to be both sensitive and specific for a tear of the subscapularis tendon (21). Originally, this test was described as being positive (poor subscapularis function) when a patient could not lift his hand posteriorly off the lumbar region (22), but has recently been modified with even greater sensitivity for subscapularis tears. In the modified lift-off test, the examiner places the arm in maximum internal rotation by passively lifting the patient's arm posteriorly off the lumbar region. The test is

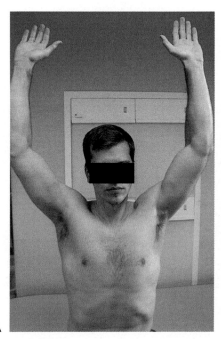

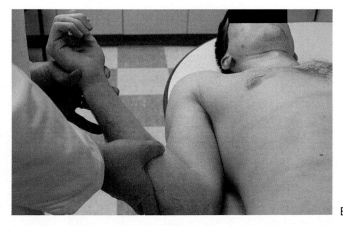

FIGURE 26.2 Range of motion is tested actively and passively by measuring forward elevation in the scapular plane **(A)**; external rotation at neutral abduction in the seated or supine position **(B)** and at 90 degrees of abduction; and internal rotation by touching the highest vertebral level posteriorly.

positive (poor subscapularis function) if the patient is unable to maintain that position and the arm falls onto the back. The internal rotation lag sign is used to assess subscapularis competency and is performed in a similar fashion to the modified lift-off test (20), except that the examiner releases the wrist at maximal internal rotation, maintains support of the elbow, and then measures the lag between maximal internal rotation. The abdominal compression test is additionally utilized to assess subscapularis weakness or deficiency, especially when passive internal rotation is difficult to perform during the lift-off test or internal rotation lag sign. A positive abdominal compression test is indicated by the patient's inability to maintain the palm of the hand compressed against the abdomen while bringing the elbow anterior to the scapular plane. A side-to-side difference between the affected and unaffected shoulders during the abdominal compression test may indicate subtle subscapularis weakness or a tear and warrants further investigation.

A thorough assessment of shoulder motion and strength must include evaluation of the scapular muscle stabilizers. Weakness in the serratus anterior muscle can cause scapular winging and a disruption of the synchronous glenohumeral motion. Scapular winging can be detected by having the patient flex to 90 degrees or do a "wall push-up," and is commonly due to a palsy of the long thoracic nerve. Trapezius muscle function is tested with a shoulder shrug, and weakness or atrophy of this muscle may be due to a palsy of the spinal accessory nerve (13). Motor strength of the rhomboid muscles is performed with the patient prone, the shoulder abducted 90 degrees, and the arms extended.

When assessing motion in overhead arm athletes, the physician should be aware of the possible existence of contractures as well as generalized ligamentous laxity (Fig. 26.3). Overhead arm athletes with subtle anterior glenohumeral instability due to repetitive microtrauma or a patient who has sustained an anterior shoulder dislocation may have a posterior capsular contracture. This can be tested by placing the shoulder in 90 degrees of elevation and internally rotating, or by placing the shoulder in 90 degrees of abduction and internally rotating. Overhead arm athletes often have a loss of internal rotation and increased external rotation, and the physician should be aware that this might exist at baseline when assessing for new pathology.

Provocative Testing

Impingement

Provocative tests are used to elicit symptoms of impingement by maneuvering the rotator cuff and biceps tendons beneath the coracoacromial arch. The Neer impingement sign (Fig. 26.4A) is performed by stabilizing the scapula with one hand and bringing the shoulder into forced elevation with the arm internally rotated (23). The Hawkins' test for impingement (Fig. 26.4B) is performed by elevation of the shoulder to 90 degrees, adduction across the chest, and internal rotation (24). Moving the shoulder through an arc of 60 to 120 degrees in the coronal plane performs a third impingement test. All of these tests are positive if they produce pain, but can be positive in other conditions besides classic subacromial impingement, including adhesive capsulitis, calcific tendonitis, and glenohumeral osteoarthritis.

Patients with classic subacromial impingement syndrome not only have pain from these impingement tests, but also frequently have symptomatic relief when a test using a sterile subacromial injection of 10 cc of 1% lidocaine is performed (23). While the injection test establishes the anatomic site of the pathology, it is not specific for the type or degree of the lesion (25). Athletes with underlying instability will have inconsistent relief from the impingement injection test, and it is thought that this test is not reliable for this group of patients (26).

The AC joint can both mimic and contribute to subacromial impingement. Pain from the AC joint can be elicited by direct palpation as well as horizontal adduction, in which the extended arm is internally rotated and ad-

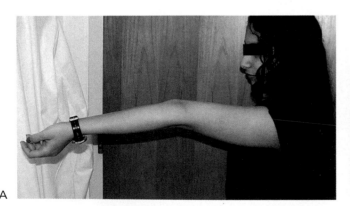
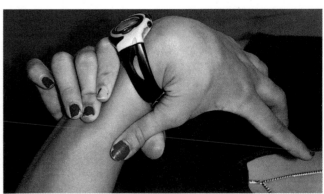

A   B

FIGURE 26.3 Each patient should be examined for generalized ligamentous laxity by evaluating elbow hyperextension **(A)** as well as the ability to appose the thumb to the forearm **(B)** and should be compared to their contralateral side.

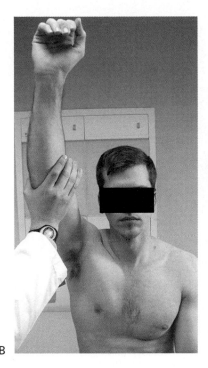
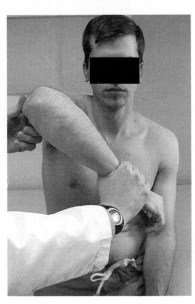

A, B

FIGURE 26.4 The Neer impingement sign **(A)** is elicited by stabilizing the scapula with one hand, and bringing the arm up into forced elevation with the other (23). This will elicit pain in patients with subacromial impingement syndrome. The Hawkins' impingement test **(B)** is performed by elevation of the shoulder to 90 degrees, adduction across the chest, and internal rotation (24).

ducted across the chest. These maneuvers are not specific for AC joint pathology and can be positive in patients with subacromial impingement. The use of selective injections to the AC joint as well as the subacromial space can be of great diagnostic value (27).

Biceps tendonitis frequently exists in both subacromial impingement as well as glenohumeral instability. The most frequently used provocative tests that are suggestive of biceps tendonitis are Speed's and Yergason's tests. Speed's test is positive if the patient experiences pain with resistance when the shoulder is abducted 90 degrees and elevated 45 degrees with the elbow extended and the forearm supinated (28). Yergason (29) described the supination sign, which localizes pain in the bicipital groove when the examiner resists active supination with the elbow flexed to 90 degrees and the forearm pronated.

Instability

Shoulder instability must be differentiated from generalized ligamentous laxity. A patient should be tested for ligamentous laxity by evaluating elbow joint hyperextension >5 degrees, the ability to touch or place the thumb parallel to the forearm, metacarpophalangeal hyperextension >60 degrees, and knee recurvatum (Fig. 26.3). Asymmetric laxity is generally not pathologic unless symptomatic (30).

The classic provocative test for anterior shoulder instability is the anterior apprehension sign (Fig. 26.5A). This test is performed with the patient supine or sitting. The arm is brought into 90 degrees of abduction, the elbow is flexed 90 degrees, and an anteriorly directed force is applied to the posterior aspect of the humeral head while the arm is externally rotated. The test is positive if the patient becomes apprehensive of being placed in this unstable position. Pain experienced by patients placed in the abducted, externally rotated position may not be specific for shoulder instability, as other conditions such as primary rotator cuff disease may also be symptomatic in this position. In this position, the examiner may be able to assess the degree of anterior translation.

The relocation test is performed with the patient in the supine position and after eliciting symptoms with the apprehension maneuver in maximal external rotation (Fig. 26.5A); a posteriorly directed force is placed on the anterior humeral head (Fig. 26.5B) (5). If the patient's pain (or apprehension) is relieved with this relocating force, the test is positive. Others have shown that patients with primary rotator cuff pathology whose primary complaint is pain may obtain relief with this maneuver, and that the relocation test is nonspecific for instability unless true apprehension is eliminated (31).

There are several tests designed to assess anteroposterior laxity of the shoulder joint. The load and shift test can be performed with the patient in the seated or supine position. In the seated position, the examiner stands behind the patient and with one hand stabilizes the scapula, while the other hand cups the proximal humerus along the joint line and loads the humeral head by pushing into the glenoid fossa. The head is then moved relative to the glenoid in the anteroposterior direction (shifting) while the degree of translation, pain, crepitation, and apprehension is recorded. In the supine position, the arm is abducted 45 degrees in the

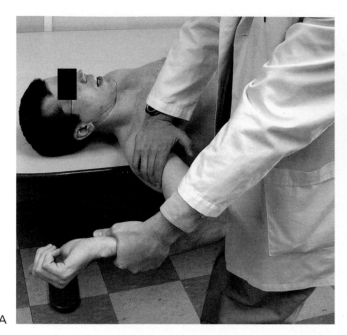
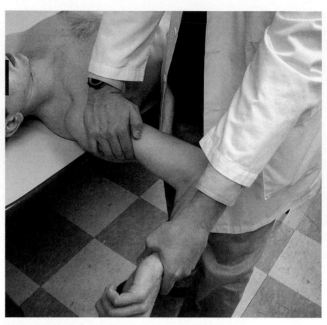

A   B

FIGURE 26.5 The relocation test is performed to test for anterior shoulder instability. With the patient in the supine position, symptoms are elicited with the apprehension maneuver **(A)**, and relieved with a relocating maneuver that is performed by placing a posteriorly directed force **(B)** on the anterior humeral head (5).

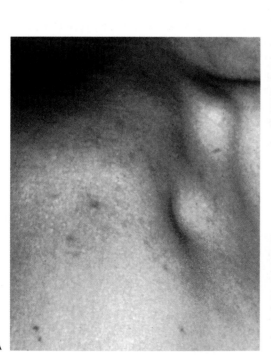
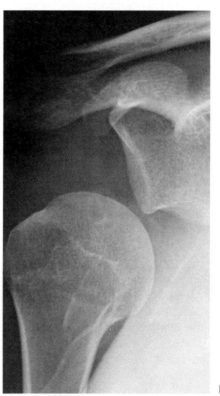

A   B

FIGURE 26.6 Clinically **(A)** and radiographically **(B)** a positive sulcus sign is exhibited.

scapular plane with neutral rotation. An axial load is applied to the humerus to compress the head into the glenoid fossa, while the other hand shifts the proximal humerus in the anteroposterior direction (32).

A shoulder drawer sign (33) is performed to assess anteroposterior translation. Stabilizing the scapula and attempting to subluxate the shoulder anteriorly performs an anterior drawer. A posterior drawer is performed with the patient supine and measures posterior excursion by flexing the arm forward while directing a posterior force with the other hand. The drawer tests have also be described as "push-pull" tests by others when performed supine (32).

Posterior shoulder instability is best assessed using the posterior stress test. To perform this test, the examiner stabilizes the medial border of the scapula with one hand while the other hand applies a posteriorly directed force to the patient's humerus, which is flexed to 90 degrees, adducted, and internally rotated (11). The test is positive if this maneuver produces pain or simulates the patient's instability symptoms.

Inferior shoulder instability is frequently combined with either anterior or posterior instability and must be thoroughly assessed in patients suspected of having inferior subluxation, multidirectional instability, or hyperlaxity. The sulcus sign (Fig. 26.6) is performed with the patient seated. The examiner applies a traction force along the longitudinal axis of the humerus by pulling inferiorly. If the distance between the acromion and the humeral head is greater than 2 cm or asymmetrical to the other side, then the test is positive for inferior subluxation or laxity. Another aspect of the sulcus test is to caudally direct a force on the 90 degree abducted arm, which if positive produces excessive inferior translation and a sulcus defect. External rotation of the shoulder in this position tightens the anterior capsule and rotator interval and should reduce the amount of inferior translation and sulcus.

Accurately defining labral pathology on physical examination is thought to be difficult by many investigators. There are several tests that have been described for evaluating labral pathology, such as the labral joint compression test (Savoie), O'Brien's sign, the labral click (Andrews), the labral crank test (Liu), the anterior slide test (Kibler), and the biceps load test (Kim).

DIAGNOSTIC MODALITIES

The diagnostic modalities are listed in Table 26.3.

Plain Radiographs

Plain radiographs are part of a comprehensive history and physical examination. All patients should have anteroposterior views in the scapular plane in neutral and in internal and external rotation, a lateral in the scapular plane, and an

TABLE 26.3 DIAGNOSTIC MODALITIES

Routine blood studies
  CBC, ESR, serum chemistries, latex fixation
  Others as indicated

Radiographs, routine
  Anteroposterior view in internal rotation, external rotation, neutral
  "Outlet" view
  Axillary

Radiographs, special
  Anteroposterior view and cephalic tilt anteroposterior with "soft tissue technique" to demonstrate AC joint
  Special views (e.g., Stryker, Hermodssen) to demonstrate Hill-Sachs defect
  Modified axillary views (e.g., "Velpeau axillary")
  Cervical spine

Special diagnostic modalities
  Arthro-CT scan
    Labral pathology
    Glenoid bone changes
  Three-dimensional CT reconstruction
  Arthrogram
  Ultrasonography
  Magnetic resonance imaging
  Arthro-MRI
  Electrodiagnostic studies (e.g., electromyogram, SSEP)
  Isokinetic muscle testing

CBC, complete blood count; CT, computed tomography; ESR, erythrocyte sedimentation rate; SSEP, somatosensory evoked potential.

axillary view (Fig. 26.1). While these radiographs in early rotator cuff disease or glenohumeral instability are usually normal, they are essential to the diagnosis of tumors, fractures, or dislocations. Cervical spine films should be ordered in patients with concomitant neck and shoulder pain.

With more advanced rotator cuff disease, anteroposterior (AP) radiographs may demonstrate degenerative changes of the greater tuberosity, AC joint, or anterior acromion (34), as well as the glenohumeral joint. Radiographic criteria for evidence of a rotator cuff tear, such as the acromiohumeral interval, can also be assessed on AP view, and if decreased less than 7 mm (Fig. 26.1A) is considered abnormal and suggestive of chronic cuff pathology (35).

Rotational AP views are of value in detecting calcium deposits in the rotator cuff (Fig. 26.1B). External rotation AP view shows the greater tuberosity on profile, which may reveal sclerosis, cysts, or excrescences. Glenohumeral instability may be evident on radiographic AP view if a bony Bankart lesion is present and an internally rotated AP view may reveal a Hill-Sachs defect (Fig. 26.7E,F) (36).

Acromial morphology may be best appreciated on a lateral or "supraspinatus outlet" view (Fig. 26.1C,D), especially when taken with slight caudal tilt (37). The shape of the acromion is an important radiographic feature, as a majority of rotator cuff tears occur in patients with a hooked (type III) acromion (38), an anterior acromial spur, or an os

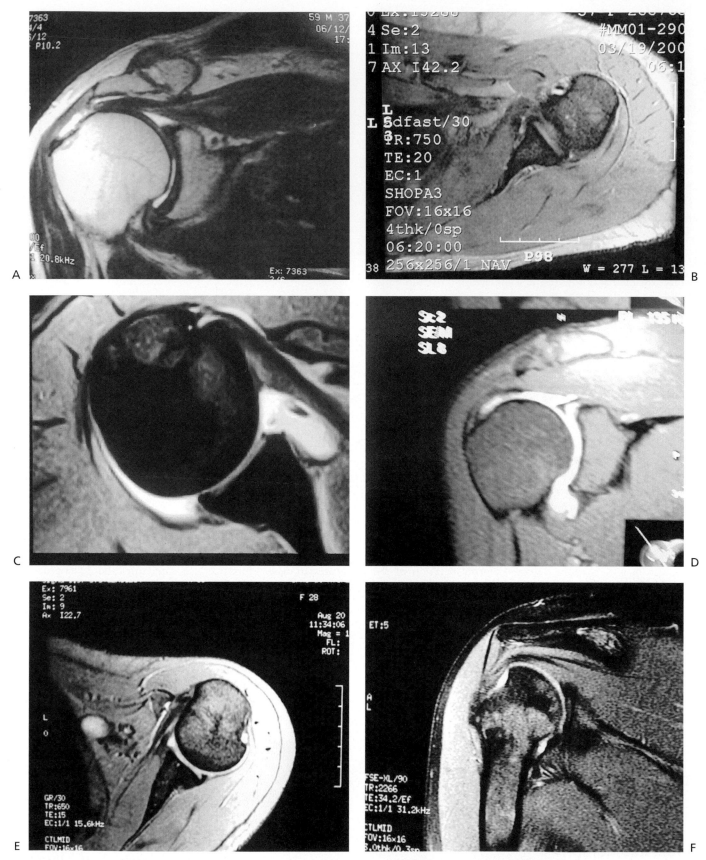

FIGURE 26.7 Magnetic resonance imaging (MRI) is an excellent, noninvasive, radiation sparing diagnostic modality useful for diagnosing rotator cuff pathology as well as glenohumeral instability. **A:** Coronal T2 image demonstrates a full-thickness tear of the supraspinatus tendon that was confirmed and primarily repaired at surgery. **B:** An axillary T1 image demonstrates a tear of the subscapularis tendon, which was repaired primarily. Gadolinium enhanced MR arthrography is useful in diagnosing glenohumeral instability as shown by the anterior labral (Bankart) tear **(C)**, the superior labral anterior posterior (SLAP) type II tear **(D)**, and the Hill-Sachs impression fractures on the posterolateral humeral head **(E,F)**.

acromiale. An AP view of the shoulder angled 30 degrees caudally demonstrates an anteroinferior acromial spur or calcification of the coracoacromial ligament (39).

Axillary radiographs are useful in demonstrating glenoid reactive changes (Fig. 26.1E) or fractures associated with instability, as well as posterior dislocations that may be overlooked on routine AP views. An unfused acromial epiphysis, or os acromiale, may be best seen on an axillary view (40). Additional modified axillary views have been described to visualize glenohumeral pathology, such as the Stryker notch view to visualize a Hill-Sachs defect, West Point view, the Velpeau view, the Didiee view, as well as Hermodsson's view (41).

Special views to visualize the AC joint are often performed with underpenetrated or "soft tissue technique," in AP and cephalic tilt AP views. These views often demonstrate osteolysis of the distal clavicle, arthritic changes, and inferior osteophyte formation, as well as fractures. Weighted stress views can be used for comparison in patients with AC joint separations.

Arthrography

Long considered the gold standard for imaging full-thickness rotator cuff tears, the arthrogram is an invasive procedure with significant risk, such as infection, allergic reaction, radiation exposure, and pain. Double-contrast arthrography is inexpensive and easily performed, but is limited in accurately diagnosing partial cuff tears as well as in providing information regarding their size and location. Despite this, arthrography remains an excellent modality for the diagnosis of full-thickness rotator cuff tears.

Ultrasound

Ultrasonography has been utilized since the 1980s to diagnose rotator cuff pathology. The advantages of ultrasonography are that it is inexpensive, noninvasive, painless, free of radiation, and dynamic, and it yields rapid results (42). The most consistent ultrasound findings of a full-thickness rotator cuff tear are nonvisualization, focal thinning, and complete discontinuity of the cuff (43). While ultrasound may be accurate in diagnosing full-thickness tears, it is not as reliable in detecting partial-thickness tears and is highly radiologist dependent.

Computed Tomography

Computed tomography (CT) arthrograms can be utilized in patients suspected of having glenohumeral instability to delineate bony and soft tissue intraarticular pathology (44). A CT arthrogram can additionally be useful in distinguishing instability from impingement, and in assessing the predominant direction—anterior, posterior, or multidirectional. Three-dimensional CT scans (Fig. 26.8) can further delineate complex proximal humerus fractures as well as other bony anomalies (45).

Magnetic Resonance Imaging

Magnetic resonance imaging (MRI) is an excellent, noninvasive, radiation-sparing modality that is useful in the diagnosis of rotator cuff pathology and glenohumeral instability (46). Performed in three orthogonal planes, MRI provides anatomic detail of the soft tissue and bony anatomy of the shoulder (Fig. 26.7). MRI can detect midsubstance and bursal-sided partial cuff tears, allowing for earlier detection and treatment of pathology. Changes in the signal intensity and morphology of the rotator cuff, fat atrophy of the muscle, or subacromial-subdeltoid bursae are significant findings consistent with the presence of a cuff tear (Fig. 26.7A,B). MRI can give information as to the size of the tear, which tendon is involved, and the degree of retraction. Bony pathology is also well visualized with MRI and is useful in detecting type III hooked acromions on coronal or sagittal oblique cuts (Fig. 26.1D), as well as degenerative changes of the AC joint.

MR arthrography with the use of gadolinium contrast has greatly improved imaging patients with shoulder instability (Fig. 26.7C,D). This modality has generally replaced arthro-CT scans and is used to delineate rotator cuff pathology and instability, as well as superior labral anterior posterior (SLAP) lesions (47).

Other Modalities

When systemic disorders are suspected, routine blood tests to evaluate rheumatologic disorders, infection, and tumors should be considered. A complete blood count with differential, a sedimentation rate, a C-reactive protein, chemistry profile, latex fixation test, serum protein electrophoresis, and an acid phosphatase level are obtained as indicated.

Electromyograms and nerve conduction studies are obtained when peripheral neuropathy, brachial plexus disorders, and cervical radiculopathies are suspected. Somatosensory evoked potential testing may be indicated with predominantly sensory pathology.

CONCLUSION

The success of shoulder arthroscopy as a therapeutic modality is dependent on proper patient selection through a comprehensive history, physical examination, and appropriate use of diagnostic modalities. A thorough understanding of the broad range of pathology that can affect the shoulder is essential in formulating the correct diagnosis and treatment plan. Recent technical advances in shoulder arthroscopy have elucidated many pathologic conditions, allowing the physician to understand, diagnose, and appropriately treat underlying pathology.

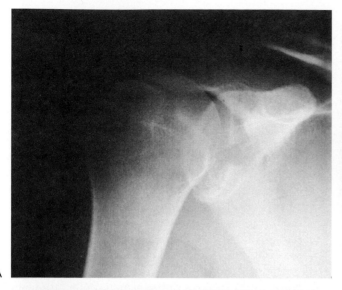

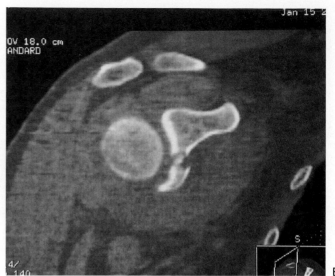

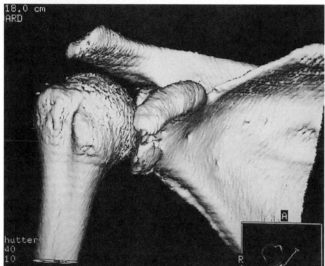

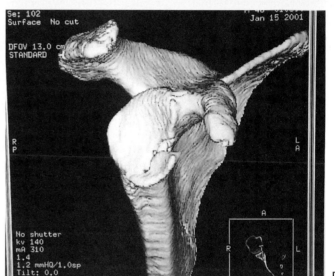

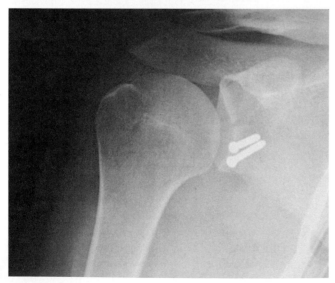

FIGURE 26.8 Computed tomography (CT) scans are useful in delineating bony pathology, especially in trauma patients. An AP radiograph demonstrates an acute fracture of the glenoid associated with a shoulder dislocation **(A)**. A CT scan shows the significant displacement of the articular surface **(B)**, and three-dimensional reconstructions **(C,D)** further delineate the fracture. An AP radiograph shows a reduced articular surface after arthroscopic reduction and internal fixation **(E)**.

REFERENCES

1. Johnson LL. Arthroscopy of the shoulder. *Orthop Clin North Am* 1980;11:197–204.
2. Cofield RH. Arthroscopy of the shoulder. *Mayo Clin Proc* 1983;58:501–508.
3. Rockwood CA Jr. Shoulder arthroscopy [editorial]. *J Bone Joint Surg* 1988;70A:639–640.
4. Neer CS II. Impingement lesions. *Clin Orthop* 1983;173:70–77.
5. Rubenstein DL, Jobe FW, Glousman RE, et al. Anterior capsulolabral reconstruction of the shoulder in athletes. *J Shoulder Elbow Surg* 1992;1:229–237.
6. Hawkins RJ, Misamore GW, Hobeika PE. Surgery for full thickness rotator cuff tears. *J Bone Joint Surg* 1985;67A:1349–1355.
7. Cahill BR. Osteolysis of the distal part of the clavicle in male athletes. *J Bone Joint Surg* 1982;64A:1053–1058.
8. Neer CS II, Foster CR. Inferior capsular shift for involuntary inferior and multidirectional instability of the shoulder: a preliminary report. *J Bone Joint Surg* 1980;62A:897–908.
9. Jobe CM, Pink M, Jobe FW, et al. Anterior shoulder instability, impingement, and rotator cuff tear. In: Jobe FW, ed. *Operative techniques in upper extremity sports injuries*. St. Louis: Mosby, 1996:164–176.
10. Arroyo JS, Flatow EL. Management of rotator cuff disease: intact and repairable cuff. In: Ianotti JP, Williams GR, Jr, eds. *Disorders of the shoulder: diagnosis and management*. Philadelphia: Lippincott Williams & Wilkins, 1999:31–56.
11. Pollock RG, Bigliani LU. Recurrent posterior shoulder instability. Diagnosis and treatment. *Clin Orthop* 1993;291:85–96.
12. Rowe CR. Recurrent transient anterior subluxation of the shoulder: the dead arm syndrome. *Clin Orthop* 1987;223:11.
13. Bigliani LU, Perez-Sanz J, Wolfe IN. Treatment of trapezius paralysis. *J Bone Joint Surg* 1985;67A:871–877.
14. Codman EA. *The shoulder. Rupture of the supraspinatus tendon and other lesions in or about the subacromial bursa*. Boston: Thomas Todd, 1934.
15. Altchek DW, Carson EW. Arthroscopic acromioplasty. *Orthop Clin North Am* 1997;28:157–168.
16. Brems JJ. Digital muscle strength measurement in rotator cuff tears. *Orthop Trans* 1988;12:735.
17. Jobe FW, Jobe CM. Painful athletic injuries of the shoulder. *Clin Orthop* 1983;173:117–124.
18. Neer CS II, Flatow EL, Lech O. Tears of the rotator cuff. Long term results of anterior acromioplasty and repair. *Orthop Trans* 1988;12:735.
19. Gerber C, Hersche O. Tendon transfers for the treatment of irreparable rotator cuff defects. *Orthop Clin North Am* 1997;28:195–204.
20. Hertel R, Ballmer F, Lombert SM, et al. Lag signs in the diagnosis of rotator cuff rupture. *J Shoulder Elbow Surg* 1996;5:307–313.
21. Gerber C, Hersche O, Farron A. Isolated rupture of the subscapularis tendon: result of operative repair. *J Bone Joint Surg* 1996;78A:1015–1023.
22. Gerber C, Krushell RJ. Isolated tears of the subscapularis muscle. Clinical features in sixteen cases. *J Bone Joint Surg* 1991;73B:389–394.
23. Neer CS. Impingement lesions. *Clin Orthop* 1983;173:70–77.
24. Hawkins RJ, Abrams JS. Impingement lesions in the absence of rotator cuff tear (stages 1 and 2). *Orthop Clin North Am* 1987;18:373–382.
25. Kessel L. *Clinical disorders of the shoulder*. Edinburgh: Churchill Livingstone, 1982.
26. Shaffer B, Jobe FW. Subacromial impingement: clinical assessment and treatment. In: Jobe FW, ed. *Operative techniques in upper extremity sports injuries*. St. Louis: Mosby, 1996:210–222.
27. Butters KP, Rockwood CA Jr. Office evaluation and management of the shoulder impingement syndrome. *Orthop Clin North Am* 1988;19:755–765.
28. Crenshaw AH, Kilgore WE. Surgical treatment of bicipital tenosynovitis. *J Bone Joint Surg* 1966;48A:1496–1502.
29. Yergason RM. Supination sign. *J Bone Joint Surg* 1931;13A:60.
30. Emery RJH, Mullaji AB. Glenohumeral joint instability in normal adolescents. *J Bone Joint Surg* 1991;73B:406–408.
31. Speer KP, Hannifan JA, Altchek DW, et al. An evaluation of the shoulder relocation test. *Am J Sports Med* 1994;22:177–183.
32. Hawkins RJ, Bokor DJ. Clinical evaluation of shoulder problems. In: Rockwood CA, Matsen FA, eds. *The shoulder*. Philadelphia: WB Saunders, 1990:164–196.
33. Gerber C, Ganz R. Clinical assessment of instability of the shoulder with special reference to anterior and posterior drawer tests. *J Bone Joint Surg* 1984;66B:551–556.
34. Gold RH, Seeger LI, Yao L. Imaging shoulder impingement. *Skel Radiol* 1993;22:555–561.
35. Norwood LA, Barrack R, Jacobson KE. Clinical presentation of complete tears of the rotator cuff. *J Bone Joint Surg* 1989;71A:499–505.
36. Hill HA, Sachs MD. The grooved defect of the humeral head. *Radiology* 1940;35:690–700.
37. Neer CS II, Poppen NK. Supraspinatus outlet. *Orthop Trans* 1987;11:234.
38. Bigliani LU, Morrison DS, April EW. The morphology of the acromion and its relationship to rotator cuff tears. *Orthop Trans* 1986;10:228.
39. Ono K, Yamamuro T, Rockwood CA. Use of a thirty degree caudal tilt radiograph in the shoulder impingement syndrome. *J Shoulder Elbow Surg* 1992;1:246–252.
40. Edelson JG, Zuckerman J, Hershkovitz I. Os acromiale: anatomy and surgical implications. *J Bone Joint Surg* 1993;75B:551–555.
41. Rockwood CR Jr. Subluxations and dislocations about the shoulder. In: Rockwood CA Jr, Green DP, eds. *Fractures in adults*, vol 1, 2nd ed. Philadelphia: JB Lippincott, 1984:722–985.
42. Collins RA, Gristina AG, Carter RE, et al. Ultrasonography of the rotator cuff: surgical correlation. *Ultrasound* 1984;12:487–492.
43. Middleton WD, Reinus WR, Totty WG, et al. Ultrasonographic evaluation of the rotator cuff and biceps tendon. *J Bone Joint Surg* 1986;68A:440–450.
44. Bigliani LU, Singson R, Feldman F, et al. Double contrast CT arthrography in the evaluation and treatment of shoulder instability. *Surg Rounds Orthop* 1987;1:37–45.
45. Kuhlman JE, Fishman EK, Ney DR, et al. Complex shoulder trauma: three dimensional CT imaging. *Orthopedics* 1988;11:1561–1563.
46. Iannotti JP, Zlatkin MB, Esterhai JL, et al. Magnetic resonance imaging of the shoulder. Sensitivity, specificity, and predictive value. *J Bone Joint Surg* 1991;73A:17–29.
47. Flannigan B, Kursunoglu-Brahme S, Snyder S, et al. MR arthrography of the shoulder: comparison with conventional MR imaging. *Am J Radiol* 1990;155:829–832.

Operative Arthroscopy, third edition. Edited by John B. McGinty, Stephen S. Burkhart, Robert W. Jackson, Donald H. Jackson, and John C. Richmond. Lippincott Williams & Wilkins © 2003.

ARTHROSCOPY OF THE SHOULDER: INDICATIONS AND GENERAL PRINCIPLES OF TECHNIQUES

AUGUSTUS D. MAZZOCCA
MAYO NOERDLINGER
BRIAN COLE
ANTHONY ROMEO

INTRODUCTION

The concept of shoulder arthroscopy was introduced in 1931 by Burman (1) when he reported on the direct visualization of cadaver joints. Although access to the joint may be more challenging than in knee arthroscopy, shoulder arthroscopy has become increasingly more popular over the last two decades. Compared with open surgery, shoulder arthroscopy allows a more complete examination of the structures about the shoulder with a low rate of complications. The anatomic structures of the shoulder can be examined in a manner that allows a greater appreciation of their structure and form than with open surgery. Less soft tissue dissection results in decreased postoperative pain and generally improved early rehabilitation.

This chapter reviews the equipment required, its use, and an overall technique of shoulder arthroscopy. The anatomy of arthroscopic portals and complications are also reviewed.

PREOPERATIVE CONSIDERATIONS

The beginning of a successful shoulder arthroscopy takes place in the office with the obtaining of an adequate medical history. The surgeon, anesthesiologist, and primary care physician can coordinate the care of the patient based on the patient's physical well-being. Patients with a history of coro-

nary artery disease or vertebral artery stenosis need special attention, because shoulder arthroscopy is optimally performed with hypotensive anesthesia. Maintenance of a mean arterial pressure of about 90 mm Hg or a systolic blood pressure of 100 mm Hg improves visualization of the shoulder, specifically the subacromial space (2).

Obesity is another factor to consider before shoulder arthroscopy. The patient in a beach-chair position who has a large abdomen runs a risk of superior vena cava compression, which could decrease venous return and cause uncontrollable hypotension. The physician must be willing to lower the back of the table to facilitate proper return of blood flow to the heart and to restore adequate cardiac output if this difficulty arises. Another consideration for the obese patient is that most operating room beds are rated for 400 lb. For a patient who weighs more than 400 lb, two beds are placed together and the patient is placed in the lateral position with a distraction device.

The role of the anesthesiologist is important to the success of shoulder arthroscopy. Regional anesthesia can be used with success, but the addition of general anesthesia can allow for more precise control of blood pressure and easier use of paralytic agents in case the procedure needs to be converted to an open procedure.

PREPARING FOR POSITIONING

With the patient in a supine position in the operating room, an examination under anesthesia (EUA) is performed. Particular attention is paid to the range of motion and stability of the affected shoulder. Comparison between the affected and unaffected limbs should be carried out before the patient is positioned. The EUA is used to support the diagnosis achieved with the preoperative history, physical examination, and radiographic studies.

A. D. Mazzocca: University of Connecticut, Department of Orthopaedic Surgery, Farmington, Connecticut.

M. Noerdlinger: Atlantic Orthopaedic Sports Medicine, Portsmouth, New Hampshire.

B. Cole: Rush Cartilage Restoration Center, Rush–Presbyterian–St. Luke's Medical Center, Chicago, Illinois.

A. Romeo: Shoulder Section, Department of Orthopaedic Surgery, Rush–Presbyterian–St. Luke's Medical Center, Chicago, Illinois.

COMMON FINDINGS ASSOCIATED WITH THE EXAMINATION UNDER ANESTHESIA

An increase in external rotation with the arm at the side may indicate a subscapularis tear, and an increase of internal rotation of the arm abducted to 90 degrees may indicate a posterior rotator cuff tear (infraspinatus or teres minor). Limited external rotation with the arm at the side is seen in patients with osteoarthritis or adhesive capsulitis. Limited internal rotation with the arm abducted is evidence of a tight posterior capsule. Labral pathology can be detected with the EUA. A click or grinding with loading of the glenohumeral joint can often be elicited in an anesthetized patient who previously was too apprehensive to allow this physical finding in the office. Increased pathologic translation can also be detected with the EUA. Posterior instability testing can be carried out with the shoulder flexed to 140 degrees (allowing the greater tuberosity to clear the acromion), and adducted to 15 degrees as a posterior-directed axial force is applied. The scapula must be stabilized with the opposite hand while this test is performed (Fig. 27.1). Anterior instability can be demonstrated with the arm abducted to 90 degrees by applying an axial and anterior force while stabilizing the scapula. Some other forms of instability may not be apparent with these maneuvers, because such extremes of motion tend to tighten the shoulder capsule. In this case, the arm should be held in neutral position with the capsule relaxed, and the humeral head should be grabbed by the examiner's fingers and translated anteriorly and posteriorly. Translation to the glenoid rim is classified as grade I, translation over the glenoid rim with spontaneous reduction is grade II, and translation over the rim that is locked and irreducible is classified as grade III instability (3). Once the EUA is completed, the patient is positioned.

POSITIONING FOR SHOULDER ARTHROSCOPY

Beach-Chair Position

In the beach-chair position (Fig. 27.2), the patient is aligned onto the edge of the table so that the affected shoulder is not supported by the table. Placing a folded towel on the medial border of the scapula may facilitate exposure of the shoulder. Some operating room tables are equipped with head rests with removal of the back so the entire posterior superior quadrant of the patient is easily accessible. The operating room table is flexed approximately 45 degrees, and the legs are lowered so that they are parallel to the floor. Lowering the legs beyond horizontal would allow any operative equipment that is placed on the patient's thighs to slide down to the floor. This is easily overcome by having a Mayo stand positioned over the patient's thighs to hold any operative equipment. The back of the table is completely elevated, which positions the acromion at approximately 60 degrees to the floor and places the glenohumeral joint in an anatomic position. If the procedure is converted to an open anterior procedure, the back of the table is lowered to 30 degrees to facilitate soft tissue retraction.

Lateral Decubitus

In the lateral position the patient needs to be placed on a bean bag or other stabilizing device with all bony prominences padded. The patient's torso is rolled posterior 25 to 30 degrees to position the glenoid parallel to the floor (Fig. 27.3). This also opens up the joint and facilitates access into the shoulder joint with the arthroscope. An axillary roll is placed under the thorax distal to the axilla to protect the

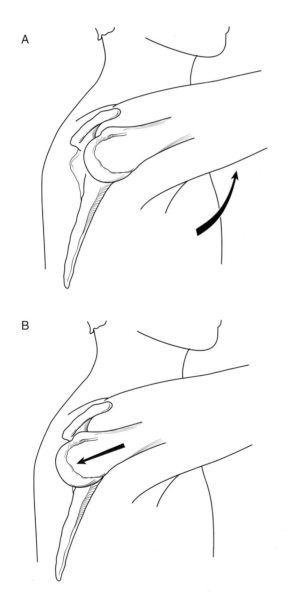

FIGURE 27.1 A: The arm is flexed to 140 degrees and adducted 15 degrees, allowing the greater tuberosity to clear the acromion. **B:** Posterior-directed axial force with stabilization of the scapula allows testing of posterior restraints.

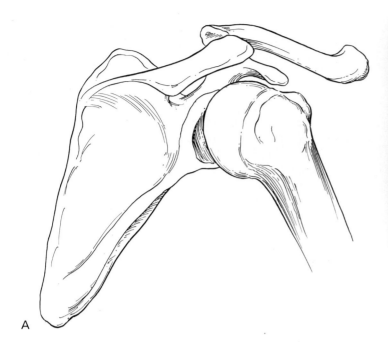

A

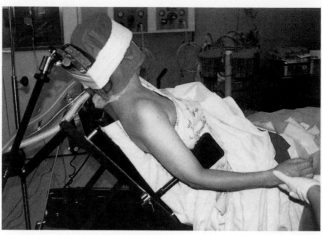

B

FIGURE 27.2 A: Illustration of the scapular humeral articulation and position in the beach-chair position. **B:** This patient in beach-chair position is supported by a McConnell head rest and side plate.

brachial plexus. Once positioned, the arm is suspended so that it can be prepped and draped in a sterile surgical fashion. With a lateral decubitus position the arm is placed in a foam traction sleeve and connected to the traction device (Fig. 27.4). It is positioned in 45 degrees of abduction and 15 degrees of forward flexion. This arm position is adequate

for visualization of both the glenohumeral joint and the subacrosomal space, alleviating the need for repositioning during the procedure. Traction is then applied with the arm in neutral position. If the arm is rotated, traction should not be placed. Ten pounds is placed for arm distraction, and 10 pounds is placed for abduction traction. The humerus is allowed to float away from the glenoid. Optimal traction is achieved when the arm is in neutral position so that the shoulder capsule ligaments are relaxed. More than 20 lb of weight is not recommended, because a neuropraxia may develop as traction increases (4,5).

Equipment Setup

After completion of patient positioning, equipment setup should be considered. A tower containing a video monitor, control box, light source, shaver power source, video tape recorder, and irrigation pump is placed opposite the surgeon at the level of the shoulder on the opposite side of the patient (Fig. 27.5A). This positioning provides for viewing of the video monitor and allows servicing of equipment without interference with the arthroscopist. A Mayo stand is placed distal to the first assistant and should contain the basic or more frequently used instruments and equipment necessary to complete the procedure (Fig. 27.5B). A back table is then positioned within easy reach behind the first assistant; it should contain procedure-specific equipment on large trays (Fig. 27.5C).

Positioning of the operative team is also important in the setup for shoulder arthroscopy. With the patient in the beach-chair position, the surgeon stands slightly behind the shoulder, and the operating room table is moved slightly away from the anesthesiologist to provide the surgeon with more room. The arthroscopic monitor is positioned on the opposite side of the patient, at the level of the shoulders, for

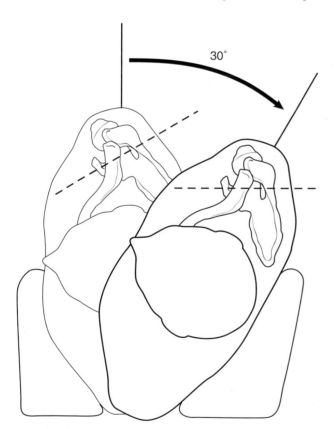

30°

FIGURE 27.3 Lateral decubitus position with the patient posteriorly angled 30 degrees to allow the glenoid to be parallel to the floor.

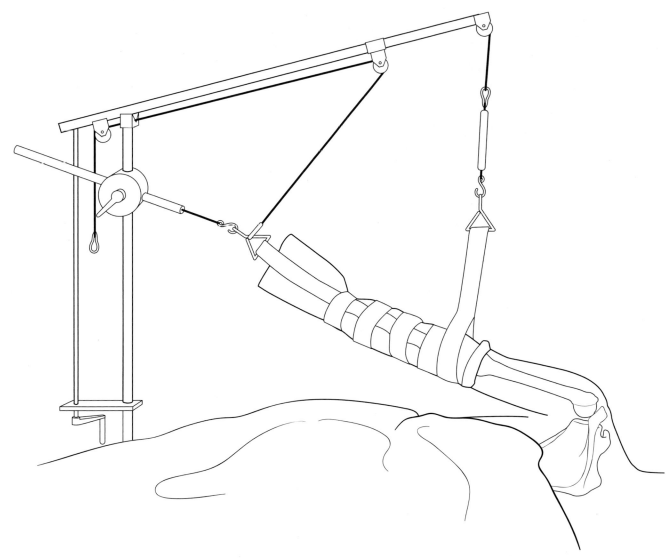

FIGURE 27.4 Lateral decubitus position with the arm in a foam sleeve. For glenohumeral surgery, the arm is abducted to 45 degrees. For subacromial surgery, the arm is abducted only 20 to 30 degrees. (Courtesy of Arthrex, Naples, FL.)

easy viewing by the surgeon. The arthroscopic pump and electrocautery unit are positioned just distal (toward the patient's feet) from the arthroscopic tower. The assistant surgeon stands next to the operating surgeon in front of the shoulder. The assistant's role is to manipulate the arm into favorable positions for the surgeon. Surgical scrub technicians stand behind the surgeon and the assistant.

With the patient in the lateral position, the head of the table is also turned away from the anesthesiologist. The surgeon stands above the shoulder, and the assistant is below the surgeon. The surgical scrub technician is positioned behind the surgeon. The table maybe rotated 180 degrees so that the anesthesiologist is situated at the patient's feet. The anesthesiologist needs to be comfortable with this technique. Its benefit is to allow the surgeon complete access to the anterior and posterior aspects of the shoulder by walking around the head of the table.

For diagnostic arthroscopies, a 30-degree arthroscope, cannula tubing, and probe are all that is needed. For any debridement work, a motorized shaver, bur, and electrocautery or ablation device are used. For any reconstructions procedures, the necessary cannulas and fixation devices must be available.

PUMPS AND FLUID SYSTEM

Fluid management is critical to shoulder arthroscopy. Despite the success of laparoscopy, fears of pneumomediastinum have made isotonic fluid the preferred choice over carbon dioxide (6–11). Glycine is another fluid that is predominantly used in Europe and allows excellent visualization. A systolic blood pressure of 100 mm Hg and a pump pressure of about 40 mm Hg assists in the control of subacromial bleeding. Increasing the pressure and/or flow too

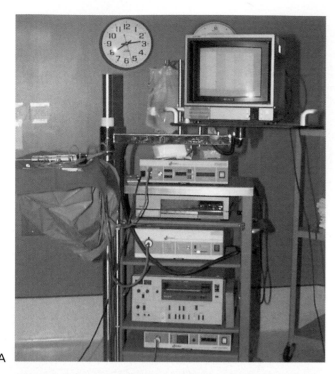

A

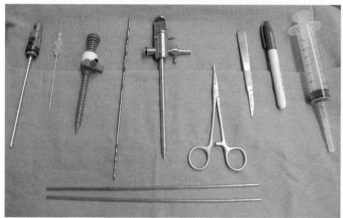

B

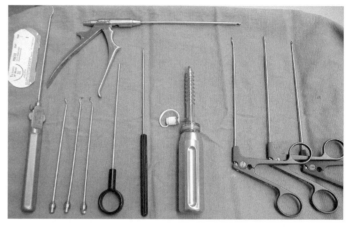

C

FIGURE 27.5 A: Arthroscopy tower. **B** and **C:** Basic arthroscopic instrumentation.

much can cause extravasation of fluid into the soft tissues and consequent distortion of the anatomy.

Fluid dynamics in shoulder arthroscopy is critical to visualization and, depending on the length of the case, to postoperative morbidity. Four basic terms are used in discussing fluid management. The first term is *flow*. Flow is determined by Pouiseuille's relation (flow = pressure ÷ resistance) (12). *Flow rate* is the second term; it is the amount of fluid that moves past a specific point over a specified time period. Flow rate is measured in liters per minute and consists of the inflow (flow of fluid into the space) and the outflow (flow of fluid out of the joint space.) *Resistance* is based on the diameter of the tube and the diameter of the cannula. The final term is *pressure,* which is a measure of force over a certain area. It is measured in millimeters of mercury. When the inflow is equal to the outflow, the pressure is stable and is said to be equilibrium. Flow in shoulder arthroscopy is

important for keeping the field of view clear as it flushes blood and debris from the field. It also increases blade-cutting efficiency. Pressure in shoulder arthroscopy distends the joint and helps control bleeding. The two main goals of fluid management systems are to maintain the desired pressure to provide for adequate distention and to control bleeding by means of flow rates to keep the surgical field clear.

There are two main systems that can be used: a pump system, in which fluid is "pumped" into the joint, and a gravity system. The gravity system works on hydrostatic pressure (1 ft = 22 mm Hg). Increasing the height of the bags or decreasing the height of the joint being worked on (i.e., the shoulder joint) increases the pressure in the system. The advantages of a gravity system are that it is simple and relatively inexpensive. A potential disadvantage is that, when there is a large flow demand, gravity cannot keep up and the system can "drain the joint."

The second type of system is the peristaltic pump. This system works by "pinching" and trapping inflow tubing as the pump head turns, causing introduction of discrete fluid quanta (individual packets of fluid). This allows for positive fluid displacement, so that flow and pressure are regulated by controlling the pump head revolutions per minute (rpm). One of the problems with this type of pump system is that it leads to a pulsing type of action, and when the flow rate is high it may produce a pressure spike. Another type of pump is a centrifugal pump, which employs a rotating impeller by which a continuous volume of fluid is sent. This continuous flow of fluid allows for a smoother control of pressure without any spiking. The problem is that there is a constant fluid flow, so that an uncontrolled or potential space (e.g., the subacromial space) may lead to distension of the surrounding soft tissue.

The control of fluid into and out of the joint is critical for shoulder arthroscopy. In basic glenohumeral shoulder arthroscopy, inflow is connected to the camera and outflow is usually regulated through the anterior portal. The relationship between inflow and outflow is especially important in the subacromial space.

PORTAL PLACEMENT AND ANATOMY

The importance of accurate portal placement cannot be overstated. Because the operative field is limited to the view of a 30-degree or 70-degree lens, the angle at which that the lens is inserted is critical. This is true for all portals but especially for the posterior portal, which is the main visualization portal for most procedures.

Accurate tracing of the patient's bony anatomic landmarks is necessary. The anterior and posterior borders of the acromion are reproducibly palpated. Marks can be placed at each of these landmarks and then, with the use of an index finger, a line can be drawn between them delineating the lateral border of the acromion. Next, an index finger can be placed in the soft spot between the posterior aspect of the distal clavicle and the anterior aspect of the scapular spine. The outline of the clavicle, as well as the scapular spine, can be drawn from this point. The acromioclavicular joint should be palpated and drawn along with the coracoid process. The coracoid usually lies 2 to 3 cm inferior to the acromioclavicular joint. The acromioclavicular joint and coracoid mark the level of the glenohumeral articulation. A line marking the path of the coracoacromial ligament is then placed. After all of these anatomic areas are palpated and drawn, portal placement can commence.

POSTERIOR PORTAL

Shoulder arthroscopy begins with the creation of the posterior portal. Through this portal the arthroscope will be inserted into the shoulder joint and subacromial space. De-

pending on the findings observed through this portal, certain accessory portals may be added during the procedure.

Typical posterior portal placement for shoulder arthroscopy is described as being approximately 2 cm inferior and 1 cm medial to the posterolateral acromion (13). Although relatively specific coordinates have been reported in the literature, it is important to use all anatomic landmarks as well as various coordinate systems to maintain ideal position of this portal. The posterior portal is extremely important, because it is the initial viewing portal. This portal "sets the tone" for the rest of the procedure. It is also important to realize that coordinate systems are given for the "normal" shoulder. In extremely small or large shoulders, such coordinates must be modified.

A method for ensuring correct placement of the posterior portal involves palpation of the bony landmarks with the same hand as the shoulder being operated on. The middle finger is placed on the coracoid process, and the index finger is placed into the notch directly posterior to the acromioclavicular joint and anterior to the scapular spine. The thumb then feels for the "soft spot," which is the muscular interval between the infraspinatus and teres minor muscle groups (Fig. 27.6). Another useful method is to grasp the

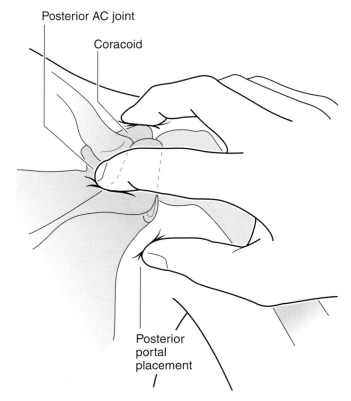

Posterior AC joint

Coracoid

Posterior portal placement

FIGURE 27.6 The Romeo Three-Finger Shuck. A method for ensuring correct placement of the posterior portal involves palpation of the bony landmarks with the same hand as the shoulder being operated on. The middle finger is placed on the coracoid process, the index finger is placed into the notch directly posterior to the acromioclavicular joint and anterior to the scapular spine, and the thumb then feels for the "soft spot," which is the muscular interval between the infraspinatus and teres minor muscle groups.

proximal humerus with one hand while stabilizing the scapula with the other and feel the motion interface at the glenohumeral joint. Once all anatomic landmarks and localization systems have confirmed correct portal placement, a mark is made where the posterior portal should go. The skin is injected with a local anesthetic, and a 1-cm incision is made through the dermis with a no. 11 or no. 15 blade.

Depending on the surgeon's preference, a sharp or dull trocar within the cannula for the arthroscope is used next. If a sharp trocar is used, it is advanced only past the deltoid musculature before it is exchanged for the dull trocar. A constant steady pressure is used to advance the trocar from the posterior skin puncture in line with the tip of the coracoid process, which is being palpated. The amount of resistance encountered at this point varies from shoulder to shoulder. Patients who have adhesive capsulitis or thick posterior capsules may have quite a bit of resistance to entering the joint capsule, and those with multidirectional instability or thin posterior capsules may have little resistance. If the trocar does not "pop in," it should not be forced, because doing so may cause iatrogenic injury. To help with the insertion, an assistant rotates the patient's arm and the surgeon palpates the moving humeral head compared with the stationary glenoid, to localize the joint space. In another method, the assistant grabs the patient's arm just distal to the axilla, creating an abduction distraction force. This in essence creates slightly more glenohumeral space, to allow the trocar to be easily slipped into the joint. Ideally, the cannula is introduced into the shoulder joint at the midequator of the glenoid, to provide visualization of the intraarticular structures at the top and bottom of the joint. An upward motion should be used at this time to avoid iatrogenic injury to the articular cartilage of the posterior humeral head. Any bony resistance encountered during insertion should be considered to be either the posterior aspect of the humeral head or the posterior glenoid. If bony resistance is experienced, it is safer to take a moment to reassess the anatomic landmarks and then reapply steady pressure at a slightly different angle, rather than continuing to use forceful insertion, which risks possible iatrogenic cartilage injury.

Creation of the posterior portal in the lateral decubitus position is slightly different. There is a natural tendency to enter the joint medially. This forces the arthroscopist to come over and around the glenoid to view the joint, which could be troublesome with some procedures. It is recommended to place this portal 3 cm inferior and in line with the posterolateral corner of the acromion (Fig. 27.7).

There is a dichotomy in the technique of predistending the glenohumeral joint with fluid before entering. The theoretical advantage is that the humeral head and glenoid are separated by the fluid, leaving a wider glenohumeral space and allowing the medial trocar to be inserted with less iatrogenic damage. Filling the joint with fluid also puts the posterior capsule in tension and may make entering the joint easier. The drawback to this technique is that the fluid may obscure the anatomy of the shoulder and make it more dif-

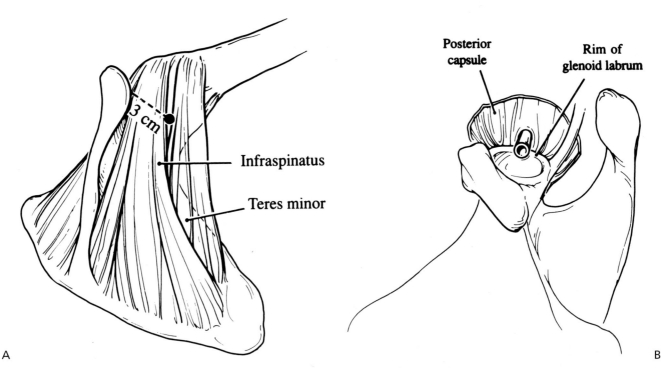

FIGURE 27.7 A: Posterior portal placement through the infraspinatus and teres minor interval in the lateral decubitus position. **B:** Intraarticular view of posterior portal in the lateral decubitus position.

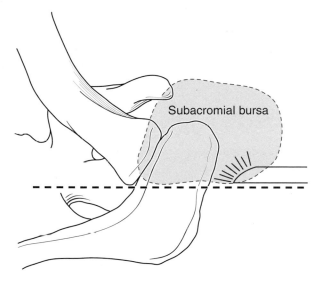

FIGURE 27.8 The subacromial bursa is an anterior structure.

ficult to place the cannula in the proper location, and iatrogenic damage to the humeral head may occur with the act of placing the needle for joint distention.

The entrance for the posterior portal for diagnostic glenohumeral arthroscopy is the same skin incision that is used for the posterior entry into the subacromial space. There are many ways to enter the subacromial space. However, the prime factor involved is visualization. The technique described here is based on the "room with a view."

After complete glenohumeral arthroscopy, the posterior portal cannula and trocar are withdrawn through the in-

terval between the infraspinatus and teres minor muscle. The trocar is withdrawn so as not to bring in any of the rotator cuff musculature when entering the subacromial space. The trocar and cannula are angled more superiorly than with glenohumeral arthroscopy, and the posterior border of the acromion is palpated with the trocar. The trocar is then placed underneath the acromion and inserted in an anterior direction. Palpation of the anterior joint with the opposite hand aids in understanding how large the acromion is in relation to the length of the cannula. This gives the surgeon feedback as to how far the trocar has been placed into the space. The subacromial bursa is an anterior structure (Fig. 27.8). After initially aiming anteromedially, the trocar is then placed as lateral as possible (Fig. 27.9A). The trocar is removed, and the arthroscope is inserted. When fluid is allowed to distend this potential space, a "room with a view" should be seen (Fig. 27.9B). If soft tissue obscures the view, the surgeon must withdraw and reposition the arthroscope. There is a tendency to be either too medial or too anterior. The anatomic references should once again be reassessed and the procedure repeated. The posterior portal must be low enough to allow smooth transition into and out of the subacromial space. If the posterior portal is too close to the scapular spine, a shaver placed through this portal will have to be aimed inferiorly to get under the acromion before it can be aimed superiorly to perform the anterior acromioplasty. Also, if an arthroscopic distal clavicle excision is part of the planned procedure, the posterior portal can be made slightly medial so that the angle of attack will be more in line with the acromioclavicular joint.

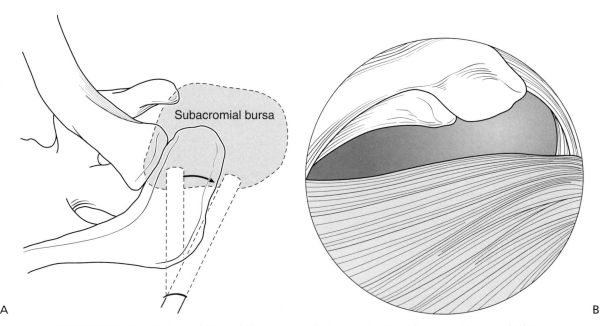

FIGURE 27.9 A: Initial angulation of the trocar medially to enter the subacromial bursa, which is followed by manipulation of the trocar laterally. **B:** "Room with a view": the arthroscopic view inside the subacromial bursa.

ANTERIOR PORTAL

The standard anterior portal (Fig. 27.10) is usually placed in the rotator interval or triangle created by the subscapularis tendon, the humeral head, and the biceps tendon superiorly. It is important before creating this portal to assess the superior glenohumeral ligament (SGHL) as well as the coracohumeral ligament (CHL) and the stability of the long head of the biceps tendon. The CHL along with the SGHL forms the medial sling of the biceps, thereby creating medial stability for the long head of the biceps tendon. The supraspinatus creates a bumper for the biceps on its lateral side (Fig. 27.11).

Creation of the anterior portal can be done with an inside-out or outside-in technique. The inside-out technique involves "driving" the arthroscope into the anterior triangle and placing it with some force into that area so that it does not move. The arthroscope is then removed, and a stout Wissinger rod is placed through the cannula. The rod is forcefully pushed through the interval tissue, tenting the skin anteriorly. This tented skin should be directly lateral to the projection of the coracoid process. If it is medial, the rod should be immediately withdrawn and reassessment of the anatomic structures performed. The musculocutaneous nerve has been found to exit 1 cm medial and 3 cm distal to the coracoid process. A scalpel (no. 11 blade) is used to create a 1-cm incision, and the Wissinger rod is pushed through this incision. A plastic cannula can then be placed over the Wissinger rod; the arthroscope is advanced into the space, and its position is checked visually (Fig. 27.12).

The outside-in technique uses direct visualization (Fig. 27.13). A spinal needle is placed from the lateral aspect of

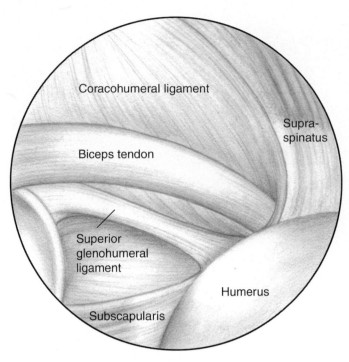

FIGURE 27.11 Biceps sling anatomy. This is a right shoulder with the arthroscope in the posterior portal, illustrating the arthroscopic view of the anterior shoulder anatomy and biceps sling.

the coracoid process in through the rotator interval. The spinal needle is then removed, and a no. 11 blade is used to make the 1-cm skin incision. Under direct visualization, the plastic cannula and plastic trocar are advanced through this tissue bounded by the long head of the biceps tendon superiorly, the humeral head laterally, and the subscapularis in-

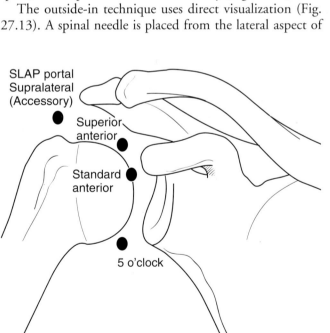

FIGURE 27.10 Anterior portals.

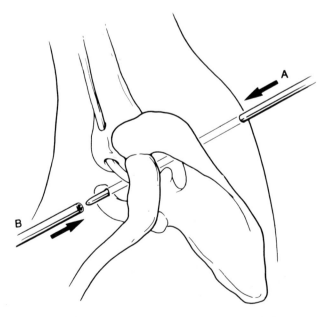

FIGURE 27.12 A: Rod being directed anteriorly through the skin. **B:** Retrograde placement of an arthroscopic cannula into the joint over a Wissinger rod.

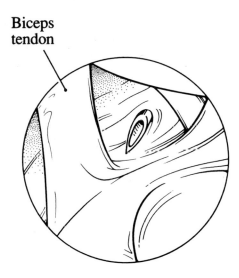

FIGURE 27.13 Intraarticular view of a spinal needle entering the anterior capsule at the proper site for the anterior portal.

feriorly. Care should be taken not to place the portal through the subscapularis tendon. Depending on pump systems and fluid dynamics, the outflow can be changed from the posterior portal to this anterior portal to improve visualization of the shoulder joint.

When the patient is in the lateral decubitus position, the tendency again is to make the anterior portal too medial. Attention must be paid to make the anterior portal more lateral. Also, if in establishing the portal there is difficulty in determining the correct site for needle insertion, the anterior aspect of the shoulder may be palpated with concomi-

tant viewing through the arthroscope to observe capsular indentation caused by the palpating finger.

In a diagnostic arthroscopic procedure, the anterior portal may be placed anywhere in the rotator cuff interval. If according to the preoperative plan various procedures are going to be performed, special attention should be given to placement of the initial anterior portal. Locating the portal slightly medial for arthroscopic distal clavicle excision is useful to provide access to the acromioclavicular joint. For arthroscopic labral stabilizations, the anterior portal may be put slightly higher than usual, because a second anterior portal will be needed. With two anterior portals, crowding can occur; increasing the distance between these portals helps with triangulation and decreases congestion.

If a selected procedure will require two anterior portals, both can be placed into the rotator interval. The superior anterior portal is close to the acromion and the standard anterior portal is next to the coracoid (Fig. 27.14).

STANDARD LATERAL PORTAL

The standard lateral portal (Fig. 27.15) is strictly a subacromial space portal, because the supraspinatus and infraspinatus tendons, depending on internal and external rotation, protect the glenohumeral joint from access by this portal. The axillary nerve anatomy is an important consideration when establishing the direct lateral portal. Many descriptions of the axillary nerve in relation to the lateral edge of the acromion have been put forth. Hollinsehead (14) stated that the axillary nerve lies 1.5 to 2.0 inches (3.81 to 5.08 cm) below the acromion. Hoppenfeld and deBoer (15) described the axillary

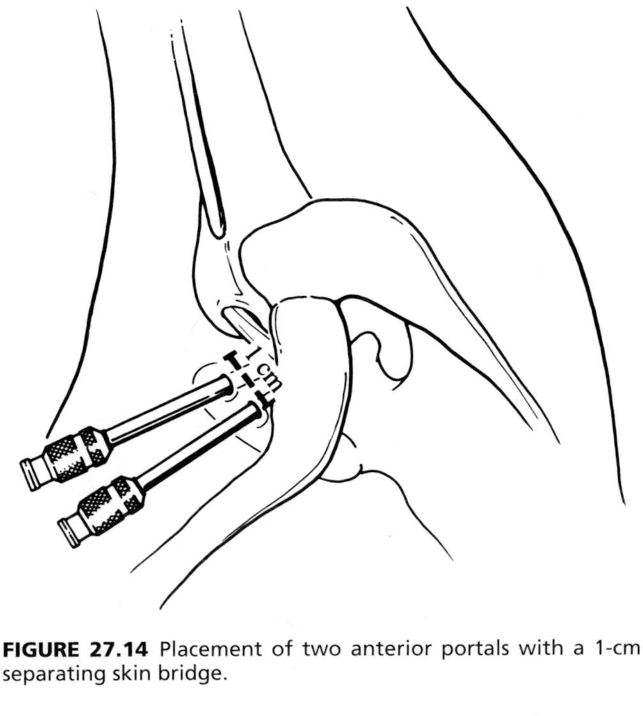

FIGURE 27.14 Placement of two anterior portals with a 1-cm separating skin bridge.

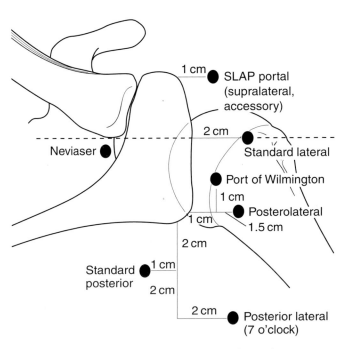

FIGURE 27.15 Posterior and lateral portals.

nerve as being 7 cm from the acromion. Beals et al. (16) describes the mean distance from all points of the acromion to the axillary nerve as averaging approximately 5 cm.

To localize this portal, an index finger can be placed in the notch between the posterior aspect of the clavicle and the spine of the scapula. A line can be drawn from this notch laterally, past the lateral edge of the acromion for approximately 2 cm. This places the line in the midportion of the acromion. A spinal needle is used to localize this portal under direct visualization. The needle is placed in the position, and once it is seen and manipulated to demonstrate that all areas of the subacromial space can be accessed with it, a 1-cm incision is made either vertically or horizontally, depending on surgeon preference. A dull trocar is used to enter the subacromial space first, and once again position is checked. If this portal is placed too close to the acromion, then, as the shoulder swells with fluid, visualization and application of instruments will become more difficult because they will be forced in a caudad direction. Such a placement will also raise the relative position of the portal, making contact with the medial acromion difficult. These factors should always be considered when making this portal.

ACCESSORY ANTERIOR PORTALS

To aid in the multitude of arthroscopic shoulder procedures, various portals have been described (Fig. 27.10). As already noted, correct placement of portals is critical to the success of the procedure. A spinal needle can be used in the glenohumeral joint to localize and ascertain the correct angle and position of the proposed portal site. One can then reproducibly create a portal site that is specific to both the patient's anatomy and the proposed procedure. When creating an accessory portal, it is important to consider the neurovascular anatomy. The musculocutaneous nerve exits usually 2 cm inferior and 1 cm medial to the coracoid process (Fig. 27.16). The cephalic vein is found in the deltopectoral interval, and the anterior humeral circumflex vessel travels along the inferior border of the subscapularis tendon to send branches into the biceps sheath and humeral head. Beals et al. (15) reported that the axillary nerve is an average of 5 cm from the acromion. This distance can be thought of as a "safe zone" for the application of accessory portals.

Superior Lateral Portal

The superior lateral portal (Fig. 27.10) was defined by Laurencin et al. (17). It is placed at a position just lateral to the acromion on a line drawn from the acromion to the coracoid. A spinal needle is placed to enter the subacromial space or joint obliquely. This portal is useful for anterior shoulder procedures and is especially important in arthroscopic rotator cuff repair for anchor placement and suture shuttling (Fig. 27.17).

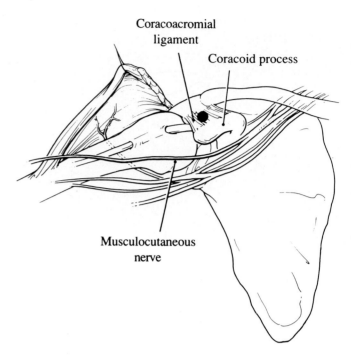

FIGURE 27.16 Anterior portal placement in relation to the coracoid process and the musculocutaneous nerve.

Neviaser Portal

The Neviaser portal (Fig. 27.15) is placed in the notch between the posterior acromioclavicular joint and the spine of the scapula. It is useful in the repair of anterior supraspinatus rotator cuff injuries and for arthroscopic distal clavicle resection (Fig. 27.18). The suprascapular nerve and artery traverse the floor of the supraspinatus fossa. They are located in the fossa, approximately 3 cm medial to the portal.

Anterior Inferior or 5 O'Clock Portal

This portal is especially useful for glenohumeral reconstructive procedures such as arthroscopic labral stabilization. Davidson and Tibone (18) described the anterior inferior portal for shoulder arthroscopy (Fig. 27.10). This portal at the 5 o'clock position provides direct linear access to the glenoid rim at the critical anterior inferior site of Bankart capsulolabral detachment (Fig. 27.19). The portal passes lateral to the musculocutaneous nerve and superolateral to the axillary nerve. The mean portal-to-nerve distance for the musculocutaneous nerve has been reported to be 22.9 mm, and for the axillary nerve, 24.4 mm (14). This portal passes within 10 mm of the deltopectoral groove, slightly lateral to the conjoined tendon in the lower third of the subscapularis muscle. This portal can be placed from inside-out or from outside-in. With an inside-to-outside technique, the humerus is maximally adducted, the upper one third of the subscapularis is pierced, and the Wissinger rod is passed through the capsule with the exiting tip directed as far later-

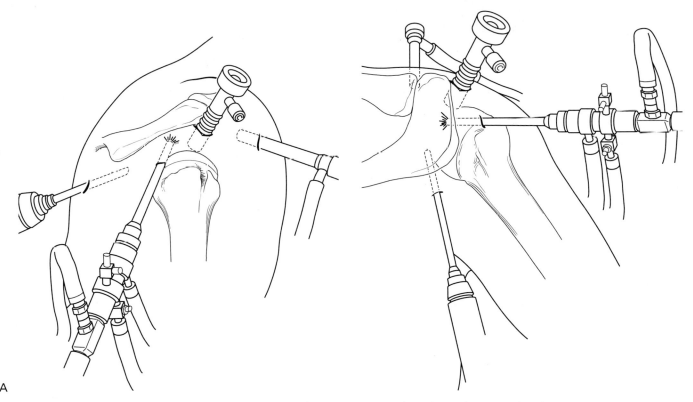

FIGURE 27.17 A: Lateral view of accessory superior lateral portal. **B:** Posterior view.

Superior view

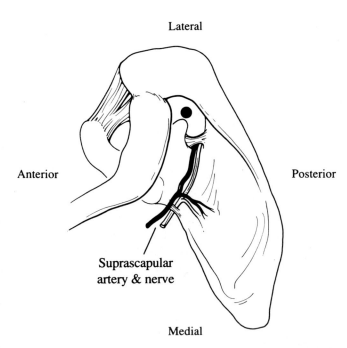

FIGURE 27.18 Neviaser portal in relation to the suprascapular nerve and artery, the acromion, the clavicle, and the spine of the scapula.

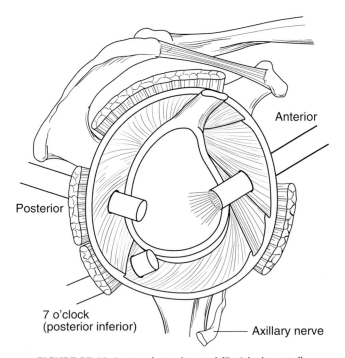

FIGURE 27.19 Posterolateral portal (7 o'clock portal).

ally as possible. A plastic cannula is then placed over the rod anteriorly to provide access to the 5 o'clock position.

Anterior Lateral (SLAP) Portal

This is a useful portal for placing anchors to repair anteriorly located superior labral tears. It is placed 1 cm lateral to the anterior acromion. Accessing the glenohumeral joint from this position does violate the supraspinatus tendon. Recent advances in anchor placement have allowed smaller incisions to be made. Anchor cannulas are smaller than the standard arthroscopic cannulas. Small incisions in the supraspinatus tendon have not been reported to cause difficulties; however, damage to the rotator cuff tendon should be minimized (Fig. 27.15).

POSTERIOR PORTALS

The anterior portals do not provide a satisfactory angle of approach for placement of suture anchors in the posterior aspect of the superior or inferior labrum.

The Port of Wilmington

This portal is used for labral repair in the posterior superior quadrant of the glenoid (19). The skin incision is made 1 cm lateral and 1 cm anterior to the posterolateral corner of the acromion. The portal is made with a 45-degree angle of attack. Usually no cannula is placed in this portal site, to avoid iatrogenic injury to the infraspinatus tendon. Once the spinal needle is localized to the correct trajectory, the labral fixation device is placed percutaneously under direct visualization (Fig. 27.15).

Posterolateral or 7 O'Clock Portal

Placement of plication sutures or anchors into the posterior inferior glenoid can be difficult, necessitating the use of an accessory posterior portal. Morrison et al. (20) described a portal that was placed 2 cm inferior to the standard posterior portal at approximately the 7 o'clock position. It facilitated easy access to the axillary pouch by entry to the joint below the equator of the glenoid. The average distance from the accessory posterior portal to the axillary nerve was 3.7 cm, and the distance to the suprascapular nerve was 2.88 cm. Another accessory posterior lateral portal was described by Goubier et al. (21). The incision for this posterolateral portal was placed 1.5 cm lateral to the acromion at its posterior third. The reported average distance between the posterior inferior portal and the axillary nerve was 14.4 to 24.1 mm. Although these coordinates are helpful, a spinal needle for localization of the portal is essential (Fig. 27.15).

Once multiple portals have been established, care must be taken to not excessively widen the portal openings. Can-

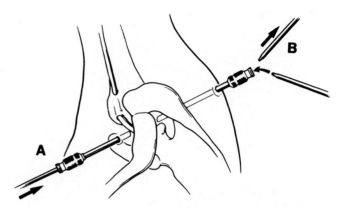

FIGURE 27.20 Use of switching sticks **(A, B)** to interchange working portals.

nulas help in keeping a standard size portal. If portal distention occurs, it can lead to extravasation of fluid into the soft tissues. Switching sticks or rods can be used to move the arthroscope from one portal to another while maintaining the same portal configuration (Fig. 27.20).

ARTHROSCOPIC ANATOMY OF THE SHOULDER: DIAGNOSTIC ARTHROSCOPY AND ANATOMY AT RISK

Diagnostic arthroscopy of the shoulder starts with the insertion of the arthroscope into the glenohumeral joint through the posterior portal. The arthroscope passes through the skin, the posterior deltoid, and the infraspinatus–teres minor interval. The quadrangular and triangular spaces are areas to avoid. These spaces are located 7 to 8 cm inferior to the posterolateral corner of the acromion. The quadrangular space is formed by the teres minor superiorly, the teres major inferiorly, the long head of the triceps medially, and the humeral shaft laterally (Fig. 27.21). The posterior humeral circumflex vessels and the axillary nerve pass through the quadrangular space. The triangular space contains the circumflex scapular vessels, and the triangular interval contains the radial nerve and the profunda brachial artery. The triangular space is bounded by the long head of the triceps laterally and the two teres muscles medially.

The anterior cannula is inserted and can be used for outflow. On entering the joint, the surgeon should see the triangle formed by the biceps tendon superiorly, the humeral head laterally, and the subscapularis inferiorly. The biceps tendon attaches to the supraglenoid tubercle at the posterior superior aspect of the glenoid rim. The biceps origin either is attached to the superior labrum or sends fibers to the anterosuperior and posterosuperior labrum (Fig. 27.22). The diagnostic glenohumeral arthroscopy then proceeds with a systematic approach.

The arthroscope is placed in the posterior portal with the 30-degree angle facing laterally. The rotator interval and the

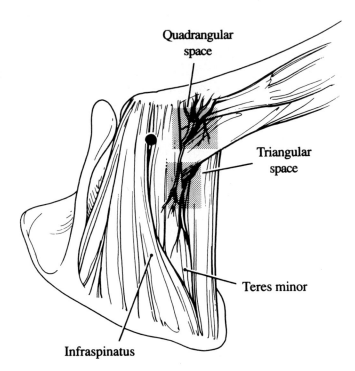

FIGURE 27.21 View of the posterior portal in relation to the infraspinatus, teres minor, quadrangular space, and triangular space.

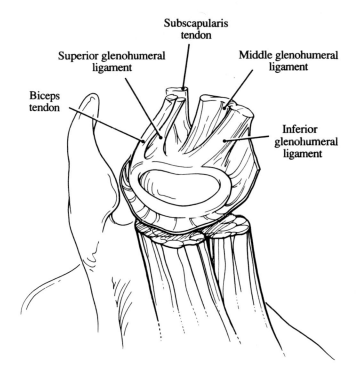

FIGURE 27.23 Anterior capsular ligaments and their relationship to the subscapularis and biceps.

rolled upper edge of the subscapularis are examined. Intersecting the subscapularis at a 60-degree angle is the middle glenohumeral ligament (MGHL) (Fig. 27.23). The MGHL varies in its thickness (22). Sometimes it is a veil of tissue, and other times it represents a cord of tissue termed the Buford complex. This complex occurs when the MGHL takes a high origin off the glenoid at the base of the biceps tendon and is a single cord-like structure. In these instances, the anterior superior labrum may be absent (23). The MGHL arises from the anterior humeral neck just medial to the

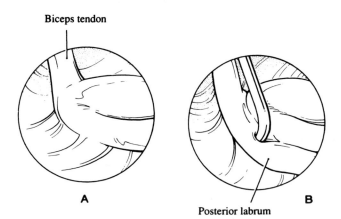

FIGURE 27.22 Attachment of the biceps tendon to the supraglenoid tubercle **(A)** and the intimate relationship of the posterior labrum **(B)**.

lesser tuberosity and inserts on the medial and superior glenoid rim and scapular neck. Its function is to resist anterior translation of the humeral head at 45 degrees of abduction (24). The SGHL runs from the anterior superior aspect of the glenoid to the upper part of the lesser tuberosity and is considered by some to be the floor of the bicipital groove. The SGHL works with the CHL in preventing anterior translation of the humeral head with the arm adducted and externally rotated. The ligament also prevents inferior subluxation to the humeral head (Sulcus sign). In diagnostic glenohumeral arthroscopy, it is also important to examine the subscapularis recess. Loose bodies can be found in this recess and will not be discovered unless the area is actually visualized. Inferiorly, the anterior and anterior inferior labrum can be inspected. Sublabral defects of the anterior superior labrum can be seen in 60% of patients. In 10% the defect is a complete hole and communicates with the subscapularis recess. These cases are normal variants and should not be mistaken for labral pathology. Any detachment of the labrum below the glenoid equator (the level of the rolled edge of the subscapularis) is pathologic.

Inferiorly, with the assistant holding traction at 20 to 30 degrees of abduction on the arm in a beach-chair position, the anterior band of the inferior glenohumeral ligament (IGHL) can be inspected. The anterior band of the IGHL prevents anterior translation of the humeral head when the arm is abducted 90 degrees and externally rotated. It also restricts inferior translation when the arm is abducted and internally rotated. The IGHL runs from the glenoid to the anatomic neck of the humerus. The humeral attachment of the anterior band is best visualized from the anterior portal. It is from this view that a humeral avulsion of the glenohumeral ligament (HAGL lesion) can be seen.

The axillary pouch is then inspected, and the posterior inferior labrum and the posterior band of the IGHL can also be inspected sequentially. The capsule of the axillary pouch is thin, and beneath it lies the axillary nerve. This relationship should always be considered when placing capsular plication sutures in this area or performing thermal capsulorraphy. The posterior band of the IGHL prevents inferior translation of the humeral head when the arm is abducted 90 degrees and externally rotated. It also prevents posterior translation when the arm is abducted and internally rotated (9).

A probe can be inserted through the anterior portal, as previously described, and this probe can be used to examine all labral and ligamentous structures. The biceps can be followed distally into the bicipital groove. Forward elevation with the elbow flexed, combined with external rotation of the arm, may assist in viewing the biceps as it passes underneath the transverse humeral ligament. The CHL originates at the base of the coracoid and inserts into the intertubercular groove of the humerus. It surrounds the biceps tendon. The subscapularis tendon represents the medial aspect of the groove, and the supraspinatus tendon represents the lateral aspect. The SGHL and CHL form the medial sling of the biceps. The supraspinatus tendon can be seen adjacent to the biceps with abduction and external rotation. Observing posteriorly and inferiorly from this point down the posterior humerus, the bare area can be viewed. This is an area of bare bone with remnants of old vascular channels. This bare area also correlates to the attachment of the infraspinatus tendon. It can be used as a landmark in rotator cuff surgery to align the infraspinatus to its footprint.

COMPLICATIONS RELATED TO SHOULDER ARTHROSCOPY

Shoulder arthroscopy is a minimally invasive procedure, and postoperative pain is significantly diminished compared with many comparable open procedures. The decreased pain with shoulder arthroscopy is a consequence of the lack of layer-by-layer dissection, which results in minimal soft tissue damage. Proper portal placement avoids most of the complications of shoulder arthroscopy. With use of the lateral decubitus position, traction in the operative limb may cause a stretch neuropraxia (25). The position that seems to place the greatest traction on the brachial plexus is 30 degrees of forward elevation and 70 degrees of abduction (25).

One disadvantage of arthroscopy is the visual distortion caused by the parallax of the 30- or 70-degree arthroscope. This distortion makes it difficult to determine the smooth-

ness of certain surfaces, especially when dealing with the anterior acromion.

Bleeding in the subacromion space is a problem and has been studied extensively. Morrison et al. (2) reported that maintaining a pressure difference (systolic blood pressure minus subacromial space pressure) equal to or less than 49 mm Hg can prevent bleeding. The acromial branch of the coracoacromial artery is a vessel that is usually transected just lateral to the acromioclavicular joint as the coracoacromial ligament is being resected. Thermal ablation electrocautery devices have facilitated the coagulation of these vessels and helped with control of generalized subacromial bleeding. If bleeding does obscure the field of view, the arthroscope should be advanced up to the suspected area of bleeding so that the fluid coming from the inflow sheath dilutes the blood, providing enough visualization of the bleeding vessel to allow control of the hemorrhage with the electrocautery device.

Another difficulty with shoulder arthroscopy includes extravasation of fluid into the soft tissues (26). Older patients with poor tissue quality have a greater chance of extravasation because their fascial and capsular tissues are not strong enough to contain the fluid in the glenohumeral or subacromial space.

Infection is rare in shoulder arthroscopy, and the risk has been reported to be less than 1% of the cases (27).

Another generalized area of concern is that of arrhythmias caused by placement of epinephrine into the arthroscopic irrigation solution. This potentially could cause an arrhythmia or generalized vasoconstriction, increasing the systemic vascular resistance, increasing the pulmonary pressure, and causing pulmonary edema.

If in large individuals with very thick necks extubation is performed too quickly, some laryngospasm may occur, causing coughing. The force generated by the accessory muscles of inspiration can cause a negative-pressure pulmonary edema.

Other complications can be caused by anesthesia. Interscalene blocks have proved to be a successful mode of pain control. Reported complications include hematoma formation, phrenic and recurrent laryngeal nerve blockade, vasovagal attack, pneumothorax, total spinal anesthesia, high epidural blockade, Horner's syndrome, and cardiac arrest (25).

Articular damage can be caused by the sharp corners of the arthroscope or by thermal ablation devices. Such damage can be caused on entrance to the joint and is more likely if there is inaccurate portal placement.

Dietzel and Ciullo (28) reported four cases of spontaneous pneumothorax after shoulder arthroscopy. All patients had a history of smoking or asthma, and all were in the lateral decubitus position.

Deep venous thromboembolism in one patient was reported by Burkhart (29). This patient had pain and swelling 3 days after surgery, and venography showed thrombosis of the basilic vein, where it was being compressed by an unsuspected Hodgkins lymphoma. The author reported that deep venous thromboembolism is so rare that its occurrence should prompt investigation into a hypercoagulable state.

REFERENCES

1. Burman MS. Arthroscopy or direct visualization of joints: experimental cadaver study. *Bone Joint Surg* 1931;13:669–695.
2. Morrison DS, Schaefer RK, Friedman RL. The relationship between subacromial pressure, blood pressure, and visual clarity during arthroscopic subacromial decompression. *Arthroscopy* 1995;11:557–560.
3. Altchek DW, Warren RF, Skyhar MJ, et al. T-plasty modification of the Bankart procedure for multi-directional instability anterior and inferior types. *J Bone Joint Surg Am* 1991;73:105–112.
4. Hennrikus WL, Mapes RC, Bratton MW, et al. Lateal traction during shoulder arthroscopy: its effect on tissue perfusion measured by pulse oximetry. *Am J Sports Med* 1995;23:444–446.
5. Klein AH, France JC, Mutschler TA, et al. Measurement of brachial plexus strain in arthroscopy of the shoulder. *Arthroscopy* 1987;3:45–52.
6. Bert JM, Posalaky Z, Snyder S, et al. Effect of various irrigating fluids on the ultrastructure of articular cartilage. *Arthroscopy* 1990;6:104–111.
7. Gradinger R, Träger J, Klauser RJ. Influence of various irrigation fluids on articular cartilage. *Arthroscopy* 1995;11:263–269.
8. Hamada S, Hamada M, Nishiue S, et al. Osteochondritis dissecans of the humeral head [Case report]. *Arthroscopy* 1992;8:132–137.
9. Jobe FW, Giangarra CE, Kvitne RS, et al. Anterior capsulolabral reconstruction of the shoulder in athletes in overhand sports. *Am J Sports Med* 1991;19:428–434.
10. Johnson LL, Schneider DA, Austin MD, et al. Two-percent glutaraldehyde: a disinfectant in arthroscopy and arthroscopic surgery. *J Bone Joint Surg Am* 1982;64:237–239.
11. Johnson LL. *Arthroscopic surgery: principles and practice,* 3rd ed. St Louis: CV Mosby, 1986.
12. Morgan C. Fluid delivery systems for arthroscopy. *Arthroscopy* 1987;3:288–291.
13. Matthews LS, Fadale PD. Techniques and instrumentation for shoulder arthroscopy. *Instr Course Lect* 1989;38:169–176.
14. Hollinsehead WH. *Anatomy for surgeons,* 2nd ed, vol 3. Philadelphia: Harper and Row, 1969:316.
15. Hoppenfeld S, deBoer P. Surgical exposures. In: *Orthopaedics,* 2nd ed. Philadelphia: JB Lippincott, 1994:25–29.
16. Beals TC, Harryman DT, Lazarus MD. Useful boundary of the subacromial bursa. *Arthroscopy* 1998;14:465–470.
17. Laurencin CT, Detsh A, O'Brien SJ, et al. The superior lateral portal for arthroscopy of the shoulder. *Arthroscopy* 1994;10:255–258.
18. Davidson PA, Tibone JE. Anterior inferior (5 o'clock) portal for shoulder arthroscopy. *Arthroscopy* 1995;11:519–525.
19. Morgan CD, Burkhart SS, Palmeri M, et al. Type II SLAP lesions: three subtypes and their relationships to superior instability and rotator cuff tear. *Arthroscopy* 1998;14:553–555.
20. Morrison DS, Schaefer RK, Friedman RL. The relationship between subacromial space pressure, blood pressure, and visual clarity during arthroscopic subacromial decompression. *Arthroscopy* 1995;11:557–560.
21. Goubier JN, Iserin A, Augereau B. The posterolateral portal: a new approach to shoulder arthroscopy. *Arthroscopy* 2001;17:1000–1002.
22. Gohlke F, Essigkrug B, Schmitz F. The pattern of the collagen fiber bundles of the capsule of the glenohumeral joint. *J Shoulder Elbow Surg* 1994;3:111–128.
23. Williams MM, Snyder SJ, Buford D. The Buford complex—the "cord-like" middle glenohumeral ligament and absent anterosuperior labrum complex: a normal anatomic capsulolabral variant. *Arthroscopy* 1994;10:241–247.
24. Jobe CM. Posterior superior glenoid impingement: expanded spectrum. *Arthroscopy* 1995;11:530–536.
25. Schaffer BS, Tibone JE. Arthroscopic shoulder instability surgery complications. *Clin Sports Med* 1999;4:737–767.
26. Jurvelin JS, Jurvelin JA, Kiviranta I, et al. Effects of different irrigation liquids and times on articular cartilage: an experimental, biomechanical study. *Arthroscopy* 1994;10:667–672.
27. Armstrong RW, Bolding F, Joseph R. Septic arthritis following arthroscopy: clinical syndromes and analysis of risk factors. *Arthroscopy* 1992;8:213–223.
28. Dietzel DP, Ciullo JV. Spontaneous pneumothorax after shoulder arthroscopy: a report of four cases. *Arthroscopy* 1996;12:99–102
29. Burkhart SS. Deep venous thrombosis after shoulder arthroscopy. *Arthroscopy* 1990;6:61–63.

ARTHROSCOPIC KNOT TYING

K. CASEY CHAN
STEPHEN S. BURKHART

Arthroscopic knot tying is a necessary skill that an arthroscopic surgeon must acquire in order to do shoulder reconstruction using suture anchors. The original knot-tying instruments attempted to recreate tying of square knots by hand. Attempts to tie square knots arthroscopically have largely been abandoned because square knots tend to "flip" into half-hitch knots with the slightest unequal tension on the suture limbs. Currently, the most popular knots for arthroscopic surgery are compound sliding knots and stacked half-hitch knots. Single-lumen knot tiers are simple and effective instruments for use with sliding knots. This chapter deals mainly with techniques using the single-lumen knot tier. There is also a brief discussion of "self-locking" knots, because of recent interest in the use of this class of knots in arthroscopic surgery. In addition, there is a brief discussion of static (nonsliding) knots, their uses, and techniques of tying them.

TERMINOLOGY AND CONCEPTS

A clear understanding of terminology helps the reader to grasp key concepts in arthroscopic knot tying. In general a knot is formed by wrapping the limbs of the suture around each other in a predetermined fashion. However, not all knots are suitable for arthroscopic knot tying. Knots used in arthroscopic surgery are generally formed outside the joint with the suture already passed through both the anchoring device and the tissue to be repaired.

Definitions

The externally formed knot must be transferred to the repair site, usually by sliding it along a substantially straight portion of the suture limb called the *post limb* (Fig. 28.1). The post limb is the straight portion of the suture limb, around

K. C. Chan: Department Of Orthopaedic Surgery, National University Hospital, National University of Singapore.

S. S. Burkhart: Department of Orthopaedics, University of Texas Health Science Center at San Antonio, and Baylor College of Medicine, Houston, Texas.

which the second limb wraps to form a *sliding knot*. A loosely equivalent term for the post limb that is sometimes used in the art of knot tying is the "standing part." The free portion of the suture that wraps around the post limb to form the sliding knot is termed the *wrapping limb*. Some loosely equivalent terms for the wrapping limb sometimes used in the art of knot tying are "working end," "running end," or "free end." When one is forming a sliding knot outside the joint, the post limb must be the shorter limb, and the length of the wrapping limb should be about half the length of the whole suture.

What is generally termed the "knot" actually consists of two portions, the knot proper and the loop. The *knot proper* is defined as the *wrappings* plus the *post* contained within the wrappings. The *loop* is defined as the loop portion of the suture distal to the knot proper. It is important to distinguish between these two portions of the knot when discussing the security of arthroscopic repair. *Knot security* is the effectiveness of the knot proper at resisting slippage when load is applied. Knot security depends on three factors: friction, internal interference, and slack between throws (1). Friction is greater for braided multifilament suture than for monofilament suture. Internal interference refers to the "weave" of the two suture limbs relative to each other; it is increased by reversing the direction of the half-hitches or by switching posts, or both. For a compound sliding knot, internal interference is increased by increasing the length of contact and the complexity of the "weave" between the two suture limbs. Slack between throws is eliminated by removing any twists between suture limbs before advancing a half-hitch and by past-pointing (running the knot pusher past the knot to tension the two limbs at 180 degrees to each other) (Fig. 28.2). *Loop security* is the ability to maintain a tight suture loop as a knot is tied (1,2). It is possible to have an ineffective repair despite good knot security if the suture loop is loose and does not adequately approximate the edges of the tissue to be repaired.

Half-Hitch Versus Compound Sliding Knot

The *half-hitch* knot is the simplest of all the sliding knots. It is formed by wrapping the suture limb once around the post

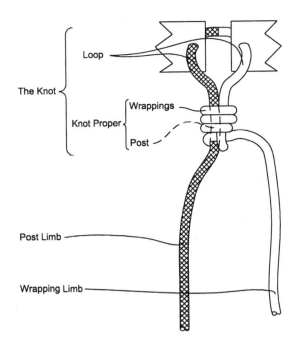

FIGURE 28.1 Definitions of various components of a generic sliding knot.

limb of the suture (one turn). The half-hitch is commonly described as either *"under-over"* or *"over-under"* according to the position of the wrapping limb relative to the post limb, as viewed by the surgeon during the knot-forming process. The direction of the half-hitch knot refers to whether the half-hitch is formed in the over-under sequence or the under-over sequence (Table 28.1). If the first half-hitch is an

over-under half-hitch and the second half-hitch is an under-over half-hitch, the second half-hitch is said to be in the *reverse direction* to that of the first half-hitch. The term *reversed half-hitches* refers to two sequential half-hitches tied in reversed direction, either on the same post or on the opposite post. *Reversed half-hitches on alternate posts (RHAP)* are commonly used to lock a sliding knot in place. These definitions are summarized in Table 28-1.

A compound sliding knot is a sliding knot that has more than one turn of the wrapping limb around the post limb (i.e., any sliding knot other than a half-hitch is a compound sliding knot). The advantage of a compound sliding knot is that, once it is properly formed, it can be made to slide down the post limb without unraveling or jamming prematurely.

The sliding knot, such as the modified Duncan loop (3), is preferably advanced along the post limb of the suture by pushing the knot forward with the knot tier. The surgeon pulls on the post limb to take up the slack of the suture in the loop of the knot (Fig. 28.3) created by the advancing knot. In order for the slack to be taken up, the suture must be able to slide easily through the tissue and the suture anchor.

Compound sliding knots cannot be used in situations in which the suture cannot easily slide through the tissue and the suture anchor. The loop of the half-hitch knot can be tightened, just as the compound sliding knot is, by advanc-

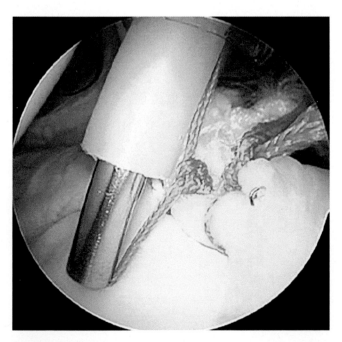

FIGURE 28.2 The Surgeon's Sixth Finger knot tier (Arthrex, Naples, FL) is used to past-point in order to maximally tighten a knot by applying opposing tension in the two suture limbs.

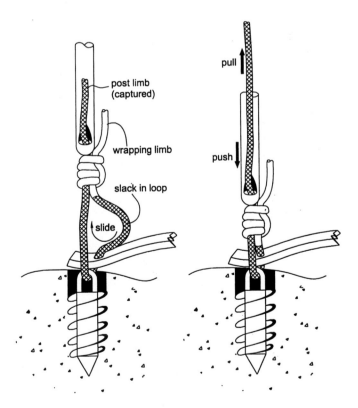

FIGURE 28.3 The compound sliding knot is advanced by pushing the knot forward, and the slack in the loop is taken up by pulling on the post limb.

TABLE 28.1 DEFINITION AND SYMBOLIC REPRESENTATION OF HALF-HITCH CONFIGURATIONS

Symbol	Schematic Representation	Description
S	under-over OR over-under	Denotes a half-hitch. The direction of the knot is determined by the relative position of the wrapping limb around the post, as viewed by the surgeon from above.
S=S		Denotes two sequential half-hitches formed in the same direction around the same post, defined here as "identical half hitches on the same post."
SxS		Denotes two sequential half-hitches formed in opposite directions around the same post, defined here as "reversed half-hitches on the same post."
S//S		Denotes two sequential half-hitches formed in reversed directions around opposite posts, defined here as "reversed half-hitches on alternate posts" (RHAP).

ing the knot along the post limb, with the slack in the loop taken up by pulling on the post limb, as shown in Fig. 28.3. If the suture does not slide through the tissue and the suture anchor, it is still possible to advance the half-hitch along the post limb and take up the slack in the loop by pulling on the wrapping limb in one of two ways, as shown in Fig. 28.4. The half-hitch can be advanced by pushing (Fig. 28.4A) or by pulling (Fig. 28.4B) the knot forward. This is possible because the single turn around the post limb allows the wrapping to slide around the post limb. This ability of the half-hitch to take up the slack in the loop by sliding in the wrapping as opposed to the knot's sliding along the post limb has prompted some arthroscopic surgeons (Snyder SJ, Southern California Orthopedic Institute, Van Nuys, CA; personal communication, 2000) to call the half-hitch a "nonsliding" knot, or static knot.

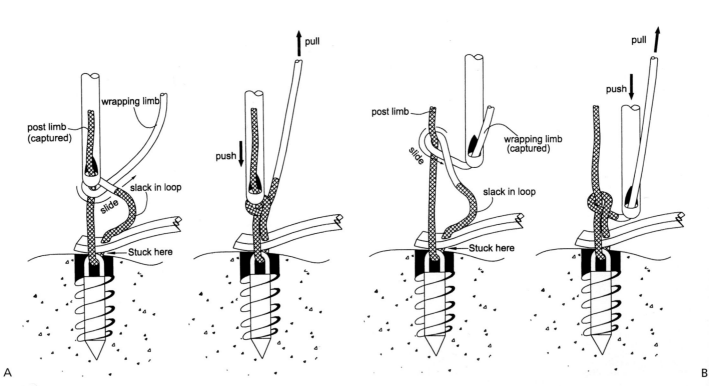

FIGURE 28.4 A: The half-hitch is advanced by pushing the knot forward, and the slack is taken up by pulling on the wrapping limb. **B:** The half-hitch is advanced by pulling the knot forward, and the slack is taken up by pulling on the wrapping limb.

Static (nonsliding) knots are very useful and represent the only type of knot that can be tied when the suture will not slide through the suture anchor or the tissue. The biggest problem with the static knot as tied by the single-lumen knot tier is the propensity for the tissue loop to loosen before the second half-hitch is seated to the point at which it provisionally "locks" the knot. One of us (SSB) has devised a knot pusher (Surgeon's Sixth Finger, Arthrex, Naples, FL) that reliably holds a tight tissue loop as it advances sequential half-hitches, providing excellent loop security (2) as well as knot security (1). One advantage of the static knot is that its formation does not result in suture damage from abrasion against the suture anchor eyelet, as can occur with sliding knots.

Switching Posts

The reader needs to be familiar with the concept of switching posts when working with half-hitches (5). It is possible to flip the half-hitch (Fig. 28.5) by simply releasing tension

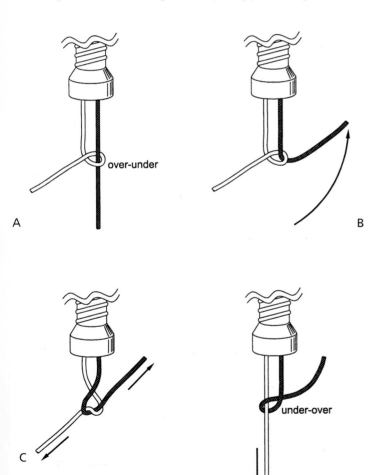

A   over-under

B

C

under-over

D

FIGURE 28.5 Switching posts. **A:** Form an over-under half-hitch outside the joint. **B:** Advance the post limb ahead of the half-hitch. **C:** Pull gently on both suture limbs. **D:** Pull axially to complete the switching of post.

from the post limb and pulling on the wrapping limb. A reliable way of flipping the half-hitch to switch posts is to release tension on the post limb and move it forward and ahead of the half-hitch (Fig. 28.5B). Gentle traction on both post limb and wrapping limb at the same time, in opposite and diagonal directions (Fig. 28.5C), transforms the half-hitch to a flat knot with symmetric throws. Axial traction on the original wrapping limb converts it to a post (Fig. 28.5D). Note that when the post is switched, the direction of the half-hitch is also reversed. With a little practice, the surgeon will be able to flip the posts back and forth with ease.

TYPES OF KNOTS

All arthroscopic surgeons who wish to do shoulder reconstruction using suture anchors should be adept at tying stacked half-hitch knots and one compound sliding knot. This section is a compendium of popular knots from which the surgeon can choose his or her favorites.

Stacked Half-Hitch Knot

The stacked half-hitch knot is a basic knot, and it is essential that arthroscopic surgeons be familiar with it. This is a static (nonsliding) knot. It can be used generally, and in particular it is most useful in situations where sliding of suture through the tissue is not possible or desired. The original Revo knot, popularized by Snyder (6), is a series of four reversing half-hitches with the post switched once after the second half-hitch. A recent study showed that other configurations of stacked half-hitches are just as strong, so long as the stack is locked by three RHAPs (7). In fact, a "base" knot of two or three stacked half-hitches can always be optimized by stacking three RHAPs on top of it. The base knot with three RHAPs always changes the knot's mode of failure from one of slippage to one of breakage, evidence that knot security has been maximized (7).

How to Tie and Lock Stacked Half-Hitch Knots

The first half-hitch has a tendency to unravel. If the second half-hitch is on the opposite post, the knot may lock prematurely, resulting in a loose loop. Therefore, as a general principle, the first two or three half-hitches should be stacked on the same post, preferably with the direction reversed. Once security of the loop is achieved, the initial stack of half-hitches is locked with three RHAPs.

An efficient technique of tying stacked half-hitches and locking with RHAPs without the need for rethreading the knot tier is detailed in Fig. 28.6. After two reversed half-hitches are formed on the same post, three RHAPs are alternately pushed and pulled into the joint. Note that with this technique of tying stacked half-hitches, the half-hitches

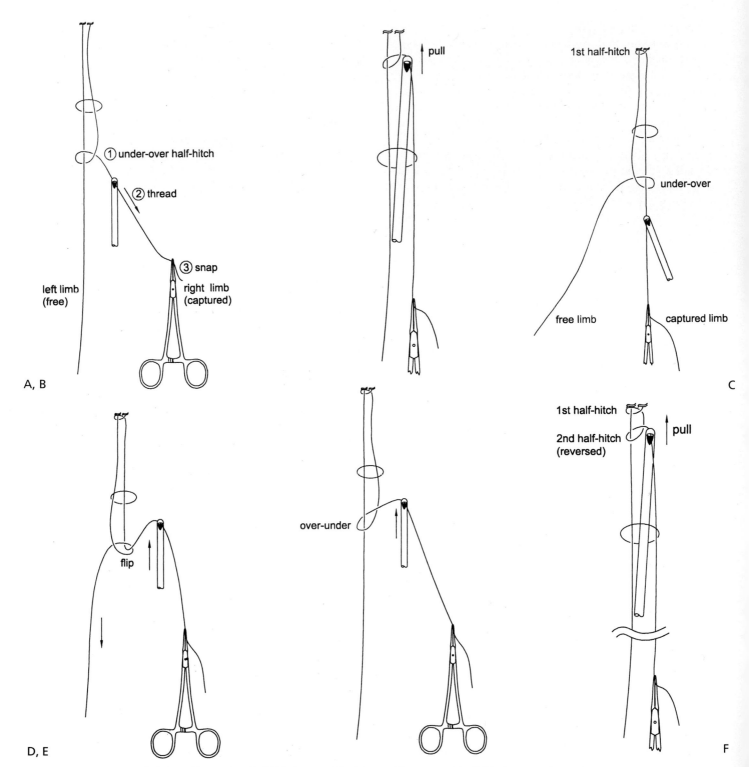

FIGURE 28.6 Tying half-hitches and locking with reversed half-hitches on alternate posts (RHAPs). **A:** Wrap the right limb around the left limb to form the first half-hitch (under-over). Then thread the right limb through the single-lumen knot tier and apply a snap to this right limb. The right limb is now the captured limb, and the left limb remains free throughout the rest of the knot-tying process. **B:** Advance the first half-hitch along the free limb by pulling this half-hitch into the joint. **C:** Form a second half-hitch around the captured limb in an under-over configuration. The first half-hitch usually tends to loosen, so a second or even a third half-hitch on the same post is necessary. **D:** Flip the second half-hitch by advancing the knot tier ahead of the knot and pulling on the free limb at the same time. **E:** After the half-hitch is flipped, the second half-hitch has an over-under configuration around the free limb *(left)*; this second half-hitch therefore has a reverse direction to the first half-hitch. **F:** Advance the second half-hitch along the free limb by pulling this half-hitch into the joint. Tighten this second half-hitch by past-pointing. If necessary, add a third half-hitch on the free limb using the technique shown in (C) and (D).

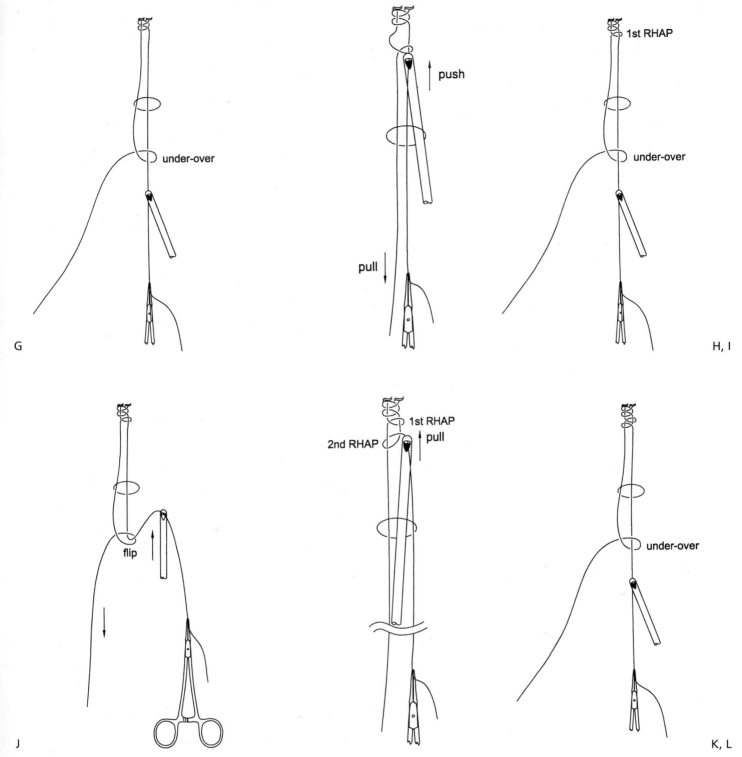

FIGURE 28.6 *(Continued).* **G:** The first RHAP is created by wrapping the free limb around the captured limb to form an under-over half-hitch. **H:** Push this first RHAP into the joint along the captured limb. Advance it 1 cm at a time, and pull on the free limb to take up slack in the loop distal to the knot before advancing it another centimeter. Snyder referred to this stepwise advancement of the half-hitch as "walking" the knot. **I:** Form another under-over half-hitch around the captured limb. **J:** Advance the knot tier ahead of the half-hitch while pulling on the free limb at the same time, causing the knot to flip and thus forming the second RHAP. This second RHAP now has a reverse direction to the first RHAP. **K:** Advance the second RHAP along the free limb by pulling this half-hitch into the joint. Tighten this second RHAP by past-pointing. **L:** Form a third RHAP by making an under-over half-hitch around the captured limb. *(cont'd)*

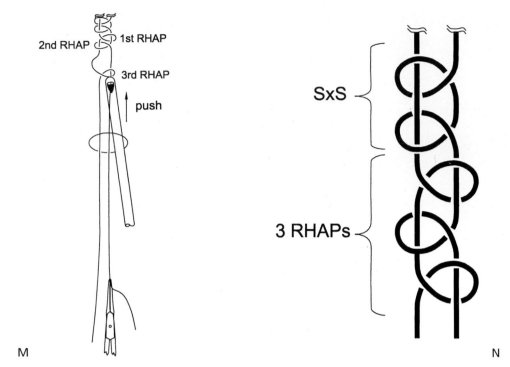

FIGURE 28.6 *(Continued).* **M:** Push this third RHAP into the joint along the captured limb and tighten the knot. **N:** Schematic representation of the completed stacked half-hitch knot.

are always formed in the same direction (under-over in the example shown). Yet the stacked half-hitch knot always ends up in the desired configuration, owing to "flipping" of the post. This configuration is easy for the surgeon to remember.

Another way of tying a stacked half-hitch knot while simultaneously maintaining excellent loop security is by means of the Surgeon's Sixth Finger knot tier (Arthrex). This knot pusher holds the first half-hitch in place as subsequent half-hitches are stacked on top of it (Fig. 28.7). The last three half-hitches are applied as RHAPs, using a "post-flipping" technique that is very similar to the one used with the single-lumen knot tier.

Even for the simple stacked half-hitch knot just described, it will take several hours of practice before the surgeon is proficient at tying this knot. First tying should be practiced using ropes and hands. After one is fully familiar with the knot configuration, practice should continue using a knot tier, suture material, and a knot tying stand.

Modified Duncan Loop

The modified Duncan loop, popularized by Eugene Wolf (3), is the most popular compound sliding knot (Fig. 28.8). This was one of the earliest knots used for arthroscopic surgery, and over time has been proven to work well. Because the wrapping limb is wound several times around the post limb, the knot, when adequately cinched, resists backing off even with monofilament suture. If the knot is made

with braided suture and is too tightly cinched, the suture may fray when the knot is advanced along the post limb. With braided suture, three turns (rather than four) of the wrapping limb around the post limb produces less resistance to advancement of the knot and still resists backing off when the knot is seated on the soft tissues.

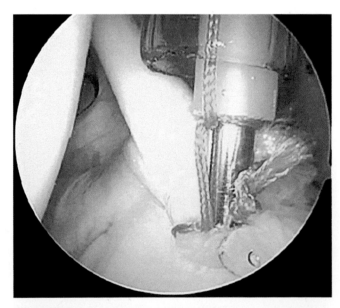

FIGURE 28.7 The Surgeon's Sixth Finger knot tier (Arthrex, Naples, FL) is used to stack sequential half-hitches while maintaining loop security through pressure on the previously thrown half-hitches.

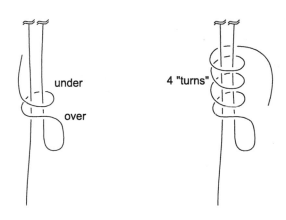

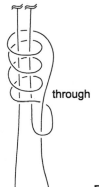

FIGURE 28.8 Modified Duncan loop.

Tautline Hitch

The modified tautline hitch is a simple compound sliding knot consisting of three turns (Fig. 28.9). It was introduced by De Beer et al. (8) for use in arthroscopic surgery. The authors gave it a catchy name, "Nicky's knot." The construction of the knot is easy to remember, and because of its simplicity it can be formed quickly at surgery.

Buntline Hitch

The buntline hitch was popularized by Snyder and Getelman (9) as the "Tennessee slider" (Fig. 28.10). It is the simplest of all compound sliding knots. The figure-of-eight configuration makes the construction easy to remember. This knot is in fact two reversed half-hitches formed on the same post in a proximal-to-distal sequence.

Modified Roeder Knot

The Roeder knot (Fig. 28.11) was originally used in ear, nose, and throat surgery and later was introduced into pelvic and laparoscopic surgery. This sliding knot is also suitable for use in arthroscopy surgery. There are several versions of this knot (4,10–13). All versions have two steps in common: wrapping around a single post, followed by wrapping one or more turns around two "posts."

Samsung Medical Center (SMC) Knot

The SMC knot (Fig. 28.12) consists of two identical half-hitches formed around the post limb (14). The wrapping limb is then passed through the space between the two half-hitches. This knot, like the buntline hitch, has a low profile.

Weston Knot

The Weston knot is not much known outside of the field of obstetrics and gynecology. The original description by Weston (15) on how the knot is formed is rather complex and may be one of the reasons why this knot is not widely adopted. A simplified construction of this knot is depicted in Fig. 28.13. A unique feature of the Weston knot is the ease with which the knot can be locked by pulling on the wrapping limb. To prevent premature locking, care must be taken to keep tension on the post limb and avoid pulling on the wrapping limb, especially during advancement of the knot into the joint.

Techniques Related to Compound Sliding Knots

It is not necessary to learn all the compound sliding knots listed here. One needs to be facile with one configuration of

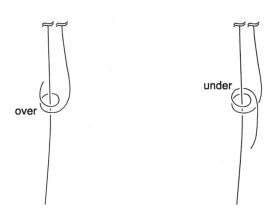

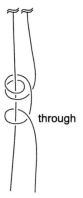

FIGURE 28.9 Tautline hitch.

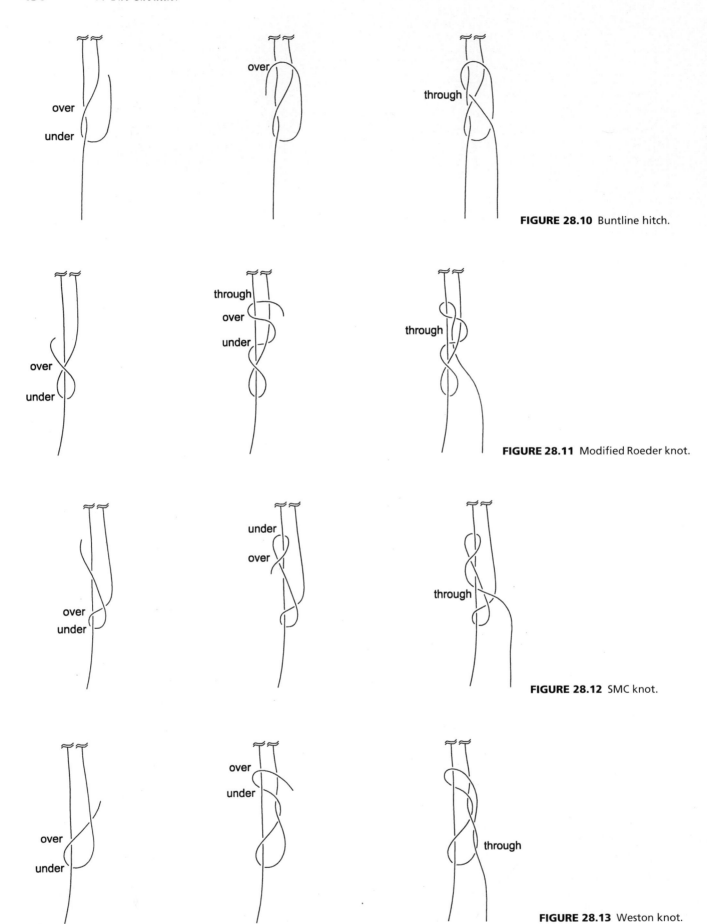

FIGURE 28.10 Buntline hitch.

FIGURE 28.11 Modified Roeder knot.

FIGURE 28.12 SMC knot.

FIGURE 28.13 Weston knot.

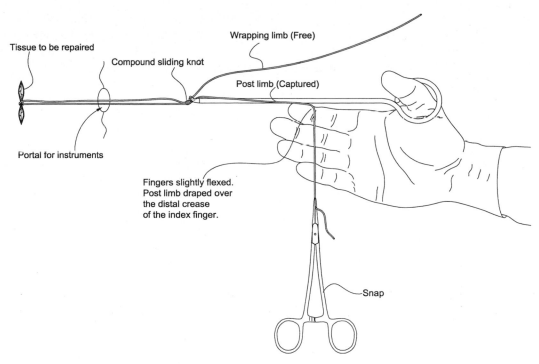

FIGURE 28.14 Thread the post limb through the lumen of the knot tier.

stacked half-hitch knots and one compound sliding knot from this group. It will on average take 4 to 8 hours of practice with a knot-tying stand to acquire sufficient skill to execute knot tying smoothly during surgery.

In forming a compound sliding knot, the post should be kept short and the wrapping limb should be approximately half the total length of the suture. When the knot slides into the joint toward the repair site, the knot takes the wrapping

limb into the joint with it, and the post limb lengthens correspondingly.

It is possible to transport a compound sliding knot toward the repair site by simply pulling on the post limb. However, this can cause undue tension at the repair site. The delivery of the knot is best controlled by pushing the knot ahead with a knot tier and pulling on the post limb at the same time (Figs. 28.3, 28.14, 28.15 and 28.16).

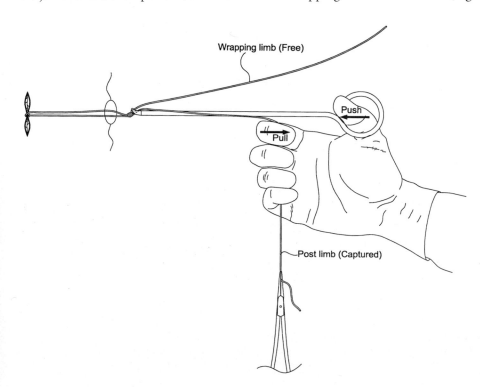

FIGURE 28.15 Advance the compound sliding knot by alternately flexing and extending the fingers. The sliding knot is advanced by gripping the post limb within the crease of the index finger, flexing all fingers and pushing the loop handle forward with the thumb. By alternately flexing and extending fingers and pushing loop handle forward with the thumb, the compound sliding knot is progressively advanced forward.

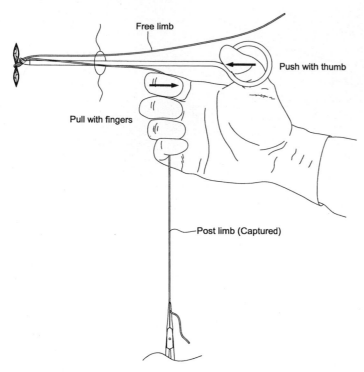

FIGURE 28.16 Tighten the loop by pulling the post limb and pushing with the knot tier.

After the compound sliding knot is properly seated at the repair site, the wrapping limb must be tensioned to ensure loop security and to prevent the knot from backing off. In the case of the modified Duncan loop, this results in tightening of the wrappings around the post, producing a tighter grip. For the other compound sliding knots such as the tautline hitch, buntline hitch, Roeder knot, SMC knot, and the Weston knot, tensioning of the wrapping limb distorts the post, resulting in a kink in the post that increases the resistance of the knot to backing off. This locking effect is variously known as the "one-way ratchet effect" and the "self-locking effect." Note that excessive tension on the post can impede the distortion by the wrapping, making the locking effect difficult to achieve.

How to Tie and Lock Compound Sliding Knots

As with stacked half-hitch knots, we recommend that all compound sliding knots be locked with three RHAPs. We believe that the initial locking, made with the technique previously described, is insufficient to provide reliable loop security. Experimental studies have shown that the maximum strength of the knot is most reliably achieved with three RHAPs (13,16,17).

Figures 28.14 through 28.24 show an efficient technique to deploy and lock a compound sliding knot. The technique has many features in common with that used for arthroscopic tying of the stacked half-hitch knot. The need for rethreading the knot tier is avoided.

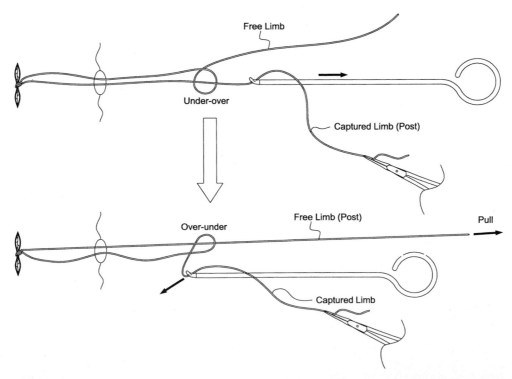

FIGURE 28.17 Top: Form half-hitch around the captured limb. Withdraw knot tier to outside of joint, then form half-hitch by wrapping free limb around the captured limb. **Bottom:** Switch post by flipping the half-hitch. To flip the half-hitch, pull gently on the free limb and move the tip of the knot tier ahead of the half-hitch.

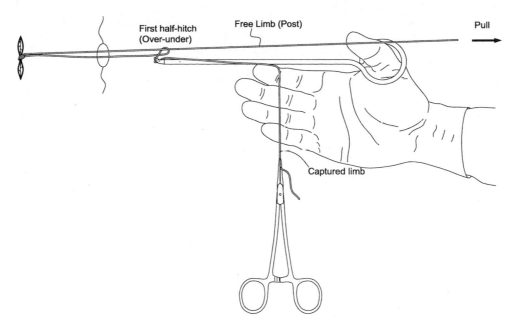

FIGURE 28.18 Pull the first half-hitch forward. Advance half-hitch by flexing and extending fingers and pushing knot tier forward. Keep tip of knot tier ahead of half-hitch to pull it forward.

A surgical snap is used as dead weight to enable the compound sliding knot to be advanced with one hand. By alternately flexing and extending the fingers, the surgeon advances the knot in a ratchet fashion. For this to occur efficiently, the powder on the glove is cleaned off and the glove is then dried. This improves the traction between the suture and the glove, enhancing suture manipulation.

The steps depicted in Figs. 28.14 through 28.24 should be followed closely. The ratchet advancement of the knot can be described as follows. The post limb is threaded through the distal hole of the knot tier, and a surgical snap is attached to the end of this captured limb as a deadweight. The knot tier is held in the right hand with the thumb through the loop handle of the knot tier, and the shaft of the knot tier is balanced on top of the slightly flexed index finger, as shown in Fig. 28.14. The post limb is draped over the distal crease of the index finger. The post limb of the suture is gripped by flexing the fingers

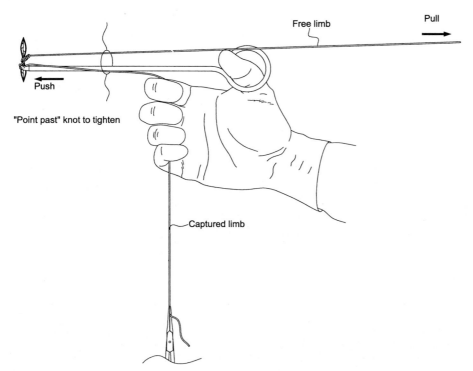

FIGURE 28.19 Tighten the first half-hitch.

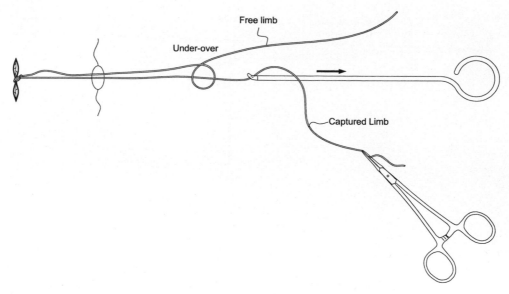

FIGURE 28.20 Form the second half-hitch around captured limb. Withdraw knot tier to outside of joint, then form second half-hitch by wrapping free limb around the captured limb.

(Fig. 28.15). By further flexing the fingers and pushing the loop of the handle of the knot tier forward, the knot is advanced along the post limb. When the fingers are reextended, the slack of the post limb around the fingers is taken up by the weight of the snap. The post limb is again gripped by the flexed fingers, and the knot is advanced further by again flexing the fingers and pushing the loop handle of the knot tier forward. In this manner (i.e., by alternately flexing and extending the fingers and pushing the loop handle forward with the thumb), the knot is progressively advanced forward and into the joint. There is the tendency for the beginner to tightly grip the captured limb, but this will not allow the slack of the captured limb to be taken up by the deadweight of the surgical snap.

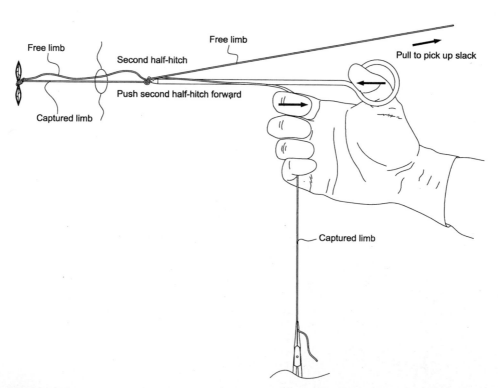

FIGURE 28.21 Push the second half-hitch forward. Maintain tension by pulling on captured limb with flexed fingers while the half-hitch is advanced one centimeter at a time.

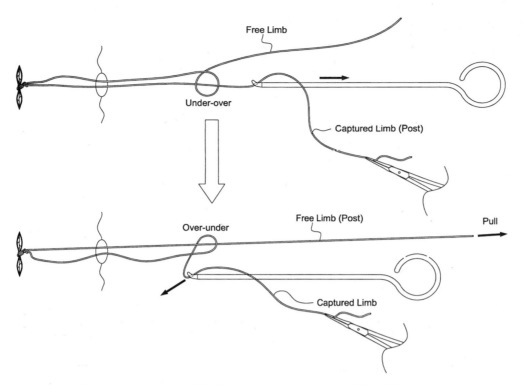

FIGURE 28.22 Top: Form the third half-hitch around the captured limb. Withdraw knot tier to outside of joint, then form third half-hitch by wrapping free limb around the captured limb. **Bottom:** Switch post by flipping the half-hitch. To flip the half-hitch, pull gently on the free limb and move the tip of the knot tier ahead of the half-hitch.

When the knot abuts against the repair site, tissue edges are urged into coaptation by increasing the tension in the loop of the knot. The tension in the loop is increased by pulling the post limb (captured limb) with the flexed fingers and pushing the knot tier against the sliding knot (Fig. 28.16). The free limb, which is the wrapping limb in this case, is pulled to tighten the wrappings of the knot to ensure loop security.

Once loop security is achieved, the knot is then locked with three RHAPs. This is achieved by forming three successive under-over half-hitches using the free limb. The first and the third half-hitch are flipped and pulled into the joint

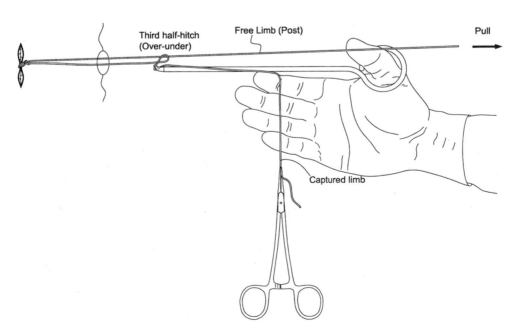

FIGURE 28.23 Pull the third half-hitch forward. Advance half-hitch by flexing and extending fingers and pushing knot tier forward. Keep tip of knot tier ahead of half-hitch to pull it forward.

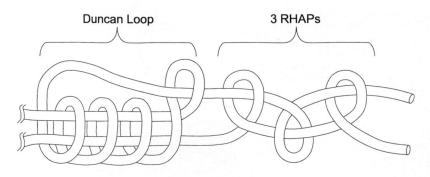

Duncan Loop   3 RHAPs

FIGURE 28.24 Schematic representation of compound sliding knot locked with three reversed half-hitches on the alternate post (RHAPs).

(Figs. 28.18 and 28.23). Note that once the half-hitch is flipped, not only is the post switched but the direction is also reversed. In this example, the under-over half-hitch becomes an over-under half-hitch, as shown in Figs. 28.17 and 28.22. The second half-hitch is pushed into the joint (Fig. 28.21). The three sequential identical half-hitches are thus converted into three RHAPS (Fig. 28.24).

This technique of locking a compound sliding knot with three RHAPs (Figs. 28.17 through 28.24) is achieved without the need for rethreading, in a manner similar to the technique for stacked half-hitch knots (Fig. 28.6G–N). The key steps are as follows:

1. The half-hitches are always formed in the same direction (under-over in the example shown) with the captured limb as the post limb.
2. The half-hitches are alternately flipped onto the opposite post.
3. The half-hitches are alternately pulled and pushed to lock the compound sliding knot.

CONCLUSION

Simply reading this article is not enough. Skill in knot tying is achieved by repetitive practice with a knot-tying stand using a knot tier that the surgeon intends to use in the operating room. There is no shortcut.

REFERENCES

1. Burkhart SS, Wirth MA, Simonich M, et al. Knot security in simple sliding knots and its relationship to rotator cuff repair: how secure must the knot be? *Arthroscopy* 2000;16:202–207.
2. Burkhart SS, Wirth MA, Simonich M, et al. Loop security as a determinant of tissue fixation security. *Arthroscopy* 1998;14:773–776.
3. Wolf EM, Wilk RM, Richmond JC. Arthroscopic Bankart repair using suture anchors. *Operative Techniques in Orthopaedics* 1991;1:184–191.
4. Nottage WM, Lieurance RK. Arthroscopic knot tying techniques. *Arthroscopy* 1999;15:515–521.
5. Chan KC, Burkhart SS. How to switch posts without rethreading when tying half-hitches. *Arthroscopy* 1999;15:444–450.
6. Snyder SJ. *Technical manual for the Revo screw and knot.* Largo, FL: Linvatec, 1994.
7. Chan KC, Burkhart SS, Thiagarajan P, et al. Optimization of stacked half-hitch knots for arthroscopic surgery. *Arthroscopy* 2001;17:752–759.
8. De Beer JF, van Rooyen K, Boezaart AP. Nicky's knot: a new slip knot for arthroscopic surgery. *Arthroscopy* 1988;14:109–110.
9. Snyder SJ, Getelman MH. Arthroscopically assisted rotator cuff evaluation and repair using threaded anchors. In: Parisien JS, ed. *Current techniques in arthroscopy.* New York: Thieme, 1998:87–101.
10. Semm K. Tissue-puncher and loop-ligation: new ideas for surgical therapeutic pelviscopy (laparoscopy) endoscopic intra-abdominal surgery. *Endoscopy* 1978;10:119–124.
11. Shimi SM, Lirici M, Vander V-G, et al. Comparative study of the holding strength of slipknots using absorbable and nonabsorbable ligature materials. *Surg Endosc* 1994;8:1285–1291.
12. Sharp HT, Dorsey JH, Chovan JD, et al. A simple modification to add strength to the Roeder knot. *J Am Assoc Gynecol Laparosc* 1996;3:305–307.
13. Mishra DK, Cannon WD, Lucas DJ, et al. Elongation of arthroscopically tied knots. *Am J Sports Med* 1997;25:113–117.
14. Kim SH, Ha KI. The SMC knot: a new slip knot with locking mechanism. *Arthroscopy* 2000;16:563–565.
15. Weston PV. A new clinch knot. *Obstet Gynecol* 1991;78:144–147.
16. Loutzenheiser TD, Harryman DT, Ziegler DW, et al. Optimizing arthroscopic knots using braided or monofilament suture. *Arthroscopy* 1998;14:57–65.
17. Loutzenheiser TD, Harryman DT, Yung S-W, et al. Optimizing arthroscopic knots. *Arthroscopy* 1995;11:199–206.

SLAP LESIONS

RONALD P. KARZEL
MEHRDAD GANJIANPOUR
STEPHEN J. SNYDER

Before the routine use of shoulder arthroscopy for the evaluation of shoulder disorders, injuries to the glenoid labrum were often difficult to diagnose and treat. Visualization of the labrum with the arthroscope has allowed advancement in knowledge of the labrum, as have recent biomechanical and cadaver studies. Arthroscopy has also led to an improved understanding of the normal variations of the glenoid labrum. These advances have been aided recently by improved imaging techniques, such as magnetic resonance imaging (MRI) and magnetic resonance arthrography. This understanding has led, in turn, to improved techniques for the treatment of labral pathology, and these lesions may now be treated using arthroscopic methods with a high success rate. This chapter discusses normal and pathologic labral anatomy, biomechanical aspects of labral function, the diagnosis and management of injuries to the superior labrum from anterior to posterior (the so-called SLAP lesions), and associated pathologic lesions commonly found with SLAP lesions. Furthermore, mechanisms of injury and treatment of the associated lesions in the throwing athlete are discussed.

NORMAL LABRAL ANATOMY

In 1953, Gardner and Gray (1) performed extensive investigations on the prenatal development of the shoulder and glenoid labrum. They studied the glenohumeral joints of 65 embryos at 8 weeks' gestation, as well as fetuses at full term, and noted that at a crown–rump length of 12 mm, the humerus and the glenoid are a mass of precartilage cells. Although no joint space is discernible, there is a condensed layer of cells, called the interzone, that demarcates the future joint line. Subsequent development of the interzone gives

rise to the glenoid labrum, the biceps tendon, the capsule, and the subscapularis muscle. At a crown–rump length of 38 mm, a clearly defined joint space and a typical triangular labrum superiorly, inferiorly, and posteriorly are noted. The anterior labrum is routinely less developed.

Snyder et al. (2) examined 21 fresh-frozen cadavers grossly and microscopically. Their studies showed a more conspicuous labrum posteriorly than anteriorly. Histologic sections revealed that the glenoid labrum consists of dense fibrous tissue and some elastic fibers. On the inner side the labrum is continuous with the hyaline cartilage of the glenoid, and on the outer side the labrum is continuous with the fibrous tissue of the capsule. The capsule covers the periphery of the labral base and is broadly attached to the scapular neck. A fibrocartilaginous interzone between the glenoid and labrum was routinely noted in the superior, anterior, and posterior labrum, but no fibrocartilage was noted inferiorly.

Detrisac and Johnson (3) performed a series of shoulder dissections and recorded the labral appearance. They originally described five variations in labral anatomy, but more recently Detrisac (4) has changed his classification to just two basic types. In the type A labrum, the superior labrum is detached centrally but attached peripherally, whereas the inferior, posterior, and anterior labra are all attached both centrally and peripherally. The second type of labrum is attached centrally and peripherally along the entire labrum.

Dissections by Snyder et al. (2) showed similar findings with a few variations. The inferior labrum had the most consistent appearance, with a triangular shape and attached central edge. The posterior labrum was similar in appearance and generally had its undersurface attached to the glenoid, although on occasion the undersurface was not attached. In contrast, the superior labrum was consistently attached peripherally, with a central free edge of varying degrees. The anterior labrum was typically attached both centrally and peripherally but did not have the usual triangular shape. Instead, the anterior labrum appeared as a thickened band distinguishable from the capsule both microscopically and macroscopically.

R. P. Karzel and **S. J. Snyder:** Southern California Orthopedic Institute, Van Nuys, California.

M. Ganjianpour: Tower Orthopaedics and Sports Medicine Medical Group, Los Angeles, California.

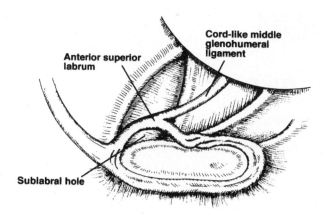

FIGURE 29.1 Sublabral foramen. (Reprinted with permission from Stephen J. Snyder.)

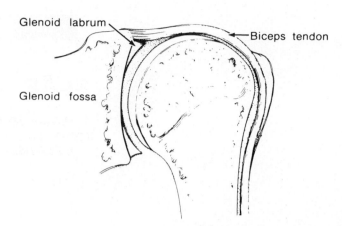

FIGURE 29.3 The glenoid fossa is deepened by the glenoid labrum. S, superior; SA, superior-anterior; IA, inferior-anterior; I, inferior; IP, inferior-posterior; SP, superior-posterior. (From Perry J. Anatomy and biomechanics of the shoulder in throwing, swimming, gymnastics and tennis. *Clin Sports Med* 1983;2:247–270, with permission.)

A more recent study by Williams et al. (5) documented the arthroscopic variations of the anterior-superior labrum. In their study, 12% of the population had a sublabral foramen below the anterior-superior labrum (Fig. 29.1). A smaller group of patients (1.5%) demonstrated a Buford complex, described as a cord-like middle glenohumeral ligament that originated directly from the superior labrum at the base of the biceps tendon and crossed the subscapularis tendon (Fig. 29.2). No anterior-superior labral tissue was identified between this attachment and the midglenoid notch. Inadvertent repair of this normal anatomic variant to the glenoid may cause severe loss of motion.

BIOMECHANICAL ASPECTS OF LABRAL FUNCTION

There is more freedom of movement at the shoulder joint than at any other joint in the body. Because of this large range of motion and the shallow configuration of the joint itself, soft tissue structures around the shoulder play an important role in providing shoulder stability. Normally the stability of the glenohumeral joint is maintained by complex interactions of the muscles and ligaments that cross the joint. No single structure is primarily responsible for stability at all positions of the shoulder. The labrum, along with other fibrous structures, helps give stability to the shoulder joint (4). The encircling labrum increases the depth of the glenoid around the humeral head (the bumper effect), thus providing increased stability (Fig. 29.3). With the addition of the labrum, the diameters of the glenoid surface are increased to 75% of the humeral head vertically and to 57% in the transverse direction (6). Reeves (7) and Perry (8) showed that the bonding strength of the labrum to the glenoid increases with maturity. Therefore, bonding strength at later ages tends to be

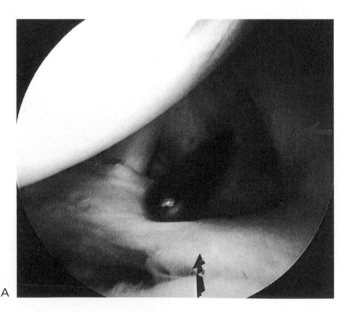

A

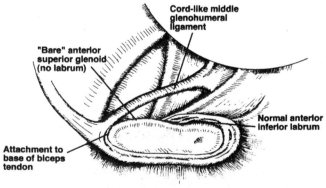

B

FIGURE 29.2 A: Buford complex. Small arrow, subscapularis; wide arrow, biceps tendon; large arrow, thickened middle glenohumeral ligament. **B:** Drawing of Buford complex. (Reprinted with permission from Stephen J. Snyder.)

greater than the strength of the capsule and subscapularis tendon. The increased strength of labral attachment with maturity may be the reason that younger patients are more likely to sustain Bankart lesions with avulsion of the glenoid labrum after a shoulder dislocation, whereas older patients are more likely to sustain a tear in the capsule.

Karzel et al. (9) performed biomechanical testing of cadaver shoulder specimens. In a position of 90 degrees abduction, the labrum affects the distribution of contact stresses when a compressive load is applied. In particular, the posterior inferior labrum seems to absorb contact stresses in much the same way as the meniscus in the knee joint does.

Another cadaveric study, by Davidson et al. (10), demonstrated that impingement of the rotator cuff onto the superior labrum may occur and lead to tearing. Cadaver specimens were positioned in 70 degrees of abduction and maximum external rotation. When the arm was fixed in this position, a permanent impression on both sides of the joint occurred where the humeral head contacted the superior labrum. The posterior superior labrum was compressed and distorted by the tuberosity of the humeral head and the interposed rotator cuff. When anterior instability was also present, the posterior labral impingement appeared to increase. These observations may help to explain posterior labral tears that are observed in throwers, as well as the articular side rotator cuff tears that occur in these individuals.

Two studies have evaluated the vascularity of the glenoid labrum. Burkhead (11) found that the vascular supply to the labrum is abundant around the entire glenoid attachment, except in the area of the superior labrum. Similar findings were noted by Cooper et al. (12), who showed that the superior and anterior superior labral segments have less vascularity than the posterior and inferior segments. These findings may help to explain the increased superior labral deterioration that is observed with advanced age (13). The limited vascularity of the superior labrum may also help to explain the development of the SLAP lesion. The lack of vascularity in this area could impede tissue healing after repeated microtrauma or after a single, isolated traumatic event.

PATTERNS OF INJURY

In addition to functioning as a load-sharing structure, the glenoid labrum is also a point for ligamentous attachment. It can be postulated that there are several potential mechanisms of injury from a biomechanical standpoint, including compression, avulsion, traction, shear, and chronic degenerative changes. These injury mechanisms can occur in isolation or in various combinations, resulting in a complex pattern of labral damage. Included can be local disruptions in any one or more of six labral areas (Fig. 29.4): 1, the superior labrum; 2, the anterior labrum above the midglenoid

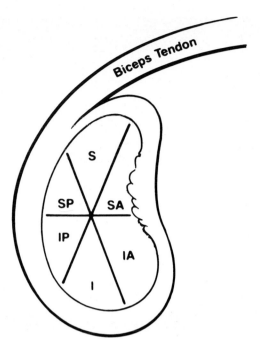

FIGURE 29.4 The glenoid and its respective labrum have been divided into six sections. (From Detrisac DA, Johnson LL. *Arthroscopic shoulder anatomy: pathologic and surgical implications.* Thorofare, NJ: SLACK, Inc., 1986, with permission.)

notch; 3, the anterior labrum below the midglenoid notch; 4, the inferior labrum; 5, the posterior inferior labrum; and 6, the posterior superior labrum. The tear pattern can be described by its arthroscopic appearance, similar to a meniscus tear in the knee. Examples of tear types include flap tears, bucket-handle tears, split nondetached tears, degenerative lesions, and SLAP lesions.

SLAP LESIONS

A SLAP lesion is a tear in the superior labrum, which occurs between areas 2 and 6 on the labrum. SLAP lesions always include the area of the biceps tendon anchor onto the superior labrum. The superior labrum in this area is the anchor of the biceps tendon to the glenoid; as noted previously, the labrum in this area is most likely to be large and to have a "meniscoid" appearance. A review of the arthroscopic appearance of these lesions resulted in a classification into four basic types of SLAP tears (14).

Type I—The superior labrum is frayed and degenerative in appearance. However, the attachment of the labrum to the glenoid and the biceps tendon anchor is intact (Fig. 29.5). This may represent a normal finding in the older patient.

Type II—The labrum may have a degenerative appearance similar to type I lesions. However, in type II lesions, the superior labrum is also detached from its insertion on the superior glenoid, and it, along with the biceps tendon,

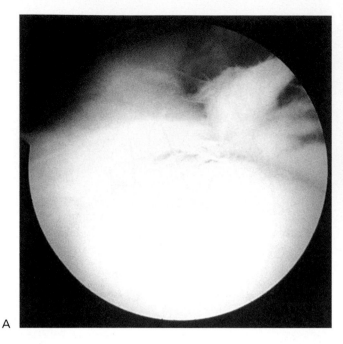

A

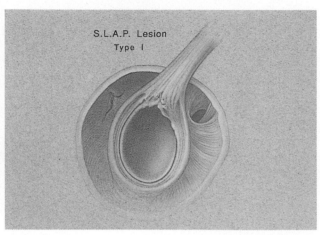

B

FIGURE 29.5 A: SLAP type I lesion. **B:** Drawing of SLAP type I lesion, degeneration of superior labrum, occasionally with rotator cuff tear.

arches away from the underlying glenoid neck. This makes the biceps–labral complex unstable (Fig. 29.6).

Type III—The superior labrum has a bucket-handle tear analogous to that seen in the knee meniscus. The biceps tendon is intact, as is the labral rim attachment of the peripheral portion of the labrum (Fig. 29.7).

Type IV—A bucket-handle tear of the superior labrum is present and extends up as a split tear of variable degrees into the biceps tendon. The torn biceps tendon is displaced with the labral flap into the joint (Fig. 29.8).

Complex and combined lesions—Frequently, a combination of two or more of the SLAP types may be seen. The most common is the combination of a type II and a type IV SLAP lesion (Fig. 29.9). Maffet et al. (15) described other variations of SLAP lesions, which they labeled types V through VII. These include an anterior-inferior Bankart lesion continued superiorly to include the biceps anchor (Type V), an unstable flap tear of the labrum with detachment of the anchor (Type VI), and biceps anchor separation extending anteriorly beneath the middle glenohumeral ligament (Type VII).

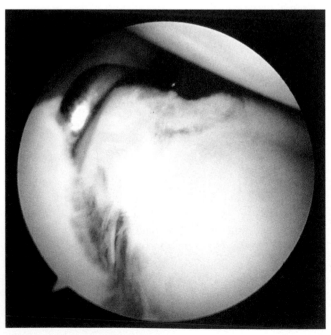

A

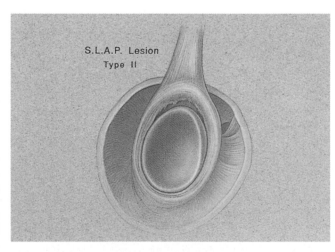

B

FIGURE 29.6 A: SLAP type II lesion. **B:** Drawing of SLAP type II lesion, avulsion of labrum and biceps anchor.

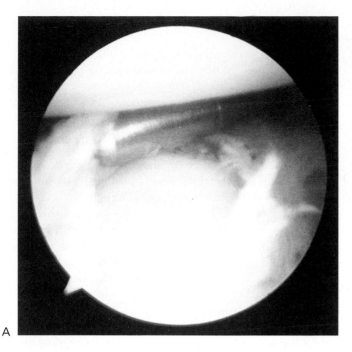

A

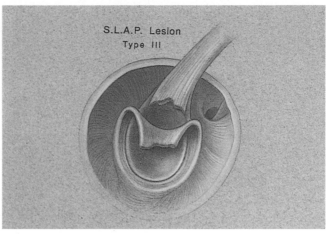

B

FIGURE 29.7 A: SLAP type III lesion. **B:** Drawing of SLAP type III lesion, which can be seen with anterior instability.

ETIOLOGY OF SLAP LESIONS

Although at present, there is no biomechanical proof to support the etiology of SLAP lesions, it appears that there are several different potential mechanisms of injury. The initial study on SLAP lesions noted that in many patients a fall had occurred onto an abducted and forward-flexed arm (14). This appeared to cause impaction and compression of the superior joint surface, as the humeral head was proximally subluxed (Fig. 29.10). In many of these cases, damage to the superior articular surface of the humeral head was seen in association with the SLAP lesion, with an appearance analogous to Hill–Sachs defect associated with injury to the anterior labrum.

In another study (16), the most common mechanism of injury was a fall or direct blow to the involved shoulder, which was seen in 31% of the patients. Nineteen percent of the patients had an episode of glenohumeral subluxation or

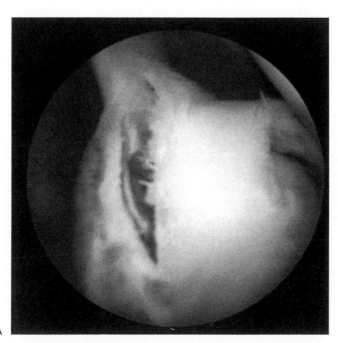

A

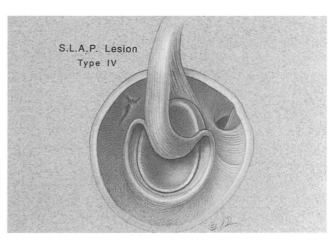

B

FIGURE 29.8 A: SLAP type IV lesion. **B:** Drawing of SLAP type IV lesion, split labrum and biceps tendon, often with partial rotator cuff tear.

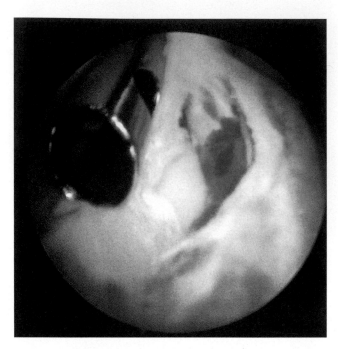

FIGURE 29.9 Complex SLAP lesion.

dislocation, and 16% noted initial pain while lifting a heavy object. Fourteen percent had the insidious onset of pain. Participation in overhead racquet sports accounted for the onset of symptoms in 6%, and an additional 6% noted pain while involved in repetitive throwing activities.

Rodosky et al. (17) pointed out the role of the biceps–superior labrum complex in maintaining anterior stability of the shoulder. When the superior labrum was experimentally detached from the glenoid in a cadaver model, anterior instability resulted. SLAP lesions, particularly type II, are frequently associated with anterior instability. Successful treatment of these patients may require anterior stabilization in addition to treatment of the SLAP lesion.

SLAP LESIONS IN THROWING ATHLETES

The mechanism responsible for injury to the superior labrum in throwing athletes may be different than for the rest of the population. Andrews and Carson (18) described tearing of the anterior superior labrum in high-level throwing athletes. These lesions were believed to be secondary to eccentric loading of the biceps during the follow-through phase of throwing, as the elbow comes into extension. It was postulated that the resulting force leads to avulsion of the biceps anchor. Many of these patients had associated lesions, including supraspinatus tendon tears and partial biceps tendon ruptures.

Morgan et al. (19) reported on a subgroup of throwing athletes with type II SLAP lesions. These patients did not have any other lesions associated with anterior instability, but they had a "drive-through" sign that was eliminated after the SLAP repair. They postulated that these patients have posterior-superior instability with a secondary anterior-inferior pseudolaxity. They also observed significant loss of internal rotation (average, 45 degrees) in those throwing athletes with type II SLAP lesions. Therefore, they proposed that a tight posterior capsule with marked lack of internal rotation greater than 40 degrees compared with the nonthrowing shoulder predisposes the athlete to develop a type II SLAP lesion. Burkhart and Morgan (20) subsequently described the dynamic peel-back sign with the shoulder in abduction and external rotation (cocking phase of throwing) as the prime arthroscopic indicator of this type of lesion. They observed this peel-back sign arthroscopically in throwers with posterior and combined anterior and posterior SLAP lesions. During arthroscopy, as the arm is removed from traction and brought into abduction and external rotation, the biceps tendon assumes a more vertical and posterior angle, which produces a twist at the base of the biceps. This causes the posterior-superior labrum to rotate medially over the corner of the glenoid. This finding was consistent in patients with posterior SLAP lesions and was absent in normal shoulders.

PATHOLOGIC CONDITIONS ASSOCIATED WITH SLAP LESIONS

In the original study describing the SLAP lesions, Snyder et al. (14) reported 40% rotator cuff pathology in their patient population. Fifteen percent of the patients had a full-thickness rotator cuff tear. Other associated pathologies included anterior instability (15%), humeral head chondromalacia/indentation fracture (15%), and acromioclavicular joint arthritis (11%).

In a follow-up study at our institution, we performed a retrospective study of all SLAP lesions we have treated (16). A total of 2,375 shoulder arthroscopic procedures were performed between 1985 and 1993 at the Southern California Orthopedic Institute. Superior glenoid labral injuries were

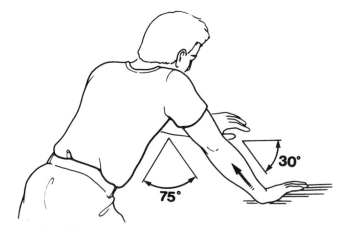

FIGURE 29.10 Proposed mechanism of injury for SLAP lesions.

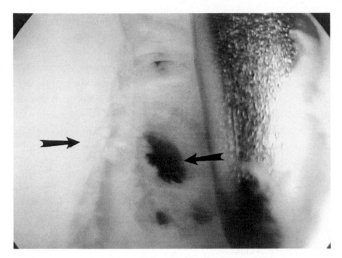

FIGURE 29.11 Arthroscopic view of paralabral ganglion cyst. Arrows point to the glenoid and the stalk of the cyst.

seen in 140 patients, or approximately 6% of all shoulder arthroscopic procedures. The average patient age was 38 years, and 91% were men. Fifty-five percent of all SLAP lesions were type II; 21% were type I, 10% were type IV, 9% were type III, and 5% were complex. Twenty-eight percent of the superior labral lesions were considered to be isolated lesions, and the remainder had associated rotator cuff or anterior labral pathology. Twenty-two percent of the patients had an associated Bankart lesion. The average time from injury to surgery was 20 months for all lesions and 13 months for isolated labral lesions.

Morgan et al. (19) reported rotator cuff pathology in 31% of their population. All patients with rotator cuff pathology had chronic SLAP lesions, and there was no evidence of rotator cuff tear with an acute SLAP lesion. Furthermore, the tears were lesion specific in that the anterior type II SLAP lesions demonstrated undersurface rotator cuff tear at the anterior rotator crescent, whereas the posterior type II SLAP lesions had more posterior undersurface rotator cuff tears. Eleven percent of rotator cuff tears were full thickness, and they were all located at the midportion of the rotator crescent. Although half of their study population consisted of throwing athletes, only one full-thickness rotator cuff tear was identified among the throwers.

Recently, paralabral cysts have become identified as a source of discomfort, disability, and loss of strength (21–24). These cysts have been identified in close proximity to SLAP lesions and posterior capsulolabral tears (21–25) (Fig. 29.11).

In our review of paralabral ganglion cysts of the shoulder, the cyst was associated with a SLAP lesion or a posterior-superior labral lesion in 67% of the cases. In order to minimize the chance of recurrence of the cyst and to alleviate patients' symptoms, all concomitant intraarticular pathologies such as SLAP lesions or posterior labral lesions should be addressed at the time of cyst excision.

Although the exact cause of ganglion cysts is unclear, some have suggested that trauma to the capsular tissue causes areas of weakness (25–27), with subsequent leakage of joint fluid into the weakened capsule in a one-way valve mechanism as the probable etiology of the cysts. The history may be variable, including vague pain and discomfort in the posterior shoulder, weakness, and loss of motion. If the cyst encroaches on the suprascapular nerve, physical findings including weakness of external rotation, impingement, and even muscle atrophy may be identified. However, given its rarity, the lack of reproducible signs on physical examination, and the overlapping symptoms with other shoulder problems, this disorder is easily overlooked. MRI is an accurate tool for demonstrating the presence and size of a ganglion cyst, and it is helpful in identifying associated labral tears (Fig. 29.12). However, the presence of a ganglion cyst does not necessarily cause suprascapular neuropathy. Therefore, electromyography and nerve conduction velocity are excellent adjuncts to physical examination in the diagnosis of suprascapular neuropathy associated with a ganglion cyst (22–29).

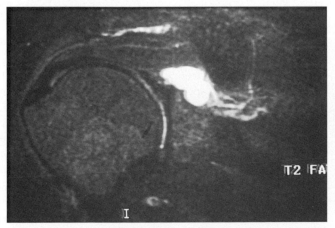

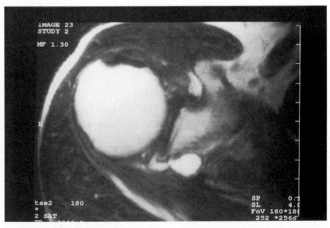

A   B

FIGURE 29.12 Coronal **(A)** and axial **(B)** views of T2-weighted magnetic resonance image showing the location of paralabral ganglion cyst.

CLINICAL PRESENTATION OF SLAP LESIONS

History

The patient's history of injury may be suggestive of a possible labral tear. A history of a fall on an abducted arm with complaints of subsequent pain associated with cracking, locking, snapping, and mechanical-type symptoms is consistent with possible labral tearing. However, given the multiple possible causes of injury to the labrum, history alone is not specific. Also, the patient may have significant associated pathology and may give a history consistent with impingement, biceps tendinitis, or instability. Particularly important are questions related to the presence or absence of subluxation or dislocation and the activities that cause the patient to have pain. The throwing athlete may complain of a "dead arm" in the cocking phase of throwing (abducted and externally rotated position) (30,31). The dead arm is a condition in which the athlete is unable to throw with preinjury velocity and control because of pain and subjective unease in the shoulder (30). In general, however, the history is nonspecific for the diagnosis of labral injury.

Physical Examination

A thorough physical examination of the shoulder is essential in the diagnosis of labral pathology. It is important to diagnose the presence of impingement and/or instability. Many patients with superior labral tears also demonstrate irritation of the biceps tendon, particularly with biceps tension testing. The biceps tension test is performed by resisting shoulder flexion with the shoulder in a 90 degrees forward-flexed position, the elbow extended, and the forearm supinated. A positive test may suggest irritation either in the biceps anchor or within the tendon itself.

The compression rotation test, popularized by Andrews and Gidumal (32), is similar to the MacMurray test in the knee. It is performed by abducting the shoulder to 90 degrees and, while applying a compression load across the joint, internally and externally rotating the humerus on the glenoid. A labral tear may be trapped within the joint during this maneuver, causing pain. Occasionally, patients have palpable catching or popping within the joint with range of motion, which may also be caused by labral damage.

The anterior slide test, as described by Kibler (33), is performed with the patient's hand on his or her hip. One of the examiner's hands is on the patient's acromion and the other hand is behind the patient's elbow. A superior force is applied to the elbow while the patient resists the force. A positive test results in pain, a pop, or a click in front of the shoulder.

The active compression test, as described by O'Brien et al. (34), has recently gained popularity because of its reported high sensitivity. With the arm flexed forward to 90 degrees, adducted 10 to 15 degrees, and maximally internally rotated, the patient resists a downward force applied to the arm. Pain in the shoulder that is reduced or eliminated by repeating the test with the arm maximally supinated is considered a positive test.

Mimori et al. (35) reported on a new pain provocative test for the diagnosis of SLAP lesions with high sensitivity and specificity. This test is performed with the patient in the sitting position and the arm abducted 90 to 100 degrees with the shoulder externally rotated. This maneuver is performed in maximal pronation and supination. As with O'Brien's test, increased pain and discomfort with pronation as opposed to supination is considered a positive finding. However, as is the case with all findings on physical examination, none of these tests is specific for labral pathology.

Imaging Studies

Conventional radiographs, routinely obtained on patients with shoulder problems, may reveal characteristic findings suggestive of impingement syndrome, degenerative arthritis, or shoulder instability. They also assist in ruling out other disorders, such as neoplasm or infection. However, radiographs generally are not helpful in diagnosing labral pathology. Iannotti and Wang (36) described a rare variation of SLAP lesions in which a fracture of the superior glenoid tubercle is present with a SLAP lesion. In these cases, findings on radiographs are suggestive of a SLAP lesion (36).

Computerized tomographic (CT) arthrography has improved the detection of labral pathology compared with conventional radiographs, particularly in cases involving a Bankart lesion (37,38). In general, CT arthrography is better for defining bony abnormalities than soft tissue abnormalities.

Although MRI has been helpful for visualizing the rotator cuff, biceps tendon, and surrounding soft tissues, it is often difficult to evaluate the glenoid labrum and capsule adequately with conventional MRI techniques. A technique has been developed that involves injecting a magnetic contrast agent, gadolinium, intraarticularly into the shoulder in an attempt to increase the efficacy of MRI evaluation (39–42). This technique, which has been labeled magnetic resonance (MR) arthrography, may be able to detect SLAP lesions in instances in which conventional MRI scanning is negative (Fig. 29.13). In one study, MR arthrography had a sensitivity of 89%, a specificity of 91%, and an accuracy of 90% (41). Furthermore, MR arthrography may be better at detecting isolated labral tears and at distinguishing normal labral variations such as a sublabral hole from a SLAP lesion (43). Although these results are encouraging, MR arthrography still tends to overdiagnose labral pathology, particularly in those patients with normal labral variations. For example, in case of a meniscoid superior labrum, dye may track under the well-anchored but thickened superior labrum. This is readily confused with a SLAP lesion. In such instances, the superior labrum demonstrates a smooth con-

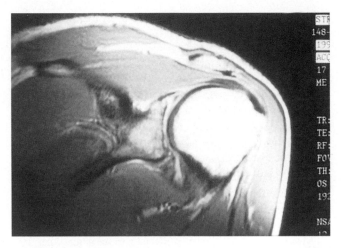

FIGURE 29.13 SLAP lesions may be demonstrated by a magnetic resonance imaging arthrogram.

tour and is well attached to the glenoid rim in other images. In other cases, the technique may give a false-negative result. Therefore, it is not possible to completely rely on MRI scanning to diagnose or exclude labral pathology.

Because of the limitations of the history, physical examination, and diagnostic studies in diagnosing labral pathology, it is important to maintain a high degree of suspicion for these lesions. In patients with persistent shoulder pain whose symptoms do not fit readily into one of the more commonly diagnosed etiologies of shoulder pain, it is important to consider labral pathology. The definitive diagnosis of labral pathology, in most cases, can be made only by performing an accurate diagnostic shoulder arthroscopy.

Arthroscopic Diagnosis of Type II SLAP Lesions

A difficult arthroscopic problem in many cases is to differentiate correctly a type II SLAP lesion from a normal variant. A type II SLAP lesion, in our opinion, is frequently overdiagnosed. The superior labrum frequently has a meniscoid appearance with a corresponding free edge, which may give the appearance of pathologic detachment. Also, as has been noted previously, in the meniscoid labrum it is common for the superior labrum to attach medial to the level of the glenoid articular surface, and this may be misdiagnosed as a labral avulsion. In the case of acute trauma, the diagnosis is fairly evident because of the hemorrhage noted around the avulsed labral tissue. In contrast, chronic lesions may be more difficult to diagnose because the natural healing process may result in fibrous tissue, which conceals a pathologic detachment that has occurred on the superior glenoid neck. In a normal shoulder, the articular cartilage of the superior glenoid extends to the labral attachment. In a chronic type II SLAP lesion, in contrast, space usually exists between the edge of the glenoid articular cartilage and the attachment of

the biceps anchor. Also, in a detached superior labrum, the superior labrum can be seen to arch away from the underlying bone by approximately 3 to 4 mm as tension is applied to the biceps tendon during arthroscopic observation. If the labrum is somewhat loosely attached but in the normal position, this is generally not considered to be a SLAP lesion, but rather a normal variation.

TREATMENT OF LABRAL LESIONS

Many labral tears occur in association with glenohumeral instability, and shoulder stability should always be carefully evaluated by examination under anesthesia before proceeding with diagnostic shoulder arthroscopy. Truly isolated labral tears occurring in otherwise stable shoulders may be treated effectively with debridement of the labral tear alone. All damaged labral tissue is removed, taking care to preserve the periphery of the labrum and the attachment of the capsule to the glenoid. Vertical split tears may be resected in a manner similar to a bucket-handle tear in the meniscus, using a combination of basket forceps, shaver blades, and, in some cases, electrocautery. If instability is present concomitantly, the labral tissue is debrided to prevent mechanical catching within the joint, and then shoulder stabilization procedures are performed.

Glasgow et al. (44) reported the results of arthroscopic glenoid labral resection in 28 overhead athletes. In patients with normal shoulder stability, results were 91% good or excellent at 2-year follow-up. In contrast, 75% of the patients had fair or poor results when debridement was performed in the presence of glenohumeral instability without shoulder stabilization. Similarly, Altchek et al. (45) studied 40 athletes who underwent labral debridement. Forty percent of the group had instability on examination at the time of surgery, but 72% reported significant pain relief during the first year postoperatively. However, their results deteriorated steadily over time, and only 7% of the patients had significant long-term relief. Both Glasgow and Altchek concluded that labral debridement alone does not generally give satisfactory results in overhead athletes, and that treatment in these individuals needs to focus on the underlying glenohumeral instability.

Payne and Jokl (46) studied 14 patients treated with arthroscopic labral debridement. These patients all had shoulder pain with overhead activity but had stable glenohumeral joints on preoperative examination. Results were initially quite good, with 93% excellent or good results at 6 months. However, at an average follow-up of 2 years, results had deteriorated to 71% excellent or good. The best results were noted in the superior and anterior inferior labral segments. They found that patients with anterior-superior labral lesions particularly were at risk for delayed development of glenohumeral instability. In general, in the high-level overhead athlete, glenohumeral instability should be considered present until proven otherwise if labral tears are observed at the time of arthroscopy.

Treatment of Types I and III SLAP Lesions

Treatment of SLAP lesions depends on the type of SLAP lesion encountered. Type I SLAP lesions may occur as part of the normal aging process. The superior labrum is debrided back to a stable rim, similar to debridement of a degenerative tear in the knee meniscus. A type III SLAP lesion is treated with resection of the torn fragment, similar to resection of a bucket-handle tear in a meniscus. In both of these cases, it is important to make sure that the remaining superior labral tissue is well anchored to the glenoid and that the biceps anchor is intact. As was the case with isolated labral tears, SLAP lesions may occur with instability. If instability is present, it must be addressed at the same time the SLAP lesion is treated.

Treatment of Type II and Type IV SLAP Lesions

In the type II SLAP lesion, the superior labrum is detached from the underlying superior glenoid. This results in instability of the biceps anchor, which must be reattached to the glenoid to restore normal shoulder stability and normal biceps function. In our initial management of SLAP lesions, type II lesions were simply debrided of interposed fibrous tissue and the superior glenoid neck was decorticated in an attempt to promote healing. Postoperatively, the arm was immobilized in a sling for several weeks, and many of these patients did heal the superior labral avulsion. However, healing was sometimes incomplete, and in many patients early motion was desirable, particularly if the SLAP lesion was found in conjunction with additional pathology such as rotator cuff tearing. Presently, we believe that the superior labral tissue will heal more reliably to the glenoid if the tissue is anchored back into place surgically. This approach also allows earlier motion. Various arthroscopic repair techniques have been reported in the literature (14,16,20,47,48,49).

Field and Savoie (47) used the transglenoid suture fixation technique in 20 patients with type II and type IV SLAP lesions. At an average of 21 months, all 20 patients had results rated as good or excellent. Yoneda et al. (48) treated 10 young athletes with type II SLAP lesions, using abrasion followed by arthroscopic staple fixation. A second-look arthroscopic evaluation was performed at 3 to 6 months for staple removal. At the time of the second-look evaluation, all 10 lesions had healed. The authors reported 88% good or excellent results in this small series at 2 years. It was believed that those patients with unsatisfactory results had problems stemming from unrelated pathology.

In Austria, Resch et al. (49) reported results of SLAP repairs in 14 patients. They used either absorbable tacks or cannulated titanium screws. At 6 months' follow-up, eight of the patients were able to return to their overhead sports, four were improved but unable to return, and two were unimproved.

In review of 140 injuries to the superior labrum at our institution, the labral lesions were treated in variety of ways (16). Second-look arthroscopy performed on 18 shoulders revealed healing in three of five type II lesions treated with debridement and glenoid abrasion. Of five type II lesions treated with an absorbable anchor, four were healed. Three type III lesions and one type IV lesion treated with debridement had stable biceps anchors. Two type IV lesions treated with suture repair had healed completely. Five reoperations were necessary because of loose bioabsorbable tack fragments.

Morgan et al. (19) reported their experience with 102 Type II SLAP lesions treated with permanent suture-anchor repair. Preliminary clinical results at 1 year follow-up assessed by the University of California at Los Angeles rating scale were 97% good or excellent. In the subgroup of 53 overhead throwing athletes, 100% of the patients had a good or excellent result, and 84% of the pitchers had returned to their preinjury level of activity both subjectively and objectively.

Technique for Arthroscopic Fixation of Type II SLAP Lesions

At the Southern California Orthopedic Institute, we prefer to fix SLAP lesions with the use of screw-in suture anchors loaded with two nonabsorbable braided sutures. This allows fixation of the SLAP lesion with a double-sling suture technique. We prefer suture anchors to bioabsorbable tacks because of the better biomechanical properties of the suture-anchor repair (50). Also, there are concerns about possible foreign body reaction to the bioabsorbable tacks, which may cause more postoperative pain and synovitis (51). In addition, the heads of the bioabsorbable tacks may break off during the absorption process, resulting in a loose body in the joint and possible articular cartilage damage. A variety of anchors are available, including anchors made with absorbable and titanium material. To accomplish the arthroscopic repair, three portals are created. A standard posterior portal is made first. The next two portals are created in an outside-in technique under direct vision from the posterior portal. The standard anterior superior portal is created just behind the biceps tendon high in the rotator interval, and a standard midglenoid portal is placed just superior to the subscapularis tendon (Fig. 29.14).

After initial diagnostic arthroscopy has confirmed the diagnosis of a SLAP lesion, the fibrous membrane over the superior glenoid neck is debrided with a soft tissue shaver inserted through the anterior superior cannula. Torn labral and biceps tissue is conservatively debrided. Next, a 4.0-mm ball-shaped bur is used to lightly decorticate exposed bone beneath the superior labrum and the biceps anchor

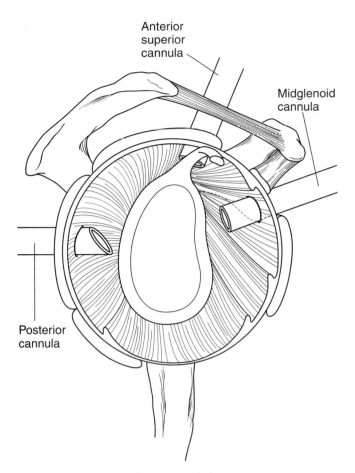

Anterior
superior
cannula

Midglenoid
cannula

Posterior
cannula

FIGURE 29.14 Portal placements.

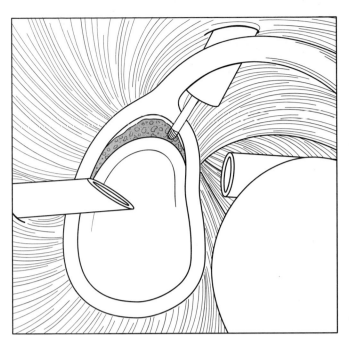

FIGURE 29.15 The superior glenoid neck is abraded to promote healing of the detached labrum.

(Fig. 29.15). Because it can be difficult to drill the superior glenoid given the angle of insertion of the anchor, it is helpful to create a pilot hole with the bur at the precise location where the suture anchor is to be implanted. This should be located directly below the normal biceps tendon insertion. The arthroscopic drill bit or punch is then inserted through the anterior superior cannula and the drill point is placed in the center of the pilot hole, adjacent to the articular cartilage and just below the biceps tendon anchor. An angle of 45 degrees to the articular surface and 45 degrees angulation posteriorly is maintained while the drill is inserted to its hub.

A screw-in suture anchor is loaded with two no. 2 braided permanent sutures and placed through the anterior-superior portal (Fig. 29.16). One suture is green and the other is white. The suture limbs closest to the biceps anchor are dyed purple using a standard sterile skin marker. After the anchor is fully seated, its stability is ensured by pulling on the suture strands.

The arthroscope is next placed in the midglenoid portal, and the undyed limb of the white suture is retrieved out the posterior portal with a crochet hook (Fig. 29.17). This suture is placed outside the cannula with the use of a switching rod. The arthroscope is once again placed in the poste-

rior portal for direct vision. The undyed limb of the green suture is then retrieved with a crochet hook out of the midglenoid portal and placed outside the cannula with the use of the switching rod. The purple limb of the green suture is then retrieved out of the midglenoid cannula with a crochet hook. Finally, the purple limb of the white suture is placed outside the anterior superior portal. This stepwise process separates the sutures into a star pattern to allow ease of suture management (Fig. 29.18).

A crescent-shaped suture hook is introduced through the anterior-superior portal and placed through the labrum just

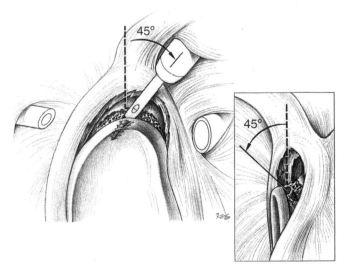

FIGURE 29.16 The suture anchor is inserted into a drill hole on the superior glenoid.

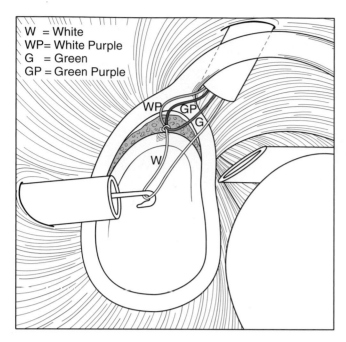

W = White
WP= White Purple
G = Green
GP = Green Purple

FIGURE 29.17 The white suture is retrieved out the posterior portal with a crochet hook. This suture is placed outside the cannula with the use of a switching rod.

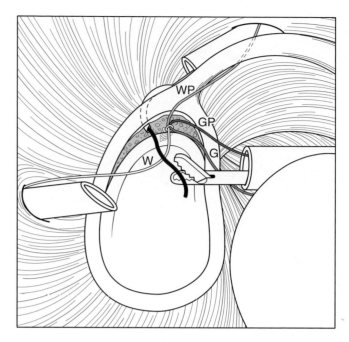

FIGURE 29.19 The suture passer is introduced under the labrum posterior to the biceps, and the shuttle is retrieved out of the midglenoid portal with an arthroscopic grasper.

posterior to the long head of the biceps tendon. The suture shuttle (Linvatec, Largo, FL) is then advanced into the glenohumeral joint and retrieved out of the midglenoid portal with a grasper (Fig. 29.19). The shuttle is then loaded with the purple limb of the green suture and carried through the labrum and out the anterior-superior portal (Fig. 29.20). The green limb of the green suture is then retrieved posterior

to the long head of the biceps tendon with a crochet hook and out the anterior-superior portal (Fig. 29.21). The green suture is tied with a sliding knot followed by three half-hitches (Fig. 29.22).

The purple limb of the white suture is then retrieved from its position outside the cannula of the anterior-superior portal out the midglenoid cannula with the use

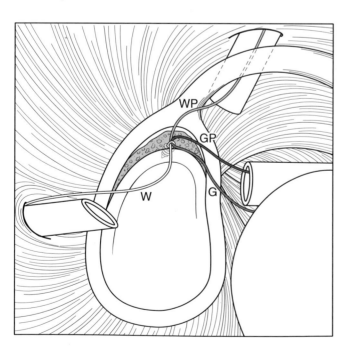

FIGURE 29.18 The sutures are separated into a star pattern to allow ease of suture management.

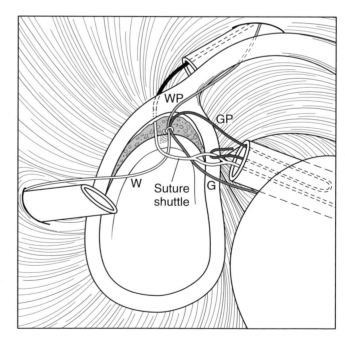

FIGURE 29.20 The purple limb of the green suture is passed through the tissue by means of the shuttle.

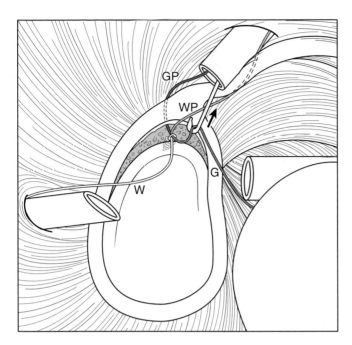

FIGURE 29.21 The other limb of the green suture is retrieved.

of a crochet hook. A crescent-shaped suture hook is again introduced through the anterior-superior cannula but just anterior to the long head of the biceps tendon. The shuttle is advanced into the joint, and a grasper retrieves it out the midglenoid cannula (Fig. 29.23). The purple limb of the white suture is loaded and is carried through the tissues and out of the anterior-superior cannula (Fig. 29.24). The undyed limb of the white suture is retrieved anterior

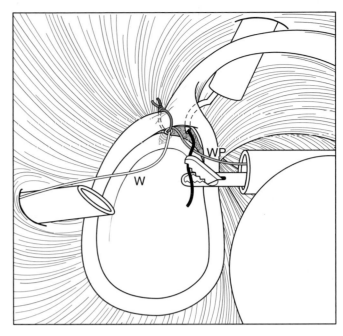

FIGURE 29.23 The purple limb of the white suture is brought back inside the midglenoid cannula with a switching stick, and the suture passer is introduced under the labrum anterior to the biceps tendon.

to the long head of the biceps tendon with the use of a crochet hook placed in the anterior-superior cannula (Fig. 29.25). The white suture is tied as described previously, completing the repair. An arthroscopic probe is then used to directly palpate the repair and check its stability (Fig. 29.26).

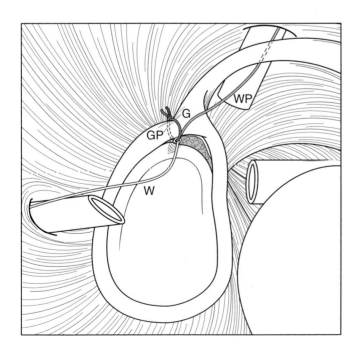

FIGURE 29.22 The purple suture is tied posterior to the biceps tendon.

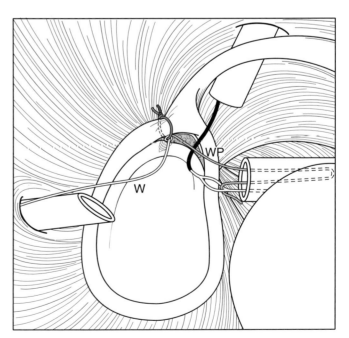

FIGURE 29.24 The purple limb of the white suture is passed through the tissue with the use of a shuttle.

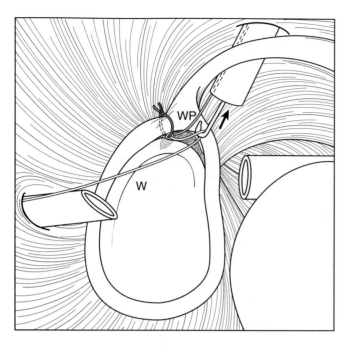

FIGURE 29.25 The other limb of the white suture is retrieved anterior to the biceps tendon out of the anterior superior cannula.

Postoperatively, the patient is immobilized with a sling for 3 weeks. During this time, the patient is allowed to perform gentle elbow, wrist, and hand exercises in the first week. After the first week, the patient may remove the sling but is instructed to avoid external rotation beyond neutral and extension of the arm behind the body with the elbow extended for an additional 4 weeks, to prevent tension on the biceps tendon. In 4 to 5 weeks, therapy is progressed with protected biceps strengthening. No stressful biceps activity is allowed for approximately 3 months.

We have reevaluated two patients at approximately 3½ months after suture anchor repair for type II SLAP lesions with a second-look arthroscopy. Both patients demonstrated excellent secure reattachment of the avulsed labrum and biceps anchor.

Technique for Arthroscopic Fixation of Type IV SLAP Lesions

In a type IV SLAP lesion, there is tearing of the biceps tendon in addition to the superior labral tear. In most cases, the remaining biceps tendon is firmly anchored to the superior glenoid. Generally, if the amount of biceps tendon that has been detached is small, then the superior labrum and biceps tendon can simply be resected. In cases where the tear encompasses 30% or more of the biceps tendon, we usually proceed with primary biceps tenodesis in an older patient, particularly if the remaining biceps tendon appears degener-

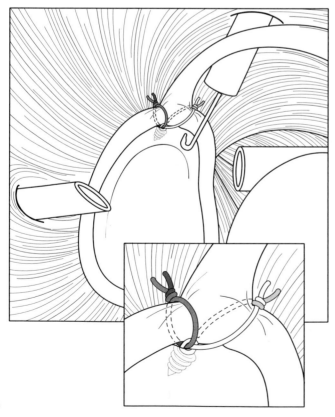

A

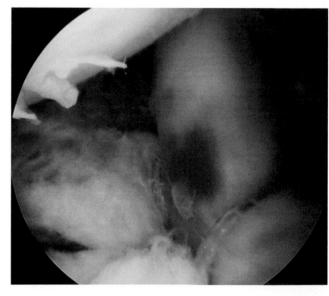

B

FIGURE 29.26 A: The white suture is tied, and the double-sling repair of biceps anchor is completed. **B:** Arthroscopic view of repaired type II SLAP Lesion.

ative. In younger patients, if there is a significant biceps tear in conjunction with a bucket-handle tear in the superior labrum, we prefer to preserve the biceps and superior labrum with a suture repair. In these cases, the sutures are placed directly through the tissues in a mattress fashion, and suture anchors are not required because the remaining labrum is well anchored to the glenoid.

The suture repair is performed with the arthroscope viewing posteriorly in the anterior-superior operating portal. A 6-inch, 17-gauge epidural needle is passed through the skin and subcutaneous tissues adjacent to the lateral acromial edge and then passed into the joint, through the biceps tendon, and across the split portion. A suture shuttle relay is passed through the needle and is retrieved with a grasping clamp from the anterior cannula. The needle is withdrawn, the shuttle is loaded with a nonabsorbable suture on the percutaneous side, and the first stitch is passed through the tendon and across the split portion as the shuttle is pulled out through the anterior-superior portal. The epidural needle is then reinserted, puncturing the biceps tendon and labrum approximately 4 mm away from the first suture site. The shuttle is passed through the needle and retrieved out the anterior-superior cannula. The suture limb that had been previously passed out the anterior cannula is then rethreaded into the eyelet of the second shuttle and pulled back retrograde through the biceps and labrum by pulling the shuttle out the percutaneous end. Now that both sutures have been placed through the biceps and brought out percutaneously, a crochet hook is inserted through the anterior cannula and is used to retrieve both limbs out the anterior cannula to be tied. An arthroscopic knot-pushing device is used to tie the suture limbs together, closing the tear on the biceps and labrum. This suturing process is repeated anterior and posterior to the biceps tendon, until the entire labral tear has been repaired. In some cases, the tear may extend posteriorly far enough that the arthroscope is shifted to the anterior portal and instruments are passed through the posterior operating cannula to effect the repair.

In some cases, a type IV SLAP lesion is seen in conjunction with a type II SLAP lesion. In these cases, the first step is to reattach the superior labrum to the glenoid. The remaining detached labrum and biceps may then be either excised or repaired in a manner similar to that described previously.

Rehabilitation after type IV SLAP repairs is similar to that described for type II repairs.

Treatment of the Associated Lesions

It is important to keep in mind that SLAP lesions are commonly associated with other pathologic conditions of the shoulder (14,16,19). These may be diagnosed before surgery with a thorough history and physical examination, or with good-quality imaging studies. Prudent attention to these associated lesions leads to a more successful surgical and clinical outcome after shoulder surgery.

Partial Rotator Cuff Tear

As discussed earlier, up to one third of patients with SLAP lesions have coexisting rotator cuff pathology (14,16). Full-thickness rotator cuff tears should be repaired by the best technique in the surgeon's armamentarium. Partial-thickness rotator cuff tears may be treated in a variety of ways depending on the size and location of the lesions. Partial-thickness articular surface tears that involve less than 50% of the thickness of the tendon may be debrided, and loose and unstable flaps may be removed (52–55). If the partial articular surface tear involves more than 50% of the rotator cuff, repair of the tendon by completing the tear or by a transtendon approach is indicated.

In the throwing athlete, care should be given to diagnose any coexisting "microinstability" in the throwing shoulder. Often, the involved shoulder has a decrease in internal rotation and an increase in external rotation. The Jobe relocation test has been helpful in diagnosing anterior instability in the throwing athlete (56). Morgan and associates used a slightly different definition of the relocation test in which posterosuperior (as opposed to anterior) pain and apprehension produced by abduction and external rotation is relieved by a posteriorly directed force applied to the humeral head (30). Jobe described internal impingement in throwing athletes as injury to the articular side of the rotator cuff, capsule, and labrum posterosuperiorly (57). He attributed this internal impingement in throwers to gradual repetitive stretching of the anterior capsuloligamentous structures and a resultant subtle anterior subluxation.

Ganglion Cysts

The association between glenoid labral tears and paralabral ganglion cysts has been documented in a number of studies over the last decade (22,23,26,27,58). Traditionally, open surgical techniques have been employed for treatment of symptomatic cysts that are compressing the suprascapular nerve and the surrounding structures (21). However, open surgical resection would preclude the surgeon from treating the frequent intraarticular pathology associated with the cyst unless it is combined with shoulder arthroscopy. Furthermore, open techniques are difficult, and complications such as acromion nonunion, scapular fractures, and muscle denervation may occur. Recently, arthroscopic decompression of paralabral ganglion cyst has been described (23–25). At the Southern California Orthopaedic Institute, we have been treating paralabral ganglion cysts with arthroscopic techniques since 1996. A recent review of our experience with this technique revealed eight cases that were documented by physical examination, MRI, and electrodiagnostic studies. All patients demonstrated a ganglion cyst that was juxtaposed to the posterior glenoid in the area of the spinoglenoid notch on the MRI scan, and all had symptoms associated with suprascapular nerve compression. Three pa-

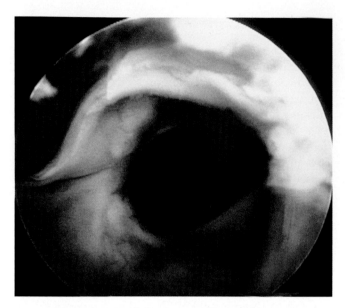

FIGURE 29.27 Cavity of a cyst after debridement.

tients had an associated SLAP lesion on preoperative MRI, and seven were diagnosed with a SLAP lesion intraoperatively. Postoperative MRI examinations of two patients revealed complete resolution of the ganglion cyst.

Technique of Arthroscopic Ganglion Cyst Decompression

After a complete diagnostic examination, an electrosurgical device is used to create a 1-cm capsulotomy posterior and superior to the glenoid neck. The capsulotomy is based on the anatomic location identified from careful study of the preoperative MRI scan. Under direct visualization from the posterior portal, a blunt dissecting tool is used to develop and probe the capsule until the cyst is located. After identification of the cyst, an arthroscopic shaver is placed within the cyst, and the characteristic amber-colored fluid is evacuated with suction. A 4.0—mm shaver is then used to remove the cyst wall along the undersurface of the supraspinatus muscle (Fig. 29.27). Careful control of the suction is maintained at all times to modulate the excision of the cyst and its contents. The shaver is kept pointing at the glenoid neck at all times, and no attempt is made to remove the capsule from the area about the spine of the scapula, in order to avoid damage to the suprascapular nerve. Dissection should not extend beyond 1 cm medial to the superior capsule attachment to avoid the nerve as it courses through the spingoglenoid notch.

The arthroscope is next moved to the anterior portal, and the shaver is introduced through the posterior portal. With the shaver again directed at the glenoid neck, the capsulotomy is further developed to remove the posterior portion of the cyst. After removal of the cyst, the remaining intraarticular pathology, such as a SLAP lesion or a posterior labral lesion, is addressed to the treatment of all associated pathologic conditions (Fig. 29.28).

Postoperatively, the patient is placed in a sling as necessary for comfort, and immediate passive and active motion is allowed as tolerated. The exact rehabilitation regimen depends on the concomitant intraarticular pathology that was addressed.

SUMMARY

Understanding of the clinical significance of superior labral pathologies has evolved significantly during the past decade.

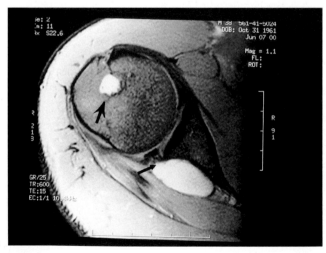
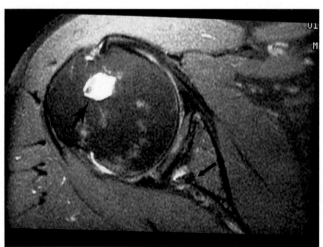

A   B

FIGURE 29.28 A: T2-weighted magnetic resonance image of a ganglion cyst. Small arrow, ganglion cyst; large arrow, incidental intraosseous bone cyst. **B:** T2-weighted image of the same patient 1 year after arthroscopic resection of a ganglion cyst and repair of the posterior labrum. Notice that the cyst is completely resolved and only the suture anchor used to repair the labrum remains (*small arrow*).

Despite new physical examination tests and advances with MRI arthrography, labral lesions are often difficult to diagnose without arthroscopic evaluation. Therefore, a high index of suspicion should be maintained in a patient with mechanical symptoms of catching or shoulder pain that do not readily fit into one of the usual patterns of shoulder pathology. Several follow-up studies have shown good clinical outcomes after arthroscopic suture anchor repair of SLAP lesions. If labral pathology is noted at the time of arthroscopy, care should be taken to ensure that the patient does not have associated intraarticular pathologies, which are commonly seen with SLAP lesions. These concomitant pathologic conditions include occult instability, rotator cuff pathologies, and paralabral ganglion cysts. These conditions may significantly alter the surgical outcome and must be addressed during the operation. The role of the superior labrum in the global stability of the shoulder is more important in the throwing athlete, in whom a tremendous amount of force must be overcome by the static and dynamic restraints of the shoulder. Longer follow-up studies and continued refinement in surgical techniques should help to further the understanding of labral lesions and to improve the results of surgical treatment.

REFERENCES

1. Gardner E, Gray DJ. Prenatal development of the human shoulder and acromioclavicular joint. *Am J Anat* 1953;92:219–276.
2. Snyder SJ, Rames RD, Wolbert E. Labral lesions. In: McGinty JB, ed. *Operative arthroscopy.* New York: Raven Press, 1991:491–499.
3. Detrisac DA, Johnson LL. *Arthroscopic shoulder anatomy: pathologic and surgical implications.* Thorofare, NJ: SLACK Inc, 1986.
4. Detrisac DA. Personal communication.
5. Williams MM, Snyder SJ, Buford D. The Buford complex—the "cord like" middle glenohumeral ligament and absent anterosuperior labrum complex: a normal anatomic capsulolabral variant. *Arthroscopy* 1994;10:241–247.
6. Howell SM, Galinat BJ. The glenoid-labral socket: a constrained articular surface. *Clin Orthop* 1989;243:122–125.
7. Reeves B. Experiments on the tensile strength of the anterior capsular structures of the shoulder in man. *J Bone Joint Surg Br* 1968;50:858–865.
8. Perry J. Anatomy and biomechanics of the shoulder in throwing, swimming, gymnastics and tennis. *Clin Sports Med* 1983;2:247–270.
9. Karzel R, Nuber G, Lautenschlager E. Contact stresses during compression loading of the glenohumeral joint: the role of the glenoid labrum. *Proc Inst Med Chicago* 1989;42:64–65.
10. Davidson PA, Elattrache NS, Jobe CM, et al. Rotator cuff and posterior-superior glenoid labrum injury associated with increased glenohumeral motion: a new site of impingement. *J Shoulder Elbow Surg* 1995;4:384–390.
11. Burkhead W. Personal communication, Nov. 13, 1992, and review of article submitted for publication: "Vascularity of the glenoid labrum."
12. Cooper DE, Arnoczky SP, O'Brien SJ, et al. Anatomy, histology, and vascularity of the glenoid labrum: an anatomical study. *J Bone Joint Surg Am* 1992;74:46–52.
13. DePalma AJ, White JB, Callery G. Degenerative lesions of the shoulder joint at various age groups which are compatible with good function. *Instr Course Lect* 1950;7:168–180.
14. Snyder SJ, Karzel RP, Del Pizzo W, et al. SLAP lesions of the shoulder. *Arthroscopy* 1990;6:274–279.
15. Maffet MW, Gartsman GM, Moseley B. Superior labrum–biceps tendon complex lesion of the shoulder. *Am J Sports Med* 1995;23:93–98.
16. Snyder SJ, Banas MP, Karzel RP. An analysis of one hundred and forty injuries to the superior glenoid labrum. *J Shoulder Elbow Surg* 1995;4:243–248.
17. Rodosky MW, Harner CD, Rudert MJ, et al. The role of the biceps–superior labrum complex in anterior stability of the shoulder. *Pittsburgh Orthop J* 1990;1:57–68.
18. Andrews JR, Carson WG. The arthroscopic treatment of glenoid labrum tears: the throwing athlete. *Orthop Trans* 1984;8:44.
19. Morgan CD, Burkhart SS, Palmeri M, et al. Type II SLAP lesions: three subtypes and their relationships to superior instability and rotator cuff tears. *Arthroscopy* 1998;14:553–565.
20. Burkhart SS, Morgan CD. The peel-back mechanism: its role in producing and extending posterior type II SLAP lesions and its effect on SLAP repair rehabilitation. *Arthroscopy* 1998;14:637–640.
21. Cummins CA, Messer TM, Nuber GW. Current concept review: suprascapular nerve entrapment. *J Bone Joint Surg Am* 2000;82:415–424.
22. Fehrman DA, Orwin JF, Jennings RM. Suprascapular nerve entrapment by ganglion cysts: a report of cases with arthroscopic findings and review of the literature. *Arthroscopy* 1995;11:727–734.
23. Chochole MH, Senker W, Meznik C, et al. Glenoid-labral cyst entrapping the suprascapular nerve: dissolution after arthroscopic debridement of an extended SLAP lesion. *Arthroscopy* 1997;13:753–755.
24. Leitschuh PH, Bone CM, Bouska WM. Magnetic resonance imaging diagnosis, sonographically directed percutaneous aspiration, and arthroscopic treatment of a painful shoulder ganglion cyst associated with a SLAP lesion. *Arthroscopy* 1999;15:85–87.
25. Iannotti JP, Ramsey ML. Arthroscopic decompression of a ganglion cyst causing suprascapular nerve compression. *Arthroscopy* 1996;12:739–475.
26. Moore TP, Fritts HM, Quick DC, et al. Suprascapular nerve entrapment caused by supraglenoid cyst compression. *J Shoulder Elbow Surg* 1997;6:455–462.
27. Tirman PFJ, Feller JF, Janzen DL, et al. Association of glenoid labral cysts with labral tears and glenohumeral instability: radiologic findings and clinical significance. *Radiology* 1994;190:653–658.
28. Padua L, LoMonaco M, Padua R, et al. Suprascapular nerve entrapment: neurophysiological localization in 6 cases. *Acta Orthop Scand* 1996;67:482–484.
29. Post M, Mayer J. Suprascapular nerve entrapment: diagnosis and treatment. *Clin Orthop* 1987; 223:126–136.
30. Burkhart SS, Morgan CD, Kibler WB. Shoulder injuries in overhead athletes: the "dead arm" revisited. *Clin Sports Med* 2000;19:125–159.
31. Rowe CR, Zarins B. Recurrent transient subluxation of the shoulder. *J Bone Joint Surg Am* 1981;63:863–872.
32. Andrews JR, Gidumal RH. Shoulder arthroscopy in the throwing athlete: perspectives and prognosis. *Clin Sports Med* 1987;6:565–571.
33. Kibler WB. Specificity and sensitivity of the anterior slide test in throwing athletes with superior glenoid labral tears. *Arthroscopy* 1995;11:296–300.
34. O'Brien SJ, Paganani MJ, Fealy S, et al. The active compression test: a new and effective test for diagnosing labral tears and

acromioclavicular joint abnormalities. *Am J Sports Med* 1998;26: 610–613.

35. Mimori k, Muneta T, Nakagawa T, et al. A new pain provocation test for superior labral tears of the shoulder. *Am J Sports Med* 1999;27:37–142.
36. Iannotti JP, Wang ED. Avulsion fracture of the supraglenoid tubercle: a variation of the SLAP lesion. *J Shoulder Elbow Surg* 1992;1:26–30.
37. Deutsch AL, Resnick D, Mink JH, et al. Computed and conventional arthrotomography of the glenohumeral joint: normal anatomy and clinical experience. *Radiology* 1984;153:603–609.
38. Rafii M, Firouznia H, Golimbu C, et al. CT arthrography of capsular structures of the shoulder. *AJR Am J Roentgenol* 1986; 46:361–367.
39. Chandnani VP, Yeager TD, DeBerardino T, et al. Glenoid labral tears: prospective evaluation with MR imaging, MR arthrography, and CT arthrography. *AJR Am J Roentgenol* 1993;161: 1229–1235.
40. Tirman PFJ, Applegate GR, Flannigan BD, et al. Magnetic resonance arthrography of the shoulder. *Magn Reson Imaging Clin North Am* 1993;1:125–142.
41. Bencardino JT, Beltran J, Rosenberg ZS, et al. Superior labrum anterior-posterior lesions: diagnosis with MR arthrography of the shoulder. *Radiology* 2000;214:267–271.
42. Karzel RP, Snyder SJ. Magnetic resonance arthrography of the shoulder: a new technique of shoulder imaging. *Clin Sports Med* 1993;1:123–136.
43. Smith DK, Chopp TM, Aufdemorte TB, et al. Sublabral recess of the superior glenoid labrum: study of cadavers with conventional nonenhanced MR imaging, MR arthrography, anatomic dissection, and limited histologic examination. *Radiology* 1996;201:251–256.
44. Glasgow SG, Bruce RA, Yacobucci GN, et al. Arthroscopic resection of glenoid labral tears in the athlete: a report of 29 cases. *Arthroscopy* 1992;8:48–54.
45. Altchek DW, Warren RF, Wickiewicz TL, et al. Arthroscopic labral debridement: a three year follow-up study. *Am J Sports Med* 1992;20:702–706.

46. Payne LZ, Jokl P. The results of arthroscopic debridement of glenoid labral tears based on tear location. *Arthroscopy* 1993;9: 560–565.
47. Field LD, Savoie FA. Arthroscopic suture repair of superior labral detachment lesions of the shoulder. *Am J Sports Med* 1993;21: 783–790.
48. Yoneda M, Hirouka A, Saito S, et al. Arthroscopic stapling for detached superior glenoid labrum. *J Bone Joint Surg Br* 1991; 73:746–750.
49. Resch H, Golser K, Thoeni H, et al. Arthroscopic repair of superior glenoid labral detachment (the SLAP lesion). *J Shoulder Elbow Surg* 1993;2:147–155.
50. Shall LM, Cawley PW. Soft tissue reconstruction in the shoulder: comparison of suture anchors, absorbable staples, and absorbable tacks. *Am J Sports Med* 1994;22:715–718.
51. Burkart A, Imhoff AB, Roscher E. Foreign-body reaction to the bioabsorbable Suretac device. *Arthroscopy* 2000;16:91–95.
52. McConville OR, Iannotti JP. Partial-thickness tears of the rotator cuff: evaluation and management. *J Am Acad Orthop Surg* 1999;7:32–43.
53. Weber SC. Arthroscopic debridement and acromioplasty versus mini-open repair in the management of significant partial thickness tears of the rotator cuff. *Orthop Clin North Am* 1997;28: 79–82.
54. Miller DV, Lewis JM. *Surgical management of partial rotator cuff tears.* Presented at the Second Annual Meeting of the American Orthopaedic Society for Sports Medicine, Lake Buena Vista, FL, June 1996.
55. Gartsman GM, Milne JC. Articular surface partial-thickness rotator cuff tears. *J Shoulder Elbow Surg* 1995;4:409–415.
56. Kvitne RS, Jobe FW. The diagnosis and treatment of anterior instability in the throwing athlete. *Clin Orthop* 1993;291:107–123.
57. Jobe CM: Posterior superior glenoid impingement: expanded spectrum. *Arthroscopy* 1995;11:530–537.
58. Ferrick MR, Marzo JM. Ganglion cyst of the shoulder associated with a glenoid labral tear and symptomatic glenohumeral instability: a case report. *Am J Sports Med* 1997;25:717–719.

PATHOPHYSIOLOGY OF SHOULDER INSTABILITY

R. SEAN CHURCHILL
DOUGLAS T. HARRYMAN II
JOHN A. SIDLES
FREDERICK A. MATSEN III

The shoulder is the most versatile articulating mechanism in the body. The typical adult shoulder sustains loads equal to the entire body weight simply for routine, everyday activities. A trained shoulder can bear loads greater than three to four times body weight, achieve tremendous flexibility, retain pinpoint precision control, and maintain perfect joint stability. These upper-extremity functions are dependent on a stable articular linkage about the shoulder and on normal joint laxity. The shoulder lacks the rigid ball-and-socket architecture of the hip on one hand and the ligamentous restraints of the knee on the other. Our focus in this chapter is to consider how the shoulder maintains its stability without limitation by bony or ligamentous constraints.

GLENOHUMERAL STABILITY AND LAXITY

Shoulder *stability* is the ability to maintain the humeral head perfectly centered within the glenoid fossa. Without this degree of precision, accurate control of the upper extremity is impossible. Instability is the inability to maintain the head centered within the glenoid fossa (1,2). Shoulder *laxity* is the amount of humeral head translation across the surface of the glenoid that is allowed by capsular and ligamentous restraints (2,3).

The difference between laxity and instability can be demonstrated easily in a living subject. When the shoulder muscles are relaxed, the clinician can translate the humeral head easily in the anterior, posterior, or inferior directions. The magnitude of this translation is the shoulder's laxity. If the shoulder muscles are tightened even slightly, it becomes impossible to translate the humeral head, demonstrating that a lax shoulder can be stable.

R. S. Churchill, J. A. Sidles, and F. A. Matsen III: Department of Orthopaedics and Sports Medicine, University of Washington, Seattle, Washington

D. T. Harryman II: Deceased.

This relationship is shown using the so-called glenoidogram, which follows the path of the humeral head center as it translates across the glenoid. The plot normally displays a "gull-wing" shape (Fig. 30.1), the depth of which aids understanding of the centering of the humeral head in the glenoid. The steeper the slope of the V on the glenoidogram, the more effective the centering of the head in the glenoid when a compressive load is applied. Glenohumeral laxity is indicated by the extent to which the humeral head can be translated across the glenoid—the straight-line distance from tip to tip of the gull wing.

Normal shoulders demonstrate laxity. Eight physicians volunteered for clinical examination after instrumentation with position sensors secured to pins drilled into their humerus and scapula (Fig. 30.2). We then recorded the actual amounts of maximal translation on tests of joint laxity (4). We found that in normal shoulders the head of the humerus translates anteriorly, posteriorly, or inferiorly an average range of 1 cm from its centered position.

The amount of translation on laxity tests alone cannot be used to determine whether a joint is unstable. Gymnasts have great laxity but very stable shoulders. Using our position sensing system, we measured the laxity in normal shoulders and in shoulders of patients who were experiencing instability after an atraumatic or traumatic onset. Unstable shoulders did not show a significant increase in laxity compared with normal shoulders (5) (Fig. 30.3).

GLENOHUMERAL MOTION: MIDRANGE OR END-RANGE?

As will be discussed later, various mechanisms are responsible for maintaining glenohumeral stability. Although most of these stability mechanisms operate throughout the entire range, the relative importance of each depends on whether the shoulder is within the midrange or end-range of motion.

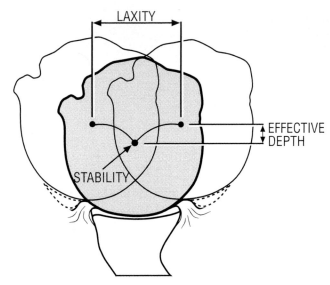

FIGURE 30.1 The center of the humeral head traces a "gull-wing" pathway as it translates across the surface of an intact glenoid and labrum (glenoidogram). Glenohumeral laxity is defined by the limit of humeral head excursion allowed by the surrounding soft tissue and is measured from end to end of the glenoidogram.

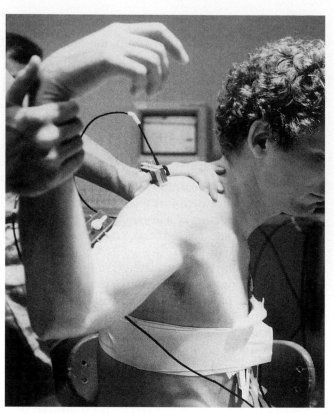

FIGURE 30.2 Spatial tracking sensors pinned to the humerus and scapula. This *in vivo* method has provided investigators the opportunity to track and accurately measure the position or rotation of the humeral head and scapula in relation to each other and to the thorax.

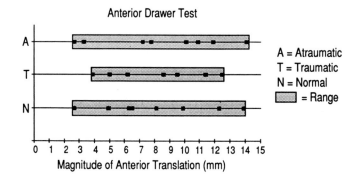

FIGURE 30.3 Comparative *in vivo* glenohumeral laxity on anterior drawer for stable shoulders (normal) and for shoulders with traumatic and atraumatic instability. Note the significant overlap among the three groups.

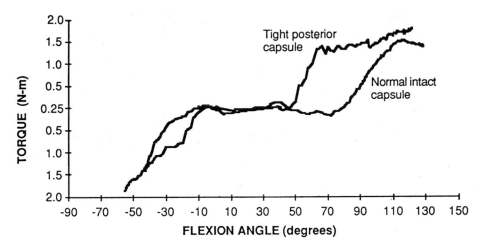

FIGURE 30.4 As the humerus is elevated perpendicular to the scapular plane (extreme flexion or extension), the cuff and capsule become tight near the end-range of motion, where torsion escalates for each incremental degree of elevation. Torsional loads become increased early in the mid-range of normal forward flexion when the posterior capsule is tight.

Activities of daily living and typical work activities are performed in humerothoracic positions that are well away from the extremes of range (6,7). We consider these positions to be within the functional midrange. During midrange motion, the capsule remains lax. When the position of the humerus is rotated or elevated toward the limit of joint motion, the capsule and its ligaments come under tension (Fig. 30.4). Cadaveric tests demonstrate that the capsule and cuff tissue remain essentially tension-free until glenohumeral motion approaches the terminal degrees of range (8). The end-range, therefore, is defined by the range in which the tensile force increases in the static restraints of the capsule and its ligaments.

STABILITY MECHANISMS
Midrange Mechanisms

There are several mechanisms of glenohumeral stability that, although active in varying degrees throughout the entire range, are most important in the midrange of motion. The ability to maintain midrange stability is critical, because it is within this range that the majority of functional, daily activities are performed (7) (Fig. 30.5). Although stability mechanisms are related and often dependent on each other, they are discussed separately here for clarity.

Concavity–Compression

Once a golf ball is placed on a tee, it is inherently stable and remains in place. However, if the tee has a chip in its surface, the golf ball may no longer remain seated. If the tee were completely flat, it would be very difficult to keep the ball in place. If a strong translating force exists (e.g., a windy day), it becomes harder to keep the ball on the tee. If the force of gravity were lessened, for example by replacing the golf ball with a ping pong ball, less displacing force would be required to displace the ball.

Two anatomic features give the glenoid a concave shape. Soslowsky et al. (10) demonstrated the thickened chondral surface on the periphery of the glenoid, which provides the fossa with depth (Fig. 30.6). In addition, Howell and Galinat (11) measured the contribution of the glenoid labrum to the depth of the glenoid fossa and found that the labrum enhances the depth by 50%. They measured the total depth of the socket as 9 mm in the superior-inferior direction and 5 mm in the anterior-posterior direction. For all glenohumeral positions, the major compressive load across the joint is provided by the action of the surrounding musculature, especially the rotator cuff (2,9).

The concavity–compression mechanism is an extremely effective glenohumeral stabilizer (9). In cadaveric shoulders, we defined glenoid concavity using the glenoidogram (9) (Fig. 30.1). The maximum lateral humeral displacement is the effective glenoid depth. In addition, we used the stability ratio, a factor defined by Fukuda et al. (12), to evaluate the contribution of concavity–compression to glenohumeral stability. The stability ratio (SR) is defined as follows:

$$SR = (\text{Dislocating force} \div \text{Compressive load}) \times 100$$

Depending on the direction of testing, Lippitt et al. (9) found stability ratios ranging from 33% to 64%. By excising the glenoid labrum and thereby decreasing glenoid depth, the stability ratio was decreased by an average of 20% (Fig. 30.7).

In more recent work performed in our laboratory, we sought to further validate the importance of concavity–compression as a stabilizing mechanism and to investigate whether this mechanism could be surgically restored in shoulders with typical findings of instability (13). In five cadaveric shoulders, a chondral–labral lesion similar to that seen in patients with recurrent traumatic instability was created in the anterior-inferior quadrant of the glenoid. Effective glenoid depths and stability ratios were measured before and after production of the lesion. Creation of this defect re-

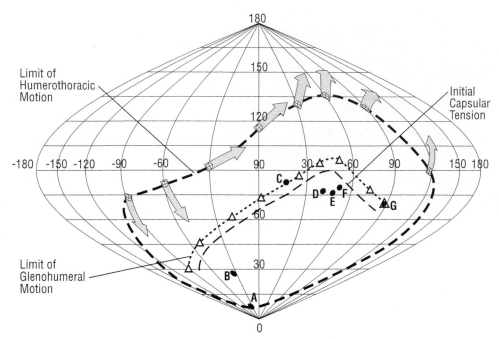

FIGURE 30.5 Mercator global graph of shoulder motion. The outer dashed line is the limit of humerothoracic motion (glenohumeral plus scapulothoracic). The dotted line is the boundary of glenohumeral motion alone. Inside the limit of glenohumeral motion is a second dashed line which, for lesser elevations without humeral rotation, represents glenohumeral positions that do not result in capsular tension. Points A through F represent glenohumeral positions for routine daily activities. The majority of these activities are recorded in the functional midrange. A, scratching the back; B, hand behind the head; C, lifting a gallon to top of head; D, placing a coin on shelf at shoulder height; E, hand to mouth; F, washing back of opposite shoulder.

Glenoid Cartilage Thickness

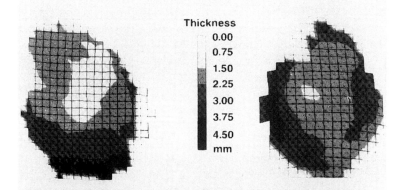

Humeral Head Cartilage Thickness

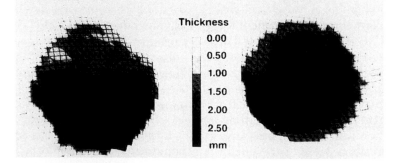

FIGURE 30.6 Articular cartilage thickness of the glenoid and humeral head of right and left shoulders. The articular cartilage on the glenoid is thin centrally, and on the humeral head it is thick centrally. The articular cartilage surfaces of the humeral head and glenoid match spherically. (Reprinted from JB Lippincott, Philadelphia, with permission.)

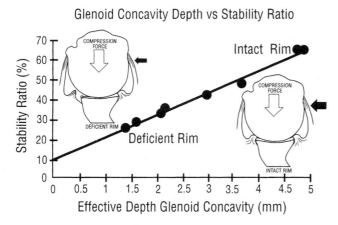

FIGURE 30.7 The stability ratio is linearly related to the maximum lateral humeral displacement (glenoid depth). As the depth of the glenoid is increased, a greater translating force is required to displace the humeral head. Left, shallow or deficient glenoid; right, intact glenoid deepened by thick cartilage and labrum.

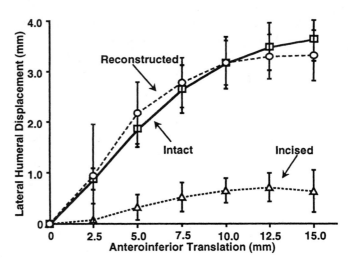

FIGURE 30.8 Path of the humeral head center in the anteroinferior direction for the normal glenoid, after an articular anteroinferior chondral–labral rim defect, and after surgical reconstruction of the lesion with a tendon autograft (mean ± 1 SD).

duced the effective glenoid depth by approximately 80% and the stability ratio by approximately 65% for translation in the direction of the lesion. Moreover, after reconstruction of the lesion using a tendon graft, both the effective glenoid depth and the stability ratio were restored to normal (Fig. 30.8, Table 30.1).

Clinically, the recreation of the glenoid concavity has been evaluated as well. Bigliani et al. (14), reported on 25 patients with glenoid rim lesions. These lesions were classified as follows: type I, a displaced avulsion fracture with attached capsule; type II, a malunited glenoid rim fracture; type III, glenoid rim erosion with less than 25% of the glenoid affected (type IIIA) or with more than 25% affected (type IIIB). Sixteen patients underwent operative repair consisting of reduction and fixation of the bony fragment if possible. Eight underwent capsular advancement to the glenoid rim, and one type IIIB lesion was treated with a coracoid transfer to fill the glenoid defect. This resulted in 88% satisfactory results without recurrent instability.

Concavity–compression is probably the most important midrange stabilizing mechanism. It also plays a significant role in the end-range of motion as well. At the end-range of motion, concavity–compression is assisted by the static capsular tensile force compressing the humeral head within the chondral dish of the conforming glenoid.

Muscle Balance

If the net joint reaction force is always directed within the confines of the glenoid fossa, the glenohumeral joint will be stable. In a dynamic cadaver shoulder model, Cain et al. (15) demonstrated that simulated contraction of the infraspinatus and teres minor acted to decrease strain in the inferior glenohumeral ligament (IGHL) by pulling the humeral head posteriorly.

The creation of a superior labral anterior and posterior (SLAP) lesion disrupting the biceps tendon insertion point resulted in a significant increase in glenohumeral inferior

TABLE 30.1 STABILITY RATIO DATA

Direction	Preparation	Stability Ratio %	Probability Value
Anterior	Intact	32.1 ± 7.8	$p < .0001^a$
	Incised	14.1 ± 1.7	
	Reconstructed	36.3 ± 7.3	$p < .0001^a$
Anteroinferior	Intact	38.4 ± 4.5	$p < .0001^a$
	Incised	13.1 ± 3.1	
	Reconstructed	46.5 ± 9.4	$p < .0001^a, p = 0.0247^b$
Inferior	Intact	45.3 ± 7.3	$p < .0001^a$
	Incised	20.0 ± 4.5	
	Reconstructed	42.7 ± 5.2	$p < .0001^a$

[a] $p < .05$ compared with incised.
[b] $p < .05$ compared with intact.

subluxation (16). To further define the importance of the biceps tendon insertion, Pagnani et al. (17) selectively sectioned the superior labrum, with or without involvement of the biceps tendon insertion. Significant increases in anterior-posterior and superior-inferior translation occurred only after the biceps tendon insertion was destabilized as well. Activation of the biceps tendon in the cocking phase of throwing has also been shown to reduce the IGHL strain and to help resist anterior humeral head translation (18).

The stabilizing effect of the muscle contractions may be the result of their ability to generate a force opposing abnormal humeral translation as well as their contribution to the concavity–compression mechanism. Howell and Kraft (19) demonstrated that selective suprascapular nerve block did not increase anterior translation in shoulders with underlying instability, implying that laxity of the shoulder is not affected by muscle action. Blasier et al. (20), in a dynamic cadaver study, also demonstrated that all rotator cuff muscles were equally effective at providing for glenohumeral stabilization in the scapular plane.

Using linear programming techniques to analyze the muscular modeling data of Bassett et al. (21), Sidles generated some interesting data regarding specific muscular activation during balanced glenohumeral motion. As one would expect, when the program is asked to display the combination of muscle activity that produces the greatest internal rotation moment for a glenohumeral position of 90 degrees of abduction and 90 degrees of external rotation (i.e., the late cocking phase of pitching), the result is complete activation of the modeled internal rotators (anterior deltoid, pectoralis major, subscapularis, latissimus dorsi, teres major, and triceps) to yield a total internal rotation moment of 752 newton-centimeters (N-cm). The resultant torque, however, also contains large adduction and flexion moments because of the line of action of these muscles.

If our program is asked to produce the muscular combination that maximizes the internal rotation moment, assuming the flexion and adduction moments must be balanced to equal zero, a very interesting result is obtained. The total internal rotation moment drops to 65.1 N-cm, "bal-anced" between 100% activity of the supraspinatus, 38.9% activity of the teres major, and 19.4% activity of the anterior deltoid. The production of a pure internal rotation moment demands maximal supraspinatus function, and the amount of internal rotation torque generated is reduced by 91%! In this model, supraspinatus activity becomes the crucial limitation for production of a pure internal rotation moment because it must balance the flexion and adduction moments.

The ability of muscle forces to maintain a stable joint despite the presence of a Bankart lesion has been demonstrated with the use of cadaveric specimens and an intricate dynamic shoulder testing apparatus (22). This reemphasizes the importance of the interplay between muscular forces and glenoid architecture within the concavity–compression model. The supraspinatus and biceps tendons were found to be the most important dynamic inferior glenohumeral stabilizers. When they were within the functional range of motion, their stabilizing effects were significantly greater than those of the coracohumeral and superior glenohumeral ligaments at resisting inferior glenohumeral translation (23).

Muscle balance is clearly an important glenohumeral stabilizing mechanism. It provides a dynamic way in which the body can ensure that the net humeral force passes through the glenoid fossa.

Joint Congruity

In general, humeral and glenoid joint surfaces have equal radii of curvature (Figs. 30.9 and 30.10). Soslowsky et al. (10) found that the deviation from sphericity for either joint surface was less than 1% in a series of cadaveric shoulders.

When the glenoid surface is flattened (i.e., has a radius of curvature greater than that of the humeral head), the humeral head is less securely centered. An extreme case is glenoid hypoplasia; 50% of patients with this condition experience symptoms of instability (24).

Flatow et al. (25), showed that the flexible labrum acts to extend the surface contact area of the glenoid without altering its radius of curvature. When capsular tension is applied

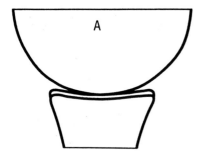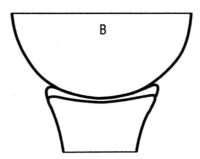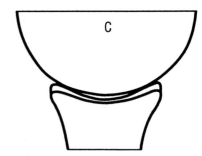

FIGURE 30.9 Saha classified the glenohumeral articulation into three types: type A, glenoid fossa with a radius of curvature greater than the humeral head; type B, glenoid fossa and humeral head with equal radii of curvature; and type C, humeral surface with a greater radius of curvature than the glenoid.

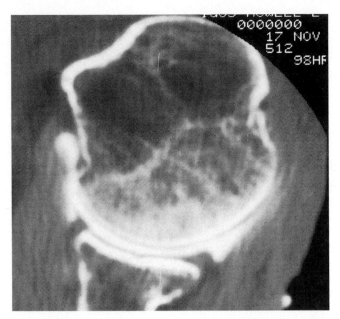

FIGURE 30.10 Computed double-contrast tomograph showing articular conformity. Note that the glenoid articular cartilage is thin centrally and thick at the periphery. The labrum deepens and extends the congruent articular surface.

to the labrum at the extremes of motion, the labrum becomes less evident (26) as it tightens to extend the glenoid depth. These conforming surfaces give the articulation much of its inherent stability.

Glenohumeral Suction Cup

When the humeral head is pressed into a compliant, conforming glenoid cavity, fluid is expressed from between them and a suction-cup effect is produced. The valve for this suction is the glenoid labrum. Similar to pulling on a depressed plunger, great force is required to break this suction (Fig. 30.11). This postulate is easily demonstrated in the operating room by gently compressing the humeral head into a congruent glenoid fossa. When a distraction force is applied, a kissing sound will be heard as the suction cup is broken.

We measured the magnitude of this force using a preparation consisting of only a saline-moistened humeral head and a glenoid with an intact labrum. The amount of force required to break the suction cup was determined in six elderly cadaveric shoulders (mean age, 76.4 years; range, 69 to 89 years). Mild degenerative changes were noted in two specimens. Each humeral head was compressed into the glenoid fossa with a 5-N force (approximately 1 lb). Direct lateral traction was applied until suction was broken. In the two shoulders with degenerative changes, no suction-cup effect could be demonstrated. In the four remaining shoulders, 20 ± 3 N (mean ± standard deviation) of force (approximately 4 lb) was required to break the suction.

Creating a defect in the labrum completely eliminated the suction effect. In younger shoulders with more compliant chondral surfaces and more robust labra, the suction effect would be expected to be greater. However, any condition in which the articular surfaces are nonconforming or the labrum is deficient would compromise this mechanism. This mechanism of stability does not consume energy, so it economizes on the need for active muscle power (27).

Negative Intraarticular Pressure and Limited Joint Volume

Any surgeon who has performed shoulder arthroscopy has heard the telltale "hiss" as air rushes into the joint when the cannula is opened. The negative pressure inside the glenohumeral joint rapidly equilibrates with atmospheric pressure. Although this mechanism was recognized well over a century ago (27), Kumar and Balasubramaniam (28) were first to measure the intraarticular pressure in the shoulder (average, -42 cm H_2O).

Capsular venting can dramatically increase the amount of joint laxity and reduce the force necessary for humeral translation. When air or other fluid is allowed to enter the glenohumeral joint, as occurs during arthroscopy or after injury, the humeral head can easily be displaced (Fig. 30.12). We studied the effect of capsular venting in our laboratory (29). Eight cadaveric shoulders underwent the equivalent of

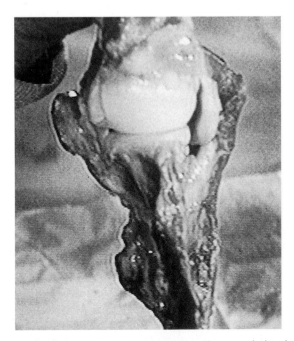

FIGURE 30.11 In this cadaveric specimen, the capsule has been completely sectioned and yet the humeral head is sealed securely against the glenolabral socket by the suction-cup effect. Here an investigator is attempting to pull the humerus away from the scapula. The weight of the entire extremity is easily supported by this mechanism.

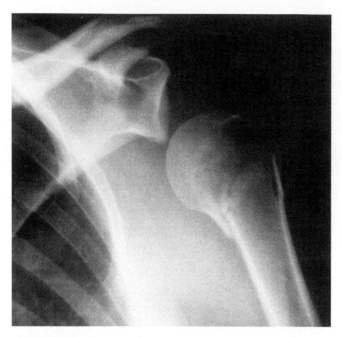

FIGURE 30.12 A joint effusion, in this case caused by a fracture, increases the intraarticular fluid volume and reduces the negative pressure within the joint. Passive stabilization by limited joint volume is lost, allowing inferior humeral head displacement, which has been termed *pseudosubluxation*.

anterior drawer, posterior drawer, and sulcus testing before and after capsular venting. Venting of the capsule reduced the force necessary to translate the humeral head by 55% for an anterior drawer, 43% for a posterior drawer, and 57% for a sulcus test.

When the joint capsule is intact, the shoulder has a finite volume. Distraction of the joint attempts to increase the joint volume, but in so doing it decreases the intraarticular pressure, according to Boyle's law:

$$P_1 \cdot V_1 = P_2 \cdot V_2$$

The greater the attempt at joint distraction, the lower the intraarticular pressure and the greater the stabilizing force from this mechanism.

Habermeyer et al. (30) measured the intraarticular pressure in cadaveric shoulders and in patients with traumatic instability or with normal shoulders. They discovered a resting pressure of -34 mm Hg (range, -25 to -42 mm Hg) in cadavers, -32 mm Hg (range, -22 to -43 mm Hg) in normal shoulders, and 0 mm Hg (range, -5 to $+5$ mm Hg) in shoulders with traumatic capsulolabral lesions. By applying traction to the cadaveric shoulders, the authors calculated that negative pressure provides a mean stabilizing force of 146 N. Moreover, when manual traction was applied in shoulders of control patients, the pressure decreased to a mean of -133 mm Hg, whereas the traumatic unstable shoulders attained a pressure of only -2 mm Hg.

Negative intraarticular pressure provides a substantial passive stabilizing force as long as the finite joint volume remains intact (Fig. 30.13).

The effectiveness of limited joint volume, however, depends not only on capsular integrity but also on capsular compliance. Patients with generalized laxity may experience multidirectional instability (31). Because the capsule is compliant, the joint volume is not fixed. As a result, attempted distraction does not result in a decrease in intraarticular pressure. Therefore, the stability deriving from limited joint volume is impaired. Perhaps the effectiveness of capsular shift procedures for atraumatic multidirectional instability results in part from limiting capsular volume (31) and diminishing capsular compliance so that appropriate negative pressure develops in response to joint distraction. Cadaveric studies have revealed that a decrease in joint volume of 57% occurs after inferior capsular shift (32).

Humeroscapular Balance and Proprioception

If the net humeral joint reaction force falls within the confines of the glenoid cavity, the joint will remain stable. Consider a marble on a wooden table top and the table is slowly tilted. Depending on the sum of the forces holding the marble steady (i.e., the weight of the marble and friction), vary-

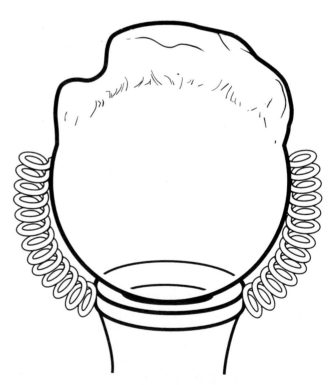

FIGURE 30.13 If apposition of the humeral head against the "labral valve" is disrupted or otherwise deficient (e.g., by simple laxity examination or trauma), negative intraarticular pressure (represented by the capsular springs) returns the humeral head to the glenoid.

ing degrees of tilt will be achieved before the marble begins to move. If the marble were placed in a depression, the table would need to be tilted further to start the marble rolling. Because so much of the discussion of glenohumeral stability revolves around the glenohumeral joint, we forget that through the scapulothoracic joint, the glenoid face can be positioned in varying degrees of "tilt," just like the table top. When the tilt becomes severe enough, the humeral head, like the marble, will tend to "fall off."

Work done in our laboratory helps us understand humeroscapular balance (33). After excision of all soft tissues, a 10-N compressive load was applied to the humeral head of ten cadaveric shoulders. The glenoid was then tilted until dislocation occurred. The total angle of balance stability in the anteroposterior direction was 37 ± 3 degrees, and that in the superoinferior (SI) direction was 57 ± 5 degrees. Excising the glenoid labrum decreased the anteroposterior balance angle of stability to 33 ± 3 degrees ($p < 0.01$). Creating a 3-mm anterior bony glenoid defect caused a decrease in the anteroposterior balance angle of stability to 12 ± 2 degrees ($p < 0.01$).

Humeroscapular balance is linked to the proprioceptive ability to position the joint in a stable alignment (Fig. 30.14). Patients with atraumatic multidirectional instability demonstrate deficient proprioception compared with normal subjects (34). Also, abnormal scapular mechanics have been demonstrated in patients with a variety of shoulder disorders (35–37), and particularly in patients with multidirectional instability (38). Electromyographic activity of the scapular stabilizers in patients with traumatic anterior insta-

bility showed significantly reduced activity in the serratus anterior muscle, one of the principal scapular stabilizers (39). Therefore, improving the humeroscapular balance through muscle coordination training and proprioception therapy should form an integral part of the treatment plan in such individuals (2).

Adhesion–Cohesion Forces

When two congruent surfaces are wet and opposed, they resist separation. The classic demonstration of this principle is a drop of water between two glass slides. The force required to pull these slides apart is surprisingly large. A similar mechanism exists in the glenohumeral joint (40). On opening of a normal human shoulder, 1 to 2 mL of viscous synovial fluid clings to the intraarticular surfaces in a thick film. Any attempt to remove the fluid from the surface is resisted by its tenacious adhesive capacity. Adhesion results from the ionic molecular attraction between the polar moieties of collagenous polymers on the articular surface and those of the mucopolysaccharides within the fluid. Cohesion results from the attraction of the molecules of joint fluid for each other.

The stabilizing effects of adhesion and cohesion are related to the surface contact area and the viscosity of the synovial fluid. Conditions that diminish the normal synovial fluid viscosity (e.g., inflammatory arthritis) would be expected to decrease the effectiveness of this mechanism (41). Conditions that diminish joint contact area would be expected to have a similar effect.

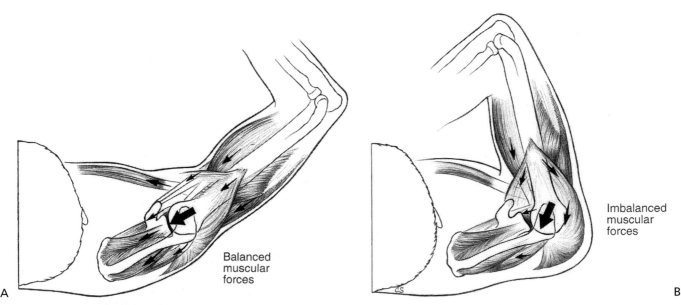

A   Balanced muscular forces   Imbalanced muscular forces   B

FIGURE 30.14 A: For the humeral head to remain stable in the glenoid fossa, the resultant joint reaction force must be directed into a sufficient glenoid concavity. **B:** Glenohumeral instability results when the patient is unable to properly sense, align, or direct scapulohumeral forces into balanced construct.

End-Range Mechanisms

Glenohumeral Ligaments and the Capsular Constraint Mechanism

Athletic upper-extremity performance relies in large part on the function of the capsulolabral ligamentous complex at the extremes of motion. The forceful transition between the phases of late cocking and early acceleration in the overhand throw could overwhelm the stabilizing mechanisms discussed previously. In such a situation, the ligamentous checkreins become of paramount importance.

The function of the capsular glenohumeral ligaments depends on the position of humeral head rotation. Whenever the joint is at an extreme position, some portion of the glenohumeral capsule becomes taut, preventing further rotation. As a capsular ligament reaches maximal tension, the resultant force vector is partly directed in opposition to translation and partly into the glenoid, adding to the concavity compression (Fig. 30.15), thus stabilizing the humeral head within the glenoid fossa (3).

There are several distinct, band-like thickenings in the anterior joint capsule (Fig. 30.16). These structures are best visualized arthroscopically. The size, origin, and insertion of these capsular modulations vary among shoulders (42,43). Let us consider the crucial function of each ligament.

The superior glenohumeral ligament (SGHL) is identified as the most consistent capsular ligament (42). It crosses the capsular portion of the rotator interval between the supraspinatus and subscapularis tendons (Fig. 30.16). Another interval capsular structure, the coracohumeral ligament (CHL), originates at the base of the coracoid, blends into the cuff tendons, and inserts into the greater and lesser

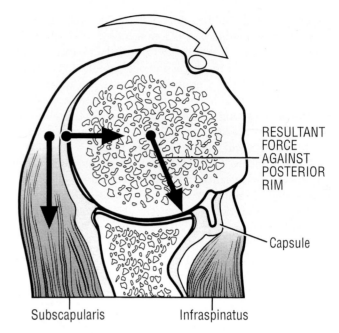

FIGURE 30.15 Rotation of the humeral head is associated with capsular tightening at the end-range of motion. The asymmetrically tight capsule opposes a load or displacement directed toward itself and attempts to translate the humeral head away from itself toward the opposite side of the glenoid. The tense capsule also applies a load to compress the humeral head into the glenoid fossa. These stabilizing forces are referred to as the capsular constraint mechanism.

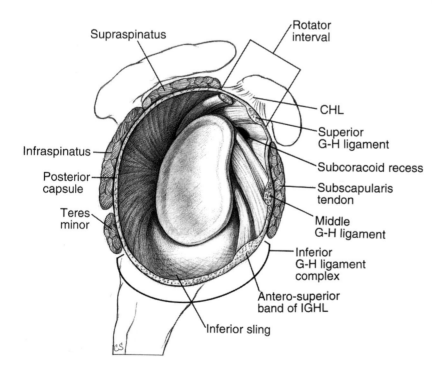

FIGURE 30.16 The capsule of the rotator interval spans the gap between the anterior border of the supraspinatus and the superior border of the subscapularis and contains the coracohumeral and superior glenohumeral ligaments (CHL and SGHL). The middle and inferior glenohumeral ligaments (MGHL and IGHL) originate proximally on the glenoid and course obliquely and inferiorly to their broad insertions on the humeral head. The IGHL blends into the inferior capsular sling.

tuberosities. Similar functions are ascribed to these ligaments. The SGHL and CHL come under tension with elevation in flexion, extension, external rotation, and adduction of the arm. In these positions, the rotator interval capsule and its ligamentous thickenings (SGHL and CHL) have been found to resist posterior and inferior displacement of the humeral head (44,45).

When the arm is unelevated, inferior and lateral translation of the head on the glenoid increases tension in the superior rotator interval capsular structures (SGHL and CHL), thereby resisting inferior translation (44–46). If, however, the humerus is abducted or the scapula adducts (drooping posture), then the superior capsular ligaments are relaxed, allowing inferior humeral head subluxation (2). Clinical and experimental data have shown that release or surgical tightening of the rotator interval capsule respectively increases or decreases the allowed posterior and inferior translational laxity (44,47,48) (Fig. 30.17). The effect of complete capsular release was examined in a cadaver model by Moskal et al. (3). They noted an increase in anterior translation from 21 to 28 mm, and in posterior translation from 14 mm to 25 mm, with complete capsular release. The intact rotator cuff myotendinous units served to limit the range of motion and translation such that no specimen could be dislocated despite the complete capsular release (3).

Anterior capsular laxity decreases with external rotation of the humerus as the anterior ligaments become tight (49). For the externally rotated, yet unelevated humerus, the rotator interval capsule (including the SGHL and CHL) becomes taut (43,44). If external rotation is maximized and the humerus is elevated (approximately 45 degrees), tension is applied to the middle glenohumeral ligament (MGHL) (50,51). The MGHL originates anterosuperior on the glenoid and inserts midway along the anterior humeral ar-

ticular surface adjacent to the lesser tuberosity. In more than one third of shoulders, the MGHL is absent or poorly defined. Some investigators believe such shoulders such are at greater risk for anterior glenohumeral instability (52).

In the fully abducted and externally rotated "apprehension" position, tension is applied to the IGHL and the inferior capsular sling (50,53). In this position, the IGHL becomes the primary ligamentous stabilizer (51). The stout IGHL originates below the sigmoid notch and courses obliquely between the anteroinferior glenoid and its humeral capsular insertion (54). O'Brien et al. (54) described an anterior thickening of the IGHL, the anterosuperior band.

Warren et al. (55) advanced the "circle concept" of shoulder instability, namely that anterior instability requires a lesion not only of the anterior superior band of the IGHL but also of the posterior portion of the IGHL.

The anterior and posterior aspects of the IGHL are said to function as a cruciate construct, alternatively tightening in external or internal rotation (45,54). When the humerus is elevated anteriorly in the sagittal plane (flexion), the posteroinferior capsular pouch and the rotator interval capsule come under tension (8,44,45,54,56). If the humerus is internally rotated while elevated in the sagittal plane, the interval capsule slackens but the posterior capsule and inferior pouch tighten.

In summary, capsular ligaments serve three functions: (a) they limit humeral rotation and absorb torsional forces which, if unchecked, would lead to tendon or bone damage by "overrotation"; (b) they compress the head into the glenoid fossa to further stabilize the glenohumeral joint for positions in which other mechanisms would be insufficient; and (c) they present a solid checkrein to restrain the humeral head and oppose the tangential displacement force with an

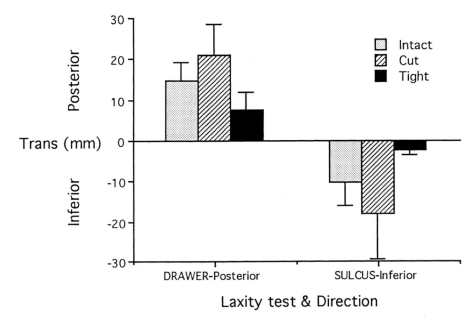

FIGURE 30.17 Posteroinferior instability may occur when a defect is present in the rotator interval capsule (RIC). Plication of the RIC may reduce or eliminate pathologic translation for patients with this type of instability (48).

oppositely directed translational force pushing the humeral head away from the tightened ligaments.

Musculotendinous Wrap

As the humeral head is rotated toward the end-range, the musculotendinous cuff develops tension passively and functions to buttress the capsular ligaments to which it is joined (49,57). Therefore, the capsule is reinforced by the tendons of the cuff and, in return, the tendon insertions are thickened, extended, and reinforced by the capsular insertions (58).

In the relaxed midrange humeroscapular position, the cuff and capsule remain slack (3,59) and do not resist glenohumeral translation except when the humeral head is displaced enough to put these tissues on stretch (4). As rotation away from the midrange increases, tension develops passively within the stretched cuff tendon as it wraps around the humeral articular surface. The musculotendinous unit, fixed between the scapular muscle origin and its point of contact on the articular surface, presents a taut barricade to humeral head translation.

Because the cuff wraps around the spherical surface of the humeral head, the effective "insertional" attachment of the muscle tendon unit becomes the tangential humeral head contact point (2) (Fig. 30.18). In the past, this muscle–tendon barricade provided the rationale for tendon-tightening procedures such as the Putti–Platt and Magnuson and Stack (60) and Osmond-Clarke (61) procedures in treatment of

Line of Force

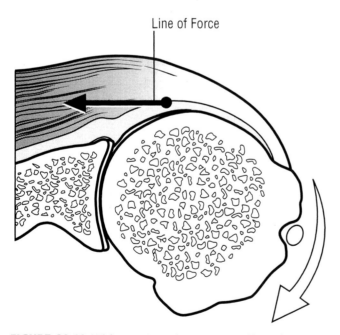

FIGURE 30.18 With rotation, the rotator cuff tendons wrap around the humeral head. Therefore, the effective force vector extends between the muscle origin and the tangential point of application where the tendon contacts the spherical head surface. For the majority of glenohumeral positions, this point is not the tendon insertion.

anterior instability. Unfortunately, the "muscular wrap" stabilizing mechanism must restrict motion or become less effective in certain extreme critical positions. When the humerus is positioned in full abduction–external rotation, the subscapularis is unable to resist anteroinferior translation because its tendon line of action only crosses the anterosuperior aspect of the humeral head (62).

Glenohumeral Instability

Patients with instability can be classified as having lost one or more stabilizing mechanisms. The treatment for these shoulders relies on identifying and correcting the deficient mechanisms.

Traumatic Instability

Traumatic instability occurs when every stabilizing mechanism is overwhelmed and the humeral head is forcibly translated from its centered position in the glenohumeral fossa, most commonly in the anteroinferior direction. Traumatic dislocations occur when the shoulder is suddenly forced beyond the range normally allowed by its ligaments.

Early in the twentieth century, detachment of the glenohumeral capsulolabral ligamentous junction from the anteroinferior glenoid rim was considered the "essential lesion" of traumatic anteroinferior glenohumeral instability (63–65), and surgical repair of this lesion remains the cornerstone of treatment (63,66–68). Attempts to duplicate this lesion traumatically in cadavers have been unsuccessful. A surgically created labral lesion alone is inadequate to allow shoulder dislocation (55,69,70). Experimentally, unless capsuloligamentous disruption extends posteriorly and/or superiorly around the glenoid or the rotator cuff is avulsed, the cadaver shoulder cannot be dislocated (69,71,72).

Some investigators claim that some degree of capsular ligament strain occurs with every traumatic anteroinferior dislocation (73–76), and that patients who experienced recurrent anterior shoulder dislocations retained excessive residual laxity in the subscapularis tendon and anterior capsule (49). Kaltsas (77) found a greater stretch capacity in the glenohumeral joint capsule than in other joints tested.

In elderly specimens, Bigliani et al. (74) found that loading the IGHL and inferior pouch to failure caused significant midsubstance strain (56%) at fast rates compared with slow strain rates (35%). The strain occurred most frequently adjacent to the bone but varied significantly along the length of each ligament. Speer et al. (78) found only small increases in anterior translation after surgical creation of a Bankart lesion in cadavers and surmised that some anterior capsular strain must occur to allow dislocation. In contrast, Reeves (79) examined the IGHL and capsule after dislocating cadaveric shoulders traumatically and found that the IGHL avulsed from the bony glenoid rim in 78% of shoulders younger than 40 years of age.

At present, it remains unclear whether significant plastic deformation of the IGHL occurs in the younger patient after a traumatic dislocation. Creating traumatic shoulder instability in a cadaver is difficult to impossible, and simply measuring translational laxity before and after creation of a Bankart lesion will never duplicate the complex *in vivo* event of a traumatic dislocation. Furthermore, it is conceivable that subsequent healing of any capsular deformation (especially after protracted immobilization) would result in a contracted rather than elongated capsule. Finally, previous clinical reports of excellent results after simple repair of the Bankart lesion without any capsular tightening suggest that plastic deformation of the IGHL may not be a clinically relevant problem (68).

Several studies have focused on the functional limitations of commonly employed reconstruction operations. Speer et al. (80) studied the effect of superior versus medial capsular shifts after Bankart reconstruction. The superior capsular shift was found to significantly reduce posterior and inferior translation in the 45-degree abducted position when compared with the medial capsular shift. Others have reported a 40% to 67% decrease in external rotation with anterior capsular shortening (81). Therefore, surgical "correction" of presumed capsular deformation may eliminate too much normal glenohumeral laxity. Recall that the capsular ligamentous mechanism provides a restraint when the joint is in a situation that is likely to overwhelm all other passive and active stabilizing mechanisms. Capsular constraint operates *only* near the limit of joint motion. In the midrange, a loose capsule accommodates normal glenohumeral motion. Formerly, shortening of the anterior capsule and subscapularis functionally was recommended for recurrent anterior instability (60,61). If too much laxity were removed, rotation would be restricted and attempts to recover full motion would invoke the capsular constraint mechanism prematurely. When the capsule becomes tight in a midrange position, it not only restricts motion but forcibly translates the head from its reduced position and applies high compressive and shear loads to the glenoid articular surface. The end result of this process has been described clinically (82) and was termed "capsulorrhaphy arthropathy" by Matsen et al. (2).

Loss of ligamentous stabilization by the IGHL is not the only deficiency in the patient with recurrent traumatic instability. These patients also have varying defects of glenoid concavity secondary to avulsion of the anteroinferior glenoid labrum, a decrease in the height of the thicker peripheral cartilage of the glenoid, and possibly even fracture of the glenoid rim (Fig. 30.19). This loss of concavity diminishes the effectiveness of all the midrange stabilizing mechanisms (Table 30.2). Simple ligamentous reattachment, therefore, may not be sufficient if the repair does not concomitantly restore the glenoid depth (Fig. 30.20). We have reported our open and arthroscopic technique of Bankart repair designed to reattach the labrum to the

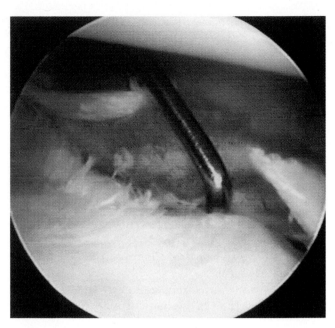

FIGURE 30.19 Traumatic dislocation of the humeral head avulses the anterior capsular and labral attachment from the glenoid rim. The depth of the glenoid concavity is further reduced by abrasive shearing of the articular cartilage and/or fracture of the bony rim. An osseous Bankart lesion occurs in one third of traumatic dislocations.

glenoid rim, deepen the glenoid concavity, and restore the capsular ligamentous constraint (68,69) (Fig. 30.21).

Atraumatic Instability

The typical patient with atraumatic instability does not have a capsulolabral avulsion (Bankart lesion) (83) but instead may have increased capsular volume, increased capsular compliance, labral insufficiency, glenoid flattening, neuromuscular imbalance, or a host of other abnormalities that are more difficult to understand and treat (Table 30.2). Again, the treating physician's goal is to assist the patient in reestablishing sufficient stabilizing mechanisms without encroaching on normal physiology.

When treating atraumatic instability surgically, the surgeon must attempt to correct for instability and not physiologic laxity. Most surgical reconstructions for atraumatic instability simply involve various designs of capsular tightening. As stated earlier, however, many normal shoulders have abundant laxity, and many unstable shoulders have less laxity than what seems "normal." In a follow-up study of patients who underwent inferior capsular shift for multidirectional instability, excessive tightness of the shoulder and pain after surgery correlated more with patient dissatisfaction than did residual instability (84). The surgeon's goal should be not only to eliminate laxity but also to optimize all active and passive stabilizing mechanisms for this multifactorial condition. The surgeon's inability to reconstruct all the normal stabilizing mechanisms leads us to prefer

TABLE 30.2 MECHANISMS OF TRAUMATIC AND ATRAUMATIC INSTABILITY

Structural Pathology	Compromised Stability Mechanism
Structural deficiency in traumatic instability	
Glenolabral concavity	Peripheral cartilage avulsion, flattening, and erosion
	Glenoid rim fracture, bony erosion, irregular subchondral bony concavity associated with a depressed, malunited fracture
	Labral avulsion from the glenoid rim and labral disruption
Capsular ligaments	Ligamentous discontinuity, avulsion from the glenoid rim
Rotator cuff (posterior mechanism)	Posterosuperior cuff tear (supraspinatus and infraspinatus tear)
	Disruption of subscapularis
Humeral head lesion	Hill–Sachs defect
Structural deficiency in atraumatic instability	
Glenolabral concavity	Flattening of the glenoid surface (glenoid plana)
	Glenoid hypoplasia
	Posterior glenoid rim rounding
	Labral instability, tears, fraying
Capsular ligaments	Absence of ligamentous structure (no anterior glenohumeral ligaments)
	Excessive capsular compliance (ligamentous laxity)
	Capsular redundancy
	Incompetent rotator interval capsule
Rotator cuff	Asymmetric weakness of cuff
	Neuromuscular dyscoordination
Scapulothoracic coordination	Abnormal humeroscapular rhythm
Loss of concavity for concavity–compression	
	Loss of joint congruity
	Loss of negative intraarticular pressure
	Decrease in balance stability angle
	Loss of labral valve for glenoid suction cup
	Loss of proprioceptive balance
	Loss of ligamentous checkrein to excessive rotation
	Loss of capsular constraint mechanism
	Loss of finite joint volume
Decrease in load for concavity–compression	
	Loss of finite joint volume
	Loss of negative intraarticular pressure
	Abnormality in muscle balance
	Loss of musculotendinous wrap
	Loss of joint congruity
	Loss of muscle balance

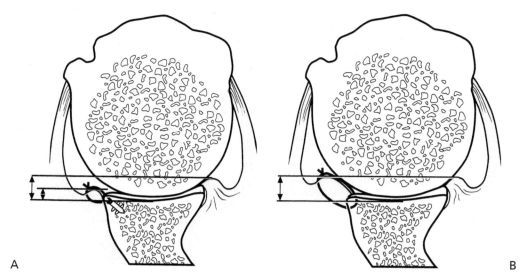

FIGURE 30.20 A: The capsular labrum must not be repaired to the anterior glenoid neck or adjacent to the deficient cartilage. **B:** The labral "valve" must be repaired up onto the glenoid rim to deepen and reconstitute the glenoid concavity and extend the congruent articular surface of the glenoid fossa.

nonoperative rehabilitation to a "laxity-reducing" capsular shift (85) that might compromise range of motion yet not restore stability.

Glenoid and Humeral Bone Loss in Instability

In some patients, glenohumeral instability has been refractory to multiple soft tissue procedures. These patients often

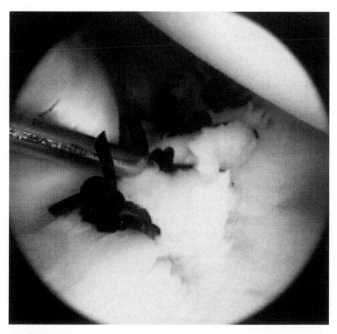

FIGURE 30.21 Arthroscopic view of an anatomic reattachment of the capsulolabral complex to the glenoid rim. Note the deepening of the glenoid concavity.

display severe deficiencies of their glenoid concavity (Fig. 30.22). As we have shown in the laboratory, reconstruction of glenoid concavity can lead to enhanced translatory stability in the "dish-deficient" glenoid (13). It may be that "dish deepening" is necessary in addition to ligamentous reconstruction or capsular tightening in these individuals. Several possible operative techniques, including anterior glenoid bone grafting (86) and posterior glenoid osteotomy, may be options for those patients who lack glenoid concavity and who experience primarily either anterior or posterior instability.

Posterior humeral head defects occur frequently in patients with traumatic instability. The impact of the Hill–Sachs lesion on further instability depends primarily on the size of the defect. Instability related to the Hill–Sachs lesion occurs as the humeral head lesion is rotated onto the anterior glenoid rim. Several options exist for treatment of this facet of the instability. If the humeral head lesion is small and contacts the anterior glenoid rim during terminal external rotation, an anterior capsular shortening procedure will produce the desired restraint. A surprisingly small amount of shortening is required to produce the desired restriction. For each 1 cm of shortening, external rotation is reduced by 20 degrees. For slightly larger deficits that would require a more significant reduction in external rotation, Connolly and Harryman (87) suggested transferring the infraspinatus tendon with a portion of the greater tuberosity into the defect. This effectively renders the humeral head defect extracapsular. When larger defects occur, which may approach 40% of the humeral head, consideration should be made toward humeral head replacement with a hemiarthroplasty.

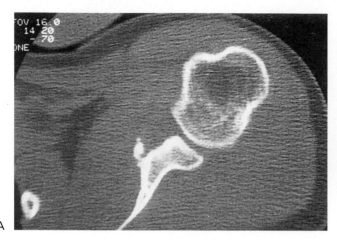
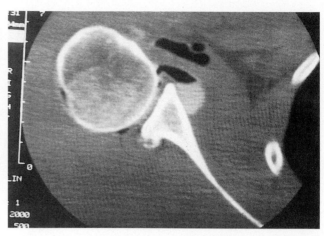

FIGURE 30.22 A: Axial computed tomograph of a patient with a large anterior glenoid deficiency resulting from chronic recurrent anteroinferior instability. **B:** Axial computed tomograph showing posterior glenoid erosion in this patient with chronic atraumatic posteroinferior

CONCLUSION

There exists in the shoulder a family of mechanisms that maintain glenohumeral stability. These mechanisms have varying degrees of importance depending on humerothoracic position and externally applied loads. Whether treating a patient with exercises or surgery, and whether operating by open or arthroscopic means, the physician must try to identify the mechanisms creating insufficient stability and provide an appropriate treatment.

Surgical reconstruction for shoulder instability should be directed at restoring the integrity or improving the function of the static restraints and rehabilitating the dynamic stabilizers that provide function to the glenohumeral joint.

REFERENCES

1. Matsen FA III. Overview and directions for future research. In: Matsen FA III, Fu FH, Hawkins RJ, eds. *The shoulder: a balance of mobility and stability.* Rosemont, IL: American Academy of Orthopaedic Surgeons, 1993:3.
2. Matsen FA III, Lippitt SB, Sidles JA, Harryman DT II. *Practical evaluation of management of the shoulder.* Philadelphia: WB Saunders, 1994.
3. Moskal MJ, Harryman DT II, Romeo AA, et al. Glenohumeral motion after complete capsular release. *Arthroscopy* 1999;15:408–416.
4. Harryman DT II, Sidles JA, Matsen FA III. Laxity of the normal glenohumeral joint: a quantitative in vivo assessment. *J Shoulder Elbow Surg* 1992;1:66–76.
5. Lippitt SB, Harris SA, Sidles JA, et al. In vivo quantification of the laxity of normal and unstable glenohumeral joints. *Orthop Trans* 1992;16:666.
6. Harryman DT II, Walker ED, Harris SL, et al. Residual motion and function after glenohumeral or scapulothoracic arthrodesis. *J Shoulder Elbow Surg* 1993;2:275–285.
7. Pearl ML, Harris SL, Lippitt SB, et al. A system for describing positions of the humerus relative to the thorax and its use in the presentation of several functionally important arm positions. *J Shoulder Elbow Surg* 1992;1:113–118.
8. Harryman DT II, Sidles JA, Clark JM, et al. Translation of the humeral head on the glenoid with passive glenohumeral motion. *J Bone Joint Surg Am* 1990;72:1334–1343.
9. Lippitt SB, Vanderhooft JE, Harris SL, et al. Glenohumeral stability from concavity–compression: a quantitative analysis. *J Shoulder Elbow Surg Am* 1993;2:27–35.
10. Soslowsky LJ, Bigliani LU, Flatow EL, et al. Articular geometry of the glenohumeral joint. *Clin Orthop* 1992;285:181–190.
11. Howell SM, Galinat BJ. The glenoid-labral socket: a constrained articular surface. *Clin Orthop* 1989;43:122–125.
12. Fukuda K, Chen CM, Cofield RH, et al. Biomechanical analysis of stability and fixation strength of total shoulder prostheses. *Orthopaedics* 1988;11:141–149.
13. Lazarus MD, Sidles JA, Harryman DT II, et al. Effect of a chondral-labral defect on glenoid concavity and glenohumeral stability: a cadaveric model. *J Bone Joint Surg Am* 1996;78:94–102.
14. Bigliani LU, Newton PM, Steinmann SP, et al. Glenoid rim lesions associated with recurrent anterior dislocation of the shoulder. *Am J Sports Med* 1998;26:41–45.
15. Cain PR, Mitschler T, Fu FH, et al. Anterior stability of the glenohumeral joint: a dynamic model. *Am J Sports Med* 1987;15:144–148.
16. Bey MJ, Elders GJ, Huston LJ, et al. The mechanism of creation of superior labrum, anterior, and posterior lesions in a dynamic biomechanical model of the shoulder: the role of inferior subluxation. *J Shoulder Elbow Surg* 1998;7:397–401.
17. Pagnani MJ, Deng XH, Warren RF, et al. Effect of lesions of the superior portion of the glenoid labrum on glenohumeral translation. *J Bone Joint Surg Am* 1995;77:1003–1010.
18. Rodosky MW, Harner CD, Fu FH. The role of the long head of the biceps muscle and superior glenoid labrum in anterior stability of the shoulder. *Am J Sports Med* 1994;22:121–130.
19. Howell SM, Kraft TA. The role of the supraspinatus and infraspinatus muscles in glenohumeral kinematics of anterior shoulder instability. *Clin Orthop* 1991;263:128–134.
20. Blasier RB, Guldberg RE, Rothman ED. Anterior shoulder stability: contributions of rotator cuff forces and the capsular ligaments in a cadaver model. *J Shoulder Elbow Surg* 1992;1:140–150.
21. Bassett RW, Browne AO, Morrey BF, et al. Glenohumeral muscle force and moment mechanics in a position of shoulder instability. *J Biomech* 1990;23:405–415.

22. Hasselman CT, Apreleva M, Debski RE, et al. A dynamic analysis of capsulolabral injury in the shoulder. *Orthop Trans* 1997;21: 103–2.

23. Malicky DM, Soslowsky LJ, Blasier RB. Inferior glenohumeral subluxation: active and passive stabilization in a biomechanical model. *Orthop Trans* 1995–1996;19(4):901.

24. Wirth MA, Lyons FR, Rockwood CA. Hypoplasia of the glenoid: a review of sixteen patients. *J Bone Joint Surg Am* 1993;75: 1175–1183.

25. Flatow EL, Soslowsky LJ, Ateshian GA, et al. Shoulder joint anatomy and the effect of subluxations and size mismatch on patterns of glenohumeral contact. *Orthop Trans* 1991;15:803.

26. Moseley HF, Overgaard B. The anterior capsular mechanism in recurrent anterior dislocation of the shoulder: morphological and clinical studies with special reference to the glenoid labrum and glenohumeral ligaments. *J Bone Joint Surg Br* 1962;44:913–927.

27. Humphry GM. *A treatise on the human skeleton (including the joints).* London: Macmillan, 1858:410:73–74.

28. Kumar VP, Balasubramaniam P. The role of atmospheric pressure in stabilising the shoulder. *J Bone Joint Surg Br* 1985;67: 719–721.

29. Gibb TD, Harryman DT II, Sidles JA, et al. The effect of capsular venting on glenohumeral laxity. *Clin Orthop* 1991;268: 120–127.

30. Habermeyer P, Schuller U, Wiedemann E. The intra-articular pressure of the shoulder: an experimental study on the role of the glenoid labrum in stabilizing the joint. *J Arthroscopy* 1992;8: 166–172.

31. Neer CS II. *Shoulder reconstruction.* Philadelphia: WB Saunders, 1990:288–298,390,398.

32. Lubowitz J, Bartolozzi A, Rubinstein D, et al. How much does inferior capsular shift reduce shoulder volume? *Clin Orthop* 1996;328:86–90.

33. Vahey JW, Lippitt SB, Matsen FA III. Humeroscapular balance: the limits of angular stability provided by glenoid geometry. *Orthop Trans* 1994;17:1021.

34. Blasier RB, Carpenter JE, Huston LJ. Shoulder proprioception: effect of joint laxity, joint position, and direction of motion. *Orthop Rev* 1994;23:45–50.

35. Inman VT, Saunders JBDM, Abbott LC. Observations on the function of the shoulder joint. *J Bone Joint Surg Am* 1994;76: 1–30.

36. Poppen NK, Walker PS. Forces at the glenohumeral joint in abduction. *Clin Orthop* 1978;135:165–170.

37. Warner JJ, Micheli LJ, Arslanian LE, et al. Scapulothoracic motion in normal shoulders and shoulders with glenohumeral instability and impingement syndrome: a study using moiré topographic analysis. *Clin Orthop* 1992;285:191–199.

38. Ozaki J. Glenohumeral movement of the involuntary inferior and multidirectional instability. *Clin Orthop* 1989;238:107–111.

39. McMahon PJ, Jobe FW, Pink MM, et al. Comparative electromyographic analysis of shoulder muscles during planar motions: anterior glenohumeral instability versus normal. *J Shoulder Elbow Surg* 1996;5:118–123.

40. Simkin PA. Synovial physiology. In: McCarty DJ, ed. *Arthritis and allied conditions.* 11th ed. Philadelphia: Lea and Febiger; 1989.

41. McCarty Jr DJ, ed. *Synovial fluid, arthritis and allied conditions,* 9th ed. Philadelphia: Lea and Febiger; 1979:51–69.

42. DePalma AF, Callery G, Bennett GA. Variational anatomy and degenerative lesions of the shoulder joint. *Instr Course Lect* 1949;6:255–281.

43. Ferrari DA. Capsular ligaments of the shoulder: anatomical and functional study of the anterior superior capsule. *Am J Sports Med* 1990;18:20–24.

44. Harryman DT II, Sidles JA, Harris S, et al. The role of the rotator interval capsule in passive motion and stability of the shoulder. *J Bone Joint Surg Am* 1992;74:53–66.

45. Warner JJ, Deng XH, Warren RF, et al. Static capsuloligamentous restraints to superior-inferior translation of the glenohumeral joint. *Am J Sports Med* 1992;20:675–685.

46. Basmajian JV, Bazant FJ. Factors preventing downward dislocation of the adducted shoulder joint. *J Bone Joint Surg Am* 1959; 41:1182–1186.

47. Neer CS II, Satterlee CC, Dalsey RM, et al. On the value of the coracohumeral ligament release. *Orthop Trans* 1989;13:235–236.

48. Nobuhara K, Ikeda H. Rotator interval lesion. *Clin Orthop* 1987;223:44–50.

49. Symeonides PP. The significance of the subscapularis muscle in the pathogenesis of recurrent anterior dislocation of the shoulder. *J Bone Joint Surg Br* 1972;54:476–483.

50. Terry GC, Hammon D, France P. The stabilizing function of passive shoulder restraints. *Am J Sports Med* 1991;19:26–34.

51. Turkel SJ, Panio MW, Marshall JL, et al. Stabilizing mechanisms preventing anterior dislocation of the glenohumeral joint. *J Bone Joint Surg Am* 1981;63:1208–1217.

52. Morgan CD, Rames RD, Snyder SJ. Arthroscopic assessment of anatomic variants of the glenohumeral ligaments associated with recurrent anterior shoulder instability. *Orthop Trans* 1992;15: 727.

53. O'Connell PW, Nuber GW, Mileski RA, et al. The contribution of the glenohumeral ligaments to anterior stability of the shoulder joint. *Am J Sports Med* 1991;18:579–584.

54. O'Brien SJ, Neves MC, Arnoczky SP, et al. The anatomy and histology of the inferior glenohumeral ligament complex of the shoulder. *Am J Sports Med* 1990;18:449–456.

55. Warren RF, Kornblatt IB, Marchand R. Static factors affecting posterior shoulder stability. *Orthop Trans* 1984;8:89.

56. Matsen FA III, Harryman DT II, Sidles JA. Mechanics of glenohumeral instability. *Clin Sports Med* 1991;10:783–788.

57. Clark JM, Sidles JA, Matsen FA III. The relationship of the glenohumeral joint capsule to the rotator cuff. *Clin Orthop* 1990;254:29–34.

58. Clark JM, Harryman DT II. Tendons, ligaments, and capsule of the rotator cuff: gross and microscopic anatomy. *J Bone Joint Surg Am* 1992;74:713–725.

59. Saha AK. Dynamic stability of the glenohumeral joint. *Acta Orthop Scand* 1971;42:491–505.

60. Magnuson PB, Stack JK. Recurrent dislocation of the shoulder. *JAMA* 1943;123:889–892.

61. Osmond-Clarke H. Habitual dislocation of the shoulder: the Putti–Platt operation. *J Bone Joint Surg Br* 1948;30:19–25.

62. McKernan DJ, Fu FH. Shoulder biomechanics. In: McGinty JB, ed. *Operative arthroscopy.* New York: Raven Press, 1991.

63. Bankart ASB. Recurrent or habitual dislocation of the shoulder joint. *Br Med J* 1923;2:1132–1133.

64. Broca A, Hartman H. Contribution a l'étude des luxations de l'épaule. *Bull Soc Anat Paris* 1890;4:312–336.

65. Perthes G. Uber operationen bei habitueller schulterluxation. *Dtsch Z Chir* 1906;85:199–222.

66. Bankart ASB. The pathology and treatment of recurrent dislocation of the shoulder joint. *Br J Surg* 1938;26:23–29.

67. Rowe CR, Patel D, Southmayd WW. The Bankart procedure: long-term end-result study. *J Bone Joint Surg Am* 1978;60:1–16.

68. Thomas SC, Matsen FA III. An approach to the repair of glenohumeral ligament avulsion in the management of traumatic anterior glenohumeral instability. *J Bone Joint Surg Am* 1989;71: 506–513.

69. Harryman DT II, Ballmer FP, Harris SL, et al. Arthroscopic labral repair to the glenoid rim. *J Arthroscopy* 1994;10:20–30.

70. Townley CO. The capsular mechanism in recurrent dislocation of the shoulder. *J Bone Joint Surg Am* 1950;32:370–380.
71. Craig EV. The posterior mechanism of acute anterior shoulder dislocations. *Clin Orthop* 1984;190:212–216.
72. Ovesen J, Nielsen S. Anterior and posterior shoulder instability: a cadaver study. *Acta Orthop Scand* 1986;57:324–327.
73. Altchek DW, Warren RF, Skyhar MJ, et al. T-plasty modification of the Bankart procedure for multidirectional instability of the anterior and inferior types. *J Bone Joint Surg Am* 1991;73:105–112.
74. Bigliani LU, Pollock RG, Soslowsky LJ. Tensile properties of the inferior glenohumeral ligament. *J Orthop Res* 1992;10:187–197.
75. Grana WA, Buckley PD, Yates CK. Arthroscopic Bankart suture repair. *Am J Sports Med* 1993;21:348–353.
76. Wolf EM, Wilk RM, Richmond JC. Arthroscopic Bankart repair using suture anchors. *Oper Tech Orthop* 1991;1:184–191.
77. Kaltsas DS. Comparative study of the properties of the shoulder joint capsule with those of other joint capsules. *Clin Orthop* 1983;173:20–26.
78. Speer KP, Deng X, Borrero S, et al. A biomechanical evaluation of the Bankart lesion. *J Bone Joint Surg Am* 1994;76:1819–1826.
79. Reeves B. Experiments on the tensile strength of the anterior capsular structures of the shoulder in man. *J Bone Joint Surg Br* 1968;50:858–865.
80. Speer KP, Deng X, Torzilli PA, et al. Strategies for an anterior capsular shift of the shoulder: a biomechanical comparison. *Am J Sports Med* 1995;23:264–269.
81. Black KP, Lim TH, McGrady LM, et al. In vitro evaluation of shoulder external rotation after a Bankart reconstruction. *Am J Sports Med* 1997;25:449–453.
82. Hawkins RJ, Angelo RL. Glenohumeral osteoarthrosis: a late complication of the Putti–Platt repair. *J Bone Joint Surg Am* 1990;72:1193–1197.
83. Cooper RA, Brems JJ. The inferior capsular-shift procedure for multidirectional instability of the shoulder. *J Bone Joint Surg Am* 1992;74:1516–1521.
84. Neer CS II, Foster CR. Inferior capsular shift for involuntary inferior and multidirectional instability of the shoulder. *J Bone Joint Surg Am* 1980;62:897–908.
85. Burkhead WZJ, Rockwood CAJ. Treatment of instability of the shoulder with an exercise program. *J Bone Joint Surg Am* 1992;74:890–896.
86. Churchill RS, Moskal M, Lippitt S, et al. Extracapsular anatomically contoured anterior glenoid bone grafting for complex glenohumeral instability. *Tech Shoulder Elbow Surg* (submitted).
87. Lazarus MD, Harryman DT II. Complications of open anterior stabilization of the shoulder. *J Am Acad Orthop Surg* 2000;8:122–132.

ARTHROSCOPIC INSTABILITY REPAIRS: ANTERIOR, POSTERIOR, MULTIDIRECTIONAL, AND MICROINSTABILITY REPAIRS

CHRISTOPHER K. JONES
LARRY D. FIELD
FELIX H. SAVOIE III

Although glenohumeral instability was once thought to occur predominantly in the anterior and inferior directions and result from a traumatic dislocation of the shoulder, it is now apparent that instability represents a wide spectrum of pathology (1–83). Glenohumeral stability is dependent on both static and dynamic forces about the joint. The dynamic stabilizers include the rotator cuff musculature and the other muscles of the shoulder girdle. The static stabilizers include the labrum, glenohumeral ligaments, coracohumeral ligament, and rotator interval capsule. Dysfunction or pathology of these dynamic or static stabilizers leads to pathologic laxity of the shoulder. This chapter addresses the pathology related to each of the defined instabilities and its arthroscopic management.

PATHOLOGY

Instability of the shoulder in any direction is due to increased translation of the humeral head on the glenoid in excess of what is considered normal for a specific individual (4–15). This is an important point because the degree of normal glenohumeral laxity can vary a tremendous amount between individuals. For instability to be clinically significant, symptoms must be present. There are several mechanisms that are responsible for maintaining the articulation (4–15). Maintenance of a negative intraarticular pressure is one of these mechanisms. This force is evident during cadaveric dissection. The shoulder remains reduced in the ab-

sence of muscle activity until the capsule is vented. The estimated stability force is relatively small at 20 to 30 pounds.

Concavity-compression is another mechanism that contributes to glenohumeral stability (11,15). This force results from the dynamic compression of the humeral head into the glenoid socket by the rotator cuff musculature. It is responsible for maintaining stability of the shoulder in the midranges of motion. Matsen et al. (11) have estimated this force to be 40% efficient, where 100 pounds of compression could withstand 40 pounds of a translating force. The concavity of the glenoid is greatly increased by the presence of the labrum at its margin. Lippitt et al. (17) have reported on the stabilizing effects of the labrum in shoulders subjected to a compressive load. The labrum also seems to act as a stress transitionary or "chock-block" between the more elastic ligaments of the capsule and the rigid bone of the glenoid (13–17). The concavity-compression force is reduced by 50% if the labrum is excised (11,16). This dynamic mechanism of maintaining stability is the main focus of the rehabilitative efforts for patients with symptomatic instability.

The most effective stabilizers of the glenohumeral joint at the end ranges of motion are the capsule and glenohumeral ligaments (4–18) (Fig. 31.1). They act as static stabilizers of the joint. These ligaments become more important in the presence of rotator cuff dysfunction when the concavity compression mechanism is not functioning (4–18). The role of these ligaments in preventing abnormal translation of the humeral head has been investigated in several studies (1,2,4–18).

The anterior band of the inferior glenohumeral ligament (IGHL) is the primary stabilizer limiting anterior translation in the 90-degree abducted shoulder (4–19) (Fig. 31.2). The role of the anterior band of the IGHL as an anterior restraint becomes less important in lesser degrees of abduction, and the middle glenohumeral ligament (MGHL) plays

C. K. Jones: Mississippi Sports Medicine and Orthopaedic Center, Jackson, Mississippi.
L. D. Field and F. H. Savoie III: Upper Extremity Service, Mississippi Sports Medicine and Orthopaedic Center; Department of Orthopaedic Surgery, University of Mississippi School of Medicine, Jackson, Mississippi.

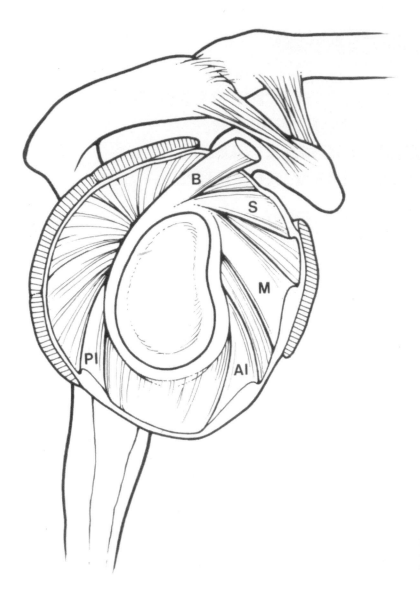

FIGURE 31.1 Glenohumeral ligaments. B, biceps tendon; S, superior glenohumeral ligament; M, middle glenohumeral ligament; AI, intrainferior glenohumeral ligament; PI, posterior inferior ligament.

a more important role (4–19) (Fig. 31.3). The entire IGHL may be avulsed during certain traumatic events (Fig. 31.4). A straight inferior dislocation tears both the anterior and posterior bands as well as the intervening sling of the IGHL (10–13,15,16). This type of tear results in multidirectional instability (MDI), which can also occur in patients without a traumatic dislocation. The underlying pathoanatomy is believed to be a redundancy of the IGHL complex, with resultant increase in capsular volume (20). Patients with MDI usually have a baseline of increased capsular volume and glenohumeral laxity. A traumatic episode may cause either gross capsular tears or microtears with plastic deformation. Following this trauma, patients develop abnormal glenohumeral mechanics and overload of rotator cuff and periscapular muscles. The dysfunctional rotator cuff fails to provide for concavity compression of the joint, which leads to increased translation. Ultimately patients develop secondary impingement or rotator cuff tendinitis, and worsen-

ing degrees of instability from mild subluxation to frank dislocation (21).

Unlike anterior instability, there does not appear to be one essential lesion responsible for producing posterior instability. Schwartz et al. (22) demonstrated that simply incising the posterior capsule alone did not result in posterior instability. For dislocation to occur in the flexed, adducted, and internally rotated shoulder, the anterior-superior capsule had to be incised in addition to the posterior capsule. The importance of the anterior-superior quadrant in posterior instability was also demonstrated by Harryman et al. (14).

The anterior-superior quadrant of the glenohumeral joint, which includes the MGHL, superior glenohumeral ligament (SGHL), coracohumeral ligament (CHL), and the rotator interval capsule, is an anatomic area that contributes significantly to shoulder stability (14,22–29) (Fig. 31.5). The MGHL shows considerable variability in its anatomic

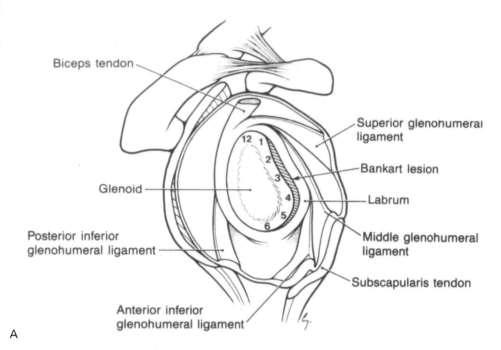

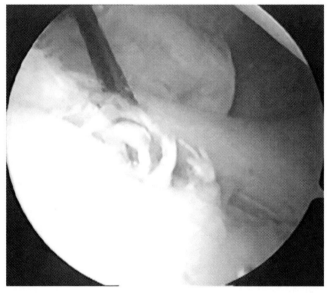

FIGURE 31.2 A: Drawing of a Bankart lesion. **B:** Arthroscopic view of a Bankart lesion.

form (27,28). One variation is a cordlike MGHL that inserts near the attachment of the SGHL along with an absent anterior-superior labrum (28) (Fig. 31.6). This was described by Snyder's group (28) and coined the "Buford complex." More commonly, two distinct forms of the middle glenohumeral ligament are noted. One is a more thickened structure similar to the anterior band of the IGHL that attaches to the anterior-superior labrum and is associated with a sublabral hole. A second variation is a less discrete band wrapping around the subscapularis and inserting into the SGHL. This dual complex of the middle and superior glenohumeral ligaments then inserts into the glenoid labrum at approximately the 1 o'clock position. It has been noted that avulsions of this MGHL attachment often result

in direct anterior instability (30). The MGHL is recognized as an important secondary restraint to both inferior and anterior translations (12,15,16). The SGHL is seen as a large structure inserting adjacent to the biceps tendon (12,15,16,30,31). This ligament resists anterior and superior translation of the humeral head in shoulder flexion and lesser degrees of abduction (12,15,16,31,32). Warner et al. (32) and Schwartz et al. (22) have also demonstrated that the SGHL plays an important role in posterior and inferior stability. The SGHL is often found avulsed in patients with symptomatic superior labral detachment lesions (1,12,15,16,30–32). This destabilization of the superior aspect of the glenohumeral joint allows an unopposed vector pull by the deltoid on the outstretched arm resulting in sec-

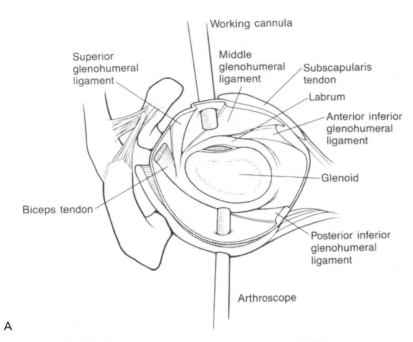

A

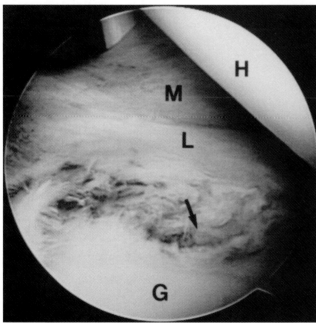

B

FIGURE 31.3 A: Illustration of middle glenohumeral ligament tear. **B:** Arthroscopic view of middle glenohumeral ligament tear. M, middle glenohumeral ligament; G, glenoid; L, labrum; H, humerus.

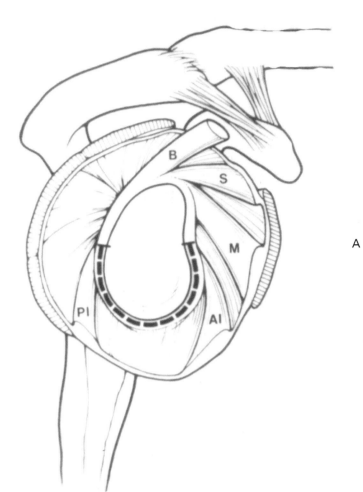

FIGURE 31.4 Disruption of entire inferior glenohumeral ligament complex results in multidirectional instability.

"Buford" Complex

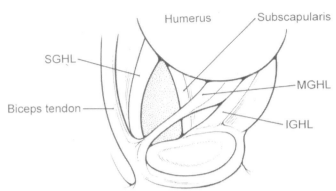

A

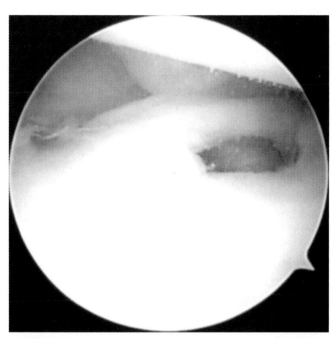

B

FIGURE 31.6 A: Illustration of the Buford complex. **B:** Arthroscopic view of cord-like middle glenohumeral ligament (MGHL) and absorb anterior-superior labrum.

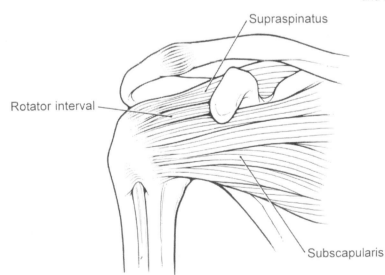

FIGURE 31.5 The rotator interval is bordered above by the supraspinatus tendon and below by the subscapularis tendon. Its medial margin is the coracoid process and the apex of this triangular-shaped interval ends laterally at the transverse humeral ligament.

ondary impingement (23,32). Tears or insufficiencies of the capsule or labrum in this area can also result in anterior-superior instability as proposed by Field and Savoie (31,33). Because of the variable anatomy in the anterior-superior quadrant, differentiating pathologic lesions from normal anatomic variants often requires putting together the information obtained from the history and physical examination with the arthroscopic findings. Patients with symptoms related to the anterior-superior quadrant often present with secondary rotator cuff tendinitis and do not have a history of frank dislocation.

ANTERIOR INSTABILITY—HISTORICAL PERSPECTIVE AND RESULTS

The anterior band of the IGHL is the primary stabilizer limiting anterior translation in the 90-degree abducted shoulder (4–19). Bankart (1) described the detachment of this ligament from the anterior margin of the glenoid articular surface as the typical lesion found with recurrent anterior shoulder dislocation. They also described the repair of the avulsed capsulolabral structures to the glenoid rim through an open approach. Repair of the Bankart lesion has become the standard form of treatment for patients with traumatic anterior instability (1–4,7–9,12,15,19,35–43). Open reconstruction has been considered the standard treatment and has success rates ranging from 80% to 97% (1–4,7–9,12,15,19,35–43). Problems associated with open reconstruction have related to motion loss and lack of ability to return to high-level activities (41–46). An important point regarding the treatment of traumatic anterior instability is that the Bankart lesion is often accompanied by interstitial damage to the capsule itself. This leads to increased capsular volume and less of a static restraint to anterior translation. A biomechanical study performed by Speer et al. (19) demonstrated that simply detaching the anterior-inferior labrum would not allow an anterior dislocation. Proponents of the open procedure state that it is easier to address the increased capsular laxity by performing a capsulorrhaphy or shift procedure. We do not think that our ability to perform a capsular shift is compromised by the arthroscopic technique.

Advances in technology have led to the development of multiple arthroscopic techniques to repair the Bankart lesion. The proposed advantages of performing the procedure via the arthroscope are less surgical morbidity, a better cosmetic result, and better overall range of motion and function. Initial attempts at arthroscopic reconstruction were performed with metallic staples (47–51). The results with this technique were unsatisfactory, with a high level of complications related to use of the metallic implants adjacent to the articular surface. The next evolution of the arthroscopic reconstruction was transglenoid suture tech-

niques (52–62). The success rates were variable, with 44% to 93% success, and there was a risk of suprascapular nerve injury with transglenoid drilling and the need for a second incision. Further, some reports suggested the procedure was not as successful in patients younger than 25 years old who would place high demands on the shoulder (55,56, 59–62).

The next technique to be developed utilized absorbable tacks to secure the labrum to the glenoid neck (43,44,56, 63,64). Success with this procedure ranged from 79% to 96% (43,44,56,63,64). Failures with this technique were attributed to the inability of the procedure to address increased capsular laxity. The previously described techniques are inherently flawed in that they repair the capsulolabral complex more medial on the glenoid neck, which essentially creates an anterior labroligamentous periosteal sleeve avulsion (ALPSA) lesion (69). More recently, the advent of suture anchors has allowed complete intraarticular repairs to be accomplished that can include a capsular shift procedure when it is necessary (28,52,65–69). Much of the success of the suture anchor technique may be attributable to the ability of the surgeon to repair the capsulolabral complex to its anatomic position at the edge of the articular margin (Fig. 31.7). However, Burkhart and DeBeer (68) have shown that significant bony defects of the glenoid or humeral head are associated with a high rate of recurrent instability following arthroscopic anterior reconstruction. Nevertheless, published reports of arthroscopic anterior reconstruction in appropriately selected patients have yielded recurrence rates similar to the open procedure (5% to 10%), but with less surgical morbidity and improved postoperative range of motion (28,65–69).

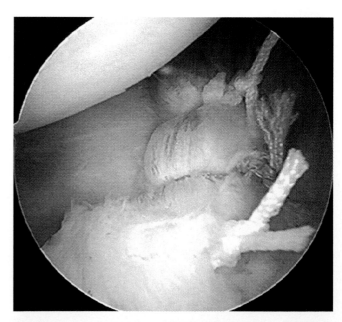

FIGURE 31.7 Suture anchors allow anatomic repair of the capsuloligamentous structures at the glenoid articular margin.

INDICATIONS FOR ARTHROSCOPIC ANTERIOR RECONSTRUCTION

The current indications for operative treatment of anterior instability include patients of all ages and all activity levels with recurrent instability who are functionally impaired by their instability and who have failed nonoperative management. Whether the procedure is performed arthroscopically or open depends on the preoperative examination and the findings at diagnostic arthroscopy. The preoperative examination should reveal isolated anterior or anterior-inferior instability for the arthroscopic anterior reconstruction to be successful. If associated instabilities exist, concomitant procedures will be necessary to address them. Diagnostic arthroscopy is performed on all patients to assess intraarticular pathology. The presence of a large bony defect in the glenoid (>30% of the articular surface) is a contraindication to performing the procedure arthroscopically. Additionally, the surgeon should be an experienced shoulder arthroscopist who is familiar with the various techniques of arthroscopic reconstruction.

BANKART RECONSTRUCTION

Surgical Technique

The patient is placed in the lateral decubitus position for the arthroscopic treatment of both MDI and Bankart lesions. Alternatively, the beach-chair position can be utilized as well. The arm is suspended with 10 to 15 pounds of traction. A standard posterior portal is established in the raphe of the infraspinatus muscle, and a diagnostic arthroscopy is performed. The presence of a Bankart lesion is confirmed, and other pathology is noted. An anterior portal is established using an outside-in technique to ensure proper orientation and access to the inferior glenoid for reconstruction. This portal should allow access at appropriate angles in all three planes to the glenoid rim for anchor placement at the 1, 3, and 5 o'clock positions (Fig. 31.8). Localization with a spinal needle before incising the skin ensures appropriate position.

The Bankart lesion and anterior capsule are evaluated from the anterior portal for associated mid-capsular or humeral-sided tears. The arthroscope is returned posteriorly, and the anterior portal is utilized for debriding and releasing the capsulolabral complex from the glenoid. The release is extended medially along the glenoid neck until the subscapularis muscle can be visualized (Fig. 31.9). The release is also performed inferiorly to the 6 o'clock position (straight inferior) of the glenoid. Care is taken to ensure complete release of the capsulolabral complex. The anterior and inferior glenoid is then abraded to a bleeding surface.

The anterior cannula is removed and a standard Linvatec (Largo, FL) suture punch cannula inserted. The drill guide is introduced through this cannula and placed just at the

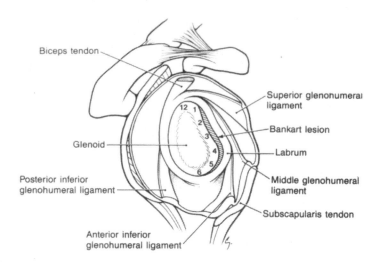

FIGURE 31.8 Schematic representation of Bankart lesion demonstrating avulsion of anterior band of inferior glenohumeral ligament and MGHL. 1, 3, and 6 demonstrate position of anchors, while 2, 4, and 6 represent position of sutures.

edge of the glenoid articular surface at the 5 o'clock position. The drill should angle 45 degrees from the articular surface and be perpendicular to the superior-inferior axis (Fig. 31.10). A suture anchor is inserted and the sutures are tagged with a hemostat. We prefer long-term absorbable anchors and either nonabsorbable or long-term absorbable braided No. 2 suture.

Following placement of the suture anchor, a nonmodified (closed-ended) Caspari suture punch is loaded with a

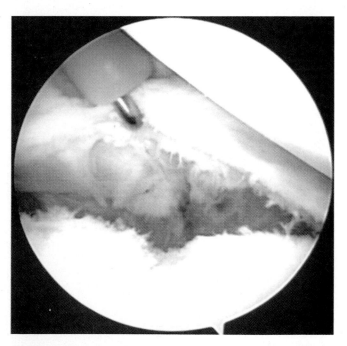

FIGURE 31.9 Arthroscopic image after complete release demonstrating visualization subscapularis muscle beneath capsule.

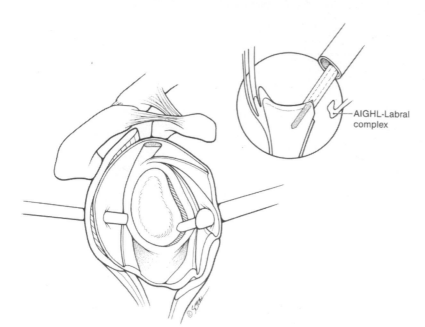

FIGURE 31.10 The drill guide is placed on the glenoid neck face junction at approximately the 5 o'clock position. This should be placed so that approximately half the diameter of the whole is on the articular surface.

48-inch-long 2-0 Prolene suture with two free ends in the punch. The punch is introduced through the anterior cannula, and the capsule at the 6 o'clock position is grasped from inside to outside. The doubled Prolene is then fed through the capsule (Fig. 31.11). As the suture punch is withdrawn through the cannula, the two free ends and the looped end of the Prolene are delivered. One limb of the anchor suture is placed through the "loop" and the two free ends of the Prolene are pulled, dragging the looped end and the anchor suture through the capsule and back out the same cannula. If a mattress stitch is desired, the steps are repeated with the other limb of the suture. Suture placement is critical at this portion of the procedure to allow for adequate tensioning of the capsule. A modified Roeder knot is tied to secure the capsule to the glenoid articular margin (Fig. 31.12).

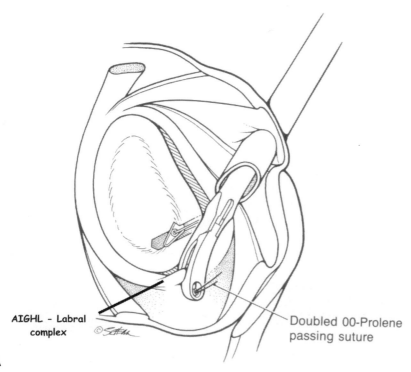

FIGURE 31.11 A: The suture punch is used to thread a 48-inch doubled 2-0 Prolene suture through the inferior glenohumeral ligament complex at approximately the 6 o'clock position.

A

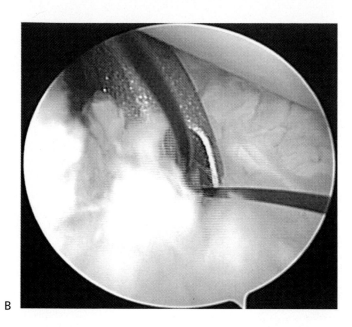

B

FIGURE 31.11 *(continued)* **B:** The suture punch is positioned on the inferior capsule as it is pulled superiorly. The two strands of the 2-0 Prolene suture are then threaded into the glenohumeral joint.

Additional anchors are placed in a similar manner at both the 3 and 1 o'clock positions. As an alternative to this technique, the anchor suture can be delivered through the labrum and capsule with a retrograde suture retriever (Innovasive Devices, Marlborough, MA) (Fig. 31.13). This device simplifies the suture passing but is unable to sufficiently reach the 6 o'-clock position for the most inferior anchor. The complete repair is assessed from both the posterior and anterior portals. The posterior capsule is also assessed and tightened if necessary by suture plication or thermal shrinkage. Prior to removing the arthroscopic equipment the anterior portal is closed and the rotator interval is plicated. This is accomplished by passing a spinal needle through the anterior edge

of the supraspinatus tendon and passing a No. 2 braided suture through this needle. A suture retriever is then passed through the anterior capsule and occasionally the middle glenohumeral ligament below the portal, and the suture is grasped (Fig. 31.14). The suture limbs are then retrieved through the anterior cannula and tied blindly using a modified Roeder knot. This completes the Bankart reconstruction.

Postoperative Management

For the first postoperative week, the patient's arm is supported in a shoulder sling with a small abduction pillow. At 1 week the patient is started on a home exercise program

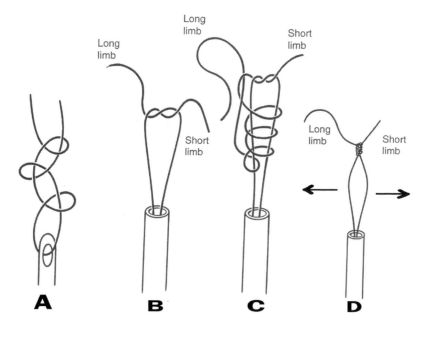

FIGURE 31.12 A: The most secure knot configuration of reversing both throws and posts. **B:** The Roeder knot is accomplished by first throwing the first half of a square knot, leaving one end long and one end short. **C:** The long end is then passed around both limbs of the suture three times, then once around the short limb. The long limb of the suture is then passed through the loop adjacent to the half square knot. **D:** The knot is then compressed by spreading the distal limbs while holding the short limb as a post.

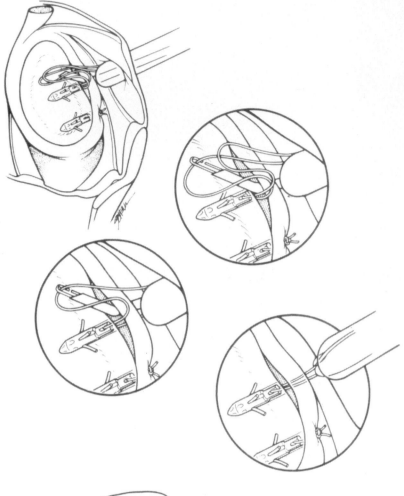

FIGURE 31.13 An alternate method of passing sutures through the labrum for the 3 o'clock and 1 o'clock anchors using the 30-degree suture retriever.

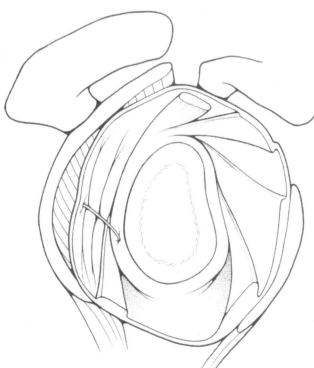

FIGURE 31.14 Lasso stitch of thermal treatment.

composed of shoulder shrugs, passive forward flexion of the shoulder, and passive external rotation, taking care not to cause pain with exercising. These exercises are continued for 2 weeks. At 3 weeks, active internal and external rotation are commenced at the waist level with a TheraBand and continued for another 3 weeks. At 6 weeks, formal physical therapy is initiated, emphasizing active range of motion with rotator cuff strengthening and no stretching. Plyometric exercises may begin at 2 months followed by return to low-velocity throwing at 3 months. Return to contact sports and aggressive sport-specific drilling is determined on an individual basis and is usually delayed until 4 months postoperatively if possible.

MULTIDIRECTIONAL INSTABILITY

Historical Perspective and Results

Multidirectional instability (MDI) of the shoulder is a condition in which symptomatic laxity is present in more than one direction: anterior, posterior, and inferior. The cause of MDI is multifactorial and not completely understood. Many shoulders with excessive laxity are asymptomatic. A traumatic event, repetitive microtrauma, fatigue, or deconditioning of the dynamic muscular stabilizers may cause a symptomatic, lax shoulder to become symptomatic. Despite an incomplete understanding of the pathophysiology of MDI, anatomic abnormalities can be recognized. At arthroscopy an abnormally increased space in the glenohumeral joint is observed. This has been referred to as a "drive-through" sign in which the arthroscope can be easily passed from the posterior to the anterior aspect of the joint. Additionally, a large inferior capsular pouch and a widened rotator interval are observed.

Since Neer and Foster (20) reported the first series of patients with MDI in 1980, it has been recognized with increased frequency. They described an inferior capsular shift procedure that produced satisfactory results in 31 of their 32 patients. The procedure is performed by shifting the medial or lateral capsule superiorly (20). Although the reports on intermediate to long-term results of inferior capsular shift procedures are few, the reported results have been satisfactory, with good or excellent outcomes occurring in 75% to 100% of cases (20,70–72). Much like the arthroscopic Bankart repair, the arthroscopic treatment of MDI has undergone its own evolution. Utilizing an arthroscopically mediated technique similar to the open procedure performed by Altchek (70), Duncan and Savoie (74) performed 10 capsular shifts between 1988 and 1990. All patients had a satisfactory result at a minimum follow-up of 1 year postoperatively based on Neer's classification. Although the results were encouraging, the procedure was not widely performed due to the advanced skill level required for the procedure. In 1992, the holmium:yttrium-aluminum-garnet (YAG) laser was found to cause shrinkage of capsular tissue at nonablative energy levels. This revived the enthusiasm for arthroscopic treatment of MDI. Subsequently in 1998, Thabit (73) presented the clinical results of 41 patients treated with laser-assisted capsulorrhaphy for MDI. All competitive athletes returned to their previous level of sports participation, and in contrast to arthroscopic suture techniques, younger patients had better outcomes than older patients. Savoie and Field (75) evaluated a new form of capsular shrinkage using a temperature-specific thermal probe. The unipolar probe was arthroscopically used to shrink shoulder capsule in 30 patients. These patients also received an arthroscopic rotator interval closure as described by Treacy et al. (76). The results were comparable to those obtained by laser capsulorrhaphy and suture capsulorrhaphy, with 28 of 30 patients having a satisfactory result.

An alternative arthroscopic technique for the treatment of MDI was described by Wichman and Snyder (77). They described a technique for arthroscopic capsular plication with multiple imbrications sutures placed to effectively decrease capsular volume. Their initial report included 24 patients with a minimum of 2 year follow-up (77). They reported 80% good or excellent results and noted that three of the five failures occurred in worker compensation cases. Our current methods of treating MDI involve a combination of these most recent advances.

Surgical Indications

The treatment of patients with MDI focuses on establishing the correct diagnosis and instituting proper physical therapy for the scapular stabilizing muscles and the rotator cuff. Rehabilitation of the larger muscles of the shoulder (deltoid, pectoralis major, and latissimus dorsi) is delayed until normal scapular and rotator cuff function is achieved. Patient education, activity modification, and patience on the part of physicians, therapists, and patients are necessary during this stage, but one can expect a rate of satisfactory results of greater than 90% with 6 months of rehabilitation. If extensive nonoperative treatment fails and symptoms of pain and functional instability persist, surgical intervention should be considered. It is important to note that the operative treatment of capsular laxity should not only address the primary area of pathology, but also correct secondary changes from the continuing symptomatic subluxation and dislocation of the shoulder. Associated capsulolabral tears or avulsions should also be repaired.

Technique of Thermal Capsulorraphy and Rotator Interval Closure for MDI

After induction of general anesthesia, examination of the affected shoulder and contralateral shoulder is performed with the patient in the supine position. Then, as with the treatment of Bankart lesions, the patient can be placed in either the lateral decubitus or the beach-chair position. The affected arm is placed in 10 to 15 pounds of traction. A standard posterior portal is established, and a complete arthroscopic evaluation of the glenohumeral joint is performed. An anterior portal is created in the rotator interval, with caution used to ensure that the anterior and inferior aspects of the capsule are easily accessible. Utilizing a spinal needle for localizing this portal is a useful technique of ensuring that all areas of concern can be reached. First, a thorough examination of the anterior structures is performed. Next, the arthroscope is switched to the anterior portal and an examination of the posterior capsule and labrum is performed. Small labral tears or avulsions are repaired, and partial-thickness rotator cuff tears are debrided at this time.

Based on the examination under anesthesia and the arthroscopic appearance of the capsular structures, the location and extent of thermal capsulorrhaphy is determined. We use a temperature-specific probe with the temperature setting of 67.5°C and power setting of 20 to 40 W. The probe is introduced through the anterior portal and placed across the joint to contact the posterior band of the inferior glenohumeral ligament. The tightening then continues across the inferior glenohumeral ligament in the anterior direction to include the anterior band. Single radial passes of the probe are made from the glenoid side to the humeral side of the capsule. The middle and superior glenohumeral ligaments are also systematically treated. The arthroscope is then switched to the anterior portal and the probe introduced through the posterior portal, with the posterior capsule being treated in a similar fashion starting on the glenoid side and making radial passes while proceeding superiorly along the posterior capsule. The amount of capsular shrinkage is frequently reassessed during the procedure. A "lasso"

suture around the posterior capsule is used to protect the area of thermal treatment (Fig. 31.14). The arthroscope is returned to the posterior portal and the area of the rotator interval evaluated. Thermal tightening of the superficial and deep layers of the interval is attempted, but shrinkage of the interval is often ineffective. If laxity persists in the rotator interval after thermal treatment, interval plication sutures are placed using the technique described by Treacy et al. (76) (Fig. 31.15).

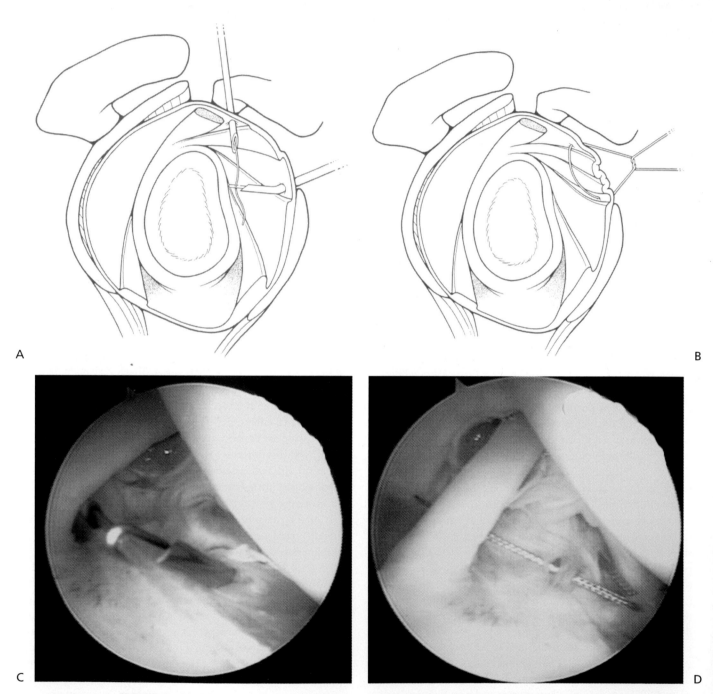

A

B

C

D

FIGURE 31.15 A,B: Schematic representation of rotator interval plication. **C,D,E:** Arthroscopic images demonstrating this technique.

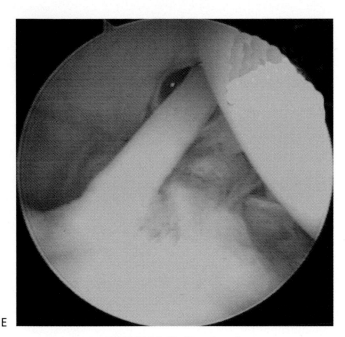

E

FIGURE 31.15 *(Continued).*

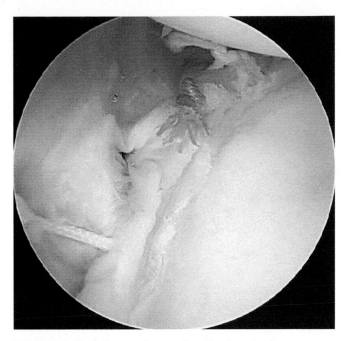

FIGURE 31.17 Arthroscopic capsular plication. Final appearance after anterior and posterior plication.

An alternative technique for the management of MDI is the arthroscopic capsular plication as described by Wichman and Snyder (77). The first step in performing this procedure is to excoriate the involved capsule with a rasp or an arthroscopic shaver. This causes bleeding and promotes healing of the two opposed tissue surfaces. The plication is then performed by placing plication sutures in the anteroinferior and posteroinferior capsule. Each suture is placed by creating a pinch stitch in the capsule 1 cm lateral to the glenoid articular margin and a second pinch stitch through the labrum. This process is repeated to form a mattress suture. Tying this arthroscopically creates a 1-cm fold between the capsule and labrum (Fig. 31.16). Additional sutures are placed anteriorly, inferiorly, and/or posteriorly as deemed necessary by history, physical examination, and arthroscopic findings (Fig. 31.17). It is important to assess range of motion following

this procedure. If less than 30 degrees of external rotation is present, one should consider revising some of the sutures.

POSTOPERATIVE MANAGEMENT FOR CAPSULAR SHRINKAGE AND ROTATOR INTERVAL CLOSURE

The patient remains in a sling with a small abduction pillow for 3 to 4 weeks. The patient begins active external rotation exercises with the arm adducted and scapular rotation exercises on the fourth week postoperative. Six weeks after surgery, a more extensive active rotator cuff and periscapular program is initiated. The exercises are progressed to proprioceptive neuromuscular facilitation patterns as tolerated,

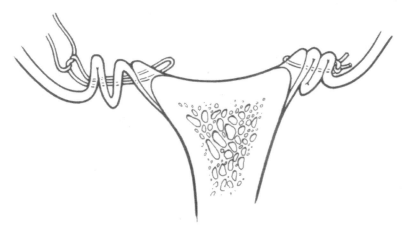

FIGURE 31.16 Arthroscopic anterior capsule plication: the mattress suture creates a 1-cm fold between the capsule and labrum.

usually at approximately 8 weeks after surgery. These are combined with progressive resistance exercises at 8 to 12 weeks after surgery. Twelve to 16 weeks postoperatively, the plyometric program and sport-specific conditioning for athletes is started and continued until normal function is achieved.

Patients are evaluated postoperatively at 1 week, 3 weeks, and each month thereafter until released without restrictions. Patients are allowed to return to unrestricted activity when range of motion and strength are equal to the contralateral shoulder. This usually occurs by 3 to 6 months postoperatively. Because of the uncertainty of the recovery of normal proprioception, no passive range of motion or capsular stretching by the physical therapist or trainer should be allowed.

POSTERIOR INSTABILITY

Historical Perspective and Results

Posterior shoulder instability has been considered to be difficult in both diagnosis and treatment. Operative management has had failure rates ranging from 30% to 72% (20,22,78–86). These high failure rates may result from there not being a single "essential" lesion that is responsible for posterior instability (15,78–86). In cases of posterior instability, laxity develops in the posterior inferior capsular ligaments as well as in the anterosuperior corner of the capsule (SGHL, CHL, rotator interval). Schwartz et al. (22) found that subluxation did occur after cutting the capsule posteriorly from 12 o'clock to 6 o'clock, but dislocation did not occur until after dividing the anterosuperior capsule as well. Additionally, many MDI patients may have a primary posterior component to their instability, further confusing the diagnosis and management process (20,73,85). Numerous surgical procedures to correct this problem have been described, including placement of a bone block at the posterior glenoid neck, glenoid osteotomy, reverse Bankart procedure, and the Neer posterior capsular shift (20,77–79). Combination procedures have tended to give better results, but the success rates reported with open procedures have not approached that reported for anterior instability. Improved arthroscopic techniques and instrumentation have allowed experienced surgeons to address this difficult problem arthroscopically. Given the fact that posterior instability can result from multiple lesions, addressing it arthroscopically has obvious advantages. Papendick and Savoie (78) reported their series of anatomy-specific arthroscopic repairs for posterior instability. They had excellent results, with a 95% success rate in their group. More recently, Savoie and Field (87) reported on their results in 61 patients. The repair technique utilized in these patients was dependent on the pathology. All patients were reexamined at 1 to 7 years postoperatively and 55 (90%) remained stable.

Operative Indications

The primary indication for operative intervention in patients with posterior instability is disabling symptoms of instability that have failed to improve with nonoperative interventions. Nonoperative measures focus on intensive physical therapy and medications.

Operative Technique

The patient is positioned in the lateral decubitus position or the beach-chair position depending on surgeon preference. Diagnostic arthroscopy is performed and all intraarticular pathology is defined, and a surgical plan is developed. Identifying the pathology responsible for the patient's symptoms is perhaps the most important part of the procedure. The type of procedure performed is dependent on this pathology.

The bioabsorbable tissue tack or a single suture anchor can be used for posterior Bankart lesions involving only the attachment of the posterior IGHL (PIGHL) (Fig. 31.18A). This is usually combined with a rotator interval plication, which addresses the anterosuperior component of the instability. In this technique the scope is placed in the anterior portal, and an end-cutting shaver is used to debride the posterior soft tissues. The glenoid neck is abraded in the region of the detached PIGHL and posterior labrum. A pilot hole is drilled at the glenoid origin of the PIGHL and adjacent to the articular margin. In the case of an absorbable tissue tack, the capsuloligamentous complex is speared with a Kirschner wire, shifted superiorly to the previously drilled hole, and the wire is inserted into this hole (Fig. 31.18B) The tack is then placed over the wire and tapped into position, securing the posterior labrum to the posterior glenoid rim (Fig. 31.18C). Alternatively, a suture anchor can be utilized as previously described for anterior reconstructions. The arthroscope is returned to the posterior portal, and the rotator interval is closed as described above.

A suture anchor technique is used for more extensive capsule labral avulsions and the posterior inferior quadrant of the shoulder (Fig. 31.19A). The debridement and abrasion of the glenoid are performed as previously described. A pilot hole is drilled at approximately the 7 o'clock position on the posterior inferior glenoid, and a suture anchor is inserted. Sutures are passed through the capsule at approximately the 6 o'clock position using the Caspari suture punch as described above for the Bankart repair. This suture is tied arthroscopically, shifting the capsulolabral complex superiorly (Fig. 31.19B). A second and third anchor is placed as needed to complete the repair. Anterosuperior labral lesions or widened rotator intervals are often encountered and require repair.

The suture punch technique is used when there is extensive damage to the posterior and inferior capsulolabral complex or in patients who have posterior and inferior capsular tears near the glenoid attachment of the ligaments. This tech-

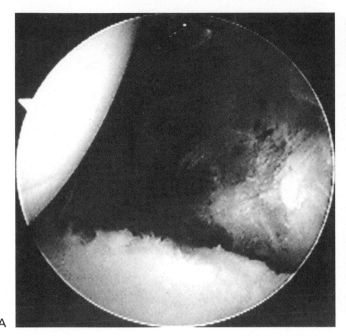

A

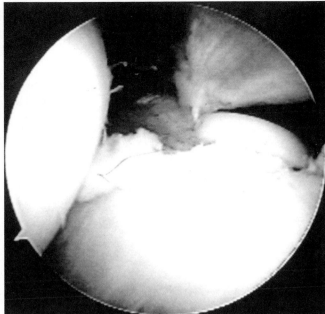

C

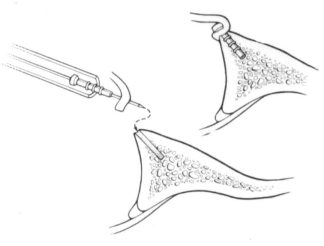

B

FIGURE 31.18 **A:** Isolated detachment of the origin of the posterior band of the inferior glenohumeral ligament from the posterior glenoid. **B:** Spearing the detached labra-ligamentous complex with the guide wire and placing the wire through the drill hole. **C:** The Suretac is then tapped into place, securing the repair.

nique provides the greatest vertical shift of the capsular structures. The soft tissue and bone are prepared as previously described. Through the posterior portal a Caspari suture punch is utilized to place between 6 and 12-0 and 2-0 polydioxanone sutures (PDSs) are placed into the inferior glenohumeral ligament, anterior band of the IGHL, PIGHL, and posterior capsule (Fig. 31.20A). Double biting with the suture punch is often used in the posterior capsule to imbricate the tissue. A superior or Neviaser portal is established, and all of these sutures are retrieved through this portal. These sutures are divided into two equal bundles and tied over fascia or bone to secure the capsular shift (Fig. 31.20B).

Thermal capsulorrhaphy or arthroscopic capsular plication can be useful in cases of mild instability where there is diffuse stretching of the entire capsular complex, but no capsular avulsions. Capsulorrhaphy is performed with the temperature-specific thermal device and supplemented by a protective "lasso" stitch around the treated capsule. Rotator interval plication is added when necessary. The technique for capsular plication, as described by Wichman and Snyder (77), is also discussed for MDI.

Postoperative Management

Postoperatively, the patient's arm is maintained in an abduction sling or gunslinger brace for approximately 3 weeks. Gentle range of motion exercises are initiated at 3 weeks. Active range of motion is initiated at 6 weeks. Functional rehabilitation begins around 8 to 10 weeks postoperatively and continues until full range of motion and normal strength are achieved. The entire rehabilitative process usually takes approximately 4 to 6 months. Patients are allowed to return to full sports participation when they achieve normal range of motion and strength.

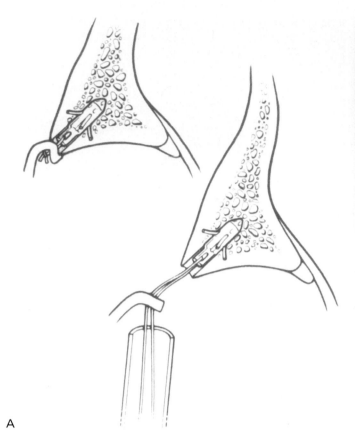

A

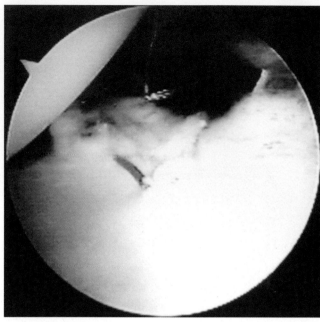

B

FIGURE 31.19 A: Illustration of the anchor being inserted into the prepared glenoid and the nonabsorbable suture retrieved through the ligaments inferior to the level of the anchor. **B:** Arthroscopic knot tying then shifts the capsule superiorly and plicates the tissue, reconstructing the posterior capsule.

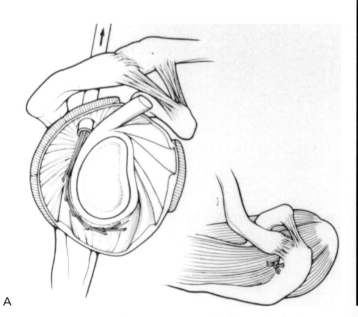

A

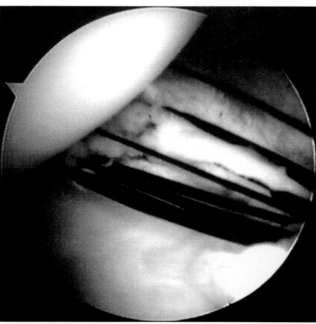

B

FIGURE 31.20 A: Global posterior laxity or severe inferior displacement of the posterior band of the inferior glenohumeral ligament may be corrected by Caspari suture punch reconstruction of the posterior capsule. Multiple polydioxan sutures are placed into the inferior and posterior capsule. These sutures are then retrieved out the superior portal and tied over fascia of the anterior aspect of the scapular spine. **B:** Arthroscopic image.

MICROINSTABILITY

Historical Perspective and Results

The term *microinstability* was coined to describe a pathologic process where abnormalities in the superior half of the shoulder joint result in abnormal translation of the humeral head on the glenoid (88). These abnormalities lead to subluxation without dislocation because of the limits to translation imposed by the coracoid, acromion, and rotator cuff. These abnormalities typically involve the middle and superior glenohumeral ligaments, the biceps anchor, the rotator interval, and rotator cuff. This abnormal translation can lead to secondary impingement of the anterior rotator cuff on the undersurface of the acromion or the posterior articular side of the cuff on the posterior superior glenoid.

Isolated or combined injuries to these structures can result in predictable pathologic translation of the humeral head. The MGHL is recognized as an important secondary restraint to both inferior and anterior translations (12,15,16,30). Avulsion of this structure can result in straight anterior instability (30) (Fig. 31.21). Savoie and colleagues (30) noted isolated avulsions of the MGHL in 33 patients with symptomatic anterior instability. Repair of the avulsion with a suture anchor resulted in decreased pain and improved function in all patients (30).

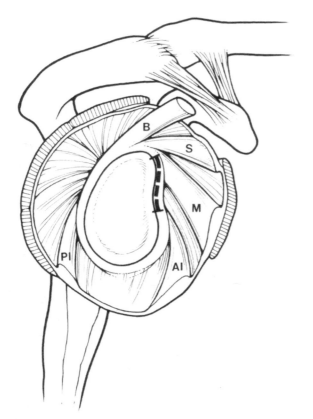

FIGURE 31.21 Illustration of the straight anterior lesion and area of detachment.

The superior glenohumeral ligament (SGHL) resists anterior and superior translation of the humeral head in shoulder flexion and lesser degrees of abduction (12,15,16,30,31). Destabilization of the SGHL can result in anterior-superior instability and secondary impingement with rotator cuff tendonitis (23,30–33) (Fig. 31.22). This association between anterosuperior labral lesions and anterior cuff pathology was coined the superior labrum–anterior cuff (SLAC) lesion by Savoie et al. (89). The classic superior labrum anterior to posterior (SLAP) lesion involving the biceps anchor can also result in symptoms of subtle instability (29).

The rotator interval occupies a triangular space of the anterior superior capsule, which is bordered superiorly by the anterior margin on the supraspinatus, inferiorly by the superior margin of the subscapularis, medially by the coracoid base, and laterally by the transverse humeral ligament. The interval consists of the glenohumeral joint capsule and is structurally enhanced by the superior glenohumeral ligament and the coracohumeral ligament. These structures become confluent at their humeral attachments. Several studies have demonstrated that lesions involving the anterosuperior quadrant or the rotator interval resulted in increased posterior and inferior translations with the arm in neutral position and increased anterior translation with the arm flexed 60 degrees (6–9,14,23,25). Patients usually present with signs and symptoms of anterior instability. However, a history of dislocation requiring manual reduction is unusual. A history and physical exam consistent with recurrent subluxation and rotator cuff tendinitis is more likely. Field et al. (25) reported on 15 patients with clinical examinations compatible with MDI in whom the only finding noted at the time of open stabilization was an isolated hole or defect in the rotator interval. Closure or imbrication of the interval was performed without any other form of stabilization. This provided for excellent intraoperative stability, and all patients had good or excellent outcomes after an average follow-up of 3.3 years (25). A rotator interval lesion is identified arthroscopically as abnormally widened or voluminous (Fig. 31.23).

Another clinical entity that falls under the classification of microinstability is internal impingement. Walch et al. (90) described impingement of the supraspinatus tendon on the posterosuperior glenoid rim with the arm positioned in 90 degrees of abduction and maximum external rotation as a cause of shoulder pain in the overhead athlete. Their patients were noted to have partial-thickness articular-sided tears of the supraspinatus/infraspinatus tendon and a "kissing lesion" of the posterior superior labrum. This lesion is thought to occur secondary to occult anterior instability, which allows the humeral head to translate anteriorly when the arm is abducted and externally rotated. In this position, the articular side of the rotator cuff impinges against the posterosuperior glenoid (Fig. 31.24). This is most commonly seen in young, athletic individuals who participate in overhead throwing sports and subject their shoulders to un-

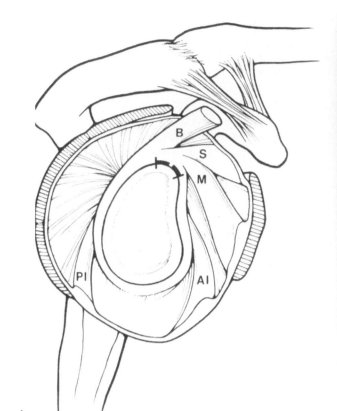

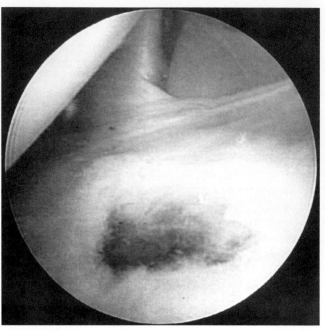

FIGURE 31.22 A: Illustration of isolated detachment of anterior-superior glenohumeral ligament. **B:** Arthroscopic view.

usually high repetitive stress. As discussed in the first section of this chapter, stability of the glenohumeral joint is dependent on static and dynamic factors. Malfunction of any one of these leads to overload of its counterpart. This overload eventually leads to injury and subsequent instability. This process is thought to account for the majority of cases of internal impingement. Therefore, to effectively treat these lesions you must not only treat the resulting pathology, but also identify and treat the inciting factor responsible for the injury process. This may be secondary to abnormal throwing mechanics, abnormally tight posterior capsule, or a functionally weak rotator cuff from chronic overload.

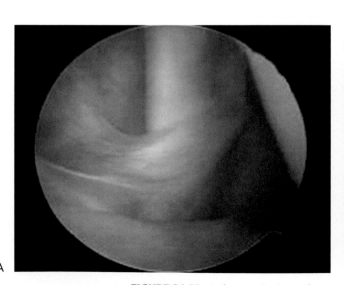

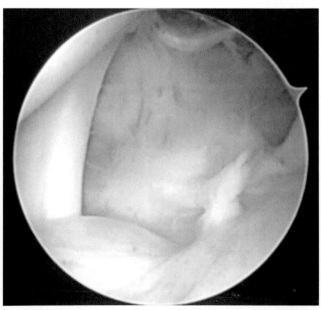

FIGURE 31.23 Arthroscopic view of normal **(A)** versus widened **(B)** rotator interval.

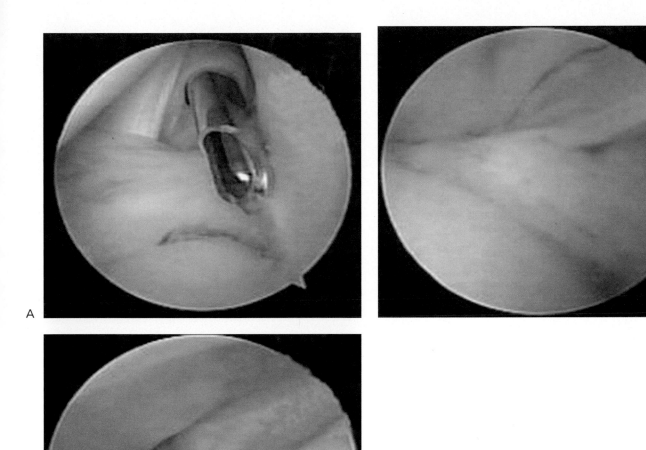

FIGURE 31.24 A: Anterior superior instability with lesion. **B:** Anterior cuff impinging against anterior-superior glenoid. **C:** Elimination of contact of cuff on labrum after repair.

Indications for Surgery

Surgery should be considered in patients who have persistent symptoms despite an extensive trial of physical rehabilitation. Because microinstability is a difficult problem to define clinically, the surgeon and the patient must be prepared to deal with whatever problem is discovered arthroscopically.

Operative Technique

A thorough understanding of the normal anatomic variants in this anterior-superior quadrant of the glenohumeral joint is paramount to treating these injuries. Stabilizing normal structures to nonanatomic locations can result in significant loss of motion and increased symptoms. Diagnosis of microinstability problems requires a high degree of clinical suspicion combined with a thorough history, physical examination, radiographic workup, and arthroscopic findings. The abnormalities seen at the time of arthroscopy should correlate with the preoperative historical and physical findings.

The exact surgical technique utilized in microinstability problems depends on the pathology that is present. Labral detachments and SLAP lesions will be repaired with either a suture anchor, as discussed above, or a bioabsorbable tack. Rotator interval lesions are repaired utilizing the technique of plication as described by Treacy et al. (76). In cases of internal impingement, the rotator cuff and posterosuperior labrum are most often addressed by simple debridement. If the cuff tear involves more than 50% of the tendon thickness, a formal repair is performed. Further, the anterior and anterosuperior quadrants of the capsulolabral complex are thoroughly examined to assess for pathologic detachments or intrasubstance injury. The most important aspect of surgically treating these problems is recognizing normal anatomic variants.

SUMMARY

Instability of the glenohumeral joint represents a wide spectrum of pathologic laxity. It can result from injury to any of the joint's stabilizing structures. With the continued development of new techniques and specialized surgical equipment, arthroscopy offers the surgeon the ability to successfully diagnose and treat the majority of these injuries.

REFERENCES

1. Bankart ASB. The pathology and treatment of recurrent dislocation of the shoulder joint. *Br J Med* 1938;23.
2. Bankart ASB. Discussion on recurrent dislocation of the shoulder. *J Bone Joint Surg* 1948;30(B):46–47.
3. Bost FC, Inman VT. The pathological changes in recurrent dislocation of the shoulder: a report of Bankart's operative procedure. *J Bone Joint Surg* 1942;24:595–613.
4. Matsen FA, Thomas SC, Rockwood CA. Anterior glenohumeral instability. In: Rockwood C, Matsen F, eds. *The shoulder.* Philadelphia: WB Saunders, 1990:526–569.
5. Andrews JR, Carson WG, McLeod WD. Glenoid labrum tears related to the long head of the biceps. *Am J Sports Med* 1985; 13:337–341.
6. Oveson J, Nielson S. Experimental distal subluxation in the glenohumeral joint. *Arch Orthop Trauma Surg* 1985;104:78–81.
7. Oveson J, Nielson S. Anterior and posterior instability of the shoulder: a cadaver study. *Arch Orthop Trauma Surg* 1986;57:324–327.
8. Oveson J, Niclson S. Stability of the shoulder joint: a cadaver study of stabilizing structures. *Arch Orthop Trauma Surg* 1986; 57:149–151.
9. Harryman DT, Sidles JA, Clark JM, et al. Translation of the humeral head on the glenoid with passive glenohumeral motion. *J Bone Joint Surg* 1990;72A:1334–1343.
10. Helmig P, Sojbjerg JE, Kjaersgaard-Anderson P, et al. Distal humeral migration as a component of multidirectional instability: an anatomical study in autopsy specimens. *Clin Orthop* 1990;252:139–142.
11. Matsen F, Harryman D, Sidles J. Mechanics of glenohumeral instability. *Clin Sports Med* 1991;10:783–788.
12. Bowen MK, Warren RF. Ligamentous control of shoulder stability based on selective cutting and static translation experiments. *Clin Sports Med* 1991;10:757–782.
13. Harris SL, Matsen FA III. Laxity of the normal glenohumeral joint: a qualitative in vivo assessment. *J Shoulder Elbow Surg* 1992;1:66–76.
14. Harryman D, Sidles J, Matsen F. The role of the rotator interval capsule in passive motion and stability of the shoulder. *J Bone Joint Surg* 1992;74A:53–66.
15. Pagnani M, Warren RJ. Stabilizers of the glenohumeral joint. *J Shoulder Elbow Surg* 1994;3:173–190.
16. Speer KP. Anatomy and pathomechanics of shoulder instability. *Clin Sports Med* 1995;14(4):751–760.
17. Lippitt SB, Vanderhooft E, Harris SL, et al. Glenohumeral stability from concavity compression: a quantitative analysis. *J Shoulder Elbow Surg* 1993;2:27–35.
18. Howell SM, Galinat BJ. The glenoid-labral socket: a constrained articular surface. *Clin Orthop* 1989;243:122–125.
19. Speer KP, Deng X, Altcheck D, et al. A biomechanical evaluation of a simulated Bankart lesion. *J Bone Joint Surg* 1994;76A: 1819–1826.
20. Neer CS, Foster CR. Inferior capsular shift for involuntary inferior and multidirectional instability of the shoulder. *J Bone Joint Surg* 1980;63:897–908.
21. Warner JJP, Micheli LJ, Arslanian LE, et al. Patterns of flexibility, laxity, and strength in normal shoulders and shoulders with instability and impingement. *Am J Sports Med* 1990;18:366–375.
22. Schwartz E, Warren RF, O'Brien S. Posterior shoulder instability. *Ortho Clin North* 1987;18:409–419.
23. Nobuhara K, Ideda H. Rotator interval lesion. *Clin Orthop* 1987;223:44–50.
24. Rowe CR, Zarins B. Recurrent transient subluxation of the shoulder. *J Bone Joint Surg* 1981;63A:863–872.
25. Field LD, Warren RF, O'Brien SJ, et al. Isolated closure of rotator interval defects for shoulder instability. *Am J Sports Med* 1995;23:557–563.
26. Cooper DE, O'Brien SJ, Arnoczky SP, et al. The structure and function of the coracohumeral ligament: an anatomic and microscopic study. *J Shoulder Elbow Surg* 1993;2:70–77.
27. Snyder SJ. *Shoulder arthroscopy.* New York: McGraw-Hill, 1994.
28. Williams MM, Snyder SJ, Buford D Jr. The Buford complex—the "cord-like" middle glenohumeral ligament and absent anterosuperior labrum complex: a normal anatomical capsulolabral variant. *Arthroscopy* 1994;10:241–247.
29. Snyder SJ, Banas MP, Belzer JP. Arthroscopic evaluation and treatment of injuries to the superior glenoid labrum. *Instr Course Lect* 1996;45:65–70.
30. Savoie FH, Papendik L, Field LD, et al. Straight anterior instability: lesions of the middle glenohumeral ligament. *Arthroscopy* 2001;17:229–235.
31. Field LD, Savoie FH. Anterosuperior instability and the rotator interval. *Oper Tech Sports Med* 1997;5:257–263.
32. Warner JP, Deng XH, Warren RF, et al. Static capsuloligamentous restraints to superior-inferior translation of the glenohumeral joint. *Am J Sports Med* 1992;20:675–685.
33. Field LD, Savoie FH. Arthroscopic suture repair of superior detachment lesions of the shoulder. *Am J Sports Med* 1993;21: 783–788.
34. Pagnani MJ, Deng XH, Warren RF, et al. Effect of lesions of the superior portion of the glenoid labrum on glenohumeral translation. *J Bone Joint Surg* 1995;77A:1003–1010.
35. Dickson JW, Devas MB. Bankart's operation for recurrent dislocation of the shoulder. *J Bone Joint Surg* 1957;39B:114–119.
36. Hovelius L. Anterior dislocation of the shoulder in teenagers and young adults: five year prognosis. *J Bone Joint Surg* 1987;69A: 393–399.
37. Pollock RG, Owens JM, Nicholson GP, et al. The anterior inferior capsular shift procedure for anterior glenohumeral instability: technique and long-term results. *Orthop Trans* 1994;17:1109.
38. Protzman RR. Anterior instability of the shoulder. *J Bone Joint Surg* 1980;62A:909–918.
39. Rowe CR, Patel D, Southmayd WW. The Bankart procedure. a long-term end-result study. *J Bone Joint Surg* 1978;60A:1–16.
40. Rowe CR, Zarins B. Recurrent transient subluxation of the shoulder. *J Bone Joint Surg* 1981;63A:863–872.
41. Rubenstein D, Jobe F, Glousman R. Anterior capsulolabral reconstruction of the shoulder in athletes. *J Shoulder Elbow Surg* 1992;1:229–237.
42. Sisto DJ, Cook DL. Intraoperative decision making in the treatment of shoulder instability. *Arthroscopy* 1998;14:389–394.
43. Cole BJ, L'Insalata J, Irrgang J, et al. Comparison of arthroscopic and open anterior shoulder stabilization. *J Bone Joint Surg* 2000;82A:1108–1114.
44. Bigliani LU, Kurzweil PR, Schwartzbach CC, et al. Inferior capsular shift procedure for anterior-inferior shoulder instability in athletes. *Am J Sports Med* 1994;22:578–584.
45. Hawkins RH, Hawkins RJ. Failed anterior reconstruction for shoulder instability. *J Bone Joint Surg* 1985;67B:709–714.
46. Hawkins RJ, Angelo RL. Glenohumeral osteoarthritis: a late complication of the putti-platt repair. *J Bone Joint Surg* 1990; 72A:1193–1197.

47. Coughlin L, Rubinovich M, Johansson J, et al. Arthroscopic staple capsulorrhaphy for anterior shoulder instability. *Am J Sports Med* 1992;20:253–266.
48. Hawkins RB. Arthroscopic stapling repair for shoulder instability: a retrospective study of 50 cases. *Arthroscopy* 1989;5: 122–128.
49. Zuckerman JD, Matsen FA III. Complications about the glenohumeral joint related to the use of screws and staples. *J Bone Joint Surg* 1984;66A:175–184.
50. Lane JG, Sachs RA, Riehl B. Arthroscopic staple capsulorraphy: a long-term follow-up. *Arthroscopy* 1993;9:190–194.
51. Field MH, Field LD, Savoie FH III. Arthroscopic labral repair with suture anchors. In: Warren RF, Craig EV, Altchek DW, eds. *The unstable shoulder.* Philadelphia: Lippincott-Raven, 1999.
52. Caspari RB. Arthroscopic reconstruction for anterior shoulder instability. In: Paulos LE, Tibone JE, eds. *Operative techniques in shoulder surgery.* Gaithersburg, MD: Aspen, 1991.
53. Morgan CD, Bodenstab AB. Arthroscopic Bankart suture repair: technique and early results. *Arthroscopy* 1987;3:11–22.
54. Savoie FH III, Miller CD, Field LD. Arthroscopic reconstruction of traumatic anterior instability of the shoulder: the Caspari technique. *Arthroscopy* 1997;13:201–209.
55. O'Neill DB. Arthroscopic Bankart repair of anterior detachments of the glenoid labrum. *J Bone Joint Surg* 1999;81A:1357–1366.
56. Grana WA, Buckley PD, Yates CK. Arthroscopic Bankart suture repair. *Am J Sports Med* 1993;21:348–353.
57. Guanche CA, Quick DC, Sodergren KM, et al. Arthroscopic versus open reconstruction of the shoulder in patients with isolated Bankart lesions. *Am J Sports Med* 1996;24:144–148.
58. Manta JP, Organ S, Nirschl RP, et al. Arthroscopic transglenoid suture capsulolabral repair: five-year follow-up. *Am J Sports Med* 1997;25:614–618.
59. Mologne TS, Lapoint JM, Morin WD, et al. Arthroscopic anterior labral reconstruction using a transglenoid suture technique: results in active-duty military patients. *Am J Sports Med* 1996; 24:268–274.
60. Pagnani MJ, Warren RF, Altchek DW, et al. Arthroscopic shoulder stabilization using transglenoid sutures: a four-year minimum follow-up. *Am J Sports Med* 1996;24:459–467.
61. Hayashida K, Yoneda M, Nakagawa S, et al. Arthroscopic Bankart suture repair for traumatic anterior shoulder instability: analysis of the causes of a recurrence. *Arthroscopy* 1998;14:295–301.
62. Arciero RA, Taylor DC, Snyder RJ, et al. Arthroscopic bioabsorbable tack stabilization of initial anterior shoulder dislocations: a preliminary report. *Arthroscopy* 1995;11:410–417.
63. Speer KP, Warren RF, Pagnani M, et al. An arthroscopic technique for anterior stabilization of the shoulder with a bioabsorbable tack. *J Bone Joint Surg* 1996;78A:1801–1807.
64. Wolf EM. Arthroscopic capsulolabral repair using suture anchors. *Orthop Clin North Am* 1993;24:59–69.
65. Hoffman F, Reif G. Arthroscopic shoulder stabilization using Mitek anchors. *Arthroscopy* 1995;3:50–54.
66. Bacilla P, Field LD, Savoie FH III. Arthroscopic Bankart repair in a high demand patient population. *Arthroscopy* 1997;13:51–60.
67. Green MR, Christensen KP. Arthroscopic Bankart procedure by suture technique: indications, technique, and results. *Arthroscopy* 1992;8:111–115.
68. Burkhart SS, DeBeer JF. Traumatic glenohumeral bone defects and their relationship to failure of arthroscopic Bankart repairs:

69. significance of the inverted-pear glenoid and the humeral engaging Hill-Sachs lesion. *Arthroscopy* 2000;16:677–694.
69. Neviaser TJ. The anterior labroligamentous periosteal sleeve avulsion lesion: a cause of anterior instability in the shoulder. *Arthroscopy* 1993;9:17–21.
70. Altchek DW, Warren RF, Skyhar MJ, et al. T-plasty modification of the Bankart procedure for multidirectional instability of the anterior and inferior types. *J Bone Joint Surg* 1991;73A:105–112.
71. Cooper RA, Brems JJ. The inferior capsular shift procedure for multidirectional instability of the shoulder. *J Bone Joint Surg* 1992;74A:1515–1521.
72. Leber RD, Alexander AH. Multidirectional shoulder instability: clinical results of inferior capsular shift in an active duty population. *Am J Sports Med* 1992;20:193–198.
73. Thabit G III. The arthroscopically assisted holmium:AG laser surgery in the shoulder. *Oper Tech Sp Med* 1998;6:131–138.
74. Duncan R, Savoie FH III. Arthroscopic inferior capsular shift for multidirectional instability of the shoulder: a preliminary report. *Arthroscopy* 1993;9:24–27.
75. Savoie FH III, Field LD. Thermal versus suture treatment of symptomatic capsular laxity. *Clin Sports Med* 2000;19:63–75.
76. Treacy SH, Field LD, Savoie FH III. Rotator interval capsule closure: an arthroscopic technique. *Arthroscopy* 1997;13: 103–106.
77. Wichman MT, Snyder SJ. Arthroscopic capsular plication for multidirectional instability of the shoulder. *Oper Tech Sports Med* 1997;5(4):238–243.
78. Papendick LW, Savoie FH III. Anatomy-specific repairs techniques for posterior shoulder instability. *South Orthop J* 1995; 4:169–176.
79. Hawkins RJ, Belle RM. Posterior instability of the shoulder. *Instr Course Lect* 1989;38:211–215.
80. Hurley JA, Anderson TE, Dear W, et al. Posterior shoulder instability. *Am J Sports Med* 1992;20:396–400.
81. Bigliani LU, Andrizzi DP, et al. Operative management of posterior shoulder instability. *Orthop Trans* 1989;13:232.
82. Tibone JE, Bradley JP. The treatment of posterior subluxation in athletes. *Clin Orthop* 1993;291:124–137.
83. Marshall JL. Joint looseness: a function of the person and the joint. *Med Sci Sports Exerc* 1980;12:189–194.
84. Tibone JE, Ting A. Capsulorrhaphy with a staple for recurrent posterior subluxation of the shoulder. *J Bone Joint Surg* 1990;72A:999–1002.
85. Hawkins JR, Coppert G, Johnston G. Recurrent posterior instability of the shoulder. *J Bone Joint Surg* 1984;66(2):169–174.
86. Pollock RG, Bigliani LU. Recurrent posterior instability. *Clin Orthop* 1993;291:85–96.
87. Savoie FH III, Field LD. Arthroscopic management of posterior shoulder instability. *Oper Tech Sports Med* 1997;5:226–232.
88. Nottage WM. Microinstability. Presented at the American Academy of Orthopaedic Surgeons AANA Specialty Day, San Francisco, 2001.
89. Savoie FH, Field LD, Atchinson S. Anterior superior instability with rotator cuff tearing: SLAC lesion. *Oper Tech Sports Med* 2000;8(3):221–224.
90. Walch G, Boileau P, Noel E, et al. Impingement of the deep surface of the supraspinatus tendon on the posterosuperior glenoid rim: an arthroscopic study. *J Shoulder Elbow* 1992;1: 238–245.

ARTHROSCOPIC ACROMIOPLASTY AND DISTAL CLAVICLE EXCISION

JAMES C. ESCH
GREGORY ALBERTON

ARTHROSCOPIC ACROMIOPLASTY

Arthroscopic subacromial decompression (ASAD) is the most frequently performed arthroscopic shoulder procedure. In terms of indications and surgical goals, it is the equivalent of the open decompression described by Neer (1,2). Advantages of the arthroscopic technique, compared with open technique, include excellent visualization of the glenohumeral joint to assess for pathology and of the rotator cuff for partial-thickness tears, less trauma to the deltoid, outpatient surgery with quicker recovery, and decreased costs. Refinements in indications and arthroscopic technique have evolved over the past 10 years to include minimal resection of the coracoacromial ligament and smoothing of the acromion from anterior to posterior, effecting a less aggressive resection. Minimal smoothing of the subacromial arch is now commonly done as advocated by Nirschl.* Complete and significant partial-thickness rotator cuff tears should be repaired, and this is also more frequently being accomplished with arthroscopic techniques.

Goal

The goal of ASAD is elimination of impingement of the rotator cuff against the anterior edge of the acromion at the attachment of the coracoacromial ligament.

Indications

Discomfort as the arm is elevated in the 90- to 120-degree arc is the main indication for ASAD. Night pain is a frequent complaint. A full range of motion and lack of re-

sponse to several months of nonoperative treatment (nonsteroidal antiinflammatory drugs, physical therapy, steroid injections) should be present before surgery is recommended. A full-thickness or partial-thickness tear expression of rotator cuff disease is usually present.

Expressions of rotator cuff disease, either partial or complete tears, are the main indication for ASAD. The complete tears are classified as small, medium, large, or massive. Massive tears may or may not be repairable. Partial tears are classified as bursal side or articular side.

Small, medium, and large tears are repaired along with ASAD. We prefer arthroscopic cuff repair followed by ASAD. Other shoulder surgeons prefer ASAD followed by either "mini-open" deltoid splitting or arthroscopic cuff repair. Massive tears should be repaired if possible. A limited bony flattening of the subacromial arch with preservation of the coracoacromial ligament should follow attempts at repair of massive rotator cuff tears. This minimal resection avoids the disaster of superior humeral migration with severe upper extremity malfunction associated with an aggressive bony resection. The surgeon should also perform this minimal resection if the rotator cuff cannot be repaired.

Bursal-side tears may consist of minimal scuffing, for which no repair is needed, or they may be flap tears requiring repair. The surgeon should always perform an ASAD for a bursal-side tear.

ASAD for articular-side tears is controversial. We prefer to perform an ASAD if we see scuffing of the acromial attachment of the coracoacromial ligament. Articular-side tears may be associated with instability and superior labral anterior and posterior (SLAP) lesions. The surgeon's options for treatment of this articular-side tear are debridement of the tear, repair of the tear, and treatment of the associated pathology, such as an unstable labrum tear (SLAP type II) or instability.

Radiology

The routine shoulder radiograph views are the anteroposterior view, the arch (or outlet) view, axillary views, and a spe-

---

* Nirschl and subacromial smoothening

J. C. Esch: Department of Orthopaedics, University of California, San Diego, School of Medicine, and Tri-City Orthopaedic Surgery, Oceanside, California.

G. Alberton: Tri-City Orthopaedic Surgery, Oceanside, California.

cific view of the acromioclavicular (AC) joint. The antero-posterior should be checked for glenohumeral arthritis and rotator cuff calcifications. The surgeon should be sure that the humeral head is not riding high and should evaluate the axillary view for a mesoacromion. The acromion shape and thickness are determined by the arch (outlet) view. The specific view of the AC joint is necessary to see joint narrowing, osteolysis, and osteophytes.

Magnetic resonance imaging of the shoulder joint is helpful for preoperative planning and discussions with the patient. The possibility of rotator cuff repair and the rehabilitation program can be discussed with the patient. Labrum and bone disease can also be evaluated.

Preoperative Patient Discussion and Results

A definite diagnosis of rotator cuff impingement associated with a full range of shoulder motion leads to the best result. If possible, any stiffness in elevation or restriction of internal rotation should be addressed before surgery. This requires diligent physical therapy and communication with the patient. Beware of patients with multidirectional instability, who frequently have secondary impingement symptoms, because the primary instability problem must be treated. Realistic discussions should include, for example, the fact that an 85% "success" rate also means a 15% "nonsuccess" or "failure" rate. Furthermore an 85% "success" rate usually means that only 35% to 50% of the patients achieve excellent results. Many patients have an "unrealistic expectation syndrome" and do not realize that they may not be perfect after surgery. An optimistic but realistic discussion about the fact that the patient must participate in the healing rehabilitation process fosters a positive surgeon–patient relationship.

Studies have demonstrated success rates for ASAD that are similar to those of open decompression. Ellman and Kay (3) reported on 2- to 5-year follow-up after ASAD in patients without full-thickness rotator cuff tears and demonstrated 89% satisfactory results on the University of California Los Angeles shoulder rating scale. Esch et al. (4) reported on 71 patients with average follow-up of 19 months and demonstrated 82% patient satisfaction for stage II disease and 88% for stage III disease (4). In a prospective randomized trial of open decompression ASAD in 20 patients with a 2-year follow-up, Lindh and Norlin (5) demonstrated similar functional results for both groups, with less time away from work and earlier restoration of motion in the ASAD group. Other studies have demonstrated success rates of ASAD between 80% and 90% (6–10).

A metaanalysis of the literature comparing results of open decompression versus ASAD was performed by Chercroun et al. and showed no significant difference (11). The objective success rates were 83.3% versus 81.4%, respectively, and the subjective success rates were 90.0% versus 89.3%, respectively.

Surgical Room Setup

The surgical technique used was originally described by Sampson (12) and later by Caspari (13–15). The lateral decubitus position is preferred. The surgeon can easily repair the rotator cuff with one surgical assistant and a scrub nurse or technician. No one needs to hold or manipulate the arm, because it is suspended.

The patient is stabilized in the lateral decubitus position with a vacuum beanbag. A rolled towel is placed in the axilla to protect the brachial plexus. The arm is suspended with a forearm sleeve wrap attached to a 10- to 15-lb weight through a shoulder-holding device. Placing the shoulder in 15 degrees of forward flexion and 30 degrees of abduction allows easy access to the subacromial space for surgical decompression and rotator cuff repair.

By turning the table 180 degrees so that the anesthesiologist is at the foot of the table, the surgeon can obtain easy access to the posterior, anterior, and superior aspects of the shoulder. The anesthesiologist lowers the systolic blood pressure to 90 to 95 mm Hg if it can be done safely. Morrison et al. (16) demonstrated that maintaining a difference of 49 mm Hg between the systolic pressure and the subacromial pressure correlated with decreased bleeding and improved visualization (16).

The shoulder is prepared with an iodine solution, then sealed and draped with a commercial U-drape and fluid pouch system. The arthroscopic camera–video–pump system is positioned above the shoulder and the shaver–suction system on the axillary side. Each system can be moved to the posterior, lateral, or anterior portal without entangling the cords and tubing.

Subacromial Bursoscopy

The subacromial bursoscopy is done before glenohumeral arthroscopy if an articular-side rotator cuff tear or labrum tear is suspected. Abnormalities of the bursa side of the rotator cuff and the acromial attachment of the coracoacromial ligament are indications for ASAD after treatment of the glenohumeral pathology. If the bursa is pristine, an arthroscopic decompression is not done. Diagnostic bursoscopy before glenohumeral arthroscopy alerts the surgeon to the extent of the total pathology and streamlines the treatment plan.

The subacromial bursa is entered from posterior with the skin portal at the posterior soft spot used for glenohumeral arthroscopy. The conical obturator of the cannula is inserted with a rapid push into the bursa located midway between the superior aspect of the cuff and the underside of the acromion near the anterior edge of the acromion. The obturator is removed from the cannula and the arthroscope is inserted. The fluid pump attached to the arthroscope is activated to distend and allow visualization of the bursa. A second or third pass should be tried if the bursa is not entered on the first attempt.

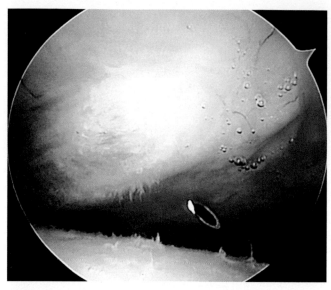

FIGURE 32.1 A needle is used to localize the lateral portal. Note the fraying of the acromial attachment of the coracoacromial ligament above and the partial-thickness bursal side rotator cuff fraying inferiorly.

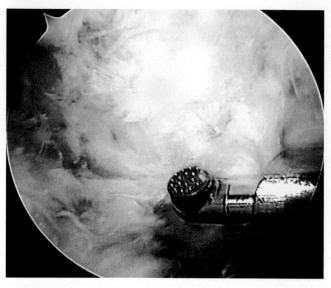

FIGURE 32.2 A bipolar cautery device (Arthrocare Corporation, Sunnyvale, CA) begins the release of the frayed coracoacromial ligament from the acromion.

An 18-gauge needle is used to locate the lateral portal, which is three fingerbreadths from the lateral edge of the acromion (Fig. 32.1). The needle is aimed perpendicular to and at the tip of the arthroscope. It is used as a probe. Later this needle can be exchanged with a cannula and tools for ASAD.

Glenohumeral Arthroscopy

The posterior portal is used to view the glenohumeral joint, with one or more anterior portals for probing and surgery. For AC resection, the anterior portal is created with the Wissinger rod technique. The surgeon has direct access to the anterior AC joint if the anterior portal is created in this manner.

A systematic evaluation of the glenohumeral joint (described in other chapters) is performed. The articular side of the rotator cuff is inspected. If there is a rotator cuff tear, its size, shape, and depth are assessed. Significant partial-thickness and complete cuff tears are repaired. SLAP type II tears, if present, are repaired before subacromial decompression is performed.

FOUR STEPS FOR ARTHROSCOPIC SUBACROMIAL DECOMPRESSION

Step 1: Detach the Coracoacromial Ligament

The bipolar radio frequency device (Fig. 32.2) (ArthroCare Corporation, Sunnyvale, CA) is used to ablate and thereby remove the portion of the coracoacromial ligament that at-

taches on the undersurface of the acromion (Fig. 32.3). The goal is clear visualization of the acromion. Any loose pieces of ligament tissue are removed with a shaver, but do not excise the ligament back to the coracoid. The troublesome bleeding vessel should be coagulated within the ligament. The ligament should not be resected in patients with massive cuff tears unless a secure repair can be done. The undersurface of the acromion is then cleaned with an end-cutting motorized shaver (Fig. 32.4).

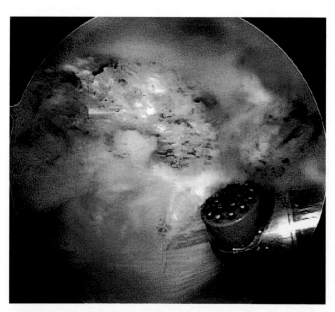

FIGURE 32.3 The undersurface of the acromion is exposed by coagulation and vaporization of the acromial attachment of the coracoacromial attachment.

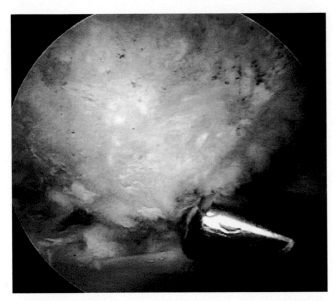

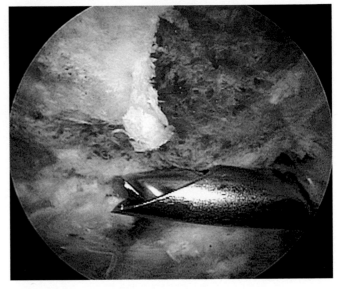

FIGURE 32.4 The undersurface of the acromion is cleaned with an end-cutting motorized shaver (Razorcut blade, Smith and Nephew Endoscopy, Andover, MA).

FIGURE 32.6 A bur from the lateral portal defines the anterior acromion.

Step 2: Define the Anterolateral Acromion

The goal of this phase of the procedure is to remove soft tissue and thereby set up the bony resection in step 3. A bur is used to remove any remaining ligament fibers. This defines the anterolateral corner of the acromion (Fig. 32.5). Enough of the lateral margin is removed to define the anterolateral resection endpoint for the posterior-to-anterior resection and smoothing of the acromion (Fig. 32.6). Any bursa tissue that prevents visualization should be removed. Perfect

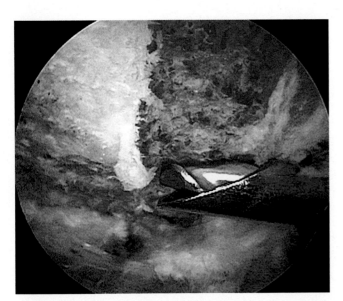

FIGURE 32.5 A bur (Helicut blade, Smith and Nephew Endoscopy, Andover, MA) is used to remove bone, defining the anterolateral corner of the acromion.

visualization of the undersurface of the acromion is necessary before proceeding to acromion resection.

Bleeding can be prevented by maintaining a proper balance between the patient's systolic blood pressure, the arthroscopic pump inflow pressure through the arthroscope, and the outflow suction in the shaver system. We use an infusion pump (IntelliJet pump, Smith and Nephew Endoscopy, Andover, MA) through the arthroscope that automatically controls and changes the inflow pump pressure and the outflow suction pressure to maintain this relationship. Special cannulas with dams prevent fluid loss and help maintain the bursa pump pressure that will prevent bleeding. The smaller, 4.5-mm shavers and burs should be used, rather than the 5.5-mm ones, to avoid excess fluid removal so that the bursa pressure is maintained to control bleeding. Any bleeding vessels are cauterized.

Step 3: Acromial Resection from Posterior to Anterior

The goal of this resection is to flatten the bone with a minimal anterior bone resection. The technique is similar for patients with a thick or a thin acromion. This technique has a known endpoint of a flat bone resection. Excessive anterior resection should be avoided, especially in patients with a large or massive rotator cuff tear, even if the tear is repairable.

The arthroscope is switched from the posterior to the lateral portal, and the shaver from the lateral to the posterior portal. A cannula system with fluid dams (IntelliJet) makes this exchange easy with minimal fluid loss. The shaver blade is used to remove the posterior bursa curtain for a wider view of

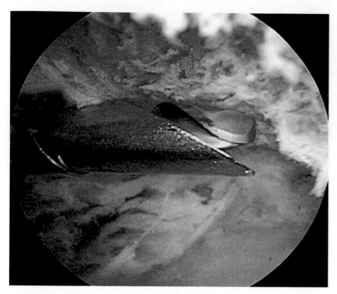

FIGURE 32.7 From the posterior portal, the bur begins the resection from posterior to anterior. Viewing is from the lateral portal.

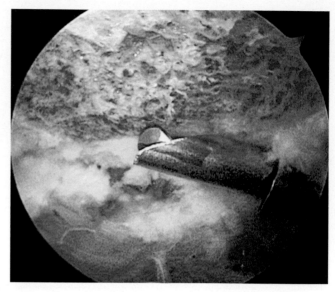

FIGURE 32.9 The acromioplasty is completed by removing any bony spurs from lateral on the right to medial on the left. Viewing is from posterior while the bur enters from the lateral portal.

the posterior acromion. Once the bone is well seen, the shaver is exchanged for a bur. The bur is placed flat on the acromion. The surgeon must be aware of the amount of bone that is to be removed to flatten the curved or hooked acromion. The bur is swept from medial to lateral as it is advanced from posterior to anterior (Figs. 32.7 and 32.8). The first centimeter of resection must be in line with the posterior acromion. The anterior spur of the acromion is removed by feathering the bone resection into the deltoid–trapezius fascia, preserving the superior periosteum. The surgeon must be aware of pre-

serving the deltoid muscle attachment, which is the distinct advantage of arthroscopic over open acromioplasty.

Step 4: Acromion Resection from Lateral to Medial

The arthroscope is moved back to the posterior portal and the shaver back to the lateral portal through the cannula system. The surgeon then should make sure that there is a smooth bony resection from lateral to medial. The bur is used to remove any lateral or medial bony prominences (Fig. 32.9).

Final Rotator Cuff Evaluation

The cuff is inspected with a probe to detect any small complete or bursal side flap tears, after which arthroscopic or mini-open cuff repair can proceed. Bleeding is less if the arthroscopic cuff repair is done before the bony decompression.

COPLANNING THE ACROMIOCLAVICULAR JOINT

Some surgeons prefer to remove large inferior AC joint spurs. Removal of the inferior aspect of the AC joint is not necessary and may be detrimental (17). The AC joint should be resected if the patient has AC joint pathology.

Acromioclavicular Joint Resection

Arthroscopic resection of the AC joint can easily be done after ASAD. Surgical indications are pain and tenderness over

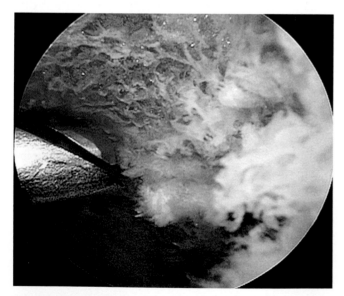

FIGURE 32.8 The bur continues the posterior-to-anterior resection, approaching the anterior bony prominence on the right.

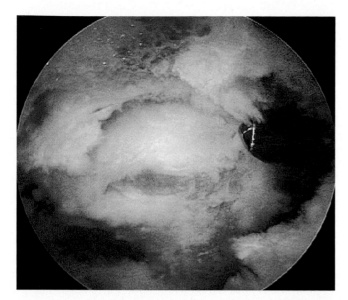

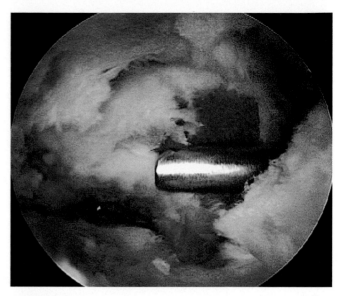

FIGURE 32.10 End-on view from the lateral portal of the acromioclavicular (AC) joint with the shaver from the anterior portal. The acromial side of the AC joint is resected at a 30-degree angle for good visualization of the AC joint.

FIGURE 32.11 Initial resection of the distal clavicle as viewed from lateral.

the AC joint, often accompanied by pain reaching across to touch the other shoulder. Radiographs may show joint narrowing, osteophytes, and osteolysis. Osteophytes should not be resected if they are not painful. The surgical goal is complete resection of the lateral 7 to 10 mm of the clavicle.

The undersurface of the AC joint is viewed from the lateral portal. The anterior portal cannula is redirected toward the AC joint. This is easily done if the anterior glenohumeral portal was created by the Wissinger rod technique. The soft tissue is removed from the anterior and inferior aspect of the AC joint with the 5.5-mm end-cutting shaver through the anterior cannula. We also use the bipolar radiofrequency cautery (ArthroCare to clean the bone and soft tissue from the lateral 1 cm of the clavicle.

The bony resection is begun on the acromial side of the AC joint with removal of 2 mm of bone and beveling of the acromion at a 30-degree angle from inferolateral to superomedial (Fig. 32.10). This resection enables a good view of the distal clavicle from the lateral portal. The 30-degree arthroscope is rotated to match the 30-degree bony resection for best viewing. Some surgeons prefer to view the AC joint resection from the posterior portal.

The clavicle is resected from anterior to posterior with a 4.5-mm bur. The bur is laid on the clavicle, and its size is used to determine the amount of bony resection. Initially the anterior one half of the oval lateral clavicle is resected (Fig. 32.11). The anterior resection is used to guide the bur posterior in a cutting block technique. This step is then repeated for another bur width (Fig. 32.12). The final view from the lateral portal shows a 7- to 10-mm distal clavicle resection. Finally, the resection is viewed from the anterior

portal (Fig. 32.13). The surgeon must be sure that no bone remains in the superior or posterior capsule and should gauge whether the anterior-to-posterior resection is parallel, and, if necessary, removing more bone.

Rehabilitation after Acromioplasty or Acromioclavicular Resection

A sling may be worn for comfort for a few days after these procedures. Pendulum exercises are begun on the evening of

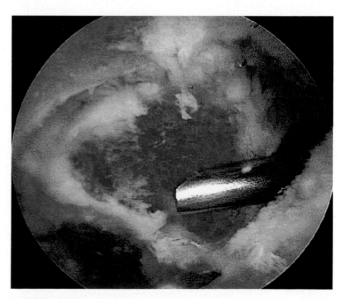

FIGURE 32.12 Continuing resection of the distal clavicle as viewed from lateral.

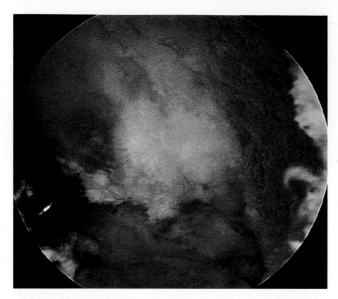

FIGURE 32.13 Anterior view of the final acromioclavicular resection with the clavicle on the right and the acromion on the left.

surgery, followed by exercises using a bar and pulley with the Shoulder Therapy Kit (BREG Inc., Vista, CA). Strengthening is begun with surgical tubing at 4 to 6 weeks if the patient is comfortable. Painless full range of motion is the initial goal; strengthening follows. The patient should go slow and work on stretching if stiffness occurs. Complete recovery takes 3 to 6 months. Of course, recovery is slower if the surgeon repairs a rotator cuff tear.

Complications

A disastrous complication is coracoacromial arch deficiency that results in superior migration of the humeral head. The cause of this complication is excessive resection of the anterior acromion and coracoacromial ligament, often coupled with AC joint resection in a patient with a massive rotator cuff tear. A limited bony flattening resection of the arch should be performed in a patient with a large repairable rotator cuff tear, and none of the acromion should be resected if the patient has a massive irreparable rotator cuff tear. Other complications include not resecting enough bone, leaving the anterior hook, heterotopic ossification, acromial fracture, and inadequate AC joint resection. Fracture or excessive resection of the distal clavicle is possible if the surgeon mistakes the distal clavicle for the acromion. Stiffness is another problem, especially if there was limited motion at the time of the bony surgery. Deltoid detachment can occur if there is aggressive anterior acromion removal without awareness of the deltoid attachment to this bone.

Isolated Acromioclavicular Arthroscopy

Direct AC arthroscopy is performed by the superior approach in young patients with a painful AC joint, radiologic evidence of osteolysis of the distal clavicle, and a normal subacromial bursa. The joint is localized with two 18-gauge needles from the anterosuperior and the posterosuperior aspect of the joint. The surgeon should use the smaller, 3.0-mm arthroscope and shaver blade/bur to view the joint, switching to the usual 4.0-mm arthroscope and shaver blade as bone is removed.

SUMMARY

ASAD is a safe and effective procedure when it is performed properly. Preoperative evaluation and careful selection of patients is important to success. Advantages of an arthroscopic approach compared with the open approach include avoidance of deltoid detachment, to facilitate more rapid recovery and less postoperative pain; improved ability to assess the glenohumeral joint and rotator cuff for associated pathology; and improved cosmesis with less scarring. The four steps required to perform this operation successfully are (a) detach the coracoacromial ligament, (b) define the anterolateral acromion, (c) resect the acromion from anterior to posterior, and (d) resect the acromion from lateral to medial.

REFERENCES

1. Neer C 2nd. Anterior acromioplasty for the chronic impingement syndrome in the shoulder: a preliminary report. *J Bone Joint Surg Am* 1972;54:41–50.
2. Neer C 2nd. Impingement lesions. *Clin Orthop* 1983;173:70–77.
3. Ellman H, Kay SP. Arthroscopic subacromial decompression for chronic impingement: two- to five-year results. *J Bone Joint Surg Br* 1991;73:395–398.
4. Esch JC, et al. Arthroscopic subacromial decompression: results according to the degree of rotator cuff tear. *Arthroscopy* 1988;4: 241–249.
5. Lindh M, Norlin R. Arthroscopic subacromial decompression versus open acromioplasty: a two-year follow-up study. *Clin Orthop* 1993;290:174–176.
6. Nutton RW, McBirnie JM, Phillips C. Treatment of chronic rotator-cuff impingement by arthroscopic subacromial decompression. *J Bone Joint Surg Br* 1997;79:73–76.
7. Olsewski JM, Depew AD. Arthroscopic subacromial decompression and rotator cuff debridement for stage II and stage III impingement. *Arthroscopy* 1994;10:61–68.
8. Petre D, et al. Treatment of advanced impingement syndrome by arthroscopic subacromial decompression. *Acta Orthop Belg* 1998;64:257–262.
9. Roye RP, Grana WA, Yates CK. Arthroscopic subacromial decompression: two- to seven-year follow-up. *Arthroscopy* 1995;11: 301–306.
10. Ryu RK. Arthroscopic subacromial decompression: a clinical review. *Arthroscopy* 1992;8:141–147.
11. Checroun AJ, Dennis MG, Zuckerman JD. Open versus arthroscopic decompression for subacromial impingement: a comprehensive review of the literature from the last 25 years. *Bull Hosp Joint Dis* 1998;57:145–151.
12. Sampson TG, Nisbet JK, Glick JM. Precision acromioplasty in arthroscopic subacromial decompression of the shoulder. *Arthroscopy* 1991;7:301–307.

13. Caspari RB, Thal R. A technique for arthroscopic subacromial decompression. *Arthroscopy* 1992;8:23–30.
14. Esch JC. Arthroscopic subacromial decompression: surgical technique. Arthroscoopy update #4. *Orthop Rev* 1989;18: 733–735,738–742.
15. Esch JC. Arthroscopic subacromial decompression and postoperative management. *Orthop Clin North Am* 1993;24:161–171.
16. Morrison DS, Schaefer RK, Friedman RL. The relationship between subacromial space pressure, blood pressure, and visual clarity during arthroscopic subacromial decompression. *Arthroscopy* 1995;11:557–560.
17. Fischer BW, et al. Incidence of acromioclavicular joint complications after arthroscopic subacromial decompression. *Arthroscopy* 1999;15:241–248.

Operative Arthroscopy, third edition. Edited by John B. McGinty, Stephen S. Burkhart, Robert W. Jackson, Donald H. Johnson, and John C. Richmond.
Lippincott Williams & Wilkins © 2003.

ARTHROSCOPIC MANAGEMENT OF ROTATOR CUFF TEARS

STEPHEN S. BURKHART

The most difficult and advanced category of arthroscopic reconstructive surgery of the shoulder is that of arthroscopic rotator cuff repair. Even so, the last decade has witnessed a rapid and dramatic evolution in the principles and techniques of arthroscopic rotator cuff repair. The arthroscopic cuff debridements of the early 1990s have yielded to the sophisticated arthroscopic cuff repairs and reconstructions of today. To the uninitiated, arthroscopic repair of a massive rotator cuff tear may seem like magic. If arthroscopic shoulder surgeons were magicians, they would keep their techniques to themselves in order to maintain the illusion, because every magician knows that to teach an act of magic is to transform it from a mysterious miracle to a simple trick. Fortunately, arthroscopic educators are more fond of tricks than miracles.

How have we been able to come so far so fast in the arthroscopic treatment of rotator cuff tears? After all, in only 10 short years we have gone from the stage of being unable to repair any rotator cuff tear arthroscopically to the current status of being able to repair virtually all rotator cuff tears, even massive tears, arthroscopically. As with any breakthrough technology, this rapid progress has been made possible by the marriage of insight to technology. Technology is a great facilitator of progress, but technology by itself cannot produce progress. The great misconception of our era is that technology alone will advance a discipline. The reality is that technology without understanding produces mere gadgets; technology guided by insight produces tools.

My goal in this chapter is to break down the magic into tricks, and to teach the reader how to systematically perform these tricks with tools rather than gadgets. One must always bear in mind that magic is the currency of ignorance, whereas tools are the instruments of understanding. This chapter is dedicated to understanding.

HISTORICAL PERSPECTIVE

It is instructive to briefly review the last 10 years of arthroscopic treatment of rotator cuff tears in order to see how certain concepts developed and enhanced our arthroscopic techniques. Much of the early literature on arthroscopic treatment of these lesions dealt with debridement of massive rotator cuff tears (1–7). In general, a massive rotator cuff tear was defined as one in which the major tear diameter was greater than 5 cm, and this definition is used throughout this chapter in referring to massive cuff tears (8,9).

The tears that did well with debridement were those that had balanced force couples in the transverse and coronal planes (Fig. 33.1). Shoulders that had balanced force couples despite large rotator cuff tears generally had good function, although they were painful; hence, they were called "functional rotator cuff tears" (3). Early reports of debridement were generally good (1,2,4–7). However, as patients undergoing debridement were monitored over time, some authors reported less than favorable results. For example, in younger, more active patients, the results of rotator cuff debridement deteriorated over time (10,11). As repair techniques developed, cuff debridement gradually fell out of favor for all tears except small partial-thickness tears.

The next phase in the history of arthroscopic rotator cuff repair was the development of an arthroscopic-assisted technique, the "mini-open" rotator cuff repair (12–15). This technique, by employing a purely arthroscopic subacromial decompression, could achieve repair of small and medium-sized rotator cuff tears through a short deltoid muscle–splitting incision without the need for detaching the deltoid from the acromion. Deltoid morbidity was thereby reduced. Repair to bone was initially performed through bone tunnels, but more recently suture anchors have been used to achieve secure fixation of tendon to bone.

The refinement of suture anchor techniques has brought us into the current era of arthroscopic repair of virtually all rotator cuff tears.

S. S. Burkhart: Department of Orthopaedics, University of Texas Health Science Center at San Antonio, and Baylor College of Medicine, Houston, Texas.

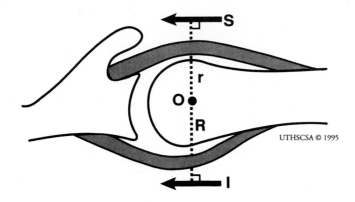

$$\Sigma M_O = O = IxR - Sxr$$
$$\therefore IxR = Sxr$$

A

FIGURE 33.1 A: Transverse (axial) plane force couple in which the anterior rotator cuff force is balanced against the posterior rotator cuff force. **B:** Coronal plane force couple in which the force from the inferior portion of the rotator cuff (both posterior and anterior) is balanced against the deltoid force.

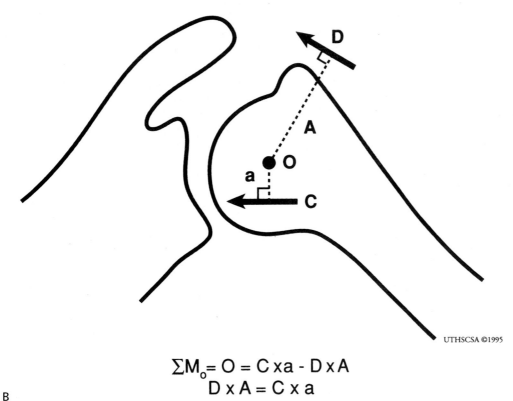

$$\Sigma M_o = O = C \times a - D \times A$$
$$D \times A = C \times a$$

B

ARTHROSCOPIC REPAIR OF ROTATOR CUFF TEARS

One of the great advantages of the arthroscope is that it frees the surgeon from spatial constraints. He or she can approach a pathologic area from anterior, posterior, medial, or lateral with equal facility. Unlike the arthroscopic surgeon, the open surgeon is restricted in approach by the position of the incision. Therefore, if the surgeon makes an anterolateral incision for cuff repair, the torn edge of the cuff must be brought to the incision so that it can be visualized and repaired. This medial-to-lateral mindset has dominated open rotator cuff surgery, in which the conventional wisdom has been that the cuff must always be mobilized sufficiently medially so that it can be pulled laterally to the humeral neck and greater tuberosity for repair (16–23). Unfortunately, in my opinion, this medial-to-lateral mindset retarded the progress of rotator cuff repair techniques by delaying the recognition of one of the most useful and powerful concepts governing the repair of massive rotator cuff tears: *margin convergence* (24).

Margin Convergence for Closure of the U-Shaped Tear: The So-Called Retracted Tear

It is critical to recognize that most so-called *retracted* massive cuff tears are not retracted at all. These large, U-shaped tears are actually L-shaped tears with a vertical split from medial to lateral; they have assumed a "U" shape by virtue of the elasticity of the involved muscle–tendon units. McLaughlin (25) recognized this tear pattern more than 50 years ago and advocated L-shaped repair utilizing a combination of side-to-side tendon-to-tendon sutures and end-on tendon-to-bone sutures. Unfortunately, McLaughlin's advice was not heeded, and mainstream orthopedic teaching went the way of medial-to-lateral mobilization regardless of the shape of the tear. The large U-shaped tears that extended far medially so that the apex of the tear was positioned above the glenoid were, in my opinion, often incorrectly designated as "re-tracted tears," and ill-advised massive mobilization of these tears guaranteed failure of the repair as a result of tension overload at the apex of the tear.

Although McLaughlin (25) recommended side-to-side repair of the vertical component of the large U-shaped tears as the anatomically correct technique of repair, he did not recognize the incredible mechanical advantage that accrued from side-to-side closure as a direct result of a biomechanical principle that we have called margin convergence (24). This term refers to the phenomenon that occurs with side-to-side closure of large cuff tears, in which the free margin of the tear converges toward the greater tuberosity as side-to-side repair progresses (Fig. 33.2). As this margin "converges," the strain at the free edge of the cuff is dramatically reduced, leaving a virtually tension-free "converged" cuff margin overlying the humeral bone bed for repair. As an ex-ample, side-to-side closure of two thirds of a U-shaped tear will reduce the strain at the cuff margin to one sixth of the strain that existed at the "preconverged" cuff margin (24). This mechanical strain reduction creates an added safety factor for the repair of tendon to bone, because decreased strain means that there will be a lower likelihood of failure of fixation to bone (for either suture anchors or bone tunnels).

The First Step: Tear Pattern Recognition

The critical first step in carrying out an arthroscopic repair of a massive tear is tear pattern recognition. Most rotator cuff tears can be broadly classified into two patterns: crescent-shaped tears and U-shaped tears (26). In my practice, U-shaped tears comprise approximately 40% of all tears and 85% of the large and massive tears (27,28). Crescent-shaped tears, even large and massive ones, typically pull away from bone but do not retract far. Therefore, they can be repaired directly to bone with minimal tension (Fig. 33.3). U-shaped tears generally extend much farther medially than crescent-shaped tears, with the apex of the tear located above the glenoid or even medial to the glenoid (Fig. 33.4). It is important to realize that this medial extension of the tear often does not represent retraction but rather represents the shape that an L-shaped tear assumes under physiologic load from its muscle–tendon components. Closing such a tear is much like closing a tent flap; one must reconstitute the two limbs of the "L" (Figs. 33.5 and 33.6). One must not make the mistake of trying to mobilize the medial margin of the U-shaped tear from the glenoid and scapular neck enough to pull it over to the humeral bone bed. The large tensile stresses in the middle of such a repaired cuff margin would doom it to failure.

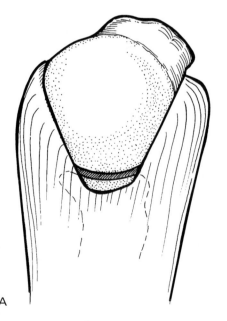

A

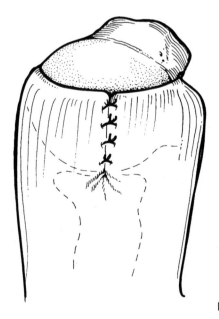

B

FIGURE 33.2 A: U-shaped rotator cuff tear. **B:** Partial side-to-side repair causes a "margin convergence" of the tear toward the greater tuberosity. This increases the cross-sectional area and decreases the length of the tear, thereby decreasing strain.

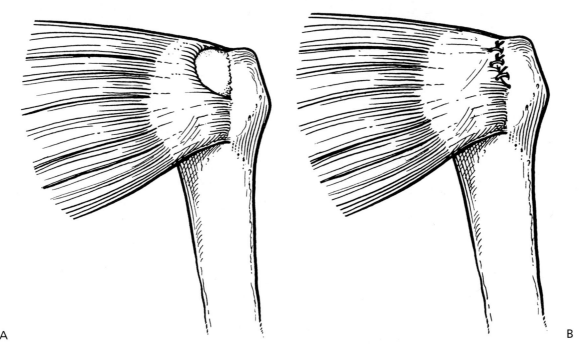

A   B

FIGURE 33.3 A crescent-shaped rotator cuff tear without much retraction **(A)** can be repaired directly to bone with minimal tension **(B)**.

Repairing the Crescent-Shaped Tear

This type of tear can easily be repaired to bone. We have previously shown that, under conditions of physiological cyclic loading, bone fixation by suture anchors is stronger than bone fixation by transosseous bone tunnels (29); therefore, suture anchors are my preferred method of fixation. I

prepare a bone bed on the humeral neck, just off the articular margin, by means of a power shaver so as not to decorticate the bone. Decortication of bone would weaken anchor fixation, so it should be avoided. A bleeding bone surface rather than a bone trough is all that is necessary for satisfactory healing of tendon to bone (30).

The suture anchors should be inserted at an angle of approximately 45 degrees to the bone surface (the so-called deadman angle) to increase the anchor's resistance to pullout (31). I prefer to use a Corkscrew or BioCorkscrew suture anchor (Arthrex, Inc., Naples, FL) but virtually all of today's permanent and biodegradable suture anchors have adequate pullout strength to resist physiologic loads (32,33).

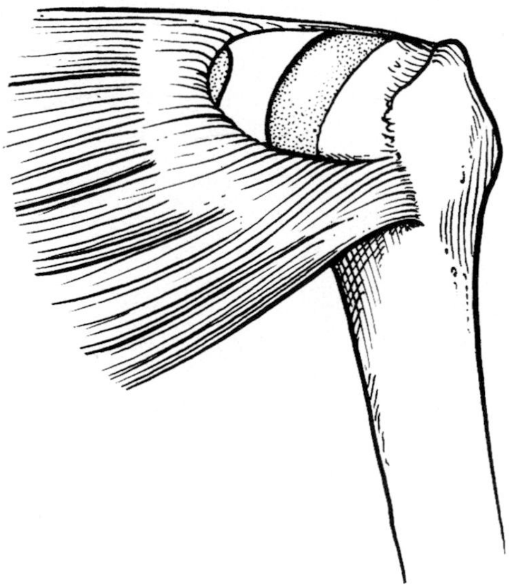

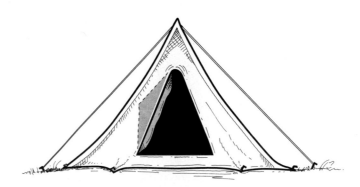

FIGURE 33.4 Large U-shaped rotator cuff tear whose apex extends to the glenoid.

FIGURE 33.5 Closing a tent flap provides an accurate analogy to closing a U-shaped rotator cuff tear by closing the vertical limb and then the horizontal limb.

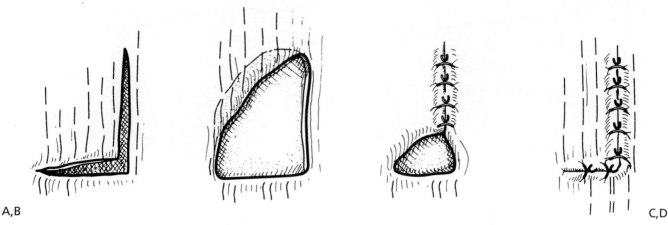

A,B   C,D

FIGURE 33.6 A: L-shaped tear. **B:** Elasticity of the musculotendinous units causes deformation of the L-shaped tear into a U-shaped tear. **C:** Closure of the vertical limb of the tear by side-to-side sutures. **D:** Closure of the horizontal limb of the tear by tendon-to-bone sutures.

The crescent-shaped margin of the tear must be respected in the repair and therefore the suture anchors should be placed in a crescent array, just 4 or 5 mm off the articular surface, to avoid tension overload at any of the fixation points (Fig. 33. 7). Tension overload has been shown experimentally to cause failure of cuff repairs subjected to physiologic cyclic loads (29,34).

Suture capture of the tendon can be done arthroscopically by either simple sutures or mattress sutures. The strength of simple sutures of no. 2 Ethibond (Ethicon, Somerville, NJ) has been shown in the laboratory to be adequate for maximal physiologic loading conditions of the rotator cuff (35,36).

Loop security is defined as the ability to maintain a tight suture loop as a knot is tied. Knot security is defined as the effectiveness of a given knot to resist slippage or breakage when load is applied. Little has been written about loop security, but it is at least as important as knot security, because a loose loop will allow loss of soft tissue fixation even if its associated knot is very strong (37) (Fig. 33.8). I prefer to tie static, nonsliding knots with an arthroscopic double-diameter knot pusher (Surgeon's Sixth Finger, Arthrex) because of the exceptional loop security, as demonstrated experimentally, that can be achieved with this device (37). Some complex sliding knots may potentially maintain adequate loop security if they are locked once they are in a set position.

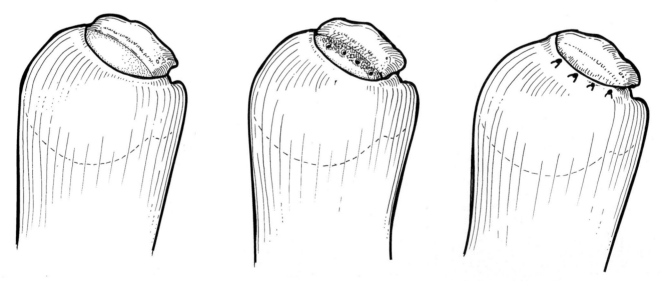

FIGURE 33.7 The surgeon must respect the crescent-shaped margin of the tear in order to avoid tension overload. Anchors are placed 4 or 5 mm off the articular surface in a crescent array.

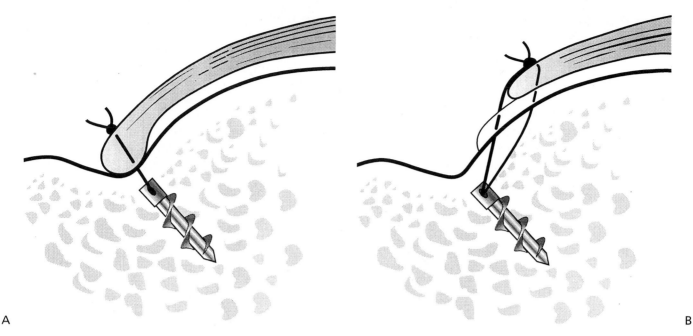

A   B

FIGURE 33.8 A: A tight suture loop keeps the tendon apposed to the prepared bone bed. **B:** A loose suture loop allows the tendon to pull away from the bone bed, even though the knot may be tight.

However, the loop security of complex sliding knots has not been investigated.

The literature pertaining to knot security is vast and confusing (38–48). We have attempted to simplify the issue of knot security by investigating its two extremes (36,49):

1. The minimal strength that a knot must possess to avoid failure under maximal physiologic load—that is, what is the weakest knot that will still be strong enough to hold a repair under all physiologic conditions?
2. The maximum strength that can be imparted to a knot, which for any given knot would necessitate converting its failure mode from failure by slippage to failure by breakage.

One must bear in mind that knot security depends on three factors: friction, internal interference, and slack between throws (36). Friction obviously will be greater for braided multifilament suture than for slick monofilament suture. Internal interference refers to the "weave" of the two suture limbs relative to each other, and it can be increased by changing posts between throws of the knot or reversing the direction of consecutive half-hitches, or both. Slack between throws is effectively removed by two maneuvers: (a) removing any twists between the two suture limbs before each half-hitch is tightened, and (b) past-pointing (running the knot pusher past the knot while tensioning the two suture limbs) to tighten each half-hitch. Therefore, one can increase knot security by using a braided suture, reversing the post suture limb and/or loop direction, removing all twists

between suture limbs to eliminate slack between throws, and past-pointing to tighten each half-hitch.

To look at the issue of suture failure, it is useful to calculate the maximal theoretical load that might be produced by a sudden forceful contraction of the rotator cuff. We have previously shown that if a 4-cm rotator cuff tear is fixed with three suture anchors loaded with two sutures each and located 1 cm apart, the load per suture during a maximal contraction is 37.75 N. We looked at the ultimate strength of all combinations of knots formed by four half-hitches (Fig. 33.9) and found that all except the same-post, same-loop configuration (S=S=S=S) withstood these forces (26,36). The other three configurations of stacked half-hitches—SxSxSxS, S//S//S//S, and S//xS//xS//xS—failed in the 38- to 50-N range, enough to withstand a maximal contraction but not by a very large margin (36). Therefore, I believe that we should consider these knots with four half-hitches to possess the minimal acceptable strength to failure.

All the above-mentioned stacked half-hitch configurations failed by slippage. However, failure by breakage rather than slippage would be preferable, because breakage always occurs at much higher loads than slippage. Failure by breakage indicates that knot security has been maximized. Therefore, we set out to determine what it takes to maximize knot security of standard knots so that they break rather than slip. In examining this issue, one must first understand that virtually all complex sliding knots (stacked half-hitches, Duncan loop, buntline hitch) fail by slippage. The conventional wisdom is that these knots can be "locked," so that they will not slip, by adding one or two half-hitches on top of the "base knot." We have investigated this concept experimentally and found that the conventional wisdom is wrong (49). One or two half-hitches will not lock the base knot in most cases. We found that the minimal configuration that will lock a base knot is three reversed-post half-hitches; that is, three half-hitches applied on top of the base knot so that the post is switched on three consecutive throws. The three reversed-post half-hitches will always lock the base knot and convert its mode of failure from slippage to breakage, thereby reliably maximizing knot security. Therefore, this is my recommended locking configuration, regardless of which base knot is used (49).

Repairing the U-Shaped Tear

Repair of massive U-shaped tears can be quite gratifying, because many of these tears appear irreparable on first view. However, one or two side-to-side sutures can often achieve such dramatic margin convergence that repair to bone becomes quite simple (Fig. 33.10).

In repairing large U-shaped tears, there are two biomechanical principles that must be sequentially followed to produce a functional rotator cuff. These principles are margin convergence (24) and balance of force couples (3).

I typically begin side-to-side closure with a combination of Penetrator and BirdBeak suture passers (Arthrex), which are used to pass permanent braided sutures through the posterior and anterior leaves of the cuff tear for side-to-side

repair, while viewing with the scope in a lateral subacromial portal. Most of the large and massive tears require three to four side-to-side sutures. These sutures are sequentially tied, the most medial suture first, to achieve margin convergence of the cuff over the prepared bone bed. Two Corkscrew or BioCorkscrew suture anchors are then placed, one for each leaf of the cuff tear. The anchor for the posterior leaf is placed approximately 1 cm anterolateral to the edge of the posterior leaf of the cuff so that the posterior leaf can be shifted proximally and anteriorly. This maneuver maximizes the moment produced by the posterior cuff in both the transverse and coronal planes, helping to create balanced force couples in both planes. The achievement of balanced force couples allows the shoulder to establish a stable fulcrum of glenohumeral motion. Loop security and knot security are vital to attaining and maintaining the shift of the posterior rotator cuff to the suture anchors (36,37). The anterior leaf is typically not as mobile as the posterior leaf, and a significant shift of the anterior leaf is usually not possible or necessary, so the anterior anchor is usually placed adjacent to the edge of the anterior leaf. Then the sutures from the anchor are passed through the anterior leaf by means of a suture passer through an anterior portal, and the sutures are tied. External rotation of the shoulder often optimizes the angle of approach of the suture passer through the anterior leaf. After suture passage, knots are tied with careful attention to knot security and loop security in order to optimize the fixation of tendon to bone.

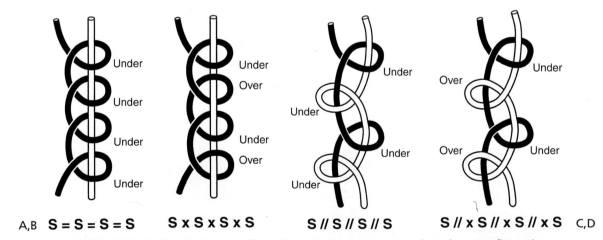

FIGURE 33.9 Half-hitch knot configurations. **A:** Same-post, same-loop knot configuration (S=S=S=S), in which the post is the same for each throw and each half-hitch is thrown in the same direction (either overhand or underhand). **B:** Same-post, reverse-loop knot configuration (SxSxSxS), in which the post is the same for each throw, but each consecutive half-hitch reverses direction (overhand to underhand, to overhand, to underhand). **C:** Reverse-post, same-loop knot configuration (S//S//S//S), in which the post is reversed with each half-hitch but each consecutive half-hitch is thrown the same way (overhand or underhand). **D:** Reverse-post, reverse-loop knot configuration (S//XS//XS//XS), in which, with each half-hitch, the post is reversed and the direction of the throw (overhand or underhand) is reversed.

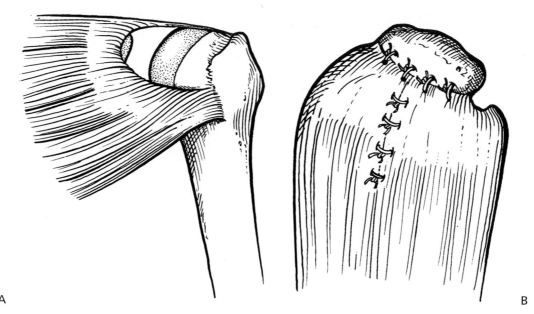

A   B

FIGURE 33.10 Repair of U-shaped cuff tears **(A)** begins with side-to-side sutures that converge the free margin toward the bone bed (margin convergence). After side-to-side sutures are placed, the free margin is repaired to bone with suture anchors **(B)**.

Partial Repair

If complete closure of cuff to bone cannot be accomplished even after margin convergence, the force couple can still be effective even though a hole is left in the superior portion of the cuff. Such partial cuff repairs have been shown to be very effective if at least half of the infraspinatus can be repaired to bone (50,51). Partial repairs are recommended whenever complete closure of the defect is not possible. I advise against transfer of rotator cuff tendons (e.g., subscapularis transfer), because such transfers change the mechanics of the shoulder and can significantly weaken the transferred muscle–tendon units.

Nonmobile Tears

In fewer than 5% of the large and massive tears in my practice, the tear is contracted and nonmobile (28). Tauro (52) advocated an arthroscopic interval slide for these patients, performing an arthroscopic release of the coracohumeral ligament (Fig. 33.11). This release sometimes achieves an additional 1 to 2 cm of lateral excursion of the supraspinatus tendon, thereby permitting a greater degree of partial repair than would have been possible without the release. My experience in doing 12 arthroscopic interval slides is that 6 patients improved their strength and motion by varying amounts and the other 6 did not improve. It is obvious that the results are quite variable, and I consider this a technique of "last resort."

Contracted nonmobile rotator cuff tears are chronic, long-standing tears with an unpredictable potential for improvement. Arthroscopic interval slide, although it may improve function, must be considered a heroic intervention for a desperate problem.

Results of Arthroscopic Repair of Rotator Cuff Tears

Published series of arthroscopic rotator cuff repair have been encouraging, reporting good to excellent results in more than 90% of patients (53,54) with small or medium-sized tears. The conventional wisdom has been that arthroscopic rotator cuff repair may be adequate for smaller tears but open repair is necessary to repair the large and massive tears. However, in my practice, I have found the conventional wisdom to be wrong. The great irony of arthroscopic cuff repair is that the larger the cuff tear, the greater the improvement compared with open techniques (9,16,21,55).

We recently reviewed the results of arthroscopic repair of 59 rotator cuff tears performed by me between September 1993 and August 1997 (28). Average follow-up was 3.5 years (range, 2 to 5 years). We subdivided these tears into groups according to tear diameter, using the classification system of DeOrio and Cofield (9), as follows: small, less than 1 cm; medium, 1 to 3 cm; large, 3 to 5 cm; and massive, greater than 5 cm) (9). Preoperative and postoperative University of California at Los Angeles (UCLA) scores were determined for each group, and intergroup comparisons

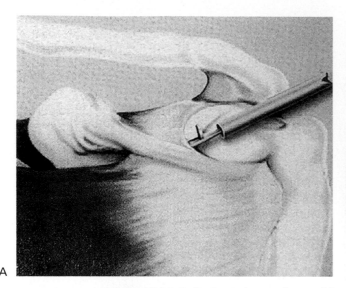
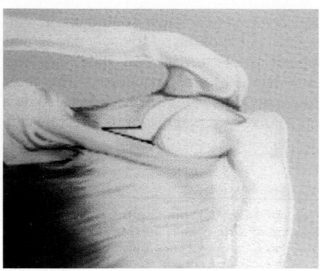

A

B

FIGURE 33.11 A: Contracted coracohumeral ligament tethers the cuff margin and prevents lateral excursion of the cuff margin. **B:** Interval slide has been performed by arthroscopically releasing the coracohumeral ligament, allowing the cuff margin to be advanced further laterally. (From Tauro JC. Arthroscopic "interval slide" in the repair of large rotator cuff tears. *Arthroscopy* 1999;15:527–530, with permission of the author.)

were done as well. Thirteen tears were in the "massive" category. Two of these were crescent-type tears that were repaired directly to bone, and 11 were U-shaped tears that were repaired by a margin convergence technique. None of these massive tears involved the subscapularis. Average UCLA scores improved from 14.0 (poor) before surgery to 29.9 (good) afterward. Forward flexion improved from 90 degrees to 132 degrees. The improvements in flexion and UCLA score were both highly significant ($p < .0001$). By UCLA criteria, good to excellent results were achieved in 92% of these patients.

Between-group comparisons for the four groups of tear sizes were made by analysis of variance (ANOVA) and confirmed by a power analysis that compared UCLA score improvements between groups to the standard deviations within groups. This analysis showed no between-group differences ($p > .005$) That is, the massive tears did as well as the small, medium, and large tears, with results independent of tear size.

Another interesting analysis was done to compare the results of all tears repaired directly to bone (crescent-shaped tears, 34 patients) with those of tears repaired by margin convergence (U-shaped tears, 25 patients). There was no difference between these two groups ($p > .05$), validating the selection criteria for repair of U-shaped tears by margin convergence. Despite the fact that the crescent-shaped tears were predominantly in the smaller categories and the U-shaped tears were mostly in the massive category, the differences in end results for forward flexion and for UCLA score between these two groups was not statistically signifi-

cant ($p > .05$). This finding is different from reported results with open cuff repair, in which larger tear sizes have been shown to have poorer outcomes than smaller ones (9,16,21,55), and it confirms the validity of repair by margin convergence.

Partial-Thickness Rotator Cuff Tears

Partial-thickness rotator cuff tears can be classified as bursal-surface tears, articular-surface tears, or interstitial tears (12). Snyder coined a clever acronym for partial articular surface tears, which he calls PASTA lesions (*p*artial *a*rticular *s*urface *t*endon *a*vulsion). Results of debridement, particularly for articular-surface tears, have been disappointing (56–58), and tear progression after debridement has been observed (59,60). It has been recommended that tears involving more than 50% of the thickness of the cuff should be repaired (57,60). The concept of the rotator cuff "footprint" is crucial to understanding what percentage thickness of the cuff is involved in a partial tear, particularly with an articular-surface tear. Tierney et al. (61) determined that the supraspinatus "footprint" in fresh-frozen cadaver shoulders had an average medial-to-lateral dimension of 16.9 mm (range, 12 to 25 mm), beginning at the articular margin. Therefore, a 50% articular-surface tear would be one with an "exposed footprint" of 8.5 mm on average from the articular margin, although an exposed footprint of 6 mm would represent a 50% tear in some patients. This exposed footprint is readily identifiable arthroscopically. This type of tear involves, at most, the supraspinatus and the upper half of the infraspinatus, because this is the only part of the cuff (other than subscapularis) whose footprint extends to the articular margin (62). The lower portion of the infraspinatus inserts lateral to the bare area of the humerus, which separates its footprint from the articular margin. (I have observed PASTA-type lesions of the subscapularis with a partially exposed footprint on the lesser tuberosity.) I advise arthroscopic repair of PASTA lesions if the exposed footprint is greater than 6 mm in width.

For the bursal-surface partial cuff tears, the unique arthroscopic characteristic is a normal intraarticular view of the cuff, with the tear being visualized only on subacromial inspection (60,63). These tears usually have an "unstable edge" consisting of a loose flap of cuff tissue that can catch under the acromion to cause symptoms. I prefer to repair bursal-surface tears that have an unstable edge, using a suture-anchor technique.

Interstitial tears are the least common of the partial tears (64). They usually can be diagnosed on magnetic resonance imaging (MRI) by a typical "bubble" appearance within the distal supraspinatus tendon, with intact cuff fibers on each side of the "bubble." Arthroscopically, the deficient tendon usually can be identified by palpation. The palpating instrument easily penetrates the thin, intact layer of tendon fibers and drops into the interstitial defect. In such cases, one should debride the "roof" of the defect to create a bursal-surface cuff tear, and then repair the resulting bursal-surface tear as described in the previous paragraph.

Results of Arthroscopic Repair of PASTA Lesions

For PASTA lesions, I have employed a transtendon suture-anchor repair technique to restore the footprint of the rotator cuff. I have evaluated 13 shoulders in 12 patients with an average of 18.5 months' follow-up after PASTA repair (range, 6 months to 5 years). The average UCLA score improved from 15.8 preoperatively to 30.8 postoperatively ($p < .0001$), with 10 of 13 scoring in the good to excellent range. Improvement in external rotation strength was often dramatic. It is my impression that low-demand patients may do well with debridement of a PASTA lesion, even though they may have persistent weakness, because their pain is decreased by the surgery. This is not the case with patients who require strength to carry out their daily activities. I have had two patients, one a mechanic and one an overhead laborer, who required revision surgery after an initial arthroscopic debridement because of persistent weakness that significantly affected their ability to perform their occupations. After arthroscopic transtendon repair of their PASTA lesions, both patients' external rotation strength improved from 50% of the normal side to approximately 90% of the normal side (as graded by manual muscle testing), and both patients rated their operated shoulders as normal after their revision surgery.

Seven of the 13 patients who underwent repair of PASTA lesions had associated superior labral anterior and posterior (SLAP) lesions that were also repaired. I have hypothesized that a SLAP lesion creates a superior instability pattern that produces excessive tensile forces in the undersurface of the cuff when the humerus subluxes proximally, and the SLAP lesion might, in this way, contribute to rotator cuff fiber failure (65).

Although I prefer a transtendon arthroscopic repair technique for PASTA lesions, there is another technique that I have used to repair these tears. This technique involves completing the tear, and then repairing the newly created full-thickness tear. When I use this approach I pay particular attention to restoring the footprint of the rotator cuff, frequently using two rows of suture anchors, one row at the edge of the articular cartilage and another row lateral to that. The reason that these types of tears require a double row of anchors is that they have an exceptionally long flap of cuff tissue. In fact, the fibers that the surgeon must cut across to complete the tear are on the lateral margin of the greater tuberosity. This long lateral extension of the cuff is in contradistinction to the majority of degenerative rotator cuff tears, which actually have loss of tendon substance within the rotator crescent (66) and therefore can be nicely repaired with one row of suture anchors.

Arthroscopic Subscapularis Repair

I performed arthroscopic subscapularis repair in 32 patients between August 1996 and May 2000 (67). Twenty-five shoulders with greater than 3 months' follow-up (average, 10.7 months) have been evaluated to assess the preliminary results.

Within that group of 25 shoulders, 17 had massive rotator cuff tears that included the subscapularis, supraspinatus, and infraspinatus, with an average tear size of 5 cm × 8 cm. Ten of these 17 shoulders had proximal humeral migration preoperatively, as demonstrated by an acromiohumeral interval of less than 5 mm and superior translation of the inferior articular margin of the humerus relative to the inferior articular margin of the glenoid of more 5 mm on anteroposterior radiographs. Eight of these ten shoulders (with preliminary follow-up of at least 3 months) had radiographically proven reversal of their proximal humeral migration (Fig. 33.12). In addition, overhead function improved in these eight shoulders from a preoperative "shoulder shrug" with attempted elevation of the arm to functional overhead use of the arm postoperatively.

Results of Arthroscopic Subscapularis Repair

We have monitored 25 shoulders with arthroscopic subscapularis repair for at least 3 months, with an average follow-up of 10.7 months (range, 3 months to 48 months) (67). The average time from onset of symptoms to surgery was 18.9 months (range, 1 to 72 months), indicating a significant delay before surgical repair. UCLA scores increased from a preoperative average of 10.7 to a postoperative average of 30.5 ($p < .0001$). Forward flexion increased from an average of 96.3 degrees preoperatively to an average of 146.1 degrees postoperatively ($p = .0016$). By UCLA criteria, excellent to good results were obtained in 92% of patients, with one fair and one poor result.

REPAIR TECHNIQUES

Mini-Open Repair Technique

Although the current trend is toward all-arthroscopic techniques, mini-open rotator cuff repair has long been considered a minimally invasive, arthroscopic-assisted technique, so it is included here for completeness. However, I expect this procedure to be largely replaced by arthroscopic repairs over the next few years.

The first stage of this procedure is to carry out an arthroscopic subacromial decompression. My preference is to use the "cutting block" technique (see Chapter 32), a variation of Sampson's "precision acromioplasty" (68). During the arthroscopic portion of the case, the cuff tear is evaluated as to its appropriateness for repair by the mini-open technique, based on the location, size, and mobility of the tear. The cuff margins are prepared arthroscopically, trimming loose flaps and fronds with a motorized shaver. The bone bed on the humeral neck and greater tuberosity can also be prepared arthroscopically with a motorized shaver or bur. At this point, the surgeon should attempt to upgrade his or her arthroscopic skills by placing suture anchors and passing sutures in order to do as much of the case arthroscopically as possible. This is the best way to make the transition from mini-open to all-arthroscopic cuff repairs.

Once the arthroscopic portion of the case is completed, the surgeon creates an anterolateral deltoid-splitting incision by extending the lateral arthroscopic portal proximally to the acromial margin and distally a couple of centimeters so that the entire deltoid split measures approximately 4 cm in length (Fig. 33.13). Deltoid retractors are used to expose the underlying rotator cuff tear. A traction suture in the cuff can be helpful in manipulating it during the repair. The humerus can be internally or externally rotated to bring other parts of the cuff into view within the mini-open incision. Suture anchors or bone tunnels are placed. Sutures are then placed through the cuff. I have found simple sutures to be adequate for most tears (Fig. 33.14). Muscle, subcutaneous, and skin layers are then repaired by standard techniques.

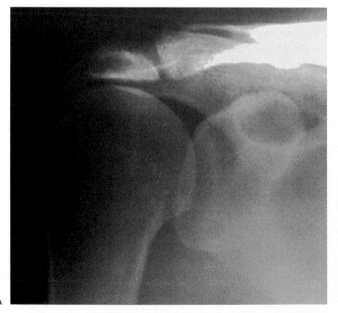
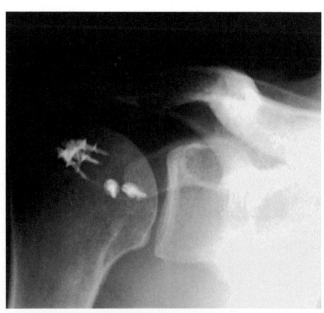

A   B

FIGURE 33.12 A: Proximal humeral migration associated with a massive tear involving the subscapularis, supraspinatus, and infraspinatus. **B:** Reversal of proximal humeral migration after repair of massive cuff tear involving subscapularis. Note that the inferior articular margins of the proximal humerus and glenoid are now at the same level.

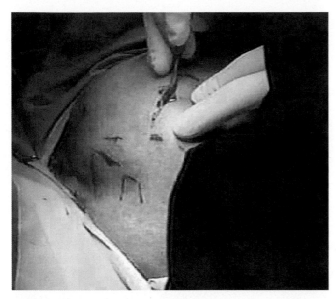

FIGURE 33.13 A 4-cm deltoid split incorporating the anterolateral portal comprises the mini-open incision. (Patient is in the lateral decubitus position.)

I prefer to perform the arthroscopic and mini-open portions of the procedure with the patient in the lateral decubitus position, with the shoulder in 20 to 30 degrees of abduction. This position allows placement of the operating room lights directly over the incision and generally allows better visualization, in my opinion, than the supine or beach-chair position.

Arthroscopic Repair of Full-Thickness Rotator Cuff Tears

I cannot overemphasize the importance of "tear pattern recognition," as discussed previously in this chapter. The

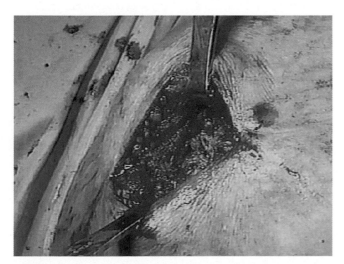

FIGURE 33.14 Final result. Cuff repair viewed through mini-open incision.

surgeon must determine whether the tear is a crescent-shaped tear or a U-shaped tear so that the proper biomechanical principles of repair can be applied. These principles were outlined in detail in an earlier section. The descriptions that follow are step-by-step instructions in the application of those principles.

Preoperative Planning

My routine radiographic series for all shoulder patients includes "true" anteroposterior views of the glenohumeral joint (30-degree posterior oblique views) in internal and external rotation, axillary view, outlet view, and 30-degree caudal tilt view (69). I obtain an MRI scan on every preoperative shoulder patient. The MRI is essential for diagnosing spinoglenoid ganglion cysts, which can produce symptoms that mimic those of rotator cuff tear and impingement. In addition, the MRI can give some clues as to whether a large or massive rotator cuff tear is repairable by margin convergence. For example, the MRI of a large U-shaped tear that can be repaired by margin convergence will show the apex of the tear located just above the glenoid, in association with an intact subscapularis and intact posterior-inferior rotator cuff (teres minor alone, or teres minor plus part of the infraspinatus).

General Technique Parameters

I perform all rotator cuff repairs arthroscopically with the patient in the lateral decubitus position. Balanced suspension of 5 to 10 pounds is used, with the arm in 30 to 40 degrees abduction and 20 degrees forward flexion, using the Star Sleeve traction system (Arthrex). The amount of abduction is set intraoperatively at the level that provides the best exposure, and it can be changed as needed during the procedure.

General anesthesia with endotracheal intubation is administered in each case. I do not use regional anesthesia such as interscalene blocks. A warming blanket is placed to prevent hypothermia. An arthroscopic pump maintains the subacromial pressure at 60 mm Hg. If bleeding causes poor visualization, the pump pressure can be temporarily adjusted up to 95 mm Hg until the bleeding is controlled, but I do not like to maintain pressures greater than 90 mm Hg for more than 15 minutes at a time because of the increased swelling that these high pressures can cause. In general, careful attention to blocking fluid flow from noncannulated portals by means of digital pressure facilitates a clear view by controlling turbulence within this closed system (70) (Fig. 33.15).

The two key elements to doing any shoulder operation arthroscopically are (a) visualization, achieved by means of electrocautery and turbulence control (70), and (b) proper angle of approach, achieved by a combination of proper por-

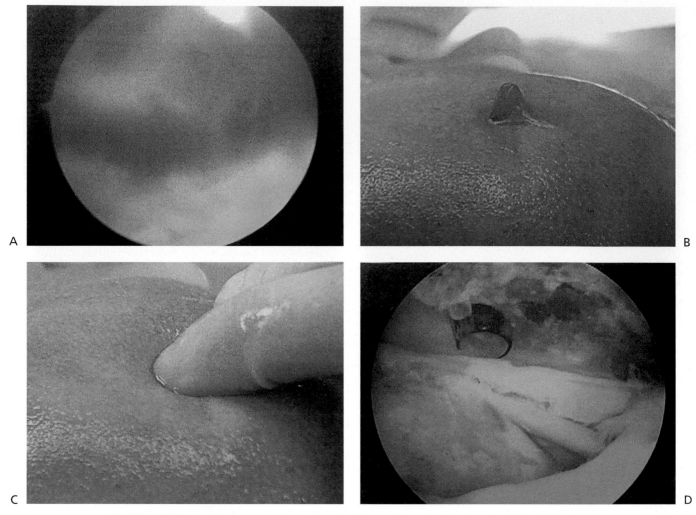

FIGURE 33.15 Turbulence control as a means of improving visualization. **A:** A bloody field of view obscures the anatomic features in this subacromial view. **B:** Turbulence associated with free egress of the fluid causes the bloody field. **C:** Digital pressure over the noncannulated portal stops the turbulent flow. **D:** Same field as (A) after 10 seconds of digital pressure over the portal. Visualization has been dramatically improved.

tal placement and proper instrument configuration. If the surgeon can see to work and can reach the pathologic area with the instruments, he or she can repair any rotator cuff tear arthroscopically.

Repair of the Crescent-Shaped Tear

After arthroscopic inspection of the glenohumeral joint and appropriate treatment of any intraarticular pathology, the arthroscope is placed in the subacromial space through a posterior portal. A lateral working and viewing portal is then established. An anterior portal is also created to function as an accessory working portal as well as an inflow portal.

The first step is to clear all bursal and fibrofatty tissues from the margins of the cuff tear in order to properly classify the tear. This is initiated with the scope posterior and the shaver lateral, but the posterior portion of a large cuff tear is best cleared of adventitial tissue by viewing through the lateral portal and bringing the shaver in through the posterior portal. After that has been done, the bone bed is prepared with a shaver through the lateral working portal.

The tear pattern is assessed by testing the mobility of the tear margin with an atraumatic tendon grasper (Arthrex). If the tear can be easily brought to the bone bed with minimal tension, then it can be repaired directly to bone with suture anchors (Fig. 33.16).

Next, I do a standard arthroscopic decompression by the cutting block technique if I am dealing with a repairable tear that is less than 5 cm in diameter. If the tear is larger than 5 cm, even if it is repairable, I do a subacromial "smoothing"

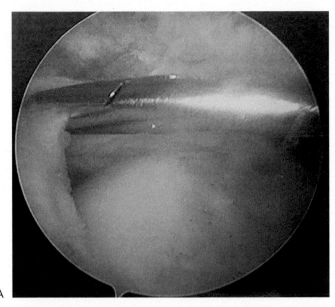
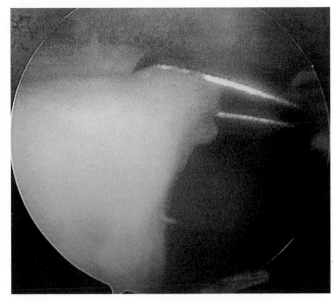

A   B

FIGURE 33.16 Right shoulder, posterior viewing portal. **A:** A tendon grasper is useful in determining tear configuration by assessing tear mobility. **B:** This tear can easily be brought laterally to the bone bed with minimal tension.

as recommended by Matsen et al. (71), rather than a true subacromial decompression.

Adequate visualization for carrying out the repair necessitates a clear view into the lateral gutter, and this requires removal of the lateral shelf of the subacromial bursa (Fig. 33.17A). I prefer to use a biodegradable DL-PLA screw-type suture anchor (BioCorkscrew). With a screw-type anchor, the suture must be passed through the tendon after the an-

chor has been placed in bone. The anchors are placed into the bone bed at a 30- to 45-degree "deadman angle" (31) approximately 5 to 10 mm from the articular margin (Fig. 33.17B). Anchors are placed 1 cm apart. A pointed bone punch with an expanded proximal section (Fig. 33.18) allows most BioCorkscrew anchors to be placed without the need for tapping a channel for the threads. However, if the bone is very hard, a tap becomes necessary (Fig. 33.19). If

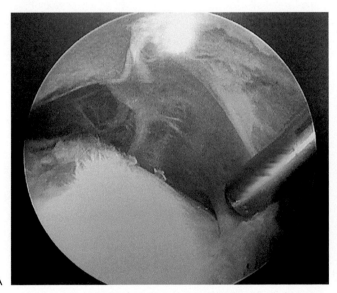
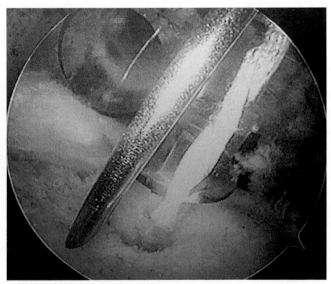

A   B

FIGURE 33.17 Right shoulder, posterior viewing portal. **A:** Lateral bursal "shelf" must be taken down to expose the "corner" of the greater tuberosity. **B:** A BioCorkscrew polylactic acid suture anchor (Arthrex, Inc., Naples, FL) is placed into bone at a 30- to 45-degree "deadman angle."

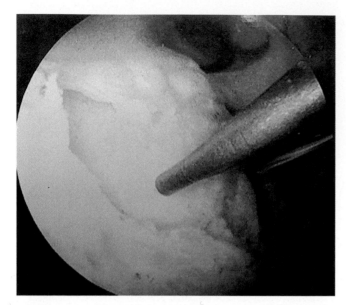

FIGURE 33.18 Right shoulder, posterior viewing portal. Bone punch with trumpet-shaped proximal section creates a bone socket for the biodegradable polylactic acid anchor (Bio-Corkscrew, Arthrex, Inc., Naples, FL).

the surgeon chooses a metallic suture anchor, the eyelet of the anchor should be directed toward the cuff margin to ensure easy sliding of the suture. In the case of the Bio-Corkscrew, the eyelet consists of a flexible loop of no. 4 Ethibond suture that is insert-molded into the body of the anchor (Fig. 33.20). The flexibility of this eyelet allows the suture to slide easily through it no matter which way it is oriented. With this flexible eyelet, "fouling" of the sutures within the eyelet has not been an issue.

Suture passage is performed by passing a suture retriever such as a Penetrator or BirdBeak through the superior aspect of the cuff in line with the sutures, which can then be easily retrieved and pulled back out through the cuff with viewing

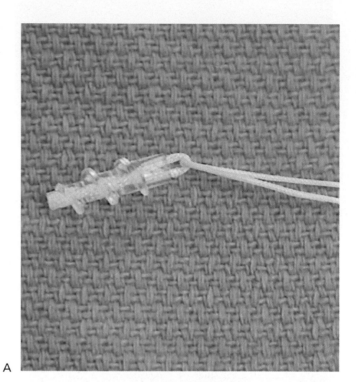

A

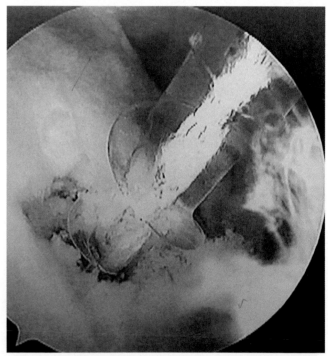

B

FIGURE 33.20 Right shoulder, lateral viewing portal. **A:** Eyelet of BioCorkscrew suture anchor (Arthrex, Inc., Naples, FL) is a flexible suture loop, which prevents fouling of suture during knot tying. **B:** Insert-molded suture that forms the eyelet can be seen through the transparent BioCorkscrew.

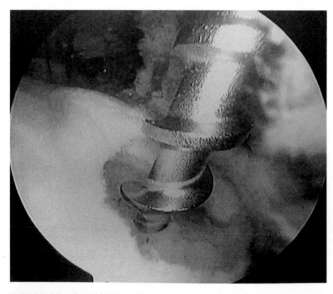

FIGURE 33.19 Right shoulder, posterior viewing portal. A tap is used on hard bone to create the channels for the screw-threads of the biodegradable suture anchor.

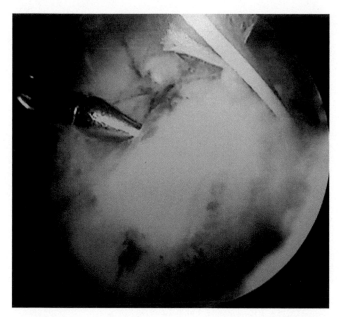

FIGURE 33.21 Right shoulder, lateral viewing portal. The Penetrator (Arthrex, Inc., Naples, FL) suture passer is brought in through a posterior portal, and the surgeon determines the proper angle of approach to the sutures by "lining up the putt" toward the sutures.

through the lateral portal. The correct angle of approach through the posterior cuff is obtained by backing the arthroscope out the lateral portal enough to obtain a panoramic view of the suture passer and sutures, then "lining up the putt" (Fig. 33.21) so that the suture retriever ends up close enough to the suture to easily capture it (Fig. 33.22). For the anterior portion of the cuff, the angle of approach is often

more easily accomplished with an angled suture passer (BirdBeak), with the shoulder held in maximal external rotation (Fig. 33.23).

For large crescent-shaped tears, the central portion of the cuff is best approached by a modified Neviaser portal as described by Nord (72). This portal consists of a small puncture wound 3 mm in length (just large enough for passage of a suture passer without a cannula), located approximately 2 to 3 cm posteromedial to the acromioclavicular joint, in the "soft spot" bordered by posterior clavicle, medial acromion, and scapular spine (Fig. 33.24). A spinal needle is used to determine the proper location of the portal, and then the suture passer is placed by "walking it down" adjacent to the needle as the surgeon arthroscopically observes its entry into the subacromial space. One limb of each suture is passed individually through the cuff in order to obtain separate soft tissue fixation points for each suture.

I prefer to pass all the sutures from the anchors before tying any knots. After suture passage, I tie knots starting with the sutures nearest the intact cuff insertions and then proceed to those that pass through the central part of the tear. In this way, I sequentially decrease the amount of tension that the central sutures will have to withstand. By passing all the sutures before tying, it is easier to manipulate the suture retriever under the cuff margin, because the cuff is not bound down by sutures that have already been tied. A potential drawback to passing all the sutures before tying any knots is that a tangled mess may result. However, the tangling is easily remedied as the suture pairs are retrieved for knot tying. By grasping suture pairs proximal to the entanglement and pulling the pairs to be tied, one pair at a time, through a dedicated cannula (usually lateral) for knot tying,

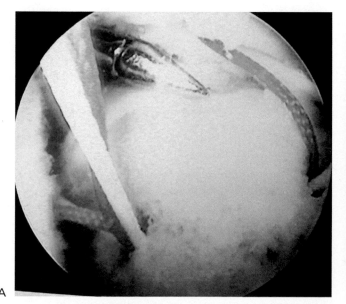

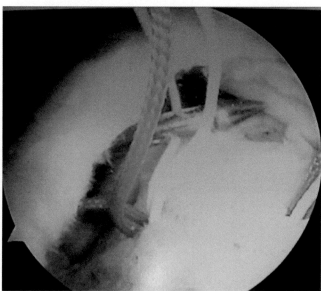

A   B

FIGURE 33.22 Right shoulder, lateral viewing portal. **A:** The Penetrator (Arthrex, Inc., Naples, FL) has passed through the cuff and is ready for suture capture. **B:** Suture has been captured in window of Penetrator for retrieval through the cuff.

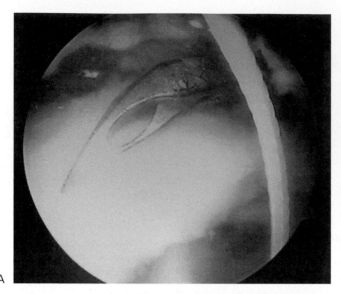
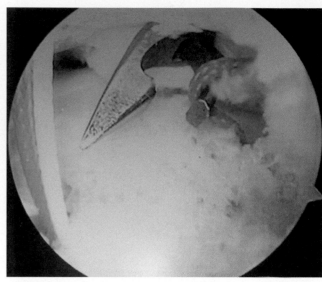

A   B

FIGURE 33.23 Right shoulder, lateral viewing portal. **A:** The angle of approach through the anterior leaf of cuff can be difficult. An angled BirdBeak (Arthrex, Inc., Naples, FL) suture passer is useful in this case. **B:** With external rotation of the arm and the use of a 45-degree BirdBeak, the suture can be easily captured.

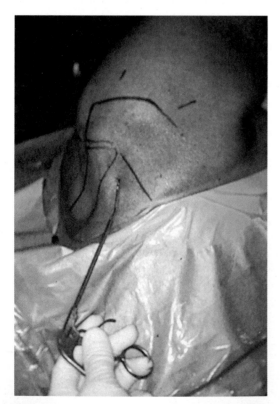

FIGURE 33.24 Right shoulder, lateral decubitus position. Modified Neviaser portal, located 2 to 3 cm posteromedial to the acromioclavicular joint, in the "soft spot" bordered by posterior clavicle, medial acromion, and scapular spine.

the entanglement is never an issue for suture pairs as they are being tied.

At this point, some surgeons would tie complex sliding knots to secure the rotator cuff to the bone bed. I prefer not to use sliding knots, in order to avoid damaging the tendon or even cutting through the tendon as the suture slides, and also to avoid abrasion of the suture against the eyelet of the anchor (especially a metal anchor), which could weaken the suture (73). I tie a nonsliding knot with a double-diameter knot pusher (Surgeon's Sixth Finger) (Fig. 33.25) to create a static locked knot composed of a base knot (consisting of three stacked half-hitches) that is locked by three additional half-hitches with the post reversed for each throw. The suture limb that passes through the cuff is threaded through the lumen of the knot pusher so that the knot will be positioned on top of the cuff rather than over the bone, for better loop security. Continuous tension is maintained in the post limb as the knot is tied to prevent loosening of the soft tissue loop. Post switching is accomplished without rethreading the knot pusher (74), simply by tensioning the wrapping suture limb at the same time that tension is released on the post suture limb (Fig. 33.26). By "flipping" the post three consecutive times in this manner, maximal knot security is ensured (49). The completed repair should produce a crescent shape to the repaired cuff margin, to avoid tension overload centrally (29), with a separate soft tissue fixation point for each suture. Tissue indentation by the suture is a good indicator of loop security (Fig. 33.27).

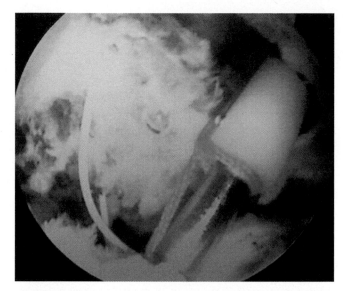

FIGURE 33.25 Right shoulder, posterior viewing portal. Double-diameter knot pusher (Surgeon's Sixth Finger, Arthrex, Inc., Naples, FL) is used to tie a static knot.

Repair of the U-Shaped Tear

After glenohumeral arthroscopy has been completed, subacromial bursoscopy is initiated through a posterior viewing portal. A lateral working portal and anterior inflow portal are established. After an initial inspection of the subacromial space through the posterior portal, the arthroscope is switched to a lateral viewing portal. With large U-shaped tears, the posterior leaf often has its margin obscured by the abundant bursal and fibrofatty tissue in the posterior por-

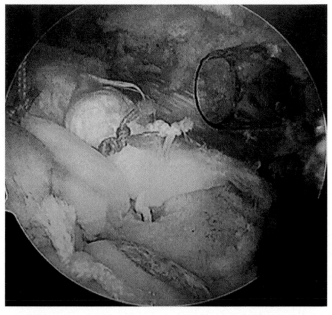

FIGURE 33.27 Right shoulder, posterior viewing portal. Crescent array of rotator cuff margin fixed by four sutures, each with a separate soft tissue fixation point. Tissue indentation by the suture confirms excellent loop security.

tion of the subacromial space. This tissue is removed by a shaver brought in through a posterior portal (Fig. 33.28). The bursal tissue can be very thick, and the surgeon may even confuse it for tendon. If there is any confusion, the surgeon must follow the edge of the ambiguous tissue as far lateral as possible. If it inserts into the humerus, it is obviously tendon. But if it continues past the humerus to "insert" into

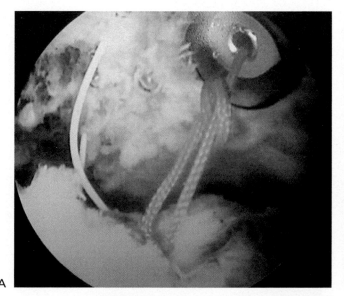

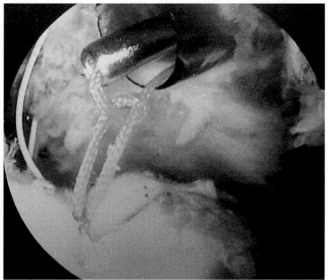

A   B

FIGURE 33.26 Right shoulder, posterior viewing portal. **A:** To "flip" the half-hitch and reverse posts without rethreading the knot pusher, the knot pusher is backed away from the unsecured half-hitch approximately 1 cm. Note that the post limb (straight suture limb under tension) is the one that is threaded through the knot pusher. **B:** After the loop limb is tensioned while tension is released on the post limb, the post has switched so that now the knot pusher is threaded on the loop limb. The post has been changed without rethreading the knot pusher.

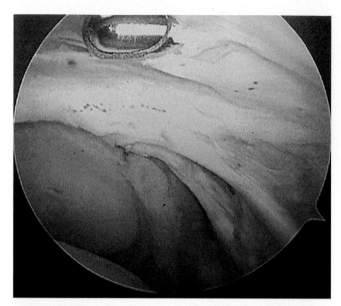

FIGURE 33.28 Left shoulder, lateral viewing portal. Power shaver is brought in through a posterior portal to remove the fibrofatty tissue that obscures the plane between posterior cuff and deltoid.

deltoid fascia, then it is bursal and must be removed (Fig. 33.29).

Once the cuff margins are totally exposed, the surgeon must determine whether the tear is a mobile U-shaped tear and therefore amenable to repair by the margin convergence technique (24). With the arthroscope lateral, the apex of the tear is visualized. If the apex is located at or medial to the glenoid margin, the tear is usually a U-shaped tear. The surgeon's next task is to determine whether it is a *mobile* tear whose anterior and posterior leaves can be approximated by side-to-side sutures to achieve margin convergence. An atraumatic tendon grasper (Arthrex) is brought in through the lateral portal to grasp the posterior leaf and test its mobility in an anterior direction. Then the grasper is used to grasp the anterior leaf and test its mobility posteriorly. If the surgeon determines that the two leaves are mobile enough to contact each other for side-to-side repair, the U-shaped configuration of the repair is confirmed (Fig. 33.30). If the configuration is not certain, the surgeon can place a single side-to-side suture approximately 1 cm from the apex of the tear, then tension the suture to see whether it achieves a partial closure of the tear (Fig. 33.31). Frequently, the margin convergence effect of a single suture is quite dramatic, causing the two leaves of the cuff to "converge" the cuff to an almost tension-free state above the bone bed that comprises the "footprint" of the rotator cuff on the humeral neck.

Cuff mobilization along the glenoid margin is not usually required, although previously operated cases may have adhesions between the cuff and the deltoid or between the cuff and the acromion that need to be lysed or excised. If the cuff is scarred to the deltoid, the proper plane of dissection be-

tween them is best located by first finding the fatty layer above the cuff at the apex of the tear, beneath the medial acromion. This fatty stripe is then followed posteriorly, using the shaver as a dissector. Because this fat layer separates the deltoid from the cuff, even in adhered cases, one can follow it to the periphery of the cuff margin, which is the portion of the cuff that is bound to the deltoid by scar. These adhesions between the deltoid and peripheral cuff are then released by a shaver or by electrocautery to fully define the leaves of the cuff to be repaired.

For large or massive U-shaped tears, I usually do not perform an arthroscopic acromioplasty. Instead, I do a subacromial "smoothing" as recommended by Matsen et al. (71). This smoothing amounts to a debridement of the soft tissues on the undersurface of the acromion, with removal of small osseous irregularities but with preservation of the coracoacromial arch, including the coracoacromial ligament. The arch is preserved to retain this last restraint against proximal humeral migration in case the repair should fail.

Next, the bone bed on the humeral neck and greater tuberosity is prepared by a power shaver through a lateral working portal. The shaver is usually adequate to prepare a bleeding bone bed without decorticating the bone. Decortication should be avoided to maximize the bone's resistance to pull-out of the suture anchors. Animal studies have demonstrated that tendon healing to a bleeding surface of cortical bone is as strong as tendon healing to cancellous bone (30).

Now the cuff is ready for the margin convergence stage of the procedure. The scope is placed through a lateral por-

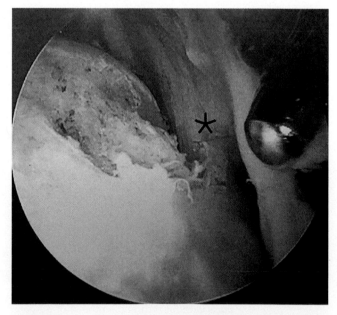

FIGURE 33.29 Left shoulder, lateral viewing portal. The shaver removes the synovialized "leader" that extends beyond the cuff margin to insert into deltoid fascia. The actual cuff insertion into bone (*) can be seen distal to this "leader."

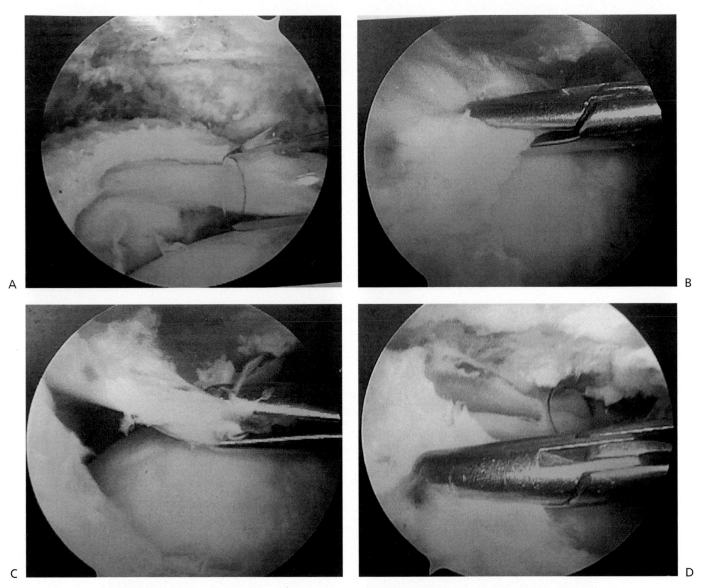

FIGURE 33.30 Right shoulder, posterior viewing portal. A through D: Testing mobility of tear. **A:** Massive rotator cuff tear with apex just above the glenoid. **B:** Tendon grasper tests medial-to-lateral mobility of cuff, and it will not reach to bone bed. **C:** Tendon grasper pulls anterior leaf posteriorly past the midline of the humeral head, confirming excellent mobility. **D:** Tendon grasper on posterior leaf demonstrates good mobility, confirming that this is a U-shaped tear requiring margin convergence.

tal for optimal viewing of side-to-side suture placement. This lateral portal gives a panoramic "Grand Canyon" view of the massive tear that is essential for passage of side-to-side sutures (Fig. 33.32). I prefer to use two suture passers (Penetrator or BirdBeak), one for each leaf of the cuff, in order to achieve a "hand-off" of the suture from one leaf to the other. A no. 2 Ethibond suture is loaded into one of the suture passers. This "loaded" suture passer is brought through the posterior portal to penetrate the posterior leaf of the cuff near the apex of the tear. A second (empty) suture passer is brought through the anterior leaf via the anterior portal, and a "hand-off" of the suture is performed from posterior to an-

terior. Then the anterior suture passer is withdrawn, pulling the suture through the anterior leaf and out the anterior portal. (Fig. 33.33). This step is repeated with additional sutures as many times as necessary, placing the sutures at intervals of 5 to 10 mm, with the most lateral suture overlying the medial portion of the bone bed. Ordinarily, if the apex of the tear overlies the glenoid, an average of four side-to-side sutures is used. White sutures are alternated with green sutures to facilitate suture management. I prefer to place all of the side-to-side sutures before tying any of them.

The sutures are then tied sequentially from medial to lateral to accomplish margin convergence (Fig. 33.34). The

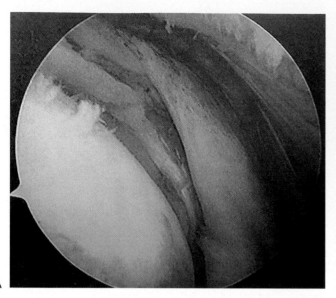
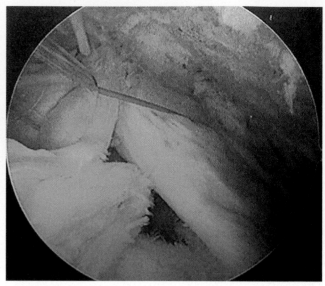

A   B

FIGURE 33.31 Left shoulder, lateral viewing portal. **A:** The apex of the tear overlies the superior glenoid rim, suggesting that this is a U-shaped tear. **B:** Placement of a single side-to-side suture accomplishes dramatic partial closure with an obvious margin convergence effect.

apex suture is tied first by bringing its two limbs out the posterior portal. All of the other suture limbs are retrieved through an alternative (usually anterior) cannula. It is important that only the two suture limbs that are being tied occupy the working cannula in order to avoid "fouling" of contiguous sutures. I prefer to use a clear, 7-mm "fish-bowl" cannula (Arthrex) for better visualization of the knot-tying, and I also prefer to tie the knots over the posterior leaf of the cuff to avoid the theoretical problem of knot impingement

under the acromion. In performing the side-to-side closure, it is important to achieve both loop security (37) (maintenance of a tight suture loop around the enclosed soft tissue) and knot security (36,49) (resistance of the knot to failure by slippage). I have been able to best accomplish those goals by means of stacked half-hitches tied with a double-diameter knot pusher (Surgeon's Sixth Finger) Other surgeons may prefer a variety of complex sliding knots (e.g., Duncan loop). With my technique, I use the knot pusher to stack two or three half-hitches (a "base knot" that comprises the simplest type of complex sliding knot), and then I add three more half-hitches, for which I consecutively switch posts for each throw. Post switching can easily be accomplished without rethreading the knot pusher simply by tensioning the wrapping suture limb at the same time that tension is released on the post suture limb. We have recently demonstrated that any sliding knot will have its strength optimized (i.e., will have its failure mode converted from slippage to breakage) by stacking three half-hitches on top of the sliding knot with reversal of the post between each half-hitch (49). I therefore recommend, no matter which basic sliding knot is used, that three reverse-post half-hitches be stacked on top of it.

As the side-to-side sutures are sequentially tied, the free margin of the cuff can be seen to converge laterally over the bone bed. However, in some cases, the margin will not converge far enough laterally for the rotator cuff to fully cover the articular surface of the humerus. In these cases, I close the cuff side-to-side as far as possible, then repair each leaf to bone with suture anchors, leaving a hole in the top of the cuff (partial repair).

After accomplishing margin convergence with side-to-side repair of the anterior and posterior leaves of the cuff, the

FIGURE 33.32 Left shoulder, lateral viewing portal. "Grand Canyon" view of a massive U-shaped rotator cuff tear.

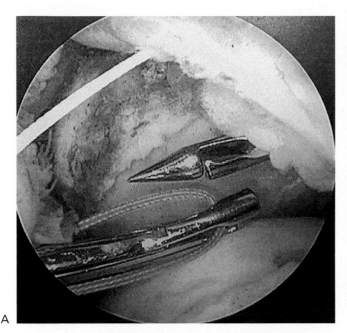
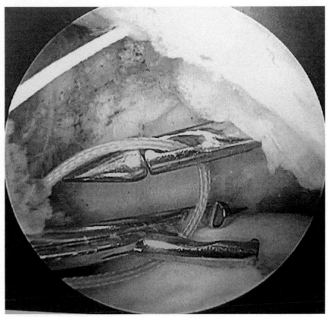

A   B

FIGURE 33.33 Right shoulder, lateral viewing portal. The "hand-off" technique of passing side-to-side sutures. **A:** A Penetrator suture passer (Arthrex, Inc., Naples, FL) delivers the suture through the posterior leaf of the rotator cuff, and another Penetrator is brought through the anterior leaf. **B:** Suture "hand-off" is accomplished.

next step is to advance the leaves on the bone bed and secure them to bone with suture anchors. Using a posterior viewing portal, I place two biodegradable DL-PLA screw-in anchors (BioCorkscrew, Arthex), one for each leaf of the cuff (Fig. 33.35). Each anchor is brought in through a 3-mm percutaneous stab wound adjacent to the lateral acromion, after first using a spiked bone punch to create sockets in the

bone bed for the anchors. A spinal needle is used to locate the optimal position of these two stab wounds. The suture anchors are placed approximately 1 cm from the posterior and anterior leaves of the cuff in order to shift the leaves to the anchors as the knots are tied. This shift optimizes the force couple provided by the repaired cuff muscles by maximizing the superior-to-inferior dimension of the bone at-

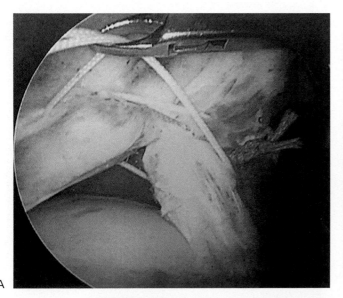
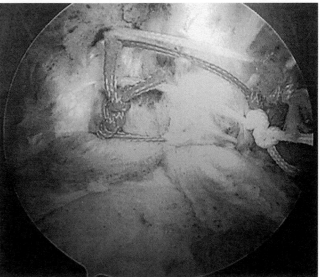

A   B

FIGURE 33.34 Margin convergence. **A:** The side-to-side sutures are sequentially tied from medial to lateral. **B:** After all of the side-to-side sutures have been tied, the "converged" margin of the rotator cuff overlies the prepared bone bed, ready for tension-free suture anchor fixation to bone.

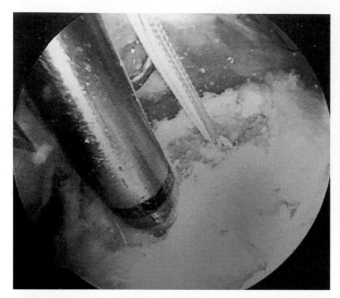

FIGURE 33.35 Left shoulder, posterior viewing portal. An anterior anchor has been placed. The punch for making the bone socket for the posterior anchor is 1 cm from the edge of the posterior leaf.

tachments of the cuff. I next place my scope laterally and pass the sutures of the posterior anchor through the posterior leaf. This is done by bringing the Penetrator suture passer through the posterior portal, withdrawing the scope enough to visualize the anchor sutures as well as the suture passer, and then "lining up the putt" to pass the Penetrator through the posterior leaf in the direction of the anchor. The Penetrator then captures one suture limb and withdraws it through the posterior leaf. This sequence is repeated for the anterior leaf, where the 45-degree BirdBeak suture passer usually provides a better angle of approach. Finally, I tie the knots through a clear cannula placed in the lateral portal while viewing through the posterior portal. In tying the knots, I shift the cuff to the anchors, maximizing contact of the cuff with the bone bed. The arm is then rotated to view the entire repair and assess its security and strength (Fig. 33.36). These repairs are quite secure with the arm at the side.

Postoperative Management after Repair of Full-Thickness Tears

I place the operated arm at the side in a sling with a small pillow attached. All procedures are performed on an outpatient basis, and the patients leave the postoperative recovery area approximately 1½ hours after surgery.

Passive external rotation is begun immediately. Elbow flexion and extension are also initiated right away. However, I do not start any overhead stretching until 6 weeks after surgery in order to avoid excessive stress on the repair, which can be significant even with passive overhead stretching. This 6-week period of immobilization maximizes tendon-to-bone healing with reestablishment of as much of the rotator cuff footprint as possible. The stiffness that comes with immobilization of open shoulder surgery patients does not seem to occur in arthroscopic patients so long as early passive external rotation is carried out. The most logical explanation is that deltoid damage is minimized by the arthroscopic approach. In addition, by avoiding massive mobilization of U-shaped tears, one does not nonphysiologically overtighten the repair.

At the end of 6 weeks, I discontinue the sling, start overhead stretches with a rope and pulley, and initiate internal rotation stretches.

I wait until 12 weeks after surgery to begin muscle strengthening. Sonnabend et al. (75) observed, in a primate study of rotator cuff repair, that strong Sharpey-type fibers did not form until 12 weeks after surgery. Therefore, to minimize the risk of early retear, I wait 12 weeks to start resistive exercises. At that point, I initiate rehabilitation of the rotator cuff, deltoid, biceps, and scapular stabilizers.

Activities are progressed as strength allows. Unrestricted activities, particularly activities that require angular acceleration of the shoulder (tennis, baseball, golf) are not allowed until at least 6 months after surgery.

Repair of the Contracted, Nonmobile Tear

Some long-standing rotator cuff tears develop a fixed, nonmobile, contracted configuration. These tears do not have enough mobility to perform either tendon-to-bone or side-to-side repair. These tears comprise less than 5% of the large and massive tears in my practice (28). Tauro advocated an arthroscopic interval slide for these cases, performing an

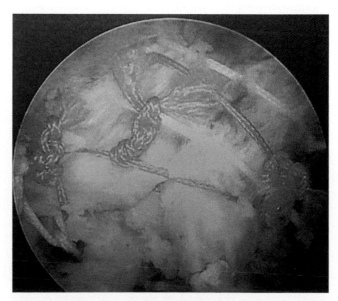

FIGURE 33.36 Left shoulder, lateral viewing portal, final result. Side-to-side sutures maintain margin convergence while the two suture anchors ensure strong fixation to bone.

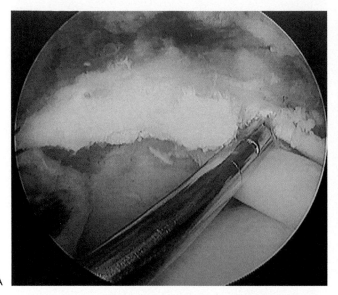

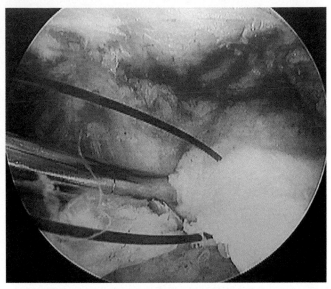

A   B

FIGURE 33.37 Right shoulder, lateral viewing portal. **A:** A basket punch is used to release the coracohumeral ligament, which overlies the root of the biceps. **B:** After coracohumeral ligament release (interval slide), the supraspinatus tendon will reach the bone bed for repair.

arthroscopic release of the corahumeral ligament (52). This release sometimes achieves an additional 1 to 2 cm of lateral excursion of the supraspinatus tendon, thereby permitting a greater degree of repair (usually partial repair) than would have been possible without the release (Fig. 33.37). Rehabilitation is the same as outlined in the previous section for full-thickness tears.

Partial Repair of Massive Rotator Cuff Tears

If complete closure of the rotator cuff tear cannot be accomplished either by tendon-to-bone repair or by margin convergence, partial repair is performed, repairing as much of the anterior and posterior cuff as possible to restore the transverse plane force couple (Fig. 33-38). Such partial cuff repairs have been shown to be very effective if at least half of the infraspinatus can be repaired to bone (50,51).

Repair of Bursal-Surface Partial-Thickness Rotator Cuff Tears

The bursal-surface partial-thickness tears have, as their defining characteristic, an intact capsule in association with a cuff tear that is visible only from a subacromial perspective (Fig. 33.39). Such tears are easily repaired by the same suture-anchor techniques that were described for full-thickness crescent-shaped tears (Fig. 33.40).

Repair of PASTA Lesions

The hallmark of the PASTA lesion is the "exposed footprint" of the rotator cuff, which is readily identifiable

arthroscopically. The rotator cuff normally inserts at the articular margin (Fig. 33.41), as seen on intraarticular inspection. In some cases, the cuff begins to tear from inside out, leaving an "exposed footprint" where the cuff would normally attach, with intact cuff fibers lateral to the "exposed footprint" (Fig. 33.42). I repair PASTA lesions that have an "exposed footprint" greater than 6 mm in width.

There are two ways to repair a PASTA lesion. The surgeon may employ a transtendon repair technique, in which suture anchors are inserted through the tendon and into bone without disruption of the intact lateral cuff fibers. Al-

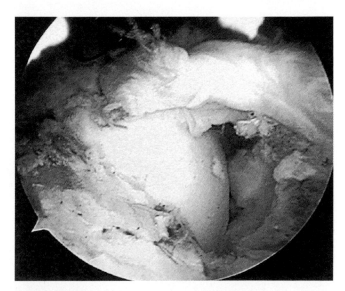

FIGURE 33.38 Left shoulder, lateral viewing portal. Partial repair of a massive cuff tear has been accomplished, repairing the subscapularis anteriorly and advancing the posterior cuff. A large hole in the superior cuff persists.

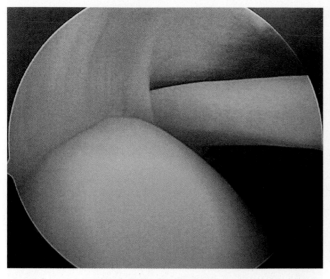
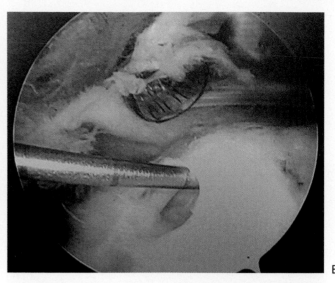

FIGURE 33.39 Left shoulder, posterior viewing portal. **A:** Intraarticular view shows normal capsular insertion at the articular margin, with no exposed "footprint." **B:** Subacromial view of the same patient shows a significant rotator cuff tear.

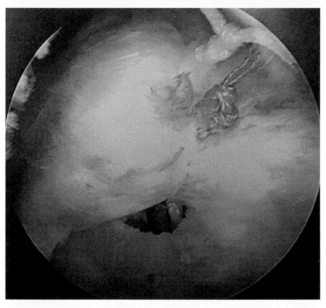

FIGURE 33.40 Left shoulder, lateral viewing portal. Rotator cuff repair has been accomplished with a single suture anchor.

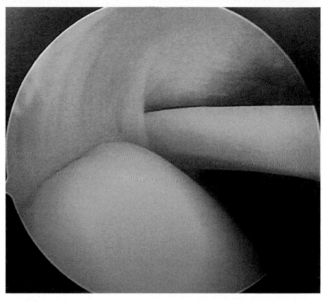

FIGURE 33.41 Left shoulder, posterior viewing portal. Normal cuff insertion extends to the articular margin of the proximal humerus.

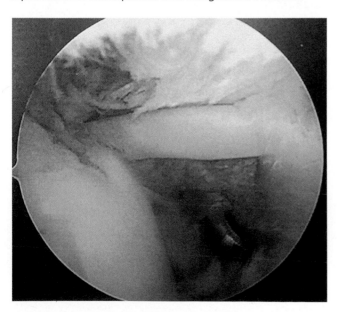

FIGURE 33.42 Left shoulder, posterior viewing portal. There is a "bare footprint" adjacent to the articular margin, with intact cuff fibers inserting into bone further laterally.

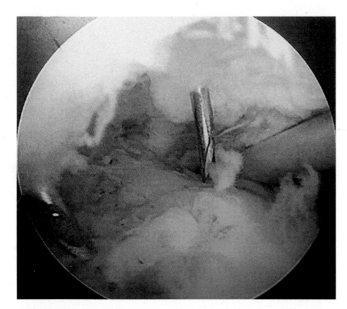

FIGURE 33.43 Left shoulder, posterior viewing portal. The bone bed has been prepared. Two transtendon spinal needles mark the angle of approach through the rotator cuff for the two suture anchors.

ternatively, the partial tear may be converted into a complete tear, and then the tear is repaired by standard arthroscopic techniques.

The transtendon approach is an advanced arthroscopic technique that usually requires two suture anchors. Before inserting the anchors, one must thoroughly clear the bursal tissue and fibrofatty tissue from the subacromial space so that the sutures will be clearly visible after anchor insertion.

If this is not done, the surgeon runs the risk of inadvertently cutting the sutures later while trying to remove the fibrofatty tissue from around them in order to visualize them adequately.

After subacromial bursectomy has been completed, the arthroscope is placed intraarticularly and the bone bed is prepared. Two percutaneous transtendon needles are used to mark the angle of approach for the transtendon insertion of suture anchors (Fig. 33.43). A bone punch is used to create a hole for the suture anchor adjacent to the articular margin (Fig. 33.44). Then the two suture anchors are placed in a transtendon fashion (Fig. 33.45). One green suture limb from each anchor is retrieved through a lateral portal, and

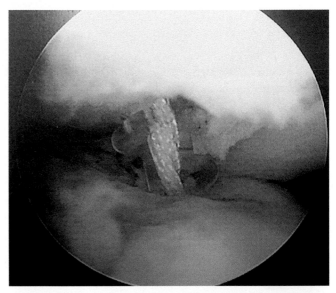

A

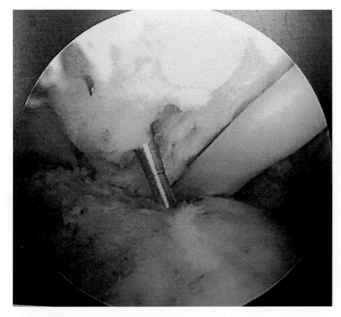

FIGURE 33.44 Left shoulder, posterior viewing portal. The transtendon bone punch creates a hole for the suture anchor directly adjacent to the articular margin.

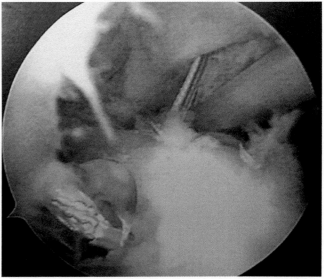

B

FIGURE 33.45 Left shoulder, posterior viewing portal. **A:** A Bio-Corkscrew suture anchor (Arthrex, Inc., Naples, FL) is placed anteriorly. **B:** A second BioCorkscrew is placed posteriorly, and the overlying cuff between the two anchors will be secured against the bone bed.

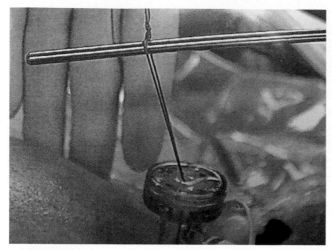

FIGURE 33.46 One green suture limb from each anchor is retrieved, and the two limbs are tied outside the body.

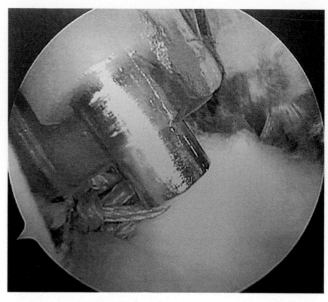

FIGURE 33.48 Double-diameter knot pusher is used to tie a static knot, completing a double-loop system that holds the cuff firmly against the bone bed.

these two limbs are tied outside the body (Fig. 33.46). By pulling on the other two green limbs, the knot is pulled into the subacromial space to the top of the cuff (Fig. 33.47). As tension is maintained in the sutures, the other two green suture limbs are tied in a static fashion with a double-diameter knot pusher (Fig. 33.48). These steps are repeated with the white sutures. These maneuvers reestablish contact of the rotator cuff with its "footprint" (Fig. 33.49).

The second technique of PASTA lesion repair is to complete the tear, turning it into a full-thickness tear. The complete tear is then repaired by standard techniques described earlier in this chapter. Because these tears often occur in younger people who require strength as well as pain relief, I prefer to maximize the rotator cuff footprint (after complet-

ing the tear) by using a double row of suture anchors: one medial, adjacent to the articular margin, and one lateral to repair the free edge of the cuff (Fig. 33.50).

The matter of subacromial decompression in association with PASTA repair is controversial. I prefer to do a standard subacromial decompression whenever I repair a PASTA lesion.

Rehabilitation is the same as outlined in the previous section for full-thickness rotator cuff tears.

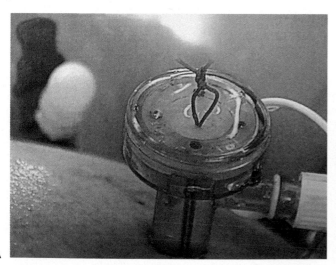

A

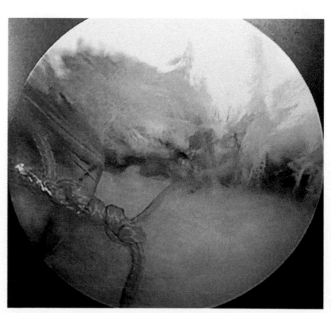

B

FIGURE 33.47 A: By pulling on the other two green suture limbs, the knot is delivered back through the cannula. **B:** The knot comes to rest over the portion of the cuff that spans between the two suture anchors.

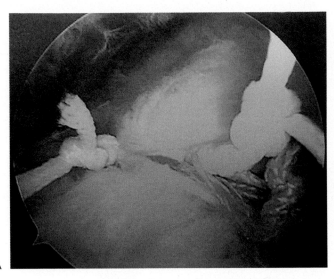
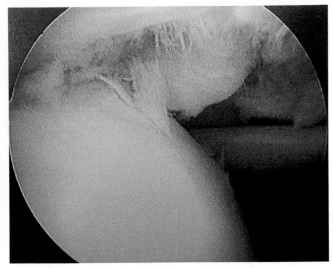

A   B

FIGURE 33.49 A: Indentation of sutures over cuff ensures good contact with the underlying bone bed. **B:** Intraarticular view shows that the cuff footprint is reestablished all the way to the articular margin.

Technique of Arthroscopic Subscapularis Repair

Tears of the subscapularis can cause a broad range of dysfunction, ranging from pain and mild weakness (for tears of the upper half of the subscapularis) to complete loss of overhead function (for tears involving more than 50% of the subscapularis as part of a massive tear that also involves the supraspinatus and infraspinatus.) The Napoleon test (67), a variant of Gerber's belly-press test (76,77), has been useful in predicting the extent of the tear (Fig. 33.51). Patients with tears of less than 50% of the subscapularis usually have a negative Napoleon sign; those with complete subscapularis tears exhibit a positive Napoleon sign; and those with tears between 50% and 100% display an intermediate Napoleon sign (67).

One can also encounter partial-thickness articular-surface tears of the subscapularis, which are analogous to the PASTA lesions that involve the supraspinatus (Fig. 33.52). These tears cause pain and some weakness but typically produce a negative Napoleon sign. These tears are likely to be missed unless the arthroscopic surgeon views the subscapularis tendon all the way to its insertion on the lesser tuberosity. When viewing through a posterior portal, this area is best seen with the arm in approximately 45 degrees of abduction and 30 degrees internal rotation.

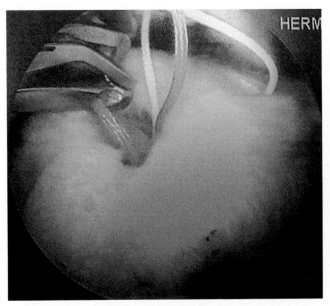
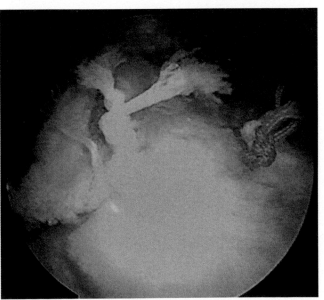

A   B

FIGURE 33.50 Left shoulder, posterior viewing portal. **A:** Sutures are being placed in two rows, medially and laterally, to maximize the rotator cuff footprint. Viper suture passer (Arthrex, Inc., Naples, FL) is prepared to pass a green suture limb. **B:** Completed two-row repair.

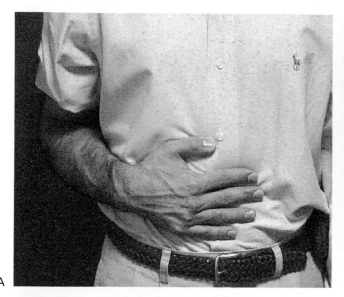

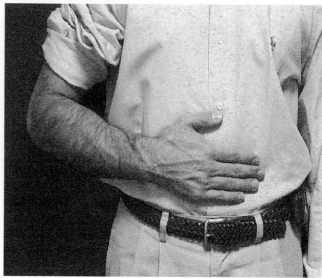

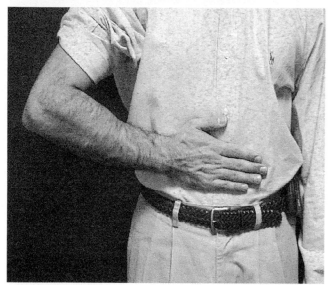

FIGURE 33.51 Napoleon test. **A:** Positive Napoleon sign, indicating a nonfunctional subscapularis. The patient can press on the belly only by flexing the wrist 90 degrees, using the posterior deltoid rather than the subscapularis to provide the power for pressing on the belly. **B:** Intermediate Napoleon sign, with wrist flexed 30 to 60 degrees as patient presses on belly, indicating partial function of subscapularis. **C:** Negative Napoleon sign, with wrist at 0 degrees while pressing on belly, indicating normal subscapularis function.

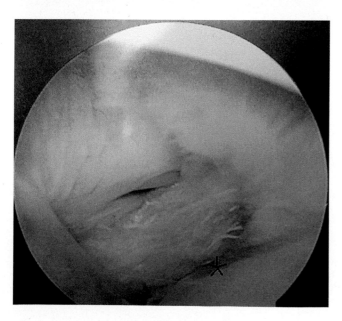

FIGURE 33.52 Right shoulder, posterior viewing portal. PASTA-type lesion of the subscapularis, with a bare footprint at the upper subscapularis insertion (*).

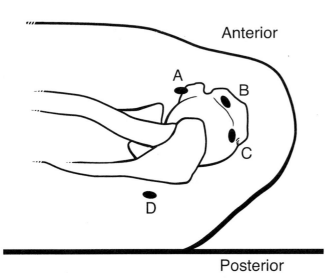

FIGURE 33.53 Portals for arthroscopic subscapularis repair. The anterior portal **(A)** is used for anchor placement and suture passage. The anterolateral portal **(B)** is used for subscapularis mobilization and preparation of the bone bed. The accessory anterolateral portal **(C)** is used for the traction sutures. The posterior portal **(D)** is used for arthroscopic viewing.

If a subscapularis tear is encountered, it is important to repair that tear before doing any other work in the shoulder, because the space available for instrumentation is very tight, and swelling of the deltoid can rapidly compromise the space even more.

Partial-thickness subscapularis tears (PASTA-type tears) should be converted to full-thickness tears by means of electrocautery or a mechanical shaver, then repaired as full-thickness tears.

The full-thickness tears may be partial (e.g., involving the upper 50% of the tendon) or complete (involving 100% of the tendon), and they may be isolated tears or combined tears (e.g., associated with tears of supraspinatus and infraspinatus). Large combined chronic tears usually require mobilization of the subscapularis tendon, whereas isolated partial tears do not.

In arthroscopically repairing the subscapularis tendon, I use four portals (Fig. 33.53). I prefer the posterior portal for viewing, bringing the bone bed into view with internal rotation of the arm. If visualization of the insertion of the subscapularis at the lesser tuberosity is difficult, one can either change to a 70-degree arthroscope and remain in the posterior portal or switch to an anterosuperolateral viewing portal. There are two anterolateral portals, one that enters the joint anterior to the biceps tendon (anterolateral portal) and one that enters the joint posterior to the biceps tendon (accessory anterolateral portal). The accessory portal is used for traction sutures, and the anterolateral portal is used for passage of instruments used in mobilizing and repairing the tendon (arthroscopic elevators, shavers, and knot pushers).

The first step is to identify the subscapularis tendon. This is easy in the case of a partial tear, but it can be very difficult with a chronic complete tear, which may be retracted to the glenoid rim and may even be scarred to the anterior deltoid. In chronic complete subscapularis tears, the tendon usually displays a "comma sign," in which the superior glenohumeral ligament avulses from its humeral attachment adjacent to the subscapularis footprint and remains attached to the lateral upper margin of the subscapularis tendon, forming a comma-shaped extension above the superolateral subscapularis (Fig. 33.54). Traction sutures (usually two

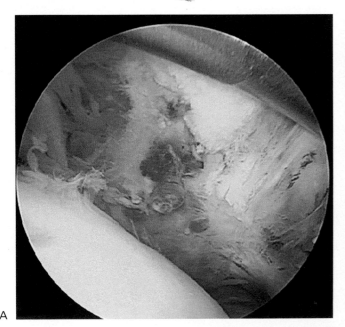

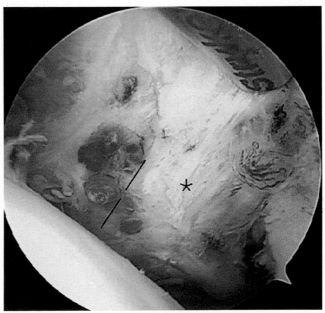

FIGURE 33.54 Left shoulder, posterior viewing portal. **A:** Retracted subscapularis tendon is difficult to identify. **B:** "Comma sign," seen in chronic retracted subscapularis tears. The arc of the comma (*) is formed by the detached superior glenohumeral ligament, which extends proximal to the superolateral border of the subscapularis tendon (——).

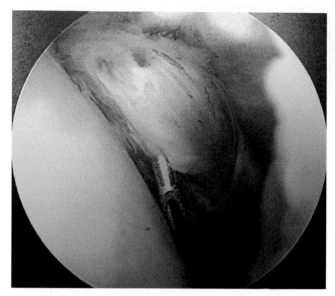

FIGURE 33.55 Left shoulder, posterior viewing portal. A spinal needle through the subscapularis is used for placement of a traction suture.

monofilament no. 1 Ethilon) are passed through the tendon by means of a spinal needle and retrieved through the accessory anterolateral portal (Fig. 33.55). In the case of a chronic retracted tear, a tendon grasper through the anterolateral portal is used to pull the tendon as far lateral as possible while the traction sutures are passed.

Next, while the surgeon pulls laterally on the traction sutures, the retracted tendon is mobilized by means of a 15-degree arthroscopic elevator (Arthrex), freeing the tendon an-

teriorly, posteriorly, and superiorly until it can be pulled laterally to its bone bed on the lesser tuberosity. I do not use the elevator inferiorly, and I do not dissect medial to the coracoid, which can easily be palpated with the elevator. Dissection posterior to the tendon, in the interface between subscapularis and glenoid neck, is quite safe, but dissection anterior to the tendon becomes dangerous if the dissection is carried medial to the coracoid. One must avoid any uncontrolled plunges medially, anteromedially, or inferomedially with the elevator.

Once the tendon has been freed enough to reach the lesser tuberosity, the bone bed is prepared with a bur through the anterolateral portal. I usually medialize the bone bed approximately 5 mm by removing the adjacent 5 mm of articular cartilage in order to provide a broad "footprint" for subscapularis healing to bone (Fig. 33.56).

At this point, I determine whether a coracoplasty will be required. I have found that in many cases of subscapularis tear, the coracoid encroaches tightly over the bone bed to which the tendon will be repaired (Fig. 33.57). To avoid coracoid impingement, the guideline that I use is that there must be at least 7 mm of space between the subscapularis tendon (when it is held reduced over its bone bed) and the coracoid. If there is less than 7 mm of space, I do an arthroscopic coracoplasty. The palpable soft tissues on the posterolateral tip of the coracoid are made up entirely of the coracoacromial ligament. These soft tissues are removed with a combination of electrocautery and power shaver, and then bone is removed in the plane of the subscapularis tendon by means of a high-speed bur until there is a 7-mm space between the coracoid and the subscapularis (Fig. 33.58).

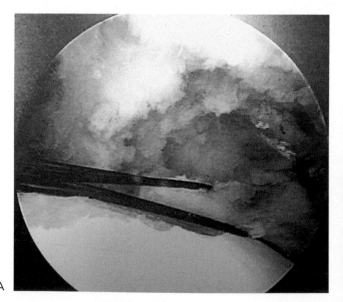
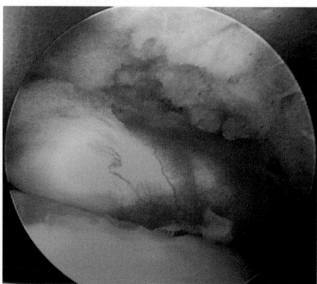

FIGURE 33.56 Left shoulder, posterior viewing portal. **A:** Bone bed on lesser tuberosity of humerus has been prepared. **B:** Lateral traction on the traction sutures brings the subscapularis tendon far over the bone bed.

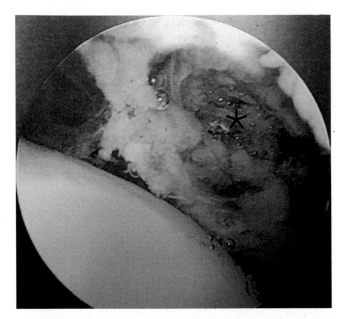

FIGURE 33.57 Left shoulder, posterior viewing portal. The coracoid (*), seen through a "window" in the rotator interval above subscapularis tendon, encroaches on the repair site for subscapularis.

An anatomic study of 18 cadaver shoulders showed that the average subscapularis tendon footprint is 2.5 cm in length, from superior to inferior (Tehrany AM, Burkhart SS, and Wirth MA, unpublished data). This information is

useful in judging how much of the subscapularis is torn. If there is an exposed footprint of 1.25 cm, for example, then 50% of the tendon has been torn.

To repair the tendon to bone, I use one or two suture anchors, depending on the percentage of tendon that has been torn. If the tear involves 50% or less of the tendon, I use one anchor; if it involves more than 50%, I use two anchors.

In placing the biodegradable screw-in anchors (Bio-Corkscrew), I use a spinal needle to determine the angle of approach to the bone bed. I try to place the anchors at a 30- to 45-degree "deadman angle," approximately 5 mm from the articular margin (Fig. 33.59).

Sutures can be passed in one of two ways. If the tendon is quite mobile and the space is not compromised excessively by swelling, a Penetrator or BirdBeak suture passer can be brought through the tendon from an anterior portal, retrieving the suture directly. Otherwise, a Viper suture passer (Arthrex) can pass the suture directly antegrade. Alternatively, if the space is very tight and visualization on both sides of the tendon is poor due to swelling, I prefer to use the "traction shuttle" technique, in which the traction sutures are used to shuttle the braided sutures from the anchor through the tendon. For the lower anchor, the posterior limb of the lowermost traction stitch is retrieved through the accessory anterolateral portal along with one limb of each suture pair from the anchor. The anterior limb of the traction stitch is retrieved out the anterolateral portal. A loop is tied in the posterior limb of the traction stitch, and the no. 2 Ethibond suture limbs from the anchor are

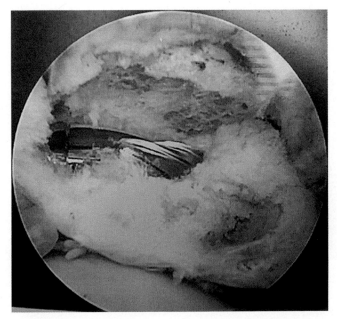

FIGURE 33.58 Left shoulder, posterior viewing portal. Coracoplasty has been performed in the plane of the subscapularis tendon, creating a 7-mm space between the remaining coracoid and the subscapularis.

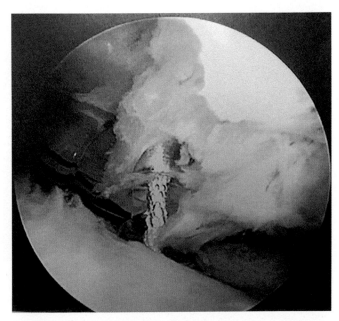

FIGURE 33.59 Left shoulder, posterior viewing portal. Bio-Corkscrew suture anchor (Arthrex, Inc., Naples, FL) is placed into lesser tuberosity at a 45-degree "deadman angle" through the anterior portal.

threaded through the loop. Then the anterior limb of the traction stitch is pulled by the surgeon in order to "shuttle" the anchor sutures through the cuff. (Fig. 33.60). At this point, the sutures are tied (Fig. 33.61). If the surgeon places the upper anchor before tying the sutures in the lower anchor, it will be very difficult to visualize the lower sutures for tying.

The upper BioCorkscrew anchor is next implanted, and the sutures are passed and tied in the same manner as for the lower anchor.

After subscapularis repair, associated rotator cuff tears are repaired in the manner described earlier in this chapter.

Postoperative Management after Subscapularis Repair

Postoperative management of subscapularis repairs differs from that of other full-thickness rotator cuff tears in one important respect: external rotation must be limited for 6 weeks, because it will stress the repair. For partial tears (in which there is no retraction), I will allow 20 to 30 degrees of external rotation during the first 6 weeks, because the tendon is supple and the repair is protected to some extent by the intact lower portion of the tendon. However, for complete tears, particularly those that have been chronically re-

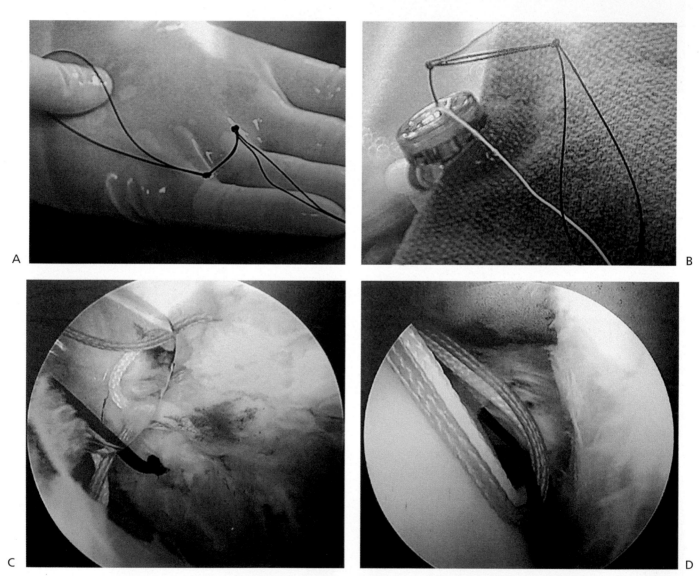

FIGURE 33.60 Traction shuttle technique. **A:** One end of monofilament traction suture has been withdrawn through the accessory anterolateral cannula, and its end has been tied into a loop. Smaller "dilator knots" are tied proximal to the loop to dilate the hole in the subscapularis tendon for easy passage of the braided suture. **B:** Traction shuttle loop is loaded with braided suture to be "shuttled" through subscapularis tendon. **C:** Dilator knot "leads the way" for trailing sutures. **D:** Braided sutures are pulled through subscapularis tendon by the loop of the traction shuttle suture.

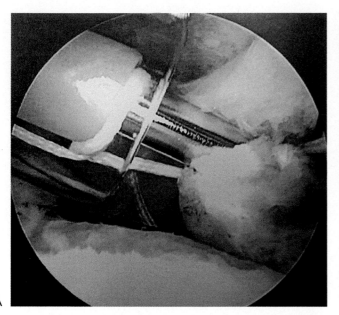 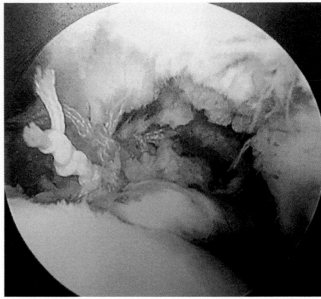

A
B

FIGURE 33.61 Left shoulder, posterior viewing portal. **A:** Sutures are tied with subscapularis tendon held firmly over the bone bed. **B:** Completed subscapularis repair.

tracted, I do not allow external rotation beyond 0 degrees for 6 weeks. After that, the patient may progress with active and active-assisted external rotation as tolerated, in addition to overhead stretching. Strengthening exercises are delayed until 12 weeks after surgery, as with other varieties of full-thickness tears.

Headed Biodegradable Implants for Sutureless Fixation

Headed biodegradable implants, both tacks and screws, are now available for rotator cuff fixation, but there are currently no clinical studies to document the efficacy of these devices. The first-generation implants, made of polyglycolic acid (PGA) with a wet-strength half-life of 2 weeks, were not appropriate for rotator cuff repair. However, the second-generation implants, made of PLA with a wet-strength half-life of up to 12 months, seem to have adequate strength and longevity for cuff repairs (78,79). These implants are usually inserted by a transtendon technique over a guide pin after a bone socket has been created with a cannulated drill, punch, or tap.

I believe that three caveats must be understood by the surgeon before these devices are used. First and most importantly, these implants are appropriate only for nonretracted rotator cuff tears that can be repaired without tension. A cuff that is repaired under tension is a setup for failure of the shaft of the implant as it weakens with degradation, potentially leaving a dissociated head above the cuff. The second caveat is that these devices cannot be used

unless the surgeon can get a straight line of approach from the entry portal (adjacent to the lateral acromion) through the rotator cuff and into the bone bed. If the cuff is retracted or if the acromion has a significant lateral overhang, this angle of approach will not be possible. The amount of lateral overhang of the acromion is quite variable among individuals, and it is possible that even a nonretracted cuff tear may not be amenable to this repair technique if the acromion extends far laterally. Another drawback to this technique in the patient with a lateralized acromion is that, even if the angle of approach permits transtendon insertion into the bone bed, the head may strike the bone at such an oblique angle that it could acutely break on insertion when it is advanced into bone. If it does not break, the obliquely oriented head will provide only point contact between tendon and bone, negating the potential ability of this type of implant to maximize contact between the cuff and bone. The third caveat is that the surgeon must see the implant go into bone rather than blindly placing a guide pin and assuming that it is in bone. I have seen a case in which a metallic anchor that was blindly inserted transtendon was actually embedded into the biceps tendon but never engaged bone.

I think that the indications for headed biodegradable implants for rotator cuff fixation should be strictly limited to nonretracted tears that are not associated with a lateralized acromion, so that a straight-line transtendon approach into the bone bed is possible. In such cases, the increased contact area under the head of the device may be theoretically beneficial to optimize the rotator cuff "footprint."

Suture Anchors without Knots: The Twist-Loc Concept

The Holy Grail of arthroscopic rotator cuff repair would be a technique using a device that would allow transport of the cuff margin to the implant, even for retracted tears under some tension, and then produce firm fixation of the tendon to bone without the need to tie knots. Until recently, such a technique did not exist. However, the Twist-Loc anchor system, recently approved by the U. S. Food and Drug Administration, achieves these critical goals:

1. Tissue transport to the anchor
2. Suture fixation of tendon to bone without knot tying

The only other suture-anchor system that avoids knot tying is the Knotless Anchor (Mitek, Inc.), but at this writing it is not approved for rotator cuff repair.

The idea for the Twist-Loc system came to me during a trip to Hong Kong. Most Westerners are not aware that the great skyscrapers of Hong Kong were constructed with the use of bamboo scaffolding that extended up to 100 stories high (Fig. 33.62). The remarkable characteristic of the bamboo scaffolding is that the bamboo sticks were held together with lashings that were wrapped and twisted in such a way that they created extremely secure fixation without ever tying a knot (Fig. 33.63). Friction (both wedge friction and cable friction) and internal interference between

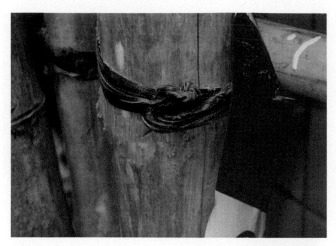

FIGURE 33.63 Close-up of the lashings supporting individual bamboo poles of the scaffolding.

the two limbs of each lashing were solely responsible for the stability of this construct that safely supported workmen far above the ground (80). The strength and simplicity of this technique were so impressive that I immediately began experimenting with ways to adapt it to a tissue-transport suture fixation system for rotator cuff repair that would not require knots. The Twist-Loc system is the product of those efforts.

Technique of Twist-Loc Repair

The concept behind this technique is that the two limbs of a suture (which has been placed through the rotator cuff) are threaded through an eyelet on the leading end (buried end) of an anchor (Fig. 33.64); the suture limbs are twisted by

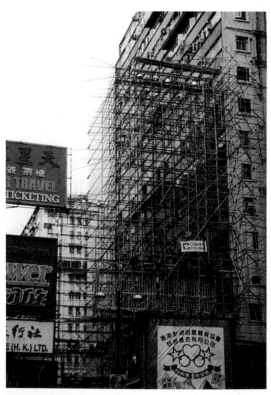

FIGURE 33.62 Bamboo scaffolding surrounds a building undergoing renovation in Hong Kong.

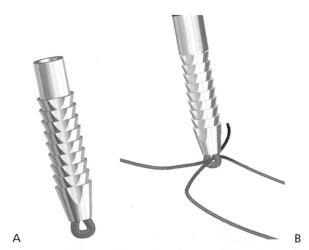

FIGURE 33.64 A: Twist-Loc anchor has an eyelet on its leading end which will be buried on insertion. **B:** Suture limbs from rotator cuff suture are passed in opposite directions through the eyelet.

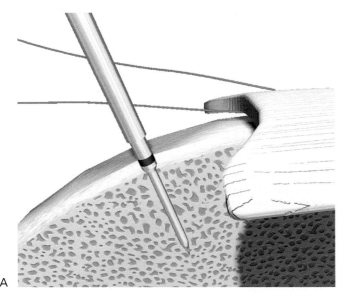
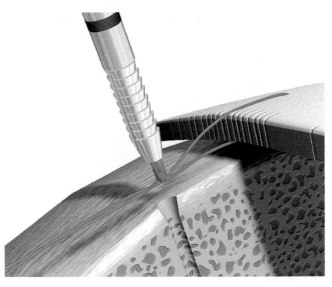

A   B

FIGURE 33.65 A: Bone punch creates socket in bone for anchor. **B:** The anchor inserter is turned three turns or more to twist the suture below the eyelet, thereby increasing the internal interference between the suture limbs.

turning the anchor three turns or more in order to increase the internal interference between suture limbs (Fig. 33.65); then the anchor is impacted into the bone (into a bone socket previously created by a punch), and the suture is pulled into the bone socket until the cuff lies adjacent to the bone socket (Fig. 33.66). The bulk of twisted suture produces a wedge effect to resist both suture slippage and anchor pullout.

Results of Twist-Loc Repair

The Twist-Loc technique is a new concept and a new technique without any long-term or intermediate-term follow-up. It is presented strictly as an illustration of the rapid and innovative developments that are taking place in the exciting field of arthroscopic rotator cuff repair.

EPILOGUE: THE VIEW FROM HERE

Ordinarily, a chapter in a surgical text ends with a section entitled *Conclusion.* I have chosen not to stigmatize my parting comments with that nomenclature because it sounds much too final for a subject that is undergoing such rapid development, in terms of both theory and technique.

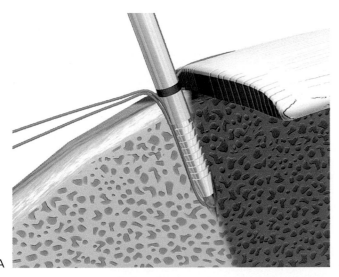
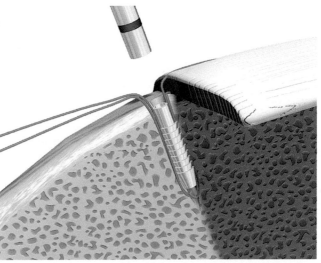

A   B

FIGURE 33.66 A: Anchor is impacted into bone, pulling the suture and the attached rotator cuff with it. **B:** Final configuration. Note that the cuff margin has been pulled to the edge of the bone socket.

For a new surgical technique to supplant the old, it must accomplish three things. First, the technique must be possible to perform on a routine basis. Arthroscopic cuff repair, although not universally done by all orthopaedic surgeons, is certainly reproducible and is done on a routine basis by an ever-increasing number of orthopaedic surgeons. Second, the results of the new technique must be at least as good as those of the old technique. The emerging literature on arthroscopic rotator cuff repair would indicate not only that the results are as good as open repair, but for the large and massive tears the results are significantly better. Third, the technique must be simple enough that the majority of surgeons can perform it. This is the area that is still evolving, but the evolution is rapid, and the new developments are exciting.

Despite this rapid progress, one must recognize that many of the large and massive rotator cuff tears will never be amenable to a simple-minded approach. Every massive tear requires a thoughtful analysis centered on basic anatomic and biomechanical principles.

I hope that, in this chapter, I have accomplished my goal of demystifying the magic of arthroscopic rotator cuff repair and exposing it for what it really is, a series of tricks. Despite this exposure, the magic is elusive, and the key to successfully performing these tricks is to practice the requisite arthroscopic skills until they are second nature, and to use tools rather than gadgets to perform these repairs. As we continue to upgrade our arthroscopic skills and tools, we will see that ignorance and inconsistency will yield to insight, and insight will lead to understanding. Thanks for understanding.

ACKNOWLEDGMENT

The author wishes to thank Peter M. Parten, M.D., for his assistance in preparation of the arthroscopic photographs for this chapter.

REFERENCES

1. Burkhart SS. Arthroscopic treatment of massive rotator cuff tears: clinical results and biomechanical rationale. *Clin Orthop* 1991;267:45–56.
2. Burkhart SS. Arthroscopic debridement and decompression for selected rotator cuff tears: clinical results, pathomechanics, and patient selection based on biomechanical parameters. *Orthop Clin North Am* 1993;24:111–123.
3. Burkhart SS. Reconciling the paradox of rotator cuff repair vs. debridement: a unified biomechanical rationale for the treatment of rotator cuff repairs. *Arthroscopy* 1994;10:1–16.
4. Ellman H. Arthroscopic subacromial decompression: analysis of one- to three-year results. *Arthroscopy* 1987;3:173–181.
5. Ellman H, Kay SP, Wirth M. Arthroscopic treatment of full-thickness rotator cuff tears: 2- to 7-year follow-up study. *Arthroscopy* 1993;9:195–200.
6. Esch JC, Ozerkis LR, Helgager JA, et al. Arthroscopic subacromial decompression: results according to the degree of rotator cuff tear. *Arthroscopy* 1984;4:241–249.
7. Gartsman GM. Arthroscopic acromioplasty for lesions of the rotator cuff. *J Bone Joint Surg Am* 1990;72:169–180.
8. Post M, Silver R, Singh M. Rotator cuff tear: diagnosis and treatment. *Clin Orthop* 1983;173:78–92.
9. DeOrio JK, Cofield RH. Results of a second attempt at surgical repair of a failed initial rotator-cuff repair. *J Bone Joint Surg Am* 1984;66:563–567.
10. Zvijac JE, Levy HJ, Lemak LJ. Arthroscopic subacromial decompression in the treatment of full thickness rotator cuff tears: a 3- to 6-year follow-up. *Arthroscopy* 1994;10:518–523.
11. Melillo AS, Savoie FH 3rd, Field LD. Massive rotator cuff tears: debridement versus repair. *Orthop Clin North Am* 1997;28:117–124.
12. Snyder SJ. Evaluation and treatment of the rotator cuff. *Orthop Clin North Am* 1993;24:173–192.
13. Levy HJ, Uribe JW, Delaney LG. Arthroscopic assisted rotator cuff repair: preliminary results. *Arthroscopy* 1990;6:55–60.
14. Liu SH, Baker CL. Arthroscopically assisted rotator cuff repair: correlation of functional results with integrity of the cuff. *Arthroscopy* 1994;10:54–60.
15. Paulos LE, Kody MH. Arthroscopically enhanced "mini-approach" to rotator cuff repair. *Am J Sports Med* 1994;22:19–25.
16. Bigliani LU, Cordasco FA, McIlveen SJ, et al. Operative treatment of massive rotator cuff tears: long term results. *J Shoulder Elbow Surg* 1992;1:120–130.
17. Codman EA. Complete rupture of the supraspinatus tendon: operative treatment with report of two successful cases. *Boston Med Surg J* 1911;164:708–710.
18. Cofield RH. Rotator cuff disease of the shoulder. *J Bone Joint Surg Am* 1985;67:974–979.
19. Ellman II, Hanker G, Bayer M. Repair of the rotator cuff: end result study of factors influencing reconstruction. *J Bone Joint Surg Am* 1986;68:1136–1144.
20. Harryman DT, Mack LA, Wang KY, et al. Repairs of the rotator cuff: correlation of functional results with integrity of the cuff. *J Bone Joint Surg Am* 1991;73:982–989.
21. Iannotti JP, Bernot MP, Kuhlman JR, et al. Postoperative assessment of shoulder function: a prospective study of full-thickness rotator cuff tears. *J Shoulder Elbow Surg* 1996;5:449–457.
22. Neer CS, Flatow EL, Lech O. Tears of the rotator cuff: long term results of anterior acromioplasty and repair. *Orthop Trans* 1988;12:735.
23. Neviaser JS. Ruptures of the rotator cuff of the shoulder: new concepts in the diagnosis and operative treatment of chronic ruptures. *Arch Surg* 1971;102:483–485.
24. Burkhart SS, Athanasiou KA, Wirth MA. Margin convergence: a method of reducing strain in massive rotator cuff tears. *Arthroscopy* 1996;12:335–338.
25. McLaughlin HL. Lesions of the musculotendinous cuff of the shoulder: the exposure and treatment of tears with retraction. *J Bone Joint Surg* 1944;26:31–51.
26. Burkhart SS. A stepwise approach to arthroscopic rotator cuff repair based on biomechanical principles. *Arthroscopy* 2000;16:82–90.
27. Burkhart SS. Arthroscopic repair of massive rotator cuff tears: concept of margin convergence. *Tech Shoulder Elbow Surg* 2001;1:232–239.
28. Burkhart SS, Danaccau SM, Pearce CE. Arthroscopic rotator cuff repair: analysis of results by tear size and by repair technique, margin convergence versus direct tendon-to-bone technique. *Arthroscopy* 2001;17:905–912.

29. Burkhart SS, Diaz-Pagan JL, Wirth MA, et al. Cyclic loading of anchor based rotator cuff repairs: confirmation of the tension overload phenomenon and comparison of suture anchor fixation with transosseous fixation. *Arthroscopy* 1997;13:720–724.

30. St. Pierre P, Olson EJ, Elliott JJ, et al. Tendon-healing to cortical bone compared with healing to a cancellous trough: a biomechanical and histological evaluation in goats. *J Bone Joint Surg Am* 1995;77:1858–1866.

31. Burkhart SS. The deadman theory of suture anchors: observations along a South Texas fence line. *Arthroscopy* 1995;11:119–123.

32. Barber FA, Herbert MA, Click JN. The ultimate strength of suture anchors. *Arthroscopy* 1995;11:21–28.

33. Barber, FA, Herbert MA, Click JN. Internal fixation strength of suture anchors: update 1997. *Arthroscopy* 1997;13:355–362.

34. Burkhart SS, Johnson TC, Wirth MA, et al. Cyclic loading of transosseous rotator cuff repairs: tension overload as a possible cause of failure. *Arthroscopy* 1997;13:172–176.

35. Burkhart SS, Fischer SP, Nottage WM, et al. Tissue fixation security in transosseous rotator cuff repair: a mechanical comparison of simple versus mattress sutures. *Arthroscopy* 1996;12:704–708.

36. Burkhart SS, Wirth MA, Simonich M, et al. Knot security in simple sliding knots and its relationship to rotator cuff repair: how secure must a knot be? *Arthroscopy* 2000;16:202–207.

37. Burkhart SS, Wirth MA, Simonich M, et al. Loop security as a determinant of tissue fixation security. *Arthroscopy* 1998;14:773–776.

38. Brouwers JE, Dosting H, deHaas D, et al. Dynamic loading of surgical knots. *Surg Gynecol Obstet* 1991;173:443–448.

39. Gerber C, Schneiberger AG, Schlegel U. Mechanical strength of repairs of the rotator cuff. *J Bone Joint Surg Br* 1994;76:371–380.

40. Gunderson PE. The half-hitch knot: a rational alternative to the square knot. *Am J Surg* 1987;154:538–540.

41. Herrman JB. Tensile strength and knot security of surgical suture materials. *Am J Surg* 1971;37:209–217.

42. Holmlund DE. Knot properties of surgical suture materials. *Acta Chir Scand* 1974;140:355–362.

43. Loutzenheiser TD, Harryman DT II, Yung SW, et al. Optimizing arthroscopic knots. *Arthroscopy* 1995;11:199–206.

44. Loutzenheiser TD, Harryman DT II, Ziegler DW, et al. Optimizing arthroscopic knots using braided or monofilament suture. *Arthroscopy* 1998;14:57–65.

45. Mishra DK, Cannon WD Jr, Lucas DJ, et al. Elongation of arthroscopically tied knots. *Am J Sports Med* 1997;25:113–117.

46. Rodeheaver GT, Thacker JG, Edlich RF. Mechanical performance of polyglycolic acid and polyglactin 91D synthetic absorbable suture. *Surg Gynecol Obstet* 1981;153:835–841.

47. Taylor FW. Surgical knots. *Ann Surg* 1938;107:458–468.

48. Van Rijssel EJC, Trimbos JB, Booster MH. Mechanical performance of square knots and sliding knots in surgery: a comparative study. *Am J Obstet Gynecol* 1990;162:93–97.

49. Chan KC, Burkhart SS, Thiagarajan P, et al. Optimization of stacked half-hitch knots for arthroscopic surgery. *Arthroscopy* 2001;17:752–759.

50. Burkhart SS. Partial repair of massive rotator cuff tears: the evolution of a concept. *Orthop Clin North Am* 1997;28:125–132.

51. Burkhart SS, Nottage WM, Ogilvie-Harris DJ, et al. Partial repair of irreparable rotator cuff tears. *Arthroscopy* 1994;10:4–19.

52. Tauro JC. Arthroscopic "interval slide" in the repair of large rotator cuff tears. *Arthroscopy* 1999;15:527–530.

53. Gartsman GM, Khan M, Hammerman SM. Arthroscopic repair of full-thickness tears of the rotator cuff. *J Bone Joint Surg Am* 1998;80:832–840.

54. Tauro JC. Arthroscopic rotator cuff repair: analysis of technique and results at 2-and 3-year follow-up. *Arthroscopy* 1998;14:45–51.

55. Hawkins RJ, Misamore GW, Hobeika PE. Surgery for full-thickness rotator-cuff tears. *J Bone Joint Surg Am* 1985;67:1349–1355.

56. Ogilvie-Harris DJ. Arthroscopic surgery of the shoulder: a general appraisal. *J Bone Joint Surg Br* 1986;68:201–207.

57. Ellman H. Diagnosis and treatment of incomplete rotator cuff tears. *Clin Orthop* 1990;254:64–74.

58. Snyder SJ, Pachelli AF, DelPizzo WD. Partial thickness rotator cuff tears: results of arthroscopic treatment. *Arthroscopy* 1991;7:1–7.

59. Yamanaka K, Matsumoto T. The joint side tear of the rotator cuff: a follow-up study by arthrography. *Clin Orthop* 1994;304:68–73.

60. Weber SC. Arthroscopic debridement and acromioplasty versus mini-open repair in the treatment of significant partial-thickness rotator cuff tears. *Arthroscopy* 1999;15:126–131.

61. Tierney JJ, Curtis AS, Kowalik DL, et al. The footprint of the rotator cuff. *Arthroscopy* 1999;15:556–557 (abstr).

62. Minagawa H, Itio E, Konno N, et al. Humeral attachment of the supraspinatus and infraspinatus tendons: an anatomic study. *Arthroscopy* 1998;14:302–302.

63. Grant LB. Full thickness supraspinatus tendon tears with intact superior glenohumeral capsule. *Arthroscopy* 1993;9:186–189.

64. Fukuda H, Craig EV, Yamanaka K. Surgical treatment of incomplete thickness tears of the rotator cuff: long-term follow. *Orthop Trans* 1987;11:327–328.

65. Morgan CD, Burkhart SS, Palmeri M, et al. Type II SLAP lesions: three subtypes and their relationships to superior instability and rotator cuff tear. *Arthroscopy* 1998;14:553–565.

66. Burkhart SS, Esch JC, Jolson RS. The rotator crescent and rotator cable: an anatomic description of the shoulder's "suspension bridge." *Arthroscopy* 1993;9:611–616.

67. Burkhart SS, Tehrany A. Arthroscopic subscapularis tendon repair: technique and preliminary results. *Arthroscopy* 2002;18:454–463.

68. Sampson TG, Nisbet JK, Glick JM. Precision acromioplasty in arthroscopic subacromial decompression. *Arthroscopy* 1991;7:301–307.

69. Greenway G, Fullmer JM. Imaging of the rotator cuff. In: Burkhead WZ Jr., ed. *Rotator cuff disorders.* Baltimore: Williams & Wilkins, 1996:73–78.

70. Burkhart SS, Danaceau SM, Athanasiou KA. Turbulence control as a factor in improving visualization during subacromial shoulder [Technical note]. *Arthroscopy* 2001;17:209–212.

71. Matsen FA III, Lippitt SB, Sidles JA, et al. Surgical approach to roughness at the non-articular humeroscapular motion interface. In: *Practical evaluation and management of the shoulder.* Philadelphia: WB Saunders, 1994:176–178.

72. Nord K. Modified Neviaser portal and subclavian portal in shoulder. Presented at the 19th Annual Meeting of the Arthroscopy Association of North America, Miami, Florida, April 14, 2000.

73. Bardana DD, Burks RT, West JR. The effect of suture anchor design and orientation on suture abrasion: an in-vitro study. *Arthroscopy* (in press).

74. Chan KC, Burkhart SS. How to switch posts without rethreading when tying half-hitches [Technical note]. *Arthroscopy* 1999;15:444–450.

75. Sonnabend, DH. Jones D, Walsh WR. Rotator cuff repair in a primate model: observations and implications. In: Proceedings of

the 14th annual Closed Meeting, American Shoulder and Elbow Surgeons, Manchester, VT, September, 1997:27.

76. Gerber C, Krushell RJ. Isolated rupture of the tendon of the sub-scapularis muscle. clinical features in 16 cases. *J Bone Joint Surg Br* 1993;73:389–394.

77. Gerber C, Hersche O, Farron A. Isolated rupture of the sub-scapularis tendon. *J Bone Joint Surg Am*1996;78:1015–1023.

78. Athanasiou KA, Agrawal CM, Barber FA, et al. Current concepts: orthopaedic applications for PLA-PGA biodegradable polymers. *Arthroscopy* 1998;14:726–737.

79. Burkhart SS. The evolution of clinical applications of biodegradable implant in arthroscopic surgery. *Biomaterials* 2000;21: 2631–2634.

80. Burkhart SS, Athanasiou KA. The twist-lock concept of tissue transport and suture fixation without knots: observations along the Hong Kong skyline. *Arthroscopy* (in press).

ADHESIVE CAPSULITIS

JO A. HANNAFIN

Primary adhesive capsulitis or frozen shoulder is a condition characterized by gradual loss of active and passive shoulder motion. The etiology of frozen shoulder remains elusive, but our understanding of the pathophysiology has recently improved. Factors associated with adhesive capsulitis include female gender (1), age greater than 40 years (2), trauma (3), diabetes (3,4,5,6,7), prolonged immobilization (8), thyroid disease (9), stroke or myocardial infarction (6,10), and the presence of autoimmune diseases (11,12). The prevalence of frozen shoulder in the general population is slightly greater than 2% (1).

The diagnosis of adhesive capsulitis encompasses primary adhesive capsulitis; secondary adhesive capsulitis which has a similar histopathologic appearance but results from a known intrinsic or extrinsic cause; and secondary shoulder stiffness after surgical intervention. In primary adhesive capsulitis, an insidious onset of pain causes the individual to gradually limit the use of the arm. Subsequently, motion is lost and the individual finds it increasingly difficult to perform activities of daily living that require overhead movement of the arm, reaching out to the side, or humeral rotation. Pain and muscular inhibition result in compensatory movements of the shoulder girdle to minimize pain. With time, there is resolution of pain and the individual is left with a stiff shoulder with severe limitation of function.

For any disease process treatment decisions should be based on the pathophysiology of the disease. However the natural history of the adhesive capsulitis remains controversial. Miller and Rockwood (6) reported on 50 patients during a 10-year period and found that the majority of the patients regained motion with minimal pain after home therapy, moist heat, antiinflammatory medications, and physician-directed rehabilitation. In contrast, Shaffer et al. (13) reported that 50% of patients had pain or residual stiffness at 7 years followup.

The treatment of patients with adhesive capsulitis remains controversial. Treatment options documented in the literature include: benign neglect (6), supervised physical rehabilitation (1,14,15,16), nonsteroidal antiinflammatory medications (17,18), oral corticosteroid (19), intraarticular injections (14,20,21,22,23), distension arthrography (24), closed manipulation (25,26,27,28,29), open surgical release (30), and more recently, arthroscopic capsular release (29,31,32,33,34). It is difficult to compare the results reported in these studies because of the lack of documentation of the stage of adhesive capsulitis being treated. It is the author's belief that the stage of adhesive capsulitis is critical in determining the appropriate treatment and predicting the response to treatment.

PATHOGENESIS

To formulate a logical and scientific approach to the treatment of patients with adhesive capsulitis, it is necessary to understand the pathophysiology of this disease. A review of the literature reveals a multitude of strategies for treatment of patients with adhesive capsulitis, with extremely variable results provided. The lack of consistency in the published literature reflects a lack of understanding of the stages of adhesive capsulitis, which play a significant role both in diagnosis and in formulation of a treatment plan. In 1945, Neviaser (35) introduced the term *"adhesive capsulitis"* and described pathologic changes in the synovium and subsynovium. There continues to be significant disagreement in the literature as to whether the underlying pathologic process is an inflammatory condition (36,37,38) or a fibrosing condition (39). There is significant evidence in support of the hypothesis that the underlying pathology in adhesive capsulitis is synovial inflammation with subsequent reactive capsular fibrosis (11,37,38,40). Thus adhesive capsulitis is both an inflammatory and a fibrosing condition, dependent on the stage noted at the time of evaluation and treatment.

Cytokines have recently been implicated in the inflammation and fibrosis described in adhesive capsulitis. Cytokines are involved in the initiation and termination of repair processes in multiple musculoskeletal tissues and their sustained production has been shown to result in tissue fi-

J. A. **Hannafin:** Sports Medicine and Shoulder Service, Hospital for Special Surgery, Department of Orthopaedic Surgery, Weill Medical College of Cornell University, New York, New York.

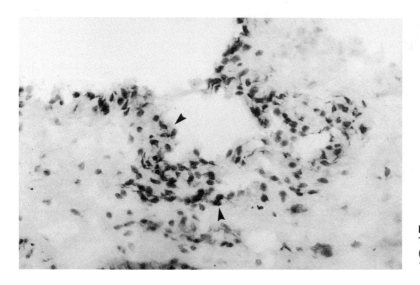

FIGURE 34.1 Immunohistochemical localization of TGF-beta in the subsynovium in frozen shoulder. (Reprinted with permission from the *J Orthop Res* 1997:15:427–436.)

brosis (41,42). Rodeo et al. (37) reported an increase in transforming growth factor-β, platelet-derived growth factor, and hepatocyte growth factor staining in capsular biopsy specimens of patients with primary and secondary adhesive capsulitis and proposed that these cytokines are involved in the inflammatory and fibrotic cascades seen in adhesive capsulitis (Fig. 34.1). A potential role of matrix metalloproteases, enzymes involved in extracellular matrix remodeling, in adhesive capsulitis has recently been described. In a series of 12 patients with inoperable gastric cancer treated with a synthetic matrix metalloproteinase inhibitor, 6 developed a frozen shoulder or a Dupuytren's-like condition (43). Three cases of acute adhesive capsulitis were recently reported in patients treated with protease inhibitors for the human immunodeficiency virus (HIV) (44).

STAGES OF ADHESIVE CAPSULITIS

Neviaser (45,46) described the arthroscopic stages of adhesive capsulitis and stressed the importance of an individualized treatment plan based on an understanding of the clinical stages of the disease. Hannafin et al. (36) have described a correlation between the arthroscopic stages described by Neviaser, the clinical examination and the histologic appearance of capsular biopsy specimens taken from patients with stages 1, 2, and 3 adhesive capsulitis. Adhesive capsulitis can be broken down into four stages as outlined in Table 34.1, however it is critical to remember that these stages represent a continuum of disease rather than discrete stages.

In Stage 1, patients will present with pain, which may be achy at rest and sharp at extremes of range of motion (ROM). Symptoms have generally been present for less than 3 months; however, the patient will report a progressive loss of motion. Loss of internal rotation, forward flexion, and abduction are apparent with a more subtle loss of external

TABLE 34.1 STAGES OF ADHESIVE CAPSULITIS

Stage 1:
Duration of symptoms: 0 to 3 months
Pain with active and passive ROM
Limitation of forward flexion, abduction, internal rotation, external rotation
EUA: Normal or minimal loss of ROM
Arthroscopy: diffuse synovitis, most pronounced in the anterosuperior capsule
Pathology: hypertrophic, hypervascular synovitis, inflammatory cell infiltrates, normal capsule

Stage 2 ("Freezing Stage"):
Duration of symptoms: 3 to 9 months
Chronic pain with active and passive ROM
Significant limitation of forward flexion, abduction, internal rotation, external rotation
EUA: ROM essentially identical to awake ROM
Arthroscopy: diffuse, pedunculated synovitis
Pathology: hypertrophic, hypervascular synovitis, perivascular, subsynovial and capsular scar

Stage 3 ("Frozen Stage"):
Duration of symptoms: 9 to 15 months
Minimal pain except at end ROM
Significant limitation of ROM with rigid "end feel"
EUA: ROM identical to awake ROM
Arthroscopy: remnants of fibrotic synovium, diminished capsular volume.
Pathology: minimal synovium, underlying capsule with dense scar formation

Stage 4 ("Thawing Phase"):
Duration of symptoms: 15 to 24 months
Minimal pain
Progressive improvement in ROM
Examination under anesthesia: data not available

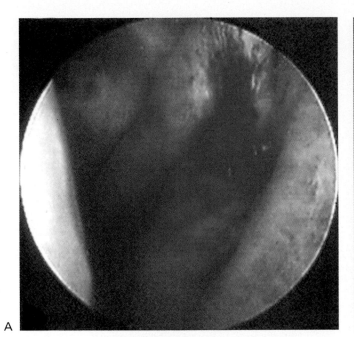

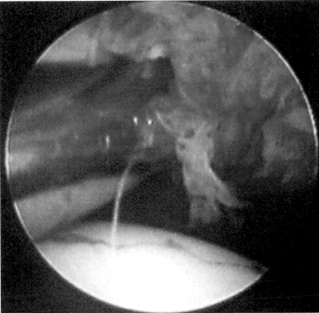

A   B

FIGURE 34.2 Arthroscopic appearance of the anterior capsule in stage 1 adhesive capsulitis. **A:** the anterior capsule is diffusely covered with a thin layer of beefy red synovium. **B:** synovitis in the region of the rotator interval is demonstrated. This region often demonstrates a more pedunculated appearance.

rotation. Examination of a patient with Stage 1 adhesive capsulitis after injection of the glenohumeral joint with local anesthetic or examination of the patient under scalene block anesthesia will reveal a significant improvement in ROM. In this early stage, the majority of motion loss is secondary to the painful synovitis rather than a true capsular contracture. Arthroscopic examination reveals a hypertrophic vascular synovitis that coats the entire capsular lining. This synovitis is often more pronounced in the rotator interval area of the capsule (Fig. 34.2). Pathology specimens show rare inflammatory infiltrates, a hypervascular synovitis and normal underlying capsular morphologic characteristics (Fig. 34.3).

In Stage 2, symptoms have been present for 3 to 9 months with progressive loss of ROM and persistence of pain. Examination of the patient after local anesthetic infiltration or scalene block reveals relief of pain, with partial improvement in ROM. The motion loss in Stage 2 adhesive

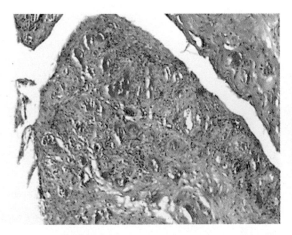

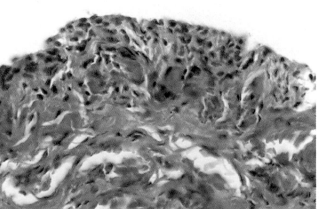

A   B

FIGURE 34.3 Histologic appearance of the synovium and underlying capsule in a biopsy specimen obtained from a patient with Stage 1 adhesive capsulitis. **A:** Typical appearance of the synovium. There is a hypervascular synovitis, rare inflammatory cell infiltrates and a normal underlying capsule (20x magnification). **B:** A high power view of the synovium (40x). There is no evidence of perivascular scar formation.

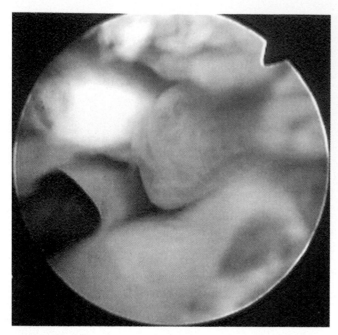

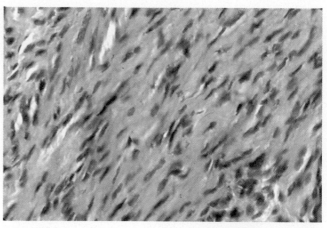

FIGURE 34.6 Histologic, appearance of the capsule in a biopsy specimen from a patient with Stage 3 adhesive capsulitis. There is dense scar formation and capsular fibroplasia (40x magnification).

FIGURE 34.4 Arthroscopic appearance of the anterior-superior capsule in Stage 2 adhesive capsulitis. The synovium remains hyperemic and is significantly thicker with a "tree-like" appearance.

capsulitis reflects both a loss of capsular volume and a response to the painful synovitis. Arthroscopic examination reveals a dense, proliferative, hypervascular synovitis (Fig. 34.4). Capsular biopsy reveals hypervascular synovitis with perivascular scar formation and capsular fibroplasia (Fig. 34.5). There is new collagen deposition with disorganized collagen fibrils and a hypercellular appearance (Fig. 34.2). No inflammatory infiltrates have been reported in Stage 2.

In Stage 3, patients will present with a history of painful stiffening of the shoulder and significant loss of ROM. Symptoms have been present for 9 to 15 months and have

been observed to change with time. Patients often report a history of an extremely painful phase that has resolved, followed by a stage characterized by a relatively pain-free but stiff shoulder. ROM examination is unchanged by injection of local anesthetic or examination under anesthesia, reflecting the persistent loss of capsular volume and fibrosis of the glenohumeral joint capsule. Arthroscopic examination of a patient with Stage 3 adhesive capsulitis is somewhat unremarkable when compared with examination of patients with Stages 1 and 2 adhesive capsulitis. A residual filmy synovial layer is visible with patches of synovial thickening without hypervascularity. Rare synovial adhesions are noted in the inferior capsular recess. Capsular biopsies reveal a dense, hypercellular collagenous tissue (Fig. 34.6). Stage 4, the "thawing stage" of adhesive capsulitis, is characterized by the slow, steady recovery of ROM resulting from capsular remodeling in response to use of the arm and shoulder. No arthroscopic

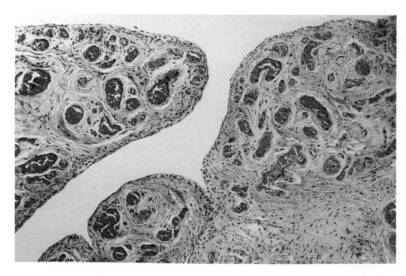

FIGURE 34.5 Histologic appearance of the synovium and underlying capsule in a biopsy specimen obtained from a patient with late Stage 2 adhesive capsulitis. The synovium remains hypervascular with striking perivascular scar formation. The underlying capsule demonstrates capsular fibroplasia and a disorganized appearance of the collagen structure (20x magnification). (Reprinted with permission from the *J Orthop Res* 1997:15:427–436.)

or histologic data are available in the literature for patients with Stage 4 adhesive capsulitis because these patients rarely undergo surgery. It is essential to consider these stages when examining a patient with adhesive capsulitis because the stage should direct the treatment options.

DIAGNOSIS

Primary and Secondary Adhesive Capsulitis

The diagnosis of primary adhesive capsulitis is made from the history and physical examination. This is an idiopathic condition and the diagnosis is made when other causes of pain and motion loss are eliminated (45,46,47,48). The physical examination should include an evaluation of the cervical spine and the shoulder. In Stages 1 and 2 patients often have pain on palpation of the anterior and posterior capsule, and describe pain radiating to the deltoid. Night pain and pain at rest are common. Evaluation of active and passive ROM should be performed because documenting the initial ROM is critical in determining the efficacy of the treatment plan. "Pure" glenohumeral motion is measured while limiting scapulothoracic motion. Active and passive forward flexion, abduction, internal rotation (measured by having the patient place the thumb to the highest point possible on the spinous process) and external rotation in neutral abduction are measured and recorded with the patient standing. Passive glenohumeral motion then is measured with the patient supine with constraint of scapulothoracic motion by manual pressure on the acromion. Supine passive internal and external rotation at 0°, 45°, and maximal glenohumeral abduction are measured and recorded.

Routine radiographic evaluation should include anteroposterior (AP) views in internal and external rotation, axillary and outlet views to rule out glenohumeral arthritis, calcific tendinitis, or longstanding rotator cuff disease. Radiographs are usually negative in patients with frozen shoulder, although there may be evidence of disuse osteopenia. Leppala et al. (49) have documented significant decreases in bone mineral density (BMD) associated with active phase adhesive capsulitis with recovery of normal bone density when measured 9 years after disease. Historically, arthrography, which shows a decreased joint capacity in Stages 2 to 4, has been used for diagnostic purposes; however, it is no longer used routinely (50,51). If the clinical diagnosis is unclear, magnetic resonance imaging (MRI) may be useful in evaluation of the rotator cuff or labrum but is not routinely recommended for the diagnosis of adhesive capsulitis. Capsular thickening and synovitis consistent with adhesive capsulitis can however be documented on MRI (Fig. 34.7). MRI has been used for investigational purposes in patients with adhesive capsulitis and has demonstrated increased blood flow to the synovium, a finding consistent with the observed histologic appearance (52).

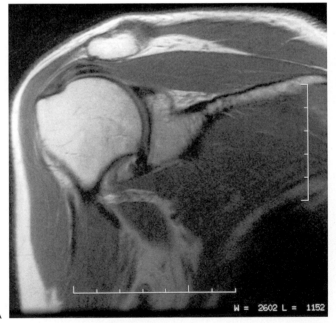
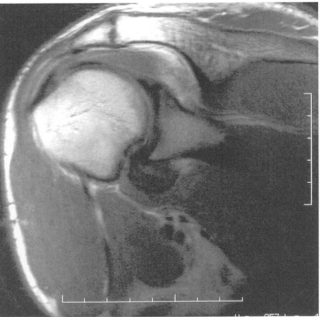

FIGURE 34.7 A: Magnetic resonance imaging of a patient with Stage 1 adhesive capsulitis. There is no significant capsular thickening or decrease in the axillary recess. Synovitis can be visualized in the axillary recess in this coronal oblique view. **B:** Magnetic resonance imaging of a patient with Stage 2 adhesive capsulitis. Synovitis and significant thickening and contracture of the axillary recess is demonstrated in this coronal oblique view. (MRI images courtesy of Hollis Potter, MD.)

TREATMENT: STAGES 1 AND 2

Patients presenting in different stages of primary adhesive capsulitis should have individualized treatment. However, certain basic principles apply to all stages. Patients who present with a painful limitation of motion are given oral nonsteroidal antiinflammatory medications which are supplemented with other analgesics as necessary. An intraarticular injection of steroid and local anesthetic is extremely useful in the diagnosis and treatment of adhesive capsulitis. The injection of the glenohumeral joint in adhesive capsulitis is analogous to injection of the subacromial space in impingement syndrome. Review of the stages outlined above provides the rationale for this approach. Injection of a local anesthetic and corticosteroid in a patient with Stage 1 adhesive capsulitis can be both diagnostic and therapeutic. The glenohumeral joint is injected via a posterior approach using traditional posterior arthroscopic portal landmarks using a 20 gauge spinal needle. The skin is lightly anesthetized using ethyl chloride spray and the needle is advanced until the capsule is palpated. When the needle enters the joint, the patient will have a brief, but sharp pain that resolves quickly upon injection of a solution containing 5cc of 1% lidocaine, 3 cc of 0.25% marcaine and 80mg depomedrol. The patient is instructed in simple pendulum exercises and is reexamined 15 minutes following the injection to evaluate pain and determine passive glenohumeral ROM. If the patient has significant improvement in pain and normalization of motion, this confirms the diagnosis of Stage 1 adhesive capsulitis. If the patient has a significant improvement in pain but a partial improvement in ROM, a Stage 2 adhesive capsulitis is present. Again, it must be reinforced that these stages represent a continuum of the inflammatory and scarring processes. A late stage 2 will be reflected in a stiffer joint than an early stage 2 despite a positive pain response to the steroid injection.

There is extensive information in the orthopaedic and rheumatologic literature regarding the efficacy of intraarticular corticosteroid in the treatment of adhesive capsulitis (15,21,22,23,24). In interpreting the results of published studies, it is critical to note the stage of adhesive capsulitis being treated. Bulgen et al. (15) randomized patients to treatment with steroid, physical therapy (PT), ice or benign neglect. The initial response to treatment was most marked in patients treated with steroid; however, no significant difference in final long-term outcome was reported when treatment groups were compared. Hazelman (53) summarized numerous studies on the use of intraarticular corticosteroid and reported that success of treatment is dependent on the duration of symptoms. Patients treated within 1 month of onset of symptoms recovered in an average of 1.5 months. Patients treated within 2 to 5 months of onset of symptoms recovered in 8.1 months; patients treated 6 to 12 months after onset of symptoms required an average of 14 months for full recovery. The author has observed a similar pattern in

treatment of patients with adhesive capsulitis at the Hospital for Special Surgery. Patients treated with intraarticular corticosteroid during Stage 1 (0–3 months) had a rapid and striking recovery of a pain-free shoulder within 6–8 weeks. Patients treated during Stage 2 had a significant improvement in night pain and pain at rest, but the time necessary for recovery of ROM was dependent on the duration of symptoms prior to treatment as reported by Hazelman. These data and others present in the literature support the hypothesis that adhesive capsulitis is both an inflammatory and fibrotic condition (15,20,37,39,40). The hypervascular synovitis present in the early stages results in subsequent fibrosis of the subsynovium and capsule. We hypothesize that early treatment with intraarticular corticosteroid provides a chemical ablation of the synovitis, thus limiting the subsequent development of fibrosis and shortening the natural history of the disease. The self-limiting nature of adhesive capsulitis also supports the role of the synovium in initiation and regulation of the fibrotic process in the capsule. With resolution of the synovitis and cessation of scar formation, capsular remodeling and recovery of ROM occurs.

Patient education and instruction in a home exercise program are mainstays of rehabilitation of the patient with adhesive capsulitis. An understanding of the diagnosis of adhesive capsulitis will encourage patient compliance and decrease patient frustration.

The primary goal of rehabilitative treatment of patients with Stage 1 adhesive capsulitis is to interrupt the inflammation-pain cycle; therefore activity modification is an important consideration. The individual is encouraged to use pain as a guide to limit activities of daily living because inflammation and pain can alter shoulder mechanics. The optimal resting posture with the arm positioned in comfortable abduction for improved vascularization of the cuff is demonstrated to the patient (54). Postural training is incorporated to discourage thoracic kyphosis and a forward humeral head position during forward elevation. Therapeutic modalities are used to reduce pain (high voltage galvanic stimulation, transcutaneous electrical nerve stimulation (55) (TENS), iontophoresis, and cryotherapy), reduce inflammation (iontophoresis, phonophoresis, and cryotherapy), and to promote relaxation (moist heat, ultrasound) (56). Gentle joint mobilizations and physiologic movements using the opposite extremity are performed. Hydrotherapy can be used to break the cycle of pain and muscle spasm. The buoyancy of the water provides an environment for active-assistive exercise and helps facilitate the return of normal scapulohumeral rhythm.

The second phase of rehabilitation is used to treat patients with Stage 2 adhesive capsulitis. The continuum of symptoms progresses in this stage to include pain in the upper trapezius and periscapular musculature. Painful spasm of these muscles may extend to the neck additionally altering shoulder mechanics. If the individual has responded successfully to intraarticular corticosteroid, capsular pain will be noted only at extremes of movement. Hiking of the shoulder girdle is evident with elevation of the arm as a result of capsular contracture and inhibition of the rotator cuff musculature. Anterior translation of humeral head may result from a decrease in capsular volume associated with adhesive capsulitis (57). The limitation of ROM is in a capsular pattern with external rotation most limited, followed by abduction, then internal rotation. In this stage, ROM evaluation reveals a rigid, capsular end-feel.

The goal of the second phase is to decrease pain, inflammation and capsular restriction thereby minimizing loss of motion. It is important to educate the patient regarding the improvement in ROM because the patient will continue to perceive pain at the end of the range, and may not recognize the objective improvement in function. In this phase, modalities are used to decrease pain and inflammation and to increase tissue extensibility. ROM exercises including passive joint mobilizations are used to restore joint glide and separation. The goal is to stretch the capsule sufficiently to allow restoration of normal glenohumeral biomechanics. Although most patients will have significant improvement by 12 to 16 weeks, some patients do not improve or have worsening of symptoms. The options at this point include continued home or supervised therapy or surgical intervention.

OPERATIVE TEATMENT

The options at this point include closed manipulation; or arthroscopy, capsular release, and manipulation; or open capsular release. The risks and benefits of these approaches are described, including fracture, neurovascular injury, residual stiffness, instability, and infection. The author's preference is to proceed with arthroscopic assessment before manipulation. If one accepts the hypothesis that the glenohumeral synovitis is an essential factor in the development of adhesive capsulitis, then an arthroscopic examination is critical to rule out residual synovitis or allow synovectomy before manipulation with or without capsular release. This will be discussed in more detail later in the chapter.

STAGE 3 AND STAGE 4

Patients who present for evaluation in Stage 3 and 4 often will report a history of longstanding pain at rest and pain at night that have resolved spontaneously (59). Physical examination will reveal a stiff shoulder, with striking alteration of scapulohumeral mechanics and a limited use of the arm during activities of daily living. As has been observed in Stages 1 and 2, treatment should be individualized to each patient. There is no indication for the use of intraarticular corticosteroid in stages 3 and 4 as the inflammatory phase of the

disease has passed. The decision to proceed with operative versus nonoperative treatment is dependent on the degree of functional disability and the patient's response to a rehabilitative program designed to improve capsular flexibility and ROM. Patients in Stage 4 are infrequently treated surgically as they have entered the "thawing" phase of the disease and are recovering range of motion.

PT for patients with Stage 3 adhesive capsulitis is designed to treat the significant loss of motion and abnormal scapulohumeral rhythm that is characteristic of this stage. There is dominance of the upper trapezius resulting in hiking of the shoulder girdle. This is attributed to decreased inferior glide of the glenohumeral joint, which prevents glenohumeral abduction (60). The primary goal of treatment is to increase ROM. In this phase, aggressive stretching will be tolerated and should be the focus of treatment. Stretching can be taken to the limits of the available ROM, and beyond. Cryotherapy may be used to reduce discomfort after stretching. Strengthening of the scapula musculature continues in this phase to reestablish effective force couples. As ROM improves, and if rotator cuff weakness persists, isolation of the cuff can be initiated to address strength and endurance. The home exercise program includes ROM and flexibility exercises and training of the scapular musculature.

OPERATIVE TREATMENT OF ADHESIVE CAPSULITIS

Closed Manipulation

Closed manipulation is contraindicated in patients with significant osteopenia, recent surgical repair of soft tissues about the shoulder, or in the presence of fractures, neurologic injury and instability. Closed manipulation is performed as described previously (27) after institution of scalene block or general anesthesia. The scapula is stabilized with one hand while the humerus is grasped just above the elbow with the other hand. Initially, the adducted shoulder is externally rotated and then abducted in the coronal plane. Next, the shoulder is externally rotated in abduction and then internally rotated while maintaining abduction. The shoulder then is flexed and finally brought back into adduction and internally rotated. There frequently is palpable and audible yielding of the soft tissue as motion is restored in the different planes. The author does not advocate closed manipulation of the shoulder for patients with adhesive capsulitis, but prefers arthroscopic inspection before any manipulative treatment.

Arthroscopic Evaluation and Treatment

Historically, arthroscopy has been reported to be of little diagnostic and therapeutic value in patients with adhesive capsulitis of the shoulder (2). However, it has been suggested that the arthroscope may be helpful for delineation of disorders, documentation of the result of closed manipulation, and treatment of concomitant intraarticular and subacromial disease (34,35,39,61). For this reason, the author recommends arthroscopy, synovectomy, capsular release and manipulation if there are no suspected extraarticular factors contributing to the motion loss. This approach has the advantage of allowing detection of concomitant disease, performing synovectomy in Stage 2, and permitting a precise capsular release. Furthermore, the force of manual manipulation required to regain motion is greatly reduced by arthroscopic capsular release before manipulation (30).

It is essential to document glenohumeral and total ROM before initiation of the surgical procedure. The timing of arthroscopy and manipulation remains controversial. Some surgeons prefer to manipulate the shoulder first and follow with the arthroscopic evaluation; however, rupture of the capsule with manipulation will greatly increase the risk of fluid extravasation in the soft tissues surrounding the shoulder joint. The author performs a diagnostic arthroscopy and synovectomy prior to manipulation of the shoulder to minimize fluid extravasation into the soft tissues.

Although it may be difficult to insert the arthroscope into a stiff shoulder because of the capsular contracture and decreased joint volume (32,39), chondral damage is avoided by inserting the arthroscope over the humeral head. The capsule is more difficult to penetrate with the blunt trocar because of the capsular fibrosis and thickening and it is helpful to distend the capsule with fluid via spinal needle before insertion of the arthroscope. The smaller 3.8-mm arthroscope has been recommended (39) but is not used routinely at our institution. The arthroscopic appearance of the joint is dependent on the stage of adhesive capsulitis as outlined previously. Surgical treatment of stage 1 adhesive capsulitis is not indicated unless the patient fails intraarticular corticosteroid injection. In Stage 1, a diffuse hypervascular synovitis is observed which may have areas of focal thickening in the anterosuperior capsule and along the proximal biceps tendon. An arthroscopic cannula is inserted just inferior to the biceps tendon and this synovium is removed atraumatically with a 4.5 mm motorized shaver. The synovium can be easily removed with minimal pressure and a steady gliding motion. It is important to perform a thorough synovectomy; thus, it is necessary to view the shoulder from anterior and posterior portals. An attempt should be made to resect any areas of synovitis in the inferior pouch. This is technically feasible in a patient with Stage 1 adhesive capsulitis, but often is extremely difficult in patients with Stage 2 adhesive capsulitis. A capsular biopsy is routinely taken to confirm the histologic stage of the syndrome. In Stage 2, the synovial lining remains hypervascular but is thicker and more pedunculated in appearance. Again, a thorough synovectomy is indicated and a capsular biopsy is obtained. In Stage 3, residual synovial thickening or scarring is seen, but the hypervascular appearance has resolved. A sheet of capsular scar, which can be debrided, may obscure the rotator cuff interval and the tendon of the subscapularis.

At this point, the arthroscopic instruments are removed and a gentle manipulation is performed. Patients with late Stage 1 or early Stage 2 adhesive capsulitis who have mild scarring and thickening of the capsule often will regain full ROM with gentle manipulation. The manipulation is performed in the following order: forward flexion, extension, abduction, and internal and external rotation. In the early stages of adhesive capsulitis, a series of small pops are heard as the anterior and inferior capsule ruptures. If the arthroscope is placed back into the shoulder, a capsular rupture is seen that runs from approximately 2 o'clock to 6 o'clock (in a right shoulder) then passes obliquely across the inferior axillary pouch. In late Stage 2 and Stage 3 adhesive capsulitis, the capsular scarring is dense and an arthroscopic capsular release is performed prior to manipulation. The capsular scar is divided using an electrocautery device. The capsular division is performed just medial to the labrum at the capsular labral junction. The capsule is incised through its full thickness using an anterior-superior portal, beginning just inferior to the biceps tendon and continuing inferiorly until the discrete upper edge of the subscapularis tendon is encountered. This constitutes a surgical release of the rotator interval region of the capsule (62). Ozaki et al. (63) have reported that an open release of this area usually is successful in restoring external rotation in shoulders with refractory adhesive capsulitis. As the capsule is released, the humeral head moves inferiorly and laterally, creating more room in the joint for the arthroscope to be moved into the anterior and inferior region of the joint. The capsular release then is continued inferiorly to 5 o'clock (Fig. 34.8). The subscapularis tendon is not routinely released. Release of the inferior recess from 5 to 7 o'clock is not performed because of potential risk to the underlying axillary nerve. After this anterior capsular release, the arthroscope is removed and a closed manipulation is performed. In most cases, external rotation in adduction is restored with minimal manipulation force. The shoulder can be manipulated with minimal force and with audible and palpable yielding of tissue. If an assistant is available, the author recommends placing one set of hands proximally and one distally when performing the manipulation to diminish the lever arm on the proximal humerus. If the patient still lacks internal rotation in abduction or extension, the arthroscope is reinserted into the joint via the anterior portal and a posterior capsular release is performed from 7 to 11 o'clock. The author has had no cases of axillary nerve injury with this technique.

The goal of treatment following surgery is to maintain the range of motion achieved under anesthesia, and to decrease pain and inflammation. In the recovery room, passive range of motion is initiated using cpm or the patient's contralateral arm. The decision to admit the patient or perform the surgery on an ambulatory basis is individualized. If the

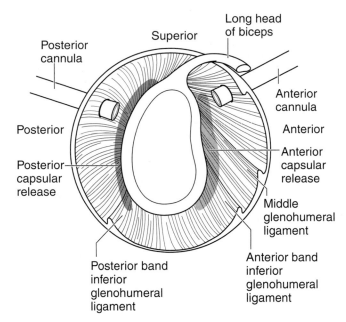

FIGURE 34.8 Landmarks for capsular release in the operative treatment of adhesive capsulitis. A schematic representation of a right shoulder is shown. The arthroscopic cannula is inserted just inferior to the long head of the biceps and the capsule is released from 1 to 5 o'clock while viewing from the posterior portal. If necessary, the arthroscope can then be inserted into the anterior portal and a release performed from 7 to 11 o'clock.

patient is to be hospitalized, a long acting scalene block is placed and CPM (continuous passive motion) is maintained while the patient is awake (64,65). Patients who are treated on an ambulatory basis begin physical therapy on postoperative day 1 with the use of appropriate narcotic analgesia. The patient is seen as an outpatient for 5 days per week for the first 2 weeks, then 3 times per week until treatment is completed. Treatment includes aggressive ROM, CPM, modalities for pain and inflammation, and hydrotherapy. Hydrotherapy is instituted as soon as possible with the use of a water-impermeable dressing to keep the suture sites dry (67). Strengthening exercises are gradually incorporated into the program as outlined previously.

CONCLUSION

Treatment of patients with adhesive capsulitis of the shoulder requires an individualized approach that considers the stages and natural history of the disease. In Stages 1 and 2, a conservative approach including the use of intraarticular corticosteroid and a supervised physical therapy program is the initial method of treatment. This approach is very successful in patients with Stage 1 adhesive capsulitis. This conservative treatment approach will often be successful in patients with Stage 2 adhesive capsulitis; however, some

patients may have a refractory motion loss. In these patients, arthroscopy, synovectomy, and closed manipulation are offered to the patient. In patients with late Stage 2 and Stage 3 adhesive capsulitis, an arthroscopic release technique is performed to successfully restore motion. This technique is demanding, and proper patient selection, anesthesia, and postoperative analgesia are critical to its success. Patients with Stage 4 adhesive capsulitis are generally managed with a home program to facilitate recovery of range of motion, as by definition, the capsular contracture is resolving during this stage. Continued clinical research in the treatment of patients with adhesive capsulitis is clearly needed to identify the biologic trigger responsible for the development of synovitis and subsequent capsular fibroplasia. The development of specific agents designed to eliminate the synovitis, capsular fibroplasia, and scar formation may make the surgical treatment of patients with adhesive capsulitis obsolete in the future. Well-controlled prospective clinical trials will be needed to determine the efficacy of these treatment regimens for women and men, and to transform the treatment of adhesive capsulitis into a clearly defined science.

REFERENCES

1. Binder A, Bulgen DY, Hazelmlan BL, et al. Frozen shoulder: A long-term prospective study. *Ann Rheum Dis* 1984;43:361–364.
2. Lloyd-Roberts GG, French PR. Periarthritis of the shoulder: A study of the disease and its treatment. *Br Med J* 1959;1:1569–1574.
3. Bridgman JF. Periarthritis of the shoulder and diabetes mellitus. *Ann Rheum Dis* 1972;31:69–71.
4. Janda DH, Hawkins RJ. Shoulder manipulation in patients with adhesive capsulitis and diabetes mellitus. A clinical note. *J Shoulder Elbow Surg* 1993;2:36–38.
5. McClure PW, Flowers KR. Treatment of limited shoulder motion: A case study based on biomechanical considerations. *Phys Ther* 1992;72:929–936.
6. Miller MD, Rockwood CA Jr. Thawing the frozen shoulder: The "patient" patient. *Orthopedics* 1997;19:849–853.
7. Pal B, Anderson J, Dick WC. Limitations of joint mobility and shoulder capsulitis in insulin and non-insulin dependent diabetes mellitus. *Br J Rheum* 1986;5:147–151.
8. DePalma AF. Loss of scapulohumeral motion (frozen shoulder). *Ann Surg* 1952;135:193–197.
9. Bowman CA, Jeffcoate WJ, Patrick M. Bilateral adhesive capsulitis, oligoarthritis and proximal myopathy as presentation of hypothyroidism. *Br J Rheumatol* 1988;27:62–64.
10. Mintner WT. The shoulder-hand syndrome in coronary disease. *J Med Assoc GA* 1967;56:45–49.
11. Bulgen DY, Binder A, Hazelman BL. Immunological studies in frozen shoulder. *J Rheum* 1982;9:893–898.
12. Rizk TE, Pinals RS. Histocompatibility type and racial incidence in frozen shoulder. *Arch Phys Med Rehab* 1984;65:33–34.
13. Shaffer B, Tibone JE, Kerlan RK. Frozen shoulder. A long-term follow-up study. *J Bone Joint Surg* 1992;74:738–746.
14. Bulgen DY, Binder A, Hazelman BL, et al. Frozen shoulder: Prospective clinical study with an evaluation of three treatment regimens. *Ann Rheum Dis* 1984;43:353–360.
15. Mao CY, Jaw WC Frozen shoulder: Correlation between the re-

sponse to physical therapy and follow-up shoulder arthrography. *Arch Phys Med Rehab* 1997;78:857–859.

16. Placzek JD, Roubal PJ, Freeman DC, et al. Long-term effectiveness of translational manipulation for adhesive capsulitis. *Clin Orthop Rel Res* 1998;356:181–191.

17. Huskisson EC, Bryans R. Diclofenac sodium in treatment of the painful stiff shoulder. *Curr Med Res Opin* 1983;8:350–353.

18. Owens-Burkhart H. Management of frozen shoulder. In Donatelli RA Ed *Physical Therapy of the Shoulder*. New York; Churchill Livingstone, 1991;91–116.

19. Binder A, Hazelman BL, Parr G, et al. A controlled study of oral prednisone in frozen shoulder. *Br J Rheum* 1986;25:288–292.

20. D'Acre JE, Beeney N, Scott DL. Injections and physiotherapy for the painful stiff shoulder. *Ann Rheum Dis* 1989;48:322–325.

21. DeJong BA, Dahmen R, Hogeweg JA, et al. Intraarticular triamcinolone acetonide injection in patients with capsulitis of the shoulder: A comparative study of two dose regimes. *Clin Rehab* 1998;12:211–215.

22. Quigley TB. Indications for manipulation and corticosteroids in the treatment of stiff shoulder. *Surg Clin North Am* 1975;43:1715–1720.

23. Steinbrocker O, Argyros TG. Frozen shoulder: Treatment by local injection of depot corticosteroids. *Arch Phys Med Rehabil* 1974;55:209–213.

24. Laroche M, Ighilahriz O, Moulinier LI. Adhesive capsulitis of the shoulder: An open study of 40 cases treated by joint distension during arthrography followed by intraarticular corticosteroid injection and immediate physical therapy. *Rev Rheum Engl Ed* 1998;65:313–319.

25. Andersen NH, Sojbjerg JO, Johannsen HV, et al. Frozen shoulder: Arthroscopy and manipulation under general anesthesia and early passive motion. *J Shoulder Elbow Surg* 1998;7:218–222.

26. Haines JF, Hargadon EJ. Manipulation as the primary treatment of frozen shoulder. *J R Coll Surg Edin* 1982;27:271–275.

27. Helbig B, Wagner P, Dohler R. Mobilization of frozen shoulder under general anesthesia. *Acta Orthop Belg* 1983;49:267–274.

28. Lundberg J. The frozen shoulder: Clinical and radiographic observations: The effect of manipulation under general anesthesia: Structure and glycosaminoglycan content of the joint capsule. *Acta Orthop Scan* 1969;119:1–59.

29. Olgilvie-Harris DJ, Biggs DJ, Fitsialos JP, et al. The resistant frozen shoulder: Manipulation versus arthroscopic release. *Clin Orthop Rel Res* 1995;319:238–248.

30. Kieras DM, Matsen FA III. Open release in the management of refractory frozen shoulder. *Orthop Trans* 191;15:801.

31. Bradley JP. Arthroscopic treatment for adhesive capsulitis. *Op Tech Orthop* 1991;1:248–252.

32. Ogilvie-Harris DJ, Myerthall S. The diabetic frozen shoulder: Arthroscopic release. *Arthroscopy* 1997;13:1–8.

33. Pollock RG, Duralde XA, Flatow EL, et al. The use of arthroscopy in treatment of resistant frozen shoulder. *Clin Orthop* 1994;304:30–36

34. Segmuller HE, Taylor DE, Hogan CS, et al. Arthroscopic treatment of adhesive capsulitis. *J Shoulder Elbow Surg* 1995;4:403–404.

35. Neviaser JS. Adhesive capsulitis of the shoulder. Study of pathological findings in periarthritis of the shoulder. *J Bone Joint Surg* 1945;27:211–222.

36. Hannafin JA, DiCarlo EF, Wickiewicz TL, et al. Adhesive capsulitis: capsular fibroplasia of the glenohumeral joint. *J Shoulder Elbow Surg* 1994;3:5.

37. Rodeo SA, Hannafin JA, Tom J, et al. Immunolocalization of cytokines and their receptors in adhesive capsulitis of the shoulder. *J Orthop Res* 1997;15:427–436.

38. Wiley AM. Arthroscopic appearance of frozen shoulder. *Arthroscopy* 1991;7:138–143.

39. Bunker TD, Anthony PP. The pathology of frozen shoulder. A Dupuytren-like disease. *J Bone Joint Surg* 1995;77B: 677–683.

40. Grubbs N. Frozen shoulder syndrome: A review of literature. *J Orthop Sports Phys Ther* 1993;18:479–487.

41. Border WA, Noble NA. Transforming growth factor beta in tissue fibrosis. *N Engl J Med* 1994;331:1286–1292.

42. Alman BA, Greel DA, Ruby LK, et al. Regulation of growth and platelet-derived growth factor expression in palmar fibromatosis (Dupuytren's disease) by mechanical strain. *Trans Combined ORS Meeting* 1995;108.

43. Hutchinson JW, Tierney GM, Parsons SL, et al. Dupuytren's disease and frozen shoulder induced by treatment with a matrix metalloproteinase inhibitor. *J Bone Joint Surg* 1998;80B: 907–908.

44. Zabraniecki L, Doub A, Mularczyk M. Frozen shoulder: A new delayed complication of protease inhibitor therapy. *Rev Rheum Engl Ed* 1998;65:72–74.

45. Neviaser RJ. Painful conditions affecting the shoulder. *Clin Orthop* 1983;173:63–69.

46. Neviaser RJ, Neviaser T. The frozen shoulder. Diagnosis and management. *Clin Orthop* 1987;223:59–64.

47. Neviaser JS. Adhesive capsulitis and the stiff and painful shoulder. *Orthop Clin North Am* 1980;11:327–331.

48. Reeves B. The natural history of the frozen shoulder syndrome. *Scand J Rheum* 1975;4:193–196.

49. Leppala J, Kannus P, Sievanen H, et al. Adhesive capsulitis of the shoulder (frozen shoulder) produces bone loss in the affected humerus, but long-term bony recovery is good. *Bone* 1998;22:691–694.

50. Reeves B. Arthrographic changes in frozen and post-traumatic stiff shoulder. *Proc R Soc Med* 1966;59:827–830.

51. Neviaser JS. Arthrography of the shoulder joint. *J Bone Joint Surg* 1942;44A:1321–1326.

52. Tamai K, Yamato M. Abnormal synovium in the frozen shoulder: a preliminary report with dynamic magnetic resonance imaging. *J Shoulder Elbow Surg* 1997;6:534–543.

53. Hazelman BD. The painful stiff shoulder. *Rheum Phys Med* 1972;11:413–421.

54. Rathbun JB, McNab I. The microvascular pattern of the rotator cuff. *J Bone Joint Surg* 1970;52B:540–553.

55. Rhind V, Downie WW, Bird HA, et al. Naproxen and indomethacin in periarthritis of the shoulder. *Rheumatol Rehab* 1982;21:51–53.

56. Wadsworth CT. Frozen shoulder. *Phys Ther* 1986;66:1878–1883.

57. Roubal PJ, Dobritt D, Placzek JD. Glenohumeral gliding manipulation following interscalene brachial plexus block in patients with adhesive capsulitis. *J Orthop Sports Phys Ther* 1966;24:66–77.

58. Ayub E. Posture and the upper quarter. In Donatella RA Ed: *Physical Therapy of the Shoulder,* second edition. New York, Churchill Livingstone, 1991;81–90.

59. Boyle-Walker KL, Gabard DL, Bietsch E, et al. A profile of patients with adhesive capsulitis. *J Hand Ther* 1997;10:222–228.

60. Hjelm R, Draper C, Spencer S. Anterior-superior capsular length insufficiency in the painful shoulder. *J Orthop Sports Phys Ther* 1996;23: 216–222.

61. Hsu SYC, Chan KM. Arthroscopic distension in the management of frozen shoulder. *Int Orthop* 1991;15:79–83.

62. Harryman DT III, Sidles JA, Harris SL, et al. The role of the rotator interval capsule in passive motion and stability of the shoulder. *J Bone Joint Surg* 1992;74A:53–66.

63. Ozaki J, Kakagawa Y, Sakurai G, et al. Recalcitrant chronic adhesive capsulitis of the shoulder: Role of contracture of the coracohumeral ligament and rotator interval in pathogenesis and treatment. *J Bone Joint Surg* 1989;71:1511–1515.

64. Brown AR, Weiss R, Greenberg C, et al. Interscalene block for shoulder arthroscopy: Comparison with general anesthesia. *Arthroscopy* 1993;9:295–300.

65. Kinnard P, Truchon R, St-Pierre A. Interscalene block for pain relief after shoulder surgery. *Clin Orthop Rel Res* 1994;304:22–24.

66. McCarthy MR, O'Donoghue PC. The clinical use of continuous passive motion in physical therapy. *J Orthop Sports Phys Ther* 1992;15:132.

67. Speer KP, Cavanaugh JT, Warren RF, et al. A role for hydrotherapy in shoulder rehabilitation. *Am J Sports Med* 1993;21:850–853.

STIFF SHOULDER: POSTTRAUMATIC STIFFNESS AND POSTSURGICAL STIFFNESS

ARIANE GERBER AND JON J.P. WARNER

DEFINITION AND CLASSIFICATION

Posttraumatic and postsurgical stiffness, also defined as *acquired or secondary shoulder stiffness,* is a condition in which a limitation of active and passive range of motion occurs after a traumatic event or a surgical procedure. Basically, three different forms of acquired shoulder stiffness, differing in their natural history, can be defined, as follows:

- Stiffness after trauma or surgery in the context of capsulitis
- Stiffness after trauma or surgery in the context of scarring of the capsule or the extraarticular soft tissue planes
- Stiffness after trauma or surgical procedures in patients with skeletal or articular deformity

Although features of more than one category are often encountered in the same patient with acquired shoulder stiffness, this classification is useful to structure a rational therapeutic approach.

ETIOPATHOGENESIS
Posttraumatic or Postsurgical Capsulitis

Idiopathic adhesive capsulitis is characterized by inflammation and subsequent scarring of the joint capsule, as well as by decreases in intraarticular volume and capsular compliance limiting motion in all planes. Inflammation of the joint capsule and subsequent scarring may also occur after trauma or surgical procedures. It is not clear whether the cause of posttraumatic or postsurgical capsulitis is different from that of idiopathic adhesive capsulitis or whether some patients simply develop adhesive capsulitis in the context of trauma or surgery. Age, longer periods of immobilization, and endocrine, neurologic, and psychologic disorders, all recog-

nized to be important in the pathogenesis of idiopathic adhesive capsulitis, also seem to play a role in the development of shoulder stiffness after trauma or surgical treatment.

Stiffness after surgical excision of calcific tendinitis of the rotator cuff has been reported to affect 6% to 20% of patients. The pathologic mechanism is unknown, but the clinical symptoms are those of adhesive capsulitis (1).

Unpublished reports on thermal capsulorrhaphy suggests that stiffness is the most common complication of this procedure (2). It has been our experience that patients showing stiffness after capsular shrinkage present, to some extent, with the same symptoms as patients with idiopathic adhesive capsulitis. Although the etiologic factor is different, inflammation and scarring also occur as repair mechanisms after thermal injury and may induce a capsulitis-like syndrome in some patients. In most cases, however, acquired stiffness is associated with alterations of extraarticular soft tissues in addition to the glenohumeral capsule, although this depends on the nature of the injury or prior surgical procedure.

Acquired Capsular Shortening or Contracture

A relative capsular laxity in the midrange of motion has been shown to be a feature of normal shoulder motion. Scarring or shortening of specific regions of the capsule is known to lead to specific patterns of motion limitation (3–5). Involvement of the rotator interval, which is composed of the coracohumeral and superior glenohumeral ligaments, typically limits flexion, extension, and external rotation when the shoulder is in an adducted position. The anteroinferior capsuloligamentous complex is a restraint for external rotation in abduction, whereas the posteroinferior capsule limits internal rotation and forward flexion. Experimental studies have demonstrated that soft tissue contracture causes increased translation of the humeral head on the glenoid socket in a direction opposite to the contracture during at-

A. Gerber and J. J. P. Warner: Harvard Shoulder Service, Massachusetts General Hospital, Boston, Massachusetts.

tempted shoulder motion. Anterior and posterior capsular contractures have been shown to increase translation in the superior direction. This can result in compression of the rotator cuff as the humeral head is pushed superiorly by the contracture and induces a "nonoutlet"-type impingement (6–8). Furthermore, an asymmetric anterior contracture tends to cause the humeral head to move posteriorly on the glenoid with attempted external rotation. This has been associated with the development of arthritis and has been termed *capsulorrhaphy arthropathy* (6) (Fig. 35.1).

Loss of glenohumeral motion also influences normal kinematics of the scapulothoracic joint. A compensatory increase of scapulothoracic motion is often seen in patients with glenohumeral contracture, and this can cause pain in the periscapular region (9). Furthermore, in osteoarthritis, global thickening and scarring are typical features of the joint capsule and are probably the consequence of dysfunctional synoviocytes (10).

Scarring of Gliding Surfaces

Another requirement for normal shoulder mobility is free gliding between tissue planes. In the normal shoulder, the rotator cuff glides underneath the coracoacromial arch and the deltoid muscle. Trauma and prolonged immobilization or surgical procedures can lead to scarring between the deltoid and the proximal humerus, the rotator cuff and the acromion, and the rotator cuff and the joint capsule. Promi-

nent implants used to stabilize proximal humeral fractures almost always lead to scarring of the subdeltoid bursa.

Rotator Cuff Dysfunction

Some degree of stiffness is not rare in patients with symptomatic rotator cuff tears and has been shown to be a predisposing factor for limitation of motion after repair, even if contracture is addressed at the time of the surgical procedure (11). Unopposed action of the normal innervated muscles in the paralyzed shoulder leads to restriction of not only active but also passive range of motion because of soft tissue contracture.

Skeletal and Articular Deformity

Smooth, normally shaped articular surfaces, properly oriented to each other, represent the osteoarticular requirement for normal glenohumeral range of motion. Skeletal deformity is always associated with soft tissue scarring.

Displaced fractures of the proximal humerus treated conservatively or in which anatomic reduction could not be achieved or maintained are usually associated with stiffness resulting from not only soft tissue contracture but also skeletal deformity. Intraarticular fractures with loss of the normal relationship between the humeral head and tuberosities are usually associated with poor function, partly because of stiffness but mostly because of malpositioning of the tuberosity. Extraarticular deformities are usually better tolerated.

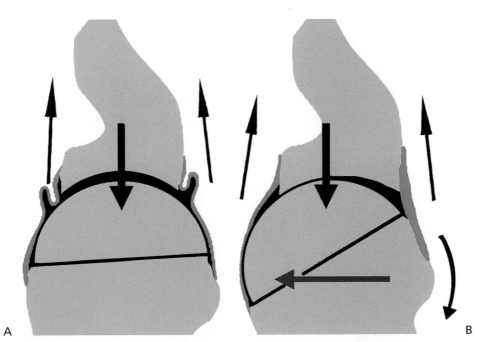

FIGURE 35.1 A: In the normal flexible shoulder, the joint reaction force *(large black arrow)* to the balanced action from the anterior and posterior rotator cuff muscles *(small black arrows)* is centered. **B:** If the anterior soft tissue sleeve is scarred and shortened, posterior translation of the humeral head will occur when the arm is rotated externally and the joint reaction force is shifted posteriorly.

Stiffness resulting from articular incongruity (and capsular contracture) is the leading feature of osteoarthritis. Except for selected cases in the early stage of the degenerative process in which only the soft tissue contracture can be addressed, correction of the articular deformity, through corrective osteotomy or replacement arthroplasty, is required in the majority of the cases. In the case of replacement arthroplasty, stiffness can be the result of nonanatomic reconstruction, such as oversizing and poor orientation of the components, and tuberosity-related problems such as nonunion or malunion (Fig. 35.2).

The muscular imbalance seen in patients with brachial plexus birth palsy has been shown to lead to an age-related articular deformity if the condition is not addressed early. Once humeral head flattening and glenoid dysplasia have developed, soft tissue release alone, either arthroscopically or as an open procedure, cannot increase mobility (12).

Bony block procedures to treat instability, such as the Bristow, Latarjet, and Trillat procedures, are techniques that distort the skeletal and soft tissue anatomy. Subscapularis entrapment or impingement and articular incongruity may lead to limitation of motion after these procedures (13).

CLINICAL PRESENTATION AND THERAPEUTIC OPTIONS

Acquired shoulder stiffness depends on the nature of the injury or surgical procedure, and clinical presentation varies from case to case. Nevertheless, careful analysis of the patient's history and accurate physical examination may help to categorize the different disorders.

Whereas the natural history of idiopathic shoulder stiffness is relatively favorable (14), shoulder stiffness after trauma or surgery is more resistant to conservative treatment. Only a few reports are available in the literature regarding surgical indications and optimal treatment of acquired shoulder stiffness. Most of the reports have addressed loss of external rotation after surgical procedures for instability, and some have shown that extreme loss of external rotation, as with an internal rotation contracture, is associated with the development of arthritis (Fig. 35.1). When conservative treatment fails, most recommended approaches have involved open release. In selected cases, an arthroscopic or a combined open and arthroscopic approach has been reported to be reliable and safe (15,16). Furthermore, one report has shown a less favorable outcome after arthroscopic

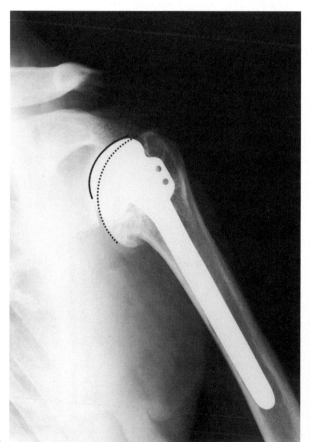
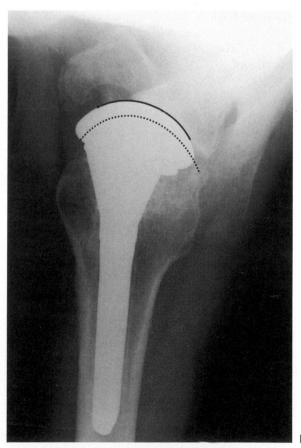

A   B

FIGURE 35.2 Stiffness after replacement arthroplasty with nonanatomic reconstruction. **A:** Anteroposterior view demonstrating malpositioning of the prosthetic head *(black line)* compared with the humeral head *(dotted line)*. **B:** Axillary view demonstrating posterior glenoid erosion.

treatment for acquired stiffness than for idiopathic stiffness (17). It is our opinion that the treatment should be tailored to each patient, and the surgeon should take into account the pathologic factors, the expected natural history, and the potential risk of a secondary articular injury.

Acquired Stiffness in the Context of Capsulitis

Clinical Symptoms

Typically acquired capsulitis is seen after minor traumatic incidents, repetitive overuse injuries, surgical treatment of calcifying tendinitis (1), or arthroscopic thermal capsulorrhaphy (2), but it can be observed after trauma or surgical procedures, such as the Bankart procedure and capsular shift. After trauma or surgery of the shoulder, some patients develop severe pain that cannot be explained by the underlying condition. The symptoms usually do not occur immediately after trauma or surgery, but after a time lag of 2 to 6 weeks. The patient localizes the pain "deep in the joint" with radiation down the arm. The pain is constant and is especially severe at night. Attempts at regaining motion rapidly with physical therapy often lead to exacerbation of the chronic discomfort. Regular pain medication prescribed after the traumatic event or operation or subacromial infiltration with 1% lidocaine (Xylocaine) does not help to control the pain. On physical examination, any manipulation of the shoulder is extremely painful to the patient. At this stage, loss of passive range of motion may be discrete, but passive rotation amplitude, especially in abduction, is already decreased and is very painful. Active range of motion is limited by pain as well as by soft tissue shortening.

Treatment

As for the early stage of idiopathic adhesive capsulitis, any aggressive manipulation or surgical approach is contraindicated for the management of acquired capsulitis (9,18). Optimal pain management and physical therapy in the form of gentle stretching are usually effective. Some patients with intractable pain may, depending on their primary diagnosis, be candidates for an intraarticular steroid injection. Furthermore, subcutaneous administration of salmon calcitonin for 21 days has been shown to decrease pain in patients with posttraumatic capsulitis (19). The prognosis is usually good if the condition is recognized and the patient is treated adequately.

Acquired Stiffness with Scarring of the Capsule or Soft Tissue Planes

Clinical Symptoms

Acquired capsular contracture, with or without scarring between tissue planes, is usually seen after fractures or postop-

eratively. The prolonged immobilization often required for healing of injured or repaired structures plays an important role in the development of this type of stiffness. Unlike patients in the group described earlier, pain is usually present especially in the end-range of motion, but limitation of motion is the leading factor. Pain mimics the symptoms of subacromial impingement, limits active range of motion, and is localized on the lateral side of the arm. Subacromial injection with 1% lidocaine may decrease the symptoms but usually does not improve active range of motion. Depending on the underlying problem, specific patterns of motion restriction are observed.

Persistent loss of motion after rotator cuff repair may be the result of inadequate operative technique or inadequate postoperative rehabilitation (13), and it is more likely to happen in patients demonstrating preoperative stiffness (20,21). Incorrect operative technique includes poor release, especially of the coracohumeral ligament, or tight closure of the rotator interval in internal rotation leading to loss of external rotation and flexion (4,5). Excessive advancement of a musculotendinous unit to achieve repair is characterized by loss of internal rotation if the posterosuperior rotator cuff is concerned or by a decrease in external rotation as seen after subscapularis repair (22). Failure to address associated pathologic processes such as acromioclavicular arthropathy or biceps tendon disease, as well as complications such as deltoid insufficiency or nerve injury, will usually result in postoperative pain and increased risk of stiffness (13). Adequate mobilization immediately after the surgical procedure is important to maintain glenohumeral flexibility. Optimization of postoperative pain management is also mandatory to allow efficient physical therapy, especially in patients with low tolerance to pain (20). Stiffness after rotator cuff repair can occur in the presence of a recurrent rupture as well. In this situation, limited active and passive range of motion is associated with weakness.

Stiffness is a potential complication of all capsuloligamentous procedures to treat instability. Traditional procedures, such as the Putti-Platt and Magnuson-Stack procedures, are designed to restrict external rotation by shortening the anterior capsule and the subscapularis tendon (23). The Bankart or capsular shift procedure, considered to address the soft tissue disorder specifically and therefore to restore stability without limitation of motion, can also be associated with severe limitation of external rotation if the capsule is overtightened (24).

Global restriction of motion is a common feature of fractures of the proximal humerus. If open reduction is indicated to achieve anatomic reduction, capsular and subdeltoid scarring can be very important, especially if postoperative immobilization is required. Prominent humeral prosthetic implants impair gliding in the subdeltoid space.

In the absence of skeletal and articular deformity, stiffness after shoulder replacement is rare and is usually a consequence of inadequate capsular and subscapularis release, characterized by a loss of forward flexion and external rotation. Limitation of postoperative mobilization to avoid secondary displacement of the tuberosity after fracture treated with hemiarthroplasty may lead to stiffness.

Although complete recovery can be expected in the majority of patients with brachial plexus birth palsy, some have persistent weakness because of a partial upper trunk lesion leading to weakness in abduction and external rotation. These patients typically present with internal rotation contracture, as the result of unopposed action of the normally innervated internal rotators (12).

Treatment

Regardless of the underlying pathologic process, supervised physical therapy should be the first treatment approach. If no improvement occurs with 12 to 16 weeks, surgical treatment should be considered.

Closed manipulation and arthroscopic or open release of adhesions have been proposed to treat the stiff shoulder after rotator cuff repair. Our experience has been that closed manipulation is rarely helpful for these patients (13). Adhesions involve not only the plane between the capsule and the rotator cuff, but also the subdeltoid space. Furthermore manipulation may pose a risk to the integrity of the repair. In the majority of the cases, arthroscopic release of the contracted capsule and adhesions is successful and allows selective release of intraarticular and subacromial adhesions. The technique of arthroscopic release is illustrated in Figs. 35.3 and 35.4. If the contracture is resistant to an arthroscopic release, the procedure should be converted to an open release. If stiffness is associated with a recurrent rupture of the rotator cuff, it is our opinion that release should be performed first, and repair, if required, should be performed as a second procedure. Dr. Warner's experience of combining both repair of the tendon and release of the contracture has been that stiffness recurs as the rotator cuff heals.

Specific guidelines regarding a minimal, "low-risk" limitation of motion after surgical procedures for instability remain unclear. Dr. Warner has suggested that a limitation of external rotation to less than 60% of that of the contralateral shoulder should be treated aggressively, especially in young patients (9). When stiffness is the result of a capsular contracture only, arthroscopic release (Figs. 35.3 and 35.4) has proven to be a reliable option (15,17). When the subscapularis is known to be shortened, as in a Putti-Platt or Magnuson-Stack procedure, open release (Figs. 35.5 and 35.6) and, sometimes, subscapularis lengthening are required (Fig. 35.7).

After nonoperative treatment of a proximal humeral fracture or after minimally invasive surgical treatment such as percutaneous pinning, conservative treatment of stiffness is usually successful, even though recovery may take several months (25). After plate fixation, osteosynthesis material removal and release of subdeltoid adhesions (Fig. 35.5) may

be necessary to improve motion effectively. Capsular release is usually not required.

Treatment of the stiff shoulder after replacement arthroplasty is challenging. This condition is usually resistant to therapy, and arthroscopic release of stiff arthroplasty has been very disappointing in the hands of Dr. Warner. The reason for these poor results is that other factors usually require treatment by an open method. These may include glenoid arthritis, component malpositioning, and inadequate release of adhesions at the time of the original surgical procedure (Fig. 35.2).

Stiffness in patients with residual brachial plexus birth palsy is resistant to physical therapy. Arthroscopic release is contraindicated, because the problem is clearly extraarticular. In younger patients with minimal articular deformity, release of the pectoralis major and transfer of the latissimus dorsi and teres major to the insertion of the posterior rotator cuff may correct the muscle imbalance (12).

Acquired Stiffness with Skeletal or Articular Deformity

Stiffness in the presence of a skeletal or articular deformity is typically found after bone block procedures to treat instability, malunited fractures of the proximal humerus, nonanatomic replacement arthroplasty, and neglected residual plexus birth palsy. A comprehensive analysis of each clinical entity is beyond the scope of this chapter, and only few specific situations are addressed here.

Stiffness after instability procedures using a bone block affects mobility either by entrapping the subscapularis tendon—the Bristow (26) and Trillat procedures (27)—or by resulting in articular incongruence—the Eden-Hybbinette (28) and Latarget procedures (29). An open approach with release of the subscapularis or correction of the articular deformity is required (9,26,30).

In their study, Gerber et al. reported on a heterogenous group of patients with major structural distortion (17). Of 15 patients, three had a malunited fracture of the greater tuberosity after dislocation, four had a malunited proximal humeral fracture, and one had avascular necrosis after fracture. Arthroscopic release did improve the range of motion significantly in this group of patients compared with their preoperative conditions. The results were inferior compared with a group of patients treated with arthroscopic release for idiopathic stiffness. When stiffness is associated with nonanatomic reconstruction after replacement arthroplasty, a complex open approach includes global soft tissue release and implant revision with or without tuberosity osteotomy (31).

Neglected residual plexus birth palsy may be associated with skeletal or articular deformity in adolescents. Release and tendon transfer are contraindicated in this situation, and humeral derotation osteotomy is the treatment of choice (12).

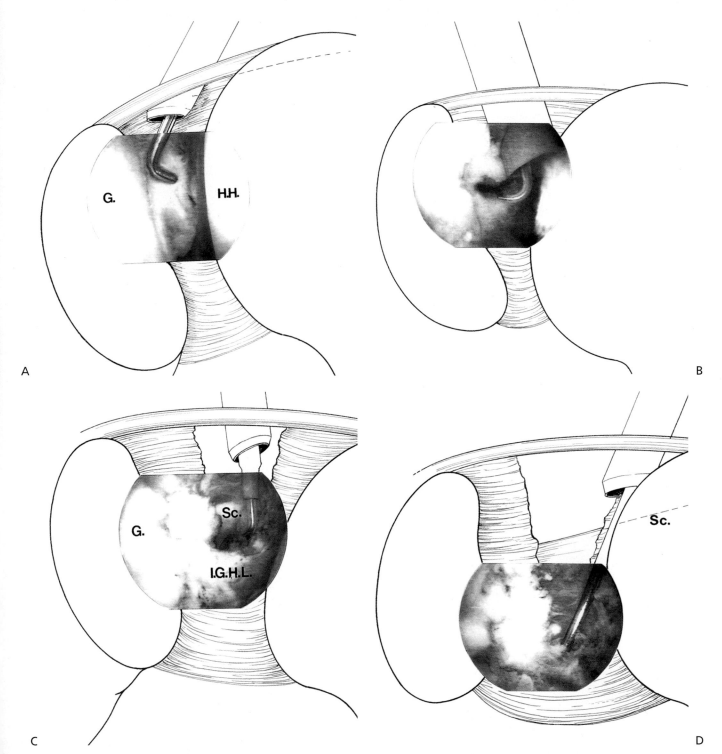

FIGURE 35.3 Arthroscopic release: anterior release. **A:** Arthroscopic view of the rotator interval and anterior capsule of a right shoulder. The arthroscope is in the posterior portal and the probe in the anterosuperior portal. G, glenoid; HH, humeral head. **B:** The electrocautery device is placed in the anterosuperior portal. **C** and **D:** The anterior capsule is released from the superior part of the rotator interval down to the 5 o'clock position including the inferior glenohumeral ligament (IGHL). The subscapularis tendon (Sc) is exposed but not damaged by the electrocautery device. The release is performed 1 cm from the anterior glenoid edge (G).

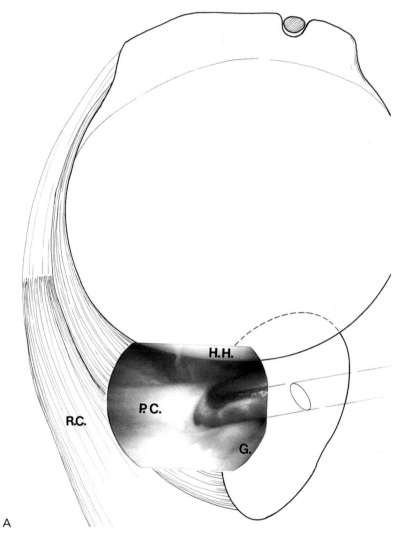

FIGURE 35.4. Arthroscopic release: posterior release. **A:** Arthroscopic view of the posterior capsule (PC) of a left shoulder. The arthroscope is in the anterosuperior portal. The metallic scope sheath is seen coming through the thick posterior capsule. RC, posterior rotator cuff.

A

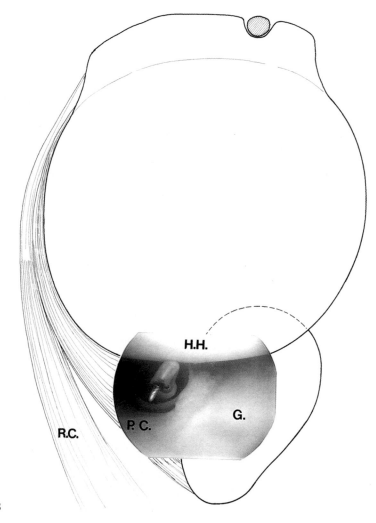

B

FIGURE 35.4. *(Continued).* **B:** The scope sheath is replaced by the plastic cannula using a switching stick, and the electrocautery device is placed in the posterior portal.

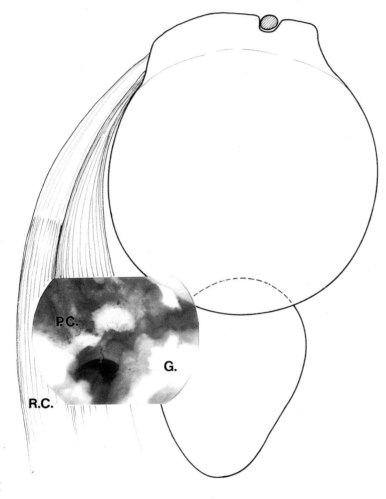

C

FIGURE 35.4. *(Continued).* **C:** The capsule is released when the posterior cuff muscles are visible in the cleft of the capsulotomy.

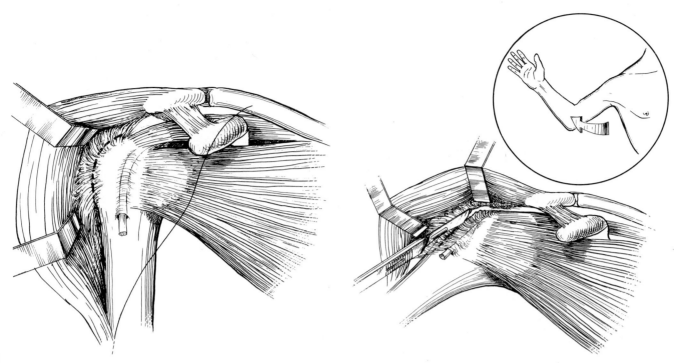

A

B

FIGURE 35.5. Open release of subdeltoid adhesions. **A:** Adhesions between the deltoid and rotator cuff restrict free motion of the humeral head under the deltoid muscle. **B:** Sharp release is facilitated when the patient's arm is placed in abduction and forward flexion to relax the deltoid muscle. (From Warner JJP. Frozen shoulder: diagnosis and management. *J Am Acad Orthop Surg* 1997;5:130–140, with permission.)

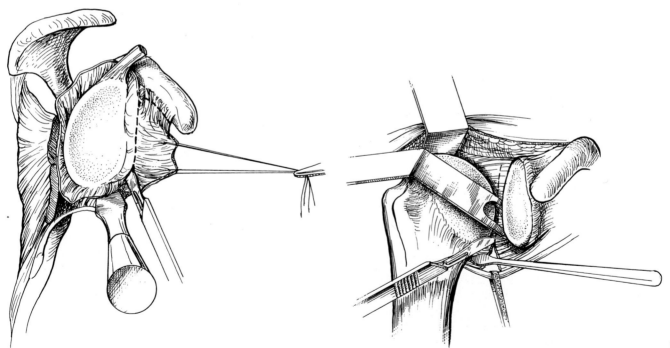

A

B

FIGURE 35.6. Open capsular release. **A:** After subdeltoid release is performed, the intraarticular side of subscapularis tendon is released by incising the joint capsule. Complete release of the subscapularis tendon requires release of the rotator interval including the coracohumeral ligament. For safe release of the lower border of the subscapularis, the axillary nerve must be protected. **B:** If required, inferior and posterior release can be performed through this approach. (From Warner JJP. Frozen shoulder: diagnosis and management. *J Am Acad Orthop Surg* 1997;5:130–140, with permission.)

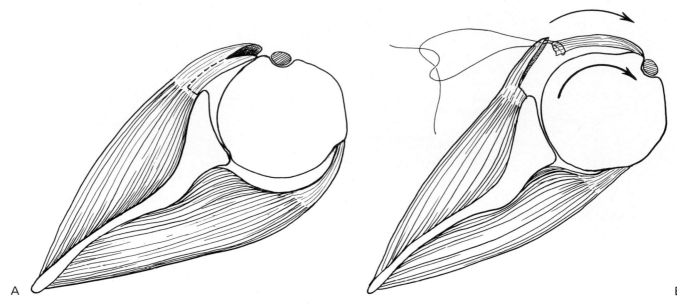

FIGURE 35.7. Technique of subscapularis tendon lengthening. **A:** Coronal Z-pasty of the subscapularis tendon and anterior capsule. **B:** The deep capsulotendinous flap is detached from the glenoid and is sutured to the superficial flap after circumferential capsular release. (From Warner JJP. Frozen shoulder: diagnosis and management. *J Am Acad Orthop Surg* 1997;5:130–140, with permission.)

POSTOPERATIVE TREATMENT

When an operative approach is chosen to treat instability, anesthetic technique and postoperative management are important parts of the therapeutic plan. General anesthesia is an adequate method, but postoperative pain interferes with therapy required immediately after the procedure. Therefore, we use an interscalene block with a long-acting agent administered through an indwelling interscalene catheter (9).

The physical therapy program depends on the type of release performed. Whereas aggressive active and passive stretching in all planes is performed immediately after arthroscopic release, restrictions are required when soft tissue repair has been performed.

SUMMARY

A logical approach to specific pathologic features and distorted anatomy gives the patient the best chance for success when surgical management of shoulder stiffness is necessary after trauma or surgical procedures. In general, arthroscopic release is most effective when it is applied to contractures that involve the capsule of the glenohumeral joint as well as the tissue gliding planes around the shoulder. This includes trauma without fracture, rotator cuff repair, arthroscopic or open Bankart or capsular shift repair, and thermal capsulorrhaphy with stiffness.

Open release of the shoulder is most appropriate when shortening of tendons around the shoulder is extreme, when distortion of extraarticular soft tissues is severe, or when bony deformity or component malpositioning in arthroplasty also forms a block to rotation. Examples include the stiff total shoulder, malunited fractures, and the Bristow, Putti-Platt, and Magnuson-Stack procedures.

REFERENCES

1. Mole D, Kempf JF, Gleyze P, et al. Results of endoscopic treatment of non-broken tendinopathies of the rotator cuff: part II. Calcifications of the rotator cuff. *Rev Chir Orthop Reparatrice Appar Mot* 1993;79:532–541.
2. Gerber A, Warner JJP. Thermal capsulorrhaphy to treat shoulder instability. *Clin Orthop* 2002;400:105–116.
3. Warner J, Deng X, Warren R, et al. Static capsuloligamentous restraints to superior-inferior translation of the glenohumeral joint. *Am J Sports Med* 1992;20:675–685.
4. Harryman D, Slides J, Harris S, et al. The role of the rotator interval capsule in passive motion and stability of the shoulder. *J Bone Joint Surg Am* 1992;74:53–66.
5. Jost B, Koch P, Gerber C. Anatomy and functional aspects of the rotator interval. *J Shoulder Elbow Surg* 2000;9:336–341.
6. Harryman DT, Slides JA, Clark J, et al. Translation of the humeral head on the glenoid with passive glenohumeral motion. *J Bone Joint Surg Am*1990;72:1334–1343.
7. Harryman DT, Matsen FA, Sidles JA. Arthroscopic management of refractory shoulder stiffness. *Arthroscopy* 1997;13:133–147.
8. Warner JJP, Allen AA, Marks PH, et al. Arthroscopic release of postoperative capsular contracture of the shoulder. *J Bone Joint Surg Am* 1997;79:1151–1158.

9. Warner JJP. Frozen shoulder: diagnosis and management. *J Am Acad Orthop Surg* 1997;5:130–140.

10. Rinaldi N, Barth T, Leppelmann-Jansen P, et al. Normal synoviocytes and synoviocytes from osteoarthritis and rheumatoid arthritis bind extracellular matrix proteins differently. *Immun Infekt* 1995;23:62–64.

11. Neer CS. *Shoulder reconstruction.* Philadelphia: WB Saunders, 1990:41–142.

12. Waters PM, Smith GR, Jaramillo D. Glenohumeral deformity secondary to brachial plexus birth palsy. *J Bone Joint Surg Am* 1998;80:668–677.

13. Warner JJP, Greis PE. Instructional course lecture: the treatment of stiffness of the shoulder after repair of the rotator cuff. *J Bone Joint Surg Am* 1997;79:1260–1269.

14. Griggs SM, Ahn A, Green A. Idiopathic adhesive capsulitis: a prospective functional outcome study of nonoperative treatment. *J Bone Joint Surg Am* 2000;82:1398–1407.

15. Warner JJP, Allen AA, Marks PH, et al. Arthroscopic release of postoperative capsular contracture of the shoulder. *J Bone Joint Surg Am* 1997;79:1151–1158.

16. Goldberg BA, Scarlat MM, Harryman DT. Management of the stiff shoulder. *J Orthop Sci* 1999;4:462–471.

17. Gerber C, Espinosa N, Perren TG. Arthroscopic treatment of shoulder stiffness. *Clin Orthop* 2001;390:119–128.

18. Neviaser RJ, Neviaser TJ. The frozen shoulder: diagnosis and management. *Clin Orthop* 1987;223:59–64.

19. Waldburger M, Meier JL, Gobelet C. The frozen shoulder: diagnosis and treatment. Prospective study of 50 cases of adhesive capsulitis. *Clin Rheumatol* 1992;11:364–368.

20. Gazielly DF, Gleyze P, Montagnon C. Functional and anatomical results after rotator cuff repair. *Clin Orthop* 1994;304:43–53.

21. Gazielly DF, Gleyze P, Montagnon C, et al. Functional and anatomical results after surgical treatment of ruptures of the rotator cuff: part I. Preoperative functional and anatomical evaluation of ruptures of the rotator cuff. *Rev Chir Orthop Reparatrice Appar Mot* 1995;81:8–16.

22. Warner JJP, Higgins L, Parsons M, et al. Diagnosis and treatment of anterosuperior rotator cuff tears. *J Shoulder Elbow Surg* 2001;10:37–46.

23. Matsen FA, Thomas SC, Rockwood CA. Glenohumeral instability. In: Rockwood CA, Matsen FA, eds. *The shoulder.* Philadelphia: WB Saunders, 1998:689–720.

24. Ticker JB, Warner JJP. Selective capsular shift technique for anterior and anterior-inferior glenohumeral instability. *Clin Sports Med* 2000;19:1–17.

25. Jaberg H, Warner JJP, Jakob RP. Percutaneous stabilization of unstable fractures of the humerus. *J Bone Joint Surg Am* 1992;74:508–515.

26. Young DC, Rockwood CA. Complications of a failed Bristow procedure and their management. *J Bone Joint Surg Am* 1991;73:969–981.

27. Gerber C, Terrier F, Ganz R. The Trillat procedure for recurrent anterior instability of the shoulder. *J Bone Joint Surg Br* 1988;70:130–134.

28. Niskanen RO, Lehtonen JY, Kaukonen JP. Alvik's glenoplasty for humeroscapular dislocation. 6-year follow-up of 52 shoulders. *Acta Orthop Scand* 1991;62:279–283.

29. Allain J, Goutallier D, Glorion C. Long-term results of the Latarjet procedure for the treatment of anterior instability of the shoulder. *J Bone Joint Surg Am* 1998;80:841–852.

30. MacDonald PB, Hawkins RJ, Fowler PJ, et al. Release of the subscapularis for internal rotation contracture and pain after anterior repair for recurrent anterior dislocation of the shoulder. *J Bone Joint Surg Am* 1992;74:734–737.

31. Boileau P, Trojani C, Walch G, et al. Shoulder arthroplasty for the treatment of the sequelae of fractures of the proximal humerus. *J Shoulder Elbow Surg* 2001;10:299–308.

THROWER'S SHOULDER: TWO PERSPECTIVES

A. PERSPECTIVE 1

CRAIG D. MORGAN

America's fascination with baseball, especially the pitcher, spans more than a century. During this time, the orthopaedist's fascination with the inability to determine why the throwing shoulder breaks down and to develop predictable successful treatment has been reminiscent of the search for the Lost Ark or the Holy Grail. Until recently, a similar situation existed regarding treatment for the anterior cruciate ligament–deficient knee. Paramount to our failure to understand what, in professional baseball circles, used to be called " the glass shoulder" has been our search for one single reason rather than several related reasons that the throwing shoulder becomes dysfunctional (1). As arthroscopic surgeons, we are currently reliving in the shoulder what we previously learned and accomplished in the knee. As such, the mysteries of the glass shoulder in the overhead-throwing athlete will ultimately be solved as they have been with the anterior cruciate ligament–deficient knee.

In the 1980s and 1990s, the painful throwing shoulder or "dead arm syndrome" seen in overhead-throwing athletes was attributed solely to acquired anterior glenohumeral instability (2–7). Repetitive capsular microtrauma caused by high tensile loads placed on the anterior capsule during the late cocking and early acceleration phases of the throwing cycle was believed to be the essential lesion (2–7). Once the shoulder became lax anteriorly, all other problems such as subacromial and internal impingement, muscular weakness, and imbalance between the rotator cuff and scapular stabilizers were believed to be secondary to the acquired anterior instability (3,5–7). I believe that anterior capsular laxity is not the essential or primary problem. Instead, the cause of the painful throwing shoulder is a multifactorial spectrum with anterior instability more than likely a secondary or tertiary problem within this spectrum (1).

As the title implies, this chapter presents my perspective, based on 20 years of clinical experience with overhead-throwing athletes regarding a spectrum of acquired shoulder problems. My intent is to organize and present a list of throwing shoulder disorders previously thought to be isolated unrelated entities into a spectrum of acquired problems that are interrelated by three simple pathophysiologic processes: the asymmetric malpositioned scapula, an acquired internal rotation deficit and, acquired external rotation excess. The perspective includes pathology, clinical presentation, and treatment. Emphasis is placed on pathophysiologic causation and treatment protocols for prophylactic prevention. As opposed to single traumatic events seen in nonthrowers, most throwing-related acquired shoulder problems are of insidious onset as a result of the unique repetitive stress patterns created during the throwing cycle. Although the pathomechanic features come on slowly, the clinical presentation may be acute with one throw. Whereas the symptoms may be acute, on persistent questioning, most throwers with acute onset of shoulder pain with decreased velocity and performance level admit to a prior period of prodromal lesion-specific low-grade symptoms, which they ignored. Recognition of the prodrome and institution of effective preventive protocols during the prodrome are important issues in this chapter. Finally, individual topics within the spectrum are presented according to anatomic location of the pathologic problem and are divided into two main categories: (a) extracapsular or muscular control issues and (b) capsular and intraarticular issues.

EXTRACAPSULAR MUSCULAR CONTROL ISSUES: SICK (SCAPULA INFERA CORACOID DYSKINESIS) SCAPULA SYNDROME

This previously unreported overuse muscular fatigue syndrome, the SICK (scapula infera coracoid dyskinesis)

C. D. Morgan: Department of Orthopaedic Surgery, University of Pennsylvania, Philadelphia, Pennsylvania; The Morgan Kalman Clinic, Wilmington, Delaware.

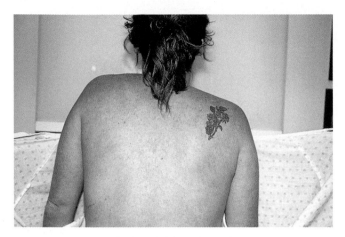

FIGURE 36A.1 A right-handed female pitcher with a SICK right scapula. The right shoulder is markedly lower than the left shoulder, despite the absence of scoliosis, pelvic tilt, or lower limb length discrepancy.

scapula syndrome, in repetitively overhead-throwing athletes presents with a dropped scapula (scapula infera) in the dominant symptomatic shoulder compared with the contralateral shoulder's scapular position. With the patient standing and the arms relaxed at the side, the involved shoulder appears lower than the nondominant side when it is viewed from either anteriorly or posteriorly (Fig. 36A.1). The visual appearance in superior height of the dermal superior surface of the shoulder is directly related to position of the acromion and thus scapular position. As the scapula drops from overuse muscular fatigue of the scapular suspensory musculature, the acromial contour superiorly also drops and gives the appearance that one shoulder is lower than the other. This is best seen by viewing the patient from posteriorly with the examiner at a distance of at least 5 feet from the patient. Scapular malposition in this syndrome is easily missed if the examiner is either too close to the patient or is not directly looking for this problem.

Symptomatic patients with an isolated SICK scapula may complain of anterior shoulder pain, posterior superior pain, superior pain, lateral pain, or any combination of these. In addition, pain may radiate posteriorly into the paraspinus neck region on the affected side, or the patient may complain of radicular or thoracic outlet–type symptoms into the affected arm, forearm, and hand or any combination of the foregoing.

The onset of symptoms (pain) with the SICK scapula syndrome is almost always insidious. By far the most common complaint is anterior shoulder pain in the region of the coracoid, with posterior scapular pain at the medial superior angle of the scapula radiating into the paraspinus neck area next in frequency. Proximal lateral arm pain (subacromial) and superior (acromioclavicular [AC] joint) shoulder pain are much less frequent, and radicular (thoracic outlet) symptoms are rare. Of 39 overhead-throwing athletes recognized

and treated for this syndrome, 24 were baseball pitchers, three were baseball catchers, eight were tennis players, and four were volleyball players. In this series, presenting pain location was as follows: 80% had anterior (coracoid) shoulder pain, 70% had both anterior (coracoid) and posterior periscapular pain in the region of the superomedial scapular angle radiating into the paraspinus neck area, 10% presented with isolated anterior (coracoid) pain, 20% had isolated superomedial scapular angle and neck pain, 20% proximal lateral (impingement) pain, and only 5% had mild radicular or thoracic outlet pain radiating into the arm, forearm, and hand.

In throwers presenting with the SICK scapula syndrome, static scapular malposition versus the nonthrowing shoulder was objectively measured in three categories: infera, lateral protraction, and abduction. All measurements were made statically with the patient standing erect with the arms relaxed in adduction at the side. *Infera* is the difference in vertical height of the superomedial scapular angle of the dropped scapula in centimeters compared with the contralateral superomedial angle (Fig. 36A.2). This assessment is most accurately done using a carpenter's level. *Lateral protraction* is the difference in centimeters of the superomedial scapula angle from the midline between the SICK and contralateral scapula (Fig. 36A.3). Scapular *abduction* is the difference in degrees of the medial scapular margin in reference to vertical plumb midline between the SICK and contralateral scapula measured with a goniometer (Fig. 36A.4). Most throwers with the SICK scapula syndrome present with static scapular malposition in all three categories, but single malpositions or combinations of any two have been seen. On average, throwers with symptomatic SICK scapula syndrome present with 2 to 3 cm of infera, 2 to 3 cm of lateral protraction, and 10 to 20 degrees of abduction.

On physical examination, patients presenting with anterior shoulder pain and a SICK scapula are found with marked coracoid tenderness more medially than laterally on the coracoid tip at the point of insertion of the pectoralis minor tendon. Throwers with anterior coracoid pain can easily be confused with throwers with other causes of anterior shoulder pain, such as anterior instability and superior labral anterior and posterior (SLAP) lesions, unless the coracoid is meticulously examined. Patients with SICK scapula syndrome who have coracoid pain usually lack full forward flexion compared with the uninvolved shoulder and have accentuated coracoid pain with attempts at maximum forward flexion. With manual relocation of the scapula done when the patient is supine (the scapular relocation test), usually full forward flexion without coracoid pain is attained, and this is diagnostic (Fig. 36A.5). The pathophysiology of the presentation of dropped SICK scapula with coracoid pain is as follows. Because of the curved conical shape of the upper chest in both the sagittal and coronal planes, as the scapula drops

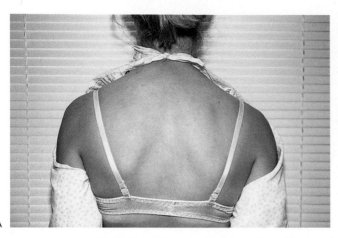
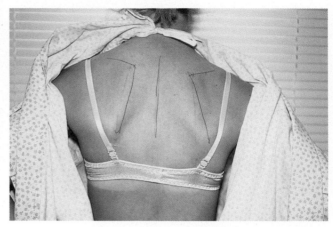

FIGURE 36A.2 Scapula infera. **A:** A right-handed female tennis player with a SICK right scapula with infera, lateral protraction, and abduction. **B:** The components of scapular malposition are best seen and measured with the medial scapular margin and the superior and inferior scapular angles outlined with a pen.

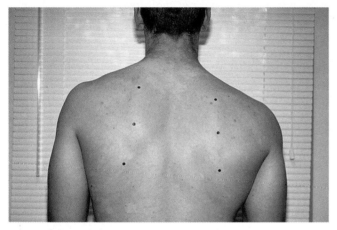
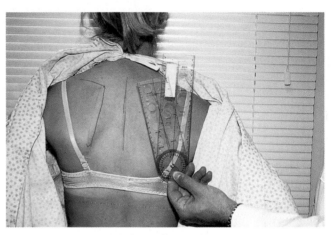

FIGURE 36A.3 Lateral scapular protraction: a right-handed professional baseball pitcher with a SICK right scapula. Note the increased distance between the superior medial scapular angle and the midline on the affected right versus the left.

FIGURE 36A.4 Scapular abduction: the same patient seen in Fig. 36A.2 with scapular abduction measured with a goniometer and expressed in degrees as the angle between the medial scapular margin and the vertical plumb midline.

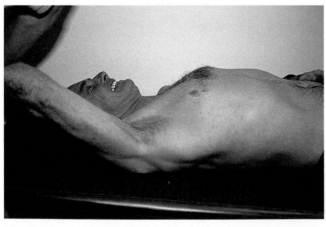
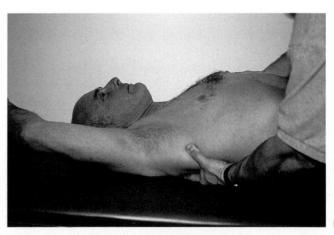

FIGURE 36A.5 A: Pseudo–pectoralis minor muscle tightness with lack of full forward flexion and coracoid pain with attempted full forward flexion resulting from scapula infera with a compensatory rise in the coracoid anteriorly. **B:** The scapular relocation test: manual anatomic scapular repositioning (superior and medial) resolves the pseudo–pectoralis minor tightness and allows full forward flexion without coracoid pain.

and protracts posteriorly, the coracoid rises and lateralizes anteriorly, and this motion, in turn, places traction on the pectoralis minor muscle and tendon, which cannot move freely with the coracoid as a result of the fixed proximal origin on the anterior chest wall. The result is coracoid pain caused by traction tendinopathy of the pectoralis minor insertion on the medial tip of the coracoid (Fig. 36A.6). This theory also explains the lack of full forward flexion resulting from to pseudotightness of the pectoralis minor caused by coracoid malposition that resolves with the supine manual scapular relocation test.

Overhead-throwing athletes with SICK scapulas who present with posterior periscapular and lower paracervical pain are usually found to have marked tenderness at the superomedial angle of the affected SICK scapula in the area of insertion of the levator scapula and uppermost rhomboid. The explanation of these findings is similar to that described for the pectoralis minor traction tendinopathy at the cora-

coid previously described. As the scapula drops, protracts, and abducts posteriorly, the levator scapula, upper rhomboid, and upper trapezius cannot move with the scapula because they are tethered by their proximal origins to the axial spine (Fig. 36A.7). As a result, the tendinous insertions of these muscles at the superior medial angle of the scapula are overtensioned, and this condition causes painful traction tendinopathy with referred pain into the muscle belly and results in secondary neck pain.

Patients with pain of subacromial origin in the throwing SICK scapula syndrome present with positive subacromial impingement tests, which bring out proximal lateral arm pain. However, the true cause of this problem is a malpositioned acromion during all phases of the throwing cycle as an extension of scapular malposition and dyskinesis. Likewise, AC joint pain is caused by a relatively discongruous position of the clavicle in reference to the acromion at the AC joint caused by scapular malposition. As the scapula

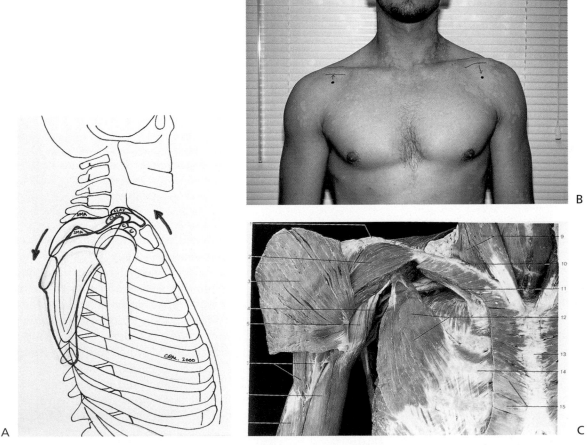

FIGURE 36A.6 Pathophysiology of coracoid pain with the SICK scapula syndrome: as the scapula drops, abducts, and protracts posteriorly, the coracoid rises anteriorly **(A)**, which can be seen as a decreased distance between the tip of the coracoid and the inferior clavicular border in the affected SICK shoulder **(B)**. Cephalization and lateralization malposition of the coracoid produces pectoralis minor traction tendinopathy at its coracoid insertion because the muscle is tethered to the anterior chest wall at its origin and cannot move with the malpositioned coracoid **(C)**.

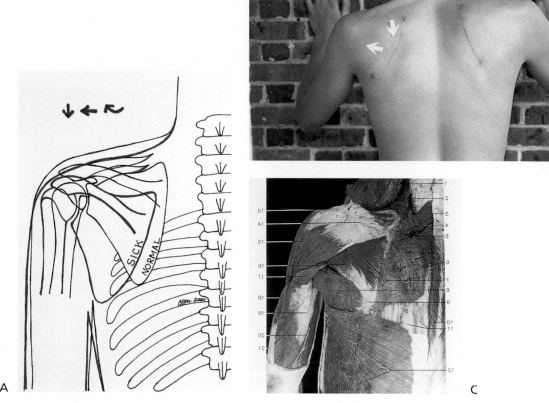

FIGURE 36A.7 Pathophysiology of levator scapula pain with the SICK scapula syndrome. As the scapula drops, protracts, and abducts **(A** and **B)**, all the muscles that insert at the superior medial scapular angle (levator scapula, upper trapezius, and upper rhomboid) are placed under tension because of their fixed origins to the axial spine **(C)**. This results in insertional tendinopathy and pain at the superomedial scapular angle, with secondary referred pain into the respective muscle bellies (neck pain).

drops, protracts, and abducts, the clavicle, tethered at its sternal attachment, cannot accommodate the altered kinematics at the AC joint, and this results in a painful AC joint with repetitive overhead activities.

Finally, the rare thrower with radicular and thoracic outlet symptoms associated with a malpositioned scapula has a shift in position of the clavicle in reference to the upper chest wall, particularly the first rib. As the scapula shifts into infera, protraction, and abduction posteriorly, the lateral clavicle also shifts posteriorly while at the same time is tethered at its sternal attachment; this situation results in a decreased space between the inferior clavicle and the first rib (Fig. 36A.8). This space restriction is believed to impinge the brachial plexus in this zone and to result clinically in radicular symptoms and the picture of thoracic outlet syndrome.

A 20-point clinical rating scale for the SICK scapula syndrome has been developed to assess the severity of the syndrome at the time of presentation and to monitor clinical

improvement during the treatment phase (Table 36A.1). The rating scale awards points for subjective and objective symptoms and signs in the categories previously stated as well as the presence and severity of scapular malposition in the three modes (infera, lateral protraction, and abduction). A patient with a healthy symmetric asymptomatic scapula has a score of 0, and one with the worst SICK malpositioned scapula with all clinical symptoms present has a score of 20.

In an attempt to determine whether components of scapular malposition could be a normal adaptive phenomenon in the throwing athlete, a group of asymptomatic professional baseball pitchers who denied any prior shoulder problems was evaluated and scored on the SICK shoulder rating scale during spring training and at the end of two successive pain-free baseball seasons. Nineteen pitchers meeting these criteria were studied and were found to have scores of 0 during the entire testing period. These findings support the concept that the healthy throwing shoulder exhibits no component of the SICK scapular syndrome, and this syn-

A 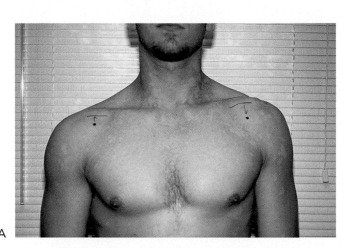 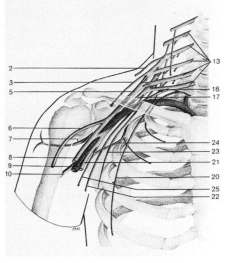 B

FIGURE 36A.8 Pathophysiology of thoracic outlet symptoms with the SICK scapula syndrome. **A:** As the scapula drops, abducts, and protracts posteriorly, the distance of the coracoid tip to the clavicle decreases anteriorly, and the sagittal vector of the clavicle shifts posteriorly and inferiorly. **B:** The change in clavicular position in reference to the stationary chest wall, particularly the first rib, results in a space restriction between the clavicle and the first rib that impinges the brachial plexus in this zone and produces thoracic outlet symptoms.

TABLE 36A.1 SICK SCAPULA RATING SCALE, STATIC MEASUREMENTS: 0–20 POINTS

Date_____   Sport_____

Name_____   Position_____

Age _____   Presenting symptoms_____

Subjective	Pain	Yes	No	Score
	Coracoid	1	0	
	Acromioclavicular joint	1	0	
	Periscapular	1	0	
	Proximal lateral arm	1	0	
	Radicular	1	0	
Objective				
	Coracoid	1	0	
	Acromioclavicular joint	1	0	
	Superior medial scapular angle	1	0	
	Impingement test	1	0	
	Scapular asst. test	1	0	
	Tos paresthesias	1	0	

Scapular Malposition	0 cm	1 cm	2 cm	3 cm	Score
Infera	0	1	2	3	
Lateral protraction	0	1	2	3	
Abduction	0°	5°	10°	15°	
	0	1	2	3	
			Total score		

Adapted from Morgan Kalman Clinic, Wilmington, Delaware, with permission.

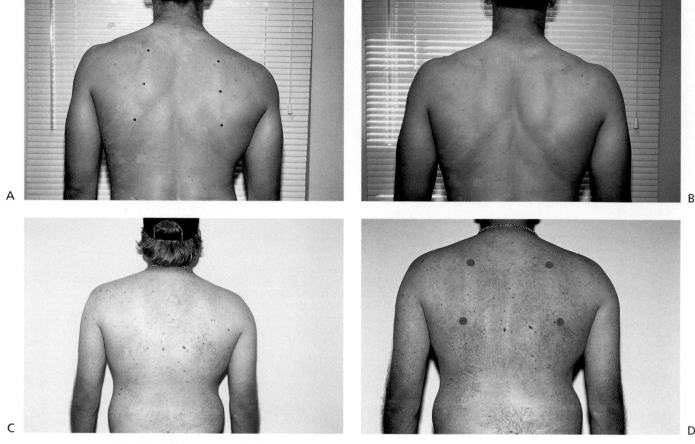

FIGURE 36A.9 Before and after SICK scapular rehabilitation. **A:** A professional right-handed baseball pitcher with a SICK right scapula with superomedial angle scapular and coracoid pain. **B:** The same patient seen in (A) now symptom free with a symmetric right scapula after 6 weeks of daily scapular rehabilitation. **C:** A professional baseball pitcher with a SICK right scapula with levator insertion and coracoid pain. **D:** The same patient seen in (C) now symptom free with a nearly symmetric scapula after 6 weeks of scapular rehabilitation.

drome is abnormal and predisposes the throwing shoulder to pathologic symptoms, as previously defined.

Treatment of the SICK scapula syndrome, regardless of presenting symptoms or the severity of scapula malposition, is nonoperative and is focused on scapular muscular rehabilitation. Initially, the thrower is restricted from all throwing and is begun on a regimented daily strengthening and reeducation program for all the scapular stabilizer muscles (1,8,9). Scapular position is monitored on a weekly basis. When the affected scapula is 50% or more improved in position from its initial state, the thrower is begun on an interval throwing program if asymptomatic and continues the scapular program until the scapula is symmetric with the other side. At this time, return to sport and unrestricted throwing is allowed (Fig. 36A.9). In general, most throwers with symptomatic SICK scapula syndrome present with scores between 10 and 14. Interval throwing usually begins with scores between 3 and 6, and return to sport at full activity occurs with scores between 0

and 2. In a compliant patient who commits to the rehabilitation exercises three times a day, the 50% repositioned scapula can be routinely attained within 2 to 3 weeks. Completion of the interval throwing program usually takes 4 to 6 weeks, and complete symmetric scapular repositioning usually takes 3 to 4 months. In general, the infera component is the first to resolve, the lateral protraction goes away second, and the abduction component is the last to resolve.

Of 39 throwers treated for this syndrome, all were successfully returned to asymptomatic throwing at their preinjury level of activity by 4 months. Resolution of symptoms during the treatment period was directly proportional to the rehabilitation program's ability to reposition the scapula symmetrically to the nonthrowing side. In addition, maintenance of an alternate-day long-term scapular stabilization muscle-strengthening program prevented recurrence of the scapular malposition and symptoms related to the SICK scapula syndrome.

CAPSULAR ISSUES: ACQUIRED POSTERIOR INFERIOR CAPSULAR CONTRACTURE WITH GLENOHUMERAL INTERNAL ROTATION DEFICIT

I am now convinced, based on a large series of throwers (124 baseball pitchers) with arthroscopically proven intraarticular disease associated with throwing dysfunction, that a throwing-related acquired posterior inferior capsular contracture seen in all patients with a resultant internal rotation deficit is the first and primary pathologic event that occurs in a pathologic cascade that secondarily produces SLAP lesions, undersurface rotator cuff tears, and the "internal impingement" spectrum, as well as acquired anterior capsular laxity, with or without Bankart pathologic features, as a tertiary event in the throwing shoulder. *Glenohumeral internal rotation deficit* (GIRD) is defined as the difference in degrees of internal rotation seen in the throwing shoulder versus the nonthrowing shoulder measured with the patient supine, the arm abducted 90 degrees in the plane of the body, and the scapula stabilized with downward pressure from anteriorly (Fig. 36A.10). With the patient's elbow flexed at 90 degrees and the arm internally rotated until the scapula starts to move on the chest wall posterior, internal rotation is measured. At this point, the degrees of internal rotation are measured with a goniometer and are compared with internal rotation measured in the contralateral shoulder using the same methods.

In my group of 124 pitchers with symptomatic type II SLAP lesions, all had GIRDs of greater than 25 degrees versus their nonthrowing shoulder; the average was 53 degrees (range, 25 to 80 degrees). These findings are in contradis-

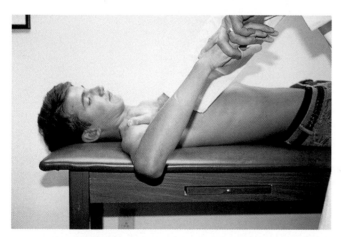

FIGURE 36A.10 Methods for measurement of glenohumeral internal rotation deficit. The patient is positioned supine, the arm is abducted 90 degrees in the plane of the body with the elbow flexed 90 degrees, and the scapula is stabilized against the examination table by downward pressure by the examiner from anteriorly. The patient's arm is internally rotated from the neutral position until the scapula starts to move on the chest wall. At this point, internal rotation is measured and is expressed in degrees from neutral measured with a goniometer.

tinction to 29 asymptomatic, healthy throwing shoulders in professional pitchers who were studied during spring training and at the end of two professional baseball seasons. These asymptomatic pitchers averaged only 13 degrees of GIRD at spring training and 16 degrees at the end of each season during the study period. Results in this group showed that GIRD in the healthy asymptomatic throwing shoulder is present but minimal compared with significantly greater deficits, which averaged 53 degrees in those who developed dysfunction secondary to operative SLAP lesions. Other investigators have reported similar findings with regard to internal rotation deficit in throwing athletes. Verna (10) was the first to associate GIRD with dysfunction in the throwing athlete. He followed 25 professional pitchers during a single baseball season who were identified at spring training with 25 degrees or less of total internal rotation and found that 60% of these athletes developed shoulder problems requiring discontinuance of pitching during the study period. Kibler (11), in a series of 38 arthroscopically proven SLAP lesion in overhead-throwing athletes, found significant GIRD in all; the average was 33 degrees (range, 26 to 58 degrees). In another study, Kibler et al. (12,13) prospectively evaluated high-level tennis players followed for 2 years who were divided into two groups: one group performed daily posterior capsular stretching to minimize GIRD, and the other group did not stretch. Over the 2-year study, the stretching group had a 38% decrease in shoulder problems compared with the symptom-free stretching group. Finally, Cooper (14) manually stretched 22 major league pitchers daily to minimize GIRD during the 1997, 1998, and 1999 professional baseball seasons. During that time, he reported no innings lost, no intraarticular problems, and no surgical shoulder procedures in the study group.

Based on the findings of both Kibler et al. and Cooper, it is believed that prophylactic posterior capsular stretching is successful in minimizing GIRD and prevents the development of secondary intraarticular problems, particularly SLAP lesions and the spectrum of internal impingement disorders (Fig. 36A.11).

Most throwers with symptomatic GIRD initially present with a prodrome of mild symptoms usually described as a sense of "tightness" or "stiffness" in the back of their shoulders. If these athletes continue to throw and ignore these prodromal signs, posterior superior soreness and pain come next, without mechanical symptoms or loss of velocity. If GIRD is identified and treated with focused posterior capsular stretching (Fig. 36A.11) during this prodromal phase, 80% to 90% of these throwers will respond by dramatically decreasing the GIRD, and their prodromal symptoms will resolve. In contrast, if they continue to pitch with prodromal pain and GIRD continues to increase, a type II SLAP event will occur, at which point their posterior superior pain in the cocking phase dramatically increases, mechanical symptoms begin, and performance and velocity suddenly decrease. In my experience, once the thrower develops me-

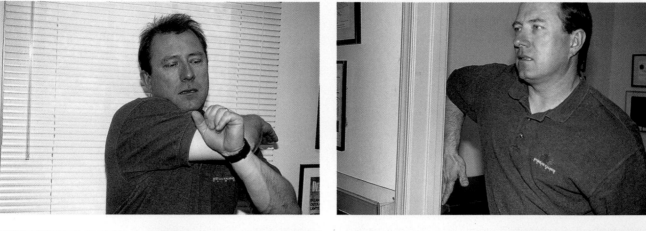

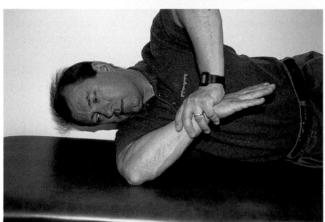
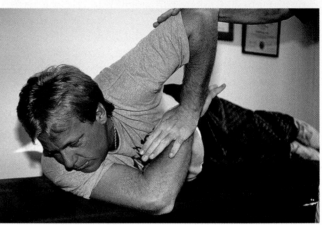

FIGURE 36A.11 Posterior capsule stretching exercises. **A:** Cross-body stretch with the shoulder adducted and forward flexed 90 degrees and the elbow flexed 90 degrees with maximum passive adduction. **B:** Doorway stretch with the shoulder abducted 90 degrees, the elbow flexed 90 degrees, and the patient leaning into the doorway to create passive shoulder internal rotation. **C:** Sleeper stretch with the patient side lying and the shoulder forward flexed 90 degrees, the elbow flexed 90 degrees, and passive internal rotation applied by the other arm at the wrist. **D:** Rollover sleeper stretch: similar to the sleeper stretch, but the shoulder is forward flexed only 45 degrees, and the patient rolls forward 45 degrees with passive internal rotation applied to the wrist.

chanical symptoms, the SLAP event has occurred, and the problem becomes a surgical issue. At this point, the thrower exhibits all the clinical examination findings shown by Morgan et al. (15) to be associated with posterior or combined posterior to anterior type II SLAP lesions: positive posterior superior pain with abduction and external rotation reduced by a relocation maneuver, positive Speed's test, positive O'Brien's test, and positive bicipital groove tenderness.

Once this sequence becomes a surgical issue, arthroscopic findings reveal a type II SLAP lesion with a hypermobile biceps root anchor (1,15,16). In all cases, the posterior superior labrum is involved, and in about 40%, the anterior superior labrum has also separated from the glenoid (1,15) (Fig. 36A.12). If the patient's arm is taken out of traction at the time of arthroscopy and the shoulder is dynamically abducted and externally rotated, one can arthroscopically visualize the posterior superior labrum "peelback" from the posterior superior glenoid rim and scapular neck while at

the same time the biceps anchor can be seen to shift medially from the supraglenoid tubercle, as described by Burkhart and Morgan (16) (Fig. 36A.13). In addition, Morgan and Burkhart reported a positive anterior inferior "drive-through" sign associated with these posterior type II SLAP lesions despite visual absence of abnormalities in the anterior inferior labrum or capsule. This condition has been described as pseudolaxity in an otherwise normal anterior inferior capsule, which resolves once the posterior superior labrum is fixed anatomically (15). In most cases, the GIRD documented at examination while the patient is under anesthesia is confirmed arthroscopically as a contracted and thickened posterior band of the inferior glenohumeral ligament with a markedly decreased space in the posterior inferior capsular recess (Fig. 36A.14).

Based on the degree of capsular thickening and contracture seen in this zone, the amount of GIRD present, and whether the patient's GIRD responded to stretching, a de-

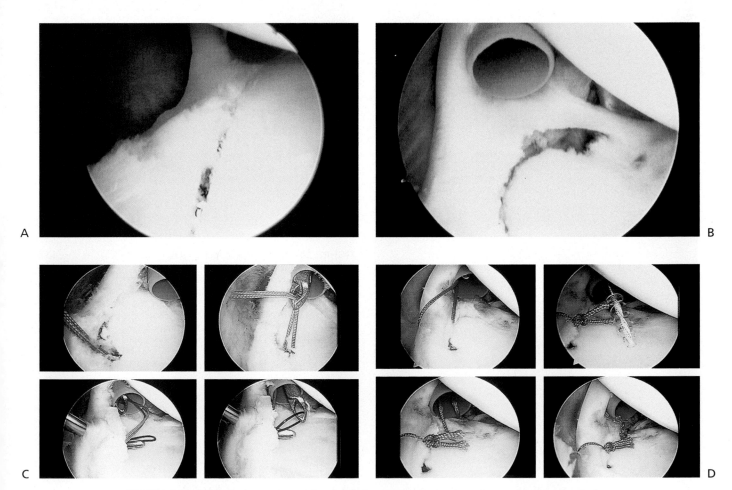

FIGURE 36A.12 Posterior and combined anterior and posterior type II superior labral anterior and posterior (SLAP) lesions with repair. **A:** A pure posterior type II SLAP lesion. **B:** A combined anterior and posterior type II SLAP lesion. **C** and **D:** A combined lesion repair being fixed with two bioabsorbable Fastak suture anchors (Arthrex, Inc., Naples, FL), one placed posteriorly and tied from anteriorly (C) and one placed and tied from anteriorly (D).

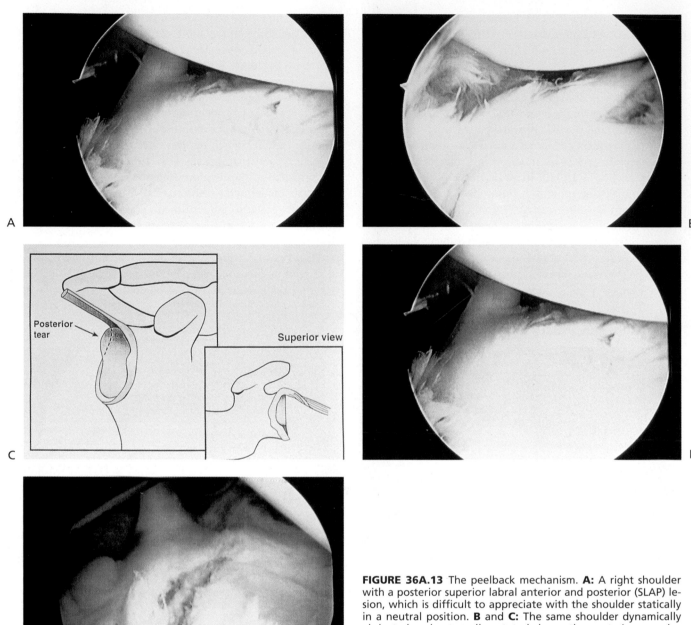

FIGURE 36A.13 The peelback mechanism. **A:** A right shoulder with a posterior superior labral anterior and posterior (SLAP) lesion, which is difficult to appreciate with the shoulder statically in a neutral position. **B** and **C:** The same shoulder dynamically abducted and externally rotated shows the posterior superior labrum peeling from its attachment to the posterior superior glenoid margin. **D** and **E:** Another patient with a posterior type II SLAP lesion seen with the shoulder in neutral (D) and with the arm abducted 90 degrees and externally rotated 90 degrees illustrating peelback of the posterior superior labrum (E).

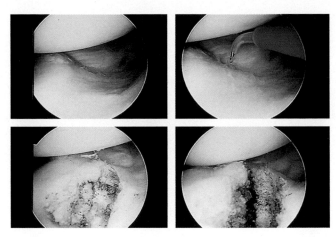

FIGURE 36A.14 Severe glenohumeral internal rotation deficit (GIRD) with a thickened and contracted posterior inferior capsule. A right shoulder viewed from posteriorly in a thrower with advanced GIRD unresponsive to stretching; note the contracted appearance of the posterior inferior recess in the upper pictures. After initiation of a posterior inferior capsulotomy, note the markedly thickened capsule (1/4 inch) posteroinferiorly *(lower two pictures)*.

cision is made at this time whether to perform a selective posterior inferior capsulotomy concomitantly with the SLAP lesion repair. In general, when a patient has not responded to preoperative posterior inferior capsular stretching and has less than 20 degrees of total internal rotation, I perform the posterior inferior quadrant capsulotomy (Fig. 36A.15). If a capsulotomy is performed, one can expect an average 65-degree immediate increase in internal rotation as measured with the arm abducted 90 degrees in the plane of

the body (Fig. 36A.16). Finally, 60% of these surgical patients who present with posterior type II SLAP lesions have variable amounts of undersurface rotator cuff involvement in the posterior portion of the supraspinatus crescent despite a normal- or pristine-appearing subacromial space (1,15) (Fig. 36A.17).

In summary, the arthroscopic findings, including posterior superior labral tears, undersurface posterior superior partial thickness rotator cuff disease, and a positive drive-through sign indicative of anterior inferior capsular laxity, were similar to those described by Jobe (7) as "internal impingement." In Jobe's description of internal impingement (7), he believed that the main causative factor was acquired anterior capsular laxity, which produced excessive external rotation and, in turn, secondarily injured the posterosuperior labrum and undersurface of the rotator cuff by excessive direct contact of the two. I disagree with that concept and believe that an acquired posterior inferior capsular contracture with resultant GIRD is the first and essential problem that produces the pathologic cascade resulting in posterior type II SLAP lesions and secondarily the picture of internal impingement. In the presence of a contracted or shortened posterior inferior capsule, as the shoulder attempts to go into the cocked positioned, the contracted posterior band of the inferior glenohumeral ligament will not allow the head to rotate fully externally. It acts as a checkrein or tether, which causes a posterior superior shift of the glenohumeral rotation point on the face of the glenoid. Once this shift occurs, the humeral head can then abnormally excessively externally rotate for two reasons: the new posterior superior rotation point and the laxity, as a result of the new rotation point, of the anterior capsular structures, which were nor-

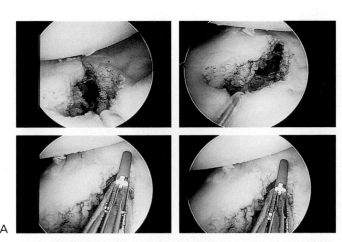

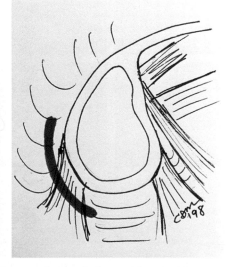

A   B

FIGURE 36A.15 Posterior inferior selective capsulotomy. The capsulotomy is done with a combination of electrocautery and basket forceps, as seen in a right shoulder, and is positioned 1/4 inch off the glenoid labrum and is extended from 6 o'clock inferiorly to 3 or 9 o'clock posteriorly **(B)**.

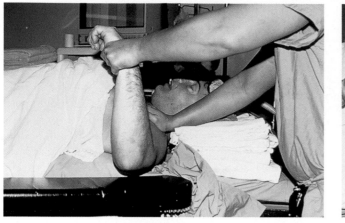
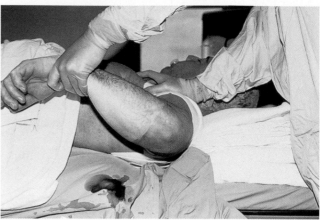

FIGURE 36A.16 A left-handed professional baseball pitcher with a type II superior labral anterior and posterior (SLAP) lesion and severe glenohumeral internal rotation deficit unresponsive to stretching seen before capsulotomy with no internal rotation **(A)** and immediately after capsulotomy and SLAP repair with 60 degrees of internal rotation **(B)**.

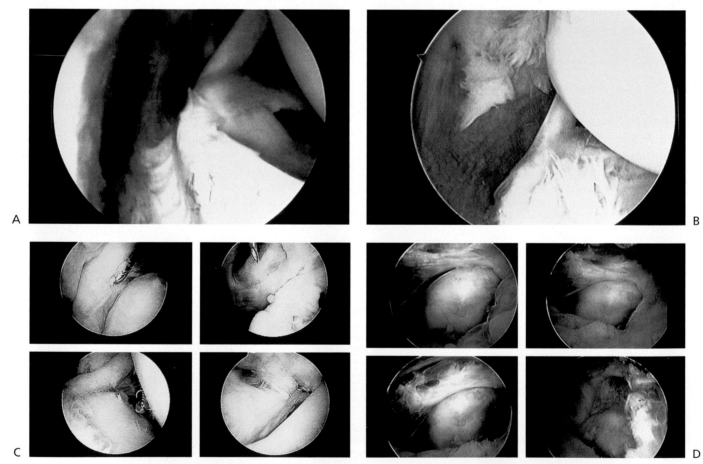

FIGURE 36A.17 Rotator cuff disease associated with superior labral anterior and posterior (SLAP) lesions and glenohumeral internal rotation deficit (GIRD). **A:** An acute type II SLAP lesion with GIRD in a right-handed pitcher; note the hemorrhagic bruise seen in the undersurface of the rotator cuff near the posterior rotator interval. **B:** A right-handed second baseman with a chronic posterior SLAP and an undersurface partial-thickness rotator cuff tear located in the posterior portion of the supraspinatus crescent. **C** and **D:** A right-handed pitcher with GIRD and a chronic combined SLAP seen 2 years after "debridement" of his anterior labrum who now has a full-thickness rotator cuff tear transversely oriented through the posterior rotator interval seen from inside the joint (C) and from the subacromial space (D). All these patients had otherwise pristine subacromial spaces and coracoacromial ligaments, a finding implying that their rotator cuff tears came from internal superior instability secondary to GIRD and their unstable biceps tendon origins, rather than from classic subacromial impingement.

mal. Because the shoulder now abducts and excessively externally rotates around the new posterior superior contact point on the glenoid, distractive forces at the biceps and posterior superior labral attachment increase, and both structures begin to fail at their attachments by tension and the peelback mechanism that produce a posterior type II SLAP lesion (1,15) (Fig. 36A.18). Once the SLAP lesion occurs, the posterior superior shift is magnified, and the cascade continues. Excessive external rotation in the cocked position caused by GIRD also causes increased undersurface contact in the posterior superior rotator cuff quadrant that presents as undersurface fiber failure, as described by Jobe (7) and as seen in 60% of my series of SLAP lesions in throwers (1,15).

In support of the concept that an acquired posterior capsular contracture produces superior shift of the glenohumeral rotation axis with resultant superior instability in the elevated shoulder, Harryman et al. in 1990 (17), in an elegant study, showed that "operative tightening of the posterior part of the capsule resulted in significant superior translation with flexion of the glenohumeral joint." In another cadaveric kinematic study, Pagnani et al. (18) showed increased superior glenohumeral translation in the presence of an unstable biceps anchor.

With regard to issues of acquired anterior capsular laxity, I used to believe (before 2000) that surgical patients with throwing shoulders with symptomatic SLAP lesions and GIRD all had normal anterior capsules, and appropriate treatment included SLAP lesion repair, minimizing GIRD by stretching or selective posterior inferior capsulotomy, and leaving the anterior capsules alone. With this approach, I obtained 86% University of California Los Angeles (UCLA)–rated excellent results at 1 year in a published se-

ries of 53 SLAP lesions in baseball pitchers. Subsequent to that series, I repaired an additional 71 SLAP lesions in baseball pitchers, of which four patients had concomitant anterior inferior Bankart lesions. These findings caused me to rethink this issue. In this later series, five additional patients had external rotation under anesthesia that exceeded 130 degrees, and this was believed to be pathologically excessive in the absence of Bankart lesions. Moreover, in four patients in the original series of 53 pitchers with less than excellent results, a second arthroscopy procedure was done more than 1 year postoperatively for persistent anterior symptoms. These patients were treated with anterior inferior thermal capsulorraphy with success in all four patients. Based on these experiences, I now believe that approximately 10% of all throwers who present with surgical type II SLAP lesions and GIRD also have a component of acquired anterior inferior capsular laxity caused as a tertiary problem by persistent throwing in the presence of a SLAP lesion with GIRD and secondary posterior superior shift of the glenohumeral rotation point that allowed excessive external rotation and eventually stretched the previously normal anterior inferior capsules. My decision to perform an anterior inferior capsular shortening procedure at the time of SLAP lesion repair is now based purely on clinical grounds, depending on the degree of external rotation present at the time of examination while the patient is under anesthesia. If external rotation of the affected shoulder exceeds 130 degrees with the patient's arm abducted 90 degrees in the plane of the body and the scapula stabilized, then I will perform a thermal capsulorraphy of the anterior band of the inferior glenohumeral ligament. Using this approach, my UCLA-rated results at 1 and 2 years in 71 pitchers were 95% excellent and 5% good. The

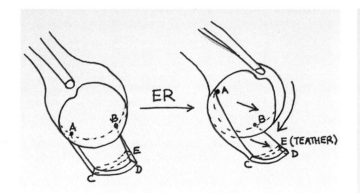 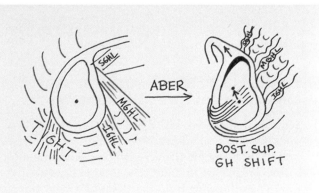

A   B

FIGURE 36A.18. Pathophysiology of a glenohumeral internal rotation deficit (GIRD) producing posterior type II superior labral anterior and posterior lesions. In a healthy shoulder with normal kinematics, the finite lengths of the anterior and posterior bands of the inferior glenohumeral ligament (IGHL) complex are equal, and this situation allows the shoulder to "wind up" and "unwind" in abduction around a relatively fixed central glenoid rotation point. In the presence of a shortened posterior band of the IGHL with GIRD, as the shoulder abducts and externally rotates, the glenohumeral rotation point shifts posterosuperiorly, which begins the cascade of failure in tension of the biceps and superior labrum from their origins, as seen schematically from the humeral side **(A)** and from the glenoid side **(B)**.

TABLE 36A.2 POSTOPERATIVE SUPERIOR LABRAL ANTERIOR AND POSTERIOR LESION REPAIR REHABILITATION PROGRAM FOR BASEBALL PITCHERS

Week 1	Sling immobilization at all times
Weeks 2–3	Codman circumduction, PROM: 0–90 degrees flexion, abduction; no external rotation in abduction because of the peelback mechanism; sling immobilization when not doing PROM regimen
Weeks 3–6	Discontinue sling; progressive PROM to full as tolerated in all planes; begin passive posterior capsular and internal rotation stretching; begin passive and manual scapulothoracic mobility program; begin external rotation in abduction; allow use of the operative extremity for light activities of daily living
Weeks 6–16	Continue all stretching and flexibility programs as above; begin progressive strengthening of the rotator cuff, scapular stabilizers and biceps
4 Months	Begin interval throwing program on level surface; continue stretching and strengthening regimen, with particular emphasis on posterior capsular stretching
6 Months	Begin throwing from the mound
7 Months	Allow full-velocity throwing from the mound; continue strengthening and posterior capsular stretching long term (indefinitely); remember an occult tight posterior capsule caused the lesion to begin with, and recurrence of the tightness can be expected to place the repair at risk in a throwing athlete

PROM, passive range of motion.

5% of patients who had good results all had significant undersurface rotator cuff partial-thickness tears.

Postoperative Rehabilitation for SLAP Lesion Repairs in Throwing Athletes

My general protocol for SLAP lesion repair in pitchers' throwing shoulders is outlined in Table 36A.2. In general, the interval throwing program, which begins at 4 months, emphasizes progressive distance toss on level ground up to 200 feet. Then throwing from the elevation of the mound begins usually at 6 months postoperatively.

REFERENCES

1. Burkhart SS, Morgan CD, Kibler WB. Shoulder injuries in overhead athletes: the "dead arm" revisited. *Clin Sports Med* 2000;19:125–158.
2. Garth WP, Allman FL, Armstrong NS. Occult anterior subluxation of the shoulder. *Am J Sports Med* 1987;15:579–585.
3. Jobe FW, Tibone JE, Jobe CM, et al. The shoulder in sports. In: Rockwood CA Jr, Matsen FA III, eds. *The shoulder.* Philadelphia: WB Saunders, 1990:963–967.
4. Jobe FW, Giangarra CE, Kvitne RS, et al. Anterior capsulolabral reconstruction of the shoulder in athletes in overhead sports. *Am J Sports Med* 1991;19:428–434.
5. Jobe CM, Pink MM, Jobe FW, et al. Anterior shoulder instability, impingement and rotator cuff tear: theories and concepts. In: Jobe FW, ed. *Operative techniques in upper extremity sports injuries.* St. Louis: CV Mosby, 1996:164–176.
6. Glousman RE, Jobe FW. Anterior shoulder instability, impingement and rotator cuff tear: anterior and multidirectional glenohumeral instability. In: Jobe FW, ed. *Operative techniques in upper extremity sports injuries.* St. Louis: CV Mosby, 1996:191–209.
7. Jobe CM. Posterior superior glenoid impingement: expanded spectrum. *Arthroscopy* 1995;11:530–537.
8. Kibler WB. The role of the scapula in athletic shoulder function. *Am J Sports Med* 1998;26:325–337.
9. Kibler WB, Livingston B, Chandler. Shoulder rehabilitation: clinical application, evaluation, and rehabilitation protocols. *Instr Course Lect* 1997;46:43–52.
10. Verna C (Seattle Mariners minor league trainer). Shoulder flexibility to O3 reduce impingement. Presented at the Professional Baseball Athletic Trainers Meeting, Mesa, Arizona, 1991.
11. Kibler W. Personal communication, 1999. Submitted for publication.
12. Kibler WB, Chandler TJ, Livingston B, et al. Shoulder rotation in elite tennis players: effect of age and tournament play. *Am J Sports Med* 1996;24:229–285.
13. Kibler WB. Relationship of glenohumeral internal rotation deficit to shoulder and elbow injuries in tennis players: a prospective evaluation of posterior capsular stretching. Presented at the annual closed meeting of the American Shoulder and Elbow Surgeons, 1998. Submitted for publication.
14. Cooper J (Philadelphia Phillies head trainer). Personal communication, 1999.
15. Morgan, CD, Burkhart SS, Palmeri M, et al. Type II SLAP lesions: three subtypes and their relationships to superior instability and rotator cuff tears. *Arthroscopy* 1998;14:553–565.
16. Burkhart SS, Morgan CD. Technical Note: The "peel-back" mechanism: its role in producing and extending posterior type II SLAP lesions and its effect on SLAP repair rehabilitation. *Arthroscopy* 1998;14:637–640.
17. Harryman DT, Sidles JA, Clark JM, et al. Translation of the humeral head on the glenoid with passive glenohumeral motion. *J Bone Joint Surg Am* 1990;72:1334–1343.
18. Pagnani MJ, Deng XH, Warren RF, et al. Effects of lesions of the superior portion of the glenoid labrum on glenohumeral translation. *J Bone Joint Surg Am* 1995;77:1003–1010.

THROWER'S SHOULDER: TWO PERSPECTIVES
B. PERSPECTIVE 2

JEFFREY R. DUGAS AND JAMES R. ANDREWS

Treatment of the thrower's shoulder is a constantly evolving algorithm. With the advent of new ideas and new technologies, it is necessary constantly to evaluate the standard of care and the possibility that treatment protocols require updating. In the following pages, we describe the common pathologic features of the throwing athlete's shoulder that we encounter in our practice. The diagnostic and treatment options described in this chapter are based only on our experience. We are not describing the "best" or "only" way to approach a problem. Rather, we hope to give the reader an insight into our thought processes and the methods used in treatment. Treatment protocols are constantly evolving as we try to improve our understanding of pathologic conditions. Also keep in mind the nature of the patient population that we are discussing. In our practice, most of the throwers we treat are elite-level throwers—college level and above. For many of these athletes, high-quality supervised rehabilitation is available and required. In some cases, athletes relocate for a short period to attend rehabilitation with our team of therapists. Certainly, the ability to spend that much time and effort on the rehabilitation aspect of their care, as well as improving our ability to adjust rehabilitation programs to fit individual athletes, makes return to competition more likely than it would be in a less aggressive program. In many ways, the confidence that we have in the therapists and trainers we work so closely with enables us to make the treatment decisions we make on a daily basis. We have always emphasized the need for both conservative rehabilitative treatment and postoperative rehabilitation as key to success with these athletes.

J. R. Dugas and J. R. Andrews: American Sports Medicine Institute, Birmingham, Alabama.

UNIQUE ASPECTS OF THE THROWER'S SHOULDER

The thrower's shoulder is a delicate balance of power and stability. The elite thrower must be able to generate incredible rotational torque to throw the ball at high speeds. The throwing arm has been measured at rotational velocities of more than 7,000 degrees per second [1,2]. Certainly, the ability to generate such rotational velocity places the shoulder at risk of fatigue and injury. Several authors have documented osseous changes in the thrower's shoulder [3]. Specifically, symptomatic throwers have less retroversion of the humeral head and glenoid than is seen in nonthrowers and asymptomatic throwers. This lack of osseous "spin-back" may place the soft tissues around the shoulder at increased risk of injury in some throwers. Despite these osseous changes, the total arc of shoulder motion is unchanged in throwing and nonthrowing shoulders [3–5]. The typical thrower has more external rotation in the throwing versus the nonthrowing shoulder, along with a decrease in internal rotation in the throwing shoulder. There is also more humeral head translation on examination in throwers than in nonthrowers. Despite these differences, shoulder dislocation is distinctly uncommon in the throwing athlete.

Because the thrower's humerus can be hyperexternally rotated, the biceps tendon can move from a relatively anterior direction of pull to a relative posterior direction of pull. Over the course of a thrower's season or career, this recurring change in vector may cause significant labral disease because of the traction of the biceps on the superior labrum. Like pulling a weed from the ground by changing the line of pull from one side to the other, the biceps may avulse the labrum from its glenoid attachment.

The aforementioned differences between thrower and nonthrower impart a laxity to the throwing shoulder that should not be considered pathologic. The difference between laxity and instability is a subtle but important aspect of treating the throwing shoulder. Only after repeated evaluation of throwers and nonthrowers will the clinician gain an appreciation for what is regarded as normal laxity in the thrower.

CLINICAL EXAMINATION AND DIAGNOSIS

As with any other patient, the first information that should be obtained is a thorough history. In the case of a thrower, the date of onset of symptoms, phase of throwing when pain occurs, and any loss of throwing velocity, loss of accuracy, or loss of endurance should be documented. Among the more useful of these points of history is the phase of throwing during which the athlete experiences pain. In the majority of cases, the athlete notices pain at the top of the windup, as the humerus reaches maximal external rotation. In other patients, the pain is experienced during the follow-through phase or deceleration phase. In these cases, the disorder usually resides in the posterior rotator cuff because these muscles are the most active during the deceleration phase (1,2). In patients with pain at maximal external rotation, rotator cuff, labrum, and articular surface injuries are frequently the cause. Understanding which structures are under the most stress during the various phases of the throwing motion provides the clinician with early insight into the problem and allows a better-directed approach to accurate diagnosis. Documentation of any previous treatment rendered and of the subsequent outcome of that treatment is very important. Any medications, injections, previous operations, or enforced periods of rest (e.g., disabled list) may affect the current recommendations for treatment. Another important piece of the history is any change in throwing mechanics that has taken place in the period preceding the onset of symptoms.

Once the history is completed, the physical examination should commence. We begin with inspection of both shoulders, to look specifically for muscle wasting posteriorly. We next proceed to range-of-motion examination, both active and passive. In most cases, the athlete has a full and nearly symmetric active range of shoulder motion. The throwing shoulder typically possesses more external rotation in abduction and less internal rotation versus the nonthrowing shoulder. In all, however, the total arc of motion is not significantly different between the two shoulders. Any loss of active motion may herald a loose body within the joint, a full-thickness rotator cuff tear, or a neurologic injury. On passive examination, it is particularly important to document the maximum internal and external rotation on both sides.

Pain in the posterior superior aspect of the shoulder with maximal external rotation is considered a positive test for internal impingement (4) (Fig. 36B.1). Walch was the first to

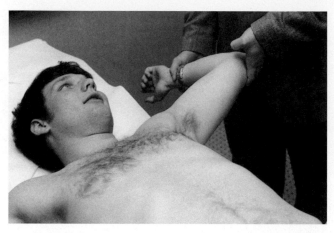

FIGURE 36B.1 Internal impingement sign. This test is done with the patient supine and the upper arm in the plane of the scapula. The shoulder is then maximally externally rotated. Pain in the posterior aspect of the shoulder in the region of the infraspinatus is considered a positive test.

describe the condition of internal impingement (5). He described the condition in which the undersurface of the rotator cuff becomes entrapped between the humeral head and the posterosuperior glenoid with the humerus in maximal external rotation. With repeated impingement, fraying of the undersurface of the cuff or even partial-thickness tearing may occur. Tests for subacromial impingement are undertaken at this time as well. After range-of-motion testing, strength testing should be performed. Specific attention should be paid to any side-to-side difference in rotator cuff strength as well as any deltoid strength. Objective data can also be obtained using an isometric testing apparatus and compared with normative data for throwing athletes. Any rotator cuff weakness should be noted because it may indicate tendinitis, tendinosis, partial-thickness or full-thickness tear, or neurologic injury.

When the strength examination is completed, we proceed to an examination for stability with the patient in the supine position. With the patient relaxed, the arm is abducted 90 degrees and is externally rotated. The patient's arm is held in the plane of the scapula and is translated anteriorly and posteriorly. This *Lachman examination* of the shoulder should have a firm endpoint anteriorly (Fig. 36B.2). Posteriorly, the humeral head should translate to the rim but should not dislocate. It is also not uncommon for the throwing shoulder to have a sulcus sign in the sitting position, but true multidirectional instability is uncommon. In throwers with anterior pain on the stability examination, an apprehension test is performed by applying anteriorly directed pressure on the abducted externally rotated arm with the patient in the prone position.

Once the stability examination is completed, we test for labral disease. We save provocative maneuvers to look for

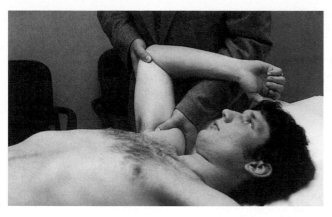
A

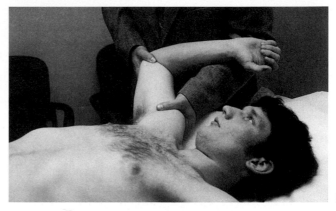
B

FIGURE 36B.2 Lachman examination of the shoulder. With the patient's arm relaxed in the plane of the scapula, the examiner first attempts to translate the patient's humeral head posteriorly **(A)**, followed by anterior translation **(B)**. The end feel and amount of translation should be noted.

labral disease for the end of the examination because significant pain may be elicited by these tests. We commonly use two tests for labral disease: the *clunk test,* as described by Andrews, and the *active compression test,* described by O'Brien (7,11). The O'Brien test is performed by placing the patient's arm in 90 degrees of forward flexion and 20 degrees of cross-body adduction. The patient's humerus is then internally rotated so the thumb points toward the ground with the elbow straight. The patient is then asked to resist a downward force applied by the examiner. Reproduction of the patient's symptoms with pain deep inside or in front of the shoulder is considered a positive test for labral disease. Pain on top of the shoulder at the acromioclavicular joint may indicate some pathologic process within this articulation, but it does not herald any labral disease. As with other tests for labral disease, we find this test very sensitive but not very specific. We are cautious about making treatment decisions based solely on the outcome of this test. The clunk test is performed with the patient supine. The examiner's hand is placed posteriorly on the patient's humeral head while the other hand is placed on the patient's elbow to create a rotational force. The patient's arm is maximally forward flexed while the posterior hand of the examiner provides an anterior force. At the same time, the examiner's other hand rotates the humerus. A "clunk" or grind can be felt in the shoulder as the humeral head snaps on or over the torn labrum.

Finally, neurologic and vascular examinations are carried out, with particular attention to the color and capillary refill in the fingertips and the quality of the radial and ulnar pulses. Sensation is tested to light touch in all distributions.

In the majority of cases, a limited differential diagnosis can be established on the basis of clinical history and examination. Although many players arrive in our office with radiologic studies from previous evaluations, we typically begin with plain radiographs, which include anteroposterior

views of the shoulder in internal and external rotation, an axillary view, and Stryker views of both shoulders. We call this the *thrower's series* of radiographs. In many players, these studies are noncontributory. However, in patient's with a thrower's exostosis (Bennett's lesion) on the posterior inferior glenoid rim, plain radiographs are typically diagnostic (Fig. 36B.3). Although no data exist to demonstrate the origin of the exostosis, we believe that these lesions originate from traction from the posterior band of the inferior glenohumeral ligament. Glenohumeral arthritis, acromioclavicular joint disease, acromial morphologic features, and os acromionale can easily be diagnosed based on these radiographic views. If rotator cuff, articular surface, or labral disease is suspected on the basis of clinical examination, contrast-enhanced magnetic resonance imaging is the study of

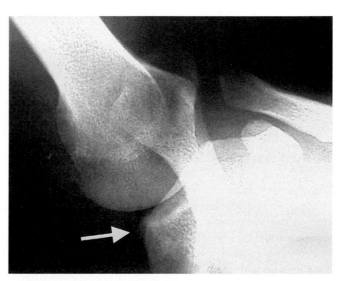

FIGURE 36B.3 Radiographs of the thrower's exostosis. The exostosis is best visualized on the West Point view, shown here.

choice in our institution for confirmation of the diagnosis. Although noncontrast magnetic resonance imaging is certainly acceptable, our radiologists are more comfortable with the diagnostic accuracy associated with the use of injected contrast. If bony disease is suspected, then a computed tomography scan is the test of choice.

EARLY TREATMENT

Once the diagnostic workup is completed, a treatment decision is made. These decisions are complex in many throwers because of the length of rehabilitation necessary after surgical intervention. For some procedures, a period as long as 12 months may be necessary to return to competition. Significant loss of playing time and, for professional players, loss of income are certainly possibilities for these injured throwers. Every attempt is made to avoid surgical intervention in throwing athletes because of the potential for such losses. Additionally, no procedure guarantees return to play. Many athletes who are referred to us for evaluation have already undergone prolonged conservative treatment for their injuries without success. Regardless, continued conservative treatment is always considered. Antiinflammatory medications, rest from throwing, strengthening of the rotator cuff musculature, and subsequent return to throwing in an interval throwing program are the hallmarks of our conservative management. We use the term *active rest* to describe the rehabilitation process for throwing athletes. In rare occasions, oral or injected steroids are used for inflammatory conditions, typically rotator cuff tendinitis. We are particularly careful about injected steroids during the playing season and typically require our patients to have a short-term rest from throwing after an injection.

If a player responds well to nonoperative management and returns to throwing, it is not uncommon for symptoms to recur as the shoulder fatigues over the course of a season or an entire career. In these patients, repeated periods of rest and rehabilitation may be necessary. As long as these methods are successful, no surgical intervention is considered. However, many players fail to improve with conservative management and become surgical candidates.

SURGICAL TREATMENT

The decision to proceed with surgical treatment is one best made by the patient after a lengthy discussion about the nature of the indicated procedure and the likelihood of success. To most throwers, success equals return to play at the same or higher level. Every thrower should understand that the rate of return to competition is not 100%, regardless of surgeon or procedure. The capacity for a player to return to competition is only partly the result of the technical aspects of the surgical procedure. However, the goals of surgical treatment are to enable the player to regain normal throwing mechanics without pain and to return to competition. The surgeon must keep in mind the underlying pathologic process in each individual athlete. In many of these patients, the problem lies in the pathologic laxity present in the capsule and ligaments around the shoulder. If this underlying pathologic process is not addressed, then fixing the secondary disease alone will be unlikely to improve the athlete's situation.

Every surgical procedure performed at our institution is preceded by an examination while the patient is under anesthesia. This is the most accurate way to document true passive range of motion and stability in both shoulders. After the examination, the patient is placed in the lateral decubitus position for shoulder arthroscopy. Diagnostic arthroscopy is performed through the standard posterior portal. We begin by documenting the status of the articular surfaces of the humerus and glenoid. A standard anterior portal is then established in the rotator interval. The biceps tendon and its origin on the glenoid labrum are then examined using a probe. The entire glenoid labrum is then visualized, with particular attention to the superior and anterior labrum. At this point, it is very important to recognize the morphologic variants of the labrum, including the sublabral foramen and the cord-like middle glenohumeral ligament. Next the rotator cuff is visualized in its entirety, including the superior border of the subscapularis. The axillary recess is inspected, and the position of the humeral head relative to the glenoid is noted. An attempt to drive through the glenohumeral joint is then made, to judge the laxity present in the capsular tissues more clearly.

For rotator cuff disorder, the obvious distinction is between partial-thickness and full-thickness injury. For any degree of partial-thickness tear, the first option is to debride the frayed and degenerative tissue. Unless a player has already had a failed debridement of a partial-thickness tear, the tear is not taken down and repaired. Along with debridement of the cuff tissue, abrasion of the greater tuberosity may be undertaken to encourage healing of the tissue back to bone. If a full-thickness tear is present, arthroscopic subacromial decompression followed by mini-open rotator cuff repair is our procedure of choice. Although arthroscopic techniques continue to improve and evolve, we have not felt confident enough in these techniques to use them in the elite thrower because of the stresses placed by these athletes on their shoulders. For undersurface fraying of the cuff, such as in internal impingement, debridement of the frayed tissue is the first order of business (Fig. 36B.4).

Labral disease comes in many forms in the throwing athlete. The most common situation we encounter is the labral detachment from the anterosuperior glenoid, including the biceps anchor (Fig. 36B.5). Other labral disease includes isolated superior labral fraying and detachment, posterosu-

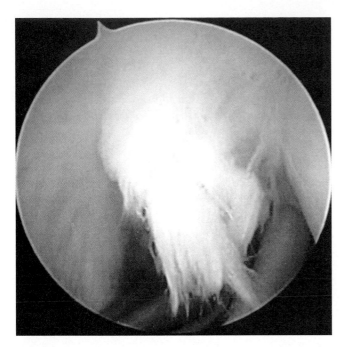

FIGURE 36B.4 Arthroscopic pictures of internal impingement. The undersurface fraying of the posterior superior rotator cuff or labrum is indicative of internal impingement. The shaver is used to debride the frayed tissue.

perior labral fraying, anterior labral detachment, and posterior labral detachment. For fraying of the labrum in any location, debridement is carried out without detaching the labrum. The detached labrum is repaired to the glenoid with arthroscopic techniques. For superior labral lesions, it is difficult to insert an anchor through the standard anterior cannula. In most cases, an accessory portal is necessary to insert the fixation device. In these cases, we use the smallest cannula possible to minimize the trauma to the rotator cuff, which must be traversed to insert the device. Ever effort should be made to repair any detached portion of the labrum to the bony glenoid. We typically use a shaver or bur to obtain a fresh bony surface in the region of repair, to enhance the healing potential.

Anterior inferior labral detachments present a dilemma because of the difficulty of inserting a fixation device through the anterior cannula. We have not made accessory portals through or below the subscapularis. We make every attempt to freshen the bone beneath the detached labrum and insert an anchor as far down the front of the glenoid as is possible. Posterior labral detachments are repaired with the arthroscope in the anterior portal and the device inserted through the posterior portal. Again, an arthroscopic technique is preferred. Flap tears of the labrum and loose bodies are all removed, including chondral and osteochondral fragments.

In cases of glenoid osteochondral injury, once the fragment is removed, the edge of the lesion is debrided back to

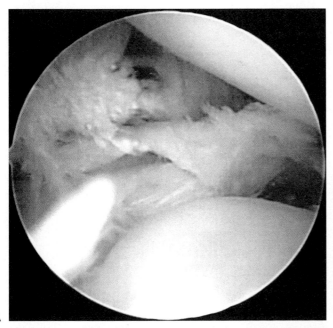

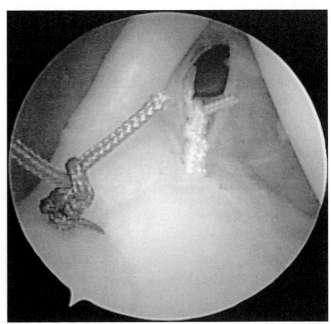

A　　　　　　　　　　　　　　　　　　　　　　　　　　　　　B

FIGURE 36B.5 Arthroscopic pictures of common labral diseases and treatment. **A:** Typical superior labral disease seen in the throwing athlete. The superior labrum surrounding the biceps anchor is detached from the glenoid. **B:** Two suture anchors have been placed to fix the labrum–biceps complex back to the glenoid.

a stable rim, and the bony surface is debrided with a shaver until the entire surface bleeds evenly when the fluid flow is turned off (Fig. 36B.6). Thrower's exostoses are removed arthroscopically by elevating the overlying labrum with a rasp or sharp elevator through the posterior cannula with the arthroscope in the anterior cannula. The shaver or bur is then used to remove the bony prominence. We have not repaired the labrum overlying the lesion back to the glenoid in these cases. Because it is suspected that the exostosis is a traction phenomenon, it seems appropriate to leave the labrum free at the location of the pathologic lesion and to allow it to heal on its own to the freshened bony surface. Anecdotally,

we have had no recurrence of symptoms following such a technique.

Finally, a decision regarding the laxity or instability of the shoulder must be made. In many patients with internal impingement, chronic tendinitis, and labral detachment, excessive humeral translation and capsular laxity are present. Previous reports of rotator cuff debridement or labral repair without addressing pathologic capsular laxity have demonstrated return-to-competition rates from 50% to 76% (9,10). In our experience, the addition of thermal shrinkage to other standard surgical treatment in the thrower's shoulder has improved the rate of return to play (8). In a group of

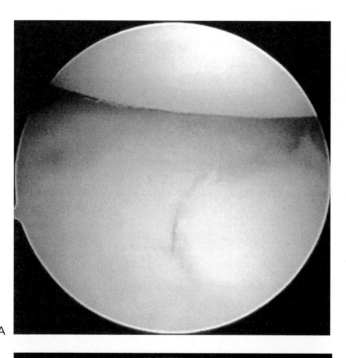

A

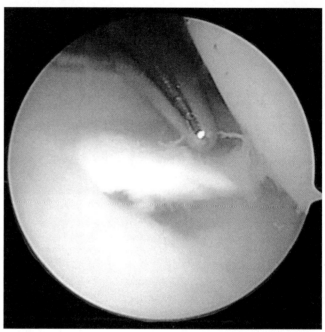

B

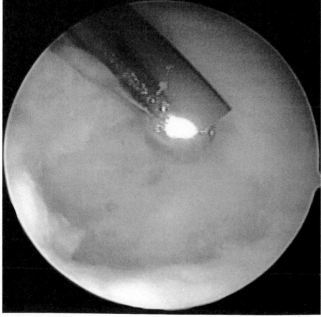

C

FIGURE 36B.6 Arthroscopic pictures of glenoid osteochondritis dissecans (OCD). The typical glenoid OCD is posterior on the glenoid. The lesion seen here is typical in that it is loosely attached to the surrounding tissue, with fibrous tissue between the articular cartilage and the underlying subchondral bone. The fragment is removed either whole or in pieces, and the bed is debrided until bleeding is noted uniformly throughout.

similar patients not undergoing thermal shrinkage, only 80% returned to play at the same or higher level versus 93% in the group receiving thermal shrinkage. Although our data collection is ongoing, results published in 2001 indicated an increased percentage of throwers still competing 30 months after thermal shrinkage (90%) when compared with a similar group without thermal shrinkage (67%) (8).

In some patients, selective shrinkage of certain portions of the capsule is done based on the clinical findings. In others, the capsule is shrunk from the posterior portal through the axillary pouch and up to the insertion of the middle glenohumeral ligament. At this point, we have not used the striping technique, in which normal capsular tissue is left in between the stripes of shrunken tissue. We have not encountered any significant long-term complications related to the thermal capsulorrhaphy, although other surgeons have reported adverse outcomes. Finally, in throwers with evidence of tendinosis or subacromial impingement, the arthroscope is inserted through the posterior portal into the subacromial space, and the space is inspected for acromial impingement and bursitis. If necessary, a lateral portal is established, and decompression of the space is performed. Typically, a mini-acromioplasty is carried out if any spur exists. Every effort is made to leave the deep deltoid fascia and coracoacromial ligament intact.

POSTOPERATIVE CARE

The postoperative management of the thrower's shoulder is as important as the intraoperative care. Although each patient receives an individualized program, the basic goals are the same. The early postoperative period is spent regaining motion in a controlled environment. In those athletes who have undergone thermal capsulorrhaphy, frequent physician–patient interaction is mandatory to ensure that the shoulder is neither too tight nor too loose. For these patients, the arm is immobilized at the side for 2 to 4 weeks. During this period, the athlete is allowed to begin limited passive range-of-motion exercises in the plane of the scapula. After the period of immobilization, the range of motion is gradually increased, with a goal of obtaining the 90–90 position (90 degrees of abduction and 90 degrees of external rotation) by the end of the sixth week. From there, the patient's arm is gradually stretched into increasing external rotation, with a goal of 115 to 120 degrees. In our study of baseball players with internal impingement, the operative shoulder lost an average of 7 degrees of external rotation in abduction after thermal capsulorrhaphy (8). Once the range of motion is complete, plyometric exercises are initiated, and throwing exercises follow. Every thrower completes an interval throwing program with stepwise increases in distance, effort, and number of throws before return to competition. In patients who undergo thermal shrinkage alone, the average length of time to return to com-

petition is 8.4 months. In patients who undergo thermal shrinkage in addition to labral repair, this time is increased to an average of slightly more than 11 months (8).

In those patients who do not undergo thermal shrinkage, aggressive range of motion is generally initiated in the early postoperative period. When range of motion is regained, strengthening and plyometric exercise is initiated, followed by return to throwing through an interval throwing program. It is not uncommon for throwers to move through the interval throwing program with occasional setbacks along the way. When discomfort occurs, the athlete is encouraged to "take a step back" in the throwing program after resting for 2 to 3 days. Before and during the interval throwing program, the athlete is encouraged to use proper throwing mechanics. Trainers and coaches are often heavily involved at this stage of the recovery.

SUMMARY

The thrower's shoulder is a delicate balance of power and stability. The stresses experienced by the soft tissues around the shoulder are extreme and are certainly capable of causing significant injury. A stepwise approach to examination of the shoulder along with a thorough thrower's history will frequently enable the clinician to diagnose the disorder correctly. Every attempt should be made to return the athlete to competition without the need for surgical treatment. All conservative options should be exhausted before surgery is considered. Active rest should be the hallmark of conservative management for most shoulder disorders. If conservative means fail, surgical treatment is indicated. At the time of surgery, every effort is made to restore normal soft tissue and bony anatomy. If pathologic laxity exists, thermal capsulorrhaphy is used to tighten the shoulder capsule. The success of thermal capsulorrhapy, as well as any surgical treatment of the thrower's shoulder, highly depends on the quality of postoperative therapy. Careful attention by the clinician and the therapist to issues such as range of motion, stability, strength, and throwing mechanics is necessary to ensure a successful return to competition.

REFERENCES

1. Dillman CJ, Fleisig GS, Andrews JR. Biomechanics of pitching with emphasis upon shoulder kinematics. *J Orthop Sports Phys Ther* 1993;18:402–408.
2. Fleisig GS, Andrews JR, Dillman CJ, et al. Kinetics of baseball pitching with implications about injury mechanisms. *Am J Sports Med* 1995;23:233–239.
3. Crockett HC, Gross LB, Wilk KE, et al. The elite throwers: etiology of increased glenohumeral external rotation. Presented at the American Orthopedic Society for Sports Medicine meeting, Sun Valley, ID, 2000.
4. Meister K, Batts J, Gilmore M. The posterior impingement sign:

evaluation of internal impingement in the overhand athlete. *Orthop Trans* 1998.

5. King JW, Brelsford HJ, Tullos HS. Analysis of the pitching arm of the professional baseball player. *Clin Orthop* 1969;67:116–123.

6. Walch G, Boileau P, Noel E, et al. Impingement of the deep surface of the supraspinatus tendon on the posterosuperior glenoid rim: an arthroscopic study. *J Shoulder Elbow Surg* 1992;1:238–245.

7. O'Brien SJ, Pagnani MJ, Fealy S, et al. The active compression test: a new and effective test for diagnosing labral tears and acromioclavicular joint abnormality. *Am J Sports Med* 1998;26:610–613.

8. Levitz CL, Dugas JR, Andrews JR. The use of arthroscopic thermal capsulorrhaphy to treat internal impingement in baseball players. Arthroscopy 2001;17:573–577.

9. Andrews JR, Broussard TS, Carson WG. Arthroscopy of the shoulder in the management of partial tears of the rotator cuff: a preliminary report. *Arthroscopy* 1985;1:117–122.

10. Payne LZ, Altchek DW, Craig EV, et al. Arthroscopic treatment of partial rotator cuff tears in young athletes: a preliminary report. *Am J Sports Med* 1997;25:299–305.

11. Andrews JR, Gillogly S. Physical examination of the shoulder in throwing athletes. In: Zarins B, Andrews JR, Carson WG, eds. *Injuries to the throwing arm.* Philadephia: WB Saunders, 1985.

THERMAL CAPSULORRHAPHY: BASIC SCIENCE

SIMON P. FROSTICK

That collagen shrinks in response to the application of heat has been known for several decades. The clinical application of this phenomenon for the treatment of shoulder instability has been reported since the mid-1990s. The clinical use of this characteristic has required the development of appropriate devices for the application of the heat.

When considering the basic science of thermal capsulorrhaphy, certain factors need to be considered:

- The effects of heat on collagen
- The clinical entities that would benefit from such techniques
- The devices available to apply heat by arthroscopic methods
- The changes in joint capsule that occur in response to the application of heat
- The outcome of using the techniques
- The possible and actual complications

It is an unfortunate aspect of thermal capsulorrhaphy that it has been greeted by excessive enthusiasm and, consequently, abuse. It is already falling into disrepute before a real role for the technique has been established. This is partly because of a lack of understanding of the phenomenon of shoulder instability. It also results from a lack of knowledge of the *in vivo* effects of applying heat to shoulder joint capsule. However, another reason is that surgeons have mistakenly regarded thermal capsulorrhaphy as an easy option in treating patients with unstable shoulders.

This chapter is written on the basis that a limited amount of published knowledge exists about thermal capsulorrhaphy. Moreover, it is based on a philosophy that thermal capsulorrhaphy is an adjunct to the treatment of a specific type of patient and indeed may well have a temporary effect, with the long-term stability of the shoulder determined mostly by reestablishing dynamic control. I have used this technique in 150 patients with multidirectional instability of the shoulder in whom a highly structured rehabilitation program had failed. Patients undergo the surgical procedure to provide a temporary constraint to shoulder subluxation that enables them to undertake the rehabilitation program without pain and so, one hopes, improves compliance.

Both laser devices and radiofrequency generators are in clinical use. Each specific type of device has its advocates. Published data on the possible relative safety of the devices are scant. Only early reports are available about the efficacy of the technique and the devices that are used.

EFFECTS OF HEAT ON COLLAGEN

Type I and type III collagen are the major constituents of interstitial collagen. Type I collagen provides considerable tensile strength, whereas type III collagen provides some compliance to the tissue (1). The fibrils of type I collagen are found to be between 100 and 500 nm in diameter. Type III collagen has a maximum diameter of 60 nm. Type I procollagen is formed from two pro α1 (I) chains and one pro α2 (I) chain. The genes for both chains are found on chromosome 17 and consist of 51 and 52 exons, respectively. Assembly of the fibrils occurs extracellularly, and a triple helix is formed with a periodicity of 67 nm. Intermolecular crosslinks are formed from lysine and hydroxylysine residues (through hydrogen bonds). Type III collagen is formed from three pro α1 (III) chains, and, as in type I, the chains are assembled in the extracellular space. The chains are linked by disulfide bonds. Fleischmajer et al. (2) suggested that an interaction between type I and type III collagen is an important part of collagen fibril assembly. Mutations of the type I collagen genes result in osteogenesis imperfecta and type VII Ehlers-Danlos syndrome. A type III collagen mutation results in Ehlers-Danlos syndrome type IV.

Types I and III collagen have been shown to be the major components of the joint capsule in human interphalangeal joints (3) and in bovine metacarpophalangeal joints (4). Further, even in major structural abnormalities such as

S. P. Frostick: Department of Musculoskeletal Science, University of Liverpool, Royal Liverpool University Hospital, Liverpool, United Kingdom.

clubfoot deformities, the capsular structure seems to be the same as normal (5). Shoulder joint collagen is similar in content to collagens found in other joints. Kaltsas (6) examined the shoulder, elbow, and hip. In a cadaver study of specimens aged between 42 and 80 years, the predominant collagen types were I, III, and V. Kaltsas also showed that the strength of the capsule decreased with age. Moreover, he showed that when the shoulder capsule ruptured, the anteroinferior part ruptured first. A variation in collagen fibril diameter with age was demonstrated by Parry et al. (7). These authors showed that fibril size distribution was unimodal at birth; in mature individuals, the mass-average diameter was larger but the distribution could be either unimodal or bimodal, and in old age, the average fibril diameter was less than in mature individuals and the distribution was unimodal. These authors suggested a direct correlation between connective tissue tensile strength and the mass-average diameter. Further, the tensile strength was also correlated with the types of intrafibrillar bonds. High-tensile strength was associated with more intrafibrillar covalent bonds, whereas more elastic connective tissue had more noncovalent crosslinks. Joint immobilization did not result in any increase in type I and type III collagen in an experiment on dog glenohumeral joints (8). Rodeo et al. (9) demonstrated that the major difference between "normal" capsule and "unstable" capsule is in the increase in stable crosslinks in the "unstable" capsule.

Shrinkage of collagen in response to heating is a phenomenon that has been known for several decades. Finch and Ledward (10) reported that the main stabilizing bonds within collagen are intramolecular H-bond. However, they also showed that these were heat-labile crosslinks that ruptured in an exothermic process. Nagy et al. (11) examined thermal denaturation in rat tail tendons and demonstrated variations in response that were related to age. The authors discussed the presence of age-related changes from heat labile H-bond crosslinks in young animals to heat-stable crosslinks of a covalent nature in mature tendons. Allain et al. (12) showed an increase in the tension that developed when collagenous structures were heated to between 65°C and 67°C, and it increased with age. The age-related differences were associated with an increase in heat-stable intermolecular crosslinks within the collagen. Variations in the concentration of reducible and nonreducible crosslinks may be found in different tendons and within different parts within the same tendon (13). These authors also demonstrated that the thermal properties of the collagen were strongly correlated with the presence of nonreducible crosslinks. Smith and Judge (14) also showed that thermal stability of collagen found within muscle increased with age and was related to the increased presence of pyridinoline crosslinks.

The response of collagenous tissues to heat may vary between those tissues that are loaded and those that are not. In an experiment using a technique known as isothermal free-shrinkage in which collagen was heated in the absence of load, Chen et al. (15) were able to demonstrate certain characteristics of response. The characteristics included a single correlation between free-shrinkage and duration of heating; the effect is cumulative, and some recovery occurs once the tissue is returned to normal body temperature. In a shoulder with lax capsular structures, it is very difficult to be certain about the type and extent of loading at any point in the tissue and at any position in three-dimensional space. The application of heat to the inferior capsule arthroscopically, with the patient in the beach-chair position, may be similar to the isothermal free-shrinkage reported by Chen et al.; that is, the heat is applied in the absence of load or at least minimal loading. This, in turn, presumably, will influence the amount of shrinkage that can be achieved. Moreover, it may be difficult to extrapolate data from *in vitro* experiments on tissues such as patella tendon when the experiments are performed under preloaded conditions to the *in vivo* shrinkage of human capsular collagen.

CLINICAL CONSIDERATIONS

It appears that thermal capsulorrhaphy has been used as either an adjunct to or treatment for several different forms of instability. Some surgeons perform thermal capsulorrhaphy to try to deal with the plastic deformation found in the capsule after an anterior (traumatic) recurrent dislocation. My view is that thermal capsulorrhaphy is a technique that should be restricted as a surgical alternative to an open anterior inferior capsular shift procedure in patients with multidirectional instability. What little evidence there is suggests that, after shrinkage of the collagen, gradual restoration and, indeed, possible elongation (in some animal models) of the collagen structure occur. Therefore, thermal capsulorrhaphy may only have a temporary effect. In the Liverpool Upper Limb Unit, all patients undergo a structured rehabilitation program before thermal capsulorrhaphy; they are considered for surgery only if that rehabilitation program fails, and they return to the program postoperatively. The approach is based on a concept that thermal capsulorrhaphy is providing a temporary static constraint to shoulder subluxation in a group of patients who have a lax shoulder capsule and who depend almost entirely on dynamic constraint to contain the humeral head central on the glenoid. It is an interesting observation that if the humeral head is in an inferiorly subluxed position, the patient will often experience quite severe pain. Centering the humeral head on the glenoid seems to reduce that pain and allows the patient to pursue the rehabilitation program. Further, many of the patients who eventually undergo thermal capsulorrhaphy are involved in overhead sports. These patients may well need to have capsular laxity to ensure that they can perform their sport.

The application of thermal energy has certain physical characteristics (see later). One of these characteristics is distance from the heating source. In terms of application to a clinical situation, this has both safety and efficacy implications, safety from the point of view that the depth of penetration of effect needs to be known to prevent collateral damage. The efficacy depends on whether sufficient tissue has been "shrunk" in appropriate anatomic localities. It is therefore important to have a reasonable knowledge of the structure and thickness of the shoulder joint capsule. Ciccone et al. (16) studied variations in the thickness of human shoulder joint capsule. Their results show a significant decrease in capsular thickness from the glenoid laterally to its insertion on the humeral head. These authors were also able to show that, in the specimens examined, the capsular thickness ranged from 2.76 to 3.18 mm in the areas closest to the axillary nerve. An earlier study on the arrangement of collagen fibers within the capsule showed a homogeneous collagen fibril arrangement, except in the area of the rotator interval (17).

For thermal capsulorrhaphy, the important anatomic region and structures are the inferior capsule and the elements of the inferior glenohumeral ligament complex (IGHLC). O'Brien et al. (18) were able to show, by both gross and histologic anatomy, that three distinct areas could be distinguished in the area of interest. In all of their 11 cadaver specimens, O'Brien et al. described anterior and posterior bands of the IGHLC with an intervening axillary pouch. The anterior and posterior bands were found to be distinct thickenings in the inferior capsule. Functionally, with the arm in 90 degrees of abduction and external rotation, the anterior band of the IGHLC and the inferior pouch are important elements in preventing excessive anterior translation. Similarly, in 90 degrees of internal rotation, the posterior band and inferior pouch cradle the head posteriorly.

Bigliani et al. (19) showed variations in the tensile strength of different areas of the IGHLC. These authors argued that the variations in the stress–strain curves found in the different regions may reflect some differences in the microarchitecture of the collagen fibers, although more grossly they are of similar arrangement in all regions.

That the stability of the shoulder depends on a complex of structures was highlighted by O'Brien et al. (20), who suggested the following five intrinsic mechanical restraints:

1. Articular surface geometry
2. Passive soft tissue capsular connective structures
3. Joint compressive forces
4. Complex muscular forces
5. Negative intraarticular pressures

The role played by each of these "intrinsic mechanical constraints" is far from clear in different types of instability. Purely from the point of view of clinical observation, it is evident that tremendous variations occur in the degree of shoulder laxity from one person to another. Moreover, the presence of symptoms is not correlated with the degree of laxity. In patients who suffer a traumatic anterior dislocation, the loss of the passive constraints seems to be an important component of the instability, although loss of proprioception and muscle control must play a part. In patients with symptomatic multidirectional instability, the passive constraints play a much smaller part in maintaining stability, with the converse true of the muscles. Obviously, the clinical implication is that, in symptomatic patients, it is very difficult to be certain of the exact nature of the instability, and it may therefore be difficult to decide on the most appropriate surgical procedure in an individual case. The use of thermal capsulorrhaphy is dogged by poor understanding of physiology and functional anatomy, poor clinical decision making, and application of a technique that in itself is poorly understood.

DEVICES AVAILABLE TO APPLY HEAT BY ARTHROSCOPIC METHODS

Holmium:yttrium-aluminum-garnet (Ho:YAG) lasers and both monopolar and bipolar radiofrequency generators are available to perform thermal capsulorrhaphy. Lasers were introduced first in this surgical technique, but in terms of numbers, radiofrequency devices are more commonly used now. The same basic principles apply to all devices. Each causes heating of water molecules that, in turn, causes collagen shrinkage. The other important principle is that heat deposition is controlled and does not cause total tissue destruction. All the devices can be used for tissue resection and hemostasis at device settings that are much higher than those used for shrinkage of collagen.

A laser operates by emitting a monochromatic, nondivergent beam of light in which all the light waves are in parallel and in phase (coherence, monochromicity, and collimation). Different tissues respond in different ways to the application of the light waves. The response depends on the optical properties of the tissue. The Ho:YAG laser used in thermal capsulorrhaphy emits a beam at 2.14 μm. At this wavelength, the energy is mostly absorbed by water molecules in tissue. Heat is generated by the water absorbing the infrared light energy. By appropriate control of the delivery of the energy, collateral damage can be minimized (21).

Radiofrequency devices operate on the principle that an alternating current will flow from the electrode into the tissues. This, in turn, produces friction between the molecules in the tissues (water molecules) resulting in heat production (Fig. 37.1). Unlike electrocautery, which produces heat at the tip of the electrode, radiofrequency causes the water molecules within the tissues to produce the heat and not the electrode. Organ (22) reviewed the physical characteristics of radiofrequency lesion generation. Organ suggests that the heat produced in a volume of tissue depends on:

- The distance from the tip
- The radiofrequency current density
- The duration of application of the radiofrequency current

Current through heater
element in probe

Heat flow from probe
to tissue

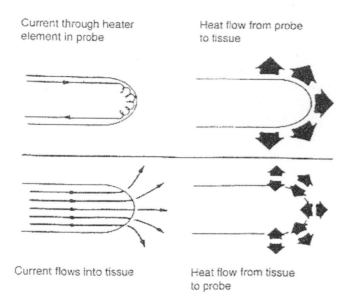

Current flows into tissue

Heat flow from tissue
to probe

FIGURE 37.1 The production and distribution of heat generated by electrocautery (A) and radiofrequency (B). (From Organ LW. Electrophysiologic principles of radiofrequency lesion making. *Appl Neurophysiol* 1976–1977;39:69–76, with permission.)

The amount of tissue heating falls rapidly as a function of $1/r^4$ (where r is radius). This means that the physical properties of radiofrequency generation limits the volume of tissue that can be heated resulting in a well-defined region of effect. The current density is a function of I^2, so within the small volume of tissue affected there will be a high current density. Organ stated that control over current density is essential. If the current density is too low, then the lesion size will be small. If the current density is too high, then this will either result in tissue charring or vaporization. The amount of heat deposited varies according to the term I^2T, where I^2 is the current density and T is time. A finite time is required to heat the tissues to an appropriate temperature for the desired effect. Obviously, different tissues respond in different ways, depending on local conditions. The amount of heat found in a volume of tissue at any one time depends on the balance between heat gain and heat loss. Heat loss depends on conduction (diffusion of heat to surrounding tissues), convection (dependent on local vascular supply), and low-resistance shunting (this will occur if there is lower resistance in some areas of the tissue than in others). The total energy applied to the tissues is given by the following equation:

$$E = PT = I^2RT$$

where E is total applied energy, P is power, I^2 is current density, R is resistance, and T is time.

The shape of a radiofrequency-generated lesion appears to be elliptical (Fig. 37.2). The size of the electrode tip has some effect on the size of the lesion. Organ stated that the

circle   ellipse

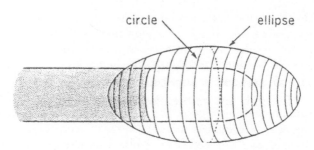

FIGURE 37.2 The shape of the radiofrequency-generated lesion—a prolate spheroid centered about the uninsulated portion of the electrode tip. (From Organ LW. Electrophysiologic principles of radiofrequency lesion making. *Appl Neurophysiol* 1976–1977;39:69–76, with permission.)

size of the lesion can be generally estimated by the following relationship:

- The long axis equals twice the length of the bare tip.
- The transverse axis equals two-thirds of the long axis.

Commercially available radiofrequency devices use either a monopolar or a bipolar principle. All the systems available can be used to perform thermal capsulorrhaphy. The monopolar device generates current that flows from the delivery electrode to a remote ground electrode (similar to the arrangement used for electrocautery). The monopolar device has a thermocouple in the probe tip that measures tissue temperature. Obviously, the accuracy of the temperature measurement depends on the position of the thermocouple in relation to the probe tip, the physical properties of the thermocouple itself, and the fluid flow through the joint. Using a traditional thermocouple may not be the most appropriate way of modulating the temperature developed at the probe tip. Shellock (23) showed, in a comparison of a monopolar probe and a bipolar probe, that the surface temperature measured in response to application of heat from the monopolar device was up to nearly 30°C higher than the temperature required for tissue shrinkage and indeed 30°C higher than the reading on the generator itself. This finding has serious safety implications for the monopolar device.

The bipolar devices operate by current flowing from the tip of the electrode in contact with the tissues to a second electrode within a few millimeters but insulated from the delivery electrode. Shellock showed that the temperature generated by a bipolar electrode was within the desirable range for tissue shrinkage throughout the course of the experiment.

CHANGES IN THE JOINT CAPSULE IN RESPONSE TO THE APPLICATION OF HEAT

It has been necessary to extrapolate data mostly from various animal models to human shoulder joint capsule to understand what may be occurring in the treatment of patients with thermal capsulorrhaphy. Some direct observations on both the acute and the longer-term effects of heat on shoulder joint capsule are available, but there are serious gaps in our knowledge. It is difficult ethically to justify second-look arthroscopic procedures in patients undergoing thermal capsulorrhaphy to gather detailed histologic data. As most data are from animal models, care must be taken in extrapolating the data. Many of the experiments have been on models in which the collagen arrangement is substantially different from that of human shoulder joint capsule. Further, in an animal model it should be possible to apply the heat in a consistent and repeatable fashion, a situation that is considerably more difficult in the human shoulder joint, where variables such as surgeon skill, equipment, and positioning, for example, come into play.

Most data on the effects of heat on collagenous structures have been derived from experiments using laser (Ho:YAG laser). It has been assumed that radiofrequency is likely to be similar in effect.

Hayashi et al. (24) showed that the degree of shrinkage, *in vitro*, in rabbit femoropatellar joint capsule directly correlated with the power used. Therefore, the reduction of capsular length for 5, 10, and 15 W was 9%, 26%, and 38%, respectively. These authors also showed some alteration in the physical properties of the tissue after shrinkage. In a further study on the same animal model, Hayashi et al. (25) reported the acute ultrastructural changes found after laser tissue shrinkage. These authors showed a power-related increase in the appearance of the collagen fibrils typified by apparent increase in the fibril diameter, a loss of the distinct edges of the fibrils, and loss of the regular cross-striations. The authors' hypothesis was that the application of heat caused denatura-

tion of the fibrillar collagen. A third study by the same authors (26) showed that although an energy-related increase in the degree of denaturation occurred, as well as fibroblast death, there was no alteration in either type I collagen content or in the nonreducible (heat-stable) crosslinks.

Naseef et al. (27) performed an *in vitro* study of thermal shrinkage. Bovine calf knee capsule was used as the experimental model. These authors showed that, at temperatures less than 57.5°C, no shrinkage effect could be observed. The maximal observed shrinkage occurred at 65°C when the tissue length was reduced to 50%. The degree of shrinkage was time and temperature dependent. Hayashi et al. (28) similarly showed that temperatures of 65°C or more were associated with shrinkage of the tissue. At 65°C, the percentage of shrinkage was 11%, and this increased to 59% at 80°C.

Vangsness et al. (29) demonstrated that a 30% decrease in length of fresh-frozen human patellar tendons occurred at about 70°C by application of laser-generated heat *in vitro*. In this model, when the tendon was shortened by 10%, there was a 33% decrease in the load to failure. Histologically, these authors showed denaturation of collagen that was well demarcated from normal collagen. These authors did not make any comment about the depth of the effect. An important observation made by Vangsness et al. is that there is a quite narrow temperature range for thermal effects. The shrinkage effect started at temperatures slightly less than 70°C, but when the temperature exceeded 80°C, the tissues "physically fell apart." Moran et al. (30) examined the kinetics of thermal shrinkage of collagen. Shrinkage of bovine knee capsule was minimal at temperatures less than 63°C and increased to 72°C. Schaefer et al. (31) used the rabbit patellar tendon to examine the effects of laser-applied heat at 4 and 8 weeks after treatment (Fig. 37.3). The initial

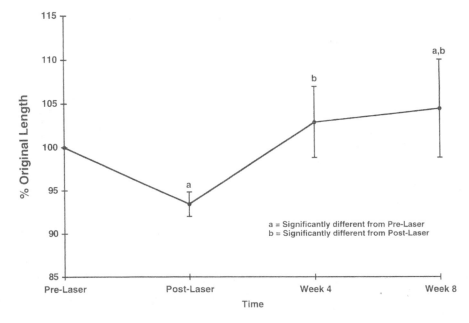

a = Significantly different from Pre-Laser
b = Significantly different from Post-Laser

FIGURE 37.3 Change in tendon length after thermal modification by laser application. (From Schaefer SL, Ciarelli MJ, Arnoczky SP, et al. Tissue shrinkage with the holmium:yttrium aluminum garnet laser: a postoperative assessment of tissue length, stiffness, and structure. *Am J Sports Med* 1997;25:841–848, with permission.)

shrinkage was 6.6±1.4%, but at 4 weeks after the treatment, the tendon length had increased to beyond the prelaser length; by 8 weeks, there had been a statistically significant increase in tendon length compared with the pretreatment length. Histologically, these authors showed increased cellularity in the tendons. Moreover, in the control tendons, a bimodal distribution of collagen fibril diameter was found that was lost in the treated tendons in which the collagen fibril diameter distribution became unimodal. The important clinical implication of this work is that the authors suggested that rehabilitation programs after shrinkage procedures must take into account the alteration in the tissues that lasted for several weeks after the treatment.

To determine further time-related changes, Hayashi et al. (32) performed thermal capsulorrhaphy on the rabbit femoropatellar joint and harvested tissues immediately after the surgical procedure and at 7 and 30 days after treatment. Immediately after the surgical procedure, denaturation of the collagen fibrils and fibroblast death were shown. At 7 days after treatment, a fibroblastic response into the areas of tissue damage was found, and at 30 days after treatment, there was evidence of collagen regeneration.

Changes in the mechanical properties of the heat-treated tissues have concerned surgeons. Selecky et al. (33) examined the changes in the load characteristics of the human IGHLC specimens immediately after laser treatment. These authors concluded that "the strength of the ligament complex was not significantly compromised by this lasing protocol." Two obvious comments about this experiment that are significant in extrapolating the data to a clinical situation are that the specimens were all elderly and there may be no relevance in knowing the mechanical properties immediately after the treatment.

In an experiment on greyhound shoulder capsule, Pullin et al. (34) showed that the intraarticular pressure was raised after laser-induced thermal shrinkage compared with normal at 6 weeks postoperatively. Of more importance, however, is these authors' observation that the effects of the laser treatment extended outside the joint capsule. The authors described pericapsular tissue reactivity. The histologic examination also showed varying degrees of "significant inflammation, necrosis, inflammatory cellular influx, and ligament destruction. . . ." In their discussion, these authors mentioned that the greyhound capsule appeared thinner, although no measurements of capsular thickness were reported. In this experiment, it would appear that the level of power deposition was closely monitored and controlled. It is therefore of concern that these researchers reported varying degrees of capsular damage including necrosis. Some reports of capsular necrosis in patients treated by thermal capsulorrhaphy have appeared. Numerous reasons may be given for this phenomenon. However, based on the experiments of Pullin et al., it may be suggested that different individuals may have marked differences in response to the applied heat. Moreover, it may not be possible to predict the level of damage that may occur in response to a known and controlled power level.

Published data on the time-related changes that occur in human shoulder joint capsule after thermal capsulorrhaphy are lacking at present. Hayashi et al. (35) reported time-related changes in the sheep femoropatellar joint. Using Ho:YAG laser energy, Hayashi et al. examined both mechanical and histologic features. Tissue stiffness decreased from the time of surgery to 7 days, but it increased again after 14 days. The tissue seemed to be weakest at 3 days postoperatively. The earliest histologic changes were collagen denaturation and cell death. Subsequently, a fibroblastic response and neovascularization were observed. These authors demonstrated that, by 60 days postoperatively, all parameters except collagen fibril diameter were normal. The collagen fibrils remained small. A further study by the same authors (36) confirmed earlier work that the main effect of applying heat to collagen by laser was to denature the collagen (Fig. 37.4).

Thermal capsulorrhaphy using radiofrequency appears to cause changes similar to those found after laser application. Lopez et al. (37) examined the acute effects of radiofrequency-applied heat on sheep femoropatellar joint capsule.

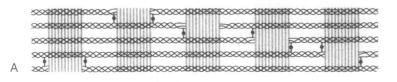

A

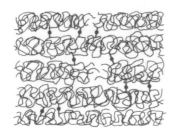

B

FIGURE 37.4 The effects of laser on the structural properties of collagen. (From Hayashi K, Peters DM, Thabit G 3rd, et al. The mechanism of joint capsule thermal modification in an *in-vitro* sheep model. *Clin Orthop* 2000;370: 236–249, with permission.)

These researchers observed an increase in fibril diameter and collagen denaturation similar to that found after laser heating. Hoad-Reddick et al. (38) demonstrated that, when using the Mitek VAPR bipolar radiofrequency generator, the depth of tissue modification immediately after shrinkage was only 40 μm; the deeper tissues were completely unaffected (Fig. 37.5).

Obrzut et al. (39) were able to show temperature-related increases in the degree of shrinkage (from 65°C to 80°C) using a monopolar radiofrequency generator. There was also a rapid reduction in tissue temperature with increasing depth through the tissues with a measured temperature of 45°C at 1.5 mm. Hecht et al. (40) showed that the effects of thermal shrinkage depend on the device power settings, but the effect is modified by perioperative joint lavage. In a comparative study of Ho:YAG laser with a monopolar radiofrequency device, Osmond et al. (41) claimed that essentially identical temperature-dependent changes in sheep glenohumeral joint capsule occurred. However, on closer examination of the data, it is apparent that a tissue temperature of more than 65°C was only achieved in the laser group set at the highest wattage. In nearly all other groups, the temperature, even at the surface, remained less than 60°C. As these authors apparently observed a shrinkage effect, it must be concluded that the measured temperature was significantly lower than the real temperature in the tissues. A study by Hecht et al. (42) showed that the mechanical properties of sheep femoropatellar joint capsule were markedly affected (weakened) for at least 2 weeks after thermal treatment. The properties improved thereafter.

OUTCOME

In a study of cadaveric shoulders, Tibone et al. (43) were able to show that, using laser-assisted thermal capsulorrhaphy, a significant reduction in both anterior and posterior translation could be achieved. Anderson et al. (44) reviewed the early use of radiofrequency thermal capsulorrhaphy. These authors strongly suggested that, because of the lack of peer-reviewed published results, surgeons must be wary of claims by companies that promote devices. Moreover, the authors emphasized the need for care when applying the technique.

Few studies are available on the short- and medium-term effects, and none are available on the long-term effects of thermal capsulorrhaphy in human tissues. Hayashi et al. (45) were able to obtain tissue samples from patients who had previously undergone laser-assisted thermal capsulorrhaphy. These authors were able to demonstrate changes similar to those found in animal tissues. In samples obtained from 7 to 38 months postoperatively, these investigators suggested that the capsule had returned to normal. In a small number of second-look procedures that I performed, the capsule returned to its normal appearance after bipolar radiofrequency thermal capsulorrhaphy after only 3 to 6 months.

A review article by Tyler et al. (46) suggests that the success of the thermal capsulorrhaphy depends on a combination of surgery, followed by a short period of immobilization, followed by rehabilitation. Frostick et al. (47) reported their minimum 2-year follow-up of patients undergoing radiofrequency thermal capsulorrhaphy (Fig. 37.6). These authors showed a continued improvement in the assessed parameters up to 12 months after the surgical procedure, followed by a plateau of the parameters thereafter (Fig. 37.7). Frostick et al. emphasized the need for the patients to return to a structured rehabilitation program to achieve long-term stability. The overall satisfaction rate for thermal capsulorrhaphy in this group of patients was 88%.

The major limitations to assessing the success of thermal capsulorrhaphy have been inconsistency in reporting results. The patient groups have often been poorly reported.

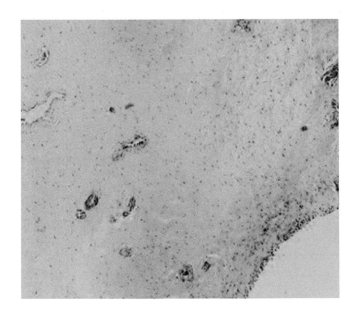

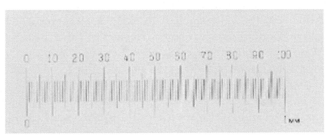

FIGURE 37.5 The depth of effect using the Mitek VAPR bipolar radiofrequency generator. The limit of tissue damage is 40 μm from the surface. Immediately after the surgical procedure, tissues more than 40 μm from the surface seem to be unaffected. (From Hoad-Reddick A, Hughes P, Brownson P, et al. Histological changes in the shoulder joint capsule following thermal capsular shrinkage for multi-directional instability. In: Proceedings of the 8th ICSS conference, Cape Town, South Africa, 2001, with permission.)

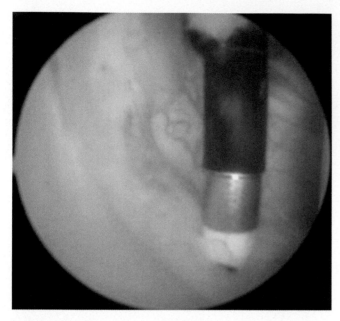

FIGURE 37.6 The arthroscopic appearance of the thermal capsulorrhaphy. The normal capsule that has blood vessels easily seen on the surface becomes white and opaque after treatment. This image shows the effect of using the Mitek VAPR bipolar system.

COMPLICATIONS

All surgical procedures are associated with complications. Thermal capsulorrhaphy is no exception. The complications or adverse events reported so far include the following:

- Failure to achieve stabilization
- Axillary nerve damage (temporary and permanent)
- Capsular necrosis
- Capsular disruption
- Shoulder stiffness

The overall rate of failure to achieve stabilization is unknown. In our series, 12% of patients failed to achieve a satisfactory outcome; this included patients with a major voluntary component to their instability. In an article sponsored by Oratec Interventions, Fanton (48) suggested that more than 90% of patients had a successful outcome at 2 years.

The two most devastating complications are axillary nerve damage and capsular necrosis. Both are anecdotally reported but, not surprisingly, generate considerable concern. It is impossible to estimate either a prevalence or an incidence of these complications. The axillary nerve injuries have been both temporary and permanent. Temperatures of 50°C to 55°C cause structural changes in peripheral nerves that result in irreversible damage (49). It seems most likely that there are two explanations for axillary nerve injuries during thermal capsulorrhaphy. The first is surgeon dependent and second is device dependent. If the surgeon leaves the activated radiofrequency probe in contact with the tis-

sues for even 1 second, then penetration of the capsule can occur. As part of a training program, I demonstrated that a bipolar probe set at 30 W can penetrate the inferior recess in a cadaver in no more than 1 second. Therefore, direct thermal injury to the nerve, which is only a few millimeters from the anteroinferior capsule, can occur (16). The damage may be device related. Shellock (23) showed that the temperature at the surface using the monopolar Oratec device may be as much as 30°C higher than the temperature shown on the generator (Fig. 37.8). In those experiments, the temperature seemed to fall rapidly deeper in the tissues. However, these experiments were conducted *in vitro* and so were well controlled. Surgeons must be cautious when using all the devices and not necessarily rely on the temperature readings from the generators.

In my experience, visual cues are very important in using the technique. In about 150 thermal capsulorrhaphies using the Mitek VAPR bipolar device, no clinically apparent axillary nerve problems were encountered. In this series, actual contraction of the deltoid was felt and seen in eight shoulders. The safety of the VAPR system was demonstrated in a series of perioperative electromyography studies performed in 12 patients undergoing thermal capsulorrhaphy and in two patients used as controls who were undergoing an arthroscopic Bankart repair (50). Electromyographic signals were recorded during the operation of the bipolar radiofrequency generator. The main "abnormality" was a slight increase in the latency, but this was detected in both the patients undergoing thermal capsulorrhaphy and in the controls, a finding possibly indicating that this was a consequence of cooling from the irrigation fluid.

Capsular necrosis has also been reported been reported in anecdotal fashion. McFarland et al. (51) reported eight patients who underwent a second arthroscopic procedure and who were found to have suffered necrosis of the capsule. Most of these patients underwent the original thermal capsulorrhaphy using the monopolar device. As clearly shown by Shellock (23), the monopolar device surface temperature is considerably higher than the output on the generator. Moreover, Shellock and Shields (52) also showed that the Mitek VAPR system increases the temperature to that which causes shrinkage and no higher. It seems likely therefore that there is unrecognized excessive power deposition in the tissues but presumably with greater depth of effect than seen in *in vitro* experiments.

Rath and Richmond (53) reported a case of "complete capsular disruption" after thermal capsulorrhaphy. These authors described the result as catastrophic. I have had one case of capsular disruption occurring 2 weeks after thermal capsulorrhaphy. This occurred after insignificant trauma to the shoulder while the patient was wearing his sling. Arthroscopic examination 1 week later showed a complete rupture of the inferior capsule; treatment was with rest. A further arthroscopic examination of the same shoulder 6 months later revealed that the inferior capsule had completely healed

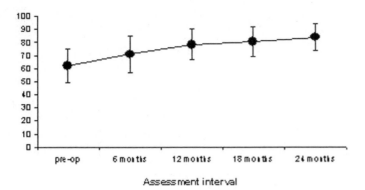

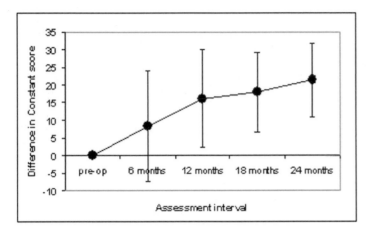

FIGURE 37.7 The change in Constant score after thermal capsulorrhaphy in patients with a minimum of 2 years of follow-up. (From Frostick SP, Sinopidis C, Al Maskari S, et al. Arthroscopic capsular shrinkage of the shoulder for the treatment of MDI: minimum of 2 years follow-up. In: Proceedings of the 8th ICSS conference, Cape Town, South Africa, 2001, with permission.)

and indeed appeared normal. During the initial postoperative period, there appears to be weakness of the capsule, as seen in the experimental situation. Therefore, appropriate protection is required; I prescribe a sling for 3 weeks postoperatively.

Shoulder stiffness is also seen after thermal capsulorrhaphy. I have seen four cases in 150 thermal capsulorrhaphies performed. All four cases occurred in the first 50 operations. Two patients mobilized, with a delay, purely with rehabilitation. The other two patients required an arthroscopic release. In all patients, full function was achieved. The origin of the shoulder stiffness is unknown. It may be caused by scarring of the capsule or by the postoperative initial immobilization. In my series, all the cases occurred in the earliest

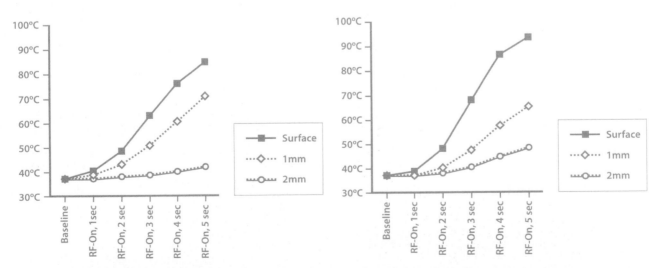

FIGURE 37.8 Temperature profiles for radiofrequency probes used in **(A)** one bipolar device (CAPSure) and **(B)** the monopolar device (TAC-S). (From Shellock FG. RF energy-induced heating of capsule tissue. *Res Outcomes Arthrosc Surg* 1999;4:2–8, with permission.)

group, and therefore it seems likely to be associated with the surgical technique.

CONCLUSIONS

Thermal capsulorrhaphy is a technique that is still searching for its place in arthroscopic shoulder surgery. Some surgeons have encountered serious complications, which are blamed on the concept of thermal capsulorrhaphy, rather than on either surgical skill or limitations of the devices available to apply heat in the arthroscopic situation. I suggest that, as part of a program for the treatment of multidirectional instability, thermal capsulorrhaphy may offer at least a short-term static constraint for the subluxing shoulder on which a structured rehabilitation program can successfully achieve dynamic stability.

REFERENCES

1. Ayad S, Boot-Handford R, Humphries M, et al. *The extracellular matrix: factsbook,* 2nd ed. New York: Academic Press, 1998.
2. Fleischmajer R, Perlish JS, Burgeson RE, et al. Type I and type III collagen interactions during fibrillogenesis. *Ann NY Acad Sci* 1990;580:161–175.
3. Lewis AR, Ralphs JR, Kneafsey B, et al. Distribution of collagens and glycosaminoglycans in the joint capsule of the proximal interphalangeal joint of the human finger. *Anat Rec* 1998;250:281–291.
4. Kleftogiannis F, Handley CJ, Campbell MA. Characterization of extracellular matrix macromolecules from bovine synovial capsule. *J Orthop Res* 1994;12:365–374.
5. van der Sluijs JA, Pruys JE. Normal collagen structure in the posterior capsule in different types of clubfeet. *J Pediatr Orthop B* 1999;8:261–263.
6. Kaltsas DS. Comparative study of the properties of the shoulder joint capsule with those of other joint capsules. *Clin Orthop* 1983;173:20–26.
7. Parry DAD, Barnes GRG, Craig AS. A comparison of the size distribution of collagen fibrils in connective tissues as a function of age and a possible relation between fibril size distribution and mechanical properties. *Proc R Soc Lond B Biol Sci* 1978;203:305–321.
8. Schollmeier G, Sarlkar K, Fukuhara K, et al. Structural and functional changes in canine shoulder after cessation of immobilization. *Clin Orthop* 1996;323:310–315.
9. Rodeo SA, Suzuki K, Yamauchi M, et al. Analysis of collagen and elastic fibers in shoulder capsule in patients with shoulder instability. *Am J Sports Med* 1998;26:634–643.
10. Finch A, Ledward DA. Shrinkage of collagen fibres: a differential scanning calorimetric study. *Biochim Biophys Acta* 1972;278:433–439.
11. Nagy I ZS, Toth VN, Verzar F. High-resolution electron microscopy of thermal collagen denaturation in tail tendons of young, adult and old rats. *Connect Tiss Res* 1974;2:265–272.
12. Allain JC, Le Lous M, Bazin S, et al. Isometric tension developed during heating of collagenous tissues: relationships with collagen cross-linking. *Biochim Biphys Acta* 1978;533:147–155.
13. Horgan DJ, King NL, Kurth LB, et al. Collagen crosslinks and their relationship to the thermal properties of calf tendons. *Arch Biochem Biophys* 1990;281:21–26.
14. Smith SH, Judge MD. Relationship between pyridinoline concentration and thermal stability of bovine intramuscular collagen. *J Anim Sci* 1991;69:1989–1993.
15. Chen SS, Wright NT, Humphrey JD. Heat-induced changes in the mechanics of a collagenous tissue: isothermal free shrinkage. *J Biomech Eng* 1997;119:372–378.
16. Ciccone WJ, Hunt TJ, Lieber R, et al. Multiquadrant digital analysis of shoulder capsular thickness. *Arthroscopy* 2000;16:457–461.
17. Steiner D, Hermann B. Collagen fiber arrangement of the human shoulder joint capsule: an anatomical study. *Acta Anat* 1989;136:300–302.
18. O'Brien SJ, Neves MC, Arnoczky SP, et al. Ligament complex of the shoulder. *Am J Sports Med* 1990;18:449–456.
19. Bigliani LU, Pollock RG, Soslowsky LJ, et al. Tensile properties of the inferior glenohumeral ligament. *J Orthop Res* 1992;10:187–197.
20. O'Brien SJ, Schwartz RS, Warren RF, et al. Capsular restraints to anterior-posterior motion of the abducted shoulder: a biomechanical study. *J Shoulder Elbow Surg* 1995;4:298–308.
21. Sherk HH. The use of lasers in orthopaedic procedures. *J Bone Joint Surg Am* 1993;75:768–776.
22. Organ LW. Electrophysiologic principles of radiofrequency lesion making: international symposium on radiofrequency making procedures, Chicago, 1976. *Appl Neurophysiol* 1976–1977;39:69–76.
23. Shellock FG. RF energy-induced heating of capsule tissue. *Res Outcomes Arthrosc Surg* 1999;4:2–8.
24. Hayashi K, Markel MD, Thabit G, et al. The effect of nonablative laser energy on joint capsular properties. *Am J Sports Med* 1995;23:482–487.
25. Hayashi K, Thabit G, Bogdanske JJ, et al. The effect of nonablative laser energy on the ultrastructure of joint capsular collagen. *Arthroscopy* 1996;12:474–481.
26. Hayashi K, Thabit G, Vailas AC, et al. The effect of nonablative laser energy on joint capsular properties: an *in vitro* histologic and biochemical study using a rabbit model. *Am J Sports Med* 1996;24:640–646.
27. Naseef GS, Foster TE, Trauner K, et al. The thermal properties of bovine joint capsule: the basic science of laser- and radiofrequency-induced capsular shrinkage. *Am J Sports Med* 1997;25:670–674.
28. Hayashi K, Thabit G, Massa KL, et al. The effect of thermal heating on the length and histologic properties of the glenohumeral joint capsule. *Am J Sports Med* 1997;25:107–112.
29. Vangsness CT, Mitchell W, Nimni M, et al. Collagen shortening: an experimental approach with heat. *Clin Orthop* 1997;337:267–271.
30. Moran K, Anderson P, Hutcheson J, et al. Thermally induced shrinkage of joint capsule. *Clin Orthop* 2000;381:248–255.
31. Schaefer SL, Ciarelli MJ, Arnoczky SP, et al. Tissue shrinkage with the holmium:yttrium aluminium garnet laser: a postoperative assessment of tissue length, stiffness and structure. *Am J Sports Med* 1997;25:841–848.
32. Hayashi K, Nieckarz JA, Thabit G, et al. Effect of nonablative laser energy on the joint capsule: an *in vivo* rabbit study using a holmium:YAG laser. *Lasers Surg Med* 1997;20:164–171.
33. Selecky MT, Vangsness T, Wei-Lee L, et al. The effects of laser-induced collagen shortening on the biomechanical properties of the inferior glenohumeral ligament complex. *Am J Sports Med* 1999;27:168–172.
34. Pullin JG, Collier MA, Johnson L, et al. Holmium:YAG laser-assisted capsular shift in a canine model: intraarticular pressure and histologic observations. *J Shoulder Elbow Surg* 1997;6:272–285.
35. Hayashi K, Hecht P, Thabit G, et al. The biologic response to

laser thermal modification in an *in vivo* sheep model. *Clin Orthop* 2000;373:265–276.

36. Hayashi K, Peters DM, Thabit G, et al. The mechanism of joint capsule thermal modification in an *in vitro* sheep model. *Clin Orthop* 2000;370:236–249.

37. Lopez MJ, Hayashi K, Fanton GS, et al. The effect of radiofrequency on the ultrastructure of joint capsule collagen. *Arthroscopy* 1998;14:495–501.

38. Hoad-Reddick A, Hughes P, Brownson P, et al. Histological changes in the shoulder joint capsule following thermal capsular shrinkage for multi-directional instability. In: Proceedings of the 8th ICSS conference, Cape Town, South Africa, 2001.

39. Obrzut SL, Hecht P, Hayashi K, et al. The effect of radiofrequency energy on the length and temperature properties if the glenohumeral joint capsule. *Arthroscopy* 1998;14:395–400.

40. Hecht P, Hayashi K, Cooley AJ, et al. The thermal effect of monopolar radiofrequency energy on the properties of joint capsule: an *in vivo* histologic study using a sheep model. *Am J Sports Med* 1998;26:808–814.

41. Osmond C, Hecht P, Hayashi K, et al. Comparative effects of laser and radiofrequency energy on joint capsule. *Clin Orthop* 2000;375:286–294.

42. Hecht P, Hayashi K, Lu Y, et al. Monopolar radiofrequency energy effects on joint capsular tissue: potential treatment for joint instability: an *in vivo* mechanical, morphological, and biochemical study using an ovine model. *Am J Sports Med* 1999;27:761–771.

43. Tibone JE, McMahon PJ, Shrader TA, ct al. Glenohumeral joint translation after arthroscopic, nonablative, thermal capsuloplasty with a laser. *Am J Sports Med* 1998;26: 495–498.

44. Anderson K, McCarty EC, Warren RF. Thermal capsulorrhaphy: where are we today? *Sports Med Arthrosc Rev* 1999;7:117–127.

45. Hayahshi K, Massa KL, Thabit G, et al. Histologic evaluation of the glenohumeral joint capsule after laser-assisted capsular shift procedure for glenohumeral instability. *Am J Sports Med* 1999;27:162–167.

46. Tyler TF, Calabree GJ, Parker RD, et al. Electrothermally assisted capsulorrhaphy (ETAC): a new surgical method for glenohumeral instability and its rehabilitation considerations. *J Orthop Sports Phys Ther* 2000;30:390–400.

47. Frostick SP, Sinopidis C, A1 Maskari S, et al. Arthroscopic capsular shrinkage of the shoulder for the treatment of patients with multidirectional instability—minimum 2 year follow up. *Arthroscopy* 2002 (in press).

48. Fanton GS. Arthroscopic electrothermal surgery of the shoulder. *Oper Tech Sports Med* 1998;6:139–146.

49. Frohling MA, Sclote W, Wolburg-Buchholz K. Nonselective nerve fibre damage in peripheral nerves after experimental thermocoagulation. *Acta Neurochir* 1998;140:1297–1302.

50. Hughes P, Hoad-Reddick A, Hovery C, et al. Does capsular shrinkage compromise axillary nerve function? In: Proceedings of the 8th ICSS conference, Cape Town, South Africa, 2001.

51. Mc Farland EG, Urquhart E, McCarthy EF. Histological evaluation of the shoulder capsule in normal shoulders, unstable shoulders and after failed thermal capsulorrhaphy. In: Proceedings of the 8th ICSS conference, Cape Town, South Africa, 2001.

52. Shellock FG, Shields CL. Temperatur changes associated with radiofrequency energy-induced heating of bovine capsular tissue: evaluation of bipolar RF electrodes. *Arthroscopy* 2000;16:348–358.

53. Rath E, Richmond J. Capsular disruption as a complication of thermal alteration of the glenohumeral capsule. *Arthroscopy* 2000;17:10.

THERMAL CAPSULORRHAPHY: INDICATIONS, TECHNIQUE, AND RESULTS

SUMANT G. KRISHNAN AND RICHARD J. HAWKINS

INDICATIONS

As the treatment of shoulder instability continues to evolve, the application of new and exciting techniques becomes commonplace. Arthroscopically assisted evaluation and management of glenohumeral instability provide appeal for both surgeons and patients (1–5). Reduced perioperative morbidity and pain, combined with less invasive tissue handling, have led to the increased popularity of arthroscopic techniques (6–9). Nevertheless, until recently, the success rate achieved with standard open stabilization techniques was not replicated by previously reported arthroscopic procedures (7,10–16). The failure to address capsular laxity adequately during routine arthroscopic shoulder stabilization has been cited as the reason for the disparity between open and arthroscopic outcomes (3,17–22). With current techniques using suture anchors and capsular plication, some authors have reported, in the peer-reviewed literature, arthroscopic results that approach and even match those achieved with open surgical procedures (7,19,23,24). Accompanying these advances in minimally invasive arthroscopic surgical techniques, the use of thermal capsulorrhaphy has risen to the forefront in the arthroscopic treatment of the increased glenohumeral capsular volume associated with shoulder instability (13,25–31).

Hippocrates first documented the use of thermal energy to reduce or eliminate glenohumeral instability in 400 BC, by applying a heated iron to the exposed axillae of soldiers who suffered recurrent shoulder dislocations (32). Current clinical applications are based on sound basic science work documenting the denaturing and shrinkage of the collagen triple helix with the application of heat (28,33–42). This procedure is followed by immediate immobilization to maintain and increase the shortening effects (26,33,28,

S. G. Krishnan: Shoulder and Elbow Service, W.B. Carrell Memorial Clinic, Dallas, Texas.
R. J. Hawkins: Steadman Hawkins Clinic, Vail, Colorado.

40,41,43.). However, the long-term biomechanical properties of this heated capsular tissue remain unknown (25,33,41,43–45). Basic science work by Markel and others documents the return of these structures to apparently normal histologic appearance by approximately 6 weeks. Surgeons still must proceed with caution in the application of this rapidly evolving technique until further peer-reviewed outcome studies clearly document clinical benefit matching that of open procedures. Nevertheless, in spite of these fears, the potential elimination of capsular laxity by the use of thermal energy provides strong promise in improving the outcomes achieved with current arthroscopic techniques for all forms of glenohumeral instability (25,26,40,46–50).

Anterior Glenohumeral Instability

Traumatic or Acute Instability

The classic capsulolabral injury (Bankart lesion) that accompanies acute traumatic anterior instability must necessarily be repaired during the arthroscopic management of such an injury (1,4,5,7–10,16,29,51–56). Bigliani et al. and Speer et al. clearly demonstrated *(in vitro)* the associated capsular stretching and plastic deformation that necessarily occurs before the traumatic labral detachment (57,58). This elongation of the inferior glenohumeral ligament after an anterior shoulder dislocation may reduce its ability to prevent pathologic humeral head translation in the abducted or externally rotated position.

As stated previously, failure to establish and recreate normal capsular tension adequately may be one of the key elements leading to poor results after the arthroscopic management of acute traumatic anterior instability (16,19,22,52). Open techniques inherently address both the labral and the capsular injuries and have been demonstrated *(in vitro)* significantly to restore the capsular strength necessary to resist pathologic anterior glenohumeral translation (57,59–62). Although early arthroscopic techniques strongly emphasized anatomic reduction and fixation of the labral injury, current arthroscopic management also includes replicating the capsular tension that is consistently gained during open surgical procedures (7,12,17,30,63).

Thermal energy has been used by several authors to shrink the inferior (and occasionally the middle) glenohumeral ligament, after completion of the labral repair (20,26,44,46). This has been reported both alone and in conjunction with suture plication of the anteroinferior capsule, in an attempt to restore normal capsular tension (7,46). Most current arthroscopic suturing instruments cannot address both the capsular tension and the labral disorder in one technical movement; consequently, instead of using two arthroscopic sutures and passes, some surgeons prefer to repair the labral injury and to add thermal capsulorrhaphy. Indications for the application of heat have varied from use in all patients with traumatic anterior instability to selective shrinkage only in those cases demonstrating intraoperative inability of the capsule to control humeral head translation after anatomic labral repair.

A less commonly encountered pathologic feature is traumatic anterior instability without a classic Bankart labral injury. In these situations, reestablishing appropriate capsular tension is paramount in the arthroscopic or open treatment of this form of instability. Again, thermal capsulorrhaphy may (either by itself or with concomitant suture plication) be a valuable technique for addressing the capsular laxity.

Atraumatic or Chronic Instability

Although less common than multidirectional or posterior causes, atraumatic anterior instability has been reported after repetitive minor traumatic events. This results in stretching of the anterior capsule, rather than frank detachment or rupture (23,47,64–66). As reported in both the orthopaedic and rheumatologic literature, certain persons are genetically predisposed to ligamentous laxity, which may lead to symptomatic glenohumeral instability by repetitive activities (21).

In these cases, reduction of capsular volume is the necessary step in surgical management, assuming that nonoperative measures fail. As mentioned before, arthroscopic suture plication of the capsule can mimic the same technique performed in open surgical procedures. Application of thermal energy to the capsule adds another potential weapon that can be used arthroscopically to reduce this capsular redundancy and to restore the normal caliber of the stretched inferior and middle glenohumeral ligaments. Furthermore, thermal capsulorrhaphy in this setting may allow the surgeon globally to restore capsular tension (with a "belt and suspenders" concept), because it can be difficult to assess adequately either the amount of volume reduction obtained with arthroscopic suture plication of the capsule or the acute effect of thermal treatment.

In the chronic situation, surgeons may be faced with a revision stabilization situation. Several reports have docu-mented that prior surgery and revision shoulder stabilization are both significant risk factors for failure of arthroscopic treatment (25,63,67). Furthermore, a history of prior surgical treatment has been documented as a risk factor for failed outcome after thermal shrinkage (25,45). In this population of patients, it is unknown whether the scarring of the capsule from previous surgical treatment responds similarly to thermal treatment as compared with native tissue.

Posterior Glenohumeral Instability

Traumatic or Acute Instability

Involuntary posterior subluxation, especially in the forward flexed, adducted, internally rotated position, can be a painful and disabling clinical problem (68–72). Posterior subluxation or dislocation can result from an isolated traumatic event. In such a case, a posterior capsulolabral injury (reverse Bankart lesion) has been documented, with associated plastic capsular deformation similar to anterior cases. Similar to the treatment of Bankart lesions, the posterior capsulolabral lesion must undergo anatomic repair to the glenoid rim before one addresses the capsular tension. Once the medial capsular anchor has been established, assessment of adequate capsular tension that would resist pathologic humeral head translation should be performed. Any associated capsular redundancy must be addressed.

Thermal energy, applied to the posterior band of the inferior glenohumeral ligament and posterior capsule, provides an appealing source for reducing pathologic posterior capsular volume (46,48). The posterior capsule of the glenohumeral joint is less stout than its anterior counterpart. Consequently, suture plication in this area may not appropriately restore the necessary thickness of the posterior static glenohumeral restraints. Heat to this capsule can provide a potential augmentation to the thickness of these posterior structures and can allow reduction in the pathologic posterior translation of the shoulder.

Atraumatic or Chronic Instability

Repetitive posterior capsular stretching leading to recurrent posterior subluxation and clinical instability is a more commonly encountered clinical situation (68–72). In these cases, the posterior subluxation may be either voluntary or involuntary. Voluntary subluxation has been shown in numerous outcome series to have the poorest surgical results, whether open or arthroscopic (68–72). Consequently, the diagnosis and treatment of symptomatic posterior instability remain tough clinical challenges, and nonoperative management is the mainstay of treatment.

In these difficult surgical cases, reduction of capsular volume is paramount. However, the often patulous nature of the posterior capsule makes open techniques less successful than their associated anterior counterparts. In addition, suture plication is also necessarily less assuring, because of the relatively decreased collagen density in the posterior (especially midposterior and posterosuperior) capsule. Although thermal energy should be applied with caution to relatively thin tissue, application of heat to the posterior capsule can be an extremely useful therapeutic endeavor in reducing symptomatic posterior subluxation (46,48). Such thermal treatment and shrinkage may aid in restoring an adequate amount of collagen to the posterior capsule and may thus allow this static structure appropriately to resist pathologic posterior humeral head translation.

Again, in the revision situation, a scarred posterior capsule may not respond similarly to nonoperatively treated collagen. Caution must be exercised in this situation.

Multidirectional Glenohumeral Instability

The classification of multidirectional instability (MDI) includes those patients with excessive and symptomatic inferior glenohumeral translation accompanying both anterior and posterior excessive translations (18,73). This terminology becomes confusing when one attempts to evaluate the results obtained from various published series in the treatment of these patients. Despite these difficulties in classification and terminology, most authors remain concerned with the potential genetic predisposition of these patients to glenohumeral hyperlaxity and potential pathologic plastic deformation of the collagenous capsule (14,49,73–75).

The origin of MDI is most commonly atraumatic, although traumatic capsulolabral injury and concomitant capsular deformation may also be causative (73,74). The capsular laxity and capsulolabral injury, if present, contribute to documented alterations in glenohumeral mechanics and lead to a spectrum from subluxation to dislocation. Although the initial management of these patients is always nonoperative, failure of conservative management suggests that surgical management may be attempted (18,73,76–78). As described by Neer and Foster, the abnormal capsular laxity and volume must be addressed at the time of surgical management (73). Furthermore, beginning with Neer, many authors have documented the associated widening of the rotator interval in the multidirectionally unstable shoulder, a condition that likely contributes both to excessive capsular volume and to inferior laxity in the neutral position (49,73,79–84). Classically, the abnormal capsular volume and pathologic laxity have been reduced through an open inferior capsular shift and superior rotator interval plication or closure (14,18,73).

Several reports have documented acceptable success rates with arthroscopic capsular shift procedures in the treatment of MDI (67,75,85). However, reported studies after thermal capsulorrhaphy for MDI (either alone or in conjunction with arthroscopic capsular shifts) remain sparse (49,86–89). Nevertheless, the adjunctive use of thermal capsulorrhaphy in these patients holds much appeal, because the thermal energy potentially can reduce global capsular laxity and vol-

ume. Accompanied by arthroscopic rotator interval capsular closure or thermal treatment of the rotator interval (and possibly suture plication of the redundant capsule), thermal energy can effectively address the voluminous axillary pouch lateral to the glenoid anteriorly, inferiorly, and posteriorly.

Despite the negative prejudicial effect of a multiply operated shoulder with MDI, thermal capsulorrhaphy may still grant the surgeon a viable option for addressing abnormal capsular tissue even in a revision situation. Nonetheless, until further reports are published in the peer-reviewed literature, surgeons must exercise caution when using thermal capsulorrhaphy alone in the treatment of MDI.

Athletes

Contact Athletes

Regardless of the direction or cause of instability, caution should be exercised in the application of thermal energy to the capsule of a contact athlete. O'Neill suggested that contact sports participation is a risk factor for treatment failure in previous reports on arthroscopic stabilization procedures (90). Because the long-term biomechanical properties of this heated tissue remain unknown, the advent of a new traumatic injury in this patient population remains a real concern. Sperling et al. suggested that, before allowing patients to return to contact sports participation, further basic research is necessary to document the fate of this altered capsular tissue (45).

Another recognized pathologic entity in this athletic population is combined anterior and posterior instability, without either inferior instability or multidirectional hyperlaxity. In this difficult situation, surgical management involves addressing both the anterior and posterior disorders. This treatment may be performed with standard open techniques, with combined open surgery on one side and arthroscopic surgery on the other, or with completely arthroscopic techniques. Thermal capsulorrhaphy may be very useful in these challenging cases, to address capsular tension in one or both directions.

Throwing Athletes

The adaptive changes in the shoulder of the throwing athlete have been thoroughly documented (47,64,65). Most of these athletes demonstrate increased external rotation and decreased internal rotation in their throwing shoulder in abduction, compared with the nondominant extremity. This may lead to a physiologic increase in anterior capsular laxity without symptomatic instability, owing to the repetitive throwing motion. Such an increase in anterior capsular laxity can also be accompanied by an increase in anterior glenohumeral translation, which may predispose the throwing shoulder to the disorders of internal impingement, partial-thickness tears of the rotator cuff, superior labral anterior and posterior (SLAP) lesions, and even instability in this population of patients (47,64,65,91).

Consequently, the throwing athlete may experience shoulder pain and negatively altered performance. After conservative rehabilitative measures have failed, numerous authors have also documented poor results with operative treatments in these athletes (12,47,64,66). Andrews and Dugas suggested that the increase in anterior glenohumeral capsular laxity in these patients is a strong contributor to the previous failures in surgical management, which neglected to address the capsular component of the disorder (47).

Before the advent of current arthroscopic techniques, an open capsular reconstructive procedure was the only technique affording reduction in this acquired anterior capsular laxity. However, several authors documented disappointing results, regarding return to previous level of performance, in the high-level throwing athlete after open capsular surgical procedures (47,64,65,91). Hence the use of anterior thermal capsulorrhaphy in the throwing athlete (in addition to the arthroscopic assessment and treatment of associated disorders) is extremely appealing, because this minimally invasive and less traumatic technique appears to afford the throwing athlete the best chance of returning to preinjury levels of performance.

A less commonly seen entity in the throwing athlete is symptomatic posterior glenohumeral subluxation, usually manifested during the deceleration and follow-through phases of throwing (47,64,69). Because of the relatively decreased internal rotation in the abducted position seen in the throwing shoulder, most of these athletes develop relatively tighter posterior capsular structures. However, repetitive trauma can create a pathologic increase in posterior glenohumeral translation. First-line management in these situations always involves proprioceptive retraining and strengthening of the posterior rotator cuff musculature, posterior deltoid, and scapular stabilizers (64). In the rare patient in whom such nonoperative management fails, surgical management must address the symptomatic posterior capsular laxity. Unfortunately, previously described open techniques violate both the posterior deltoid and the posterior cuff (infraspinatus) and potentially compromise the throwing athlete's ability to return to prior performance levels (47,68). The use of arthroscopic techniques in these delicate situations and of thermal energy to reduce redundant posterior capsular laxity may allow reduction of the disorder without compromising important muscular structures.

Our Current Indications

The enthusiasm for the current use of thermal energy in the shoulder likely stems from its relative ease of application, compared with other arthroscopic techniques for reducing capsular volume. However, the presence of a technology does not mandate that the technology should unequivocally be used. Inappropriate application of this technique will only lead to iatrogenic complications and dissatisfaction with its use. To this end, we outline our personal experience with thermal capsulorrhaphy.

Anterior Instability

In our early experience with thermal capsulorrhaphy, we applied laser thermal energy to the capsule of selected patients who presented with symptomatic anterior instability, whether acute or chronic. Basic science work has documented that, despite different mechanisms, laser treatment and radiofrequency energy achieve similar tissue modification; however, laser treatment produces steeper temperature increases accompanying peak temperature. As our clinical experience evolved, we used radiofrequency thermal capsulorrhaphy accompanied by anatomic reconstruction of the Bankart lesion (if present) with arthroscopic suture anchor fixation. When a Bankart lesion was not present, the anterior and inferior capsule was heated in its entirety.

Currently, we continue to use radiofrequency thermal capsulorrhaphy on a frequent basis. After arthroscopic reattachment of any capsulolabral injury, we assess the degree of capsular laxity and capsular redundancy and the amount of excessive pathologic humeral head translation. Guided by these parameters, we augment our labral repair with arthroscopic suture plication of the glenohumeral capsule, by arthroscopically shifting the anterior band of the inferior glenohumeral ligament medially and superiorly. Finally, we add thermal energy to the anterior and inferior capsule, in an attempt to shrink and thicken both the inferior and middle glenohumeral ligaments.

We continue to remain cautious with the use of thermal energy in contact athletes and seek to augment these patients with suture plication in nearly every case. Regarding the subtle anterior capsular laxity that may be present in the throwing athlete, we proceed in a logical fashion: if the thrower demonstrates no clinical symptoms of instability, we use our preoperative examination as well as our examination with the patient under anesthesia to assist in determining pathologic translation from nonpathologic hyperlaxity. After arthroscopic treatment of any concomitant intraarticular disorder, we reassess humeral translation and selectively determine whether reduction in capsular laxity (with the use of thermal capsulorrhaphy) is still necessary.

We also remain cautious with the use of thermal capsulorrhaphy in surgical revision of instability, whether or not the primary surgical procedure was open or arthroscopic. We do believe that a surgically altered capsule may not respond to thermal treatment in the same manner as an untreated capsule. Consequently, we arthroscopically assess this capsular situation and tissue response and proceed accordingly, often relying on suture plication (if proceeding arthroscopically) or open reconstruction as necessary. Our preference is an arthroscopic operation for the first revision procedure or for a failed open stabilization. For a multiple revision or a failed arthroscopic attempt, we do not hesitate to proceed to open surgical treatment.

Posterior Instability

Similarly, in our early experience, we arthroscopically applied laser thermal energy alone to the posterior capsule when attempting to reduce symptomatic posterior humeral subluxation. We have continued to encounter a reverse Bankart lesion much less commonly than we encounter a redundant and patulous posterior capsule without frank labral detachment.

Currently, we reduce and anatomically reattach any posterior capsulolabral injury and restore normal capsular tension through the combined use of arthroscopic suture plication techniques and radiofrequency thermal capsulorrhaphy. The posterior capsule is a much less robust structure than its anterior counterpart, especially in the midposterior and posterosuperior regions. However, the posterior band of the inferior glenohumeral ligament is usually thicker and more responsive to thermal treatment. We believe that the heat probe may prove to be an important tool in the comprehensive treatment of posterior instability and may help to reduce the excessive posterior capsular recess effectively without the morbidity of open reconstruction. We are also currently investigating the concomitant arthroscopic suture closure (with or without thermal treatment) of the rotator interval during the correction of isolated posterior instability.

As in revision of anterior instability, we proceed with caution during the thermal treatment of surgically altered posterior capsular tissue. In each case, we arthroscopically evaluate the redundant tissue and intraoperatively decide on appropriate arthroscopic or open management. Again, for a first revision or a failed open stabilization, we prefer an arthroscopic operation, with suture plication or heat. For a multiple revision or a failed arthroscopic procedure, we lean toward open stabilization techniques.

Multidirectional Instability

We initially began using laser thermal energy globally to treat the multidirectionally unstable shoulder. Thermal energy can be used to address the anteroinferior and the posteroinferior capsular recesses, by reducing the volume of these pathologically lax pouches. However, in our experience, the incidence of recurrent instability with either isolated laser or isolated radiofrequency thermal energy was unacceptable.

In our current practice, we arthroscopically assess the amount of laxity and the quality of tissue in the pathologic shoulder with MDI. If the capsular tissue appears amenable to arthroscopic shifting techniques (without detaching the capsule from either the humerus or the glenoid), we augment suture plication with radiofrequency thermal capsu-

lorrhaphy. We use suture plication in the areas of more symptomatic instability (whether anterior, posterior, or both anterior and posterior) and systematically add thermal treatment to the inferior capsule as well as to both the anterior and posterior capsules.

Several authors have documented the consistent presence of a rotator interval lesion in producing the inferior laxity demonstrated in MDI. Our experience with rotator interval plication or thermal treatment is early, and we have begun to combine rotation interval plication with heat treatment in the patient with MDI.

If the capsular tissue is of poor quality, either through heredity or previous surgical treatment, we use the arthroscopic assessment of that tissue to guide us in proceeding to standard open inferior capsular shift procedures. We systematically use an open inferior capsular shift (usually through an anterior approach) for any multiply operated MDI shoulder or for any shoulder with MDI and resting inferior subluxation. Occasionally, we augment this open anterior approach with arthroscopic thermal or suture plication posteriorly.

Contact Athletes

We have not encountered the same postoperative clinical difficulties reported by other authors with thermal capsulorrhaphy in contact athletes. However, even as recent reports cite return to contact sports participation as a significant risk factor for failure of open stabilization procedures, we also counsel our contact athletes on the potential risks of returning to their sport after an arthroscopic stabilization (with or without thermal treatment). We understand the theoretical fears inherent in the lack of knowledge of the ultimate biomechanical fate of thermally treated tissue, but we remain optimistic that this technique will continue to hold promise in all patients who place significant athletic demands on the glenohumeral joint.

For athletes who demonstrate both anterior and posterior instability (with no inferior component), we prefer to treat the less symptomatic side arthroscopically with suture plication and thermal capsulorrhaphy and the other side with an open procedure. Usually, this involves an arthroscopic treatment of the posterior capsule and an open anterior modified Bankart reconstruction. We have had 12 such cases and have experienced no treatment failures or recurrent instability at this time (minimum follow-up, 12 months). Four of these 12 patients have returned to their previous level of professional football play.

Throwing Athletes

This population of patients represents our strongest indication for the use of thermal capsulorrhaphy. The demands of the throwing shoulder, as well as avoiding the potential for career-threatening loss of motion, have led us to a significant increase in the arthroscopic management of instability in these athletes. Consequently, we apply the thermal probe routinely in all patients with anterior and posterior instability and MDI in the throwing shoulder.

Andrews and Dugas documented the systematic use of the heat probe adjunctively to treat subtle anterior glenohumeral laxity in all throwers with either SLAP lesions or partial-thickness articular-sided rotator cuff tears associated with internal impingement (47). We preoperatively assess the clinical symptoms and amount of glenohumeral translation, correlate this with the examination while the patient is under anesthesia, and finally factor in the intraarticular arthroscopic findings before we apply thermal capsulorrhaphy techniques. In our experience, this approach allows us to differentiate more clearly those throwing athletes manifesting symptomatic glenohumeral instability from those with mere clinically present hyperlaxity. Again, we use thermal capsulorrhaphy in those throwers who exhibit both clinical instability *and* laxity.

TECHNIQUE

Instruments

As discussed elsewhere, the transfer of thermal energy to *in vivo* tissues can be accomplished through laser light, electrical energy, or radiofrequency energy (92–95). A comprehensive documentation of the instruments available for thermal capsulorrhaphy is beyond the scope of this text. The goal of capsular shrinkage involves full-thickness alteration of the collagenous capsular tissue; commercially available devices for this purpose include the holmium:yttrium-aluminum-garnet laser, bipolar radiofrequency devices (Arthrocare Corp., Sunnyvale, CA, and Mitek Products, Johnson & Johnson, Westwood, MA), and monopolar radiofrequency devices (Oratec Interventions, Menlo Park, CA). Differences in technical design affect the depth of tissue penetration during thermal capsulorrhaphy (33–39,92–95).

Surgical Technique

Basic science work reports that the response of tissue to thermal energy depends on both temperature and time (33–39). The optimal temperature for appropriate tissue penetration and for collagen denaturation and shrinkage is 65°C. The amount of time that the heat probe is left in one place also affects tissue response.

Thermal capsulorrhaphy can be performed through standard anterior and posterior arthroscopic portals. DeFelice et al. described an accessory posteroinferior portal that reportedly provides safe access to the central portion of the inferior

axillary recess, if this area cannot be reached through the typical arthroscopic portals (48).

Patient positioning can be either beach-chair or lateral decubitus, depending on the surgeon's preference. Adequate visualization and fluid flow are paramount during this procedure. Abrams raised the valid concern that water temperature and fluid flow may adversely affect the actual tissue temperature (and consequently the amount and depth of transferred thermal energy) during the arthroscopic procedure (46). Work is currently under way to determine whether traction on the arm during thermal capsulorrhaphy may also adversely affect tissue response and the amount of capsular shrinkage intraoperatively (R.J. Hawkins, *unpublished data,* 2001). Hence most surgeons reduce flow, and some reduce arm traction (if the patient is in the lateral position) during thermal capsulorrhaphy. However, with flow and traction reduced, it can prove difficult to reach the desired areas of the capsule after labral fixation.

As the probe is moved across the glenohumeral capsule, temperature is monitored, and the tissue is examined for quality of response to the thermal energy. Response is visually confirmed by alteration in color of the capsular tissue (the tissue appears yellower and flatter) and by visible shrinkage of the tissue. Thicker, more collagenous areas demonstrate more robust responses than thinner areas of the capsule. Care should be exercised to avoid overheating the capsule, either through too high a temperature or through leaving the probe in one place for too long, especially in the axillary recess.

Basic science reports have documented a more favorable capsular response and outcome with the use of a "grid" pattern during thermal capsulorrhaphy (94). This technique employs the creation of parallel "cornrows" with single passes of the thermal probe from medially to laterally, leaving strips of untreated capsule between the treated rows (Fig. 38.1).

Our Technique

Thermal capsulorrhaphy is performed using standard anterior and posterior arthroscopic portals. We have not found the use of an accessory posteroinferior or anteroinferior portal to be necessary in the majority of cases. We prefer the use of a monopolar device, which not only presets temperature but also measures contact tissue temperature at the tip of the probe. This further allows for a greater depth of penetration of thermal energy into the capsular tissue and hence must be appropriately used to avoid iatrogenic damage to either the capsule or the underlying vital structures, such as the axillary nerve.

During all cases of thermal capsulorrhaphy, temperature is closely monitored. Flow is restricted appropriately to compromise between good visualization and accurate delivery of thermal energy to the capsular tissue. We perform all

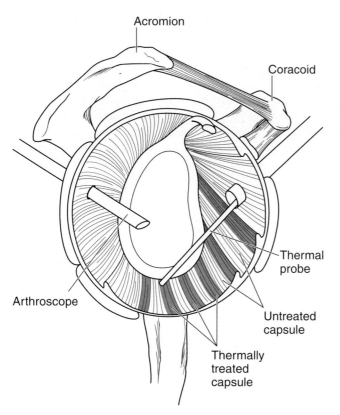

FIGURE 38.1 Drawing depicting our preferred "grid" or "corn-row" pattern that should be applied to the glenohumeral capsule during the technique of thermal capsulorrhaphy. Note the untreated strips of capsular tissue present between heated areas.

arthroscopic cases with the patient in the lateral decubitus position and have begun to study the effect of arm traction on the capsular response to thermal shrinkage.

Anterior thermal capsulorrhaphy is performed with the arthroscope in the standard posterior viewing portal and the heat probe in the anterior portal (Fig. 38.2). We bend the tip of the thermal probe 30 to 40 degrees, to allow easier access to the entire capsule. Beginning in the most anteroinferior portion of the axillary recess, the anterior capsular structures are heated from medially to laterally, progressing from inferiorly to superiorly. Rows are created, with 5-mm strips of normal tissue between the thermally treated capsular areas. Thermal treatment creates a grid of medial-to-lateral "cornrows" from the inferior axillary recess to the middle glenohumeral ligament (Fig. 38.1) Caution should be exercised in the inferior recess, where the axillary nerve is vulnerable if heating is excessively long or with an inappropriate temperature. If access is difficult, we do not hesitate to use a "paintbrush" technique to heat as much of the capsule as we can reach.

Similarly, posterior thermal capsulorrhaphy is performed using standard portals (Fig. 38.3). The arthroscope is placed in the anterior portal, and the heat probe is placed in the posterior portal. The tip of the thermal probe is bent to 90

degrees, to allow easier access to the entire posterior capsule. Again, thermal treatment is begun in the posteroinferior portion of the axillary recess, and it is continued until the entire posterior capsule has been treated in the grid or corn-row pattern.

Thermal capsulorrhaphy for MDI should proceed in an orderly fashion: initially, the heat probe is placed through the anterior portal, and the anterior and anteroinferior capsular structures are treated. Special attention should be paid to heating the inferior axillary recess completely, because inferior instability is the hallmark lesion in MDI. With switching sticks, the thermal device is subsequently placed in the posterior portal, and the posterior and posteroinferior capsular structures are addressed. Again, the inferior pouch mandates close attention to detail, as well as caution because of the proximity of the axillary nerve to the inferior capsule. Further, we avoid reheating previously treated capsular areas when we switch portals. Finally, we have begun to investigate suture plication and closure with or without thermally treating the widened rotator interval, both in the case of MDI and also in patients with chronic anterior or posterior instability with a concomitant pathologic rotator interval capsule. The rotator interval is addressed with the heat probe in the anterior portal.

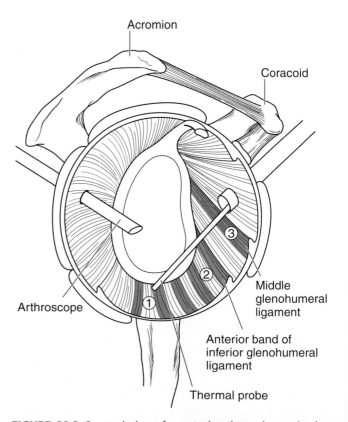

FIGURE 38.2 Our technique for anterior thermal capsulorrhaphy. The arthroscope is in the posterior portal, the heat probe is in the anterior portal, and the procedure is performed in an orderly fashion from anteroinferior to anterosuperior.

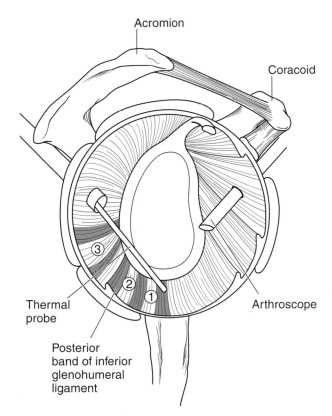

Acromion

Coracoid

Thermal probe

Posterior band of inferior glenohumeral ligament

Arthroscope

FIGURE 38.3 Our technique for posterior thermal capsulorrhaphy. Conversely, the arthroscope is now in the anterior portal, with the heat probe in the posterior portal. The procedure is again performed systematically from posteroinferior to posterosuperior.

POSTOPERATIVE REHABILITATION

Postoperative immobilization is one of the most important components of thermal capsulorrhaphy for the glenohumeral joint. Several animal studies have suggested that the fibroblastic proliferation and new collagen formation that follow thermal treatment may take several months and may not even begin for a few weeks postoperatively, although some shrinkage does occur immediately (33–39,93). Consequently, early activities or rehabilitative exercises that are too aggressive may potentially stretch the heated capsule and may create untoward laxity of the thermally treated tissue. Hence proper immobilization is necessary to maintain the acute effects of thermal capsular shrinkage. Research has demonstrated that, without a postoperative immobilization protocol, thermally treated rabbit patellar ligaments (after initial shrinkage immediately after laser heat application) stretched to their pretreatment length after 4 weeks and beyond that pretreatment length by 8 weeks (96). These reports seem to emphasize that too much early postoperative movement may stretch the thermally treated capsular tissue (counterproductively) beyond the original length and may potentially lead to treatment failure and recurrent instability.

The appropriate length of immobilization after thermal capsulorrhaphy (whether for anterior or posterior or for MDI) remains controversial (86). Nevertheless, the importance of a meticulous immobilization protocol immediately after thermal capsulorrhaphy cannot be overemphasized. Intraoperative findings and postoperative follow-up seem to indicate that only 25% to 50% of the total contracture from heat capsulorrhaphy takes place at the time of heat application (86,93). The remaining 50% to 75% of shrinkage appears to occur during the first 6 postoperative weeks (86,94). This finding correlates with the previously mentioned animal studies and indicates that a firm period of immobilization should be followed by guarded and structured mobilization, to allow new fibroblastic growth into the denatured collagen network. Such a program theoretically should maintain the desired translational effects of thermal capsulorrhaphy while maintaining a functional arc of glenohumeral motion.

Our Preferred Rehabilitation Protocol

Anterior Instability

Phase I: Immobilization and Passive Range of Motion (Weeks 1 through 5)

After arthroscopic anterior reconstruction with thermal capsulorrhaphy is performed, the shoulder is placed in a sling while the patient is in the operating room. Immobilization in a sling is continued for 3 weeks, with no motion or rehabilitation allowed, except for elbow and wrist exercises. During week 4, pendulum exercises are performed for warmup; these are accompanied by passive external rotation to 0 degrees (neutral), forward elevation to 90 degrees, and internal rotation to the belt line level. During week 5, passive range of motion is advanced to 30 degrees of external rotation, with full forward elevation and full internal rotation. Pendulum exercises are performed as warmup exercises before each session of passive range of motion, and the sling is continued for the entire 5-week postoperative period (Table 38.1).

Phase II: Active Range of Motion (Weeks 6 and 7)

The sling is discarded at the commencement of active exercises, and active range of motion begins during week 6. Again, pendulum exercises begin each session. Full forward elevation and internal rotation are encouraged. External rotation is gradually progressed from 30 degrees at week 6 to full external rotation (compared with the normal contralateral shoulder) by week 12.

Phase III: Resisted Range of Motion (Strengthening, Weeks 8 through 12)

During week 8, resisted forward flexion, external rotation, and internal rotation are begun. As previously indicated, ex-

TABLE 38.1 OUR REHABILITATION PROTOCOL FOR ANTERIOR INSTABILITY TREATED WITH THERMAL CAPSULORRHAPHY[a]

Postoperative Date	Immobilization	Rehabilitation	Forward Flexion	External Rotation	Internal Rotation
Weeks 0–3	Sling	Elbow and wrist only	None	None	None
Week 4	Sling	Phase I: passive ROM	90 degrees	0 degrees (neutral)	Belt line
Week 5	Sling	Phase I: passive ROM	Full	30 degrees	Full
Weeks 6–7	None	Phase II: active ROM	Full	Gently progress	Full
Weeks 8–12	None	Phase III: resisted ROM	Full	Full	Full

[a] ROM, range of motion.

ternal rotation is advanced to full rotation by week 12. A cord-resistance program for strengthening of the glenohumeral musculature and shrugs and rows for strengthening of the periscapular muscles are also begun during week 8. By week 12, a cautious weight-training program is incorporated into the protocol. Exercises that stress the anterior capsule (wide-gripped bench press, military press behind the head, and chest fly) are not ever permitted.

Return to Activities

Patients are allowed to shower, with the arm maintained in the same position dictated by the shoulder sling, at 1 week postoperatively. Computer-related and desk activities are allowed at 4 weeks. Chipping and putting may begin at 8 weeks, but full golf strokes may not be performed until week 12. Tennis ground strokes are permitted at 12 weeks, with no overhead strokes until 4 months postoperatively. Contact sports are not allowed until at least 6 months after the surgical procedure. Overhead throwing and stress in the provocative "late-cocking" position are restricted until 4 months postoperatively and are gradually progressed.

Posterior Instability

Immediate Postoperative Period: Strict Immobilization (Weeks 1 through 6)

After arthroscopic posterior reconstruction with thermal capsulorrhaphy is performed, the shoulder is placed in a "gunslinger" harness brace, which maintains the arm in the neutral to slightly externally rotated position, while the patient is in the operating room (Fig. 38.4). No rehabilitation is performed during the first 6 weeks after the surgical procedure (Table 38.2).

Phase I: Passive Range of Motion (Week 7)

During postoperative week 7, the "gunslinger" brace is removed, and a sling is used for 1 week longer. Passive range-of-motion exercises are allowed with full elevation in the

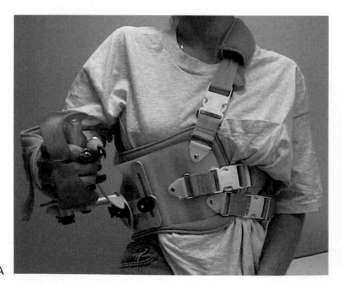

A

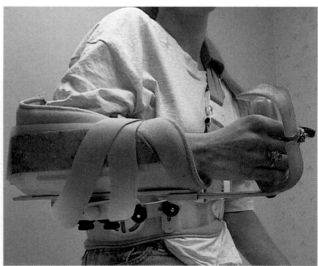

B

FIGURE 38.4 Patient in a "gunslinger" postoperative harness brace.

TABLE 38.2 OUR REHABILITATION PROTOCOL FOR POSTERIOR INSTABILITY TREATED WITH THERMAL CAPSULORRHAPHY[a]

Postoperative Date	Immobilization	Rehabilitation	Forward Flexion	External Rotation	Internal Rotation
Weeks 0–6	"Gunslinger" brace	Elbow and wrist only	None	None	None
Week 7	Sling (comfort)	Phase I: passive ROM	Full (scapular plane only)	Full	Belt line
Week 8	None	Phase II: active ROM	Full (scapular plane only)	Full	Gently progress
Weeks 9–12	None	Phase III: resisted ROM	Full (scapular plane only)	Full	Full

[a] ROM, range of motion.

scapular plane (forward elevation in the true sagittal plane is avoided, to prevent excessive stress caused by forward elevation on the posterior capsule). This is accompanied by full external rotation and internal rotation to the belt line level.

Phase II: Active Range of Motion (Week 8)
The sling is discarded at the commencement of active exercises, and active range of motion is begun in postoperative week 8. Motion is progressed to full elevation in the scapular plane (for the reasons previously detailed) and full external rotation. Internal rotation is gradually increased over weeks 8 through 12.

Phase III: Resisted Range of Motion (Strengthening, Weeks 9 through 12)
A cord-resistance program for strengthening of the glenohumeral musculature and shrugs and rows for strengthening of the periscapular muscles are begun during week 9. By week 12, a cautious weight-training program is incorporated into the protocol, with careful avoidance of posterior capsular stresses (including narrow-grip bench presses and pushups).

Return To Activities
Computer and desk activities are allowed by 8 weeks postoperatively. Golf chipping and putting are permitted in the ninth week, with restriction of full swings until 4 full

months after the surgical procedure. Tennis strokes are not allowed until at least 4 months postoperatively. Contact sports are restricted until at least the sixth postoperative month.

Multidirectional Instability

Immediate Postoperative Period: Strict Immobilization (Weeks 1 through 8)
After thermal capsulorrhaphy for MDI, the shoulder is placed in a "gunslinger" harness brace, while the patient is in the operating room. This brace maintains the arm in neutral rotation, with the brace adjusted to gently push superiorly on the arm (thereby supporting the rotator interval and the shifted inferior capsule). No rehabilitation is performed during the first 8 weeks after the surgical procedure. During early rehabilitation, all passive range-of-motion exercises and stretching are strictly avoided. We believe that *passive* stretching of the capsule is extremely detrimental in the early rehabilitation of the multidirectionally unstable shoulder. Range of motion should be recovered only through *active* exercises that use muscular cocontractions to center the humeral head on the glenoid through concavity–compression (Table 38.3).

Phase I: Passive Range of Motion
Passive range of motion is strictly avoided.

TABLE 38.3 AUTHORS' REHABILITATION PROTOCOL FOR MULTIDIRECTIONAL INSTABILITY TREATED WITH THERMAL CAPSULORRHAPHY

Postoperative Date	Immobilization	Rehabilitation	Forward Flexion	External Rotation	Internal Rotation
Weeks 0–8	Gunslinger brace	Elbow and wrist only	None	None	None
Week 9–10	Sling (comfort)	PHASE II: active ROM	Full (scapular plane only)	Full	Full
Weeks 11	None	Phase III: resisted ROM	Full (scapular plane only)	Full	Full

Note: No passive range-of-motion (ROM) or stretching exercises.

TABLE 38.4 RESULTS OF THERMAL CAPSULORRHAPHY IN THE TREATMENT OF ANTERIOR INSTABILITY

Author	Number of Patients	Bankart	Heat Source	Suture Plication	Minimum Follow-up	Recurrence of Instability
Fanton	54	N/A	RF	18/54 (33%)	24 months	10%
Hawkins	47	N/A	Laser	None	24 months	3%
Karas and Hawkins	40	16/40 (40%)	RF	None	24 months	21% (no Bankart); 31% (with Bankart)
Abrams	30	All	RF	ALL	24 months	6%
Gartsman	53	48/53 (91%)	Laser	ALL	24 months	7.5%

Phase II: Active Range of Motion (Weeks 9 and 10)

The "gunslinger" brace is discarded at the commencement of active exercises, and a sling is used for comfort only. Again, no passive range-of-motion or pendulum exercises are permitted. Active range of motion begins, with no limits on scapular plane elevation, internal rotation, and external rotation. Again, scapular plane elevation (instead of forward elevation) is preferred to prevent stress on the posterior capsule. Terminal range of motion is gradually increased throughout the entire active program

Phase III: Resisted Range of Motion (Strengthening, Week 11)

During postoperative week 11, a cord-resistance program for strengthening of the glenohumeral musculature and shrugs and rows for strengthening of the periscapular muscles are begun. At this time, terminal passive stretching and pendulum exercises are used *only* if the shoulder is very stiff on clinical examination.

Return to Activities

Recreational sporting activities of any type are not allowed until at least 3 months after the surgical procedure. Contact sports are strictly prohibited until at least 6 months postoperatively.

RESULTS

As the initial outcomes reported after thermal capsulorrhaphy begin to enter into the peer-reviewed literature, surgeons must interpret these results with caution. The relative technical ease and availability of this procedure may produce inappropriate indications that could potentially cloud what may otherwise be more favorable results. Furthermore, as basic science work continues to clarify both the role of postoperative immobilization and the eventual biomechanical properties of the thermally treated capsule, the indications and technique for this procedure will concomitantly evolve, to produce consistently favorable or unfavorable outcomes that will ultimately define the place of thermal capsulorrhaphy in the management of glenohumeral instability.

Anterior Glenohumeral Instability

Little exists in the peer-reviewed literature regarding the outcomes of thermal capsulorrhaphy for the treatment of anterior instability. Several unpublished reports and non–peer-reviewed articles form the basis of current indications and conclusions (Table 38.4).

Thabit (in *Operative Techniques in Sports Medicine*) reported on the results of 41 shoulders treated with laser-assisted capsulorrhaphy for both unidirectional instability and MDI (40). Anterior instability was present in 27 shoulders, with follow-up ranging from 2 to 12 months. Although the population is heterogeneous, the Rowe score averaged 88.2 postoperatively, and there was a strong positive inverse outcome with age. All competitive athletes returned to their preinjury level of sports participation.

Fanton (in *Operative Techniques in Sports Medicine*) reported on the results of a heterogeneous population of 54 patients with unidirectional instability and MDI, with a minimum follow-up of 2 years (20). Thirty-six patients underwent radiofrequency thermal capsulorrhaphy alone, and 18 required supplemental capsulolabral suture fixation. The success rate was reported to exceed 90%, with only six patients having fair or poor results. Two complications (one postoperative adhesive capsulitis, and one transient axillary neuritis) occurred.

Hawkins et al. (at the annual meeting of the American Shoulder and Elbow Surgeons [ASES]) reported on the results of 47 laser-treated patients operated on between 1994 and 1997, with a minimum follow-up of 2 years (27). Failure of the procedure, defined as recurrence of symptomatic instability or recalcitrant pain or stiffness, occurred in one patient (3%). The ASES score improved from a preoperative average of 63 (out of a possible 100) to 94 postoperatively. Average postoperative patient satisfaction was 9 (on a 10-point scale). No patients suffered axillary nerve neuritis or neuropraxia or postoperative adhesive capsulitis.

Karas et al. (at the annual meeting of the American Academy of Orthopaedic Surgeons [AAOS]) reported on the results of 40 patients treated with radiofrequency thermal capsulorrhaphy between 1997 and 1998, with a minimum follow-up of 2 years (including five contact athletes) (88). Sixteen patients underwent an associated arthroscopic Bankart reconstruction at the time of heat treatment for anterior instability. Failure (symptomatic instability, recalcitrant pain, or intractable postoperative stiffness) occurred in five patients (31%). In the 24 patients managed without a Bankart lesion, treatment failure occurred in another five patients (21%). The preoperative ASES score (with a Bankart reconstruction) improved from an average of 71 to 98 postoperatively. The preoperative ASES score (without a Bankart lesion) rose from 69 to 94 postoperatively. Patient satisfaction averaged 9.6 out of 10 points (with an associated Bankart lesion) and 8.8 (without a Bankart lesion).

Abrams (in *Instructional Course Lectures*) has also reported on 30 patients treated for symptomatic anterior instability with a Bankart lesion, with a minimum follow-up of 2 years (46). All patients underwent arthroscopic treatment of the instability, and, according to the reporting surgeon, this population represents the approximately 20% of anterior shoulder reconstructions requiring additional capsular tension after anatomic capsulolabral fixation. In these 30 shoulders, arthroscopic suture anchor repair of the labral injury was followed by capsular tensioning of the inferior and middle glenohumeral ligaments with radiofrequency thermal treatment and, if necessary, suture plication for poorly responding capsular tissue. Success rate for this combined approach was reported at 94%.

Gartsman et al. (in the *Journal of Bone and Joint Surgery*) reported on the arthroscopic treatment of anteroinferior glenohumeral instability in 53 patients, with a minimum follow-up of 2 years (7). Bankart lesions were addressed in 48 patients. Laser-assisted thermal capsulorrhaphy supplemented suture plication in the restoration of capsular tension in 48 patients. The overall mean ASES score improved from 45.5 to 91.7 points. According to the system of Rowe et al., no patients demonstrated a good or excellent preoperative rating; postoperatively, 92% of patients (49 of 53) demonstrated good or excellent Rowe scores at follow-up. The University of California Los Angeles shoulder score improved from 17.6 to 32.0 (out of 35 points) at final review. Four patients (7.5%) demonstrated failure of the procedure because of recurrent instability.

Posterior Glenohumeral Instability

Even less has been published regarding the treatment of posterior shoulder instability with thermal capsulorrhaphy. Because of the relatively rare nature of the lesion, reported series have small numbers of patients (Table 38.5).

Hawkins et al. (at the annual meeting of the ASES) reported on nine patients with posterior instability treated with isolated laser capsulorrhaphy (27). Minimum follow-up was 2 years. No recurrences of instability were reported. One patient underwent capsular releases for excessive capsular tightness refractory to conservative management.

Karas et al. (at the annual meeting of the AAOS) reported on 12 patients, with a minimum follow-up of 2 years, who were treated solely with radiofrequency thermal capsulorrhaphy for recalcitrant posterior instability (88). Failure of this management occurred in two patients (16%). The preoperative ASES average score of 58 improved to 90 postoperatively. Patient satisfaction after surgery averaged 9 points out of 10.

Abrams (in *Instructional Course Lectures*) reviewed 25 cases of posterior instability treated with a combination arthroscopic suture plication and radiofrequency thermal capsulorrhaphy (46). Minimum follow-up was 2 years. The success rate was reported at 92% for this combined technique. The role of rotator interval capsular plication (rotator interval arthroscopic capsular closure between the superior band of the middle glenohumeral ligament and the superior glenohumeral ligament) was emphasized in this series.

Multidirectional Glenohumeral Instability

Among the earliest applications of thermal capsulorrhaphy was the arthroscopic management of MDI, which gave surgeons a technically easier procedure for reducing abnormal capsular laxity and volume. Reports detailing the outcome of these procedures have produced widely varied results (Table 38.6).

Karas et al. (at the annual meeting of the AAOS) reported on 17 patients treated only by radiofrequency thermal capsulorrhaphy for MDI, with a minimum follow-up of 2 years (88). Nine patients (53%) experienced clinical failure of the procedure. Nevertheless, the preoperative ASES score of 59.5 significantly improved to 97 postoperatively. Moreover, average patient satisfaction was nine points out of ten. No complications were reported.

Miniaci et al. (at the annual meeting of the AAOS) documented a review of 19 patients with MDI who were treated with radiofrequency thermal capsulorrhaphy (89). Minimum follow-up was 2 years or until failure of the index procedure required surgical revision. Postoperative immobilization was 3 weeks. In nine patients (47%), thermal

TABLE 38.5 RESULTS OF THERMAL CAPSULORRHAPHY IN THE TREATMENT OF POSTERIOR INSTABILITY

Author	Number of Patients	Heat Source	Suture Plication	Minimum Follow-up	Recurrence of Instability
Hawkins	9	Laser	None	24 months	0%
Karas and Hawkins	12	RF	None	24 months	16%
Abrams	25	RF	ALL	24 months	8%

TABLE 38.6 RESULTS OF THERMAL CAPSULORRHAPHY IN THE TREATMENT OF MULTIDIRECTIONAL INSTABILITY

Author	Number of Patients	Heat Source	Suture Plication	Rotator Interval Closure	Minimum Follow-up	Recurrence of Instability
Karas and Hawkins	17	RF	None	None	24 months	53%
Miniaci	19	RF	None	None	24 months	47%
Jones and Paulos	20	Laser	None	None	24 months	25%
Lyons and Savoie	27	Laser	None	ALL	24 months	4%

capsulorrhaphy failed. Four patients (21%) demonstrated postoperative axillary nerve dysfunction (one) or axillary nerve neuritis (three); all four patients recovered within 9 months. The reporting authors did not comment on whether these axillary nerve injuries occurred early in the operative experience with this technique or later in the patient series.

Jones and Paulos (at the annual meeting of the AAOS) reported on the clinical outcome of 20 patients treated with laser-assisted thermal capsulorrhaphy for MDI, with a mean follow-up of 3 years (87). Five patients (25%) experienced clinical failures. Two patients (10%) suffered postoperative adhesive capsulitis requiring manipulation under anesthesia to regain full range of motion.

Lyons et al. (in the *Journal of Arthroscopy and Related Surgery*) published the results of laser-assisted thermal capsulorrhaphy in the treatment of 27 patients with MDI, with a clinical follow-up ranging from 24 to 35 months (49). The average age of the patients was 25 years. One patient (4%) experienced recurrence of instability. Twelve patients (86%) postoperatively returned to their previous level of sports participation. In all cases, arthroscopic closure of the rotator interval was performed in addition to heat shrinkage of the capsule.

Throwing Athletes

Grana et al. (in the *American Journal of Sports Medicine,* 1999) reported on 14 throwers who were treated with thermal capsulorrhaphy at the time of superior labral debridement or debridement of internal impingement lesions (47). All patients remained asymptomatic at final review, but only

eight (57%) returned to throwing. No results are reported regarding return of these eight athletes to their preinjury level of participation (Table 38.7).

Andrews and Dugas (in *Instructional Course Lectures*) documented the results of a dual-armed retrospective review of elite-level throwers, followed for a minimum of 2 years (47). Fifty-one consecutive athletes with internal impingement and partial-thickness undersurface rotator cuff tears were reviewed. Forty-nine of these patients (96%) demonstrated increased glenohumeral laxity during examination under anesthesia. No patient underwent thermal capsulorrhaphy at the time of surgical treatment. Eighty percent returned to play, but only 61% were competing at the same level at final review.

The second group of 30 throwers underwent thermal capsulorrhaphy at the time of debridement of the internal impingement lesion. Increased laxity was not documented in these athletes preoperatively. At 2 years postoperatively, 93% were competing, and 86% had reached their same preinjury level of competition.

Andrews and Dugas (in *Instructional Course Lectures*) similarly reported retrospectively on results of thermal capsulorrhaphy in addressing capsular laxity at the time of debridement of an internal impingement lesion and SLAP repair (47). Fifty percent of throwers who underwent debridement and SLAP repair without heat shrinkage were competing 2 years postoperatively, compared with 73% who underwent thermal capsular treatment in addition to debridement and SLAP repair.

Hawkins et al. (at the annual meeting of the ASES) also reported on the beneficial effect of reducing anterior capsular laxity with thermal capsulorrhaphy in the elite thrower

TABLE 38.7 RESULTS OF THERMAL CAPSULORRHAPHY IN THE TREATMENT OF THE THROWING ATHLETE

Author	Number of Patients	Anterior Thermal Capsulorrhaphy	Treatment of SLAP or Internal Impingement	Minimum Follow-up	Return to Pre-Injury Level of Play
Grana	14	Yes	Debridement	24 months	57%
Andrews	51	No	Debridement	24 months	61%
Andrews	30	Yes	Debridement	24 months	86%

with either internal impingement or SLAP lesions, when examination with the patient under anesthesia demonstrated pathologic laxity compared with the contralateral shoulder (27).

CONCLUSIONS

As we cautioned previously, the early results reporting thermal capsulorrhaphy for the treatment of glenohumeral instability should be interpreted critically. The ease and ready availability of this technique may confound the appropriate indications for the procedure. Furthermore, as we have begun to learn more about the tissue and collagen response to this thermal treatment, we continue to modify both our surgical technique and our postoperative rehabilitation. This includes determining the appropriate length of postoperative immobilization and subsequent therapeutic mobilization that correctly create a compromise between maintenance of stability and restoration of functional glenohumeral motion. These questions remain controversial, and hence they affect the ability to compare results obtained by different authors, who may use different postoperative protocols.

In all types of instability, whether unidirectional (anterior or posterior) or MDI, the results obtained using arthroscopic management have begun to approach the outcomes obtained with open reconstructive procedures. The published incidence of recurrent instability using open surgical techniques for anterior instability ranges from 0% to 12% (6,8,30,97,98). The most current reported series of arthroscopic management (including both suture plication and a component of thermal capsulorrhaphy) documented failure rates ranging from 6% to 10% (6,7,29). These studies report improved outcomes compared with previous arthroscopic series that documented up to a 50% failure rate (8,10,99,100). As the learning curve has progressed with these arthroscopic techniques, the incidence of recurrent instability has progressively decreased during the evolution of arthroscopic management.

Despite the relative lack of knowledge regarding the eventual biomechanical fate of the thermally treated glenohumeral capsule, we remain optimistic regarding the use of thermal shrinkage to aid in restoring normal capsular tension in the treatment of instability. We continue to investigate and are encouraged by the combined role of both suture plication and thermal capsular shrinkage in the arthroscopic management of instability. We believe that the heat probe is an effective adjunct, but it may not replace suture repairs, either open or arthroscopic.

In the throwing athlete, we remain encouraged by our results obtained using the heat probe to treat any excessive glenohumeral laxity that may be associated with internal impingement or SLAP lesions. The low morbidity and potential restoration of appropriate capsular tension make this technique very appealing for the throwing athlete, in the proper clinical setting. Consequently, we combine the clinical history and physical examination, the examination with the patient under anesthesia, and the diagnostic arthroscopic examination before we add thermal capsulorrhaphy to our treatment regimen for the symptomatic thrower. We again caution that, until further research clarifies the fate of the thermally treated tissue, surgeons should continue to maintain a very current fund of knowledge regarding the indications, use, and results of this easily applicable technique in the management of their patients.

ACKNOWLEDGMENTS

We wish to thank Marilee P. Horan, B.S., for her invaluable assistance in the preparation of this manuscript.

REFERENCES

1. Abrams JS. Arthroscopic shoulder stabilization for recurrent subluxation and dislocation. *J Shoulder Elbow Surg* 1993;2:25.
2. Arciero RA, Taylor DC, Snyder RJ, et al. Arthroscopic bioabsorbable tack stabilization of initial anterior shoulder dislocations: a preliminary report. *Arthroscopy* 1995;11:410–417.
3. Bacilla P, Field LD, Sawoie FH. Arthroscopic bankart repair in a high demand patient population. *Arthroscopy* 1997;13:51–60.
4. Benedetto KP, Glotzer W. Arthroscopic Bankart procedure by suture technique: indications, technique, and results. *Arthroscopy* 1993;8:111–115.
5. Caspari RB, Savoie FH, Meyers JF. Arthroscopic stabilization of traumatic anterior shoulder instability. In: Post M, Morres B, Hawkins R, eds. *Surgery of the shoulder.* Chicago: Year Book, 1990.
6. Cole BJ, L'Insalata J, Irrgang J, et al. Comparison of arthroscopic and open anterior shoulder stabilization: a two to six year follow-up study. *J Bone Joint Surg Am* 2000;82:1103–1114.
7. Gartsman GM, Roddey TS, Hammerman SM. Arthroscopic treatment of anterior-inferior glenohumeral instability: two to five-year follow-up. *J Bone Joint Surg Am* 2000;82:991–1003.
8. Geiger DF, Hurley JA, Tovey JA, et al. Results of arthroscopic versus open Bankart suture repair. *Clin Orthop* 1997;337:111–117.
9. Grana WA, Buckley PD, Yates CK. Arthroscopic Bankart suture repair. *Am J Sports Med* 1993;21:348–353.
10. Green MR, Christensen KP. Arthroscopic Bankart procedure: two- to five-year follow-up with clinical correlation to severity of glenoid labral lesion. *Am J Sports Med* 1995;23:276–281.
11. Glasgow SG, Bruce RA, Yacobucci GN, et al. Arthroscopic resection of glenoid labral tears in the athlete: a review of 29 cases. *Arthroscopy* 1992;8:48–54.
12. Jobe FW, Giangarra CE, Kwitne RS, et al. Anterior capsulolabral reconstruction of the shoulder in athletes in overhand sports. *Am J Sports Med* 1991;19:428–434.
13. Nottage WM. Laser-assisted shoulder surgery. *Arthroscopy* 1997;13:635–638.
14. Pollock RG, Owens JM, Flatow EL, et al. Operative results of the inferior capsular shift procedure for multidirectional instability of the shoulder. *J Bone Joint Surg Am* 82;7:919–928.
15. Speer KP, Warren RF, Pagnani M, et al. An arthroscopic technique for anterior stabilization of the shoulder with a bioabsorbable tack. *J Bone Joint Surg Am* 1996;78:1801–1807.

16. Torchia ME, Caspari RB, Asselmeier MA, et al. Arthroscopic transglenoid multiple suture repair: 2 to 8 year results in 150 shoulders. *Arthroscopy* 1997;13:609–619.

17. Abrams JS. Shoulder stabilization and evolving trends in arthroscopic repair. *Sports Med Arthrosc Rev* 1999;7:104–116.

18. Altchek DW, Warren EF, Skyhar MJ, et al. T-plasty modification of the Bankart procedure for multidirectional instability of the anterior and inferior types. *J Bone Joint Surg Am* 1991;73:105–112.

19. Cole BJ, L'Insalata J, Irrgang J, et al. Comparison of arthroscopic and open anterior shoulder stabilization: a two to six year follow-up study. *J Bone Joint Surg Am* 2000;82:1103–1114.

20. Fanton GS. Arthroscopic electrothermal surgery of the shoulder. *Oper Tech Sports Med* 1998;6:139–146.

21. Marshall JL, Johanson N, Wickiewicz TL, et al. Joint looseness: a function of the person and the joint. *Med Sci Sports Exerc* 1980;12:189–195.

22. Walch G, Boileau P, Levigne C, et al. Arthroscopic stabilization for recurrent anterior shoulder dislocation: results of 59 cases. *Arthroscopy* 1995;11:173–179.

23. Kvitne RS, Jobe FW, Jobe CM. Shoulder instability in the overhand or throwing athlete. *Clin Sports Med* 1995;14:917–935.

24. Snyder SJ, Strafford BB. Arthroscopic management of instability of the shoulder. *Orthopedics* 1993;16:993–1002.

25. Anderson K, McCarty EC, Warren RF. Thermal capsulorrhaphy: where are we today? *Sports Med Arthrosc Rev* 1999;7:117–127.

26. Fanton GS, Wall MS. Thermally assisted arthroscopic stabilization of the shoulder joint. In: Warren RF, Craig EV, Altchek DW, eds. *The unstable shoulder*. Philadelphia: Lippincott–Raven, 1999:329–343.

27. Hawkins RJ, Noonan TJ, Horan M. Arthroscopic laser capsulorrhaphy for the treatment of shoulder instability: a minimum two-year follow-up. Presented at the annual meeting of American Shoulder and Elbow Surgeons, 2000.

28. Hayashi K, Massa KL, Thabit G, et al. Histologic evaluation of the glenohumeral joint capsule after the laser-assisted capsular shift procedure for glenohumeral instability. *Am J Sports Med* 1999;27:162–167.

29. McIntyre LF, Caspari RB, Savoie FH. The arthroscopic treatments of anterior and multidirectional shoulder instability. *Instr Course Lect* 1996;45:47.

30. Roberts SN, Tayloer DE, Brown JN, et al. Open and arthroscopic techniques for the treatment of traumatic anterior shoulder instability in Australian rules football players. *J Shoulder Elbow Surg* 1999;8:403–409.

31. Treacy SH, Field LD, Savoie FH. Rotator interval capsule closure: an arthroscopic technique. *Arthroscopy* 1997;13:103–106.

32. Adams F, ed. *The genuine works of Hippocrates*. New York: William Wood, 1886.

33. Hayashi K, Markel MD. Thermal modification of joint capsule and ligamentous tissues. *Oper Tech Sports Med* 1998;6:120–125.

34. Hayashi K, Thabit G, Bigdanske JJ, et al. The effect of nonablative laser energy on the ultrastructure of joint capsular collagen. *Arthroscopy* 1996;12:474–481.

35. Hayashi K, Thabit G, Massa KL, et al. The effect of thermal heating on the length and histologic properties of the glenohumeral joint capsule. *Am J Sports Med* 1997;25:107–112.

36. Hecht P, Hayashi K, Cooley AJ, et al. The thermal effect of monopolar radiofrequency energy on the properties of joint capsule: an *in vivo* histologic study using a sheep model. *Am J Sports Med* 1998;26:808–814.

37. Hecht P, Hayashi K, Lu Y, et al. Monopolar radiofrequency energy effects on joint capsular tissue: potential treatment for joint instability: an *in vivo* mechanical, morphological, and biochem-

38. Naseef GS, Foster TE, Trauner K, et al. The thermal properties of bovine joint capsule: the basic science of laser- and radiofrequency-induced capsular shrinkage. *Am J Sports Med* 1997;25:670–674.

39. Obrzut SL, Hecht P, Hayashi K, et al. The effect of radiofrequency energy on the length and temperature properties of the glenohumeral joint capsule. *Arthroscopy* 1998;14:395–400.

40. Thabit G. The arthroscopically assisted holmium:YAG laser surgery in the shoulder. *Oper Tech Sports Med* 1998;6:131–138.

41. Vangsness CT, Mitchell W, Nimni M, et al. Collagen shortening: an experimental approach with heat. *Clin Orthop* 1997;337:267–271.

42. Wall MS, Deng XH, Torzilli PA, et al. Thermal modification of collagen. *J Shoulder Elbow Surg* 1999;8:339–344.

43. Schaefer SL, Ciarelli MJ, Arnoczky SP, et al. Tissue shrinkage with the holmium:yttrium aluminum garnet laser: A postoperative assessment of tissue length,stiffness,and structure. *Am J Sports Med* 1997;25:841–848.

44. Abelow SP. Use of lasers in orthopedic surgery: current concepts. *Orthopedics* 1993;16:551–556.

45. Sperling JW, Anderson K, McCarty EC, et al. Complications of thermal capsulorrhaphy. *Instr Course Lect* 2001;50:37–41.

46. Abrams JS. Thermal capsulorrhaphy for instability of the shoulder: concerns and applications of the heat probe. *Instr Course Lect* 2001;50:29–36.

47. Andrews JR, Dugas JR. Diagnosis and treatment of shoulder injuries in the throwing athlete: the role of thermal-assisted capsular shrinkage. *Instr Course Lect* 2001;50:17–21.

48. Giffin JR, Annunziata CC, Bradley JP. Thermal capsulorrhaphy for instability of the shoulder: multidirectional and posterior instabilities. *Instr Course Lect* 2001;50:23–28.

49. Lyons TR, Griffith PL, Savoie FH, et al. Laser-assisted capsulorrhaphy for multidirectional instability of the shoulder. *Arthroscopy* 2001;17:25–30.

50. Savoie FH, Field LD. Thermal versus suture treatment of symptomatic capsular laxity. *Clin Sports Med* 2000;19:63–75.

51. Bigliani LU, Kurzweil PR, Schwartzbach CC, et al. Inferior capsular shift procedure for anterior-inferior shoulder instability in athletes. *Am J Sports Med* 1994;22:578–584.

52. Pagnani MJ, Warren RF, Altchek DW, et al. Arthroscopic shoulder stabilization using transglenoid sutures: a four-year minimum follow-up. *Am J Sports Med* 1996;24:459–467.

53. Rowe CR, Patel D, Southmayd WW. The Bankart procedure: a long-term end-result study. *J Bone Joint Surg Am* 1978;60:1–16.

54. Savoie FH, Miller CD, Field LD. Arthroscopic reconstruction of traumatic anterior instability of the shoulder: the Caspari technique. *Arthroscopy* 1997;13:201–209.

55. Warner JJ, Miller MD, Marks P, et al. Arthroscopic Bankart repair with the Suretac device: part I. Clinical observations. *Arthroscopy* 1995;11:2–13.

56. Wolf EM. Arthroscopic anterior shoulder capsulorrhaphy. *Tech Orthop* 1988;3:67–73.

57. Bigliani LU, Pollock RG, Soslowsky LJ, et al. Tensile properties of the inferior glenohumeral ligament. *J Orthop Res* 1992;10:187–197.

58. Speer KP, Deng X, Borrero S, et al. Biomechanical evaluation of a simulated Bankart lesion. *J Bone Joint Surg Am* 1994;76:1819–1826.

59. O'Brien SJ, Neves MC, Arnoczky SP, et al. The anatomy and histology of the inferior glenohumeral ligament complex of the shoulder. *Am J Sports Med* 1990;18:449–456.

60. Pollock RG, Bigliani LU. Glenohumeral instability: evaluation and treatment. *J Am Acad Orthop Surg* 1993;1:24–32.

61. Ungersbock A, Michel M, Hertel R. Factors influencing the re-

sults of a modified Bankart procedure. *J Shoulder Elbow Surg* 1995;4:365–369.

62. Zabinski SJ, Callaway GH, Cohen S, et al. Revision shoulder stabilization: 2- to 10-year results. *J Shoulder Elbow Surg* 1999;8:58–65.

63. Mologne TS, McBride MT, Lapoint JM. Assessment of failed arthroscopic anterior labral repairs: findings at open surgery. *Am J Sports Med* 1997;25:813–817.

64. Abrams JS. Special shoulder problems in the throwing athletes: pathology, diagnosis, and nonoperative management. *Clin Sports Med* 1991;10:839–861.

65. Halbrecht JL, Tirman P, Atkin D. Internal impingement of the shoulder: comparison of findings between the throwing and nonthrowing shoulders of college baseball players. *Arthroscopy* 1999;15:253–258.

66. Jobe CM. Posterior superior glenoid impingement: expanded spectrum. *Arthroscopy* 1995;11:530–536.

67. Wichman MT, Snyder SJ. Arthroscopic capsular plication for multidirectional instability of the shoulder. *Oper Tech Sports Med* 1997;5:238–243.

68. Bigliani LU, Pollock RG, McIlveen SJ, et al. Shift of the posteroinferior aspect of the capsule for recurrent posterior glenohumeral instability. *J Bone Joint Surg Am* 1995;77:1011–1020.

69. Bowen MK, Warren RF. Recurrent posterior subluxation: open surgical treatment. In: Warren RF, Craig EV, Altchek DW, eds. *The unstable shoulder.* Philadelphia: Lippincott–Raven, 1999:237–247.

70. Boyd HB, Sisk TD. Recurrent posterior dislocation of the shoulder. *J Bone Joint Surg Am* 1972;54:779–786.

71. Fronek J, Warren RF, Bowen M. Posterior subluxation of the glenohumeral joint. *J Bone Joint Surg Am* 1989;71:205–216.

72. Wirth MA, Groh GI, Rockwood CA. Capsulorrhaphy through an anterior approach for the treatment of atraumatic posterior glenohumeral instability with multidirectional laxity of the shoulder. *J Bone Joint Surg Am* 1998;80:1570–1578.

73. Neer CS II, Foster CR. Inferior capsular shift for involuntary inferior and multidirectional instability of the shoulder: a preliminary report. *J Bone Joint Surg Am* 1980;62:897–908.

74. Schenk TJ, Brems JJ. Multidirectional instability of the shoulder: pathophysiology, diagnosis, and management. *J Am Acad Orthop Surg* 1998;6:65–72.

75. Treacy SH, Savoie FH, Field LD. Arthroscopic treatment of multidirectional instability. *J Shoulder Elbow Surg* 1999;8:344–349.

76. Cooper RA, Brems JJ. The inferior capsular shift procedure for multidirectional instability of the shoulder. *J Bone Joint Surg Am* 1992;74:1516–1621.

77. Cordasco FA, Bigliani LU. Multidirectional shoulder instability: open surgical treatment. In: Warren RF, Craig EV, Altchek DW, eds. *The unstable shoulder.* Philadelphia: Lippincott–Raven, 1999:249–261.

78. McIntyre LF. Arthroscopic capsulorrhaphy for multidirectional instability. *Oper Tech Sports Med* 1997;5:233–237.

79. Field LD, Warren RF, O'Brien SJ, et al. Isolated closure of rotator interval defects for shoulder instability. *Am J Sports Med* 1995;23:557–563.

80. Harryman DT II, Sidles JA, Harris SL, et al. The role of the rotator interval capsule in passive motion and stability of the shoulder. *J Bone Joint Surg Am* 1992;74:53–66.

81. Nobuhara K, Ikeda H. Rotator interval lesion. *Clin Orthop* 1987;223:44–50.

82. Pagnani MJ, Warren RF. Stabilizers of the glenohumeral joint. *J Shoulder Elbow Surg* 1994;3:173–190.

83. Warner JJ, Deng XH, Warren RF, et al. Static capsuloligamentous restraints to superior-inferior translation of the glenohumeral joint. *Am J Sports Med* 1992;20:675–685.

84. Bowen MK, Warren RJ. Ligamentous control of shoulder stability based on selective cutting and static translation experiments. *Clin Sports Med* 1991;10:757–782.

85. Duncan R, Savoie FH. Arthroscopic inferior capsular shift for multidirectional instability of the shoulder: a preliminary report. *Arthroscopy* 1993;9:24–27.

86. Hawkins RJ, Karas SG. Arthroscopic stabilization plus thermal capsulorrhaphy for anterior instability with and without Bankart lesions: the role of rehabilitation and immobilization. *Instr Course Lect* 2001;50:13–15.

87. Jones D, Paulos L. Thermal capsular shrinkage for shoulder instability: a prospective study comparing electrocautery and laser heat sources. Presented at the 17th open meeting of the American Shoulder and Elbow Surgeons, San Francisco, CA, 2001.

88. Karas SG, Noonan, TJ, Hawkins RJ, et al. Electrothermal arthroscopic capsulorrhaphy for the treatment of shoulder instability: a minimum two-year followup. Presented at the annual meeting of the American Academy of Orthopaedic Surgeons, San Francisco, CA, 2001.

89. Miniaci A, McBirnie J, Miniaci S. Thermal capsulorrhaphy for the treatment of multi-directional instability of the shoulder. Presented at the 17th open meeting of the American Shoulder and Elbow Surgeons, San Francisco, CA, 2001.

90. O'Neill DB. Arthroscopic Bankart repair of anterior detachments of the glenoid labrum: a prospective study. *J Bone Joint Surg Am* 1999;81:1357–1366.

91. Walch G, Boileau P, Noel E, et al. Impingement of the deep surface of the supraspinatus tendon on the posterosuperior glenoid rim: an arthroscopic study. *J Shoulder Elbow Surg* 1992;1:238–245.

92. Wallace AW, Hollinshead RM, Frank CB. The scientific basis of thermal capsular shrinkage. *J Shoulder Elbow Surg* 2000;9:354–360.

93. Tibone JE, Lee TQ, Black AD, et al. Glenohumeral translation after arthroscopic thermal capsuloplasty with a radiofrequency probe. *J Shoulder Elbow Surg* 2000;9:514–518.

94. Lu Y, Hayashi K, Edwards RB, et al. The effect of monopolar radiofrequency treatment pattern on joint capsular healing. *Am J Sports Med* 2000;28:711–719.

95. Lopez MJ, Hayashi K, Fanton GS, et al. The effect of radiofrequency energy on the ultrastructure of joint capsular collagen. *Arthroscopy* 1998;14:495–501.

96. Schlegel T, Hawkins RJ. Thermal shrinkage of rabbit patellar ligaments: the role of immobilization. Unpublished data, 1999.

97. Guanche CA, Quick DC, Sodergren KM, et al. Arthroscopic versus open reconstruction of the shoulder in patients with isolated Bankart lesions. *Am J Sports Med* 1996;24:144–148.

98. Levine WN, Arroyo JS, Pollock RG, et al. Open revision stabilization surgery for recurrent anterior glenohumeral instability. *Am J Sports Med* 2000;28:156–160.

99. Koss S, Richmond JC, Woodward JS. Two- to five-year followup of arthroscopic Bankart reconstruction using a suture anchor technique. *Am J Sports Med* 1997;25:809–812.

100. Youssef JA, Carr CF, Walther CE, et al. Arthroscopic Bankart suture repair for recurrent traumatic unidirectional anterior shoulder dislocations. *Arthroscopy* 1995;11:561–563.

Operative Arthroscopy, third edition. Edited by John B. McGinty, Stephen S. Burkhart, Robert W. Jackson, Donald H. Johnson, and John C. Richmond. Lippincott Williams & Wilkins © 2003.

THERMAL CAPSULORRHAPHY: COMPLICATIONS

STEPHEN C. WEBER

Open treatment for shoulder instability has remained the standard for multidirectional instability of the shoulder (1–8). Arthroscopic suture capsulorrhaphy has been reported and used since the 1980s (6,9–13). Outcomes have varied among surgeons, but complications have primarily related to recurrence of instability. Other types of complications are rare, and revision of these instability complications is not generally viewed as technically difficult. Neurologic injury remains unreported. Significant capsular damage is also unreported.

Thermal shrinkage of the lax capsule was first proposed in the early 1990s, encouraged by the visual appearance of shrinkage of the tissue with the application of laser heat. Thermal shrinkage became more popular with the advent of radiofrequency energy applications, which were significantly cheaper and safer that the application of laser energy. Multiple early *in vitro* studies showed time zero shrinkage of about 10% (14–18,20–28). Based on this *in vitro* information, various devices were marketed to alter the joint capsule thermally. Ease of application and shorter recovery were the purported advantages of these techniques. *In vivo* data have been limited. Schaefer et al. (25) and Hecht et al. (29) showed that the *in vivo* shrinkage is replaced by extensive capsular necrosis and significant structural alteration with marked inflammation and degradation of the mechanical properties that persists for months. It appears that the type of energy is irrelevant, a view consistent with Arnoczky and Aksan's (15) review suggesting that the mechanism by which the tissue is thermally necrosed is independent of the heating technique. Because the shrunken tissue is necrosed and replaced, these investigators pointed out that the "exact mechanism for this (thermal) clinical improvement has yet to be clearly defined" (15). These data have been widely accepted and have led to general recognition that rehabilitation should be, if anything, more cautious and slower than with more established procedures, to accommodate the

structural alterations caused by thermal treatment. This leaves the only purported advantage of thermal capsulorrhaphy to be ease of application. Thermally treating unattached tissue has not seemed logical. Therefore, two broad treatment patterns have been established: thermal treatment alone for patients with multidirectional instability and thermal treatment in combination with some type of fixation for patients with structural lesions such as Bankart or superior labral anterior and posterior lesions (SLAP lesions).

Published complications have remained rare. Anecdotal reports of complications have surfaced, some consistent with those previously faced by arthroscopic surgeons and some new. Only three studies deal to any degree with complications related to thermal capsulorrhaphy. Jensen (30) reported on a small series of patients explored open after complications related to recurrence of instability after thermal capsulorrhaphy. Miniaci et al. (31) carefully followed complications during a prospective series of thermal capsulorrhaphy for patients without associated structural lesions. The series by Miniaci et al. showed a high rate of complications, and their review was thorough in assessing these complications. I presented a series of 15 patients, 13 of whom had surgical revision related to complications of thermal capsulorrhaphy performed elsewhere (32). Patient demographics in this study are shown in Table 39.1. Outcomes of subsequent treatment are shown in Tables 39.2 and 39.3. This study documented the difficulties that could be encountered with surgical revision of failed thermal capsulorrhaphy, such as capsular necrosis and stiffness refractory to further treatment. Many of these complications were unreported with traditional arthroscopic or open repair. Postsurgical residual pain remained a concern, with a mean University of California Los Angeles score of only 24 (fair) after surgical revision. Incidence rates for complications related to thermal modification of tissue remain difficult to estimate, because only the work of Miniaci et al. allows any estimation of the percentage of patients who had each complication. Complications highlighted in these three studies can be divided into five categories: (a) recurrence, (b) cap-

S. C. Weber: Sacramento Knee & Sports Medicine Medical Corporation, Sacramento, California.

TABLE 39.1 PATIENT DEMOGRAPHICS

Mean patient age (yr)	30.13
Gender (male/female)	10/5
Dislocator	6
"Subluxator"	9
Duration index thermal to second Procedure (mos)	21.3
Final follow-up (mos)	10.07

sular necrosis, (c) axillary nerve injuries, (d) stiffness, and (e) biceps subluxation.

RECURRENCE

Anecdotal reviews (17,33) and non–peer-reviewed presentations (34–38) have shown mixed results. Success rates for pure thermal techniques have varied from 70% (39), 76% (36), 83% (40), 92% (37), to 100% (35). The study by Miniaci et al. showed a 47% recurrence rate, increasing to 80% in patients with posterior instability (31). Many of these outcomes are inferior to prior reports of either arthroscopic suture capsulorrhaphy (9,10,11,13) or open procedures (1–5,7,8). Results with mixed thermal and fixation techniques have fared better (41–45), but because no control group was present comparing thermal techniques with either arthroscopic or open capsulorrhaphy, it is difficult to

ascribe the beneficial results to the thermal procedure alone, especially given that similar good results have been obtained using standard suture techniques without thermal treatment of the capsule (13,46). Only the study of Levitz et al. (43) assessed the results of thermal treatment compared with any control group; as could be expected, the patients who received no treatment of capsular laxity fared worse than those patients who had at least some treatment of capsular laxity with heat.

CAPSULAR ALTERATION AND NECROSIS

Basic science information confirms that the temperatures required to shrink collagen (65°C) far exceed the temperatures required for cell death (45°C) (18,20–23). Because cell death in the treated area is universal, necrosis of the treated tissue is perhaps not unexpected. Capsular alterations after thermal treatment in patients with recurrent instability after failed thermal capsulorrhaphy were varied in my study (32). Modest scarring with a bland histologic appearance did occur in this study, and in two cases it allowed arthroscopic shifting of tissue at the revision procedure. Marked scarring was the rule, with significant stiffness and adhesion to the extracapsular tissue that did not allow arthroscopic shifting and required open repair. Jensen (30) reported "capsular friability" in several of his patients treated with open revision; autogenous tissue was not required. Miniaci et al. noted

TABLE 39.2 PATIENT LIST WITH COMPLICATIONS AND DEVICE USED, IF KNOWN

Patient	No.	Age	Type of Device	Other Procedures Besides Capsulorrhaphy	Complication	Second Complication	Revision Procedure
sc	1	27	monopolar	Cuff repair	Stiffness	Pain	Lysis
jw	2	27	monopolar	Acromioclavicular, labral debridement	Stiffness	Pain, impingement	Lysis, acromioclavicular
jl	3	39	monopolar	None	Stiffness	Failed manipulation	Lysis
rv	4	34	monopolar	Slap	Stiffness	Impingement	Acromioclavicular
Rn	5	31	bipolar	None	Necrosis	Recurrence	Open Bankart
cg	6	35	bipolar	None	Recurrence	Pain	Open anterior shift
kv	7	31	Laser	Anterior Bankart	Necrosis	Recurrence	Open Bankart
ap	8	22	monopolar	Prior capsular shift	Subluxing biceps	None	Biceps tenodesis
mi	9	53	bipolar	Debridement	Pain, DJD	None	Hemiarthroplasty
lc	10	23	bipolar	Open Bankart	Necrosis	Recurrence	Open shift
mk	11	26?		Bankart, acromioclavicular	Recurrence	Loose body	Open Bankart
ej	12	33	bipolar	None	Recurrence	None	Open capsular shift rerepair SLAP
ia	13	19	monopolar	SLAP repair	Recurrence	Failed SLAP	Arthroscopic capsular shift
mj	14	35	monopolar	Prior open repair	Recurrence	None	Pending
jg	15	17	Laser	Prior open repair	Recurrence	None	Pending

DJD, degenerative joint disease; SLAP, superior labral anterior and posterior lesion.

TABLE 39.3 PREOPERATIVE AND POSTOPERATIVE SCORES FOR PATIENTS IN SERIES

Patient	No.	Pre-UCLA Score	Post-UCLA Score	Post-Neer
sc	1	12 P	22 F	U
jw	2	10 P	26 F	S
jl	3	10 P	14 P	U
rv	4	18 P	26 F	U
Rn	5	16 P	28 F	S
cg	6	8 P	9 P	U
kv	7	16 P	33 E	E
ap	8	20 P	33 G	E
Ml	9	16 P	26 F	S
lc	10	12 P	17 P	U
mk	11	19 P	31 G	S
ej	12	21 F	21 F	S
ia	13	20 P	28 G	S
mj	14	16 P		
jg	15	16 P		
		Mean = 15.3	Mean = 24.0	

UCLA, University of California Los Angeles.

frank capsular necrosis (31) and believed that, if time were permitted to elapse between the thermal procedure and revision, the thermally damaged tissue could reconstitute, thus allowing easier open revision. This series included three patients with severe capsular necrosis, one requiring autogenous tissue during surgical revision (32) (Fig. 39.1). Frank

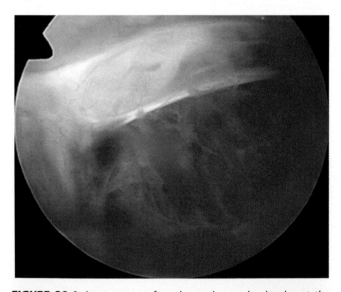

FIGURE 39.1 Appearance after thermal capsulorrhaphy at the time of revision arthroscopy, 22 months after the initial thermal treatment. The view is of a right shoulder seen from posteriorly. The subscapularis muscle belly is easily visible through the massive capsular defect including the entire anterior inferior glenohumeral ligament complex.

capsular necrosis after thermal treatment was also noted by Romeo, Snyder, Harryman, and Savoie (Romeo A, Snyder S, Harryman D, Savoie F, *personal communication,* 2000). The suggestion by Miniaci et al. that time would correct capsular necrosis was not supported by my study, because the worst case was revised at 21 months.

Laser and electrical sources were equally implicated in causing thermal necrosis (32). Necrosis of thermally treated tissue has also been reported in the knee (47). Capsular necrosis remains unreported with arthroscopic suture techniques. The occurrence of capsular scarring requiring open rather than arthroscopic revision and of capsular necrosis, especially to the extent of requiring off-site tissue, remains a serious concern in the use of thermal capsulorrhaphy. Good but not excellent ultimate results were obtained with surgical revision in my series of patients, even those with frank capsular necrosis (32). Planning for possible capsular necrosis is important for the surgeon contemplating surgical revision of failed thermal capsulorrhaphy. Recurrence of instability after revision in my series was high, but perhaps it was consistent with other series of surgical revision for instability.

AXILLARY NERVE INJURY

Axillary nerve injury has been the most widely reported complication, related to the proximity of the axillary nerve to the inferior capsule. Gryler et al. showed that temperatures could easily be raised to dangerous levels with routine thermal treatment of this area of the capsule (48). Nerve injuries have been difficult to document, because early axillary sensory dysesthesias have been easy to confuse with postoperative pain. Temporary injury to the sensory branches has predominated in those series reporting this complication, with an 8% rate in one series (36) and a 21% rate in another (31). Miniaci et al. (31) reported temporary motor palsy. My review identified no axillary nerve injuries (32); nine of 15 patients had postthermal electromyographic studies that were negative. Anecdotal reports of permanent nerve injuries continue to circulate. These reports have led some surgeons to suggest avoiding heating the axillary fold (31). Treatment has usually been expectant, but it is often associated with stiffness in patients with associated nerve injuries (31). Neurologic injury with arthroscopic capsulorrhaphy is unreported, and experimentally it is almost impossible to produce (49). The risk of neurologic injury not reported with other more established techniques is alone enough to raise concerns.

STIFFNESS

Persistent late stiffness was studied by one of the principal proponents of this technique, with capsular alterations at the microscopic level for at least 2 years in some patients (19). The reasons for this complication were unclear; these investigators noted considerable difficulty in regaining motion even with arthroscopic release. The long-term histologic changes documented by Hayashi et al. that are associated with thermally treated tissue may be responsible for this persistent stiffness (19). Miniaci et al. (31) noted that 21% of their patients became stiff as a result of thermal capsulorrhaphy. My study documented four patients with severe stiffness (32). Persistent pain in this group was the rule rather than the exception, and the patients in my series responded poorly to arthroscopic release. Stiffness continues to be unreported in most other series. The outcome of these thermally treated patients is at odds with other studies reporting good results with arthroscopic treatment of post-capsulorrhaphy stiffness created by arthroscopic suture or open capsulorrhaphy. Stiffness in reported series on arthroscopic suture capsulorrhaphy has been minimal (6,9–13). Stiffness refractory to capsular release with arthroscopic suture capsulorrhaphy remains unreported.

BICEPS SUBLUXATION

Both Jensen (30) and I (32) reported biceps subluxation as a complication of arthroscopic thermal capsulorrhaphy. The cause of this complication is unknown, but it may be related to thermal treatment of the biceps anchor at the proximal bicipital groove. Both reported cases were treated successfully with biceps tenodesis.

Incidence rates for these serious complications are difficult to determine because of the absence of data. Clearly, the addition of thermal energy may not be the only reason for the complications seen in these patients, and distinguishing asymptomatic capsular laxity from pathologic instability remains one of the most important and difficult clinical judgments. Thermal treatment of asymptomatic capsular laxity may have been a factor in some of the patients my series (32). That these complications do occur with some frequency means that recognition and management of these complications are crucial for the surgeon either doing these procedures or managing these complications. Early reports of serious complications not present with more traditional arthroscopic or open techniques led several authors to advise caution with thermal capsulorrhaphy (16,31,34,49,50,51). The only purported advantage of thermal capsulorrhaphy is ease of application at this time. Although new technology is always appealing, both the basic science and early clinical results of this technology are worrisome. The available reports do not answer the question of the incidence rates for these serious complications, nor do they address whether these complications can be avoided by alteration of application of thermal energy such as decreasing time of application, temperature, or pattern of application. They do raise concerns about the widespread use of this technology until these questions are answered.

REFERENCES

1. Altchek DW, Warren RF, Skyhar MJ, et al. T-plasty modification of the Bankart procedure for multidirectional instability of the anterior and inferior types. *J Bone Joint Surg Am* 1991;72: 105–112.
2. Bigliani LU, Kurzweil PR, Schwartzbach CC, et al. Inferior capsular shift procedure for anterior-inferior shoulder instability in athletes. *Am J Sports Med* 1994:22:578–584.
3. Jobe FW, Jobe CM. Painful athletic injuries of the shoulder. *Clin Orthop* 1983;173:117–124.
4. Jobe FW, Giangara CE, Kvitne RS, et al. Anterior capsulolabral reconstruction of the shoulder in athletes in overhand sports. *Am J Sports Med* 1991;19:428–434.
5. Jobe FW, Tibone JE, Pink MM, et al. The shoulder in sports. In: Rockwood CW, Matsen FA, eds. *The shoulder.* Philadelphia: WB Saunders, 1998.
6. Mallon WJ, Speer KP. Multidirectional instability: aurrent concepts. *J Shoulder Elbow Surg* 1995;4:54–64.
7. Montgomery WH, Jobe FW. Functional outcomes in athletes after modified anterior capsulolabral reconstruction. *Am J Sports Med* 1994;22:352–358.
8. Neer CS II, Foster CR. Inferior capsular shift for involuntary inferior and multidirectional instability of the shoulder: a preliminary report. *J Bone Joint Surg Am* 1980;62:897–908.
9. Altchek DW, Wickiewicz TL, Warren RF, et al. Arthroscopic capsular shift: a retrospective analysis of 21 patients. *Arthroscopy* 1992;8:411–412.
10. Duncan R, Savoie FH III. Arthroscopic inferior capsular shift for multidirectional instability of the shoulder: a preliminary report. *Arthroscopy* 1993;10:24–27.
11. Loren GJ, Snyder SJ, Karzel RP, et al. Extended success of arthroscopic capsular plication for glenohumeral instability in the absence of a Bankart lesion. *Arthroscopy* 1999;15:573.
12. Tauro JC, Carter FM. Arthroscopic capsular advancement for anterior and anterior-inferior shoulder instability: a preliminary report. *Arthroscopy* 1994;10:513–517.
13. Weber SC. Arthroscopic suture capsulorrhaphy in the management of type 2 and type 3 impingement. *Arthroscopy* 2000;16: 428.
14. Arnoczky SP. Basic science of thermal capsulorrhaphy. Presented at the fall course of the Arthroscopy Association of North America, Palm Desert, CA, 2000.
15. Arnoczky SP, Aksan A. Thermal modification of connective tissues: basic science considerations and clinical implications. *J Am Acad Orthop Surg* 2000;8:305–313.
16. Arnoczky SP, Hawkins RJ, Bradley JP. Symposium: thermal capsular shrinking for shoulder instability. *Pract Arthrosc* 2000;4: 484–487.
17. Fanton GS. Thermal shoulder surgery: an exciting new alternative. *Inside AANA* 1999;15:4–5.
18. Hayashi K, Markel MD, Thabit G III, et al. The effect of nonablative laser energy on joint capsular properties: an *in vitro* mechanical study using a rabbit model. *Am J Sports Med* 1995:23: 482–487.
19. Hayashi K, Massa KL, Thabit G, et al. Histologic evaluation of the glenohumeral joint capsule after the laser-assisted capsular shift procedure for glenohumeral instability. *Am J Sports Med* 1999;27:162–167.
20. Hayashi K, Thabit G III, Massa KL, et al. The effect of thermal

heating on the length and histologic properties of the glenohumeral joint capsule. *Am J Sports Med* 1997;25:107–112.

21. Hayashi K, Thabit G III, Bogdanske JJ, et al. The effect of non ablative laser energy on the ultrastructure of joint capsular collagen. *Arthroscopy* 1996;12:474–481.

22. Lopez JM, Hayashi K, Fanton GS, et al. The effect of radiofrequency energy on the ultrastructure of joint capsular collagen. *Arthroscopy* 1998;14:495–501.

23. Naseef GS III, Foster TE, Trauner K, et al. The thermal properties of bovine joint capsule: the basic science of laser and radiofrequency-induced capsular shrinkage. *Am J Sports Med* 1997; 25:670–674.

24. Obrzut SL, Hecht, Hayashi K, et al. The effect of radiofrequency energy on the length and temperature properties of the glenohumeral joint capsule. *Arthroscopy* 1998;14:395–400.

25. Schaefer SL, Ciarelli MJ, Arnoczky SP, et al. Tissue shrinkage with the holmium yttrium aluminum garnet laser: a postoperative assessment of tissue length, stiffness and structure. *Am J Sports Med* 1997;25:841–848.

26. Tibone JE, McMahon PH, Shrader TA, et al. Glenohumeral joint translation after arthroscopic nonablative thermal capsuloplasty with a laser. *Am J Sports Med* 1998;16:495–498.

27. Wallace AL, Hollinshead RM, Frank CB. The scientific basis of thermal capsular shrinkage. *J Shoulder Elbow Surg* 2000;9: 354–360.

28. Vangsness TC Jr, Mitchell W III, Mimni M, et al. Collagen shortening: an experimental approach with heat. *Clin Orthop* 1997;337:267–267.

29. Hecht P, Hayashi K, Cooley AJ, et al. The thermal effect of monopolar radiofrequency energy on the properties of joint capsule: an *in vivo* histologic study using a sheep model. *Am J Sports Med* 1998;26:808–814.

30. Jensen K. Management of complications associated with thermal capsulorrhaphy. Presented at the American Shoulder and Elbow Surgeons open meeting, Orlando, FL, 2000.

31. Miniaci A, McBirnie J, Miniaci SL. Thermal capsulorrhaphy for the treatment of multi-directional instability. Presented at the American Shoulder and Elbow Surgeons closed meeting, Austin, TX, 2000.

32. Weber SC. Surgical treatment of complications associated with thermal capsulorrhaphy. Presented at the 20th annual meeting of the Arthroscopy Association of North America. Seattle, WA, 2001.

33. Fanton GS. Arthroscopic electrothermal surgery of the shoulder. *Oper Tech Sports Med* 1998:6:139–146.

34. Anderson K, Warren RF, Altchek DW, et al. Risk factors for poor outcome after thermal capsulorrhaphy. Presented at the American Orthopedic Society for Sports Medicine specialty day, Orlando, 2000.

35. Ceballos C, Zvijac JE, Uribe JW, et al. Arthroscopic thermal capsulorrhaphy in multidirectional glenohumeral instability. *Arthroscopy* 2000;16:428.

36. D'Alessandro DF, Bradley JP, Fleischli JF, et al. Prospective evaluation of electrothermal arthroscopic capsulorrhaphy (ETAC) for shoulder instability: indications, technique, and preliminary results. *J Shoulder Elbow Surg* 1999;8:1999.

37. Wells J, Kohl JL, Warren RF, et al. Oratec RF–assisted capsular shrinkage of the shoulder: preliminary results. *J Shoulder Elbow Surg* 1999;8:663.

38. Wong KL, Williams GR, Ramsey ML, et al. Thermal capsulorrhaphy for glenohumeral instability. Presented at the 16th annual closed meeting of the American Shoulder and Elbow Surgeons, Philadelphia, PA, 1999.

39. Noonan TJ, Horan M, Hawkins RJ. Outcomes of shoulder instability treated with radiofrequency thermal capsulorrhaphy. *Arthroscopy* 2000;16:428–429.

40. Levy O, Wilson M, Williams H, et al. Thermal capsular shrinkage for shoulder instability: mid-term longitudinal outcome study. Presented at the 67th annual meeting of the American Academy of Orthopaedic Surgeons, Orlando, FL, 2000.

41. Griffith PL, Field LD, Savoie FH. Laser-assisted capsulorrhaphy in multidirectional shoulder instability: a two-year comparison with arthroscopic capsular shift. *Arthroscopy* 1998;14:429.

42. Levitz CL, Andrews JR. The use of arthroscopic thermal shrinkage in the management of internal impingement. *Arthroscopy* 1999;15:569.

43. Levitz CL, Andrews JR, Dugas, C. The use of thermal capsular shrinkage in the management of labral detachments in elite throwing athletes. Presented at the American Orthopedic Society for Sports Medicine specialty day, Orlando, FL, 2000.

44. Mishra DK, Fanton GS. Two-year outcome of arthroscopic Bankart repair and electrothermal assisted capsulorrhaphy for recurrent traumatic anterior shoulder instability. *Arthroscopy* 2000;16:429.

45. Noonan TJ, Briggs K, Hawkins RJ. Outcomes of shoulder instability treated with radiofrequency thermal capsulorrhaphy. Presented at the American Orthopedic Society for Sports Medicine specialty day, Orlando, FL, 2000.

46. Van der Reis W, Wolf EM. Arthroscopic capsulo-labral and superior capsular closure for anterior shoulder instability. *Arthroscopy* 1999;15:571.

47. Perry JJ, Higgins LD. Anterior and posterior cruciate ligament rupture after thermal treatment. *Arthroscopy* 2000;16:732–735.

48. Gryler EC, Greis PE, West JR, et al. Temperatures along the axillary nerve during radiofrequency induced thermal capsular shrinkage of the shoulder. Presented at the 67th annual meeting of the American Academy of Orthopaedic Surgeons, Orlando, FL, 2000.

49. Eakin CL, Dvirnak P, Miller CM, et al. The relationship of the axillary nerve to arthroscopically passed capsulolabral sutures: an anatomic study. *Am J Sports Med* 1998;26:505–509.

50. Anderson K, McCarty EC, Warren RF. Thermal capsulorrhaphy: where are we today? *Sports Med Arthrosc Rev* 1999;7:117–127.

51. Vangsness TC Jr. Thermal capsulorrhaphy: proceed with caution. *Inside AANA* 1999;15:7.

ARTHROSCOPIC TREATMENT OF FRACTURES ABOUT THE SHOULDER

STEPHEN S. BURKHART AND PETER M. PARTEN

The literature on arthroscopic treatment of fractures about the shoulder is sparse, and it is mostly in the form of case reports (1–4).The reason for the paucity of clinical studies in this area is, at least in part, that fractures about the shoulder, in contradistinction to fractures about other major joints such as the hip and knee, are often amenable to nonoperative treatment. Therefore, the shoulder presents less opportunity for the surgeon to consider operative intervention by any means, much less arthroscopic.

This chapter relates our arthroscopic experience in three areas of fracture care for the shoulder:

1. Arthroscopic reduction and internal fixation of acute fractures
2. Arthroscopic approaches to late sequelae of fractures (i.e., malunion, bone deficiency)
3. Arthroscopic treatment of postfracture stiffness

The surgical approaches described here are largely anecdotal and were devised in response to specific situations. They are not necessarily applicable to all fractures in the same category. However, these cases do serve to demonstrate how arthroscopic techniques and principles can be applied in a customized fashion to achieve good results with minimally invasive techniques for problems that otherwise would have required extensive open dissections.

ARTHROSCOPIC REDUCTION AND INTERNAL FIXATION OF ACUTE FRACTURES

Intraarticular Glenoid Fractures

Glenoid fractures that involve more than 25% of the diameter of the inferior glenoid have been shown to constitute a significant bone deficiency that, if ignored, will lead to a high rate of recurrent dislocation, even if the labrum is re-

S. S. Burkhart: The University of Texas Health Science Center at San Antonio, Director of Medical Education, The Orthopaedic Institute, San Antonio, Texas.

P .M. Parten: The San Antonio Orthopaedic Group, San Antonio, Texas.

paired to the rim of the remaining glenoid (5,6). Most glenoid rim fractures are small flecks of bone that can be ignored when performing an arthroscopic or open Bankart repair. However, we have had a few patients with acute anteroinferior dislocations who had such large displaced glenoid fracture fragments that they were unable to keep the shoulder reduced, even in a sling. In our opinion, this type of patient, with an acute injury, is the ideal candidate for arthroscopic reduction and internal fixation of the fracture fragment.

Zamudio (7) reported his experience with arthroscopically guided fixation of comminuted glenoid fractures using percutaneous Kirschner wire (K-wire) fixation. Although his results were anecdotally good, the risk of neurovascular injury with this approach seems significant.

Technique

The operation is carried out with the patient in the lateral decubitus position. After initial inspection of the joint through a posterior portal, we establish an anterosuperior portal as our primary viewing portal, as well as an anterior working portal. This portal affords the best view for assessing the fracture, its reduction, and its fixation. The anteroinferior fracture fragment is typically depressed and requires reduction (Fig. 40.1). Through the anterior portal, a 15-degree elevator (Arthrex, Inc., Naples, FL) is introduced. The elevator is used to lever the displaced fragment to its anatomic position (Fig. 40.2). Next, the fragment is fixed with a K-wire to the main body of the glenoid (Fig. 40.3). This step has several critical points. The angle of approach must be almost parallel to the glenoid articular surface. If the K-wire is aimed more than 30 degrees medially, it likely will not engage the glenoid body, because the anterior glenoid neck forms an acute angle of approximately 40 degrees to the glenoid face. To place the K-wire at the proper angle, its entry point on the skin will be a couple of centimeters medial to the standard anterior portal, so it is essential to minimize abduction of the shoulder to less than 20 degrees, to decrease the risk of injury to the musculocutaneous nerve.

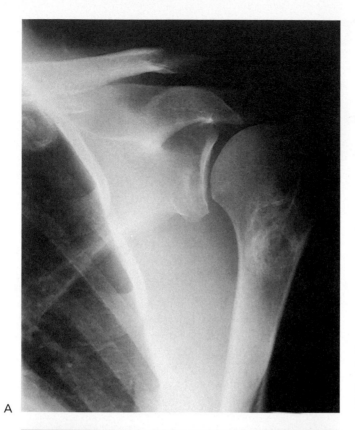

A

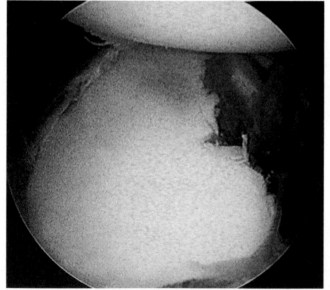

B

FIGURE 40.1 Intraarticular glenoid fracture, left shoulder.
A: An anteroposterior radiograph showing a large displaced anteroinferior glenoid fracture. **B:** An arthroscopic view of a
glenoid fracture through the anterosuperior portal shows a displaced anteroinferior glenoid fragment. **C:** A close-up view of
the displaced fragment.

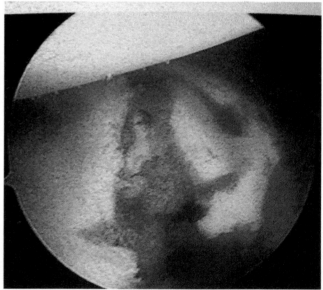

C

Abduction of more than 20 degrees carries the musculocutaneous nerve laterally and can place it dangerously close to
the path of the K-wire. It is best to determine the proper angle of approach with a spinal needle and then to introduce a
small-diameter guide (Spear or BioSpear, Arthrex, Inc.) for
K-wire insertion. The K-wire alone is too flexible for introduction without a guide. The small guide (Spear or Bio-
Spear) is preferable to a standard cannula because the guide
and K-wire must go through the subscapularis tendon,

which is so thick that introduction of a standard cannula can
be quite difficult. If there is room for placement of a second
K-wire to stabilize the fragment further, it is best to place it.
However, the fragment is often small enough that there is
no room for a second K-wire. For fixation, we have used
cannulated 4.0-mm cancellous AO screws (Synthes, Inc.,
Paoli, PA). The Spear guide is removed, leaving only the K-
wire in place. The AO cannulated drill is then introduced
over the K-wire to create the hole for the screw. A depth

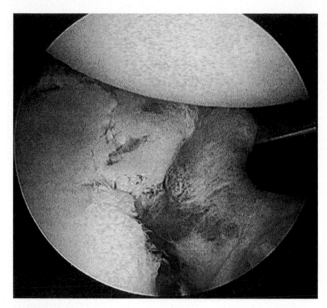

FIGURE 40.2 An arthroscopic elevator confirms that anatomic reduction is possible.

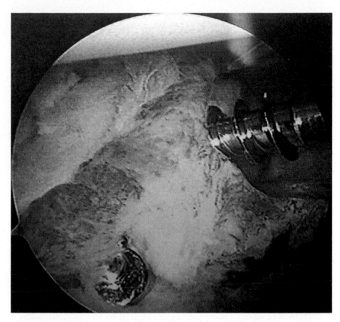

FIGURE 40.4 The second cancellous screw is inserted, to provide rigid fixation of the fracture.

gauge measures the required length of the screw. Then the cannulated 4.0-mm screw is placed over the K-wire (Fig. 40.4). If the proper angle of approach has been chosen, the screw head in its fully seated position will not be "sitting proud" as a potential source of damage to the humeral head. A single screw usually provides excellent fixation. If there is enough room, a second screw is inserted. We have not

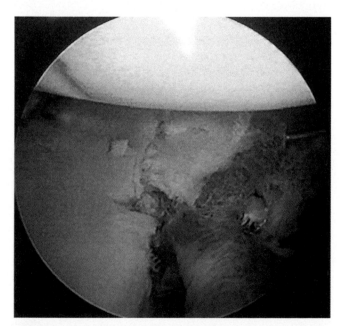

FIGURE 40.3 The most inferiorly placed Kirschner wire (K-wire) is visible distal to a cannulated cancellous screw that has been inserted over the upper K-wire.

arthroscopically fixed any fragments that were large enough to require more than two screws. After the fragment has been fixed to the body of the glenoid, any residual labral disruption from the rim of the glenoid should be repaired with suture anchors (Fig. 40.5).

Humerus: Greater Tuberosity Fractures

There is currently some controversy over the indications for reduction and fixation of displaced fractures of the greater tuberosity. Some authorities have recommended nonoperative treatment if there is less than 1 cm of displacement (8–11). However, Weber brought that recommendation into question, by reporting poor results in several patients with less than 1 cm of displacement who were treated nonoperatively (12). Kim and Ha (4) reported on an arthroscopic approach to the treatment of greater tuberosity fractures. However, they simply debrided the area around the fracture and did not perform any fixation.

If the greater tuberosity heals in a proximally displaced position, it will become a source of subacromial impingement. We have performed arthroscopic subacromial decompression in such cases, and this is quite successful if the tuberosity is not excessively displaced. However, if it is displaced 1 cm or more and heals in that position, then subacromial decompression alone may not be enough to relieve the impingement. In fractures that involve the entire greater tuberosity, the external rotators also produce a deforming force, so the net effects are proximal migration, external rotation, and posteromedial translation of the tuberosity. A fracture that heals in this position will produce not only impingement symptoms, but also weakness of the external

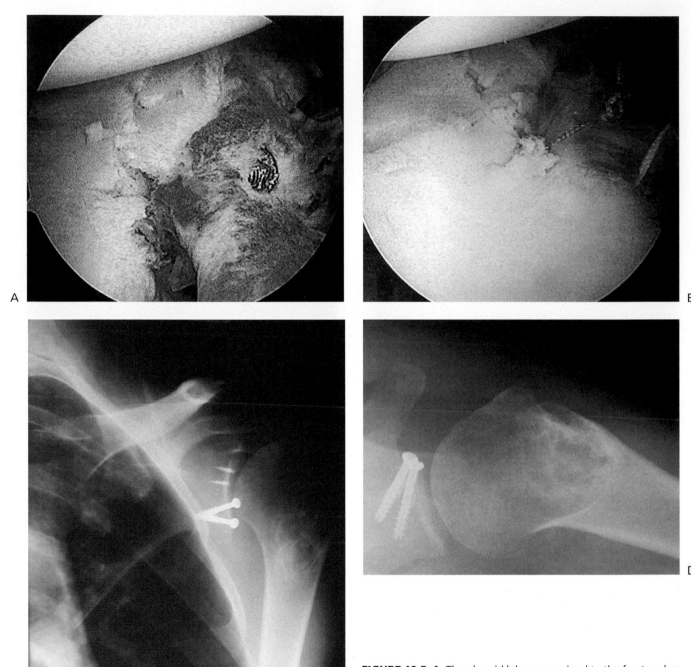

FIGURE 40.5 A: The glenoid labrum proximal to the fracture has been avulsed from the bone and will require repair. **B:** The labral disruption has been repaired with suture anchors. **C:** An antero-posterior radiograph shows anatomic healing of the fracture. The patient has regained a full painless range of shoulder motion, and the shoulder is stable. **D:** An axillary radiograph shows restoration of the glenoid articular arc.

rotators as a result of shortening of their muscle–tendon units caused by the medial translation of their insertion points on the greater tuberosity. To avoid the aforementioned problems, arthroscopic reduction and internal fixation of the greater tuberosity seem reasonable.

Technique

The procedure is performed with the patient in the lateral decubitus position. Glenohumeral arthroscopy is first performed, and the fracture is assessed (Fig. 40.6).

After intraarticular inspection, the scope is placed in a posterior subacromial viewing portal. Through a lateral working portal, a shaver is used to perform a subacromial bursectomy as well as to remove clots and debris from around the fracture site. The surgeon must remove the lateral bursal shelf to afford a clear view into the lateral gutter for optimal visualization of the fracture. The arthroscope is alternated between the posterior and lateral portals for the best view. A spinal needle is used to determine the best angle of approach to the fracture fragment for instrumentation, and accessory lateral or posterolateral portals are established as needed, with care taken to place them above the axillary nerve.

As with open treatment of fractures, the hematoma at the fracture site must be cleared or it may block anatomic reduction. A 15-degree arthroscopic elevator (Arthrex, Inc.) is wedged into the fracture site to hinge it open, and a curette and 4-mm shaver are used to clean out the fracture hematoma (Fig. 40.7). An arthroscopic elevator is used to manipulate the fracture fragment into an anatomic position, and then a percutaneous K-wire is placed for temporary fixation. Next, a second K-wire is placed to serve as the guide for a cannulated screw. This K-wire is overdrilled to provide

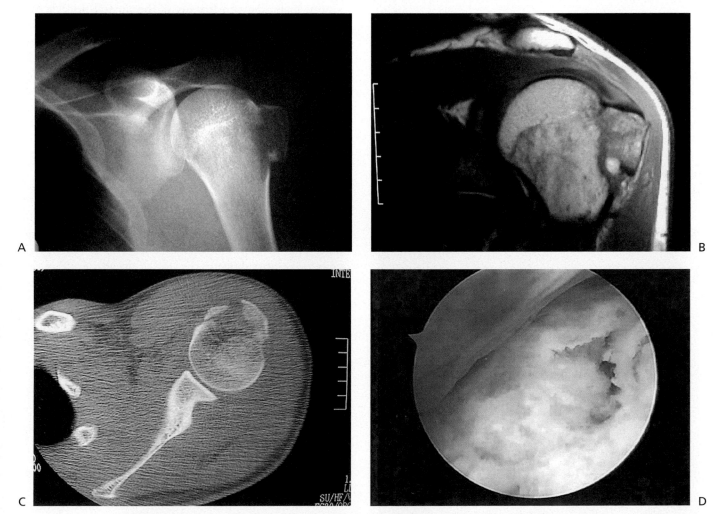

FIGURE 40.6 A: An anteroposterior radiograph of the left shoulder in a 34-year-old man shows a displaced fracture of the greater tuberosity. **B:** Magnetic resonance imaging (MRI) scan shows displacement and rotation of the greater tuberosity fragment. **C:** The axial MRI projection shows external rotation of the greater tuberosity fragment. **D:** The fracture site is identified arthroscopically.

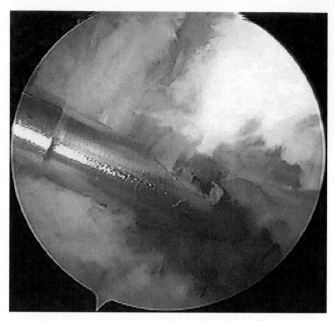

FIGURE 40.7 After the fracture site has been hinged open, a power shaver is used to clean out the fracture hematoma.

a hole for the screw (Fig. 40.8), the channel is measured with a depth gauge, and then a cannulated 4.0-mm AO cancellous screw with a washer (Synthes, Inc.) is inserted over the K-wire (Fig. 40.9). Bicortical fixation is usually possible for the larger fracture fragments because the screw is placed at the metaphyseal level. However, for a small fragment, the obligate obliquity of the screw placement may preclude bicortical fixation.

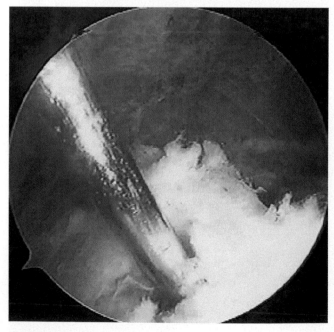

FIGURE 40.8 The transfixing Kirschner wire has been overdrilled to create a hole for the screw.

We have had one patient with an extremely comminuted fracture of the greater tuberosity in whom screw fixation was not possible because of the comminution. Interestingly, the radiograph underestimated the degree of comminution. In that case, we arthroscopically excised the tuberosity bone fragments using pencil-tip electrocautery. This left a free margin of rotator cuff, which we repaired to the bone bed with suture anchors (Fig. 40.10).

ARTHROSCOPIC TREATMENT OF LATE SEQUELAE OF FRACTURES

This section contains anecdotal cases that we have treated arthroscopically.

Varus Malunion of Proximal Humerus Fracture

A varus malunion of a fracture of the surgical neck of the humerus often causes pain. We think that the pain results from two factors. First, we believe that there is impingement pain because the varus rotation of the humeral head, neck, and tuberosity have positioned the tuberosity at a high level, above the humeral head, and in close proximity to the lateral acromion (Fig. 40.11). Second, the medial rotation and translation of the greater tuberosity have effectively shortened the supraspinatus and infraspinatus muscle–tendon units, have caused them to function at less than maximal efficiency, and have predisposed them to muscle fatigue.

For the surgical treatment of varus malunion of the proximal humerus, we have used the following arthroscopic approach. We initially use pencil-tip electrocautery to detach the supraspinatus and infraspinatus insertions from the bone. Then a high-speed bur is brought in to flatten the greater tuberosity down to the level of the articular surface, as well as to perform an arthroscopic subacromial decompression. Finally, we repair the rotator cuff *laterally* onto the bone bed to reestablish the normal length of the supraspinatus and infraspinatus muscle–tendon units (Fig. 40.12).

Malunion of "Head-Splitting" Intraarticular Fracture of the Proximal Humerus

We have had three cases of nondisplaced or minimally displaced greater tuberosity fractures associated with a "head-splitting" fracture that healed with displacement and an intraarticular step-off. The step-off creates a painful catching sensation and sometimes an audible clunk. We have been able to relieve the painful catching by arthroscopically sculpting the humerus to eliminate the step-off and to create a smooth arc in its place. Even though this procedure requires some removal of articular cartilage and creates a fairly large area of exposed bone intraarticularly, patients

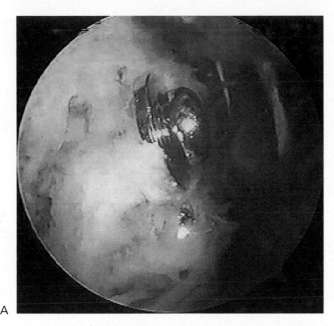
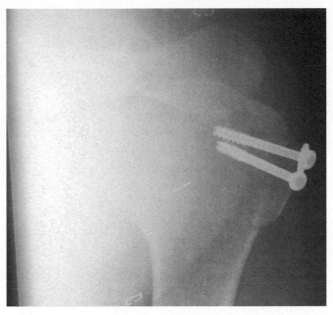

A

B

FIGURE 40.9 A: Screws have been placed to maintain anatomic reduction. **B:** An anteroposterior radiograph confirms anatomic reduction with two AO screws.

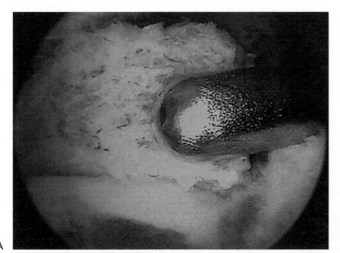
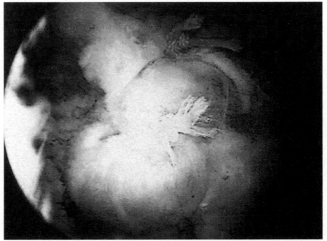

A

B

FIGURE 40.10 A: Left shoulder, lateral viewing portal. Comminuted bone fragments, still attached to the rotator cuff, overlie the humeral articular surface. **B:** Lateral viewing portal. Comminuted bone fragments have been removed, and the cuff margin has been repaired to the humerus with suture anchors.

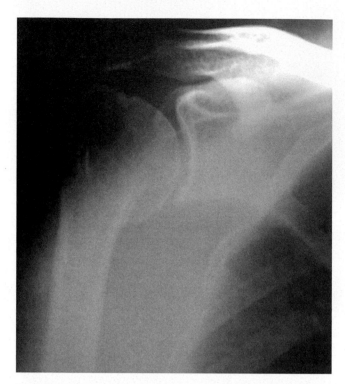

FIGURE 40.11 This anteroposterior radiograph of a right shoulder demonstrates that the varus malunion of the proximal humeral fracture has created two effects: (1) subacromial impingement by upward rotation of the greater tuberosity and (2) shortening of the distance to the supraspinatus and infraspinatus insertion that causes the length–tension relationship to be less than optimal.

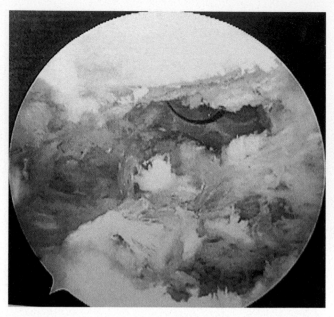

FIGURE 40.12 Right shoulder, posterior viewing portal (same patient as in Fig. 40.11). The subacromial space has been well decompressed by a combination of standard arthroscopic acromioplasty and arthroscopic tuberosityplasty, in which the height of the tuberosity was reduced 6 mm. The rotator cuff was then repaired in a lateralized position on the bone bed to reestablish the length–tension relationship of the supraspinatus and infraspinatus.

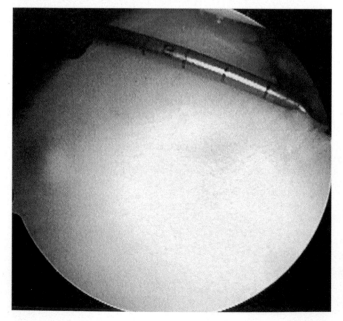

FIGURE 40.13 Left shoulder, anterosuperior viewing portal. This arthroscopic view shows the "inverted pear" appearance of the glenoid with an estimated 30% bone loss of the inferior glenoid diameter based on the location of the glenoid bare spot. The tip of the probe is hooked over the anteroinferior portion of the glenoid, in the area of bone deficiency.

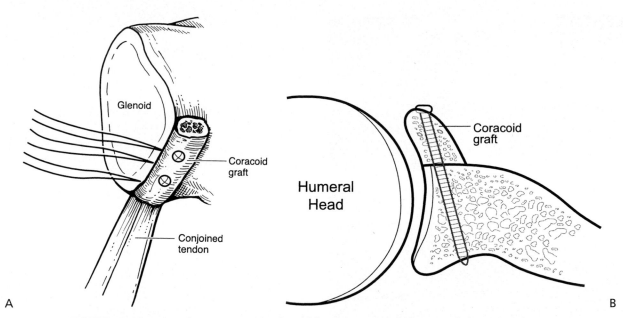

FIGURE 40.14 A: Latarjet reconstruction in which a large coracoid bone graft is used to reconstitute a bone-deficient glenoid. **B:** The axillary projection shows the proper position of the coracoid graft to extend the glenoid articular arc.

report a great deal of pain relief after this surgical procedure.

Arthroscopic Bone Grafting for Glenoid Bone Deficiency

In patients with acute intraarticular glenoid fractures comprising more than 25% of the diameter of the inferior glenoid, we perform arthroscopic reduction and internal fixation as described earlier in this chapter. In patients with chronic recurrent anteroinferior instability as a result of the repetitive dislocations, one frequently finds traumatic compressive bone loss of the anteroinferior glenoid as a result of

the repetitive dislocations, and this bone loss frequently comprises more than 25% of the diameter of the inferior glenoid (Fig. 40.13). This degree of glenoid bone loss predisposes to a high failure rate if arthroscopic Bankart repair is performed (5,6). We have used the open Latarjet reconstruction in this situation, because it uses a large coracoid bone graft to reconstitute the glenoid platform (Fig. 40.14). We have been able to perform a modified Latarjet reconstruction arthroscopically by using a tricortical autogenous bone graft from the scapular spine (rather than the coracoid). The bone graft is easily harvested with the patient in the lateral decubitus position through a 4-cm mini-incision (Fig. 40.15). The graft is transported into the joint and is

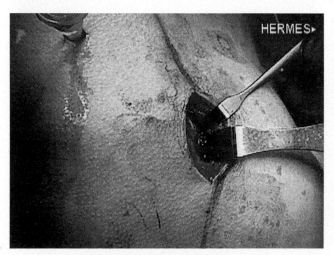
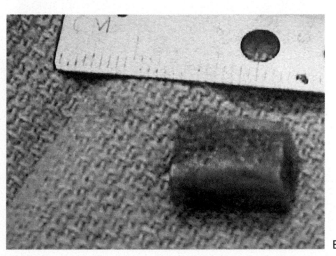

FIGURE 40.15 A: Tricortical bone graft is harvested from the scapular spine through a 4-cm mini-incision. **B:** The harvested scapular bone graft is 12 mm in length.

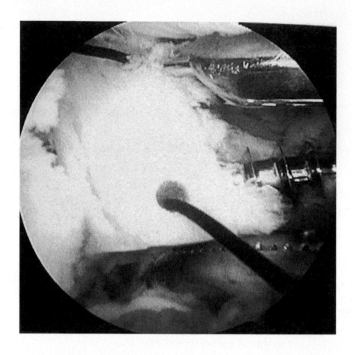

FIGURE 40.16 Left shoulder, anterosuperior viewing portal. Steering sutures, which were used to introduce the graft into the joint, also help to control it within the joint. Kirschner wires (K-wires) hold the graft in place as a 4.0-mm cannulated AO screw is inserted over one of the K-wires.

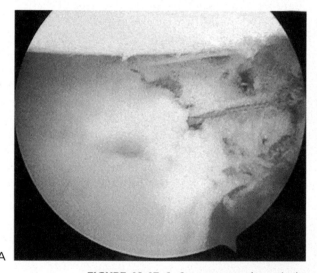

A

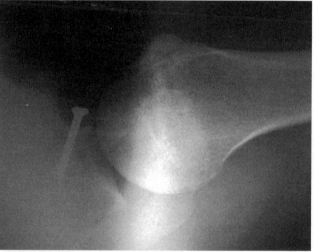

B

FIGURE 40.17 A: Sutures cross the articular surface of the bone graft and traverse from suture anchors placed in the native glenoid to fix the glenohumeral ligaments firmly against the bone graft. We prefer not to place anchors in the graft itself. **B:** The axillary projection shows that the graft has created an anterior extension of the glenoid articular arc.

manipulated into place with steering sutures. Provisional fixation by K-wires and permanent fixation with a cannulated 4.0-mm cancellous AO screw (Synthes, Inc.) are performed in the same manner as for acute glenoid fractures (Fig. 40.16). Suture anchors are placed in the native glenoid to secure the capsule (Fig. 40.17). This is an extremely demanding arthroscopic procedure, and it is mentioned here only as an example of the complexity of what can be done arthroscopically.

ARTHROSCOPIC TREATMENT OF POSTFRACTURE STIFFNESS

For completeness, arthroscopic capsular release for postfracture stiffness is mentioned here. The full technique is outlined in Chapter 35. The stiffness that develops in some patients after fractures about the shoulder may be refractory to stretching exercises in physical therapy as well as resistant to manipulation under anesthesia. The only way to regain motion in these patients is by arthroscopic release, which should be done anteriorly, inferiorly, and posteriorly. We usually release all but a small bridge of capsule spanning the 6 o'clock position, and then we release that most inferior section of capsule by manipulation, to minimize risk to the axillary nerve. The surgeon should be prepared to find a very thick capsule in these postfracture cases, often 8 to 10 mm thick.

CONCLUSION

The advantages of arthroscopic reduction and internal fixation of acute fractures are the same as for arthroscopic treatment of other shoulder conditions, namely, the avoidance of deltoid damage and dysfunction and the prevention of stiffness that results from obliteration of tissue planes by scar formation, as can occur with open surgery. Chronic postfracture reconstructive situations such as malunion and bone deficiency can sometimes be addressed as well. Capsular release for postfracture stiffness can dramatically increase motion and improve function.

Despite the potential for arthroscopy to improve the results of fracture care about the shoulder, the overall percentage of patients who have shoulder fractures is quite small, and therefore we expect that advancement in this area will lag behind the pace of advancement in shoulder arthroscopy in general. Even so, we envision a steady transition over the next few years from open to arthroscopic techniques for treatment of fractures about the shoulder.

REFERENCES

1. Cameron SE. Arthroscopic reduction and internal fixation of an anterior glenoid fracture. *Arthroscopy* 1998;14:743–746.
2. Carro LP, Nuñez MP, Llata JI. Arthroscopic-assisted reduction and percutaneous external fixation of a displaced intra-articular glenoid fracture. *Arthroscopy* 1999;15:211–214.
3. Gartsman GM, Taverna E, Hammerman SM. Case report: arthroscopic treatment of acute traumatic anterior glenohumeral dislocation and greater tuberosity fracture. *Arthroscopy* 1999;15: 648–650.
4. Kim SH, Ha KI. Arthroscopic treatment of symptomatic shoulders with minimally displaced greater tuberosity fracture. *Arthroscopy* 2000;16:695–700.
5. Burkhart SS, DeBeer JF. Traumatic glenohumeral bone defects and their relationship to failure of arthroscopic Bankart repairs: significance of the inverted-pear glenoid and the humeral engaging Hill–Sachs lesion. *Arthroscopy* 2000;16:677–694.
6. Bigliani LU, Newton PM, Steimann SP, et al. Glenoid rim lesions associated with recurrent anterior dislocation of the shoulder. *Am J Sports Med* 1998;26:41–45.
7. Zamudio A. Arthroscopically assisted percutaneous pinning of displaced intra-articular glenoid fractures. Presented at the annual meeting of South American Arthroscopy Association, Santiago, Chile, 1997.
8. Bigliani LU. Fractures of the proximal humerus. In: Rockwood CA II, Green DP, eds. *Fractures*. Philadelphia: JB Lippincott, 1991:899.
9. DePalma AF, Cautilli RA. Fractures of the upper end of the humerus. *Clin Orthop* 1961;20:73–93.
10. Mc Laughlin HL. Dislocation of the shoulder with tuberosity fracture. *Surg Clin North Am* 1963;43:1615–1620.
11. Neer CS. Four-segment classification of proximal humeral fractures. *Instr Course Lect* 1975;24:160–168.
12. Weber SC. The ten millimeter rule revisited: recent experience with the outcome of minimally displaced greater tuberosity fractures. Presented at the 17th annual open meeting of American Shoulder and Elbow Surgeons, San Francisco, CA, 2001.

41

ARTHROSCOPIC MANAGEMENT OF ARTHRITIS AND SYNOVITIS OF THE SHOULDER

SANDRA J. IANNOTTI
RICHARD G. LEVINE
LESLIE S. MATTHEWS

INTRODUCTION

The "shoulder" anatomically refers to the glenohumeral joint, the acromioclavicular (AC) joint, the scapulothoracic articulation, and the musculotendinous and soft tissue structures surrounding these articulations. The focus of this chapter is on the arthritic and synovitic conditions that affect these structures.

Osteoarthritis is relatively uncommon in the shoulder compared with the weight-bearing joints of the body; however, when it is present and symptomatic, can be quite disabling. It is often the result of a local process such as trauma or muscular imbalance that develops over a period of time. In contrast, inflammatory arthritis and synovitis of the shoulder are most commonly local manifestations of a systemic disease process. The more common etiologies are shown in Table 41.1. Appropriate management can be divided into two parts. First, medical treatment of the underlying disease process is essential for the long-term health of the patient. Second, symptom-specific treatment is often necessary to combat local progression of the disease and/or provide symptomatic relief.

Shoulder arthritis can often be successfully managed nonoperatively, but for those cases refractory to conservative treatment, arthroscopic surgical techniques provide an excellent alternative to conventional surgical approaches. In considering surgical treatment of these disorders, the arthroscopic surgeon must have a thorough knowledge of the various disease entities and their patterns of shoulder involvement. Familiarity and experience with the arthroscopic techniques suited to these disorders are also important. This chapter presents an overview of the arthritic and synovitic conditions that can affect the shoulder joint and describes in detail the techniques of arthroscopic management of these disorders.

Diagnosis

Successful management of shoulder disorders begins with obtaining the proper diagnosis. Most patients with shoulder pain do not have arthritis or synovitis but, rather, an impairment of the soft tissues of the shoulder, such as bursitis, tendonitis, capsulitis, or rotator cuff conditions. Other diagnostic considerations must include referred pain from cervical nerve root irritation, abdominal sources (e.g., cholecystitis), the lungs (e.g., Pancoast's tumor), and the heart (e.g., angina). Obtaining the proper diagnosis is essential to formulating an appropriate treatment plan. Knowledge of the presenting signs and symptoms in combination with examination and investigative studies will aid the clinician in accurate diagnosis.

History

Certain historical features are helpful in developing the differential diagnosis. For example, pain at rest rarely occurs in rheumatoid arthritis (RA) or the seronegative spondyloarthropathies. If pain at rest is present, septic arthritis, gout, or a neoplastic process should be considered. A complete medical and musculoskeletal history should be obtained to aid in diagnosis, in addition to a quantitative and qualitative description of the chief complaint. Symptom onset, duration, and association with other complaints (e.g., involvement of multiple joints) should be elicited.

Physical Examination

Physical examination should be performed in a systematic fashion to identify the pathology and evaluate the overall

S. J. Iannotti, R. G. Levine, and L. S. Matthews: Department of Orthopaedic Surgery, The Union Memorial Hospital, Baltimore, Maryland.

TABLE 41.1 INFLAMMATORY ARTHRIDITIES

Seronegative spondyloathridities	Polymyalgia rheumatica
Ankylosing spondylitis	Amyloid arthritis
Reiter's syndrome	Pigmented villonodular synovitis
Psoriatic arthritis	Synovial chondromatosis (osteochondromatosis)
Enteropathic arthritis	Hemophilic arthritis
Rheumatoid arthritis	Reactive synovitis
Juvenile rheumatoid arthritis	
Crystalline arthritis	
Gout	
Pseudogout	
Apatite gout	

shoulder function. Inspection, palpation, active and passive range of motion (ROM), neurologic status, vascular status, muscle strength testing, and cervical spine examination must be included in the evaluation, as well as disease-specific maneuvers (Table 41.2). Examination of the sternoclavicular joint, AC joint, and scapula must also be included.

Radiographic Analysis

A standard radiographic shoulder series should be obtained for the routine initial evaluation of a patient with shoulder pathology. This consists of anteroposterior (AP) and lateral views in the plane of the scapula and an axillary view. Additional radiographic evaluation should be obtained according to the specific indications based on a working diagnosis. Advanced imaging modalities such as magnetic resonance imaging (MRI), bone scan, sonography, arthrography, and computed tomography (CT) can assist in confirmation of the diagnosis.

Laboratory Analysis

Initial laboratory screening for a patient with a shoulder complaint is not necessary. Tests should be obtained to as-

TABLE 41.2 COMMONLY PERFORMED EXAMINATION MANEUVERS OF THE SHOULDER

Maneuver	Indication
Impingement sign	Subacromial impingement
Adson's maneuver	Thoracic outlet
Spurling's test	Cervical radiculopathy
Cross arm adduction test	Acromioclavicular joint
O'Briens test	SLAP lesion and acromioclavicular joint
Drop arm test	Rotator cuff—supraspinatus
Lift-off test	Subscapularis
Napolean's test	Subscapularis
Anterior Apprehension	Instability
Jobe's relocation test	Instability
Posterior stress test	Instability
Sulcus sign	Instability

sist with confirmation of the diagnosis formulated from a thorough history, physical examination, and radiologic evaluation. However, serologic and synovial fluid evaluation is often helpful in the diagnosis of inflammatory arthritis.

Synovial aspirate should be placed in an anticoagulated tube, because inflammatory synovial fluid contains clotting proteins. The traditional classifications of the leukocyte (WBC) count to classify fluid as inflammatory (2,000 to 40,000 cells/μL) or infectious (more than 40,000/μL) have too many exceptions to be considered valid (1). Typically, a WBC count of less than 2,000/μL with less than 50% neutrophils is found in noninflammatory disorders such as osteoarthritis, amyloidosis, and sickle cell disease. In uncomplicated osteoarthritis, the WBC count is usually less than 1,000/μL with less than 30% neutrophils. If the WBC count is greater than 100,000/μL, infection should be considered present until proven otherwise (1). If the WBC count is between 50,000 and 100,000/μL, the diagnosis could be sepsis or a crystal-induced or inflammatory condition such as RA or Reiter's syndrome.

The WBC differential count also aids in diagnosis. Typically, the neutrophil count is greater than 95% in infectious fluids, although gouty arthritis can have a similar presentation. (1). A Gram's stain and culture should be done if infection is suspected. Examination under routine microscopy and polarized light microscopy will demonstrate crystals in cases of crystal-induced synovitis. There is little, if any, benefit in measuring glucose, lactate, or protein levels or in performing immunologic testing on synovial fluid in the clinical setting.

Treatment

Treatment of inflammatory arthritis or synovitis is disease specific. Both the inflamed joint and the underlying disease process need to be addressed, and this often necessitates systemic treatment. The majority of these disorders require medical intervention as primary therapy, with adjunctive surgical management for progressive disease or to control symptoms. Exceptions include septic arthritis, which requires early surgical intervention, and osteochondromatosis and reactive synovitis, which require removal of the offending source. In contrast, osteoarthritis can often be managed with antiinflammatory medications or local corticosteroid injection.

DEGENERATIVE ARTHRITIS OF THE GLENOHUMERAL JOINT

The primary presentation of arthritis is pain and loss of motion of varying degrees. Of all patients who present with these complaints, degenerative arthritis is less common as the cause. Early osteoarthritis is often difficult to diagnose, and the presenting physical findings are subtle. In contrast, patients with degenerative arthritis secondary to severe rotator cuff tears (so-called cuff tear arthropathy) (2,3) usually have greater pain and dysfunction, including weakness and ankylosis. Other causes of secondary arthritis include posttraumatic arthritis, arthropathy associated with instability (4,5), and conditions such as osteonecrosis or hemochromatosis.

Glenohumeral arthritis in its early stages may be difficult to diagnose. Patients commonly complain of pain with overhead or extremes of motion and have difficulty finding a comfortable position in which to sleep. These complaints are also typically voiced by patients with inflammation of the rotator cuff and subacromial bursa, which are more common conditions. The physical examination may be confusing as well, with both conditions potentially demonstrating loss of motion and pain at extremes of motion. A sensitive indicator of intraarticular pathology is loss of external rotation (6). Tenderness over the posterior joint line has been described as a marker for osteoarthritis (7). It may be

possible to elicit catching and grinding at the glenohumeral joint when osteoarthritis is present, but this is sometimes difficult to distinguish from the crepitation produced by inflammation of the rotator cuff and subacromial bursa (8). Selective injections of a local anesthetic agent may be helpful in narrowing the diagnosis.

Early radiographic findings of osteoarthritis consist of joint space narrowing and subchondral irregularity. A small osteophyte may be present at the inferior articular border of the humeral head (8). True AP and axillary radiographs of the glenohumeral joint are essential in the identification of these abnormalities in the early stages of the disease. Standard radiographs may remain negative even when degenerative changes are significant enough to produce pain (9). MRI has not been shown to be particularly sensitive in identifying early osteoarthritis (8), but it may be useful to rule out other shoulder pathology (10). As the disease progresses, radiographic changes become obvious, with joint space narrowing and irregularity, osteophytic and cystic changes, and loose body formation (Fig. 41.1).

Diagnostic arthroscopy is a valuable adjunct to the clinical and radiographic evaluation of a patient with shoulder pain of undetermined origin. Inspection of the glenohumeral joint will demonstrate chondral damage to the humeral head and/or glenoid in cases of early osteoarthritis. Arthroscopy may also aid in determining the underlying etiologic factors in cases of secondary osteoarthritis. Early identification and treatment of a correctable disorder may halt or slow the degenerative process. Degenerative arthritis associated with chronic instability is an important example (4).

Therapeutically, arthroscopy provides an alternative midway between conservative treatment and more radical

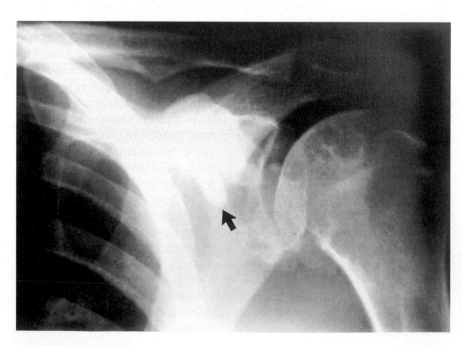

FIGURE 41.1 Radiograph demonstrating glenohumeral arthritis, with irregularity and narrowing of the joint space, inferior osteophytes, cystic changes, and a loose body *(arrow)*. The rotator cuff is intact, and the normal relationship of the humeral head to the glenoid is maintained.

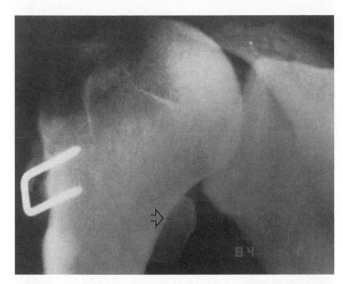

FIGURE 41.2 Radiograph demonstrating a large inferior loose body *(arrow).* Staple is from a prior failed Magnuson–Stack procedure.

surgical techniques (11,12). Traditional treatment of glenohumeral osteoarthritis has consisted of prolonged conservative treatment with oral antiinflammatory agents and physical therapy, with progression to arthroplasty or arthrodesis when conservative treatment is no longer successful (6,13). Arthroscopic treatment with joint lavage, loose body removal (Fig. 41.2), degenerative articular cartilage and labral debridement (Fig. 41.3), and subacromial bursectomy may offer pain relief with relatively low morbidity (11). Favor-

able short-term results with improved function and pain have been reported with this technique (11,14,15). Benefit appears to be greatest when the rotator cuff is intact and joint involvement is mild. Arthroscopic capsular release has been suggested for patients with substantially limited ROM, to improve motion, lessen pain, and lessen abnormal glenohumeral joint forces (6,15,16).

In the case of more advanced degenerative disease of the glenohumeral joint, arthroscopy is usually not needed for diagnostic purposes. Arthroscopic debridement offers only transient relief (Fig. 41.4) (8,15). The evidence supporting the use of abrasion of articular surfaces and microfracture techniques in the shoulder is anecdotal (6).

Patients with classic cuff tear arthropathy exhibit osteoarthritis of the shoulder secondary to a large tear of the rotator cuff and resultant loss of the primary stabilizers of the glenohumeral joint. The instability and resultant articular damage lead to crystal formation and the secretion of destructive enzymes by an inflamed synovium (3,17). The disease is more common in elderly women and is often bilateral (3). The degenerative joint disease seen in this group of patients is usually quite severe (2,18). Pain and restriction of motion may be great, and the torn rotator cuff causes demonstrable loss of strength. Radiographic changes include joint destruction, osteoporosis, and superior migration of the humeral head (Fig. 41.5).

Most patients present after failure of conservative treatment, with a degree of degenerative joint disease so severe that only fusion or arthroplasty can be considered. Arthroscopic debridement and irrigation has a limited role in the treatment of this condition, providing transient relief (3). If the patient presents at an earlier stage, with less severe de-

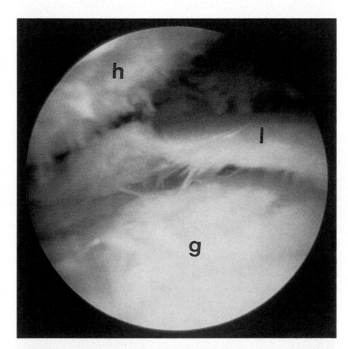

FIGURE 41.3 Arthroscopic photograph of glenohumeral arthritis with articular cartilage degeneration and a degenerative labral tear. h, humeral head; g, glenoid; l, labrum.

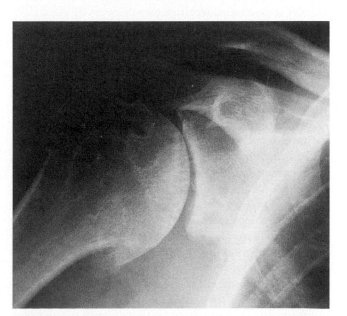

FIGURE 41.4 Radiograph demonstrating severe glenohumeral arthritis. The disease in this shoulder is advanced. Arthroscopic treatment is extremely unlikely to be helpful.

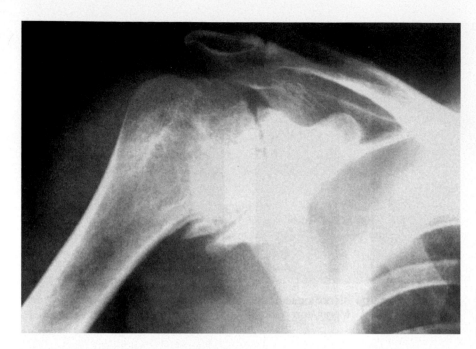

FIGURE 41.5 Radiograph demonstrating cuff tear arthropathy, with cystic changes, osteophytes, joint space obliteration, and superior migration of the humeral head.

generative joint disease, rotator cuff repair should be considered the treatment of choice. Arthroscopic subacromial decompression should be viewed with caution, because it may compromise the secondary stabilizing structures of the coracoacromial arch, preventing further superior humeral head migration.

ACROMIOCLAVICULAR JOINT ARTHRITIS

The differential diagnosis of pain referable to the AC joint includes degenerative arthritis, osteolysis of the distal clavicle, AC instability, glenohumeral arthritis, and subacromial impingement. Painful degenerative arthritis of the AC joint is often associated with prior trauma, either fracture or separation, but commonly the cause is idiopathic. Normal narrowing of the AC joint occurs with aging, is associated with heavy laborers, and is most often asymptomatic (19,20). The contribution of inferior AC osteophyte formation to the impingement syndrome is controversial.

Clinical evaluation must identify the role of the AC joint in the production of each patient's symptoms, so that the appropriate treatment is prescribed. The presenting symptom of AC arthritis is pain localized to the joint. The pain may radiate medially toward the base of the neck or laterally toward the acromion. The pain is worse with activity, especially overhead motion and cross-body adduction. The most reliable finding is localized tenderness directly over the joint (21). Pain localized to the AC joint may be elicited by cross-body adduction of the arm (Fig. 41.6). Injection of a local anesthetic into the joint should provide almost complete (albeit often temporary) relief in cases of isolated involvement. There is a pitfall: One must be careful when injecting the

AC joint to avoid penetrating the inferior AC joint capsule and injecting anesthetic into the subacromial space. Selective injections into the AC joint, subacromial space, and glenohumeral joint may be useful in determining the contribution of the AC joint to shoulder pain when impingement or combined degenerative joint disease is present.

A complete radiographic examination includes an AP view in the plane of the thorax, an axillary lateral view, a scapular "Y" view, and an AP with a 10-degree cephalic tilt. Reducing the voltage by 33% to 50% compared with a glenohumeral view improves visualization of the AC joint. Radiographic changes include sclerosis, joint space narrowing, and osteophyte and cyst formation (22) (Fig. 41.7). Symptoms at the AC joint do not necessarily correlate with

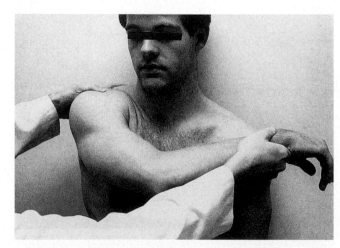

FIGURE 41.6 This cross-body adduction maneuver elicits pain in the presence of acromioclavicular joint disease.

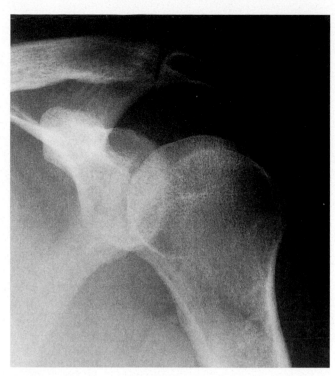

FIGURE 41.7 Radiograph demonstrating acromioclavicular degenerative disease, with inferior osteophyte formation and joint space narrowing and irregularity.

the radiographic appearance of the joint, further increasing the importance of clinical evaluation (23). MRI may show fluid and edema in the AC joint. However, these findings should be interpreted with caution, because MRI has shown findings of degenerative arthritis in 75% of asymptomatic people (19,24).

Surgical treatment is indicated if conservative treatment with nonsteroidal antiinflammatory drugs (NSAIDs) and judicious intraarticular corticosteroid injections has failed. Open resection of the distal clavicle has been shown to give consistently satisfactory results in the treatment of AC joint disorders. Arthroscopic distal clavicle resection was first described in conjunction with subacromial decompression and accordingly was performed through the subacromial bursa (25). This approach continues to be very useful, especially in cases of combined AC arthritis and impingement syndrome. If isolated AC disease is present, the joint may be accessed alternatively through the direct superior approach originally described by Johnson (26). This technique allows the surgeon to avoid acromioplasty when it is not indicated.

The bony resection of the distal clavicle obtained with arthroscopic techniques has traditionally been less that that with open techniques, which typically remove 10 to 20 mm of bone. Several studies demonstrate that arthroscopic resection of 5 to 10 mm is sufficient to prevent bony contact (27,28). Violation of either the superior or the inferior AC ligament is unlikely to increase instability of the joint unless both of these ligaments are removed (27). Successful short-

term to mid-term clinical results have been reported with either arthroscopic technique (13,23,24,29–31). Advantages of arthroscopic techniques include decreased postoperative pain, smaller scars, and the opportunity to avoid inpatient surgery. In addition, preservation of the deltoid attachment to the acromion lowers the risk of postoperative weakness and eliminates the need for lengthy postoperative protection in a sling. However, the choice of arthroscopic versus standard open techniques should be based on each surgeon's preference and experience.

INFLAMMATORY ARTHRITIS

Almost all of the approximately 100 rheumatologic diseases can affect the shoulder. Those most commonly exhibiting shoulder involvement are, in decreasing order of frequency, the seronegative spondyloarthropathies, seropositive RA, pseudogout, gout, Reiter's syndrome, and juvenile rheumatoid arthritis (JRA) (32).

Seronegative Spondyloathridities

The seronegative sypondyloarthropathies comprise a group of disorders with similar clinical manifestations and the absence of rheumatoid factor that most often involve the sacroiliac joint and the peripheral joints in an asymmetric fashion. They include ankylosing spondylitis, Reiter's syndrome or reactive arthritis, psoriatic arthritis, and enteropathic arthritis. The role of arthroscopy in the management of these conditions is limited.

Ankylosing Spondylitis

Ankylosing spondylitis primarily involves the axial skeleton, with sacroiliac joint involvement. Men are more commonly affected than women, with a ratio of 2:1 to 3:1 and a disease prevalence in most populations of 0.1% to 0.2% (33). Clinical manifestations begin in late adolescence or early adulthood, and the most common early complaints are low back pain and morning stiffness that usually improves with exercise (33). One third to one half of patients develop peripheral arthritis, most commonly involving the hip and shoulder (34,35). Shoulder involvement can be divided into three categories: (a) acute inflammatory arthropathy of the sternoclavicular or AC joint, (b) restriction of scapulothoracic motion, and (c) destructive involvement of the glenohumeral joint (36). Patients exhibit limitation of motion of the lumbar spine and expansion of the chest of less than 2.5 cm. They often have shoulder pain, but moderate restriction in ROM is more common (37).

Radiographs often show the pathognomonic advanced intervertebral ankylosis of bone in the cervical, thoracic, and lumbar spine—the "bamboo spine" of ankylosing spondylitis. The most characteristic signs of ankylosing spondylitis in the shoulder are erosion of the humeral head and the presence of enthesophytes (osteophytes arising at the attachment of tendons, muscles, or articular capsule and ligaments). The combination of an enthesophyte at the acromial attachment of the coracoacromial ligament, termed a bearded acromion, and an erosion of the superolateral area of the humeral head is often present (36). AC joint changes are also frequently seen, as is ossification of the coracoclavicular ligaments. Ankylosing spondylitis is strongly associated with the presence of the human leukocyte antigen class I antigen, HLA-B27; however, routine testing is not necessary for diagnosis. Treatment is aimed at control of pain and inflammation, with maintenance of motion to prevent deformity of the axial skeleton.

Reiter's Syndrome (Reactive Arthritis)

Reiter's syndrome is often defined as aseptic arthritis triggered by an infectious agent located outside the joint (e.g., urethritis, cervicitis, dysentery). Peripheral arthritis, enthesopathic involvement, pelvic and axial symptoms, and genitourinary or gastrointestinal involvement are often present. With the peripheral arthritis syndrome, the onset is acute; within a few days, two to four joints (oligoarthritis) are painful and swollen, with an asymmetric distribution (33). Examination is variable. Diffuse polyarticular pain, stiffness, and swelling are often accompanied by weight loss and fever. The erythrocyte sedimentation rate (ESR) and C-reactive protein (CRP) values are usually elevated. Synovial fluid analysis shows a WBC count greater than 2,000 cells/μL, with a majority of neutrophils. Urogenital swab culture is a useful diagnostic method for detection of arthritogenic infection in extraarticular-asymptomatic patients with undifferentiated oligoarthritis (38). Treatment involves management of the underlying infection and NSAIDs as needed.

Psoriatic Arthritis

Psoriatic arthritis is a seronegative inflammatory arthritis that is associated with psoriasis. It affects men and women equally, and the reported overall prevalence has ranged from 0.67% to 1% (33). Oligoarthritis affecting fewer than five joints, often in an asymmetric distribution, is considered the most common pattern of psoriatic arthritis. Patients present with pain, stiffness, and swelling of the affected joints. The inflamed joints in patients with psoriatic arthritis often have a purplish discoloration. Skin and nail changes typical of psoriasis are usually present, and involvement of the distal interphalangeal joints is common. Specific radiologic features of psoriatic arthritis include lack of juxtaarticular osteopenia, presence of the "pencil-in-cup" change, ankylosis, periosteal reaction, and spur formation (33). NSAIDS are used for symptomatic treatment of the arthritis in patients with mild or moderate disease. Slow-reacting antirheumatic drugs are used for severe cases.

Enteropathic Arthritis

Enteropathic arthritis refers to the articular manifestations seen in patients with the inflammatory bowel diseases—ulcerative colitis and Crohn's disease. The overall incidence of peripheral arthritis in these patients ranges form 2% to 20% (33). There is an equal incidence in women and men, and the age at onset ranges from 25 to 44 years. The arthritis is pauciarticular and asymmetric, usually transient, and migratory, lasting 6 to 8 weeks. However, 10% of patients go on to develop a chronic arthritis (33). Recurrences are common. The knees and ankle are the most commonly affected joints, with the shoulder involved in one third of cases. Affected joints are painful and swollen, often with an accompanying effusion. Radiographs of the peripheral joints usually do not show erosions. Synovial fluid analysis reveals low-grade to severe inflammation, with WBC counts ranging from 1,000 to 50,000 cells/μL, predominantly neutrophils (39). NSAIDs may be of benefit, but they should be used with caution because they can affect the underlying inflammatory bowel disease. Successful management of the bowel disease usually terminates the peripheral arthritis (34).

Rheumatoid Arthritis

RA, the most common form of inflammatory arthritis, is a disease of the synovial tissue that can lead to progressive joint destruction and often affects the shoulder in patients with polyarticular disease. Disease onset most frequently occurs during the fourth or fifth decade, with a prevalence of 1% that increases with age (40). Lehtinen et al. (41–43) reported on the incidence of glenohumoral, AC, and subacromial involvement with 15-year follow-up in a series of studies. They found that after 15 years more than half of the patients with RA showed definite involvement of the glenohumoral joint, and two thirds had involvement of the AC joint; among patients with shoulder involvement, diminution of the subacromial space was commonly appreciated. Previous studies have implicated shoulder involvement in up to 90% of patients with RA who were monitored over long periods (44).

Onset is insidious, with episodic exacerbations interspersed with quiescent periods. Initial involvement consists of synovitis of the glenohumeral joint, AC joint, and/or subacromial bursa. In later stages, degenerative arthropathy with involvement of the rotator cuff often develops. Clinical AC symptoms are less common than radiographic joint degeneration. Disease in the AC joint and in the glenohumeral joint may follow independent courses in both timing and severity (42,43). Patients often experience pain during periods of synovitic exacerbations and loss of motion that gradually worsens as the disease becomes more chronic. In early disease, the symptoms are often more severe in the morning.

Physical examination of the entire musculoskeletal system is necessary with care to evaluate the hips, knees, hands, feet, and cervical spine. Shoulder girdle pain and loss of ROM are often present, and they vary in severity in relation to the stage of disease progression. Warmth, diffuse swelling, and fullness may be appreciated with the presence of a mild effusion. The joint is often held in slight flexion and internal rotation to increase capsular volume. AC joint palpation and cross-arm adduction tests are often positive, and careful evaluation of the rotator cuff should be performed. Scapulothoracic motion should be evaluated to assess involvement of the scapulothoracic bursa, which is commonly inflamed.

Radiographic changes include marginal erosions of the humeral head, subchondral sclerosis, osteopenia, subchondral cysts, joint space narrowing, and osteophyte formation. Neer classified the pattern of structural destruction into wet, dry, and resorptive types (45). In the dry type, there is a diminished joint space, periarticular sclerosis, and bone cysts. In the wet type, marginal erosions and intrusion of the humeral head into the glenoid are present. The resorptive type is characterized by bone resorption. More recently, Hirooka et al. (46) classified patients with shoulder involvement into five categories based on their radiographic appearance 5 to 10 years after onset of disease and correlated these findings with prognosis and disease progression. They found that patients exhibiting subchondral cysts and bone erosion and patients with extensive or rapid bone resorption had more rapid and severe joint destruction. Lehtinen et al. reported the radiographic findings in 74 patients with seropositive RA at 15-year follow-up. The type, frequency and distribution of glenohumeral involvement are shown in Table 41.3 and Fig. 41.8 (42). AC joint involvement is most often seen on the inferior joint margin of the clavicle, followed by the inferior joint margin of the acromion (43). Bony erosions predominate, with osteophytes, pseudocysts, and subchondral sclerosis also present.

Sonography can reveal inflammatory conditions at early stages of RA when no radiographic changes are seen. Alasaarela and Alasaarela (47) performed ultrasound examinations on 44 patients (88 shoulders) with RA and found subacromial–subdeltoid bursitis in 69%, glenohumeral syn-

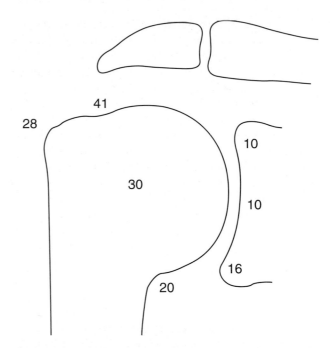

FIGURE 41.8 Distribution and frequency (%) of erosive changes in 148 rheumatoid glenohumeral joints 15 years after onset. The illustration represents the right shoulder in the anteroposterior view. (From Lehtinen JT, Belt EA, Kautiainen HJ, et al. Incidence of glenohumeral joint involvement in seropositive rheumatoid arthritis: a 15 year endpoint study. *J Rheumatol* 2000;27:347–350, with permission.)

ovitis in 58%, biceps tendonitis in 57%, and changes in the supraspinatus in 33% of shoulders. MRI is valuable in the assessment of patients with RA because it examines both the soft tissues and the bony structures of the shoulder (48). It can be particularly useful in the evaluation of the rotator cuff.

Laboratory analysis of synovial fluid demonstrates a class II inflammatory fluid with a predominance of polymorphonuclear leukocytes. Approximately 80% of patients with RA have positive serum rheumatoid factor (49).

Nonoperative management with medications such a NSAIDs or disease-modifying drugs is usually the first-line treatment for patients with RA. Corticosteroid injections may be used as symptoms dictate with significant effective-

TABLE 41.3 INCIDENCE OF RADIOGRAPHIC FINDINGS IN 148 GLENOHUMERAL JOINTS 15 YEARS AFTER ONSET OF RHEUMATOID ARTHRITIS

Radiographic Finding	Humerus, N (%)	Glenoid, N (%)	Total	
			N (%)	95% CI[a]
Erosions	71 (48)	28 (19)	71 (48)	40–56
Cysts	25 (17)	0 (0)	25 (17)	11–23
Subchondral sclerosis	13 (9)	9 (6)	14 (9)	5–15
Osteophytes	7 (5)	6 (4)	13 (9)	5–15

[a] 95% confidence interval for the total value of the percentage.
From Lehtinen JT, Belt EA, Kautiainen HJ, et al. Incidence of glenohumeral joint involvement in seropositive rheumatoid arthritis: a 15-year endpoint study. *J Rheumatol* 2000;27:347–350, with permission.

ness; however, they are not curative and do not prevent progression of joint destruction. Physical therapy plays an important role in management of the shoulder in patients with RA. Active and passive ROM exercises are valuable in maintaining function.

Operative treatment of the shoulder is indicated for those patients with RA who have persistent pain that fails to improve with nonoperative management or significant loss of shoulder function. The most common treatment options are synovectomy (open or arthroscopic), bursectomy, capsular release, and arthroplasty. Historically, synovectomy and bursectomy were offered to patients in the early stages of their disease process, in an attempt to alleviate symptoms before joint destruction occurred and perhaps to delay the natural progression of the disease. More recently, researchers have been able to categorize the patterns of disease progression by radiologic studies and offer treatment recommendations based on disease type. Wakitani et al. (50) reported results of 47 shoulder surgeries (18 arthroscopic synovectomies, 10 total shoulder replacements, 19 humeral head replacements) in relation to five different destruction patterns of RA: nonprogressive, arthrosis-like, erosive, collapse, and mutilating patterns. Arthroscopic synovectomy, which also included bursectomy, decompression, cuff debridement, and cuff repair when present, was effective in relieving pain and improving ROM in those patients in the nonprogressive category and relieving pain in those in the erosive category. Arthroscopic treatment was of no benefit for patients in the collapse category.

Arthroscopic management of RA of the shoulder allows for treatment of intraarticular pathology, rotator cuff repair, and access to the AC joint. For advanced disease, shoulder arthroplasty remains a safe and reliable method of treatment that provides patients with reliable pain relief. Postarthroplasty function is related to preoperative motion, the status of the rotator cuff, and scapulothoracic motion.

Juvenile Rheumatoid Arthritis

JRA is a systemic disease of childhood that is characterized by chronic synovial inflammation. Associated signs and symptoms include rash, iridocyclitis, cervical spine involvement, pericarditis, tenosynovitis, intermittent fever, and morning stiffness. It affects girls more commonly than boys, with disease onset at any age during childhood. There are three subtypes—pauciarticular, polyarticular, and systemic—with different attributes. Approximately one third of JRA patients have significant functional limitations at 10 years' follow-up (1). At 3 to 7 years after disease onset, 12% of JRA patients have limited ability to care for themselves or are wheelchair bound; however, the percentage with substantial disability jumps to 48% at 16 or more years after the onset of disease (1). Shoulder involvement appears uncommon in children with pauciarticular arthritis, but it occurs in 50% of children with polyarticular onset and in 80% of

children with systemic onset (51). In total, arthritis of the shoulder is present in 33% of children with JRA, as reported by Libby et al. (51).

Physical examination should include evaluation for skin rashes and eye involvement (slit-lamp examination to identify iridocyclitis), as well as a standard musculoskeletal examination. Stiffness and swelling are commonly seen, but pain is often minimal in patients with JRA. Radiographic changes consisting of erosions and joint space narrowing occur in approximately one half of patients with systemic or polyarticular disease and one third of those in the pauciarticular JRA subgroup (1). Serologic evaluation for rheumatoid factor and antinuclear antibody (ANA) should be performed to assist with diagnosis and categorization of disease type. Testing for other causes of arthritis, including infectious causes (e.g., Lyme disease, gonococcal infection), should be performed.

Treatment includes night splinting, salicylates, and NSAIDs. Synovectomy has been used for patients whose disease was refractory to conservative management. Ovregard et al. (52) reported a retrospective analysis of 212 patients who underwent a total of 512 open synovectomies in various joints. Of the 389 operations evaluated according to response to synovectomy after 3 years, 303 were classified as responders, 45 as nonclassifiable, and 41 as nonresponders. Global assessment, soft tissue swelling, and limitation of movement were the parameters used for postoperative evaluation. Glenohumeral synovectomy was performed in only three of these patients. Progression of radiologic osteoarthritic changes at 5-year follow-up after synovectomy was reported in another study (53). Therefore, the effect of synovectomy on disease progression remains unclear. Arthroscopic synovectomy of the shoulder should be considered in cases of chronic pain and swelling unresponsive to other forms of therapy. Results are likely to be better if the procedure is performed before the appearance of destructive radiographic changes (54).

Crystalline Arthritis

Although several rare forms of crystalline arthritides have been described, gout, pseudogout, and apatite gout (the "Milwaukee shoulder syndrome") are by far the most common (55). Each involves intraarticular crystal deposition. Subsequent phagocytosis and release of lysosomal enzymes and chemotactic factors produces an inflammatory reaction.

Gout

Gout encompasses a heterogeneous group of disorders that occur alone or in combination and include hyperuricemia; attacks of acute, typically monoarticular, inflammatory arthritis; tophaceous deposition of urate crystals in and around joints; interstitial deposition of urate crystals in renal parenchyma; and urolithiasis.

Acute monoarticular arthritis is often of rapid onset and extremely painful. Occasionally patients experience a prodrome or previous episodes of milder pain lasting hours. Pain is accompanied by inflammation, swelling, erythema, warmth, and tenderness and may be accompanied by a low-grade fever. If untreated, the attack usually peaks 24 to 48 hours after the initial episode and resolves over the next 7 to 10 days. Typically the attack affects only one joint, although multiple joint symptoms can occur. The peripheral joints are more commonly affected, with the first metatarsal–phalangeal joint being involved in more than 50% of first attacks and more than 90% at some time in the life of the patient with chronic gout.

Affected joints are usually exquisitely tender with painful ROM, resembling in this way a septic joint. Erythema and warmth can also be present. In patients with chronic gout, large nodular soft tissue prominences, called tophi, may be present. The classic radiographic change of gout is periarticular bony erosion. These changes are not detectable in the early stages of the disease. Joint space is often maintained until late degenerative processes occur.

Hyperuricemia is a prerequisite for gout and is defined as a plasma urate concentration greater than 420 $v$mol/L (7.0 mg/dL). This can be the result of either overproduction of uric acid, undersecretion of uric acid, or a combination of the two. Joint fluid aspirate is the most common and simple way to diagnose gout. Synovial fluid and polymorphonuclear neutrophils contain negatively birefringent monosodium urate crystals when viewed under polarized light. Joint fluid aspirate should also be evaluated for infection if clinical suspicion exists, because acute gouty arthritis and infection can coexist.

Management with either oral colchicine or NSAIDs, after infection has been ruled out, is effective in relieving symptoms of acute gouty arthritis. In those patients who are unable to tolerate oral medication, intraarticular injection of glucocorticoids may be used. Allopurinol is used in chronic gout to manage the hyperuricemia. Before starting treatment with allopurinol, the patient should be free of all signs of inflammation and should have begun colchicine for prophylaxis. The sudden drop in serum urate with the initiation of allopurinol may prolong or precipitate an acute attack. Subacromial bursitis is not uncommon in patients with gout; if it is unresponsive to conservative measures, it is an indication for arthroscopic treatment.

Pseudogout

Calcium pyrophosphate dihydrate (CPPD) crystal deposition in articular cartilage, synovium, and periarticular structures may be seen radiographically in 10% to 15% of persons 65 to 75 years of age and in 30% to 60% of those older than 85 years. In most cases, this process is asymptomatic and the cause of CPPD is uncertain (1). It may be hereditary, idiopathic, or associated with metabolic disease or trauma (including surgery). Symptoms are caused by local joint inflammation that occurs secondary to inflammatory mediators released locally by neutrophils as a result of crystal phagocytosis.

CPPD disease may be asymptomatic, acute, subacute, chronic, or superimposed on other systemic processes. Symptomatic episodes can also be exacerbated by local trauma or surgery. The knee is most often affected, but the shoulder, wrist, ankle, elbow, and hand are other common sites. Presentation of symptoms is often localized to one joint, although clinical and radiographic evidence suggests polyarticular involvement in up to two thirds of patients. The acute attack is a dose-related inflammatory response to the shedding of CPPD crystals from cartilaginous tissues into the synovial fluid. Diffuse pain and tenderness with attempted active or passive ROM are characteristic during an acute attack. Local signs of inflammation may or may not be present. In as many as 50% of cases, CPPD is associated with systemic signs such as fever (37 to 39°C [99 to 103°F]), leukocytosis of 12,000 to 15,000 cells/μL, and elevated ESR (1).

Radiographic changes include punctate or linear densities in articular, hyaline, and fibrocartilaginous tissues. Subchondral cysts and osteophyte formation are common in the pseudo-osteoarthritic form (55). Almost one half of patients demonstrate the pseudo-osteoarthritic pattern, with progressive degeneration of numerous joints, usually in a symmetric distribution (1). Polarized microscopy reveals weakly positive birefringent crystals in the extracellular fluid and within the neutrophils that are rhomboid in shape. This finding is confirmatory for CPPD disease, although concomitant infection can exist and can be the cause of the CPPD flare-up. Treatment of acute attacks include the use of NSAIDs, colchicine, or both. Aspiration of the joint may relieve intraarticular pressure, and injection with glucocorticoid may relieve symptoms.

Apatite-Associated Destructive Arthritis (Milwaukee Shoulder)

Calcium hydroxyapatite (HA) is the primary mineral of bone. Abnormal accumulation in soft tissue and joints is seen in conditions that result in hypercalcemia, such as hyperparathyroidism and metastatic disease. Although the true incidence of HA arthritis is unknown, 30% to 60% of patients with osteoarthritis have HA microcrystals in their synovial fluid (1). This chronic condition can be quite destructive and deforming. Most often it affects the dominant shoulder of elderly women. Bilateral disease occurs in about 60% of patients. Patients may have extensive joint destruction and attenuation of supporting structures and tissues, such as failure of the rotator cuff. This leads to crepitus and decreased ROM on examination, with a large effusion and glenohumeral instability (55). Intraarticular and/or periarticular calcifications as well as joint degeneration and destruction are variably seen. Joint space narrowing and irregularity, osteophyte and subchondral cyst formation, and superior subluxation of the humeral head are common (56).

The synovial fluid WBC count in HA arthritis is usually low (less than 2,000 cells/μL) but may at times be greater than 50,000/μL. Mononuclear cells predominate, but the presence of many neutrophils is not an uncommon finding. Individual crystals are nonbirefringent and are too small to be seen by standard microscopy. Clumps of crystals may be seen and can be stained bright red with alizarin red S.

Treatment is focused on reduction of inflammation. NSAIDs, aspiration, and intraarticular glucocorticoids provide symptomatic relief. Untreated, acute synovitis is generally self-limited, lasting days to several weeks. The role of arthroscopy is limited owing to the advanced degrees of destruction usually seen on presentation. Arthroplasty can be a consideration in patients with severe pain.

Polymyalgia Rheumatica

Polymyalgia rheumatica (PMR) is characterized by aching and morning stiffness in the neck, shoulders, and pelvic girdle, along with evidence of an underlying systemic inflammatory reaction (fever, anorexia, weight loss, and high ESR) (57,58). The pathogenesis is poorly understood, but involvement of the immune system in the inflammatory process is suspected. PMR affects women twice as often as men, usually occurs after 50 years of age, and has a strong association with giant cell arteritis. There is often mild swelling of the glenohumeral joint, with the presence of an effusion which may not be detectable on examination. The AC and sternoclavicular joints may also be involved.

Radiographs are typically normal. MRI of the shoulder often shows inflammation of the subacromial and subdeltoid bursae (59). The use of sonography to differentiate PMR from other inflammatory diseases has been investigated, with inconsistent results (60,61). Hematologic analysis reveals an elevated ESR in almost all cases of PMR. Histologic analysis of synovial biopsies obtained from shoulders of patients with PMR shows mild to moderate synovitis in most patients, characterized by vascular proliferation and leukocyte infiltration in the absence of relevant lining layer hyperplasia (57). Synovial fluid analysis reveals predominantly mononuclear cells with rare polymorphonuclear neutrophils present.

Shoulder corticosteroid injection was shown in a double-blind, prospective, randomized, placebo-controlled study to be an effective and safe therapy for patients with PMR (62). Oral corticosteroids can also provide highly effective treatment. Arthroscopy does not typically play a role, although it has been used for diagnostic purposes (63).

Amyloidosis

Amyloidosis may be defined as the extracellular deposition of the fibrous protein amyloid in one or more sites of the body. It was named in 1854 by Virchow based on its color after staining with iodine and sulfuric acid. Various forms of this protein disease differ both clinically and chemically and have been classified into the following types: (a) primary or idiopathic amyloidosis; (b) amyloidosis associated with multiple myeloma; (c) secondary or reactive amyloidosis, associated with chronic infectious or inflammatory disease; (d) heredofamilial amyloidosis, comprising a variety of neuropathic, renal, and cardiovascular accumulations associated with syndromes; (e) local amyloidosis; (f) amyloidosis associated with aging; and (g) amyloidosis associated with long-term hemodialysis.

The presence of associated medical conditions should be sought. Pain and stiffness are common, particularly in the morning (1). Patients with amyloid arthropathy secondary to dialysis exhibit knee swelling, carpal tunnel syndrome, and painful, stiff shoulders (64). Amyloid deposition in the soft tissue around the shoulder can lead to infiltration and prominence of this region, termed the "shoulder pad sign" (65). Examination for associated neuropathy should be performed.

Ultrasound has been found to be useful in diagnosing amyloidosis in the shoulders of patients undergoing chronic hemodialysis (66–69). Changes in the rotator cuff musculotendinous tissue, synovium, and bursa can be identified and monitored for disease progression. MRI findings in patients with amyloid arthropathy have been described (70,71), but use of MRI is not routine for establishing the diagnosis.

The synovial fluid usually has a low WBC count, a good to fair mucin clot, a predominance of mononuclear cells, and no crystals. Surgical specimens show deposition of amyloid in synovium, capsule, cartilage, and surrounding soft tissues. Definitive diagnosis is made on tissue biopsy that stains with Congo red and has green birefringence under polarized light.

Medical consultation and treatment are paramount in the management of patients with amyloid disease. The primary type and source of amyloidosis must be ascertained to allow proper evaluation and management of other affected organ systems and associated diseases. Surgical synovectomy of involved shoulders appears to be effective in decreasing pain, although relief may be temporary. In one published report, open surgery gave more lasting relief than arthroscopic synovectomy did (72).

MISCELLANEOUS SYNOVITIC CONDITIONS

Miscellaneous synovial proliferative disorders are generally considered separately from the inflammatory disorders discussed previously (Table 41.4). Pigmented villonodular synovitis and synovial osteochondromatosis appear to arise from the synovium itself. Hemophilic arthropathy occurs when repeated intraarticular hemorrhages lead to marked synovial proliferation and hypervascularity. Reactive synovi-

TABLE 41.4 CLASSIFICATION OF MAJOR SYNOVIAL DISORDERS

Inflammatory	
Idiopathic	Rheumatoid arthritis
	Systemic lupus erythematosus
	Ankylosing spondylitis
	Inflammatory bowel disease
Specific	Gout
	Pseudogout
	Infections
Reactive	Reiter's disease
	Viral arthritides
	Enteroarthritis (*Salmonella, Shigella, Yersinia, Campylobacter*)
Miscellaneous	Pigmented villonodular synovitis
	Synovial osteochondromatosis
	Neoplasm
	Hemophiliac arthropathy

From Frassica FJ, Combs JJ, Jr., Sim FH: Synovial proliferation disorders: differential diagnosis. *Arthroscopy* 1985;1:183–189, with permission.

tis is secondary to a foreign, usually biodegradable, implant. These diseases are amenable to arthroscopic treatment by synovectomy.

Pigmented Villonodular Synovitis

Pigmented villonodular synovitis (PVNS) is a nonneoplastic proliferative process involving synovial tissue in joints, tendon sheaths, and bursae. PVNS is usually seen in the knee, with only 1% of instances affecting the shoulder (32,73). Only 30 cases of PVNS of the shoulder have been reported (74). The time to diagnosis from presentation of signs and symptoms in the shoulder has been reported to average 3 to 4 years (75,76). Several case reports in the literature demonstrate initial diagnosis of PVNS made while treating other shoulder pathology, such as rotator cuff disease and instability (77). It is most commonly seen in the third and fourth decades, and women and men are equally affected (71,78). The condition is thought to be either inflammatory in origin or a manifestation of a benign neoplastic process (78,79). Three forms exist: an isolated lesion of the tendon sheath, a solitary intraarticular localized or pedunculated lesion, and diffuse involvement of the synovial membrane (73,78,79). However, most authors refer to two forms, localized and diffuse. Most shoulder PVNS is intraarticular, with occasional extraarticular extension into the bursa (74). Exclusively extraarticular PVNS of the shoulder is rare (80,81).

Patients present with diffuse joint swelling, effusions, and limited ROM. Pain is not usually a prominent feature (73,76,78,79); however, in the late stages, degenerative joint disease may be present and cause symptoms. Radiographs are often normal, but soft tissue swelling or effusion may be visualized. Late changes can include local bone invasion, pe-

riarticular cysts, and bony erosions (94) which appear to be a more prominent feature of PVNS involving the shoulder. MRI reveals hypertrophic synovium with hemosiderin pigmentation. The arthrographic appearance of PVNS of the shoulder is that of multilobulated filling defects within a normal distensible joint (82). This appearance can also be seen in hypertrophic synovitis secondary to inflammatory arthritides, hemophilia, or chronic indolent infection (82).

Aspiration yields a brownish fluid that is usually bloody, with low to moderate WBCs (73). Biopsy reveals areas of subsynovial, nodular proliferation of synovial cells and histiocytes surrounded by lipid-laden foam cells, multinucleated giant cells, and hemosiderin-laden cells. The stroma, which contains hemosiderin pigment and numerous thin-walled vascular channels, is hyalinized to varying degrees (32,76,78,79).

Resection of the involved synovium is the mainline treatment. The localized nodular form may be managed with simple resection, but the more common diffuse form requires a more extensive synovectomy. This can be performed by an open technique or arthroscopically. In addition, curettage of periarticular cysts to remove intraosseous synovial inclusions should be performed. Recurrences in the diffuse form are frequent (20% to 30%), probably because of incomplete excision of the involved synovium (73,76,78). Compared with open techniques, arthroscopic synovectomy may allow a more complete resection and decreased morbidity (74). Adjuvant radiotherapy has not proved beneficial compared with surgical excision alone (73). However, use of adjuvant therapy (radiotherapy, yttrium 90, or osmic acid) has been advocated by various authors (74). Arthroplasty and arthrodesis are reserved for advanced bony involvement.

Synovial Chondromatosis (Osteochondromatosis)

Synovial chondromatosis is a disease that arises in the synovial tissues of the joints. It is almost exclusively seen in the knee, hip, shoulder, and elbow, but may also involve the synovial membranes of bursae and tendon sheaths (83,84). Patients usually present in the third or fourth decade and men are involved two to three times more frequently than women (83,85). Multiple loose chondral bodies are formed by a metaplastic maturation of the primitive mesenchymal cells in the joint capsule. Hundreds of loose chondral bodies can be found in various stages of maturation throughout the joint. In addition, a chronic capsular inflammation is invariably present.

Pain is the most common presenting symptom, with swelling, stiffness, and mechanical symptoms occurring less often (83,86–88). Decreased ROM and palpable loose bodies may be present. Multiple loose bodies may be seen on plain radiographs (Fig. 41.9), and noncalcified densities can be visualized with arthrography or MRI. Microscopically,

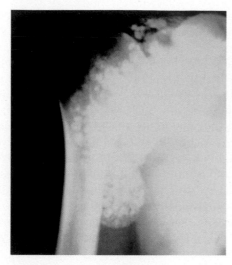

FIGURE 41.9 Anteroposterior radiograph of shoulder demonstrating synovial osteochondromatosis.

the joint capsule reveals minute nests of cartilage enmeshed in primitive mesenchymal tissue in all stages of maturation. The nuclei of the cartilaginous cells have some abnormalities, and many double nuclei may be seen (89).

Synovectomy with removal of loose bodies is the definitive treatment for symptomatic disease; however, nonoperative treatment has been shown to be successful in selected cases involving the upper extremities (90). Arthroscopic removal of loose bodies and affected synovium in the knee has produced recurrence rates comparable to those obtained with open techniques (25%) (88). Reports of arthroscopic treatment of synovial chondromatosis in the shoulder are limited to isolated cases with good results (86,91). Loose bodies and any involved synovium should be removed. A limited incision to address bicipital groove involvement is necessary in some cases (84,85,87,91). Coolican and Dandy (88) identified three distinct arthroscopic appearances: large, deep lesions with normal overlying synovium; small, superficial lesions partially attached to, or covered by, synovium; and multiple small cartilaginous fragments with normal-appearing synovium. Figure 41-10 shows the appearance of multiple loose bodies within the joint.

Hemophilic Arthropathy

Patients with congenital plasma coagulation defects commonly bleed into muscles, joints, and body cavities after injury. Hemophilia A (factor VIII deficiency) and hemophilia B (factor IX deficiency or dysfunction, also called Christmas disease) are the most common of these inherited plasma coagulation disorders. They are genetically X-linked and are caused by defects in single coagulation proteins. Hemophilic arthropathy refers to the resulting manifestations of this disease in the joints. Three stages of arthropathy are recognized: the first, characterized by acute, intraarticular bleeding, occurs during childhood; the second, a

chronic proliferative synovitis, is stimulated by the repeated hemorrhages; and the third is a destructive arthropathy (34). There is a positive correlation between the degree of joint destruction and the number of hemarthroses. However, a few cases of arthropathy have been reported after very few bleeds (92). Large joints are affected more frequently than small joints. The incidence of shoulder involvement is usually considered to be small (10% to 15%) (92,93), although one study demonstrated shoulder symptoms in 37% of 41 adult patients (94).

Those patients with severe factor deficiency are usually diagnosed in infancy. However, mild hemophiliacs may not present clinically with symptoms until they are adolescents or young adults. Joint destruction occurs through a series of intraarticular hemorrhages. Phagocytosis of the red blood cells, hemosiderin deposition, and platelet activation cause release of degradative enzymes. Chronic synovial inflammation results, with vascular proliferation, cell infiltration, and marked villus formation. Additional acute hemorrhages may produce a permanently swollen joint, with widening of the joint space and subluxation of the humeral head (49,93). In adolescence, epiphyseal arrest or acceleration may occur as a result of nutritional deficiencies or excessive blood flow (93). Rotator cuff pathology is not infrequent, with one study reporting a 50% incidence of cuff tears detected by ultrasound in symptomatic shoulders (94).

Patients present with pain followed by swelling, usually in a weight-bearing joint, after minimal trauma. Initial perception of an acute hemarthrosis often starts as an aura or a tingling sensation in the joint. The involved articulation is usually held in flexion, and active and passive motion are

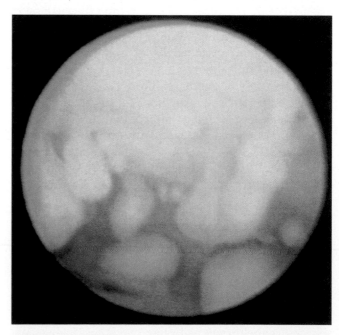

FIGURE 41.10 Arthroscopic photograph demonstrating loose bodies and synovial proliferation associated with synovial chondromatosis.

painful and very restricted (95). Those patients who have had chronic hemarthrotic episodes may present with a stiff or ankylosed joint and muscular atrophy.

The radiographic appearance varies with the extent of disease. Early degenerative changes, with subarticular cysts, osteophytes, and irregular joint surfaces, predominate. Ultrasound is a safe and precise diagnostic technique to differentiate synovial hypertrophy from effusion.

Patients with suspected hemophilia should have screening tests of hemostasis, including a platelet count, bleeding time, prothrombin time (PT), and partial thromboplastin time (PTT). Typically patients have a prolonged PTT with all other tests normal. Specific assays can then be used to determine the factor deficiency.

Treatment is initially predicated on factor replacement to control hemorrhage and avoid recurrence. Immobilization and ice are useful during an acute bleed; early active ROM is begun once bleeding is controlled (93). Aspiration of an acute bleed, after adequate factor replacement, may decrease synovial proliferation by reducing the stimulus; however, this procedure is not recommended unless the joint is unusually tense or infection is suspected (1). Continuous prophylactic clotting factor replacement has been shown to slow the natural course of hemophilic arthropathy (96).

Synovectomy has been valuable in reducing pain and controlling hemorrhage in hemophilic arthropathy of the elbow and knee (97). Arthrofibrosis is a significant aspect of advanced hemophilic arthropathy, and postsurgical loss of motion is a well established complication. Arthroscopic debridement has resulted in better preservation of motion when used in the hemophilic knee (98). However, it has also resulted in a higher incidence of postoperative hemarthrosis, presumably because of the lack of intraoperative hemostasis. Better results with synovectomy have been achieved in the younger population, probably because of the shorter duration of disease (97). Although there are no reports in the literature of shoulder synovectomy for hemophilic arthropathy, indications and results should be similar to those described for the knee. With attention to intraoperative hemostasis with electrocautery, postoperative hemarthrosis may be minimized.

Before surgery, patients must be screened for the presence of an inhibitor to factor VIII. Patients with hemophilia A who do not have an inhibitor should receive factor VIII infusions (hemophilia B patients require additional infusions) just before surgery and should be monitored daily so that the factor VIII level is maintained above 50% for 10 to 14 days after surgery. When patients undergo joint replacement or other major orthopedic surgery, therapy should be continued for 3 weeks (99).

The role of radioactive or chemical synovectomy has been defined previously by many authors, and it is a common therapeutic procedure for chronic hemophilic synovitis. However, controversy exists regarding the optimal age and stage of the disease for use of such drugs (95,100). For those patients with chronic synovitis that has caused significant joint destruction, arthroplasty is an acceptable option. Intraarticular dexamethasone in advanced disease has been advocated for management of symptoms before joint replacement (101).

Reactive Synovitis (Biodegradable Implant–Induced Synovitis)

The use of biodegradable or bioresorbable implants in orthopaedic surgery has become more common, particularly with respect to arthroscopic procedures. Research has found adverse effects related to the use of biodegradable fixation devices, such as delayed tissue reaction, foreign-body reaction, osteolysis, and synovitis (102–107). Polylactic acid (PLA) and polyglycolic acid (PGA) are presently the two most commonly used biodegradable materials in orthopaedics. PLA exists in two forms differentiated by the asymmetric molecular structure of lactic acid, L-PLA (mostly crystalline) and DL-PLA (mostly amorphous). PGA exists in only one form (108). PLA–PGA copolymers are produced in various ratios which alter the rate of degradation and mechanical characteristics of the implant.

A review of 516 patients treated with Biofix rods (PGA and PLA-PGA copolymer) for fractures revealed a late noninfectious inflammatory response requiring operative drainage in 8% of cases. Inflammatory complications were seen in 15% of patients with intraarticular knee implants and in 8% (1/13) of patients who underwent glenoid osteotomy for recurrent dislocation of the shoulder (103).

Animal studies of the use of polyglycolide (PGA) implants in knees of sheep similarly showed a reactive process histologically. The authors recommended caution when considering the use of these implants intraarticularly. Factors related to the severity of the reaction included degradation rate, shape, and crystallinity of the implant (106).

Reports of shoulder synovitis related to bioabsorbable implants are common. In one series, 4 (22%) of 18 patients treated with the Suretac device (polyglyconate polymer), 3 for fixation of superior labral anterior and posterior (SLAP) lesions and 1 patient with a Bankart repair, developed an acute synovitis. All four patients were treated successfully with local synovectomy. The authors hypothesized that mechanical failure of the device caused increased debris, resulting in an inflammatory reaction (109). The amount of reaction is related to the dose of material to which the macrophages are exposed. Implants that take longer to degrade may expose the tissues to a lower dose of material and therefore cause less reaction.

Historically PGA and PLA have been used in the production of screws, fixation pins, anchors, plates, and sutures. With recent advances in tissue engineering, new applications for these materials (e.g., scaffolding systems, carriers of bioactive agents) are being developed. The potential for reactive synovitis with these new applications should be considered.

Physical examination is variable, because the reactive synovitis often manifests in the early postoperative period. Diffuse swelling and inflammation are present, superimposed on the traumatic reaction to the recent surgery. The clinical presentation may mimic a postoperative infection. Radiographic analysis is often normal. Implants are radiolucent, and their location and integrity are difficult to assess. A nonspecific effusion is seen on MRI.

Joint aspiration and evaluation for infection must be performed to rule out postoperative septic arthritis. Synovial fluid analysis may reveal birefringent particles under polarized light, and lymphocytes are the predominant cell type (105,107). The PGA implants are relatively inert immunologically, but they do induce an inflammatory mononuclear cell migration leading to a nonspecific lymphocytic activation (105). CRP and ESR are usually mildly elevated, and the WBC count is in the normal range.

Histological analysis reveals histiocytic and giant cell inflammatory reaction to crystalline implant fragments containing phagocytosed debris. The crystalline implants break down into small particles before degradation is completed, and these fragments have been implicated as the cause of mechanical irritation or reactive synovitis (110).

Most authors have advocated local synovectomy with removal of the offending implant for the management of reactive synovitis. These recommendations are based on the clinical responses observed after this treatment in selected cases reported in the literature (102–107). However, complete resolution of symptoms has been reported in cases of reactive synovitis after removal of the offending implant alone, and also after local synovectomy adjacent to the retained implant.

SEPTIC ARTHRITIS OF THE SHOULDER IN THE ADULT

Septic arthritis is relatively uncommon in the glenohumoral joint compared with the weight-bearing joints of the lower extremities. However, the incidence of shoulder involvement has been reported to range from 3% to 12%, placing the shoulder joint third after knee and hip in occurrence (111). Affected patients are predominantly very young infants or elderly patients with chronic debilitating disease such as diabetes, malignancies, liver disease, or alcoholism (112,113). A review of 27 adult patients diagnosed and treated for septic glenohumoral arthritis identified a systemic immunocompromising condition or a local pathologic condition (or both) in 96% of patients (114). Lossos et al. (112) found in an extensive review of the literature that bacterial septic arthritis is more likely to develop in a joint with preexisting chronic arthritis than in a normal healthy joint, and a history of preceding shoulder disorders or ma-

nipulations is found in 24% of patients with septic arthritis of the shoulder. Presenting symptoms are often vague and misinterpreted as bursitis or impingement, leading to a delay in diagnosis.

Presentation in the adult is quite variable, often with minimal signs and symptoms. Painful ROM, tenderness, and swelling are the common findings on examination. Radiographs of the shoulder in septic arthritis are commonly inconclusive (115). Many patients have coexisting shoulder morbidities that are present on evaluation. Widening of the glenohumeral joint space can be caused by intraarticular fluid accumulation with inferior subluxation of the humeral head (116). More advanced or chronic cases may reveal bony erosion. A bone scan may be helpful in long-standing cases with associated osteomyelitis, but results in the acute phase may be negative. MRI has been reported to be helpful in identifying the location of associated fluid collections, including involvement of the subacromial space and the AC joint.

The most consistent laboratory finding in patients with septic arthritis is an increased ESR; the lack of sensitivity of this measurement obligates further investigation. Fever and leukocytosis with a myeloid shift to the left are often present but can be variable in patients with concomitant chronic medical conditions. Joint aspiration with cellular analysis remains the gold standard for diagnosis. Gram's stain, culture and sensitivity, cell count, and crystal analysis should be performed. The ability to isolate an organism from the aspiration is variable from study to study, averaging 88% (112). Synovial biopsy at the time of arthroscopic treatment has been reported to be more accurate. The most prevalent pathogen causing bacterial arthritis of the shoulder, accounting for 41% of all cases published in the literature, is *Staphylococcus aureus* (112,114). Other common pathogens include *Salmonella* spp. (15.6%), *Escherichia coli* (8.3%), other gram-negative bacilli (*Klebsiella pneumoniae, Proteus mirabilis,* and nonenterococcal bacilli), and *Streptococcus* spp. (8.6%) (112). In rare cases, atypical mycobacterial and tuberculous sources have reported (117).

Drainage or decompression of the involved joint, followed by the use systemic antibiotics, is necessary to adequately treat septic arthritis. This can be performed by open arthrotomy, percutaneous aspiration, or arthroscopy. Several retrospective studies have looked at the outcomes of these three methods with varying results (118–120). Final disability is more likely related to the time interval between onset of symptoms and definitive treatment than to the method of decompression (121). Arthrotomy of the glenohumeral joint allows for adequate decompression but affords higher morbidity than arthroscopy or aspiration. Aspiration of the glenohumeral joint may be incomplete if associated subacromial involvement is present (114,122). Arthroscopy allows for adequate decompression and drainage of both the glenohumeral joint and the subacromial space, as well as access to tissue for biopsy, using a relatively benign procedure (123–125).

ARTHROSCOPIC TECHNIQUES

To a large extent, shoulder arthroscopy has replaced conventional surgical approaches in the management of shoulder arthritides, especially the inflammatory disorders. Diagnostic arthroscopy may be useful when other diagnostic techniques are inconclusive, because it allows more precision and greater sample size than does a needle biopsy, and morbidity is much lower than with comparable open procedures. Additionally, arthroscopy affords a more complete inspection of the glenohumeral joint than does an open surgical exposure, enabling accurate determination of the extent of rotator cuff, synovial, and articular involvement and providing multiple sites for biopsies. In the case of infection, arthroscopy allows more complete lavage and debridement.

Operative arthroscopy is used for indications specific to each disease entity. The primary treatment for the degenerative glenohumeral joint is arthroscopic debridement of labral tears and articular flaps, removal of loose bodies, and irrigation. This procedure allows access to the glenohumeral joint, rotator cuff, subacromial space, and AC joint to treat disease in these areas. The management for the inflammatory and synovitic diseases and septic arthritis consists of synovectomy and debridement, in addition to diagnostic biopsies.

Diagnostic Arthroscopy

For diagnostic arthroscopy, we prefer the lateral decubitus position with the arm suspended in skin traction, although the semi-sitting ("beach-chair") position is an acceptable alternative. Extremes of arm position and excessive traction must be avoided to prevent complications of fracture or neurovascular injury. More than 7 to 10 lb of traction is rarely indicated or necessary. Draping allows access to the entire shoulder region. With the use of an infusion pump, standard anterior and posterior portals generally suffice. Accessory inflow portals may be created if distention cannot be maintained, although the newer infusion pumps usually make this step unnecessary.

Technique: Degenerative Joint Disease

Arthroscopic debridement of the degenerative glenohumeral joint is carried out after diagnostic arthroscopy (126,127). Debridement is done with standard arthroscopic handheld punches, grasping forceps, and motorized instruments. The newer radiofrequency devices allow tissue to be removed while minimizing bleeding. Loose bodies should be sought by a thorough and systematic exploration of the joint. Examination of the subacromial space commonly reveals thickened bursa, and a bursectomy is indicated in these cases (11). In patients with combined glenohumeral arthritis and impingement syndrome or AC arthritis, an arthroscopic subacromial decompression or distal clavicle resec-

tion (or both) is carried out after glenohumeral debridement. Newer techniques for early arthritis include arthroscopic capsular releases (128,129) to increase glenohumeral motion and microfracture techniques for degenerative cartilage (6,16); the effectiveness of these methods in glenohumeral degenerative arthritis in unknown.

Particular challenges exist when arthroscopy is attempted in the presence of a massive rotator cuff tear. The rare patient who presents early enough in the disease course that the glenohumeral arthritis is amenable to arthroscopic debridement will probably also require debridement of the rotator cuff. Because of the large rotator cuff tear, the normal compartmentalization between the glenohumeral joint and subacromial space is lost (2). This often creates difficulty with maintenance of joint distention, resulting in reduced visualization. The procedure is further compromised by fluid extravasation and the resultant soft tissue swelling.

Technique: Septic Arthritis

When considering the diagnosis of infection, aspiration of joint fluid before joint distention is recommended. This fluid is sent for Gram's stain, cultures, fluid analysis, and a crystal search. When indicated, a complete synovectomy is performed after diagnostic arthroscopy; the technique is detailed in the next section. Multiple biopsies are obtained from inflamed areas, including subacromial and AC as well as intraarticular areas. We recommend drainage of the subacromial bursa before glenohumeral arthroscopy if there is a history of recent subacromial injection as a possible cause of the infection.

Technique: Inflammatory Synovitis and Synovectomy

In general, synovectomy of the shoulder is indicated for patients with inflammatory arthritis or synovitis who have disabling pain and loss of function refractory to conservative measures, including medication, injection, and physical therapy (130). Patients best suited for synovectomy demonstrate minimal bony destruction and an intact rotator cuff. The benefits of synovectomy appear to diminish in relation to the severity of articular involvement. When considering arthroscopic synovectomy in the patient with inflammatory arthritis or synovitis, the surgeon must attempt to make an accurate estimation of the extent of involvement. Arthroscopic synovectomy, although technically challenging, offers many advantages compared with open surgical synovectomy. Results of both debridement and synovectomy appear best when the procedure is performed early in the disease process, before severe joint destruction, loss of ROM, and rotator cuff compromise occur.

Synovial disorders may involve the subacromial space, AC joint, and scapulothoracic region in addition to the

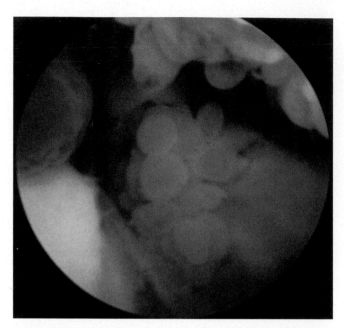

FIGURE 41.11 Abundant synovial proliferation, as depicted in this arthroscopic photograph, may create technical problems, with decreased visualization and increased bleeding.

glenohumeral joint; therefore, careful preoperative assessment is necessary.

Arthroscopic synovectomy is preceded by standard diagnostic arthroscopy. Problems with visualization may be encountered owing to marked synovial proliferation, bleeding, or both (Fig. 41.11). An additional superior portal for insertion of a large-bore inflow cannula may be necessary if extensive synovitis is present (Fig. 41.12). The hydrostatic pressure required to maintain distention is usually sufficient to control hemorrhage, and the use of an infusion pump is helpful. However, maintenance of adequate hydrostatic pressure may sometimes cause fluid extravasation and soft tissue swelling. Although complications resulting directly from this problem appear to be rare, the swelling can make manipulation of the arthroscopic instruments progressively more difficult (131,132). Hemorrhage may also be controlled in selected cases through the use of electrocautery or use of low-concentration epinephrine solutions. Epinephrine should be added only after consideration of the patient's general medical condition and consultation with the anesthesiologist.

Complete synovectomy of the glenohumeral joint can be accomplished with a two-portal technique (133). Using standard portals, the procedure is begun with the arthroscope posterior and the instruments anterior (Fig. 41.13). Access to the superior and anterior half of the joint is adequately achieved with this arrangement. The inferior and posterior half of the joint is reached with the operating instruments posterior and the arthroscope anterior. In cases of severe involvement of the inferior recess, an accessory inferior posterior portal may be necessary for instrumentation of

this area. The subscapularis bursa, between the upper border of the tendon and the glenoid, is lined with synovium and often contains loose bodies (6). A cannula system that allows for exchange of the arthroscope and instruments is helpful. Standard equipment for arthroscopic shoulder surgery is sufficient for performing a synovectomy. A radiofrequency device is extremely helpful in controlling bleeding and maintaining visualization. The subacromial space is entered by inserting the arthroscope through the same posterior portal but directing it above the rotator cuff. The anterior portal and an accessory lateral portal are used for instrumentation. The AC joint is also accessible in this manner (see later discussion).

Complications particular to synovectomy include excessive bleeding and the formation of synovial fistulae. Substantial postoperative bleeding is rare and can usually be controlled by pressure dressings and ice. Synovial fistulae usually resolve with immobilization. Excision of the fistula and closure of the joint capsule is rarely required.

Postoperative management begins with suture closure of the portals and application of absorbent dressings for the first 24 hours. Drains may be necessary in cases of excessive bleeding and are recommended for infection. The application of cold therapy (ice) is helpful in controlling both discomfort and bleeding. A sling is used for comfort, and ROM exercises are begun on the first postoperative day. Pendulum-type exercises may be performed independently, but formal physical therapy for more aggressive ROM should begin within the first postoperative week.

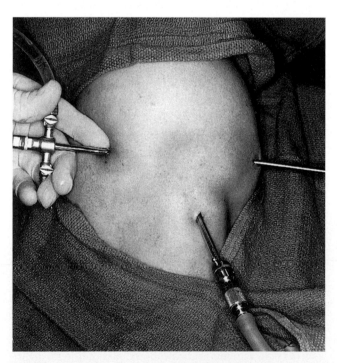

FIGURE 41.12 Photograph of the three-portal glenohumeral arthroscopy technique with the arthroscope positioned posteriorly, working instruments anteriorly, and an accessory inflow cannula superiorly.

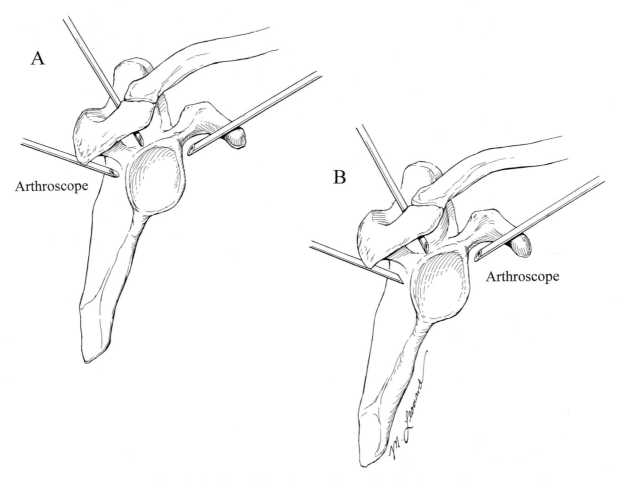

FIGURE 41.13 Schematic drawing of the arthroscopic setup for glenohumeral synovectomy. **A:** With the arthroscope positioned posteriorly, access to the superior and anterior half of the joint is possible. **B:** With the arthroscope positioned anteriorly, the inferior and posterior half of the joint is accessible. A large-bore inflow cannula is inserted through an accessory superior portal to maintain distention and improve visualization in cases of excessive bleeding.

Techniques of Distal Clavicle Resection

Subacromial Approach

The AC joint may be resected through the subacromial space, using routine posterior and lateral portals. An anterior portal is added either routinely or to facilitate difficult exposure, according to each surgeon's preference. This approach requires resection of bursal tissue and the subclavicular fat pad for identification of the undersurface of the AC joint. At the beginning of the procedure, localization is facilitated by insertion of a needle into the AC joint from above, before the onset of soft tissue swelling. This needle can later be used to identify the AC joint, with the arthroscope in the posterior portal (Fig. 41.14). Resection of the inferior capsule can be performed with a motorized synovial resector, but radiofrequency devices are more useful to minimize bleeding and expose bony landmarks. A motorized bur, inserted through the lateral portal, is used to remove the acromial facet of the AC joint and, subsequently, the bone of the distal clavicle (Fig. 41.15). Manual pressure from above is quite efficacious to depress the clavicle further into the subacromial space,

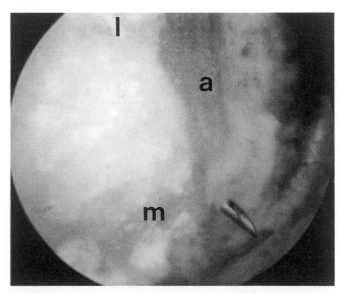

FIGURE 41.14 Arthroscopic photograph of a localizing needle in the AC joint. It is inserted from above, before the arthroscopic procedure begins. After debridement of the subacromial bursa and subclavicular fat pad, the needle is visible arthroscopically. In this case, an acromioplasty is also being performed. l, lateral border of the acromion; a, anterior border; m, medial border.

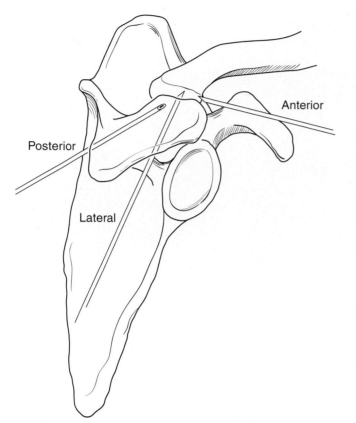

FIGURE 41.15 Schematic drawing of the setup for resection of the distal clavicle through the subacromial bursa. The arthroscope is positioned in the posterior portal, and the working instruments are inserted through the lateral portal. The anterior portal can also be used as the working portal, with the AC joint viewed from either posterior or lateral. The arthroscope can then be placed in the lateral portal with the working instruments in the anterior portal for better access to the distal clavicle.

facilitating resection of its superior aspect. An anterior portal provides better access to the AC joint, does not violate the superior joint capsule, and is useful to evaluate the often missed posterior superior clavicle. The anterior portal is directly in line with the distal clavicle, lateral to the coracoid process, and 1 to 2 cm distal to the clavicle. A 70-degree arthroscope placed in the posterior portal is also useful to assess completeness of the resection, especially to ensure that a posterior clavicular ridge does not remain.

Superior Approach

The direct superior approach to the AC joint may be used in cases of isolated disease. Patients with symptomatic osteolysis of the distal clavicle are ideal for the superior approach, because the widened joint space allows technically easier entry. Advocates of this approach report improved visualization and minimization of bleeding and edema, compared with the subacromial technique (23,134). Additionally, the coracoacromial ligament is not violated, and an acromioplasty is not needed. Arthroscopy is performed with the patient in the semisitting or lateral decubitus position,

through anterosuperior and posterosuperior portals (Fig. 41.16). The portals avoid the midportion of the joint and thus preserve the majority of the superior capsule. The portal pathway is guided by the use of needles to determine the inclination of the joint. The 2.7-mm arthroscope is used initially through the posterior portal, and the joint is debrided with a 2.0-mm resector through the anterior portal. The joint space opening can be started with curettes. After a portion of the distal clavicle is resected with a 2.0-mm bur, the standard 4.0-mm arthroscope can be inserted. Electrocautery or radiofrequency is used to subperiostially elevate soft tissue circumferentially about the distal clavicle, and a large bur is then used to complete the resection. The arthroscope and bur are switched from anterior to posterior portals to facilitate uniform resection (23,30). A contraindication to the superior approach is hypertrophic edge osteophytes, which may block entrance to the joint (13). An additional disadvantage of the superior approach is the need for two arthroscope sizes.

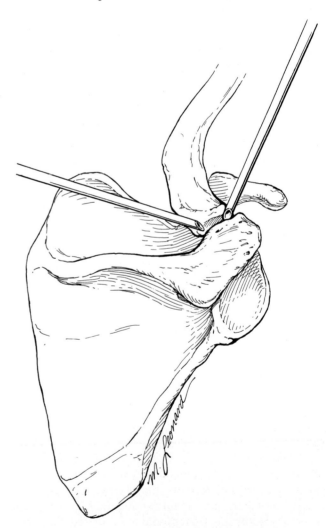

FIGURE 41.16 Schematic drawing of the direct superior approach for resection of the distal clavicle. The arthroscope and working instruments are used interchangeably in the anterosuperior and posterosuperior portals.

With either the superior or the subacromial approach, the width of bony resection can be estimated intraoperatively. This is aided by the insertion of two needles from above, one adjacent to the medial acromion and one adjacent to the resected edge of the distal clavicle, or by comparison with the width of the bur. The recommended resection is 7 to 10 mm (30,31,134). Arthroscopic AC resection is most often performed as an outpatient procedure, with the use of ice and a sling in the early postoperative period. ROM exercise is begun early and progresses as comfort allows, with rapid advancement to a strengthening program.

Complications of arthroscopic AC resection are uncommon. Intraoperative difficulties are usually secondary to poor visualization and bleeding. A failure of diagnosis is a major reason for postoperative pain (24). Complications include AC joint instability, as a result of aggressive distal clavicle resection, and inadequate resection, usually of the posterior superior aspect of the joint.

CONCLUSION

Degenerative and inflammatory disease affecting the glenohumeral and AC joints is not uncommon. If conservative treatment fails, arthroscopic techniques offer a valuable adjunct to traditional open approaches. The limitations imposed by the disease process and by the surgeon's experience and skills are important factors in the decision-making process when considering arthroscopic intervention.

REFERENCES

1. Klippel JH, ed. *Primer on the rheumatic diseases,* 11th ed. Atlanta: Arthritis Foundation, 1997.
2. Neer CS, Craig EV, Fukuda H. Cuff-tear arthropathy. *J Bone Joint Surg Am* 1983;65:1232–1244.
3. Jensen KL, Williams GR, Russell IJ, et al. Rotator cuff tear arthropathy. *J Bone Joint Surg Am* 1999;81:1312–1324.
4. Samilson RL, Prieto V. Dislocation arthropathy of the shoulder. *J Bone Joint Surg Am* 1983;65:456–460.
5. Brems JJ. Arthritis of dislocation. *Orthop Clin North Am* 1998; 29:453–466.
6. Iannotti JP, Williams GR, eds. *Disorder of the shoulder: diagnosis and management.* Philadelphia: Lippincott Williams & Wilkins, 1999.
7. Neer CS. Replacement arthroplasty for glenohumeral osteoarthritis. *J Bone Joint Surg Am* 1974;56:1–13.
8. Ellman H, Harris E, Kay SP. Early degenerative joint disease simulating impingement syndrome: arthroscopic findings. *Arthroscopy* 1992;8:482–487.
9. Kerr R, Resnick D, Pineda C, et al. Osteoarthritis of the glenohumeral joint: a radiologic-pathologic study. *AJR Am J Roentgenol* 1985;144:967–972.
10. Tirman PF, Steinbach LS, Belzer JP, et al. A practical approach to imaging of the shoulder with emphasis on MR imaging. *Orthop Clin North Am* 1997;28:483–515.
11. Weinstein DM, Bucchieri JS, Pollock RG, et al. Arthroscopic

12. debridement of the shoulder for osteoarthritis. *Arthroscopy* 2000;16:471–476.
13. Rowe CR. Arthrodesis of the shoulder used in treating painful conditions. *Clin Orthop* 1983;173:92–96.
14. Matsen FA, Rockwood CA, Wirth MA, et al. Glenohumeral arthritis and its management. In: Rockwood CA, Matsen FA, eds. *The shoulder.* Philadelphia: WB Saunders, 1998:840–942.
15. Blasier RD, Bucholz R, Cole W, et al. Bioresorbable implants: applications in orthopaedic surgery. *Instr Course Lect* 1997;46: 531–546.
16. Ogilvie-Harris DJ, Wiley AM. Arthroscopic surgery of the shoulder: a general appraisal. *J Bone Joint Surg Br* 1986;68:201–207.
17. Gartsman GM, Hasan SS. What's new in shoulder surgery. *J Bone Joint Surg Am* 2001;83:145–151.
18. Collins DN, Harryman DT. Arthroplasty for arthritis and rotator cuff deficiency. *Orthop Clin North Am* 1997;28:225–239.
19. Leffert RD, Rowe CR. Subacromial syndromes: tendon ruptures. In: Rowe CR, ed. *The shoulder.* New York: Churchill Livingstone, 1988:131–154.
20. Clarke HD, McCann PD. Acromioclavicular joint injuries. *Orthop Clin North Am* 2000;31:177–187.
21. Petersson CJ, Redlund-Johnell I. Radiographic joint space in normal acromioclavicular joints. *Acta Orthop Scand* 1983;54: 431–433.
22. Gartsman GM. Arthroscopic resection of the acromioclavicular joint. *Am J Sports Med* 1993;21:71–77.
23. Gartsman GM, Combs AH, Davis PF, et al. Arthroscopic acromioclavicular joint resection: an anatomical study. *Am J Sports Med* 1991;19:2–5.
24. Bigliani LU, Nicholson GP, Flatow EL. Arthroscopic resection of the distal clavicle. *Orthop Clin North Am* 1993;24:133–141.
25. Shaffer BS. Painful conditions of the acromioclavicular joint. *J Am Acad Orthop Surg* 1999;7:176–188.
26. Esch JC, Ozerkis LR, Helgager JA, et al. Arthroscopic subacromial decompression: results according to the degree of rotator cuff tear. *Arthroscopy* 1988;4:241–249.
27. Johnson LL. *Diagnostic and surgical arthroscopy: the knee and other joints.* Philadelphia: CV Mosby, 1981.
28. Branch TP, Burdette HL, Shahriari AS, et al. The role of the acromioclavicular ligaments and the effect of distal clavicle resection. *Am J Sports Med* 1996;24:293–297.
29. Matthews LS, Parks BG, Pavlovich LJ Jr., et al. Arthroscopic versus open distal clavicle resection: a biomechanical analysis on a cadaveric model. *Arthroscopy* 1999;15:237–240.
30. Levine WN, Barron OA, Yamaguchi K, et al. Arthroscopic distal clavicle resection from a bursal approach. *Arthroscopy* 1998; 14:52–56.
31. Flatow EL, Duralde XA, Nicholson GP, et al. Arthroscopic resection of the distal clavicle with a superior approach. *J Shoulder Elbow Surg* 1995;4:41–50.
32. Martin SD, Baumgarten TE, Andrews JR. Arthroscopic resection of the distal aspect of the clavicle with concomitant subacromial decompression. *J Bone Joint Surg Am* 2001;83:328–335.
33. Mills JA. Arthritis of the shoulder. In: Rowe CR, ed. *The shoulder.* New York: Churchill Livingstone, 1988:471–480.
34. Linden S, Heijde D. Ankylosing spondylitis. *Rheum Dis Clin North Am* 1998;24:663–676.
35. Schumacher HR, ed. *Primer on the rheumatic diseases,* 9th ed. Atlanta: Arthritis Foundation, 1988.
36. Hill JA, Lombardo SJ. Ankylosing spondylitis presenting as shoulder pain in an athlete: a case report. *Am J Sports Med* 1981;9:262–264.
37. Emery RJH, Ho EKW, Leong JCY. The shoulder girdle in ankylosing spondylitis *J Bone Joint Surg Am* 1991;73:1526–1531.

37. Will R, Kennedy G, Elswood J, et al. Ankylosing spondylitis and the shoulder: commonly involved but infrequently disabling. *J Rheumatol* 2000;27:177–182.

38. Erlacher L, Wintersberger W, Menschik M, et al. Reactive arthritis: urogenital swab culture is the only useful diagnostic method for the detection of the arthritogenic infection in extra-articularly asymptomatic patients with undifferentiated oligoarthritis. *Br J Rheumatol* 1995;34:838–842.

39. Gravallese EM, Kantrowitz FG. Arthritic manifestations of inflammatory bowel disease. *Am J Gastroenterol* 1988;83:703–709.

40. Cuomo F, Greller MJ, Zuckerman JD. The rheumatoid shoulder. *Rheum Dis Clin of North Am* 1998;24:67–82.

41. Lehtinen JT, Belt EA, Lyback CO, et al. Subacromial space in the rheumatoid shoulder: a radiographic 15-year follow-up study of 148 shoulders. *J Shoulder Elbow Surg* 2000;9:183–187.

42. Lehtinen JT, Belt EA, Kautiainen HJ, et al. Incidence of glenohumeral joint involvement in seropositive rheumatoid arthritis: a 15 year endpoint study. *J Rheumatol* 2000;27:347–350.

43. Lehtinen JT, Belt EA, Kautiainen HJ, et al. Incidence of acromioclavicular joint involvement in rheumatoid arthritis: a 15 year endpoint study. *J Rheumatol* 1999;26:1239–1241.

44. Petersson CJ: The acromioclavicular joint in rheumatoid arthritis: prevalence, clinical and radiologic features. *Scand J Reumatol* 1986;15:275–279.

45. Neer II CS. Reconstructive surgery and rehabilitation of the shoulder. In: Kelly WN, Harris ED Jr, eds. *Textbook of rheumatology.* Philadelphia: WB Saunders, 1985:1855–1870.

46. Hirooka A, Wakitani S, Yoneda M, et al. Shoulder destruction in rheumatoid arthritis: classification and prognostic signs in 83 patients followed 5–23 years. *Acta Orthop Scand* 1996;67:258–263.

47. Alasaarela EM, Alasaarela ELI. Ultrasound evaluation of painful rheumatoid shoulders. *J Rheumatol* 1994;21:1642–1648.

48. Kieft GJ, Dijkmans BA, Bloem JL, et al. Magnetic resonance imaging of the shoulder in patients with rheumatoid arthritis. *Ann Rheum Dis* 1990;49:7–11.

49. DePalma AF. Arthritides: local and systemic. In: DePalma AF. *Surgery of the shoulder.* Philadelphia: JB Lippincott, 1983:299–347.

50. Wakitani S, Imoto K, Saito M, et al. Evaluation of surgeries for rheumatoid shoulder based on the destruction pattern. *J Rheumatol* 1999;26:41–46.

51. Libby AK, Sherry DD, Dudgeon BJ. Shoulder limitation in juvenile rheumatoid arthritis. *Arch Phys Med Rehabil* 1991;72:382–384.

52. Ovregard T, Hoyerall HM, Pahle J, et al. A three-year retrospective study of synovectomies in children. *Clin Orthop* 1990;259:76–82.

53. Paus AC, Dale K. Arthroscopic and radiographic examination of patients with juvenile rheumatoid arthritis before and after open synovectomy of the knee joint: a prospective study with a 5-year follow-up. *Ann Chir Gynaecol* 1993;82:55–61.

54. Heimkes B, Stotz S. [Results of late synovectomy of the hip in juvenile chronic arthritis.] *Z Rheumatol* 1992;51:132–135.

55. McCarty DJ. Arthritis associated with crystals containing calcium. *Med Clin North Am* 1986;70:437–454.

56. Halverson PB, Carrera CF, McCarty DJ. Milwaukee shoulder syndrome: fifteen additional cases and a description of contributing factors. *Arch Intern Med* 1990;150:677–682.

57. Meliconi R, Pulsatelli L, Uguccioni M, et al. Leukocyte infiltration in synovial tissue from the shoulder of patients with polymyalgia rheumatica: quantitative analysis and influence of corticosteroid treatment. *Arthritis Rheum* 1996;39:1077–1207.

58. Chuang T, Hunder GG, Ilstrup DM, et al. Polymyalgia rheumatica: a 10-year epidemiologic and clinical study. *Ann Intern Med* 1982;97:672–680.

59. Salvarani C, Cantini F, Olivieri I, et al. Proximal bursitis in active polymyalgia rheumatica. *Ann Intern Med* 1997;127:27–31.

60. Paoletti C, Iagnocco A. Shoulder involvement in rheumatic diseases: sonographic findings. *J Rheumatol* 1999;26:668–673.

61. Lange U, Teichmann J, Stracke H, et al. Elderly onset rheumatoid arthritis and polymyalgia rheumatica: ultrasonographic study of the glenohumeral joints. *Rheumatol Int* 1998;17:229–232.

62. Salvarani C, Cantini F, Barozzi L, et al. Corticosteroid injections in polymyalgia rheumatica: a double-blind, prospective, randomized, placebo controlled study. *J Rheumatol* 2000;27:1470–1476.

63. Douglas WA, Martin BA, Morris JH. Polymyalgia rheumatica: an arthroscopic study of the shoulder joint. *Ann Rheum Dis* 1983;42:311–316.

64. Munoz-Gomez J, Gomez-Perez R, Llopaart-Buisan E, et al. Clinical picture of the amyloid arthropathy in patients with chronic renal failure maintained on haemodialysis using cellulose membranes. *Ann Rheum Dis* 1987;46:573–579.

65. Gordon DA, Ogryzlo MA, Pruzanski W, et al. Shoulder pads in amyloid arthropathy. *N Engl J Med* 1973;288:1080.

66. Kay J, Benson CB, Lester S, et al. Utility of high resolution ultrasound for the diagnosis of dialysis-related amyloidosis. *Arthritis Rheum* 1992;35:926–932.

67. McMahon LP, Radford J, Dawborn JK. Shoulder ultrasound in dialysis related amyloidosis. *Clin Nephrol* 1991;35:227–232.

68. Sommer R, Valen GJ, Ori Y, et al. Sonographic features of dialysis-related amyloidosis of the shoulder. *J Ultrasound Med* 2000;19:765–770.

69. Cardinal E, Buckwalter KA, Braunstein EM, et al. Amyloidosis of the shoulder in patients on chronic hemodialysis: sonographic findings. *AJR Am J Roentgenol* 1996;166:153–156.

70. Miyata M, Sato N, Watanabe H, et al. Magnetic resonance imaging findings in primary amyloidosis-associated arthropathy. *Intern Med* 2000;39:313–319.

71. Della Sala SW, Centonze M, Ghobert AD, et al. Role of magnetic resonance in hemodialysis patients with amyloid shoulder arthropathy. *Radiol Med* 1998;96:300–309.

72. Takenaka R, Fukatsu A, Matsuo S, et al. Surgical treatment of hemodialysis-related shoulder arthropathy. *Clin Nephrol* 1992;38:224–230.

73. Flandry F, Hughston JC. Pigmented villonodular synovitis. *J Bone Joint Surg Am* 1987;69:942–949.

74. Mahieu X, Chaouat G, Blin J, et al. Arthroscopic treatment of pigmented villonodular synovitis of the shoulder. *Arthroscopy* 2001;17:81.

75. Johansson JE, Ajjoub S, Coughlin LP, et al. Pigmented villonodular synovitis of joints. *Clin Orthop* 1982;163:159–166.

76. Schwartz HS, Unni KK, Pritchard DJ. Pigmented villonodular synovitis: a retrospective review of affected large joints. *Clin Orthop* 1989;247:243–255.

77. Cheng JC, Wolf EM, Chapman JE, et al. Pigmented villonodular synovitis of the shoulder after anterior capsulolabral reconstruction. *Arthroscopy* 1997;13:257–261.

78. Rao AS, Vigorita VJ. Pigmented villonodular synovitis (giant-cell tumor of the tendon sheath and synovial membrane). *J Bone Joint Surg Am* 1984;66:76–94.

79. Jaffe HL, Lichtenstein L, Sutro CJ. Pigmented villonodular synovitis, bursitis, and tenosynovitis: a discussion of the synovial and bursal equivalents of the tendosynovial lesion commonly denoted as xanthoma, xanthogranuloma, giant cell tumor, or myeloplaxoma of the tendon sheath, with some consideration of this tendon sheath itself. *Arch Pathol* 1941;31:731–765.

80. Konrath GA, Nahigian K, Kolowich P. Pigmented villonodular synovitis of the subacromial bursa. *J Shoulder Elbow Surg* 1997;6:400–404.

81. Mulier T, Victor J, Van Den Bergh J, et al. Diffuse pigmented villonodular synovitis of the shoulder: a case report and review of the literature. *Acta Orthop Belg* 1992;58:93–96.

82. Dorwart RH, Genant HK, Johnston WH, et al. Pigmented villonodular synovitis of synovial joints: clinical, pathologic, and radiographic features. *AJR Am J Roentgenol* 1984;143:877–885.

83. Gudmundsen TE, Siewers PB. Synovial chondromatosis of the shoulder: a case report. *Acta Orthop Scand* 1987;58:419–420.

84. Small R, Jaffe WL. Tenosynovial chondromatosis of the shoulder. *Bull Hosp Joint Dis Orthop Inst* 1981;41:37–47.

85. Volpin G, Nerubay J, Oliver S, et al. Synovial osteochondromatosis of the shoulder joint. *Am Surg* 1980;46:422–424.

86. Richman JD, Rose DJ. The role of arthroscopy in the management of synovial chondromatosis of the shoulder: a case report. *Clin Orthop* 1990;25791–93.

87. Hjelkrem M, Stanish WD. Synovial chondrometaplasia of the shoulder: a case report of a young athlete presenting with shoulder pain. *Am J Sports Med* 1988;16:84–86.

88. Coolican MR, Dandy DJ. Arthroscopic management of synovial chondromatosis of the knee: findings and results in 18 cases. *J Bone Joint Surg Br* 1989;71:498–500.

89. Enniking WF. *Clinical musculoskeletal pathology*, 3rd ed. 1990 Board of Regents of the State of Florida. Gainesville, FL:University Press of Florida, 1990.

90. McFarland EG, Neira CA. Synovial chondromatosis of the shoulder associated with osteoarthritis: conservative treatment. I: two cases and review of the literature. *Am J Orthop* 2000;29:785–787.

91. Covall DJ, Fowble CD. Arthroscopic treatment of synovial chondromatosis of the shoulder and biceps tendon sheath. *Arthroscopy* 1993;9:602–604.

92. Hogh J, Ludlam CA, Macnicol MF. Hemophilic arthropathy of the upper limb. *Clin Orthop* 1987;218:225–231.

93. Epps CH Jr. Painful hematologic conditions affecting the shoulder. *Clin Orthop* 1983;173:38–43.

94. MacDonald PB, Locht RC, Lindsay D, et al. Haemophilic arthropathy of the shoulder. *J Bone Joint Surg Br* 1990;72:470–471.

95. Rodriguez-Merchan EC. Pathogenesis, early diagnosis, and prophylaxis for chronic hemophilic synovitis. *Clin Orthop* 1997;343:6–11.

96. Nilsson IM, Bewrntorp E, Lofquist T, et al. Twenty-five years' experience of prophylactic treatment in severe haemophilia A and B. *J Intern Med* 1992;232:25–32.

97. Luck JV Jr. Surgical management of advanced hemophilic arthropathy. *Prog Clin Biol Res* 1990;324:241–256.

98. Eickhoff HH, Koch W, Raderschadt G, et al. Arthroscopy for chronic hemophilic synovitis of the knee. *Clin Orthop* 1997;343:58–62.

99. Isselbacher KJ, Martin JB, et al. Harrison's principles of internal medicine, 13th ed. New York: McGraw-Hill, 1994.

100. Caviglia HA, Fernandez-Palazzi F, Maffei E, et al. Chemical synoviorthesis for hemophilic synovitis. *Clin Orthop* 1997;(343):30–36.

101. Fernandez-Palazzi F, Caviglia HA, Salazar JR, et al. Intraarticular dexamethasone: I. Advanced chronic synovitis in hemophilia. *Clin Orthop* 1997;343:25–29.

102. Barfod G, Svendsen RN. Synovitis of the knee after intraarticular fracture fixation with Biofix. *Acta Orthop Scand* 1992;63:680–681.

103. Bostman O, Hirvensalo E, Makinen J, et al. Foreign-body reactions to fracture fixation implants of biodegradable synthetic polymers. *J Bone Joint Surg Br* 1990;72:592–596.

104. Friden T, Rydholm U. Severe aseptic synovitis of the knee after biodegradable internal fixation. *Acta Orthop Scand* 1992;63:94–97.

105. Santavirta S, Konttinen Y, Saito T, et al. Immune response to polyglycolic acid implants. *J Bone Joint Surg Br* 1990;72:597–600.

106. Weiler A, Helling H, Kirch U, et al. Foreign-body reaction and the course of osteolysis after polyglycolide implants for fracture fixation. *J Bone Joint Surg Br* 1996;78:369–376.

107. Song EK, Lee KB, Yoon TR. Aseptic synovitis after meniscal repair using the biodegradable meniscus arrow. *Arthroscopy* 2001;17:77–80.

108. Athanasiou KA, Agrawal CM, Barber FA, et al. Orthopaedic applications for PLA-PGA biodegradable polymers. *Arthroscopy* 1998;14:726–737.

109. Burkart A, Imhoff AB, Roscher E. Foreign-body Reaction to the bioabsorbable Suretac device. *Arthroscopy* 2000;16:91–95.

110. Stahelin A, Weiler A, Rufenacht H, et al. Clinical degradation and biocompatibility of different bioabsorbable Interference screws: a report of six cases. *Arthroscopy* 1997;13:238–244.

111. Le Dantec L, Maury F, Flipo RM, et al. Peripheral pyogenic arthritis: a study of one hundred seventy-nine cases. *Rev Rhum Engl Ed* 1996;63:103–110.

112. Lossos IS, Yossepowitch O, Kandel L, et al. Septic arthritis of the glenohumeral joint: a report of 11 cases and review of the literature. *Medicine (Baltimore)* 1998;77:177–187.

113. Dubost JJ, Soubrier M, Sauvezie B. Pyogenic arthritis in adults. *Joint Bone Spine* 2000;67:11–21.

114. Ward WG, Goldner RD. Shoulder pyarthrosis: a concomitant process. *Orthopedics* 1994;17:591–595.

115. Armbuster TG, Slivka J, Resnick D, et al. Extraarticular manifestations of septic arthritis of the glenohumeral joint. *AJR Am J Roentgenol* 1977;129:667–672.

116. Resnick CS. Septic arthritis: a rare cause of drooping shoulder. *Skeletal Radiol* 1992;21:307–309.

117. Rutten MJ, van den Berg JC, van den Hoogen FH, et al. Nontuberculous mycobacterial bursitis and arthritis of the shoulder. *Skeletal Radiol* 1998;27:33–35.

118. Leslie BM, Harris JM, Driscoll D. Septic arthritis of the shoulder in adults *J Bone Joint Surg Am* 1989;71:1516–1522.

119. Gristina AG, Rovere GD, Shoji H. Spontaneous septic arthritis complicating rheumatoid arthritis. *J Bone Joint Surg Am* 1974;56:1180–1184.

120. Watkins MB, Samilson RL, Winters DM. Acute suppurative arthritis. *J Bone Joint Surg Am* 1956;38:1313–1320.

121. Gelberman RH, Menon J, Austerlitz MS, et al. Pyogenic arthritis of the shoulder in adults. *J Bone Joint Surg Am* 1980;62:550–553.

122. Ward WG, Eckardt JJ. Subacromial/subdeltoid bursa abscesses. *Clin Orthop* 1993;288:189–194.

123. Parisien JS, Shaffer B. Arthroscopic management of pyarthrosis. *Clin Orthop* 1992;275:243–247.

124. Stutz G, Kuster MS, Kleinstuck F, et al. Arthroscopic management of septic arthritis: stages of infection and results. *Knee Surg Sports Traumatol Arthrosc* 2000;8:270–274.

125. Jerosch J, Hoffstetter I, Schroder M, et al. Septic arthritis: arthroscopic management with local antibiotic treatment. *Acta Orthop Belg* 1995;61:126–34.

126. Matthews LS, Terry G, Vetter WL. Shoulder anatomy for the arthroscopist. *Arthroscopy* 1985;1:83–91.

127. Matthews LS, Zarins B, Michael RH, et al. Anterior portal selection for shoulder arthroscopy. *Arthroscopy* 1985;1:33–39.

128. Zanotti RM, Kuhn JE. Arthroscopic capsular release for the stiff shoulder: description of technique and anatomic considerations. *Am J Sports Med* 1997;25:294–298.

129. Warner JJ, Allen AA, Marks PH, et al. Arthroscopic release of postoperative capsular contracture of the shoulder. *J Bone Joint Surg Am* 1997;79:1151–1158.

130. Sim FH. Synovial proliferative disorders: role of synovectomy. *Arthroscopy* 1985;1:198–204.
131. Small NC. Complications in arthroscopic surgery performed by experienced arthroscopists. *Arthroscopy* 1988;4:215–221.
132. Fu FH, Klein AH. Shoulder arthroscopy: complications and pitfalls. *Tech Orthop* 1988;3:27–32.
133. Hawkins RJ, Misamore GW, Hobeika PE. Surgery for full thickness rotator-cuff tears. *J Bone Joint Surg Am* 1985;67:1349–1355.
134. Flatow EL, Cordasco FA, Bigliani LU. Arthroscopic resection of the outer end of the clavicle from a superior approach: a critical, quantitative, radiographic assessment of bone removal. *Arthroscopy* 1992;8:55–64.

THE ELBOW

ELBOW ARTHROSCOPY: INTRODUCTION, INDICATIONS, COMPLICATIONS, AND RESULTS

ETHAN R. WIESLER
GARY G. POEHLING

Arthroscopy of the elbow is in relative infancy compared with the various other joints for which arthroscopy is currently indicated. However, with a better understanding of landmarks and improved techniques and training over the last two decades, elbow arthroscopy has become a more safe and effective treatment option for many elbow disorders.

In part because of the contour of the osseous anatomy of the elbow, with a high degree of conformity at the humerus, ulna, and radius, and in part because of the proximity of the neurovascular structures, elbow arthroscopy has been less commonly used in orthopaedic practice. Since the late 1970s, however, many surgeons have contributed to a better understanding of elbow disorders, mechanics, and pathology, facilitating the safe and effective use of arthroscopic techniques.

INDICATIONS

Morrey suggested two broad categories for surgical indications for elbow arthroscopy that help to guide surgical decision making: diagnostic and therapeutic/operative (1) (Table 42.1). There are certain clinical situations in which there is a diagnosis of an internal elbow disorder but imaging studies do not provide a clear picture. This may be seen in cases of: elbow pain with or without mechanical symptoms, pain out of proportion to the findings of a clinical examination, or joint contracture without bony injury. These clinical situations may warrant arthroscopic evaluation of the intraarticular anatomy to rule out any pathology not seen on routine radiographic evaluation. With newer and more advance imaging modalities (e.g., computed tomogra-

phy, magnetic resonance imaging), the diagnosis before arthroscopic surgery is more definite.

The most rewarding and successful indication for elbow arthroscopy is the removal of loose bodies, either posttraumatic or idiopathic, with or without associated limitations in joint range of motion (ROM) (1,11,36). In this situation, inspection of the anterior and posterior joints is performed. If the arthroscopic findings correlate with those of the physical examination, this is a very successful operative option, without the morbility of an open arthrotomy.

Another routine indication for elbow arthroscopy is for cases of either posttraumatic or inflammatory arthritis. This condition can cause progressive loss of elbow ROM, which can be simultaneously evaluated and treated through an arthroscopic synovectomy and capsular release. In the setting of inflammatory arthritis (e.g., lupus, rheumatoid arthritis), arthroscopic synovectomy and evaluation of the intraarticular anatomy can provide useful therapeutic information as well as definitive treatment (2,11–13,37).

Osteochondritis desiccans (OCD) of the elbow is defined as an inflammatory process or injury affecting the articular surface of the elbow (usually the capitellum) that involves a segment of cartilage, often with attached subchondral bone. It is differentiated from osteochondrosis (often called Panner's disease), which is a disease of the ossification center of the immature capitellar physis. When OCD involves the capitellum, magnetic resonance imaging can often help in both localizing the lesion and defining its anatomic borders (16). Loose bodies can often arise from prior or existing OCD lesions. With persistent mechanical symptoms and/or progressive loss of ROM of the elbow, plain radiographs and magnetic resonance imaging can often make the diagnosis. Arthroscopy in this setting is useful for evaluating the stability of the lesion and performing a debridement or *in situ* pinning of the lesion, thereby eliminating the need for a more extensive open procedure with associated complications.

E. R. Wiesler and G. G. Poehling: Wake Forest University Baptist Medical Center, Comprehab Plaza, Orthopaedic Surgery, Wake Forest University Baptist Medical Center, Winston-Salem, North Carolina.

TABLE 42.1 SURGICAL INDICATIONS FOR ELBOW ARTHROSCOPY

Loose bodies	Rheumatoid arthritis	Panner's disease
Synovitis	Joint contracture	Fracture management
Cartilage lesions (OCD)	Radial head excision	Valgus overload/instability
Osteoarthritis	Instability	Lateral epicondylitis

From references 1–17.

Many authors have described elbow arthroscopy for radial head resection, because radiocapitellar abnormalities can often be the cause of elbow pain and limited ROM (2,3,6,10). Arthroscopic procedures have also been described for the treatment of posterior rotatory instability of the elbow, although long-term results are still forthcoming. Finally, elbow arthroscopy can be used for lavage and debridement of acute sepsis of the joint.

COMPLICATIONS

As with any "new" procedure, there is a learning curve involved in establishing safe portals and avoiding neurovascular injury (Table 42.2).

There is no other joint for which more vigorous attention to the neurovascular anatomy needs to be observed. Descriptions in the literature of neurovascular complications of elbow arthroscopy are fortunately rare, but they do exist, and their obvious severity warrants respect.

Papilion et al. in 1988 and Thomas et al. in 1987 reported on two palsies of the posterior interosseous nerve (PIN), one in a 20-year-old and another in a 14-year-old athlete; one resolved by 6 months, and the other was incompletely resolved.

Morrey summarized anatomic proximity of nerves at the elbow to standard portals, and others have extensively studied the relationship of the cutaneous as well as median, ulnar, and radial nerves to the distended and nondistended elbow. The nerve most at risk is the radial nerve, which lies 5 to 16 mm from the lateral and anterolateral portals, depending on joint distention and exact portal placement. It has been well documented that joint distention alters anatomic relationships and does not completely protect the nerve from injury (19,22,26).

TABLE 42.2 COMPLICATIONS IN ELBOW ARTHROSCOPY

Nerve injury	Infection
Vascular injury	Tourniquet problems
Cartilage injury	Instrument failure/breakage
Compartment syndrome	Arthrofibrosis
Complex regional pain syndrome (CRPS)	Synovial fistula

From references 1, 18–28, 34.

Marshall et al. pointed out that instruments passed parallel to the joint kept the PIN safely anterior to the anterolateral portal. Verhaar recommended more anterior and more proximal portal location for the anterolateral portal (19,22).

Other potential sites for nerve injury include the ulnar nerve at the proximal medial portal, especially with procedures involving the posterior medial corner of the elbow, where the nerve can be 2 to 4 mm from the joint capsules (1,20). The median nerve can also be injured at arthroscopy, especially in the arthrofibrotic joint during anterior capsulectomy. Arthroscopic injury to the anterior interosseous nerve was reported after synovectomy in a 65-year-old patient with rheumatoid arthritis (28).

Lynch et al. (24), in 1986, did cadaveric dissection after standard portal placement and noted that the radial nerve lay in closest proximity to the joint in five cadavers (average, 5 mm), a distance that did increase with distension (to approximately 10 mm). The median nerve was similarly close to the anterior joint, at an average of 5 mm that increased to more than 10 mm with joint distension. The authors had no neurovascular complications in 21 consecutive procedures.

Lindenfeld (23) reported on the proximity of ulnar, radial, and median nerves at arthroscopy. The radial nerve was an average of 7.8 mm from the radial cannula at the anterolateral portal (which was made 3 cm distal and 1 cm anterior to the lateral epicondyle). He concluded that an anterior medial portal was the safest means to start elbow arthroscopy.

Moskal et al. (5) performed a metaanalysis of 465 elbow arthroscopies from a review of the literature. They reported a 12.6% overall complication rate, including both permanent and transient neurologic injuries, hematomas, synovial fistulae, and heterotopic ossification (5).

The general consensus on complications of most authors is the following:

1. Proximal portals are safer than distal ones.
2. Joint distension diminishes, but does not eliminate, the risk of nerve injury.
3. The radial nerve at the anterior lateral portal is most at risk.
4. Elbow flexion to 90 degrees aids in portal placement.
5. Posterior medial portals and direct anterior portals should be avoided.

RESULTS

Joint Contracture

Kim and Shin (29) reported on 63 patients with limited elbow ROM, with a total arc of motion of 79 degrees before surgery. Their results showed improved motion in 92% of patients, with an increase to 121 degrees immediately after surgery. They noted a temporary loss of ROM in the early postoperative period, but patients generally recovered to their intraoperative ROM within 1 year. They also noted that patients with a shorter duration of problems (less than 1 year) had greater improvement in ROM than did patients with a longer duration (49 versus 30 degrees), as did those who underwent anterior capsular release (23 versus 15 degrees).

Ward and Anderson (30) reported 90% improved function in 35 athletes who underwent arthroscopy for loose bodies or osteophytes of the dominant elbow. They found increases in flexion and extension of 9 and 6 degrees, respectively, with improved function (subjective functional score, 59 before versus 89 after surgery) and decreased pain (7 before versus 1 after surgery). They reported four complications (11%), including two chondral abrasions, one broken instrument, and one superficial infection.

Redden and Stanley (31) used the arthroscopic equivalent of the Outerbridge–Kashiwagi procedure to fenestrate the distal humerus. Twelve patients underwent this procedure without osteophyte excision; all patients achieved pain relief with improved ROM.

Nowicki and Shall (32) presented a case report of one volleyball player who underwent elbow arthroscopy for joint contracture and had improvement in flexion from 90 to 120 degrees after loose body removal in the anterior compartment.

Arthritis

Andrews et al. (33) reported on 62 patients who underwent elbow arthroscopy between 1979 and 1985, for a variety of pathologic entities, such as loose bodies, arthritis, synovitis, OCD, and contracture. They reported 85% good or excellent results, with 90% return to presurgical reports participation.

Moskal and Savoie (5), in 1999, reported unpublished data on 33 patients who had degenerative arthritis; 93% were satisfied with the operation. There was one ulnar nerve injury and two repeat arthroscopic procedures to maintain motion.

Schneider et al. (34) reported the results for 67 patients who underwent elbow arthroscopy between 1977 and 1991. The diagnoses included infection, posttraumatic arthritis, osteochondrosis, pain, and loose bodies. Ages ranged from 11 to 59 years (median, 26 years). The overall scores (Figgie) improved from 61 to 85. There were seven nerve injuries (four radial, two ulnar, and one median), all of which resolved by 6 months after surgery.

In 1992, O'Driscoll and Morrey (35) reviewed 70 patients who underwent elbow arthroscopy for a variety of conditions. However, 36 (64%) underwent the procedure for diagnostic purposes. The best results were in patients who had loose bodies without other secondary pathology. They reported a 10% complication rate overall; transient radial nerve palsy occurred in 3 patients (4%), persistent drainage without sepsis in 4 (6%), and minor ROM loss in 1.

Although the diagnoses in these studies range widely, there has been a definite trend for improved symptoms and function with fewer nerve injuries as experience is gained and anatomic details are elucidated (36).

CONCLUSIONS

Elbow arthroscopy, in its current practice, is a safe and effective treatment option for a variety of elbow disorders. Diligent attention to anatomic detail and clinical acumen are paramount.

REFERENCES

1. Morrey BF. Complications of elbow arthroscopy. *Instr Course Lect* 2000;49:255–258.
2. Jerosch J, Schroder J, Schneider T. Good and relative indications for elbow arthroscopy: a retrospective study on 103 patients. *Arch Orthop Trauma Surg* 1998;117:246–249.
3. Byrd JW. Elbow arthroscopy for arthrofibrosis after type I radial head fractures. *Arthroscopy* 1994;10:162–165.
4. Day B. Elbow arthroscopy in the athlete. *Clin Sports Med* 1996;15:785–797.
5. Moskal JH, Savoie FH, Field LD. Elbow arthroscopy in trauma and reconstruction. *Orthop Clin North Am* 1999;30:163–177.
6. O'Driscoll SW, Morrey BF, An KN. Intraarticular pressure and capacity of the elbow. *Arthroscopy* 1990;6:100–103.
7. Andrews JR, Carson WG. Arthroscopy of the elbow. *Arthroscopy* 1985;1:97–107.
8. Angelo RL. Advances in elbow arthroscopy. *Orthopedics* 1993;16:1037–1046.
9. Poehling GG, Ekman EF, Ruch DS. Elbow arthroscopy. *Operative Arthroscopy* 1996;57:821–828.
10. Lyons TR, Field LD, Savoie FH. Basics of elbow arthroscopy. *Instr Course Lect* 2000;49:239–246.
11. Morrey BF. Arthroscopy of the elbow. *Instr Course Lect* 1986;35:102–107.
12. Baker CL, Brooks AA. Arthroscopy of the elbow. *Clin Sports Med* 1986;15:261–281.
13. Ekman EF, Poehling GG. Arthroscopy of the elbow. *Hand Clin* 1994;10:453–460.
14. Woods GW. Elbow arthroscopy. *Clin Sports Med* 1987;6:557–564.
15. Poehling GG, Whipple TL, Sisco L, et al. Elbow arthroscopy: a new technique. *Arthroscopy* 1989;5:222–224.
16. Baker CL Jr, Salvoy RM. The prone position for elbow arthroscopy. *Clin Sports Med* 1991;10:623–628.

17. Murphy BJ. MR imaging of the elbow. *Radiology* 1992;184:525–529.
18. Gallay SH, Richards RR, O'Driscoll SW. Intraarticular capacity and compliance of stiff and normal elbows. *Arthroscopy* 1993;9:9–13.
19. Thomas MA, Fast A, Shapiro D. Radial nerve damage as a complication of elbow arthroscopy. *Clin Orthop* 1987;215:130–131.
20. Hahn M, Grossman JA. Ulnar nerve laceration as a result of elbow arthroscopy. *J Hand Surg Br* 1998;23:109.
21. Papilion JD, Neff RS, Shall LM. Compression neuropathy of the radial nerve as a complication of elbow arthroscopy: a case report and review of the literature. *Arthroscopy* 1998;4:284–286.
22. Verhaar J, Mameren H, Brandsma A. Risks of neurovascular injury in elbow arthroscopy: starting anteromedially or anterolaterally? *Arthroscopy* 1991;7:287–290.
23. Lindenfeld TN. Medial approach in elbow arthroscopy. *Am J Sports Med* 1990;18:413–417.
24. Lynch GJ, Meyers JF, Whipple TL. Neurovascular anatomy and elbow arthroscopy: inherent risks. *Arthroscopy* 1986;2:190–197.
25. Miller CD, Jobe CM, Wright MH. Neuroanatomy in elbow arthroscopy. *J Shoulder Elbow Surg* 1995;4:168–174.
26. Marshall PD, Fairclough JA, Johnson SR, et al. Avoiding nerve damage during elbow arthroscopy. *J Bone Joint Surg Br* 1993;75:129–131.
27. Stothers K, Day B, Regan WR. Arthroscopy of the elbow: anatomy, portal sites, and a description of the proximal lateral portal. *Arthroscopy* 1995;11:449–457.
28. Ruch DS, Poehling GG. Anterior interosseus nerve injury following elbow arthroscopy. *Arthroscopy* 1997;13:756–758.
29. Kim SJ, Shin SJ. Arthroscopic treatment for limitation of motion of the elbow. *Clin Orthop* 2000;375:140–148.
30. Ward WG, Anderson TE. Elbow arthroscopy in a mostly athletic population. *J Hand Surg Am* 1993;18:220–224.
31. Redden JF, Stanley D. Arthroscopic fenestration of the olecranon fossa in the treatment of osteoarthritis of the elbow. *Arthroscopy* 1993;9:14–16.
32. Nowicki KD, Shall LM. Arthroscopic release of a posttraumatic flexion contracture in the elbow: a case report and review of the literature. *Arthroscopy* 1992;8:544–547.
33. Andrews JR, St. Pierre RK, Carson WG Jr. Arthroscopy of the elbow. *Clin Sports Med* 1986;5:653–662.
34. Schneider T, Hoffstetter I, Fink B, et al. Long-term results of elbow arthroscopy in 67 patients. *Acta Orthop Belg* 1994;60:378–382.
35. O'Driscoll SW, Morrey BF. Arthroscopy of the elbow: diagnostic and therapeutic benefits and hazards. *J Bone Joint Surg Am* 1992;74:84–94.
36. O'Driscoll SW. Elbow arthroscopy for loose bodies. *Orthopaedics* 1992;15:855–859.
37. O'Driscoll SW. Operative treatment of elbow arthritis. *Curr Opin Rheumatol* 1995;7:103–106.

43

ELBOW ARTHROSCOPY: SUPINE TECHNIQUE

J. F. MEYERS
W. G. CARSON, JR.

Arthroscopy has been most commonly used to evaluate various disorders of the knee and shoulder joints. Arthroscopy of the elbow is less frequently indicated. In the past several years it has been used with increased frequency by some arthroscopists, although not by the majority of orthopaedic surgeons. Because of technical advances in arthroscopic equipment, development of various arthroscopic techniques for elbow arthroscopy, and increased knowledge of the arthroscopic anatomy of the elbow, arthroscopy of the elbow can now be performed on a reasonably routine basis (1–13).

Elbow arthroscopy is a technically demanding surgical procedure, and attention to detail is essential for a safe and reproducible arthroscopic examination. Attention to detail is particularly important with regard to the location of the neurovascular structures about the elbow. Multiple complications of elbow arthroscopy have been reported (14–25); however, many of these complications can be avoided by adhering to a strict technique (26–32). A thorough knowledge of the extraarticular portal anatomy of the elbow is necessary, because the arthroscopic instruments must be placed through deep muscle layers and near important neurovascular structures. In addition, there are other anatomic barriers, such as a tightly constructed joint that precludes marked distention and the fact that manipulation of the elbow does not improve visualization or advancement of the arthroscopic instruments within the elbow.

HISTORY OF ELBOW ARTHROSCOPY

The first mention of elbow arthroscopy in the orthopaedic literature was by Michael Burman (33) in 1931. He reported on arthroscopy performed on cadavers using a 3-mm

J. F. **Meyers:** Tuckahoe Orthopaedic Associates, Ltd., Richmond, Virginia, and Medical College of Virginia, Richmond, Virginia.

W. G. **Carson, Jr.:** University of South Florida College, Tampa, Florida, and The Sports Medicine Clinic of Tampa, Florida.

diameter endoscope. He stated that the elbow was "unsuitable for examination" and that the "anterior puncture of the elbow is out of the question." In 1971, Watanabe (34) developed the 1.7-mm, no. 24 arthroscope for use in small joints. After this development, various surgical approaches to elbow arthroscopy were described, including those of Ito (35,36) and Maeda (37) in 1979 and 1980. In 1981, Ito (38) reported a clinical study of elbow arthroscopy in the Japanese literature based on 226 cases. In 1983, Hempfling (39) described the prone position for elbow arthroscopy. In 1985, Guhl (7) reported a series of elbow arthroscopies in 45 cases. Also in 1985, Andrews and Carson (1,2,4,14) reported 12 cases of elbow arthroscopy and reviewed the arthroscopic technique and anatomy of the elbow. In the mid-1980s, elbow arthroscopy techniques were described by Eriksson and Denti (40), Boe (41), Johnson (42), and Woods (10). New arthroscopic approaches were also described by Poehling et al. (43) in 1989 and by Lindenfeld (44) in 1990.

INDICATIONS

The indications for arthroscopy of the elbow continue to evolve. At the present time, the following indications have been described for elbow arthroscopy:

1. Loose body removal
2. Evaluation and treatment of osteochondritis dissecans of the capitellum
3. Evaluation and debridement of chondral or osteochondral lesions of the radial head
4. Debridement and lysis of adhesions
5. Debridement of posttraumatic or certain degenerative processes about the elbow
6. Partial synovectomy
7. Partial excision of humeral or olecranon osteophytes
8. Flexion contracture release
9. Valgus extension overload syndrome

10. Irrigation and debridement for septic arthritis
11. Evaluation of ulnar collateral ligament instability
12. Treatment of ligament instability
13. Evaluation and treatment of elbow fractures
14. Diagnosis of chronic elbow pain
15. Treatment of lateral epicondylitis

CONTRAINDICATIONS

Contraindications for arthroscopy of the elbow include any condition in which the normal bony or soft tissue anatomy has been distorted in such a manner that the neurovascular structures are placed at risk or the intraarticular space precludes distention, visualization, and instrumentation. Conditions such as bony ankylosis and severe fibrous ankylosis are possibly contraindicated because of the difficulty in introducing instruments into the elbow. In addition, previous surgical procedures such as anterior transposition of the ulnar nerve or osteotomies may alter the normal portal anatomy and place neurovascular structures at risk.

As with any arthroscopic procedure, certain skin conditions, such as cellulitis of the overlying skin that interferes with portal placement and risks intraarticular infection, are also contraindications.

INSTRUMENTATION

Surgical techniques for elbow arthroscopy do not differ from those used in other joints, with the exception that greater care must be taken to avoid scuffing or gouging of the articular surface, particularly the distal humerus, radial head, or olecranon. The elbow joint is inherently stable, and there is little room in which to maneuver the various instruments. Elbow arthroscopy should be performed slowly and deliberately to avoid slippage of the arthroscope out of the elbow capsule. Creation of multiple entries of the various cannulas into the elbow joint can result in excessive fluid extravasation (3).

Basic arthroscopic equipment includes

- 18-gauge Spinal needles
- Marking pen
- 50-mL Syringe
- Intravenous connecting tubing
- No. 11 knife blade
- Hemostat
- Probe
- Punches
- Graspers with teeth
- Ruler
- Blunt and sharp trocars
- 4-mm, 30-degree Angled arthroscope
- 2.7-mm, 30-degree Angled arthroscope
- Interchangeable cannula systems for 4- and 2.5-mm arthroscopes

- Motorized shavers, trimmers, and burs
- Pump system (optional)
- Switching sticks
- Small osteotome
- Large-bore inflow tubing

Handheld instruments such as probes, grasping forceps, and punches are commonly used in elbow arthroscopy. Motorized instruments include synovial resectors, trimmers, cutters, and abraders. The use of motorized instruments inserted through cannulas is safer because repeated passes are avoided. Repeated passes create multiple capsular holes and increase the extravasation of fluid about the elbow, thus increasing the risk of damage to nearby neurovascular structures. Whether handheld or motorized, all instruments should be used carefully within the elbow. The instruments should not be wedged between articular cartilage surfaces, because this would cause damage to the articular cartilage. As with any arthroscopic procedure, the instruments should always be in full view.

The arthroscopic systems used in the larger joints, such as the shoulder and the knee, are also used in the elbow. A 4-mm, 30-degree angled arthroscope provides optimal visualization of the elbow. Smaller arthroscopes may be used as well. A "small joint system" arthroscopic setup is helpful for visualization of the smaller spaces within the elbow, such as the lateral compartment as seen through the direct lateral portal. However, the overall field of view is somewhat narrower in these small joint systems, and more optimal visualization is possible with the larger 4-mm arthroscope.

ANESTHESIA

General anesthesia is commonly used for arthroscopy of the elbow because it affords complete comfort for the patient and provides total muscle relaxation. Intrascalene or axillary blocks can be used, but some practitioners believe that they require considerable expertise and increase the difficulty of immediate postoperative neurovascular evaluation. Ito (45) advocated the use of local anesthesia for diagnostic arthroscopy. Intravenous regional anesthesia may also be used; however, the use of dual tourniquets about the upper arm can compromise elbow exposure and cause vascular engorgement and edema, thereby interfering with visualization of the joint.

SURGICAL TECHNIQUE: SUPINE POSITION

A properly padded tourniquet is placed as high on the upper arm and as near the axilla as possible. When tourniquet control is used, care should be taken to use a cuff of appropriate size, with underlying padding, and to limit tourniquet time to no more than 90 minutes. Others claim that 120 minutes appears to be safe (9).

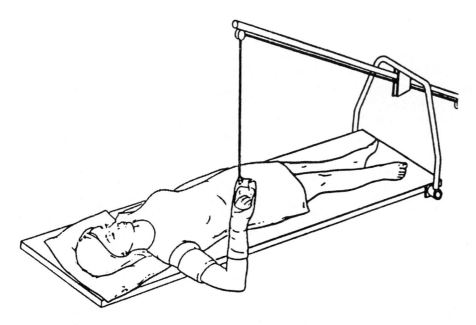

FIGURE 43.1 Supine position with suspension system for elbow arthroscopy.

The patient is placed in the supine position with the scapula at the edge of the operating table and the shoulder abducted 90 degrees. The hand or forearm is connected to a forearm splint, skin traction, or "finger trap" supports. The arm is then connected to an overhead suspension device so that the elbow is flexed to 90 degrees (Fig. 43.1). Approximately 5 lb, or only enough weight to suspend the arm, is applied through a pulley-and-weight system that suspends the arm and keeps the elbow flexed to 90 degrees. Some of the commercially available skin traction or finger traction devices, including the suspension ropes, are prepackaged sterilely and may be applied to the arm after it has been prepared. Other devices, such as forearm splints, are not sterile, so the elbow is prepared and draped after the splint is applied. A single sterile towel covered by a transparent plastic drape can be used to cover the forearm wrist support. Routine upper extremity drapes are then used on the upper arm and to cover the remainder of the patient.

This position provides ready access to both medial and lateral aspects of the elbow and eliminates the need for an extra assistant to stabilize the arm. The forearm may also be freely pronated and supinated throughout the surgical procedure.

At times the use of an overhead suspension device can make the elbow somewhat unstable as it swings on the traction apparatus. An alternative to the overhead suspension device is to place two routine operating table arm boards on the same side of the operating table and to allow the arm to rest on this support (Fig. 43.2). With this setup, an assistant keeps the elbow in 90 degrees of flexion at all times, and folded towels are placed beneath the upper arm to support the arm and to raise the actual elbow away from the underlying table. This setup appears to be somewhat more stable than that supplied by the overhead traction device, but it does require the use of an extra assistant to stabilize the arm.

After the arm has been stabilized and the upper extremity prepared and draped, the surgeon stands or sits on the radial side of the elbow and the first assistant on the axilla side. A Mayo stand can be placed at the end of the table, and the second assistant or scrub technician may stand behind it. The video equipment is placed opposite the patient on the other side of the operating table.

Whether an arm board support or an overhead traction device is used, the elbow must remain in 90 degrees of flexion at all times when the anterior structures are being examined arthroscopically, in order to maintain complete relaxation of the neurovascular structures in the antecubital fossa (1–5,14,15,26,27,41,46,47). O'Driscoll et al. (27) demonstrated that the intraarticular pressure of the elbow is lowest at 80 degrees of flexion, and capsular rupture occurs at relatively low intraarticular pressures. Rupture of the capsule can lead to extravasation of fluid about the elbow, compro-

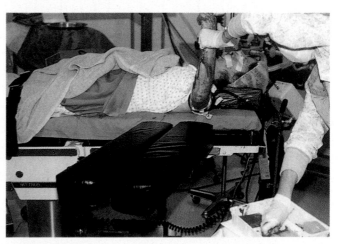

FIGURE 43.2 Example of double arm board used in elbow arthroscopy.

mising visualization and making the procedure technically more difficult. Therefore, the flexed position of the elbow should be maintained at all times.

After anesthesia has been administered and the position of the patient is stabilized, the bony landmarks are outlined with a marking pen before initiation of the procedure. Large amounts of fluid can be extravasated during the arthroscopic procedure, and marking of the landmarks facilitates their identification during surgery. Landmarks commonly marked include the radial head, lateral humeral epicondyle, olecranon tip, medial humeral epicondyle, and ulnar nerve (Fig. 43.3). The anterolateral, anteromedial, direct lateral, posterolateral, and straight posterior portals are also marked at this time.

Some surgeons have proposed placing the patient in the prone position for elbow arthroscopy (39,43,44,47). This position provides ready access to both the anterior and posterior aspects of the elbow and allows gravity to help move the neurovascular structures in the antecubital fossa away from the entering instruments. Poehling et al. (43) believe that this position improves mobility because it does not require a traction suspension device. They asserted that the prone position of the arm is more stable than the supine position with the arm suspended in the overhead traction apparatus. When used in conjunction with a proximal medial portal as the initial arthroscopic portal, the instruments enter more parallel to the neurovascular structures and possibly may protect these structures during initiation of the arthroscopic portal (44). An improved view of the anterior joint with use of this portal has also been reported (44). A more detailed description and technique of the prone position and proximal medial portals is provided in Chapter 44.

There are several advantages of the supine position compared with the prone position. No special equipment is needed, such as the foam padding that is required to suspend the arm in the prone position. The usual shoulder traction device that is used in shoulder arthroscopy, which is available in most operating rooms, can be used to support the elbow in the supine position. In addition, it is not necessary to intubate the patient, as it is in the prone position. There is excellent access to all aspects of the elbow with the supine position, and the conceptualization of the intraarticular anatomy is often easier for the surgeon who is working on the patient in the supine position rather than "upside down" in the prone position.

Disadvantages of the supine position primarily relate to the fact that it is difficult to work in the posterior compartment of the elbow when using the overhead suspension device or if the arm is supported by towels on an arm board. An assistant has to extend the elbow away from the underlying table, and even if the suspension traction device is used, the assistant still has to extend the arm more in order for work to be performed in the posterior portal. In addition, the surgeon many times feels he or she is working "upside down" when working on the posterior compartment with the patient in the supine position. Swelling in this area and extravasation of fluid can make this portal technically difficult.

PORTALS

The most commonly used portals in elbow arthroscopy are the proximal lateral, anterolateral, anteromedial, and pos-

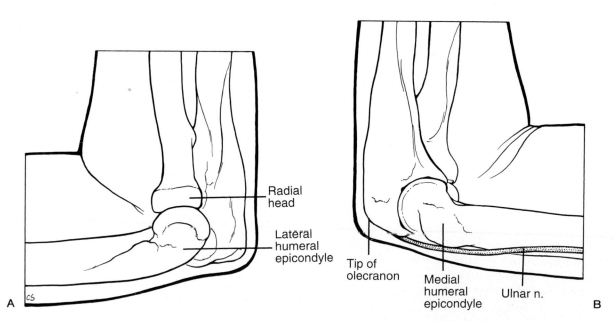

FIGURE 43.3 The lateral humeral epicondyle, radial head, and olecranon have been outlined at the beginning of the procedure.

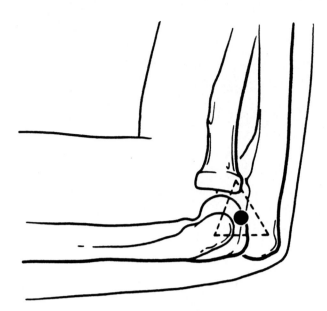

FIGURE 43.4 Insertion site for the 18-gauge spinal needle for initial distention of the elbow is located through the triangular area bordered by the lateral humeral epicondyle, the radial head, and the tip of the olecranon.

terolateral portals. Other portals have been described for elbow arthroscopy (8,324–38,40), including several lateral portals (7) and the anteromedial supracondylar or proximal medial portal (23,43,46). Two accessory portals, the midlateral portal and the direct posterior or "transtriceps" portal, can be used if required.

Before insertion of the arthroscope into any of these portals, the elbow should be maximally distended with saline solution with the use of a 50-mL syringe connected to intravenous tubing and an 18-gauge spinal needle. The most reliable insertion site for this needle is through the triangular area over the lateral aspect of the elbow, which is bordered by the radial head, the lateral humeral epicondyle, and the tip of the olecranon (Fig. 43.4). This is the "soft spot" of the elbow that is often used in aspiration of the elbow as a treatment for hemarthrosis. When this area is penetrated, the 18-gauge needle traverses skin, a thin subcutaneous layer, the anconeus muscle, and the capsule. Proper placement in the elbow joint is verified by free backflow from the needle (Fig. 43.5). After entry into the elbow is verified and approximately 20 mL of saline solution is injected, the needle is removed. When the elbow joint is fully distended, it will extend a few degrees. No further fluid should be injected, or the capsule may rupture. At this time the primary diagnostic portal of choice may be established.

Proximal Lateral Portal

With the patient in the supine position, the proximal lateral portal is usually the standard diagnostic portal for arthroscopy of the elbow and is usually established first.

As previously mentioned, the landmarks and portals are outlined with a methylene blue sterile marker at the outset of the procedure. To palpate the radial head, one places the index finger or thumb over the radiocapitellar joint line while pronating and supinating the forearm. The entire radial head is outlined with a marker.

The lateral epicondyle is palpated and outlined. The portal is 1 to 2 cm proximal to the lateral epicondyle along the anterior surface of the humerus. As described, the elbow is flexed 90 degrees and an 18-gauge needle is placed in the soft spot. The elbow joint is maximally distended with 20 mL of sterile saline through the 18-gauge spinal needle. After distention is complete, a second 18-gauge spinal needle is placed at the point previously marked as the proximal lateral portal. The needle is aimed directly toward the center of the joint. Location of this second needle in the elbow joint is confirmed by free backflow of fluid.

Once proper placement of the 18-gauge spinal needle is confirmed and the elbow is maximally distended and flexed 90 degrees, the larger arthroscopic instruments can be introduced (Figs. 43.6 and 43.7). The cannula system is introduced by making a small incision in the skin, with care taken to avoid injury to the underlying subcutaneous nerves. Close attention should be given to the subcutaneous nerves about the elbow during establishment of these portals. A no. 11 blade is laid across the skin, and the skin is then pulled across the blade. The incision and the underlying subcutaneous tissues may then be deepened with the use of a hemostat (18). The lateral and posterior antebrachial cutaneous nerves should be avoided (Fig. 43.8). The lateral antebrachial cutaneous nerve, a terminal branch of the musculocutaneous nerve, pierces the brachial fascia just lateral to

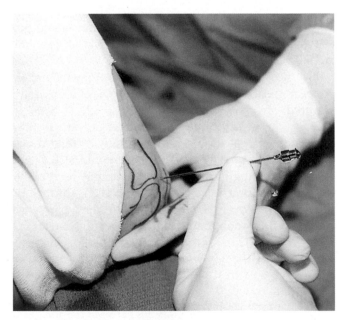

FIGURE 43.5 Proper placement into the elbow joint is verified by backflow of fluid from the 18-gauge spinal needle.

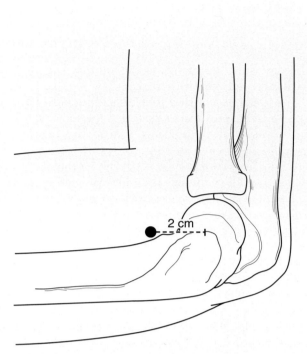

FIGURE 43.6 The proximal lateral portal is 2 cm proximal to the lateral epicondyle along the anterior border of the humerus.

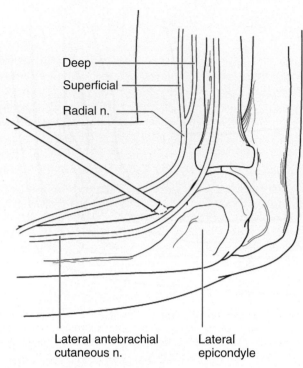

FIGURE 43.7 The arthroscope enters the joint through the proximal lateral portal, hugging the anterior border of the humerus.

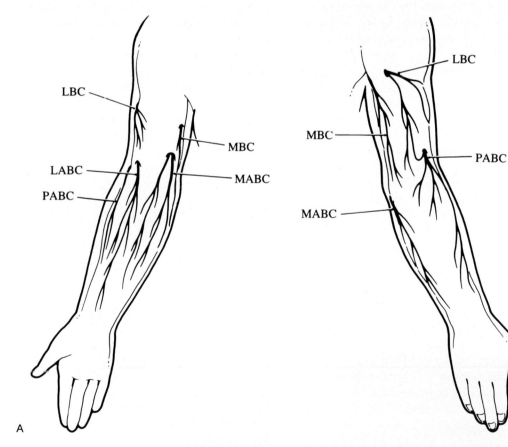

FIGURE 43.8 A: Anatomy of subcutaneous nerves of anterior aspect of arm. **B:** Anatomy of posterior subcutaneous nerves of the arm. LBC, lateral brachial nerve; LABC, lateral antebrachial cutaneous nerve; PABC, posterior antebrachial cutaneous nerve; MBC, medial brachial cutaneous nerve; MABC, medial antebrachial cutaneous nerve.

the biceps tendon proximal to the elbow joint. It then divides into an anterior and posterior branch, with the anterior branch supplying the skin over the anterior portion of the forearm. The posterior branch passes over the lateral humeral epicondyle and supplies the skin of the radial border of the forearm. The posterior antebrachial cutaneous nerve, a branch of the radial nerve, pierces the brachial fascia in the lower two thirds of the arm, supplying the skin behind the lateral humeral epicondyle and the dorsal aspect of the forearm.

A blunt trocar is used because it can be readily inserted through the subcutaneous fat and muscles. Use of the blunt trocar during insertion of the cannula minimizes damage to nearby neurovascular structures and articular cartilage.

Careful attention must be given to the angle of insertion of the trocar and cannula system. The instruments should be directed to the center of the elbow, with the elbow remaining flexed at 90 degrees at all times. As the surgeon aims the trocar and cannula toward the joint, the capsule and synovium must be "trapped" against the distal humerus to puncture it and enter the elbow joint. Once the capsule is entered, free backflow of fluid through the cannula will be evident, verifying entrance into the elbow. At this time, the arthroscope is inserted and diagnostic arthroscopy is begun.

If a single arthroscopic portal is used initially for diagnostic arthroscopy of the elbow, an arthroscopic connector or "bridge" will require both an inflow and an outflow connector. Continuous distention of the elbow is maintained by the use of two 3-L bags of normal saline or lactated Ringer's solution elevated above the patient and attached to the arthroscope, allowing distention by gravity. An alternative technique is to use an infusion pump to distend the elbow. Intermittent suction through the outflow connector is used to remove any cloudy fluid or debris. Unless cleansing is required, the sleeve is occasionally left clamped off to maintain distention pressure within the elbow. During insertion of larger instruments into the elbow joint, it is important that the elbow is kept maximally distended, because this further displaces the neurovascular structures away from the entering arthroscopic instrument (6,18). After the second arthroscopic portal is established, usually medially, a separate cannula may be inserted for inflow and fluid distention, and visualization will be greatly improved.

Proximal Lateral Portal Anatomy

This portal has been shown to be safer than the anterolateral portal, the distance from the arthroscopic sheath to the radial nerve being approximately twice as great (50,51). During the establishment of the proximal lateral portal, the sheath passes through the brachioradialis, the brachialis, and the lateral elbow capsule. The posterior branch of the lateral antibrachial cutaneous nerve is between 0 and 14 mm away,

and the radial nerve is approximately 9 mm away when the elbow is flexed and the joint distended. Capsular distention carries the radial nerve further away from this proximal portal.

Arthroscopic Anatomy of the Proximal Lateral Portal

Intraarticular structures of the elbow that can be seen from the proximal lateral portal are the distal humerus, trochlear ridges, and coronoid process of the ulna. Flexion and extension of the elbow allow visualization of the coronoid process of the ulna. Extension of the elbow provides a better view of the medial and lateral trochlear ridges and the trochlear notch of the distal humerus. By slowly retracting and angling the 30-degree arthroscope toward the radial head, the surgeon can see the radial head and the superior articulation between the ulna and radial head.

Anterolateral Portal

The anterolateral portal was the originally described lateral portal; it is no longer as popular since greater safety of the proximal lateral portal has been established. It is still a useful portal, however, and with proper attention to details it can be used safely.

The point just anterior and proximal to the radial head is marked as the anterolateral portal. This portal is usually 3 cm distal and 1 to 2 cm anterior to the lateral humeral epicondyle (Figs. 43.9 and 43.10). The key to the location of

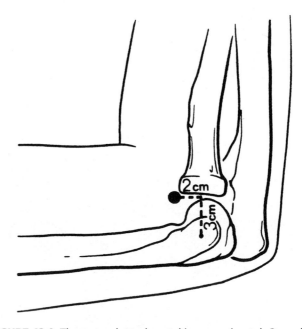

FIGURE 43.9 The anterolateral portal is *approximately* 3 cm distal and 1–2 cm anterior to the lateral humeral epicondyle.

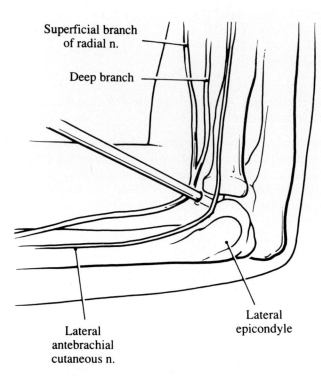

FIGURE 43.10 The arthroscope courses just anterior and proximal to the radial head to visualize the anterior structures of the elbow joint.

this portal is that it lies just anterior and proximal to the radial head. The measurement described (3 × 1 to 2 cm) is an *estimation* of this location and varies in every elbow.

Anterolateral Portal Anatomy

During the establishment of the anterolateral portal, the arthroscope passes anterior to the radial head through the extensor

carpi radialis brevis muscle and then through the lateral capsule before entering the joint (1,18) (Fig. 43.11). The arthroscope may pass from 4 mm (18) to 7 mm (1) beneath the radial nerve when establishing the anterolateral portal. The radial nerve is located between the brachialis and the brachial radialis over the distal aspect of the arm. As the nerve passes in front of the lateral humeral epicondyle, it divides into a superficial branch, which runs on the deep surface of the brachioradialis, and a deep motor branch, which pierces the supinator muscle to supply the extensor muscles of the forearm (Fig. 43.12). Lynch et al. (18) demonstrated that the arthroscopic instruments pass within a mean distance of 4 mm from the radial nerve, regardless of the flexion or extension of the elbow, when the elbow is not distended with fluid. However, if 35 to 40 mL of fluid is inserted into the elbow capsule, the radial nerve moves an additional 7 mm anteriorly (18). Therefore, maximal distention of the elbow should be maintained at all times, particularly when establishing the initial arthroscopic portals.

Arthroscopic Anatomy of the Anterolateral Portal

Intraarticular structures of the elbow that can be seen from the anterolateral portal are the distal humerus, trochlear ridges, and coronoid process of the ulna (Figs. 43.13 and 43.14). The medial aspect of the radial head and its articulation with the ulna can be seen by retracting the arthroscope (Fig. 43.15). Lateral joint visualization is somewhat better through the proximal lateral portal, but this is an excellent working portal for procedures on the radial head.

Anteromedial Portal

After the anterolateral portal has been established, the anteromedial portal is established by way of direct intraarticu-

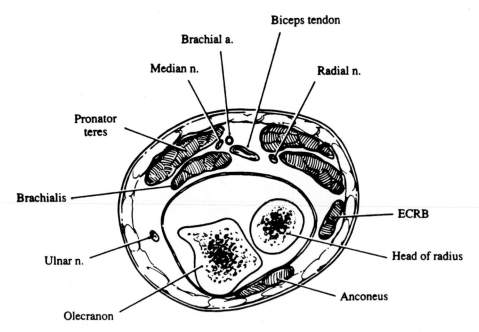

FIGURE 43.11 Cross-sectional view of elbow at level of anterolateral and anteromedial portals with joint distention. ECRB, extensor carpi radialis brevis.

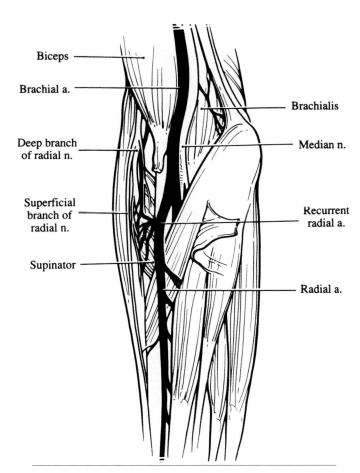

FIGURE 43.12 Neurovascular structures of antecubital fossa of the elbow.

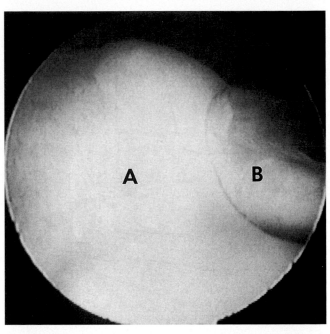

FIGURE 43.14 Arthroscopic view from the anterolateral portal in a right elbow, showing distal humerus trochlea **(A)** and coronoid process of ulna **(B).**

lar visualization. The anteromedial portal is identified approximately 2 cm anterior and 2 cm distal to the medial humeral epicondyle (Fig. 43.16). With the arthroscope in the anterolateral portal, an 18-gauge spinal needle is inserted at the entry point described previously with the elbow flexed 90 degrees. The elbow is maximally distended with fluid, and the needle is aimed directly toward the center of the

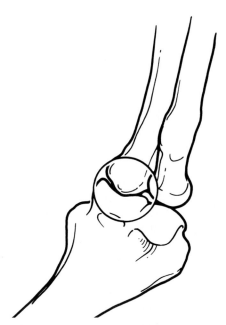

FIGURE 43.13 Intraarticular structures that can be visualized from the anterolateral portal include the distal humerus and trochlear ridges and the coronoid process of the ulna.

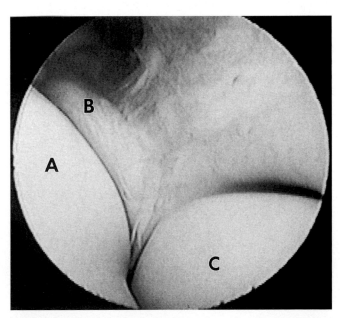

FIGURE 43.15 Arthroscopic view from anterolateral portal. If the arthroscope is retracted posteriorly and directed inferiorly, not only can the trochlea **(A)** and the coronoid process of the ulna **(B)** be seen, but also portions of the radial head **(C)** can be visualized.

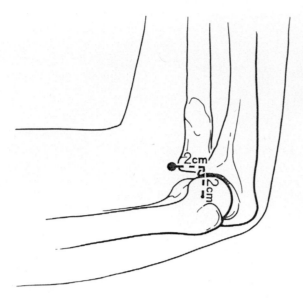

FIGURE 43.16 The anteromedial portal is located *approximately* 2 cm anterior and 2 cm distal to the medial humeral epicondyle.

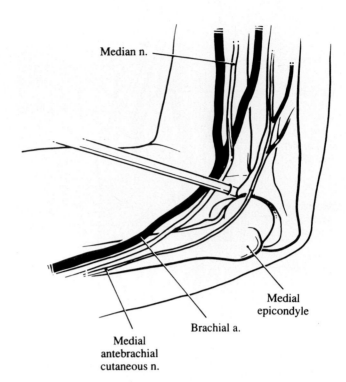

FIGURE 43.18 The arthroscope passes just anterior to the medial humeral epicondyle to view the anterior structures of the elbow joint.

joint. Confirmation that the needle is entering the joint is provided by direct visualization through the arthroscope in the anterolateral portal (Fig. 43.17). The needle passes just anterior to the medial humeral epicondyle and inferior to the antecubital structures (Fig. 43.18). The ideal position of the needle is just proximal to the humeral ulnar joint and just anterior to the humerus. The location mentioned (2 × 2 cm) is an *estimation* of the ideal position of the anteromedial portal and varies in elbows of different sizes.

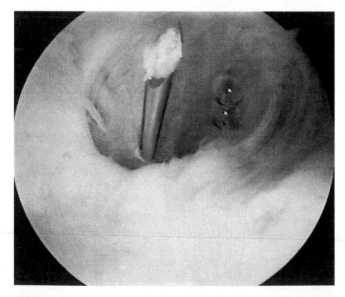

FIGURE 43.17 Arthroscopic view from the anterolateral portal in a right elbow. An 18-gauge spinal needle has been placed through the anteromedial portal. The antecubital structures are displaced anteriorly by fluid distension within the elbow.

A small incision is made in the skin, with care taken to protect the subcutaneous nerves. The arthroscopic cannula and blunt trocar system are then introduced. When establishing the anteromedial portal, the medial antebrachial cutaneous nerve should be avoided (Fig. 43.8). This nerve divides into an anterior branch, which supplies the forearm, and a smaller ulnar branch, which courses over the medial humeral epicondyle. An interchangeable cannula system is used to change freely from the anterolateral to the anteromedial portal with the various instruments. If a simple diagnostic arthroscopy is being performed, an inflow cannula can be placed through the anteromedial portal to provide better distention and visualization. Because maximal distention of the elbow is being maintained at all times, the extracapsular extravasation of the fluid should be monitored closely. Extracapsular extravasation is most often seen when repeated attempts have been made to establish the arthroscopic portals, resulting in multiple holes in the capsule and fluid leakage. When a separate inflow cannula is used for distention, the cannula should have no "side vents" because if the inflow cannula slips back somewhat during the arthroscopic procedure, the fluid will leak directly into the subcutaneous tissues.

Most arthroscopic surgical procedures in the elbow are performed because of pathologic processes located over the lateral aspect of the elbow, such as loose bodies or osteochondritis dissecans of the capitellum (11,12,48,49). Therefore, the surgeon needs to be proficient in establishing both the anterolateral and the anteromedial portal. The anteromedial portal provides excellent visualization of the lateral aspect of the anterior compartment, compared with that provided through the lateral portal.

When the anterolateral portal is used for the arthroscope, the surgeon sits at the lateral or radial aspect of the arm. If the surgeon attempts to use the anteromedial portal for the arthroscope and still sits at the lateral or radial aspect of the arm, the arthroscope will be coming backward toward the surgeon, and the orientation could be somewhat confusing when this movement is viewed on a video monitor. Therefore, if the surgeon is at the lateral aspect of the arm and uses a medial arthroscopic portal, the surgeon should change positions and sit at the medial aspect of the arm. This will greatly aid in orientation and maneuvering within the elbow joint (Fig. 43.19).

As with establishment of the anterolateral arthroscopic portal, the elbow should be flexed 90 degrees at all times and maximum fluid distention should be maintained during establishment of the anteromedial arthroscopic portal. Lynch et al. (18) demonstrated that, when 35 to 40 mL fluid is injected into the elbow, the median nerve and brachial artery are displaced anteriorly by 10 and 8 mm, respectively, from the entering arthroscopic instruments.

Anteromedial Portal Anatomy

In establishing the anteromedial portal, the arthroscope enters through the tendinous portion of the pronator teres and penetrates the radial aspect of the flexor digitorum superficialis and medial capsule. This portal is anterior to the ulnar collateral ligament. As these muscles are penetrated, the median nerve is 1 cm lateral to the arthroscope, and the brachial artery is just lateral to the median nerve. The

brachial artery divides into the radial and ulnar arteries opposite the neck of the radius. The median nerve crosses the elbow joint in the antecubital fossa and passes beneath the bicipital aponeurosis and between the two heads of the pronator teres. As the arthroscope passes deeper and closer to the joint capsule, it passes within 6 mm of the median nerve and brachial artery in a nondistended elbow. If 35 to 40 mL of fluid is injected within the elbow, the median nerve and brachial artery are displaced respectively 10 and 8 mm anteriorly from the entering arthroscopic instruments.

Arthroscopic Anatomy of the Anteromedial Portal

The capitellum and radial head are best seen from the anteromedial portal (Fig. 43.20). Examination of the radial head is facilitated by pronating and supinating the forearm. Approximately three fourths of the radial head can be seen with the use of this technique (Fig. 43.21). At times the annular ligament can be seen coursing across the radial neck (Fig. 43.22). If the arthroscope is slowly retracted and directed toward the ulna, the coronoid process will also be visible. Flexion and extension of the elbow allows visualization of most of the anterior surface of the capitellum.

Posterolateral Portal

Arthroscopic evaluation of the elbow is not complete until the posterior structures have been visualized. The posterolateral portal is established approximately 3 cm proximal to the tip of the olecranon, just proximal and posterior to the lateral humeral epicondyle, along the lateral epicondylar ridge near the lateral border of the triceps muscle (Fig. 43.23). This portal is established with the elbow in 20 to 30 degrees of flexion. Extension of the elbow relaxes the poste-

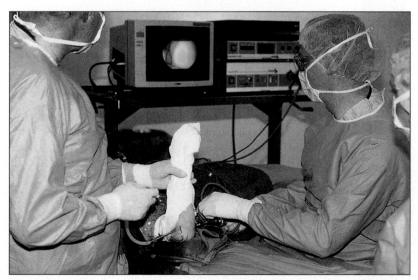

FIGURE 43.19 When using the arthroscope in the anteromedial portal, it is helpful for the surgeon to sit at the medial aspect of the arm.

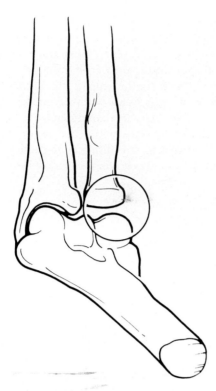

FIGURE 43.20 The capitellum and radial head are best seen from the anteromedial portal. Examination of the radial head is facilitated by pronation and supination of the forearm.

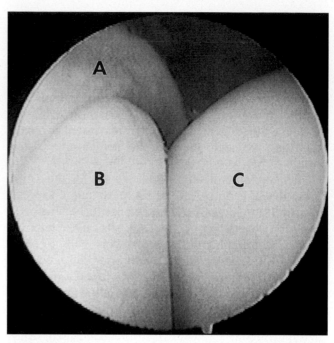

FIGURE 43.22 Anteromedial view of the annular ligament: **(A)**, radial head **(B)**, and capitellum **(C)** in a right elbow.

rior soft tissues and enlarges the space available for arthroscopy of the posterior compartment (Fig. 43.24). An 18-gauge spinal needle is placed through the previously marked posterolateral portal site and directed toward the olecranon fossa. If the joint has already been distended with fluid from the anteromedial or anterolateral portal, a capsular bulge can often be felt over the posterolateral elbow and

used to identify the insertion site for the needle. Once free backflow is visualized, the skin is sharply incised with a knife. The blunt trocar and then the arthroscope are placed.

If pathology is present in the posterior compartment of the elbow, there may be significant synovitis; visualization is sometimes obscured and can be quite difficult when the arthroscope is initially inserted into the posterior compart-

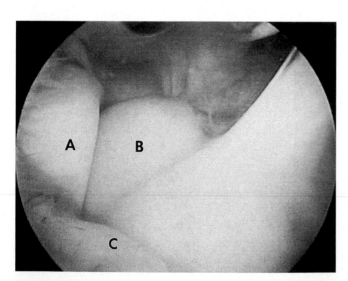

FIGURE 43.21 Arthroscopic anatomy as viewed from anteromedial portal: radial head **(A)**, capitellum **(B)**, and coronoid process of ulna **(C)**.

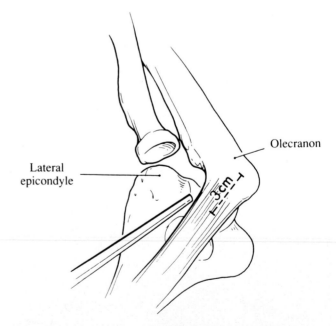

FIGURE 43.23 The posterolateral portal is located approximately 3 cm proximal to the olecranon tip just superior and posterior to the lateral border of the triceps muscle.

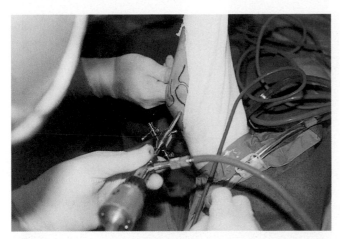

FIGURE 43.24 Extension of the elbow facilitates visualization of the posterior aspect of the elbow.

ment. At times, in order to visualize the posterior compartment properly, it is necessary to make an adjacent straight posterior portal and place a motorized instrument to shave the synovial tissues away from the tip of the arthroscope. A spinal needle is placed through the triceps muscle approximately 2 cm medial to the posterolateral portal, and once the tip of the needle is visualized arthroscopically it is kept in sight at all times. With the spinal needle still in place, the surgeon makes the skin incision and places the blunt trocar, and then the shaver, while keeping the needle in view at all times. At this time, synovial tissue or adhesions that are obscuring visualization are carefully debrided, keeping the tip of the shaver in view at all times and taking care not to injure the end of the arthroscope.

The posterior antebrachial cutaneous nerve, which courses over the posterolateral aspect of the distal humerus and the lateral brachial cutaneous nerve, is to be avoided in the establishment of the posterolateral portal (Fig. 43.8). The ulnar nerve is fairly well protected when this portal is used; it lies approximately 2.5 cm medial to the center of the elbow joint (6).

Whereas the anteromedial and anterolateral portals are primarily used to view the anterior aspects of the elbow, the posterolateral portal is used to complete the full evaluation of this joint, because loose bodies or osteophytes may be located in the olecranon fossa and the posterior aspect of the capitellum. If pathology is expected in the posterior compartment of the elbow, some prefer to establish the posterolateral portal first. Fluid extravasation during the procedure can make this compartment difficult to visualize if the anteromedial and anterolateral portals have been established first and fluid has extravasated around the posterior portal, causing subcutaneous extravasation and closing off the capsular space posteriorly.

With the arthroscope already in the lateral portal, one can occasionally follow the trochlear ridge from distal to

proximal until the posterolateral aspect of the olecranon tip is in view (46).

Posterolateral Portal Anatomy

The posterior antebrachial cutaneous nerve, which courses over the posterolateral distal humerus, and the lateral brachial cutaneous nerve, which is the terminal branch of the axillary nerve, are to be avoided when establishing this portal (Fig. 43.8). The trocar pierces the triceps musculature and then the posterolateral elbow capsule. Care must be taken to avoid the ulnar nerve, which lies approximately 2.5 cm medial to the center of the elbow joint.

Arthroscopic Anatomy of the Posterolateral Portal

Structures that can be seen from this portal are the olecranon fossa, located over the posterior aspect of the distal humerus, and the tip of the olecranon (Fig. 43.25). Flexion and extension of the elbow will help delineate the various portions of the distal humerus (Fig. 43.26).

Accessory Portals

When pathology is encountered that is not amenable to the arthroscopic portals mentioned so far, two accessory portals—the mid-lateral portal and the straight posterior portal—may be used.

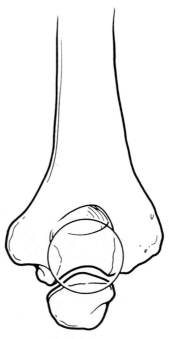

FIGURE 43.25 Structures that may be visualized from the posterolateral portal include the olecranon fossa, the distal humerus, and the tip of the olecranon.

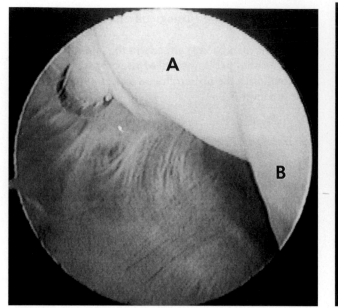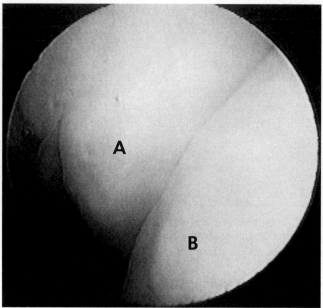

FIGURE 43.26 A: Example of area visualized arthroscopically in the posterolateral portal, showing the distal posterior humerus (A) and the tip of the olecranon (B). **B:** Another example of visualization from the posterolateral portal, demonstrating the distal humerus (A) and the tip of the olecranon (B).

Midlateral or "Soft Spot" Portal

The midlateral portal is located in the triangular area bordered by the lateral humeral epicondyle, the radial head, and the olecranon (Fig. 43.27). Through this portal, the trocar system passes through the anconeus muscle and the posterior capsule, the same area in which the 18-gauge spinal needle is inserted for initial distention of the elbow joint. This portal may be established without direct visualization by the use of an 18-gauge spinal needle and the sharp and blunt trocar system. When establishing this portal, the posterior ante-

brachial cutaneous nerve should be avoided. Occasionally a small, 2.7-mm arthroscope is placed through this portal; it has the advantage of being smaller in this tight area of the elbow joint. Alternatively, the 4-mm arthroscope may be used.

The radial–ulnar joint and the inferior surface of the radial head can be seen through the straight lateral portal (Fig. 43.28). In addition, the undersurface of the capitellum can be followed posteriorly. At times the arthroscope will slip directly into the posterior compartment providing a view of this area as well.

Straight Posterior (Transtriceps) Portal

The straight posterior or transtriceps portal is located approximately 2 cm medial to the posterolateral portal and directly traverses the triceps tendon (Fig. 43.29). The elbow is flexed 20 to 30 degrees. This portal is established by placing the 18-gauge spinal needle through the area under direct visualization. With the arthroscope in the posterolateral portal, the skin over the needle is incised in the direction of the triceps fibers. The straight posterior portal is the "working" portal posteriorly; it is useful for removing loose bodies from the posterior aspect of the elbow and for the occasional resection of an impinging olecranon osteophyte (14).

POSTOPERATIVE ROUTINE

At the completion of the arthroscopic procedure, thorough irrigation of the joint can improve the postoperative recov-

FIGURE 43.27 Structures visualized through the straight lateral portal include the radial–ulnar joint and the inferior surface of the radial head.

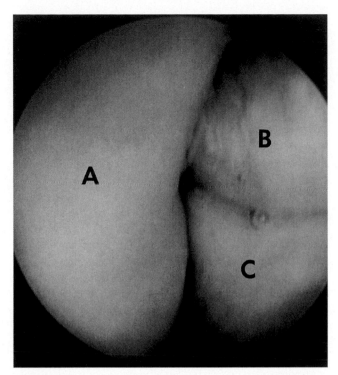

FIGURE 43.28 Arthroscopic view from the straight lateral portal in a right elbow. Structures that can be seen in this small space include the humerus **(A)**, the radial head **(B)**, and the ulna **(C)**.

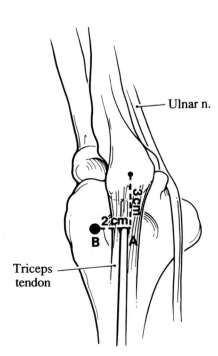

FIGURE 43.29 The straight posterior or transtriceps portal **(A)** is located 2 cm medial to the standard posterolateral portal **(B)** and passes directly through the triceps tendon.

ery. Irrigation is particularly important with debridement of adhesions or of articular surfaces. This step is often neglected because of the belief that the joint has been sufficiently irrigated during the operative procedure. With all of the instruments in place, the elbow cannot be flexed and extended completely; however, larger material can be removed from an open cannula system than from one that has an arthroscope in place. Therefore, at the end of the surgical procedure, one inflow cannula is left in place, the elbow is completely flexed and extended several times, and irrigation and suction are alternated to remove any debris. The arthroscopic portals may be closed with suture material or left open, depending on the preference of the surgeon and the amount of subcutaneous swelling. The use of local anesthetics for postoperative pain control should usually be avoided, because they may leak out of the capsular holes and cause a temporary nerve block (1,26) that would interfere with the immediate postoperative neurovascular assessment. At times a drain may be placed through the anterior or posterior portals if extensive debridement has been performed. Soft dressings are applied to the elbow, and in most cases immobilization is not required. Active range of motion of the elbow is initiated as soon as pain and swelling permit. Strengthening exercises are initiated after sufficient range of motion is achieved and when pain and swelling permit.

COMPLICATIONS

The complications of elbow arthroscopy are similar to those encountered with any arthroscopic procedure, such as infection, problems associated with the use of a tourniquet, instrument breakage, iatrogenic scuffing of articular surfaces, and neurovascular complications. Infection is infrequent with elbow arthroscopy because of the large amount of fluid passed through the joint during the surgical procedure and the small size of the incisions required for arthroscopic instrumentation.

More serious neurovascular complications, however, have been reported. In a series of 21 elbow arthroscopies, Lynch et al. (18) reported one transient low radial nerve palsy, a transient low median nerve palsy, and formation of a neuroma of the medial antebrachial cutaneous nerve. It was believed that the transient low radial nerve palsy was a result of overdistention of the joint, and the condition resolved in 8 hours. The transient low median nerve palsy was believed to be secondary to the use of a local anesthetic agent. The neuroma of the medial antebrachial cutaneous nerve ultimately required resection.

Casscells (16) described a case of irreparable damage to the ulnar nerve during abrasion arthroplasty of the elbow. Thomas et al. (21) described a radial nerve injury, and Papilion et al. (19) described compression neuropathy of the radial nerve during elbow arthroscopy. Guhl (7) reported one injury to the sensory branch of the radial nerve in a series of 45 patients, and Morrey (26) reported a transient radial nerve palsy secondary to fluid extravasation. In a series of 24 arthroscopies reported by Andrews and Carson (1), one patient experienced a transient median nerve palsy; this was believed to be secondary to leakage of local anesthetic from the capsule that caused a temporary nerve block.

In a survey of members of the Arthroscopy Association of North America, 395,556 surgical arthroscopic procedures were evaluated. Of these, 569 were elbow arthroscopies. The respondents were performing an average of 0.74 elbow arthroscopies per month and had been performing surgical elbow arthroscopy an average of 3.9 years. Of this entire group, only one reported a neurovascular complication, a radial nerve injury (34). I am also aware of undocumented cases of compartment syndrome of the forearm, complete transection of the median nerve, and complete transection of the radial nerve secondary to elbow arthroscopy.

To summarize, injuries to the subcutaneous or deeper nerves about the elbow have been reported, with the injuries occurring secondary to either actual surgical transection or possibly fluid extravasation during the surgical procedure or the use of a tourniquet. The other consideration is traction or blunt trauma to the various nerves about the elbow. Injury to the brachial artery has not been reported; it appears to be somewhat protected because it lies directly toward the middle of the joint and is lateral to the median nerve when the lateral portal is established. It appears that the radial nerve is most at risk during arthroscopy of the elbow.

INITIAL ARTHROSCOPIC PORTAL: MEDIAL VERSUS LATERAL

The anterolateral portal has been described as a portal to be established first in performing arthroscopy of the elbow (1,4,15). This anterolateral portal is approximately 3 cm distal and 1 to 2 cm anterior to the lateral humeral epicondyle and enters the elbow just anterior and proximal to the radial head. The proximal lateral portal, located 1 to 2 cm proximal to the lateral epicondyle, has become more popular because of greater safety (50,51).

More recent interest, however, has been shown in the use of the prone approach in combination with the proximal medial (43,47) or medial (44) arthroscopic portal as the initial arthroscopic portal to be established. Poehling et al. (43), Lindenfeld (44), and others who advocate a medial approach as the initial arthroscopic approach have demonstrated that the distance between the median nerve and the medial arthroscopic instruments is increased, compared with the minimal distance between the lateral arthroscopic instruments and the radial nerve in establishment of the lateral portals. Lindenfeld (44) inserted polyurethane foam to distend the elbow capsule in six cadaver specimens. The foam was allowed to harden, the specimens were dissected with the medial and lateral portals established, and the proximity of the neurovascular structures to the portals was established. It was found that the lateral portal, established 3 cm distal and 1 to 2 cm anterior to the lateral humeral epicondyle, extended on average to within 2.8 mm of the radial nerve. In contrast, the medial portal (1 cm proximal and 1 cm anterior to the medial humeral epicondyle) extended on average to within 22 mm to the median nerve. The ulnar nerve was 25 mm from the medial portal.

Verhaar et al. (22) performed cadaveric dissections of five specimens with plastic rods in place through the anteromedial and anterolateral portals. These dissections were performed without elbow distention. It was seen that in establishment of the anterolateral portal the radial nerve was on average 17 mm from the entering instruments, and the deep branch of the radial nerve was 7 mm away. In establishment of the anteromedial portal, the median nerve was on average 18 mm from the arthroscopic instruments, the brachial artery was 26 mm away, and the ulnar nerve was always at least 26 mm away. Lynch et al. (18) performed dissections of nondistended and distended elbows and found that in the anterolateral portal the radial nerve was on average 4 mm away from the elbow when the elbow was nondistended, but this distance increased to 11 mm with elbow distention. In establishment of the anteromedial portal, they found that the median nerve was 3 to 10 mm from the instruments; the distance increased to 14 mm with distention. Andrews and Carson (1), in dissections of nondistended elbows, found that the radial nerve was approximately 7 mm from the arthroscopic instruments in the anterolateral portal and the median nerve was approximately 6 mm from the arthroscopic instruments in establishment of the anteromedial portal.

Therefore, with regard to nerve injury, it appears from these cadaveric dissections that the margin of safety is greater during establishment of the medial portals than during establishment of the lateral portals. Advocates of the proximal medial portals believe that there is less risk to neurovascular structures, not only because of the greater distance between the instruments and the neurovascular structures, but also because the instruments enter parallel to the neurovascular structures as they progress toward the elbow joint, resulting in less chance of injury. With the standard anteromedial or anterolateral portals, the entering instruments approach at an angle of 60 to 90 degrees to the neurovascular structures, and in theory this would appear to place these structures at more risk.

In the clinical setting, however, the proximal lateral, anterolateral, anteromedial, and medial portals all appear to be relatively safe, provided one adheres to a strict and detailed surgical technique. The medial epicondyle is more rounded than the ridge-shaped lateral epicondyle and possibly provides a more distinct landmark (44). In establishing the anterolateral portal, it is important to remember that the "3 cm distal and 1 to 2 cm anterior" distance is *approximate* and changes slightly in each elbow. The instruments should enter just anterior and proximal to the radial head, which is easily palpated by pronation and supination of the forearm.

SUMMARY

Arthroscopy of the elbow is a technically demanding surgical procedure, and careful attention to detail is essential to performing a safe and reproducible arthroscopic examination. It is important that the skin be properly marked before initiation of the surgical procedure to maintain proper orientation at all times. Also, the use of an 18-gauge spinal needle as a precursor to the larger arthroscopic instruments is recommended. The elbow should be kept flexed at 90 degrees and maximally distended with fluid to relax the neurovascular structures and to move these structures away from the arthroscopic instruments. Complications may be avoided by adhering to a strict surgical technique.

REFERENCES

1. Andrews JR, Carson WG. Arthroscopy of the elbow. *Arthroscopy* 1985;1:97–107.
2. Andrews JR, Carson WG. Arthroscopy of the elbow. In: McGinty JB, ed. *Techniques in orthopaedics: arthroscopic surgery update.* Rockville, MD: Aspen Systems, 1985:283–290.
3. Carson WG. Arthroscopy of the elbow. In: Zarins B, Andrews J, Carson WG, eds. *Injuries to the throwing arm.* Philadelphia: WB Saunders, 1985:221–227.
4. Carson WG. Arthroscopy of the elbow. *Instr Course Lect* 1988; 37:195–201.
5. Carson WG. Arthroscopy of the elbow. In: Torg J, Welsh RP, eds. *Current therapy in sports medicine.* Philadelphia: BC Decker, 1988:426–430.
6. Carson WG, Meyers JF. Diagnostic arthroscopy of the elbow: surgical technique and arthroscopic portal anatomy. In McGinty JB, ed. *Operative arthroscopy.* New York: Raven Press, 1991: 583–594.
7. Guhl JF. Arthroscopy and arthroscopic surgery of the elbow. *Orthopaedics* 1985;8:290–296.
8. Johnson LL. Elbow arthroscopy. In: *Arthroscopic surgery: principles and practice.* St. Louis: Mosby, 1981:390–399.
9. Schonholtz GJ. *Arthroscopic surgery of the shoulder, elbow and ankle.* Springfield, IL: Charles C Thomas, 1986:73–78.
10. Woods GW. Elbow arthroscopy. *Clin Sports Med* 1987;6:557.
11. Reddy AS, Kvitne RS, Yocum LA, et al. Arthroscopy of the elbow: a long-term clinical review. *Arthroscopy* 2000;16:588–594.
12. Ogilvie-Harris DJ, Schemitsch E. Arthroscopy of the elbow for removal of loose bodies. *Arthroscopy* 1993;9:5–8.
13. Redden JF, Stanley D. Arthroscopic fenestration of the olecranon fossa in the treatment of osteoarthritis of the elbow. *Arthroscopy* 1993;9:14–16.
14. Andrews JR, St Pierre RK, Carson WG. Arthroscopy of the elbow. *Clin Sports Med* 1986;5:653–662.
15. Carson WG. Complications of elbow arthroscopy. In: Minkoff J, Sherman O, eds. *Arthroscopic surgery.* Baltimore: Williams & Wilkins, 1988:166–179.
16. Casscells SW. Neurovascular anatomy and elbow arthroscopy: inherent risks [Editor's comment]. *Arthroscopy* 1986;2:190.
17. DeLee JC. Complications of arthroscopy and arthroscopic surgery: results of a national survey. *Arthroscopy* 1985;1:214–220.
18. Lynch GJ, Meyers JF, Whipple TL, et al. Neurovascular anatomy and elbow arthroscopy: inherent risks. *Arthroscopy* 1986;2: 191–197.
19. Papilion JD, Neff RS, Shall LM. Compression neuropathy of the radial nerve as a complication of elbow arthroscopy: a case report and review of the literature. *Arthroscopy* 1988;4:284–286.
20. Small NC. Complications of arthroscopy: on knee and other joints. *Arthroscopy* 1986;2:253–258.
21. Thomas MA, Fast A, Shapiro D. Radial nerve damage as a complication of elbow arthroscopy. *Clin Orthop* 1987;214:130–131.
22. Verhaar J, VanMameren H, Brandsma A. Risks of neurovascular injury in elbow arthroscopy: starting anteromedially or anterolaterally? *Arthroscopy* 1991;7:287–290.
23. Kelly E, O'Driscoll S, Morrey BF. Complications after elbow arthroscopy. *J Bone Joint Surg Am* 2000;82.
24. Ruch DS, Poehling GG. Anterior interosseous nerve injury following elbow arthroscopy. *Arthroscopy* 1997:13:756–758.
25. Smith JB. Safe and effective arthroscopic evaluation and treatment of the elbow. *Arthroscopy* 1989;5:238–241.
26. Morrey BF. Arthroscopy of the elbow. *Instr Course Lect* 1986:35:102.
27. O'Driscoll SW, Morrey BF, Au KN. Intraarticular pressure and capacity of the elbow. *Arthroscopy* 1990;6:100–103.
28. Cohen B, Constant CR. Extension-supination sign in prearthroscopic elbow distension. *Arthroscopy* 1992;8:189–290.
29. O'Driscoll SW, Morrey BF. Arthroscopy of the elbow. *J Bone Joint Surg Am* 1992;74:84–94.
30. Tedder JL, Andrews JR. Elbow arthroscopy. *Orthop Rev* 1992;21:1047–1053.
31. Marshall PD, Faircloth JA, Johnson SR, et al. Avoiding nerve damage during elbow arthroscopy. *J Bone Joint Surg Br* 1993;75: 129–131.
32. Meyers JF. Elbow arthroscopy. In: Shahriaree H, ed. *O'Connor's textbook of arthroscopic surgery.* Philadelphia: JB Lippincott, 1992:641–648.
33. Burman MS. Arthroscopy or the direct visualization of joints. *J Bone Joint Surg* 1931;12:669–695.
34. Watanabe M. Arthroscopy of small joint [Japanese]. *J Jpn Orthop Assoc* 1971;45:908.
35. Ito K. The arthroscopic anatomy of the elbow joint [Japanese]. *Arthroscopy* 1979:4:2–9.
36. Ito K. Arthroscopy of the elbow: a cadaver study [Japanese]. *Arthroscopy* 1980:5:9–22.
37. Maeda Y. Arthroscopy of the elbow joint [Japanese]. *Arthroscopy* 1980:5:5–8.
38. Ito K. Arthroscopy of the elbow joint. *Arthroscopy* 1981;6:15–24.
39. Hempfling H. Die endoskopisch Untersuching des Ellenbogen gelenkesvom dorso-radialen Zugang. *Z Orthop* 1983;121:331.
40. Eriksson E, Denti M. Diagnostic and operative arthroscopy of the shoulder and elbow joint. *Ital J Sports Traumatol* 1985:7:165–188.
41. Boe S. Arthroscopy of the elbow: diagnosis and extraction of loose bodies. *Acta Orthop Scand* 1986;57:52–53.
42. Johnson LL. Elbow arthroscopy. In: *Arthroscopic surgery: principles and practices.* St. Louis: Mosby, 1986:1446–1477.
43. Poehling GG, Whipple TL, Sisco L, et al. Elbow arthroscopy: a new technique. *Arthroscopy* 1989;5:222–224.
44. Lindenfeld TN. Medial approach to elbow arthroscopy. *Am J Sports Med* 1990;18:412–417.

45. Ito K. Arthroscopy of the elbow joint. In: Watanabe M, ed. *Arthroscopy of small joints.* New York: Igaku-Shoin, 1985:57–84.

46. Andrews JR, Craven WM. Lesions of posterior compartment of the elbow. *Clin Sports Med* 1991;10:637–652.

47. Baker CL. Shalvoy RM. The prone position for elbow arthroscopy. *Clin Sports Med* 1991;10:623–628.

48. Ruch DS, Poehling GG. Arthroscopic treatment of Fanner's disease. *Clin Sports Med* 1991;10:629–636.

49. O'Driscoll SW. Elbow arthroscopy for loose bodies. *Orthopedics* 1992;15:855–859.

50. Field LD, Altchek DW, Warren RF, et al. Arthroscopic anatomy of the lateral portal: a comparison of three portals. *Arthroscopy* 1994;10:602–607.

51. Strothers K, Day B, Regan WR. Arthroscopy of the elbow: anatomy, portal sites, and a description of the proximal lateral portal. *Arthroscopy* 1995:11:449–457.

44

NORMAL ARTHROSCOPIC ANATOMY OF THE ELBOW: PRONE TECHNIQUE

CHAMP L. BAKER, JR.

ADVANTAGES OF THE PRONE POSITION

As the therapeutic use of the arthroscope grows, adequate visualization of and access to the posterior compartment of the elbow becomes increasingly important. Although the standard patient positions for elbow arthroscopy remain supine, decubitus, or prone, there are distinct advantages to placing the patient in either the lateral decubitus or the prone position. For the purpose of the discussion here, it can be assumed that having the patient in the lateral decubitus position and using an arm holder gives the surgeon approximately the same advantages as having the patient in the prone position. Placing the patient in the prone position facilitates access and offers several advantages over the supine position. First, no traction is required, because the weight of the arm over a bolster or commercial holder allows gravity to aid in joint distraction. Second, the arm position is stable during insertion of the arthroscope or instruments, making the procedure technically easier. When the arm is suspended with the patient supine, there is a tendency for the arm to swing to and fro like a pendulum, making entry into the joint more difficult. Third, gravity coupled with fluid distention pushes the anterior neurovascular structures further from the capsule and thus further from the operative instruments. Fourth, when necessary, conversion from the arthroscopic to an open procedure, using either a lateral or a medial exposure, is easier from the prone position. Fifth, the elbow can be fully extended, if necessary. Flexion is limited to 110 to 120 degrees by the positioning of the bolster.

The main advantage of elbow arthroscopy with the patient prone, however, is the improved visualization of the posterior compartment. Better access to the posterior compartment facilitates treatment of impingement caused by posteriorly located bony osteophytes, as sometimes occurs in throwing athletes; removal of loose bodies from the pos-

terior compartment; and the treatment of ankylosis of the elbow—particularly when lack of extension is a major component. Another advantage of the prone position is that the surgeon can either stand or sit and still look down onto the elbow, operating from a position of equal or greater height. When the patient is positioned supine, visualization of the posterior compartment necessitates suspending the elbow above the surgeon. This requires the surgeon to operate at or above shoulder level, or in an "uphill" direction. Not only is this technically demanding, but leakage of fluid from the elbow can make arthroscopy awkward and untidy.

OPERATING ROOM AND SETUP

Prone Position Setup

Surgery can be performed using a local or regional block or a general anesthetic. The advantage of using a general anesthetic is that an accurate postoperative neurovascular assessment can be made. If a block has been used, the postoperative evaluation may be inconclusive. The patient is then intubated and turned onto his or her chest. Chest bolsters are used to keep the torso elevated and the airway free. The involved arm is brought to the edge of the operating table with the forearm hanging free, and the elbow is flexed to 90 degrees. A towel, foam bolster, or commercial arm holder is used to keep the shoulder adducted to 90 degrees and the elbow stable (Fig. 44.1). Care is taken to prevent hyperextension of the arm.

The tourniquet, which may be incorporated into the commercial arm holder, is applied before the arm is prepared and draped. The surgeon flexes and extends the patient's elbow to make sure that it is clear of the table and can be mobilized during surgery. Depending on whether the surgeon prefers to stand or sit, the table can be raised or lowered. Viewing the elbow from this perspective is not unlike viewing the knee (Fig. 44.2). With the patient in this position, the elbow is stable and the surgeon can establish the various portals.

Next, the bony landmarks of the elbow—the medial and lateral epicondyles, the olecranon, and the radial head—and

C. L. Baker, Jr.: The Hughston Clinic, Columbus, Georgia, and Department of Orthopaedic Surgery, Tulane University School of Medicine, New Orleans, Louisiana.

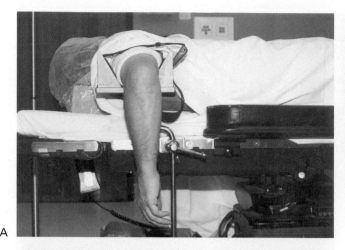

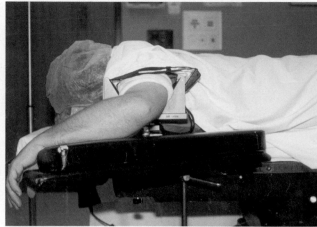

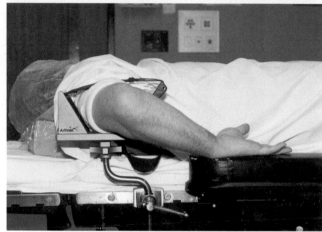

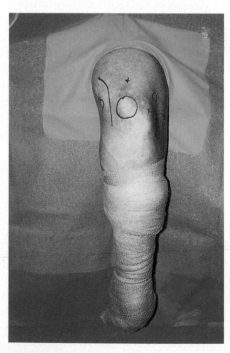

FIGURE 44.1 The patient is positioned prone. **A:** A commercial arm holder is used to position the shoulder at 90 degrees of adduction and the elbow in 90 degrees of flexion. This position allows access to both lateral **(B)** and medial **(C)** aspects of the elbow, as well as the anterior and posterior compartments of the joint, and, if necessary, it makes conversion to an open procedure possible.

FIGURE 44.2 With the patient positioned prone, the elbow is stable and the surgeon has easy access to all portal sites.

the position of the ulnar nerve are outlined (Fig. 44.3). If a tourniquet is used, the hand and forearm are exsanguinated at this time and the tourniquet is inflated. Initially, the arthroscopic technique is the same as with the patient in the supine position. The joint is distended with fluid introduced through an 18-gauge needle in the direct lateral portal (Fig. 44.4). As the fluid enters, the triceps often seems to lift off the humerus as the posterior compartment is filled. When the stylus is removed from the needle, backflow of fluid ensures that the joint is distended. Usually, the maximum joint capacity is 20 to 30 mL. The contracted arthrofibrotic joint may hold as little as 0 to 10 mL, and a pathologic joint (e.g., in a patient with rheumatoid arthritis) may hold more than 40 mL. Care must be taken in rheumatoid or tissue-compromised patients not to overdistend the joint and cause fluid to leak into the soft tissues. Doing so would compromise the injured joint and could potentially cause compartment problems.

Lateral Decubitus Position Setup

There are times when, whether because of the surgeon's preference, the medical situation, or the need to perform a

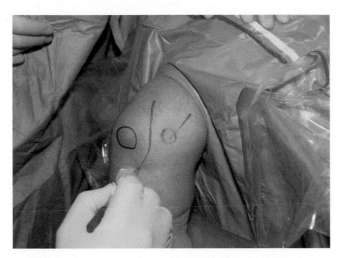

FIGURE 44.3 The bony anatomic landmarks and the course of the ulnar nerve are outlined with a marking pen before the procedure begins.

concomitant procedure, the patient is best positioned in the lateral decubitus position. After intubation or block is established, the patient is positioned and the affected arm is placed over a bolster or a commercial arm holder. The advantage of the lateral decubitus position is that it allows the patient to be awake for the procedure. If a concomitant shoulder procedure is being done, it can be accomplished without changing the patient's position. After the patient is positioned and draped, the operative technique is the same as if the patient were prone.

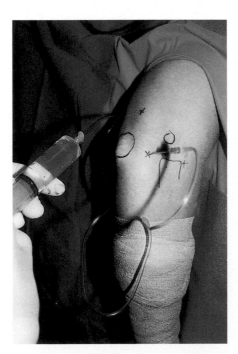

FIGURE 44.4 Joint distention through the direct lateral portal. Before the arthroscope is inserted into a portal, the joint should be maximally distended with saline solution. A 50-mL syringe connected to an 18-gauge spinal needle is used.

Conversion to an Open Procedure

As stated earlier, one advantage of the prone position is the easy conversion from an arthroscopic to an open procedure using a medial, lateral, or straight posterior approach. No changes to the setup are needed for a straight posterior approach, which can be done through a midline or midlateral incision. At the time of positioning the patient, a small arm holder is positioned next to the operating table. If a lateral open incision is planned, it is placed near the patient's head. If a medial incision is planned, the placement is inferior (Fig. 44.5).

After the arthroscopic portion has been completed, the bolster is pushed away from the table under the drapes, the arm is externally rotated, and the hand is placed on the arm holder. This creates a stable position for any open procedure. If the procedure is directly medially, the bolster is brought inferiorly away from the table. The arm is then internally rotated and the dorsum of the hand is placed on the holder. This position is particularly helpful if the combined procedure involves arthroscopy and concomitant ulnar nerve exploration and transfer.

ARTHROSCOPIC TECHNIQUE

After the extremity has been prepared and draped, the landmarks identified, the limb exsanguinated, and the tourniquet inflated (if one is used), the joint is distended through the lateral portal. I prefer the proximal medial portal for the initial viewing portal. Using my fingertip to locate the medial epicondyle, I palpate the intermuscular septum. I make a small nick in the skin proximal to my fingertip and use a hemostat to spread the subcutaneous tissues (Fig. 44.6). Either a 2.7-mm or a 4.0-mm arthroscope can be used, according to the surgeon's preference. The trocar and cannula are inserted through the skin and maintained anterior to the

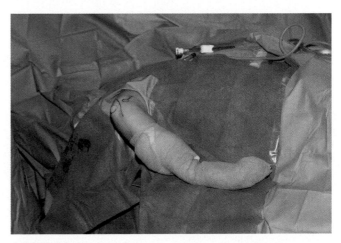

FIGURE 44.5 Conversion to an open procedure from an arthroscopic procedure. The hand is placed on the holder for stability. A medial incision is planned.

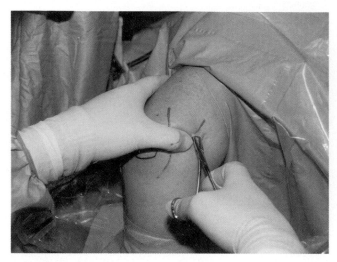

FIGURE 44.6 The "nick and spread" technique is used to create the proximal medial arthroscopic portal.

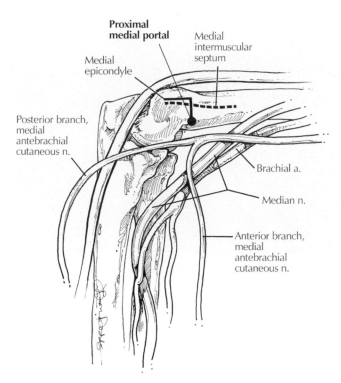

FIGURE 44.7 The proximal medial portal is established 2 cm proximal to the medial epicondyle and immediately anterior to the intermuscular septum.

intermuscular septum; they follow along the anterior aspect of the humerus, aiming toward the center of the joint. When the joint is entered, there is often a visual "give" of the arthroscope and backflow of fluid is noted, ensuring that the instrument is safely inside the joint. The trocar is removed, and the arthroscope is then placed through the sheath.

ARTHROSCOPIC PORTALS

With the patient in the prone position, the two portals most commonly used for viewing and instrumentation are the proximal medial and the proximal lateral portals. The mid-lateral portal, also known as the "soft spot" portal, is commonly used to distend the joint initially and as a viewing or operative portal for disorders of the posterior compartment. If other portals are needed to access the posterior compartment, the posterolateral and straight posterior portals can be established.

Proximal Medial Portal

In the first description of elbow arthroscopy with the patient prone, Poehling et al. (1) described a proximal medial portal located 2 cm proximal to the medial epicondyle and anterior to the intermuscular septum (Fig. 44.7). Savoie and Field called this portal the proximal anteromedial portal (2). It has become the primary viewing portal for elbow arthroscopy with the patient in either the prone or the lateral decubitus position. Lindenfeld (3) later described a similar approach, calling it the superomedial portal, and locating it 1 cm proximal and 1 cm anterior to the center of the medial epicondyle

The ulnar nerve rests 4 cm from this portal site and is out of harm's way. A caveat regarding this portal concerns the

ulnar nerve. If there has been previous surgery on the medial aspect of the elbow, the patient's history must be obtained to determine whether the nerve was superficially or transcutaneously moved. Also, the presence of a subluxating ulnar nerve must be appreciated, and the nerve must remain reduced at the time of joint entry. If the ulnar nerve has been transferred previously, the surgeon can reopen a portion of the existing incision (Fig. 44.8), identify the position of the

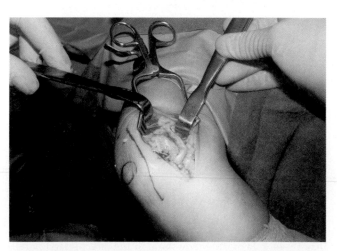

FIGURE 44.8 In a patient who has had an ulnar nerve transfer, the surgeon can open a portion of the previous incision to determine the position of the nerve before establishing the portal.

nerve, and, under direct visualization, establish the proximal medial portal away from the nerve.

Other structures at risk from this portal are the medial antebrachial cutaneous nerve, the median nerve, and the brachial artery. The proximal medial portal is the safest medial portal, because it is farther from the median nerve than other portals.

I use the proximal medial portal as the initial viewing portal (4–6). Its location is approximately one fingerbreadth proximal to the medial epicondyle and 1 to 2 cm anterior to the intermuscular septum. Variations are made depending on the patient's size, and a different angle of entry may be needed to have a clear arthroscopic field.

With the joint distended, the median nerve lies an average of 2 cm from the portal and the brachial artery is approximately 2.2 cm from the portal (see Fig. 44-7). The posterior branch of the medial antebrachial cutaneous nerve is the sensory nerve at greatest risk, and it is protected after skin incision.

After the joint has been distended, a no. 11 knife is used to make a small incision in the skin at the site of the proximal medial portal. The soft tissues are spread down to the level of the fascia with a hemostat to protect the cutaneous nerves in this area. The ulnar nerve lies posterior to the intermuscular septum and is protected as long as the trocar enters anterior to the septum.

To establish the proximal medial portal, the trocar penetrates the proximal portion of the flexor muscle mass and enters the joint capsule near the brachialis. As the trocar is introduced, the surgeon feels a pop as the distended joint is entered, and, as the trocar is removed, fluid backflow ensures that the joint has been entered.

Proximal Lateral Portal

Called the proximal anterolateral portal by Savoie and Field (2), the proximal lateral portal is located 2 cm proximal to the lateral epicondyle and roughly 1 cm anterior to the lateral epicondyle and the lateral intermuscular septum (Fig. 44.9). Stothers et al. (7,8) described the proximal lateral portal as the safest lateral viewing and instrumentation portal. They compared it with the anterolateral portal described by Andrews and Carson (9), which is 3 cm distal and 1 cm anterior to the lateral epicondyle. The portal described by Stothers et al. is more proximal. With the elbow in extension, the portal is an average of 4.8 mm away from the radial nerve, compared with 1.4 mm for the more distally located anterolateral portal of Andrews and Carson. With the elbow in flexion, the portal is an average of 9.9 mm from the nerve. This fact emphasizes the importance of maintaining elbow flexion during elbow arthroscopy. The anterolateral portal described by Andrews and Carson has been largely abandoned in favor of the proximal lateral portal or the portal that is described as a straight lateral portal.

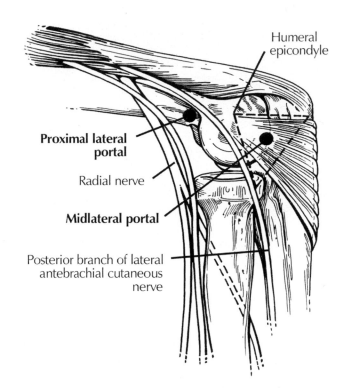

FIGURE 44.9 The proximal lateral portal is established 2 cm proximal and 1 cm anterior to the lateral epicondyle. The midlateral (soft spot) portal is located in the center of a triangle formed by the lateral epicondyle, the radial head, and the olecranon tip.

Midlateral Portal

A second commonly used operating portal when the patient is positioned prone is the midlateral, or soft spot, portal, which is a variation of the straight lateral. The portal is located in the center of a triangle formed by the radial head, the lateral humeral epicondyle, and the olecranon tip (2,9) (see Fig. 44-9), and it is the portal most often used for initial distention of the joint. Although it can be used with the patient supine to view the anterior chamber, it is most useful as a viewing and therapeutic portal for disorders in the posterior compartment. Extending the elbow as the trocar is introduced allows the trocar to penetrate the joint capsule through the soft spot (Fig. 44.10). With the elbow extended, the trocar and cannula are introduced and swept in a side-to-side manner. This maneuver clears a space in the bursa overlying the olecranon and removes any adhesions that may be present, clearing a space for distention. The arthroscope is then inserted. Next, a localizing needle is introduced into the posterior compartment through the posterocentral (straight posterior) or posterolateral portal. The midlateral and straight posterior portals can then be used alternately as diagnostic and operative portals.

Posterior Portals

The posterocentral, or straight posterior, portal is located midline through the triceps tendon, approximately 3 cm

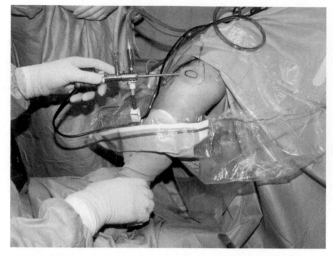

FIGURE 44.10 The surgeon extends the elbow while introducing the trocar through the soft spot portal.

proximal to the olecranon tip (Fig. 44.11). It enters directly through the triceps tendon, making it a safe portal. Care must be taken before arthroscopy to mark the course of the ulnar nerve to remind the surgeon of its location.

The second posterior portal is the posterolateral portal (see Fig. 44-11). It is also 3 cm proximal to the olecranon and is lateral to the straight posterior portal. The structures at risk, in addition to the triceps tendon, are the neurovascular structures, the posterior antebrachial cutaneous and lateral brachial cutaneous nerves.

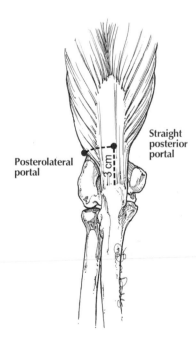

FIGURE 44.11 The straight posterior portal is established through the triceps tendon 3 cm proximal to the olecranon tip. The posterolateral portal is also 3 cm proximal to the olecranon tip and is lateral to the straight posterior portal.

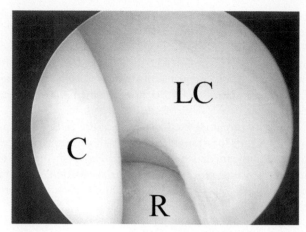

FIGURE 44.12 Viewing from the proximal medial portal. The radial head (R), capitellum (C), and lateral capsule (LC) can be seen.

ARTHROSCOPIC ANATOMY AND EXAMINATION

Intraarticular anatomy is best seen from the portal opposite the structure to be viewed. Therefore, the medial portal is best for observing the radial head and its articulation with the capitellum, and the lateral portals are best for viewing the coronoid process and the medial capsule. The lateral portals can be used to view the posterior articulation of the olecranon and the humerus and the articulation of the posterior portion of the capitellum and radial head.

When viewing from the medial portal, the surgeon can see the radial head and the radiocapitellar articulation on the anterolateral aspect of the elbow (Fig. 44.12). Because the forearm is free in the gravity-dependent, prone position, it can be pronated and supinated, allowing the surgeon to see almost three fourths of the surface of the radial head. With varus pressure on the forearm, the joint may be opened a little further, allowing more of the radial head's articular surface to be seen (Fig. 44.13). The annular ligament can be

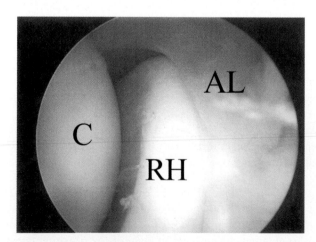

FIGURE 44.13 By placing varus pressure on the forearm, the surgeon can see the annular ligament (AL) and the articular surface of the radial head (RH). C, capitellum.

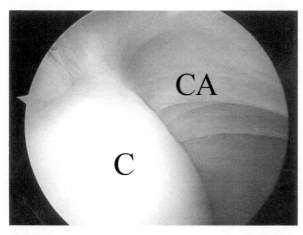

FIGURE 44.14 By pushing the arthroscope to the far side of the joint and rotating it, the surgeon can see the capitellum (C) and the capsular attachment (CA) from the proximal medial portal.

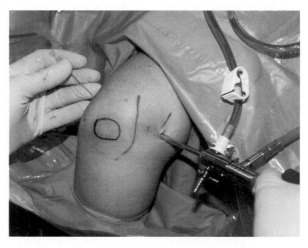

FIGURE 44.16 The outside-in technique is used to establish the proximal lateral portal.

seen coursing across the neck of the radius. If the arthroscope is pushed all the way across the joint and rotated, the undersurface of the capsule and the attachment of the extensor muscles to the lateral epicondyle are visible (Fig. 44.14). For example, if a patient has tendinosis of the extensor carpi radialis brevis, tears or ruptures of the capsule and underlying tendinous structures can be seen from the medial portal. The annular ligament is easily identified, and evidence of entrapment of the ligament or synovial proliferation can be seen.

As the arthroscope is retracted and rotated, most of the rest of the capitellum and the trochlea can be seen (Fig. 44.15), and, superiorly, the attachment of the capsule to the humerus is visible (see Fig. 44.14). The coronoid process articulation can be seen as the arthroscope is retracted farther, although it is seen best from a lateral portal. Evidence of a fracture or degenerative joint disease can be seen at this point in the examination.

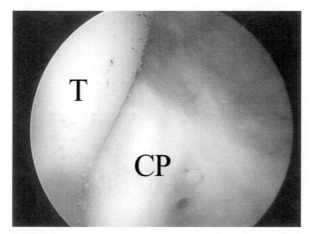

FIGURE 44.15 By rotating the arthroscope while retracting it from the proximal medial portal, the surgeon can visualize the trochlea (T) and coronoid process (CP).

When establishing the proximal lateral portal, I use the outside-in technique (Fig. 44.16), although the inside-out technique also can be used. With my fingertip, I palpate the distended lateral compartment to ensure placement of an 18-gauge needle directly opposite the joint. It is interesting to note that if needles are placed in the proximal lateral, the midlateral, and the anterolateral portals, they emerge approximately 1 cm from each other inside the joint (Fig. 44.17). My recommendation is that the more proximal the placement of the portal, the safer the portal. Next, the needle is removed, the skin is incised, and a hemostat is used to divide the tissues down to the joint. The cannula and trocar are brought into the joint. All cannulas used in elbow arthroscopy should be straight and without side holes, to avoid extravasation of fluid that could distend the soft tissue surrounding the joint and complicate the procedure.

Using a switching stick, I bring the arthroscope through the lateral portal to complete the diagnostic portion of the procedure (Fig. 44.18). When one is viewing through the anterolateral portal, the most obvious structure is the coronoid process and its articulation with the trochlea. Flexion and extension of the elbow allow the surgeon to inspect this articulation.

Studies have shown that arthroscopic visualization of the intact ulnar collateral ligament is not possible (10,11). The authors found that the bulk of the anterior bundle of the ligament could not be seen most of the time, and, when it could be seen, only a small portion (25%) was visible. The substance of the anterior bundle is parallel and in close proximity to the medial border of the trochlea, leaving no space for the arthroscope to assess the ligament if partial disruption is suspected. However, it can be viewed from across the joint by placing the elbow in 30 degrees of flexion. Gapping between the ulna and the trochlea suggests disruption of the ligament.

After examination of the anterior chamber is complete, I extend the patient's elbow to approximately 30 degrees, in-

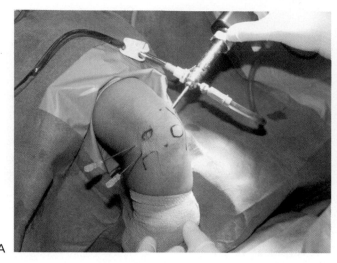

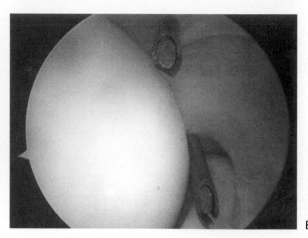

FIGURE 44.17 A: Needles are in the proximal lateral and anterolateral portals. **B:** Intraarticular view. The superior needle is in the proximal lateral portal, and the inferior needle is in the anterolateral portal.

sert the arthroscope into the midlateral portal, and establish the straight lateral portal. The midlateral portal is used to view the posterior compartment. The articulation of the olecranon with the humerus in the posteromedial compartment and the buildup of osteophytes, or spurs, in this area can be seen easily through this portal (Fig. 44.19).

The olecranon fossa must be thoroughly examined and palpated for any loose bodies and degenerative changes that could hinder elbow extension. The midlateral portal allows easy visualization of the posterior radiocapitellar joint to assess disorders, such as posterolateral instability, rotary instability, osteochondritis dissecans of the capitellum or radial head, posterior meniscoid lesions, and posterolateral synovial plicae. With the elbow flexed, I slowly withdraw the

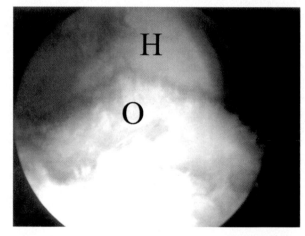

FIGURE 44.19 The midlateral portal is best for viewing the articulation of the humerus (H) and olecranon tip (O).

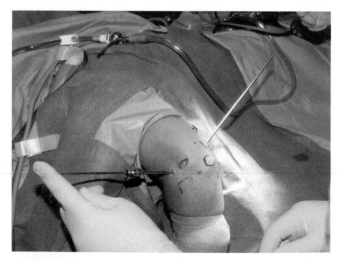

FIGURE 44.18 A switching stick is used to transfer the arthroscope to the lateral portal to complete the diagnostic portion of the arthroscopic procedure.

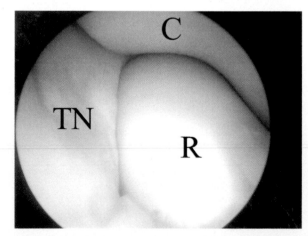

FIGURE 44.20 The capitellum (C), the posterior aspect of the radial head (R), and the trochlear notch (TN) can be evaluated with the arthroscope in the midlateral portal.

arthroscope and direct it inferiorly. As the arthroscope is retracted and turned inferiorly, the surgeon can see the entire articulation of the olecranon and the olecranon fossa. There is a small area of the trochlear notch of the ulna, the sigmoid notch, that is devoid of articular cartilage and is considered a normal finding. It should not be mistaken for arthritis or articular damage. Next, I rotate the arthroscope further and bring it inferiorly to the posterior aspect of the radiocapitellar joint and the posterior surface of the radial head (Fig. 44.20). This allows a secondary view of the articulation of the capitellum and the radial head posteriorly to look for articular damage and osteochondritis dissecans of the capitellum, synovial fringe, and plicae. It is also an excellent viewing and operating portal for any surgical procedure performed on the radial head, such as radial head excision.

SUMMARY

The prone position for elbow arthroscopy does have a few disadvantages. Its use necessitates general anesthesia to maintain a good airway, and if an open anterior approach were needed at the conclusion of the arthroscopic procedure, a change in the patient's position would be necessary. However, for most surgical indications, the prone patient position is ideal for elbow arthroscopy. In particular, the prone position is best for viewing and treating disorders of the posterior compartment, such as bony impingement or posterior compartment ankylosis, and for removing loose bodies. The proximal medial portal and the midlateral portals are used as diagnostic and therapeutic portals for the anterior and posterior compartments. With the patient prone,

arthroscopic visualization of the articulation of the radius and the capitellum, the coronoid and the trochlea, and, posteriorly, the olecranon and the humerus is improved. As experience grows with this patient position and these newer portals, elbow arthroscopy will become a safer, more predictable procedure.

REFERENCES

1. Poehling GG, Whipple TL, Sisco L, et al. Elbow arthroscopy: a new technique. *Arthroscopy* 1989;5:222–224.
2. Savoie FH III, Field LD. Portals in elbow arthroscopy. In: Morrey BF, ed. *The elbow and its disorders.* Philadelphia: WB Saunders, 2000:505–509.
3. Lindenfeld TN. Medial approach in elbow arthroscopy. *Am J Sports Med* 1990;18:413–417.
4. Baker CL, Brooks AA. Arthroscopy of the elbow. *Clin Sports Med* 1996;15:261–281.
5. Baker CL, Jones GL. Arthroscopy of the elbow. *Am J Sports Med* 1999;2:251–264.
6. Baker CL, Shalvoy RM. The prone position for elbow arthroscopy. *Clin Sports Med* 1991;10:623–628.
7. Stothers K, Day B, Regan W. Arthroscopic anatomy of the elbow: an anatomical study and description of a new portal. *Arthroscopy* 1993;9:362–363.
8. Stothers K, Day B, Regan WR. Arthroscopy of the elbow: anatomy, portal sites, and a description of the proximal lateral portal. *Arthroscopy* 1995;11:449–457.
9. Andrews JR, Carson WG. Arthroscopy of the elbow. *Arthroscopy* 1985;1:97–107.
10. Field LD, Callaway GH, O'Brien SJ, et al. Arthroscopic assessment of the medial collateral ligament complex of the elbow. *Am J Sports Med* 1995;23:396–400.
11. Timmerman LA, Andrews JR. Undersurface tear of the ulnar collateral ligament in baseball players: a newly recognized lesion. *Am J Sports Med* 1994;22:33–36.

ARTHROSCOPIC RADIAL HEAD RESECTION

CHAMP L. BAKER, JR.

Although arthroscopy has become an accepted means of treating many elbow disorders, use of the arthroscope to excise the radial head is a rather new procedure. Lo and King first described their results in the early 1990s (1). Other authors have shared their experiences with the procedure more recently (2–4). Although indications for the surgery may vary among surgeons, the traditional approach for excision of the radial head at this time requires a large arthrotomy with the use of a Kocher lateral approach. The procedure can be complicated by a difficult and lengthy rehabilitation with an increased instance of neurovascular complications. In contrast, arthroscopic radial head excision provides a straightforward means of identifying, assessing, and then resolving problems related to the radial head and its capitellar articulation, allowing for a quick and effective rehabilitation.

INDICATIONS

Acute Conditions

In the acute setting, the most common indication for excision of the radial head is a Mason type III (uncomplicated, comminuted, closed) radial head fracture (Fig. 45.1). Although long-term studies of open resection have been published (5,6), arthroscopic excision of acute radial head fractures is an expanded indication for elbow arthroscopy. The ease of the postoperative course, coupled with minimal surgical invasion, makes arthroscopic excision my preferred surgical treatment for comminuted Mason type III fractures.

An accurate diagnosis is very important for the surgeon who is considering excision of the radial head acutely. The radial head fracture must be an isolated finding. It should not be associated with a fracture–dislocation or with injury

C. L. Baker, Jr.: The Hughston Clinic, Columbus, Georgia, and Department of Orthopaedic Surgery, Tulane University School of Medicine, New Orleans, Louisiana.

to a ligamentous complex. If it is not an isolated injury, excision of the radial head, either arthroscopic or open, may be contraindicated and other treatment should be considered.

Chronic Conditions

The most common chronic conditions for which removal of the radial head is indicated are osteoarthritis with secondary ankylosis (Fig. 45.2), rheumatoid arthritis, posttraumatic radiocapitellar joint arthritis, and, in some instances, posttraumatic radiocapitellar degeneration related to chronic valgus instability. Field and Savoie (7) also list it as a treatment option in patients with chronic symptoms associated with osteochondritis dissecans of the capitellum after bone growth maturity has occurred.

In patients with degenerative joint disease, when the radial head is markedly malformed or is a block to extension or flexion, it can be removed in conjunction with capsular release and excision of loose bodies and spurs (Fig. 45.3). In a chronic condition that is the result of a fracture, the changes are usually related to loss of motion with both flexion–extension and pronation–supination. Arthroscopy affords the opportunity for joint evaluation and removal of loose bodies and cartilage flaps to determine whether the loss of motion is directly related to the radial head malformation.

CONTRAINDICATIONS

There are several relative contraindications for radial head excision in general, and for arthroscopic excision in particular. Obviously, a familiarity with elbow arthroscopy and arthroscopic anatomy is needed. If there is marked radial head deformity after a fracture, severe contracture and adherence of tissue to the radial head could place the radial nerve at risk, making it difficult to effect a safe excision. In other instances, the need to remove heterotopic bone, if present, would make a lateral arthrotomy preferable. As mentioned earlier, if associated instability is present, exci-

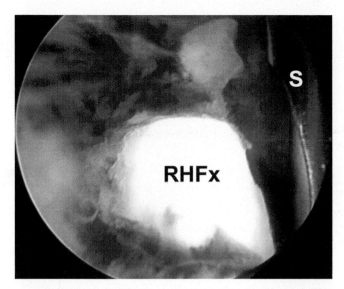

FIGURE 45.1 View of a comminuted radial head fracture from the proximal medial portal. RHFx, radial head fracture; S, shaver.

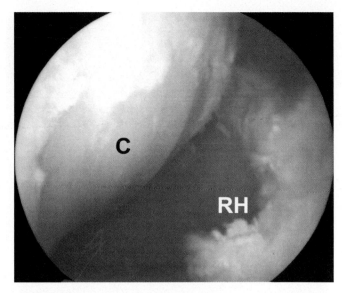

FIGURE 45.3 With the arthroscope in the proximal medial portal, grade IV degenerative joint disease of the radial head can be seen. On the articular surface of the capitellum, an area can be seen that is devoid of cartilage. C, capitellum; RH, radial head.

sion of the head, by either an arthroscopic or an open technique, may be contraindicated.

PHYSICAL EXAMINATION

Clinically, the most common objective finding in a patient who is a candidate for radial head excision is loss of motion. Patients usually experience a combination of pronation and supination loss and extension loss. The deformity of the radial head is rarely an isolated occurrence. Secondary degenerative changes are also involved in the loss of motion.

Symptoms usually consist of activity-related pain located over the lateral aspect of the elbow and radial head. Occa-

sionally, there is swelling that may lead to an inability to perform daily tasks. This inability is most often a result of the loss of motion—in particular, a loss of pronation and supination.

IMAGING STUDIES

Radiographs can be helpful in determining the cause of the problem. The presence of obvious degenerative changes, such as those seen in patients with rheumatoid arthritis, may or may not be helpful. However, anteroposterior, lateral, and specifically radial head radiographic views can determine the incongruity of the head (Fig. 45.4). Magnetic resonance imaging studies are not usually indicated, although computed tomograms can occasionally be helpful in differentiating between an acute or chronic radial head fracture and loose bodies in the joint.

SURGICAL TECHNIQUE

Arthroscopy is performed with the patient in the prone or the lateral decubitus position (Fig. 45.5). Chest bolsters are used to keep the torso elevated and the airway free. The involved arm is brought to the edge of the operating table with the forearm hanging free and the elbow flexed to 90 degrees. A towel, foam bolster, or commercial arm holder is used to keep the shoulder adducted to 90 degrees and the elbow stable. Care is taken to prevent hyperextension of the arm.

Portals used for arthroscopic radial head excision are the standard proximal medial, proximal lateral, and direct lat-

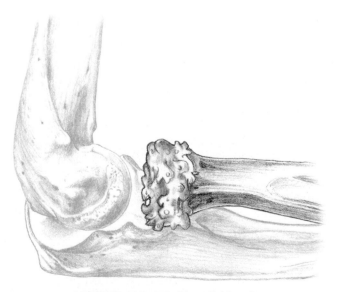

FIGURE 45.2 Arthritic radial head.

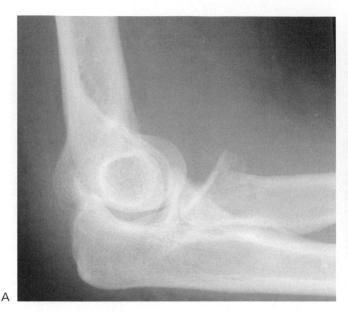
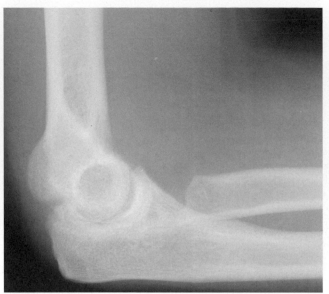

A   B

FIGURE 45.4 A: Preoperative lateral radiographic view shows a comminuted Mason type III radial head fracture. **B:** Postoperative lateral radiographic view after arthroscopic radial head excision.

eral or "soft spot" portals. As described in Chapter 44, the proximal medial portal is located a fingerbreadth above the medial epicondyle and 1 to 2 cm anterior to the intermuscular septum. The proximal lateral portal is 2 cm proximal to the lateral epicondyle, and the midlateral portal is established in the so-called soft spot, the triangular area formed by the radial head, the olecranon, and the lateral epicondyle.

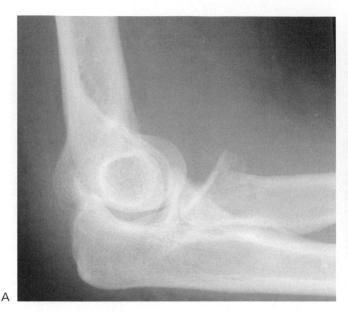

FIGURE 45.5 The patient is positioned prone for elbow arthroscopy. A commercial arm holder is used to keep the elbow stable.

The proximal medial portal is used initially for viewing the anterior aspect of the joint and, in particular, for viewing across the radiocapitellar joint. The proximal lateral portal is used initially for instrumentation for the synovectomy and finally for removal of the radial head. The posterolateral portal is used to examine the posterior compartment and to complete the removal of the radial head.

If a tourniquet is used, the landmarks are identified and marked before it is inflated. Next, the joint is distended with 20 to 30 mL of fluid through an 18-gauge needle inserted in the lateral soft spot. A markedly constricted joint with degenerative changes may hold less fluid for distention than a normal joint does.

I establish the proximal medial portal with a nick in the skin and use a hemostat to spread the tissue, to prevent injury to the medial and antebrachial cutaneous nerves. The cannula and trocar are then inserted into the joint.

Initial examination of the joint reveals the articulation of the radial head with the capitellum. I observe the radiocapitellar joint for loose bodies, malformation of the radial head and associated involvement of the coronoid, or articular changes. If the anterior portion of the capsule has adhered to the distal proximal humerus, it can be visualized and identified at this time.

The proximal lateral portal is established next, using either an inside-out or an outside-in technique. Initially, I use a radial resector to perform an anterior synovectomy, and I remove loose bodies with a basket grasper or a Schlesinger clamp. If the procedure is performed in conjunction with a synovectomy in a patient with rheumatoid arthritis, the complete anterior synovectomy is performed first. The articulation between the radial head and capitellum can be

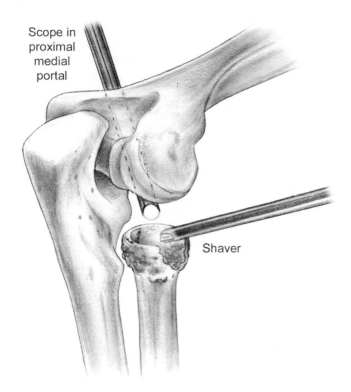

FIGURE 45.6 With the arthroscope in the proximal medial portal, the radial head is resected by a shaver introduced through the proximal lateral portal.

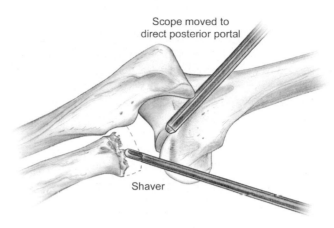

FIGURE 45.7 To complete the resection, the arthroscope is moved to the direct posterior portal and the shaver is moved to the midlateral portal.

viewed easily at this time. Initially, an ablater inserted through the lateral portal can be used to remove the cartilage from this portion of the head. Next, a burr or shaver can be used to remove the proximal anterior two-thirds or three-quarters of the radial head, including all of the remaining articular cartilage (Fig. 45.6). Usually, 2 to 3 mm of the head and neck is removed. Great care should be taken to keep the annular ligament intact. The patient's arm can be easily pronated and supinated to allow for adequate evaluation and access to the head.

Next, I move the arthroscope to the direct posterior portal and insert a trocar and cannula into the midlateral portal (Fig. 45.7). Using this portal places the shaver at the most posterior aspect of the radial head. The remainder of the excision can be accomplished with medial and lateral sweeps of the shaver, using a "cutting block" technique (Fig. 45.8). Resection is complete when I can see no impingement with full pronation and supination or with flexion and extension of the arm. Again, great care is taken not to dissect distal to the annular ligament, because of concern for injury to the radial nerve, which may be adherent or scarred to the capsule.

Excision of the radial head often is done in preparation for debridement and removal of osteophytes. After the head is excised, the arthroscope is inserted through the posterolateral or posterocentral portal to evaluate the adequacy of the excision. In patients with persistent loss of motion, the surgeon can then look through the direct lateral portal and bring a shaver through the posterocentral portal to clean out

the olecranon fossa and remove any osteophytes. If the excision is done in conjunction with a complete cleanout, the ulnohumeral arthroplasty may be done at this time.

Portals are closed with simple sutures. A dressing and a sling or splint is applied at the time of discharge. The radial head excision is usually done on an outpatient basis, and the patient usually returns for follow-up in 2 to 3 days. Use of the sling is discontinued, and the patient begins an aggressive active and passive therapy program, emphasizing range of motion and strength. Return to light duty at work is allowed within 2 to 3 weeks.

Complications

As with most arthroscopic procedures, the most serious potential complication of arthroscopic radial head resection is

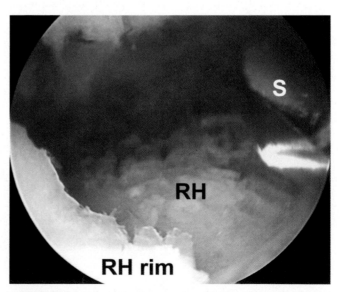

FIGURE 45.8. With medial and lateral sweeps of the shaver, the procedure is completed. RH rim, radial head rim; RH, radial head; S, shaver.

injury to neurovascular structures. The risk of injury to the radial nerve is heightened with a malunited fracture and severe deformity. Often, capsular contracture occurs in these patients, and the anterior capsule adheres to the radial head and tethers the nerve. In this instance, an injury could be caused by soft tissue release and excision of the radial head. If there is marked scarring or deformity, the procedure should be done through an open incision.

Other possible complications include inadequate excision of the radial head or osteophytes and problems related to instability. In the acutely injured patient, inadequate removal of the radial head can result in heterotopic ossification of the radial head and arthrofibrosis. Instability can occur if preoperative evaluation did not disclose concomitant ligamentous injury.

SUMMARY

Few results of arthroscopic radial head excision have been published (1,7,8). Field and Savoie (7) recently reviewed their results in 37 patients who had undergone the procedure: The outcome was successful in 34. One failure was caused by continued loss of motion and pain despite radiographic evidence of adequate excision. Another was caused by significant wrist pain and loss of motion after excision, which ultimately required a radial head replacement for radioulnar instability. The third unsuccessful result was in a patient who had arthrofibrosis and instability that returned after the surgery.

Kim et al. (8) and Lo and King (1) each reported their results with the procedure in a single patient and suggested that decrease in postoperative pain and stiffness and rapid recovery are the potential advantages of this treatment method.

In summary, arthroscopic excision of the radial head has several distinct advantages over the open procedure. Secondary procedures, such as synovectomy and removal of loose bodies and osteophytes, can be accomplished easily at the same time without an extensive arthrotomy. Arthroscopic treatment minimizes postoperative arthrofibrosis and loss of motion, allowing the patient to recover more quickly and to regain range of motion and strength sooner. The arthroscopic technique is straightforward but demands a competent arthroscopist who is experienced in elbow arthroscopy. The procedure demands great attention to detail. As for any arthroscopic procedure, the surgeon should be concerned with risk to the neurovascular structures. If there is doubt about the safety of these structures, the procedure should be avoided and converted to a lateral arthrotomy.

REFERENCES

1. Lo IKY, King GJW. Arthroscopic radial head excision. *Arthroscopy* 1994;10:689–692.
2. Poehling GG, Troum SJ, Ruch DS. Arthroscopic radial head resection. In: Chow JCY, ed. *Advanced Arthroscopy.* New York: Springer Verlag, 2000;189–191.
3. Savoie FH, Nunley PD, Field LD. Arthroscopic management of the arthritic elbow: indications, technique, and results. *J Shoulder Elbow Surg* 1999;8:214–219.
4. Menth-Chiari WA, Poehling GG, Ruch. Arthroscopic resection of the radial head. *Arthroscopy* 1999;15:226–230.
5. Coleman DA, Blair WF, Shurr D. Resection of the radial head for fracture of the radial head. Long-term follow-up of seventeen cases. *J Bone Joint Surg Am* 1987;69:385–392.
6. Janssen RPA, Vegter J. Resection of the radial head after Mason type-III fractures of the elbow. *J Bone Joint Surg Br* 1998;80: 231–233.
7. Field LD, Savoie FH. Arthroscopic radial head resection. In: Baker CL, ed. *Operative treatment of elbow disorders.* New York: Springer Verlag, 2001;185–194.
8. Kim SJ, Kim HK, Lee JW. Arthroscopy for limitation of motion of the elbow. *Arthroscopy* 1995;11:680–683.

ELBOW ARTHROSCOPY IN THE THROWING ATHLETE

E. LYLE CAIN, JR.
JAMES R. ANDREWS

Recent advances in arthroscopic equipment and surgical techniques have allowed the expansion of indications for elbow arthroscopy. With careful technique, elbow arthroscopy allows the surgeon to avoid the large capsular incisions and postoperative scarring often seen with arthrotomy. By placing small portal incisions, the surgeon can view the entire joint space with minimal risk of complications. The consequent reduction in operative trauma and wound healing concerns allows for a much more aggressive postoperative rehabilitation regimen with early return to activity.

The close proximity of neurovascular structures to portal sites makes elbow arthroscopy more technically demanding than knee or shoulder arthroscopy. A thorough understanding of anatomic relationships of neurovascular structures about the elbow is essential to avoid potential complications in elbow arthroscopy.

The throwing elbow is subjected to high forces as the arm proceeds through the late cocking and acceleration phases of the throwing motion. The combination of medial tensile stress, lateral compressive stress, and posterior shear force has been termed the "valgus extension overload syndrome" and forms the biomechanical basis of overuse injuries in the throwing elbow (1) (Fig. 46.1). This chapter presents our treatment approach to elbow arthroscopy for the various pathologic conditions seen in the overhead-throwing athlete.

INDICATIONS FOR ELBOW ARTHROSCOPY

Most injuries to the throwing elbow are a result of repetitive overuse stress to the elbow from valgus, extension, and shear stress during the throwing motion. Acute injuries to the elbow are uncommon in overhead athletes and most often represent an acute-on-chronic injury with underlying bony or soft tissue adaptive changes. Therefore, an adequate period of rest and rehabilitation is essential before any surgical intervention is considered in the throwing athlete. Injuries that seem acute may actually represent an acute exacerbation of a chronic condition, and these often respond to several weeks of cessation of throwing. We generally require throwing athletes complete a minimum of two periods of 6 weeks of rehabilitation (3 months total) before considering surgery. During this time of "active rest," the athlete works aggressively on shoulder and elbow rehabilitation exercises but avoids the throwing motion and similar movements associated with valgus stress (e.g., golf, tennis). However, this regimen may be altered somewhat by previous treatment, time of year, level of competition, and proximity of upcoming competitive events. Determining the appropriate timing of surgery often requires input not only from the patient and physician but also from parents, spouses, family, training staff, and coaches.

Elbow arthroscopy is indicated for the evaluation and treatment of various pathologic conditions of the elbow after failure of adequate conservative treatment. Common indications in the throwing elbow include excision of posteromedial olecranon osteophytes; evaluation of valgus instability, loose bodies, or osteochondritis desiccans (OCD) of the capitellum; and arthroscopic-assisted fixation of an olecranon stress fracture. Additional indications not covered in this chapter include radial head excision, lateral epicondylitis, management of arthrofibrosis, osteoarthritis, chronic synovitis, fracture evaluation and fixation, septic arthritis, synovial biopsy, and plica excision (2–7).

CONTRAINDICATIONS

Contraindications to elbow arthroscopy include infection, severe bony or fibrous ankylosis or deformity (congenital, arthritic, or posttraumatic), and any significant distortion of normal anatomy. Alterations in normal elbow bony anatomy or neurovascular relationships may be caused by trauma or surgical procedures and present challenges in portal placement. Previous elbow surgeries, particularly ulnar

E. L. Cain, Jr. and J. R. Andrews: American Sports Medicine Institute, Birmingham, Alabama

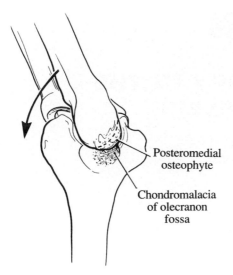

FIGURE 46.1 Valgus extension overload. (From McGinty JB. *Operative arthroscopy,* 2nd ed. Philadelphia: Lippincott-Raven, 1996:883, with permission.)

nerve transposition, may alter the preferred sites for placement of arthroscopic portal incisions or make certain portal placements (i.e., anteromedial) contraindicated.

IMAGING

Preoperative evaluation in the throwing athlete consists of a thorough throwing and injury history and physical examination, along with ancillary testing. Our standard plain radiographic series of the thrower's elbow includes anteroposterior, lateral, oblique, and axial views. Valgus stress views are obtained if injury to the ulnar collateral ligament (UCL) is suspected. Magnetic resonance imaging with intraarticular gadolinium contrast is helpful for diagnosis of associated pathology such as loose bodies or OCD of the capitellum and to rule out UCL injury (8). Computed tomography is not routinely performed but may be used to evaluate the size and extent of the olecranon osteophyte, to look for osteocartilaginous loose bodies, and to rule out an olecranon stress fracture. Intraarticular contrast-enhanced computed tomography may also be helpful to assist in the evaluation of the UCL (9). It is important to note that normal imaging studies do not rule out the presence of pathology in the throwing elbow. Olecranon osteophytes, small loose bodies, and subtle injury to the UCL may not be readily apparent on imaging studies, and the diagnostic acumen of the treating surgeon is required to reach the appropriate diagnosis.

ARTHROSCOPIC SURGICAL TECHNIQUE: SUPINE POSITION

Elbow arthroscopy has been described in the lateral decubitus, prone, or supine position (2,3,6,7). We prefer to place the patient supine with the arm suspended by an overhead traction device. Advantages of the supine position for elbow arthroscopy include ease of administering anesthesia given the accessibility of the patient's airway, simple conversion to open procedures (UCL reconstruction), and a more familiar reference position for anatomic structures in the elbow.

General anesthesia is most commonly used, although we have performed elbow arthroscopy with regional or local anesthesia. A tourniquet is routinely used and set at 250 mm Hg, and a pressure-sensitive arthroscopic pump is helpful to allow adequate visualization while preventing overdistention of the elbow. Overhead traction is applied to maintain the elbow at 90 degrees of flexion and neutral rotation with the shoulder at 90 degrees of abduction. The arm is suspended from the traction device with a Velcro gauntlet and elastic wrap. The patient's fingers remain exposed to ensure that the elastic wrap is not too tight (tourniquet effect). The room must be arranged to allow the surgeon to easily view both the arthroscopic video monitor and the pump pressure readings (Fig. 46.2). Overdistention or pressurization of the elbow is a common reason for complications and may be avoided by the surgeon's awareness and visualization of pump pressure readings.

A standard 4.0-mm arthroscope and 2.7-mm small joint arthroscope are routinely used. Initially, all bony landmarks and portal locations, as described by Andrews and Carson (2), are marked with a methylene blue pen and the elbow is injected with 30 mL of saline through the lateral soft spot (Fig. 46.3). A detailed knowledge of elbow anatomy is critical for proper portal placement and prevention of neurovascular complications (2). Marking of all bony and soft tissue landmarks before fluid distention helps the surgeon maintain a reference for safe distances between portals and critical anatomic structures. All portals should be established with the elbow flexed at 90 degrees and fully dis-

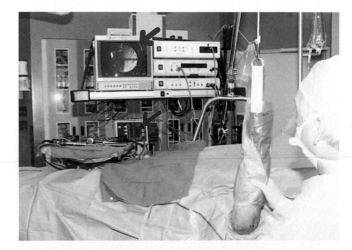

FIGURE 46.2 Supine position with the patient's arm in a traction device at neutral rotation, 90 degrees elbow flexion, and 90 degrees shoulder abduction. The surgeon should be able to view the video monitor as well as the arthroscopic pump pressure readings.

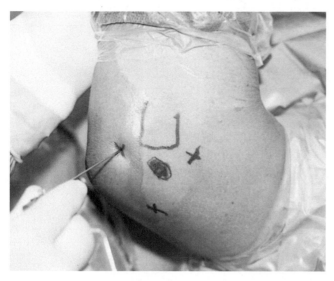

FIGURE 46.3 The lateral soft spot is injected with 30 mL of saline after marking all bony landmarks.

tended with fluid, because this has been demonstrated to increase the distance from neurovascular structures (10–12).

ARTHROSCOPIC TECHNIQUE FOR SPECIFIC LESIONS IN THROWERS

Olecranon Osteophyte Excision

Posterior elbow pain in the throwing athlete often requires surgical treatment. High valgus shear stress on the posteromedial olecranon tip and forced extension of the olecranon into the olecranon fossa during the throwing motion may result in posteromedial olecranon hypertrophy, osteophyte formation, chondral damage to the trochlea, and loose bodies. Osteophyte formation and degenerative changes in the posterior compartment may result in loss of motion and pain during overhead sporting activities, which limits effectiveness. As a result of these changes, olecranon osteophyte formation with valgus extension overload syndrome has been reported as the most common diagnosis requiring surgery in the throwing athlete (13). With careful attention to detail and meticulous surgical technique, arthroscopic management of posterior elbow impingement may be performed with minimal risk of complications.

Elbow arthroscopy is performed with the patient in the supine position, as described previously. Initially, the anterolateral portal is established by placement of an 18-gauge spinal needle to confirm fluid return, followed by careful skin incision with a no. 11-blade scalpel. A hemostat is used for blunt dissection to the anterolateral joint capsule before penetration of the capsule with a 4.0-mm blunt trocar and sheath (Fig. 46.4). Diagnostic arthroscopy of the anterior compartment is performed, and an anteromedial portal is established with the use of an 18-gauge spinal needle for

portal localization (Fig. 46.5). The anterior compartment is thoroughly evaluated for loose bodies; evidence of chondral damage to the coronoid process, capitellum, or radial head; and osteophyte formation in the coronoid fossa.

A lateral soft spot portal is then established for the 2.7-mm arthroscope at the site of initial elbow injection, the center of a triangle formed by the radial head, lateral epicondyle, and olecranon tip. A second lateral portal may be placed approximately 1 cm distal to the first lateral portal for instrumentation of the lateral compartment or removal of loose bodies (Fig. 46.6). Fluid inflow is through the 4.0-mm arthroscope in the anterolateral portal, and the posterior compartment is viewed with the 2.7-mm arthroscope in the lateral portal. A posterolateral portal is then established for placement of the 4.0-mm arthroscope for both visualization and fluid flow (Fig. 46.7).

The elbow is extended slightly by adding traction weight, until approximately 30 degrees of flexion is obtained, to increase the posterior working space. Manual axial distraction of the elbow by an assistant may also be used to facilitate viewing of the ulnohumeral joint. An accessory straight posterior portal is then established through the triceps tendon, with care taken to avoid the ulnar nerve within the cubital tunnel. It is important to keep the posterior portals as far apart as possible to allow triangulation in the posterior compartment working space. Optimal placement allows the two portals to meet at the working area (olecranon tip) at a 90-degree angle (Fig. 46.8).

A spinal needle is initially placed for proper localization of the straight posterior portal, after which an incision through the capsule is made with a no. 11 scalpel. Loose bodies from the posterior or lateral compartment often migrate to the anterior compartment or vice versa; therefore, all three compartments (anterior, posterior, and lateral) must be thoroughly inspected. With the arthroscope in the posterolateral portal, a shaver is introduced through the accessory (straight) posterior portal to debride synovitis and soft tissue from the olecranon tip and olecranon fossa, so that the entire bony margin of the olecranon tip can be visualized. Although subtle olecranon osteophytes may not be well visualized on radiographic evaluation, the margin of cartilage and bony hypertrophy is easily seen after adequate soft tissue debridement of the olecranon tip. The "kissing lesion," articular damage on the posteromedial trochlea, is also debrided. We address trochlear chondral injuries with debridement of all loose cartilage margins and abrasion chondroplasty to stimulate fibrocartilage repair.

The olecranon osteophyte is then excised with an osteotome and 5.5-mm acromionizer bur. Meticulous technique is required to avoid damage to the distal humerus articular surface with the osteotome. A small, sharp osteotome is used to complete the osteophyte removal along the articular surface. Each small piece of the bone is removed with a grasper as it is freed with the osteotome, with care taken to prevent the loss of small fragments of excised bone within

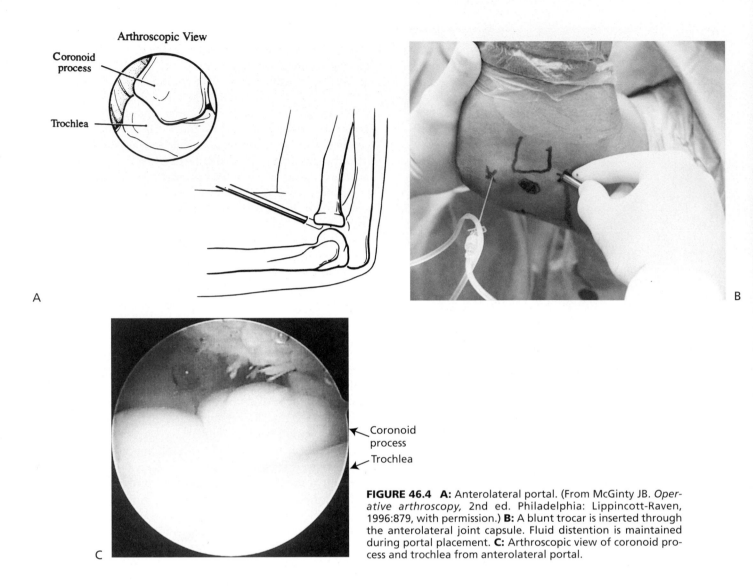

FIGURE 46.4 A: Anterolateral portal. (From McGinty JB. *Operative arthroscopy*, 2nd ed. Philadelphia: Lippincott-Raven, 1996:879, with permission.) **B:** A blunt trocar is inserted through the anterolateral joint capsule. Fluid distention is maintained during portal placement. **C:** Arthroscopic view of coronoid process and trochlea from anterolateral portal.

the elbow (Fig. 46.9). The amount of olecranon tip that can safely be excised without increasing the stress on the UCL is unknown. We remove only enough bone to begin to see into the articular space of the ulnohumeral joint and allow full elbow extension without bony impingement—approximately 3 to 5 mm.

A lateral radiograph is then performed intraoperatively to assess adequate bone removal and ensure that no bone debris remains in the soft tissues around the elbow (Fig. 46.10). A drain is placed into the elbow through the anterolateral portal, and the portals are closed with nylon suture. A compressive dressing is applied, and the arm is iced and elevated postoperatively.

Diagnosis of Valgus Instability

The diagnosis of medial elbow laxity with resultant valgus instability may be confirmed by elbow arthroscopy before UCL reconstruction. We currently perform elbow arthroscopy

with a single anterolateral portal if the diagnosis of UCL insufficiency is uncertain or if intraarticular pathology or loose bodies are suspected from preoperative diagnostic studies. We prefer open arthrotomy for excision of posteromedial olecranon osteophytes during UCL reconstruction. Surgical dissection during UCL reconstruction provides for simple evaluation of the posterior compartment through a small arthrotomy and prevents excessive fluid extravasation and surgical time needed to properly evaluate the posterior compartment arthroscopically.

After marking all bony landmarks, the elbow capsule is distended by injecting the lateral soft spot with 30 mL of saline, as previously described for elbow arthroscopy. An anterolateral arthroscopy portal is established by incising the skin and bluntly dissecting to the joint capsule, followed by penetration with a blunt trocar. The anterior compartment is evaluated for loose bodies, chondral lesions, synovitis or injury to the anterior band of the UCL, and medial capsular disruption. The anterior portion of the anterior band of

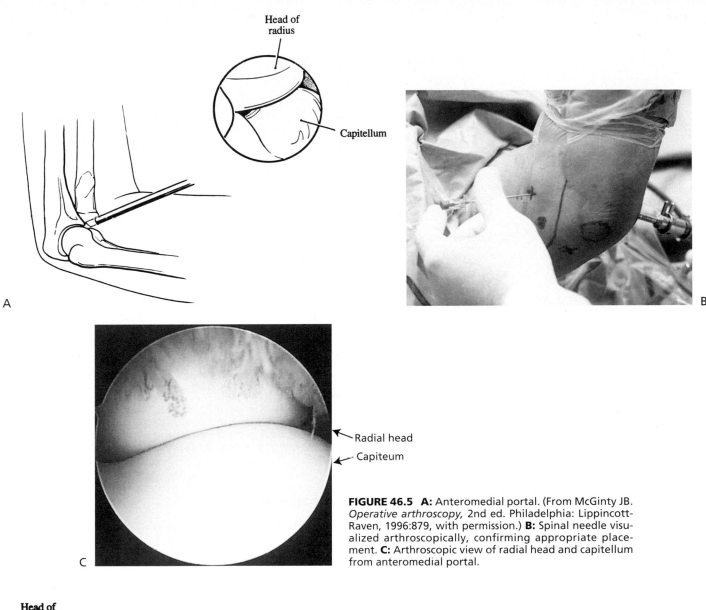

Head of
radius

Capitellum

A

B

Radial head
Capiteum

C

FIGURE 46.5 A: Anteromedial portal. (From McGinty JB. *Operative arthroscopy,* 2nd ed. Philadelphia: Lippincott-Raven, 1996:879, with permission.) **B:** Spinal needle visualized arthroscopically, confirming appropriate placement. **C:** Arthroscopic view of radial head and capitellum from anteromedial portal.

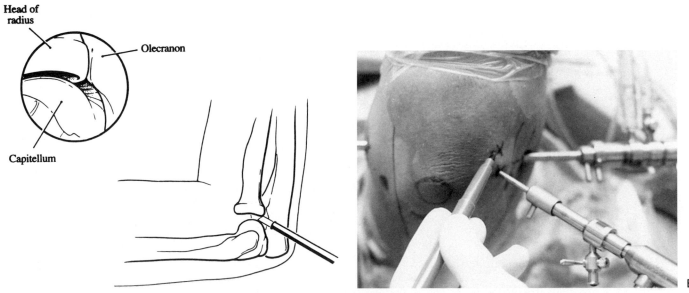

Head of
radius

Olecranon

Capitellum

A

B

FIGURE 46.6 A: Straight lateral portal. (From McGinty JB. *Operative arthroscopy,* 2nd ed., page 880, Figure 5A, with permission.) **B:** The portal is placed at the lateral soft spot. A second working portal may be placed 1 cm distal to the straight lateral portal (marking pen).

Olecranon

Olecranon fossa

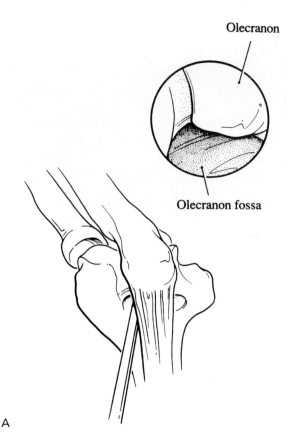

A

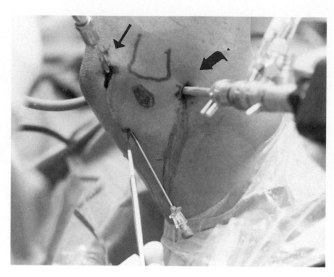

B

FIGURE 46.7 A: Posterolateral portal. (From McGinty JB. *Operative arthroscopy,* 2nd ed. Philadelphia: Lippincott-Raven, 1996:880, with permission.) **B:** The posterolateral portal is located by viewing a spinal needle from the straight lateral portal *(small arrow),* with fluid inflow through the anterolateral portal *(large arrow).*

the UCL may occasionally be viewed through the anterolateral portal (5,14). An assistant stabilizes the elbow at 70 degrees of flexion while the surgeon applies valgus stress. The opening between the coronoid process and trochlea is compared before and after the application of valgus stress. An increase of 1 to 2 mm has been reported to indicate UCL insufficiency (4) (Fig. 46.11).

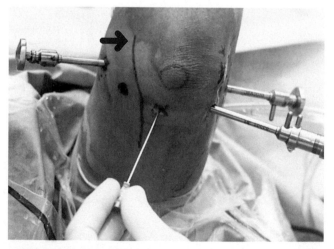

FIGURE 46.8 Accessory straight posterior portal. Placement should allow the two posterior portals to intersect at the working space at a 90-degree angle. Note the course of the ulnar nerve *(arrow).*

Loose Bodies

Loose fragments of cartilage, bone, or soft tissue are often present in the throwing elbow as a result of the overuse forces experienced during throwing. Osteochondral fragments most commonly originate from the lateral compartment due to compression stress at the radial head–capitellum articular surface, from OCD of the capitellum in the adolescent athlete, or from fractured olecranon osteophytes in the posterior compartment. Cartilaginous loose bodies may originate in any compartment as a result of excess shear stress, trauma, or synovial disease (e.g., synovial chondromatosis). Fibrous loose bodies may result from hypertrophic synovial villi or detached capsular adhesions.

Throwing athletes with loose bodies in the elbow commonly present with additional pathology, including UCL injury, olecranon osteophyte formation, and loss of motion with capsular contracture. Mechanical symptoms resulting from the loose bodies may be the cause for seeking medical attention but should trigger a thorough evaluation for additional lesions. Loose fragments should be removed to prevent third-body wear and potential chondral damage and joint destruction. However, the surgeon and patient must be aware that (a) usually, more loose bodies are present than initially suspected; (b) some loose bodies, or "joint mice," may "hide" during arthroscopy and not be visualized; and (c) additional loose bodies may be produced after complete removal owing to similar overuse stresses (recurrent loose bodies).

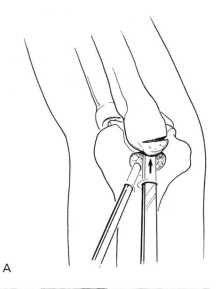

A

FIGURE 46.9 **A:** Olecranon osteophyte removal. (From McGinty JB. *Operative arthroscopy,* 2nd ed. Philadelphia: Lippincott-Raven, 1996:883, with permission.) **B:** An osteotome is used to carefully remove the olecranon tip. **C:** Arthroscopic view of osteotome against olecranon tip. **D:** Fragment removal. **E:** Arthroscopic view of final olecranon resection. Note the "kissing lesion" of the medial olecranon fossa *(arrow).*

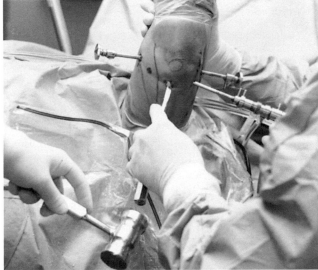

B

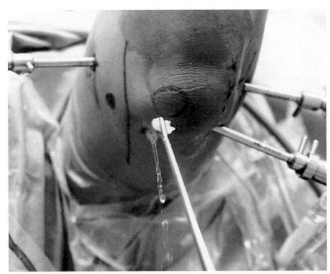

D

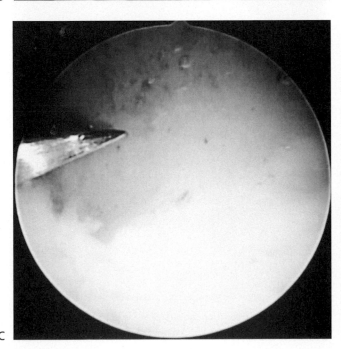

C

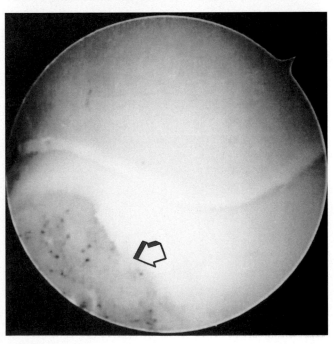

E

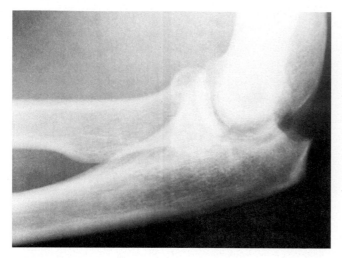

FIGURE 46.10 Postoperative lateral radiograph of the elbow showing olecranon resection.

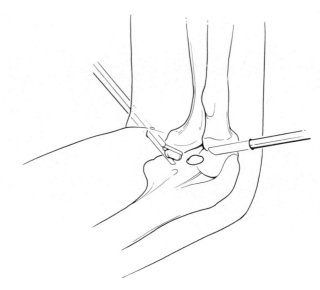

FIGURE 46.12 Removal of loose bodies from the anterior compartment. (From McGinty JB. *Operative arthroscopy.* 2nd ed. Philadelphia: Lippincott-Raven, 1996:881, with permission.)

The arthroscopic surgical approach for removal of loose bodies employs all arthroscopic portals described previously for osteophyte excision (Fig. 46.12). Because loose fragments can migrate into any portion of the elbow, a complete and thorough evaluation of the entire joint is essential. Anterior compartment evaluation must include the medial and lateral recesses. Loose bodies are often encapsulated or adherent to dense soft tissue. It is often necessary to debride hypertrophic synovium and soft tissue with a shaver to explore all potential sites of loose body entrapment, especially in the lateral (radiocapitellar) compartment. Posterior compartment evaluation should include probing of the olecra-

non fossa and the posteromedial and posterolateral recesses. Removal of a large loose body often requires extension of the capsular portal incision. Usually, this should be performed after the complete arthroscopic examination, to prevent loss of fluid distention or fluid extravasation into the soft tissues around the elbow. We generally prefer to remove anterior compartment loose fragments through the anterolateral portal because of the relatively thin lateral soft tissue envelope there, compared with the flexor muscle mass medially.

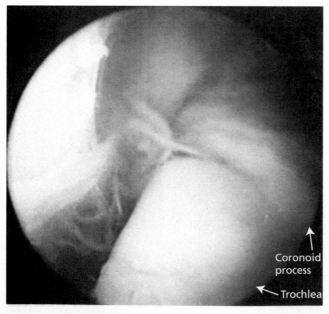

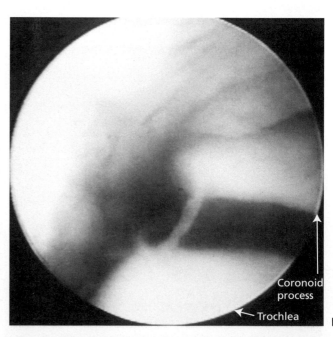

FIGURE 46.11 Arthroscopic valgus stress test: articulation between coronoid process and trochlea before **(A)** and after **(B)** application of valgus stress at 70 degrees of elbow flexion.

Osteochondritis Desiccans of the Capitellum

OCD of the capitellum with secondary degenerative changes in the radial head occurs in the adolescent throwing athlete as a result of compressive stress on the lateral compartment of the elbow with valgus torque. Compressive forces during the throwing motion are theorized to cause repetitive microtrauma to the vulnerable subchondral blood supply of the humeral capitellum, resulting in osteochondral injury, osteonecrosis, and loose bodies from the capitellum or radial head. Treatment recommendations vary based on the age of the patient, level of activity, size of the lesion, and extent of osteochondral stability. Options include rest with avoidance of throwing and surgical treatment with open or arthroscopic excision of loose bodies, capitellum debridement, or fragment fixation (15–20).

Overall, capitellar OCD in adolescents appears to be best managed conservatively unless loose bodies, mechanical symptoms, or failure of extended conservative treatment occurs. Arthroscopic debridement, loose body excision, and abrasion chondroplasty currently appear to offer the best results in terms of surgical morbidity and return of function. Fixation of loose capitellar osteochondral fragments has not been shown to offer any advantage over excision (21); however, new techniques using osteochondral plug transfer to the capitellum defect are currently being evaluated (22).

The arthroscopic treatment of OCD of the capitellum includes a thorough examination of the entire joint to search for loose bodies, as described earlier, with additional focus on the lateral compartment. The osteochondral lesion of the capitellum is best viewed through the straight lateral portal (Fig. 46.13). A second lateral portal is established for instrumentation and loose body removal. The size and stability of the osteochondral defect are assessed with a probe. Although drilling and fixation of OCD lesions of the capitellum has been described, we generally remove unstable fragments and perform limited abrasion chondroplasty to stimulate fibrocartilage filling of the defect. In our experience, simple excision of the fragmented portion of the capitellum with abrasion chondroplasty yields more consistent results than attempted fixation does (15). Complete examination of all elbow compartments is essential to search for additional loose fragments of capitellum or radial head.

Olecranon Stress Fracture

Olecranon stress fractures in throwing athletes may occur as a result of repetitive microtrauma due to olecranon impingement or excessive triceps tensile stress. Clinical findings often include posterolateral olecranon pain and tenderness during and after throwing. Early radiographs may be normal, and MRI, computed tomography, or bone scan findings are often diagnostic. Treatment initially begins with active rest, throwing cessation, and possibly bone growth stimulation. We have found that olecranon stress fractures in the competitive overhead athlete often fail extended conservative treatment and require surgical fixation, similar to stress fractures at the proximal diaphysis of the fifth metatarsal (Jones fracture). Therefore, we have been aggressive at performing early internal fixation of these lesions.

Standard elbow arthroscopy is performed as described for olecranon osteophyte debridement. This allows the surgeon to diagnose associated lesions, especially loose bodies, and to view the intraarticular portion of the olecranon stress fracture. The fracture displacement gap is usually best viewed through the posterolateral portal. Using fluoroscopy, a guide wire for a 6.5- or 7.3-mm titanium cannulated screw is placed down the intramedullary canal of the olecranon tip through a small posterior incision. The screw is placed after

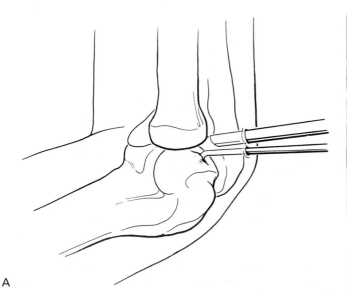

A

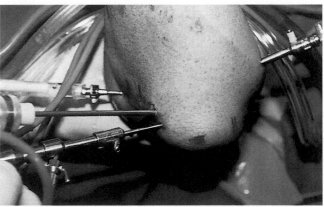

B

FIGURE 46.13 Arthroscopic evaluation of OCD of the capitellum. (From McGinty JB. *Operative arthroscopy,* 2nd ed Philadelphia: Lippincott-Raven, 1996:882, with permission.)

appropriate reaming, and fracture site compression is viewed arthroscopically. Placement is confirmed radiographically, and early postoperative motion is initiated.

COMPLICATIONS

Potential surgical complications including septic arthritis, arthrofibrosis, reflex sympathetic dystrophy, and thromboembolism appear to be less frequent in elbow arthroscopy than the published rates for shoulder and knee arthroscopy (23). Iatrogenic articular cartilage injury is probably more common than reported, owing to the limited working space in the elbow.

Injury to nearby neurovascular structures is the most common complication during elbow arthroscopy, with a prevalence ranging from zero to 14% in published reports (2,12,23–25). Complications may be the result of inexperience, poor technique, or failure to understand the relationship of portals to local anatomy. Distances of major neurovascular structures from portals have been well described (2,10,11,26). The anterolateral portal places the posterior antebrachial cutaneous nerve (2 mm), the lateral antebrachial cutaneous nerve (2 mm), and the radial (posterior interosseous) nerve (3 to 11 mm) at risk. The anteromedial portal is in close proximity to the medial antebrachial cutaneous nerve (1 mm), the median nerve (6–14 mm), and the brachial artery (17 mm), and the accessory straight posterior portal may be placed less than 10 mm from the ulnar nerve. Neurovascular injury may result from direct trauma during portal placement, instrumentation, aggressive fluid distention of the joint, tourniquet neuropraxia, or fluid extravasation and compartment syndrome. Extracapsular extravasation of local anesthetic used to infiltrate portal sites may also result in neurologic injury (2). Injury to the radial, median, medial antebrachial cutaneous, ulnar, and anterior interosseous nerves has been reported (2,11,12,23–25).

Attention to anatomic detail and surgical technique may prevent the most common complications in elbow arthroscopy. Fluid distention during portal placement has been well documented to increase the distance from neurovascular structures (10,11,24). When moving between portals, the surgeon should leave all cannulas in place to avoid repetitive puncture of the capsule and fluid extravasation. Constant monitoring of pump pressure and soft tissue swelling around the elbow is important during the entire procedure. If excessive fluid extravasation occurs, the arthroscope should be removed, the tourniquet released, and the arm wrapped from distal to proximal with an elastic bandage to dissipate fluid from the soft tissues. Formal fasciotomy for compartment syndrome is rarely necessary.

During evaluation of the posterior compartment for excision of an olecranon osteophyte, extreme caution must be used while debriding the medial olecranon tip. The ulnar nerve has been demonstrated to lie in direct contact with the posterior band of the UCL and posteromedial elbow capsule, making the ulnar nerve vulnerable to instrumentation in the posteromedial gutter (5,14). Complete transection of the ulnar nerve with a 1.5-cm defect requiring microsurgical repair has been reported after posteromedial debridement and capsular penetration (27).

RESULTS

Andrews and Timmerman (13) reported the results of elbow surgery in professional baseball players at the American Sports Medicine Institute (ASMI) over a 5-year period. Sixty-four patients underwent arthroscopic elbow procedures, with the most common procedure being debridement of posteromedial olecranon osteophytes (58%). Loose bodies were found in 16 patients (27%), although the authors noted surprisingly poor preoperative sensitivity of both plain radiographs (27%) and computed tomographic arthrography (59%) for the diagnosis of loose bodies. Seventy-three percent of the players were able to return to the same or a higher level of play; however, 19 (32%) required subsequent surgical procedures, including 41% of those initially treated with arthroscopic debridement of an olecranon osteophyte. The authors emphasized the palliative, rather than curative, nature of treatment elbow injuries in throwing athletes.

Baumgarten et al. (15) reported excellent results in a group of 17 patients treated with arthroscopic debridement and abrasion chondroplasty for capitellar OCD (15). In this group of patients with ages from 10 to 17 years, average extension increased by 14 degrees, flexion increased by 6 degrees, and 14 of 17 patients had returned their preinjury activity level at an average of 48 months' follow-up. No radiographic degenerative changes were noted, but slight residual flattening of the capitellum was seen on follow-up radiographs in 8 patients.

CONCLUSION

Elbow pain is a common problem in the throwing athlete due to adaptive bony and soft tissue changes that occur in response to the valgus extension overload syndrome. A thorough history and physical examination with appropriate ancillary diagnostic tests is required to correctly identify the cause of elbow pain. Arthroscopy is valuable in the treatment of common lesions, including posteromedial olecranon osteophytes, loose bodies, OCD of the capitellum, and olecranon stress fractures, and in the evaluation of valgus instability. With proper attention to anatomic landmarks for portal placement and meticulous surgical technique, arthroscopic evaluation and treatment of elbow pathology can be safely accomplished in the throwing athlete with a minimal risk of complications. However, the treatment of elbow pathology in the high-level athlete should be viewed as palliative, with a high rate of return to play but also a high rate of recurrence.

REFERENCES

1. Wilson FD, Andrews JR, Blackburn TA, et al. Valgus extension overload in the pitching elbow. *Am J Sports Med* 1983;11:83–88.
2. Andrews JR, Carson WG. Arthroscopy of the elbow. *Arthroscopy* 1985;1:97–107.
3. Day B. Elbow arthroscopy in the athlete. *Clin Sports Med* 1996;15:785–797.
4. Field LD, Altchek DW. Evaluation of the arthroscopic valgus instability test of the elbow. *Am J Sports Med* 1996;24:177–181.
5. Field LD, Callaway GH, O'Brien SJ, et al. Arthroscopic assessment of the medial collateral ligament complex of the elbow. *Am J Sports Med* 1995;23:396–400.
6. Moskal MJ, Savoie FH, Field LD. Elbow arthroscopy in trauma and reconstruction. *Orthop Clin North Am* 1999;30A:163–177.
7. O'Driscoll SW: Elbow arthroscopy for loose bodies. *Orthopedics* 1992;15:855–859.
8. Schwartz ML, Al-Zahrani S, Morwessel RM, et al. Ulnar collateral ligament injury in the throwing athlete: evaluation with saline-enhanced MR arthrography. *Radiology* 1995;197:297–299.
9. Timmerman LA, Schwartz ML, Andrews JR. Preoperative evaluation of the ulnar collateral ligament by magnetic resonance imaging and computed tomography arthrography. *Am J Sports Med* 1994;22:26–32.
10. Lindenfeld TN. Medial approach in elbow arthroscopy. *Am J Sports Med* 1990;18:413.
11. Lynch GJ, Meyers JF, Whipple TL, et al. Neurovascular anatomy and elbow arthroscopy: inherent risks. *Arthroscopy* 1986;2:191.
12. Rodeo SA, Forster RA, Weiland AJ. Neurologic complications due to arthroscopy. *J Bone Joint Surg Am* 1993;75:917–926.
13. Andrews JR, Timmerman LA. Outcome of elbow surgery in professional baseball players. *Am J Sports Med* 1995;23:407–413.
14. Timmerman LA, Andrews JR. Histology and arthroscopic anatomy of the ulnar collateral ligament of the elbow. *Am J Sports Med* 1994;22:667–673.
15. Baumgarten TE, Andrews JR, Satterwhite YE. The arthroscopic evaluation and treatment of osteochondritis desiccans of the capitellum. *Am J Sports Med* 1998;26:520–523.
16. Dehaven KE. Elbow problems in the adolescent. *Cleveland Clin Quart* 1975;42:297–302.
17. Lindholm TS, Osterman K, Vankka E. Osteochondritis desiccans of the elbow, ankle, and hip: a comparison study. *Clin Orthop* 1980;148:245–253.
18. Takahara M, Ogino T, Fukushima S, et al. Nonoperative treatment of osteochondritis desiccans of the humeral capitellum. *Am J Sports Med* 1999;27:728–732.
19. Torg JS. The little league pitcher. *American Family Physician* 1972;6:72–76.
20. Tullos HS, Erwin WD, Woods GW, et al. Unusual lesions of the pitching arm. *Clin Orthop* 1972;88:169–182.
21. Jobe FW, Nuber G. Throwing injuries of the elbow. *Clin Sports Med* 1986;5:621–636.
22. El Attrache N. Personal communication.
23. Small NC. Complications in arthroscopy: the knee and other joints. *Arthroscopy* 1986;2:253–258.
24. Hahn M, Grossman JAI. Ulnar nerve laceration as a result of elbow arthroscopy. *J Hand Surg Br* 1998;23:109.
25. Ruch DS, Poehling GG. Anterior interosseous nerve injury following elbow arthroscopy. *Arthroscopy* 1997;13:756–758.
26. Marshall PD, Faircloth JA, Johnson SR, et al. Avoiding nerve damage during elbow arthroscopy. *J Bone Joint Surg Br* 1993;75:129–131.
27. Reddy AS, Kvitne RS, Yocum LA, et al. Arthroscopy of the elbow: a long-term clinical review. *Arthroscopy* 2000;16:588–594.

ARTHROSCOPIC MANAGEMENT OF THE STIFF ELBOW

FELIX H. SAVOIE III

Arthroscopic rather than open management of the stiff elbow has now progressed to become the operative treatment of choice in most cases. The stiff elbow includes both the arthritic elbow with ulnohumeral, radiocapitellar, and proximal radioulnar joint deterioration and the elbow with loss of motion due to arthrofibrosis. Capsular contracture, intraarticular adhesions, and extraarticular rigidity may occur after trauma, surgery, or systemic disease. This chapter addresses management of the arthritic and the arthrofibrotic elbow. Although each of these disorders may result in a stiff elbow, the etiology and management are quite different and therefore are discussed in separate subsections.

PATHOLOGY OF FLEXION CONTRACTURE

Flexion contracture of the elbow is defined as a loss of both extension and flexion of the elbow due to fracture, dislocation, arthritic conditions, burns, head injury, or cerebral palsy (1–6). Overall, the conditions producing stiffness in the elbow may be grouped into intrinsic and extrinsic factors. Intrinsic factors include intraarticular damage, fractures, loose bodies, synovitis, and foreign bodies, whereas extrinsic factors include contractures caused by scarring of the capsule or collateral ligaments, flexor and/or extensor musculature, instability, heterotopic bone, and skin contractures. Peripheral problems including head injuries, cerebral palsy, and neurologic dysfunction may also result in muscular contracture with resultant loss of motion.

In the management of flexion contracture of the elbow, all possible causes must be considered before treatment. Patients with skin contracture or muscle spasticity must obviously be managed in a different fashion from those with intraarticular fracture or an arthritic condition. Commonly, more than one problem is involved in producing a stiff el-

bow. Each should be evaluated and managed appropriately. Arthroscopic treatment of flexion contracture of the elbow allows the surgeon to address the intrinsic intraarticular causes of elbow contracture, as well as those extrinsic causes that may be safely reached by this technique, including capsular and collateral ligament damage and problems with the extensor musculature. The risk of nerve injury, including posterior interosseous nerve (PIN) and ulnar nerve injury, is quite real in these stiff elbows and should be considered by the operative surgeon before arthroscopic management of this condition is undertaken.

Indications for Treatment

Loss of motion of the elbow may cause significant morbidity (7,8). The American Academy of Orthopaedic Surgeons defines normal flexion of the elbow as 0 to 146 degrees of flexion (8). In 1981, Morrey et al. defined a functional arc of motion of the elbow as 30 to 130 degrees of flexion (9). This 100-degree arc of motion is the arc in which most activities of daily living are performed, and motion less than this results in an inability to perform even minimal activities. Certain activities may require more motion, such as tying shoes, eating, and personal hygiene. Treatment is indicated for those contractures with a loss of extension of 30 degrees of motion, or a similar loss of flexion, and for those patients in whom a greater range of motion is required. As in all areas of the body, pain and functional impairment refractory to nonoperative management represent the primary indication for surgical treatment.

Anatomic Considerations

The altered anatomy of the contracted elbow joint makes a thorough understanding of the pathogenesis of contracture and how the anatomy is altered of paramount importance to the surgeon. Because the contracted joint does not distend normally with inflow, neurovascular structures about the elbow may not be safely displaced from the joint during insufflation.

F. H. Savoie III: Mississippi Sports Medicine and Orthopaedic Center, and Department of Orthopaedic Surgery, University of Mississippi School of Medicine, Jackson, Mississippi.

The medial epicondyle and medial intramuscular septum are preserved in most cases and can be used as a guide to the initial entrance to the elbow joint. The anterior lateral portal is usually made in an outside-in manner and superiorly, because this provides an extra margin of safety to protect the PIN from possible damage. Lateral elbow trauma or contracture can cause capsular hypertrophy that may bind the PIN. Use of the inside-out technique with an anterior superior lateral portal decreases the risk of injury to this structure. Posteriorly, an adherent medial capsule or extensive olecranon deformity may displace the ulnar nerve, increasing the risk of the initial insertion through a posterior central portal into the olecranon fossa. In these cases, it is essential to insert the cannula directly into the olecranon fossa and to avoid medial displacement that might put this neurologic structure at risk. Unlike a normal elbow, portal establishment in a contracted elbow joint requires cautious and careful placement of the cannula, not only through the skin but also during joint entrance, to prevent misdirection by the hypertrophied tissue with resultant soft tissue injury.

During the capsular release, the surgeon must remember the relationship of the capsule and the brachialis muscle to the neurovascular structures. Proximally, the brachialis muscle lies between the capsule and the anterior neurovascular structures (median nerve, radial nerve, and brachial artery). Therefore, arthroscopic capsular release and excision should be continued from within the joint until brachialis muscle fibers are visible, but no further. Shaver blades and cutting instruments must be kept in proximity to the humerus at all times, to avoid straying too far anteriorly and potentially into the neurovascular structures by brachialis muscle penetration.

On the lateral aspect of the elbow, the radial nerve courses between the brachioradialis and brachialis muscles. It divides into the superficial radial nerve and the PIN at the level of the elbow joint. The latter branch courses distally and laterally to the brachialis muscle and becomes immediately adjacent to the anterior joint capsule in the distal half of the elbow. Scar tissue and hypertrophied joint capsule secondary to injury to this area may tether the PIN and damage it during release. Those conditions that produce scar tissue in this area, such as anteriorly displaced radial head fractures, are relative contraindications to arthroscopic contracture release, because the nerve may be bound and stretched or transected during release. Lateral capsular excision should remain proximal to the radiocapitellar joint.

During medial portal placement, one must be conscious of the ulnar nerve at all times. The proximal medial portal is placed only after adequate identification of the intermuscular septum has been accomplished. Debridement of the medial gutter and release of adhesions in this area should be accomplished with a hooded, non–end-cutting shaver so that the covered portion of the blade is always directed toward the ulnar nerve and the open or cutting face toward the joint, to avoid potential damage to the ulnar nerve.

THE ARTHROFIBROTIC ELBOW

The loss of motion in arthrofibrosis centers around soft tissue trauma (10). An injury or disease process produces a synovitic reaction, hemorrhage, and inflammation of the capsule. In arthrofibrosis, the capsular tissues respond by thickening and becoming quite rigid. Attempts to aggressively stretch the capsule produces tearing, which creates more hemorrhage and increases stiffness. The elbow is held in a flexed position to accommodate the hemarthrosis and the painful swelling in the capsular tissues. Physical therapy and/or splinting in this inflammatory phase may actually result in worsening conditions rather than improvement, owing to the repeat damage inflicted on the capsule. Collateral ligament injury can further contribute to elbow contracture by allowing abnormal movement that produces further pressure on the damaged capsule (10–13).

Posttraumatic arthrofibrosis of the elbow may also be secondary to other intraarticular causes. Fractures and osteochondral lesions, articular incongruities, loose bodies, and foreign material may stimulate an inflammatory response in the capsule and result in a mechanical limitation to elbow motion. On the lateral side of the joint, this is often caused by residual deformity in the capitellum or radial head after osteochondritis or trauma. Jones and Geissler (14) found a significant incidence of elbow flexion contracture after type I radial head fractures treated with immobilization (14). They believed that this was caused by a combination of radial head incongruity and soft tissue trauma involved in the injury and subsequent fibrosis of the periarticular structures.

On the medial side of the joint, a more congruous relationship of articular surfaces exists. Less severe injures to the coronoid or olecranon may produce bony incongruity, resulting in a painful arc of motion and subsequent stiffness.

The specific components of arthrofibrosis vary according to the mechanism of injury and the history of postinjury treatment (15,16). Each factor must be considered in the management of the arthrofibrotic elbow.

Management of the Arthrofibrotic Elbow

Management options for the contracted elbow include both conservative and surgical management. All patients with this disorder should undergo an extended trial of nonoperative therapy before being considered for surgery. Selective injections of betamethasone sodium phosphate (Celestone), protected range of motion using a double-hinged elbow brace, and physical therapy including *gentle* stretching, icing, and joint mobilization may prove to be beneficial (17,18). Static splinting is often helpful in obtaining a functional arc of motion in the elbow. Caution should always be exercised during therapy to prevent additional capsular damage and worsening of the arthrofibrotic condition.

Surgical treatment is indicated for those cases refractory to conservative management. Both the surgeon and the patient should play an active role in the decision for surgical management of the stiff elbow. The cause of the condition, potential risks, expected results, and possible complications, including the risk of nerve damage, should be understood by both surgeon and patient before operative intervention is undertaken.

In the past, several authors have described surgical release techniques for the correction of elbow flexion contractures. These have included osteotomy of the medial epicondyle with complete anterior capsulectomy and lengthening of the biceps, limited lateral approach with capsulotomy, limited medial approach, and extensive posterior approach (7,8). Urbaniek et al. (19) found a decrease in preoperative flexion contracture from 48 to 19 degrees with a lateral approach. Husband and Hastings (20) reported that extension improved from a mean of 45 degrees preoperatively to 12 degrees postoperatively, and flexion increased from 116 to 129 degrees.

Open surgical release of elbow flexion contracture produces increased soft tissue trauma from the dissection, postoperative scarring of the capsule and anterior structures that may add to the risk of contracture recurrence, additional elbow trauma above and below the elbow when an external fixator is used, and potentially increased time before physical therapy may be initiated due to surgical pain and scarring. Furthermore, it is difficult to address the entire intrinsic joint pathology without a combined approach of the elbow. In contrast to open release techniques, an arthroscopic release allows the surgeon a complete examination and treatment avenue for intrinsic, intraarticular joint pathology. Removal of intraarticular adhesions, release of associated scarring, and capsular resection anteriorly and posteriorly can all be accomplished arthroscopically. Evaluation, management, and release of medial and lateral gutter adhesions as well as collateral ligament release can also be accomplished arthroscopically, reducing the risk of recurrence and allowing early initiation of a physical therapy program. The main contraindication to capsular release for arthrofibrosis is a lack of experience with elbow arthroscopy. This procedure can be extremely difficult, with a high risk of nerve injury, and should be attempted only by experienced arthroscopic surgeons.

Surgical Technique

The arthroscopic setup for surgical release of elbow flexion contracture is that of a standard elbow arthroscopy. A

TABLE 47.1 INDICATIONS FOR EXPLORATION OF THE RADIAL/POSTERIOR INTEROSSEOUS NERVE

Anterolateral heterotopic ossification
Previous radial head fracture with anterior displaced fragments

TABLE 47.2 INDICATION FOR EXPLORATION OF THE ULNAR NERVE

Preoperative ulnar nerve symptoms
Narrowed cubital tunnel due to spurs or loose bodies
Previous ulnar nerve surgery of unknown type

4.5-mm arthroscope and shaver are used along with standard camera and video recording equipment. I prefer the prone position, because it allows better access to both the anterior and posterior capsular structures, but certainly either the lateral decubitus or supine position could be used at the surgeon's preference. If the patient has quite a bit of scarring around the ulnar nerve or the PIN, each of these may be approached through a small incision, with a Penrose drain used to surround the nerve before to arthroscopy is attempted, to protect the nerve from possible intraoperative damage. Indications for this approach include anteriorly displaced radial head fracture or anterior heterotopic bone for the PIN, and large osteophytes or extraarticular fragments (or both) over the ulnar nerve.

Nerve Exploration

In high-risk situations (Tables 47.1 and 47.2), at-risk neurologic structures may be explored and tagged to forestall injury. This can be accomplished through a small incision before arthroscopy, allowing placement of an elastic band around the nerve. The band can then be used to pull the nerve away from the capsule during the procedure.

The PIN is approached via the transbrachioradialis approach of Lister with minimal damage (Fig. 47.1). The ulnar nerve is approached through a small incision posterior to the epicondyle. The initial attempt to insufflate the elbow is

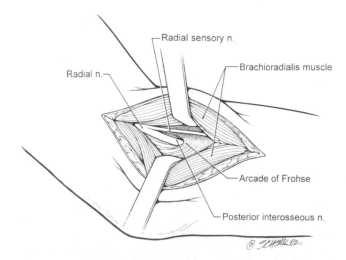

FIGURE 47.1 Lister's approach to the posterior interosseous nerve involves splitting of the transbrachioradialis or brachiorfadialis. This is a direct approach to the posterior interosseous and radial nerves in the forearm.

made through a standard soft spot portal, entering the joint between the radial head, capitellum, and ulna. A proximal medial portal is then established, using a blunt trocar only (Fig. 47.2A). The arthroscope is introduced through this cannula, and the anterior compartment of the elbow is evaluated (Fig. 47.3). An anterolateral portal is then established via an outside-in technique. The portal here should be proximal, to avoid injury to the PIN. Anterolateral or more distal portals produce an extremely high risk of injury to the PIN and should be avoided in the contracted elbow (Fig. 47.2B).

Debridement of the anterior structures is accomplished, and an anterior capsular excision is performed (Fig. 47.4A). Excision usually begins with the shaver in the lateral portal. The capsule is excised in the middle of the joint until brachialis muscle fibers can be visualized. This excision continues laterally to the intermuscular septum (Fig. 47.4B). The arthroscope is then placed in the lateral portal, and sim-

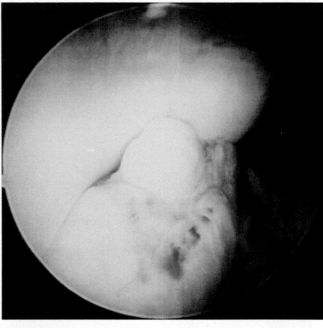

FIGURE 47.3 This view from the proximal anteromedial portal demonstrates the anterior compartment of the elbow with the damaged, contracted anterior capsule.

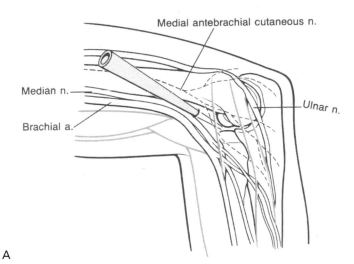

Medial antebrachial cutaneous n.

Median n.

Brachial a.

Ulnar n.

A

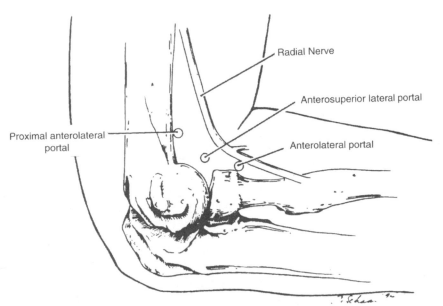

Radial Nerve

Anterosuperior lateral portal

Proximal anterolateral portal

Anterolateral portal

B

FIGURE 47.2 **A:** The portals on the medial side include the proximal anterior medial portal. **B:** Comparison of the related distances of the radial nerve from the proximal anterolateral portal, the anterosuperior lateral portal, and the anterolateral portal.

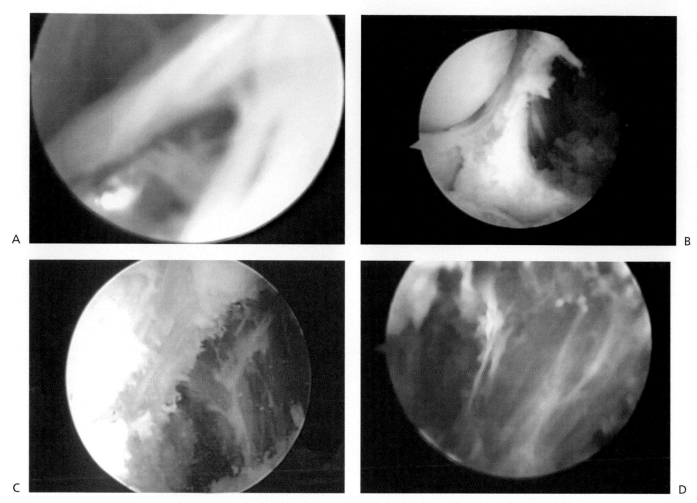

FIGURE 47.4 Steps in the anterior compartment of the elbow during capsular release. **A:** The anterior capsule is incised, and the release is begun adjacent to the humerus. **B:** As the release begins, the brachialis fibers begin to be seen through the capsule. **C:** As the release continues, approximately 1 cm of the anterior capsule is excised. The humerus, brachialis, and capsule are all well visualized. **D:** On completion of the release and partial excision of the superior aspect of the capsule, the brachialis muscle should be well visualized from medial to lateral across the anterior aspect of the elbow.

ilarly the proximal 1 to 2 cm of capsule is excised to the medial intermuscular septum (Fig. 47.4C,D). On completion of the anterior capsulotomy, the proximal 2 cm of the capsule should have been excised and the brachialis muscle should be visualized from the lateral to the medial intermuscular septum. Extension of the elbow is attempted, and range of motion is evaluated. The arthroscope is then transferred to a posterior central and proximal posterolateral portal (Fig. 47.5).

The triceps is elevated off the distal humerus, and the olecranon fossa is debrided (Fig. 47.6). An ulnohumeral arthroplasty may be performed at this point, connecting the olecranon and coronoid fossae to allow improved flexion and extension (Fig. 47.7). The medial gutter is then debrided of all loose bodies, joint adhesions, and osteophytes while the ulnar nerve is protected (Fig. 47.8). The lateral gutter is then debrided as well; the posterolateral plica is ex-

cised, and synovitis, which is quite common in this area, is also removed (Fig. 47.9). Motion is reattempted, and this time full flexion and extension should be achieved. A drain is then inserted anteriorly and a pain pump posteriorly, and the patient provided a soft tissue dressing (Table 47.3).

Postoperative Management

Continuous passive motion is initiated in the recovery room and continued for approximately the first 3 weeks. Physical therapy is started on the day of surgery for aggressive stretching and strengthening of the elbow. The patient is encouraged to use the arm as aggressively as possible in the immediate postoperative period. Therapy is provided daily for 3 weeks, and three times per week thereafter. Static splints are used after 3 weeks if full motion is not obtained by the therapist.

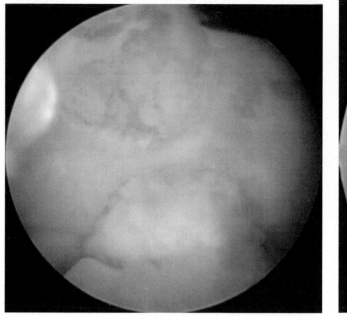

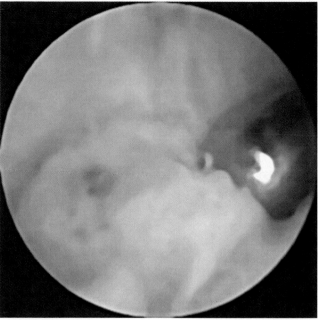

A   B

FIGURE 47.5   A: A degenerative olecranon tip producing posterior impingement. **B:** The tip of the olecranon after debridement.

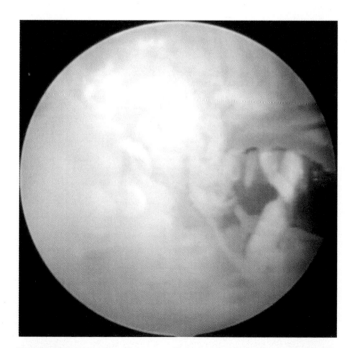

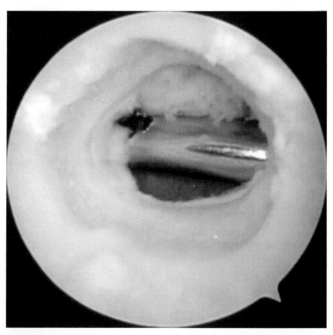

FIGURE 47.6 During the posterior capsular debridement, the triceps muscle is elevated off the humerus to allow the elbow to regain flexion.

FIGURE 47.7 An arthroscopic ulnohumeral arthroplasty is performed by drilling multiple holes in the olecranon fossa, connecting it to the coronoid fossa, and then connecting these holes to form a hole approximately 2 cm in diameter, allowing improvement in both flexion and extension.

TABLE 47.3 STEPS IN ARTHROSCOPIC MANAGEMENT OF THE ARTHROFIBROTIC ELBOW

1. Diagnostic arthroscopy
2. Anterior debridement
   a. Resect coronoid
   b. Remove adhesions
3. Proximal capsular resection
   a. Medial septum to lateral septum
   b. Expose brachialis

4. Olecranon fossa debridement
   a. Elevate triceps tendon
5. Resect olecranon
6. Medial gutter debridement
7. Lateral gutter debridement
8. Olecranon fossa fenestration

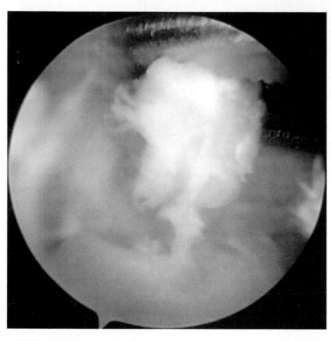

FIGURE 47.8 The medial gutter of the elbow is debrided with the shaver in the posterior central portal and the arthroscope in the posterolateral portal.

Results

The arthroscopic management of arthrofibrosis has continued since the initial report by Jones and Savoie (21). Currently, I have performed more than 200 capsular releases with 3 specific failures. Extension of the elbow increased by 46 degrees to 5 degrees, and flexion increased by 96 to 138 degrees.

Complications

In the current series there has been a single isolated nerve injury, case no. 12. However, reports by Haapaniemi et al. (22) and Jobe et al. (23) delineated the further risk of nerve damage. Morrey et al. (24) also presented the risk of elbow arthroscopy in the Mayo Clinic series, with a complication rate of approximately 10%, a level that parallel's my own experience.

THE ARTHRITIC ELBOW
Nonoperative Management

Nonoperative management includes the use of selected Celestone injections, nonsteroidal antiinflammatory medica-

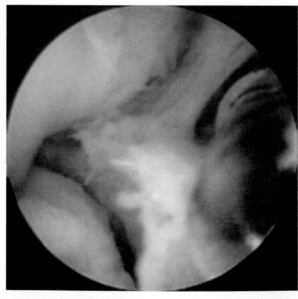
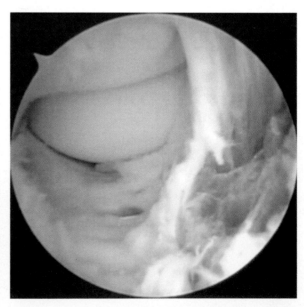

A   B

FIGURE 47.9 A: The posterolateral gutter often is the site of loose bodies and synovitis as well as capsular contractures. **B:** These contractures are debrided in the posterolateral gutter, using a combination of a posterolateral portal and a soft spot portal.

tions, and physical therapy. Surgical treatment is indicated only if nonoperative management becomes ineffective and the patient's pain and functional limitations warrant surgical intervention.

Indications for Surgery

Pain and functional impairment refractory to nonoperative management would indicate surgery for the arthritic elbow. The surgeon's skill with the arthroscope determines whether to do the procedure arthroscopically or by an open technique.

Surgical Management: History

Modern operative management for arthritis of the elbow dates back to the Outerbridge–Kashiwagi procedure (25). Through a triceps-splitting approach, the olecranon is debrided and a Cloward drill is used to bore a hole between the olecranon and coronoid fossae, improving both flexion and extension and decreasing symptoms of anterior and posterior impingement. In inflammatory arthritis, resection of the radial head has proved beneficial, especially in patients with rheumatoid arthritis. Morrey (26,27) modified the Outerbridge–Kashiwagi procedure by using a Bryan–Morrey approach and elevating the triceps rather than splitting it, believing that this approach decreased intraarticular adhesions and improved range of motion while allowing transposition of the ulnar nerve. Savoie et al. (28) modified Morrey's approach to perform the procedure arthroscopically and used the arthroscopic instruments to fenestrate the olecranon and coronoid fossa, resect the radial head as necessary, remove loose bodies, and perform synovectomy with excellent results with a minimum of 2 years of follow-up (28).

Surgical Technique

The elbow is entered through a standard proximal anteromedial portal. The proximal anterolateral portal is established, and the anterior aspect of the elbow joint is debrided. The tip of the coronoid is evaluated and is resected if necessary (Fig. 47.10). The radial head is evaluated; if radial head excision is contemplated, a straight lateral or soft spot portal is established (Fig. 47.11A). The anterior aspect of the radial head is resected first, to avoid penetrating the anterior capsule with possible *injury to the PIN* (which lies adjacent to the anterolateral capsule at the level of the radial head). Once the radial head anterior margin has been resected, the radial head is coplaned (Fig. 47.11B). In case of radiocapitellar impingement, the proximal 8 to 10 mm of the radial head may be resected; if the proximal radioulnar joint is involved, the entire radial head can be resected (Fig. 47.11C). An inflow cannula is left, anteriorly and the posterior central and posterolateral portals are established. Leaving an inflow anteriorly ensures fluid wash to the posterior compartment.

The olecranon fossa is debrided, and three 5-mm drill holes are placed in the olecranon fossa, connecting it to the coronoid fossa. These holes are connected with the use of a bur and enlarged until a fenestration of approximately 1 to 3 cm in diameter is made. This should allow seating of the coronoid process in flexion and of the olecranon in extension. The tip of the coronoid, if degenerative, may be excised, and spurs may be removed from it as well. The tip of the olecranon is then excised. Care should be taken to plane medially and laterally, to prevent impingement of the medial and lateral aspects of the olecranon on the columns of the distal humerus. Medial gutter spurs are then resected, with the suction turned off to prevent injury to the ulnar

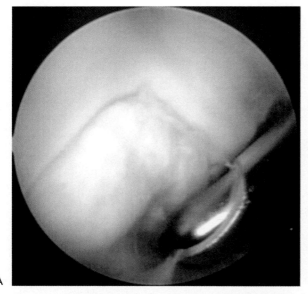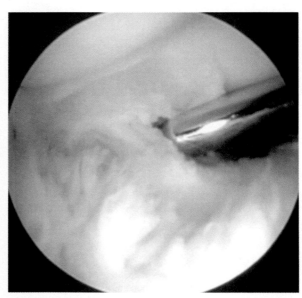

A   B

FIGURE 47.10 **A:** In the arthritic elbow, the coronoid may be grossly deformed, preventing flexion. **B:** This gross deformity of the coronoid tip should be excised.

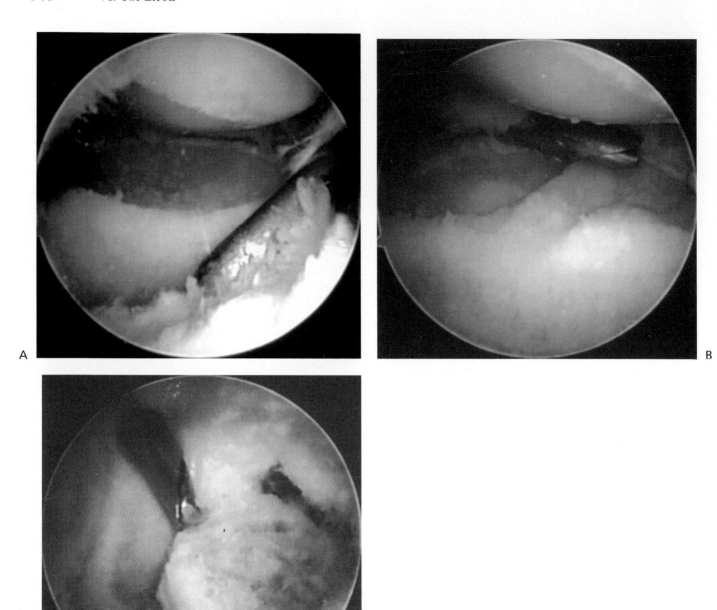

FIGURE 47.11 A: In the arthritic elbow, the radial head may be remarkably degenerative. **B:** In cases of radiocapitellar impingement, the radial head can be coplaned and excised for a distance of approximately 6 mm to allow clearance. **C:** With proximal radial–ulnar joint problems, the entire radial head can be excised down to the radial neck.

nerve. The lateral gutter is then evaluated, and any debris is removed. If a symptomatic posterolateral plica is present, it is resected. The entire elbow joint is then reevaluated, completing the procedure.

Postoperative Course

The patient is started on immediate continuous passive motion in the recovery room. Physical therapy is initiated on

postoperative day 1, and the patient is allowed to resume activities as tolerated.

Results

In a previous study, Savoie et al. (28) delineated approximately 96% good to excellent results with at least 2 years of follow-up for the arthritic elbow. This was in a degenerative population in which two thirds of the patients required radial head excision, indicating the efficacy of this procedure for the arthritic elbow.

SUMMARY

Arthroscopic management of the stiff elbow has certainly gained a foothold in the armamentarium of the operative arthroscopist. Arthroscopy can prove beneficial for intraarticular adhesions, arthritic changes, posttraumatic arthrofibrosis, and other factors causing symptoms in the elbow. Although the potential for complication is high owing to the proximity of neurovascular structures, a thorough knowledge of anatomy, competent arthroscopic skills, and meticulous attention to detail will provide satisfactory results in the stiff elbow.

REFERENCES

1. Protzman RR. Dislocation of the elbow joint. *J Bone Joint Surg Am* 1978;60:539–541.
2. Bede WB, Lefebvre AR, Rosman MA. Fractures of the medial humeral epicondyle in children. *Canadian J Surg* 1975;18:137.
3. Saito T, Koschino T, Okamoto R, et al. Radial synovectomy with muscle release for the rheumatoid elbow. *Acta Orthop Scand* 1986;57:71–73
4. Huang TT, Blackwell SJ, Louis SR. Ten years of experience in managing patients with burn contractures of the axilla, elbow, wrist and knee joints. *Plast Reconstr Surg* 1978;61:70–76.
5. Sherk HH. Treatment of severe rigid contractures of cerebral palsy to upper limbs. *Clin Orthop* 1977;125:1151–1155.
6. Freehafer A. Flexion and supination deformities of the elbow in tetraplegics. *Paraplegia* 1977;15:221–225.
7. Glynn J, Niebauer JJ. Flexion and extension contractures of the elbow. *Clin Orthop* 1976;177:289–291.
8. Wilner P. Anterior capsulectomy for contractures of the elbow. *J Int Coll Surgeons* 1948;11:359–361.
9. Morrey BF, Askew LJ, An KN, et al. A biomechanical study of normal functional elbow motion. *J Bone Joint Surg Am* 1981; 63:872–877.
10. Tucker K. Some aspects of post-traumatic elbow stiffness. *Injury* 1977;9:216.
11. Buxton JD. Ossification in the ligaments of the elbow. *J Bone Joint Surg* 1938;20:709.
12. Gutierre LS. A contribution to the study of the limiting factors of elbow extension. *Acta Anat* 1964;56:146.
13. Morrey BF, An KN. Articular and ligamentous contributions to the stability of the elbow joint. *Am J Sports Med* 1983;11:315.
14. Jones GS, Geissler WB. *Complications of minimally displaced radial head fractures.* San Francisco: American Academy of Orthopaedic Surgeons, 1993.
15. Roberts PH. Dislocation of the elbow. *Br J Surg* 1969;56:806.
16. Thompson HS, Garcia A. Myositis ossificans: aftermath of elbow injuries. *Clin Orthop* 1976;50:129.
17. Dickson RA. Reverse dynamic slings: a new concept in the treatment of post-traumatic elbow flexion contractures. *Injury* 1976;8:35–38.
18. Green DP, McCoy H. Turn buckle orthotoic correction of elbow flexion contractures after acute injuries. *J Bone Joint Surg Am* 1979;61:1092.
19. Urbaniak JR, Hansen PE, Beissinger SF, et al. Correction of post-traumatic flexion contracture of the elbow by anterior capsulotomy. *J Bone Joint Surg Am* 1985;67:1160–1164.
20. Husband JB, Hastings H. The lateral approach for operative release of post-traumatic contracture of the elbow. *J Bone Joint Surg Am* 1990;72:1353–1358.
21. Jones GS, Savoie FH. Arthroscopic capsular release of flexion contractures (arthrofibrosis) of the elbow. *Arthroscopy* 1993;9: 277–283.
22. Haapaniemi T, Berggren M, Adolfsson L. Complete transection of the median and radial nerves during arthroscopic release of post-traumatic elbow contracture. *Arthroscopy* 1999:10:784–787.
23. Miller CD, Jobe CM, Wright MH. Neuroanatomy in elbow arthroscopy. *J Shoulder Elbow Surg* 1995;4:168–174.
24. Kelly EW, Morrey BF, O'Driscoll SW. Complication of elbow arthroscopy. *J Bone Joint Surg Am* 2001:83:25–34.
25. Kashiwagi D. Osteoarthritis of the elbow joint: intra-articular changes and the special operative procedure. Outerbridge-Kashiwagi method. In: Kashiwagi D, ed. *Elbow joint.* New York: Elsevier; 1985:177–188.
26. Morrey BF. Primary degenerative arthritis of the elbow: treatment by ulnohumeral arthroplasty. *J Bone Joint Surg Br* 1992; 74:409–413.
27. Morrey BF. Post-traumatic contracture of the elbow: operative treatment, including distraction arthroplasty. *J Bone Joint Surg Am* 1990;72:601–618.
28. Savoie FH, Nunley PD, Field LD. Arthroscopic management of the arthritic elbow: indications, technique, and results. *J Should Elbow Surg* 1999;8(3):214–219.

THE WRIST

ARTHROSCOPY OF THE WRIST: INTRODUCTION AND INDICATIONS

ROBERT S. RICHARDS
JAMES H. ROTH

Arthroscopy was first reported by Professor Kenji Takagi (1) in 1920, but it was not until 1979 that small-joint instrumentation was perfected and the wrist procedure was described by Yung-Cheng Chen (2). It was the mid-1980s before wrist arthroscopy was taught on a widespread basis. Initially arthroscopy was used mainly as a diagnostic tool. Intraarticular surgery was initially performed with handheld instruments that had been developed for other joints. The introduction of suction punches and smaller motorized resectors and burs facilitated arthroscopic removal, or "ectomy," of bone and soft tissue (3,4). The therapeutic indications were extended as the principles of open surgical procedures were adapted to the arthroscope. Currently in its third decade, wrist arthroscopy is a widely used diagnostic and therapeutic tool.

The goals of arthroscopy are to provide an accurate anatomic diagnosis of wrist pathology and to treat those patients with an anatomic lesion. The magnification provided by arthroscopy allows superior visualization of the anatomy and placement of instruments with precision. New techniques and instrumentation have extended the therapeutic possibilities of wrist arthroscopy. Arthroscopy is a minimally invasive technique that enables the patient to rehabilitate quickly with less morbidity and fewer complications. Using the anatomic principles that have been developed for open surgical procedures, arthroscopic techniques are producing good long-term results.

INDICATIONS FOR WRIST ARTHROSCOPY

The indications for wrist arthroscopy are both diagnostic and therapeutic. Wrist arthroscopy has become the gold standard for diagnosis of intraarticular pathology. In addition to the magnification obtained, detailed structural assessment can be performed by palpation with the probe. No other diagnostic modality allows such a detailed dynamic and static assessment of wrist pathology. Wrist arthroscopy is indicated to confirm findings suggested by other diagnostic modalities and for the diagnosis of wrist pain of unknown origin. Wrist arthroscopy can be used to assess the severity of degenerative changes before other surgical procedures are performed. This would include assessment of the midcarpal joint before proceeding to a proximal row carpectomy, or assessment of the status of an interosseous ligament before reconstruction. A list of indications of wrist arthroscopy is presented in Table 48.1.

DIAGNOSTIC VALUE OF ARTHROSCOPY

Wrist arthrography was historically used for the diagnosis of wrist pathology. The introduction of arthroscopy and, more recently, magnetic resonance imaging (MRI) has significantly changed this situation.

Arthrography

Although it was previously widely used, arthrography is associated with a high incidence of false-negative studies because ligament perforations may be obstructed by synovitis or fibrosis. A tear may act as a flap valve and prevent communication of the contrast agent between compartments.

Cooney (5) reported a high incidence of false-positive and false-negative studies when assessing interosseous ligaments with arthrography. Arthrography does not quantify the size or type of the perforation, and it does not provide information about adjacent structures such as the articular cartilage and synovium. A further concern is that patients with a positive arthrogram have up to a 74% chance of having a positive arthrogram on the asymptomatic contralateral wrist (6).

R. S. Richards and J. H. Roth: Divisions of Orthopaedic Surgery and Plastic Surgery, Department of Surgery, University of Western Ontario, London, Ontario, Canada, and Hand and Upper Limb Centre, St Joseph's Health Centre, London, Ontario, Canada.

TABLE 48.1 INDICATIONS FOR WRIST ARTHROSCOPY

Diagnostic arthroscopy
Assessment of ligamentous injuries of the wrist
Scapholunate ligament disruption
Lunotriquetral ligament disruption
TFCC disorders
Assessment of chondral defects
Assessment of chronic wrist pain of unknown cause
Therapeutic arthroscopy
ARIF of scapholunate and lunotriquetral ligament tears
ARIF of distal radial fractures
Debridement and repair of TFCC tears
Distal ulnar resection
ARIF of scaphoid fractures
Lavage of septic arthritis
Synovectomy
Removal of loose bodies
Debridement of chondral defects
Debridement of degenerative arthritis
Excision of ganglion
Resection arthroplasty

ARIF, arthroscopic-assisted reduction and internal fixation; TFCC, triangular fibrocartilage complex.

Currently, the only area in which arthrography is superior to MRI is in detecting tears of the lunotriquetral ligament (7,8). In view of its invasiveness and its disadvantages as outlined here, arthrography has a very limited role in assessing the wrist today.

Magnetic Resonance Imaging

With the advances in MRI coils, pulse sequences, and gradient hardware, MRI is becoming as accurate in the wrist as in larger joints. However, there is still significant variation in its usefulness depending on the structure being assessed.

The sensitivity rates for diagnosis of triangular fibrocartilage complex (TFCC) tears vary from 72% to 100% (7–13). Reported specificities range from 89% to 100% (8). False-positive studies are usually caused by irregularities of the central portion of the TFCC (8). MRI advances have allowed the detection of mucoid TFCC degeneration, which can occur before a complete tear. One significant weakness of MRI is its inability to detect the cartilage erosions that can be associated with ligamentous injuries (10,11).

For scapholunate ligament tears, MRI has reported sensitivity rates of 53% to 90% and sensitivity rates of 86% to 100% (8).

MRI of the lunotriquetral ligament is difficult because of its small size and curvature. Sensitivity rates for lunotriquetral tears are only 40% to 56%, and specificity ranges from 45% to 100% (8).

Despite theoretical advantages and promising early results, MRI has not yet established itself as the wrist investigation of choice. With newer techniques, the image quality of MRI is likely to improve, but at this time neither arthrography nor MRI provides an entirely satisfactory method of identifying intraarticular ligament injuries.

Arthroscopy

In contrast, arthroscopy provides detailed anatomic information. Palpation with the arthroscopic probe allows assessment of the stability and texture of intraarticular structures and measurement of the size of defects. The stability of ligaments can be assessed under direct vision, when the joint is stressed with a probe or by external manipulation. Adjacent structures such as the synovium and articular cartilage can be clearly seen, allowing a more thorough assessment of the wrist. The surgeon can then treat the abnormalities that are observed.

THERAPEUTIC ARTHROSCOPY

Tears of the Triangular Fibrocartilage Complex

Tears of the TFCC are a common clinical problem. The patient usually presents with ulnar-side wrist pain aggravated by rotation. The diagnosis of TFCC tears can be made with arthrography or MRI. However, there are limitations of these diagnostic modalities, as outlined previously. Tears of the TFCC are well visualized with wrist arthroscopy. The arthroscopic probe can be used to assess the location, size, and stability of the tear (Fig. 48.1). These factors dictate the type of treatment indicated (14). The majority of tears are located in the central or radial avascular portions of the TFCC. Because of concerns about their potential to heal, they are often managed with debridement (Fig. 48.2A), although arthroscopic repair can be performed (Fig. 48.2B).

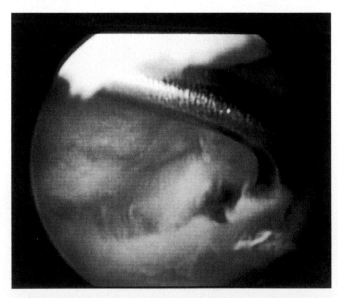

FIGURE 48.1 Examination of an acute triangular fibrocartilage complex tear with the arthroscopic hook probe.

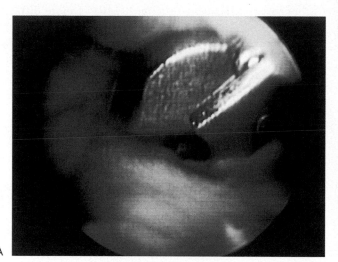
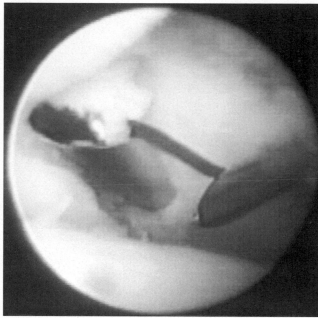

FIGURE 48.2   A: Debridement of a triangular fibrocartilage complex (TFCC) tear with the suction punch. **B:** Arthroscopic suture repair of a TFCC tear using an outside-in technique.

Osterman (15) reported good results from a prospective study of 52 consecutive patients with an isolated tear of the TFCC. Pain was completely relieved in 73% of patients, and improved in another 12%. Range of motion and grip strength improved in most patients, without clinical or radiologic evidence of instability of the distal radioulnar joint or carpus. These results are similar to the 78% good results reported for ulnar shortening (16), but arthroscopy does not involve an open surgical procedure, immobilization, or the risk of a nonunion.

Ulnar impaction syndrome is a degenerative condition characterized by ulnar wrist pain, swelling, crepitus, and limited wrist motion caused by excessive load bearing across the ulnar aspect of the wrist (15,17,18). Patients with ulnar-positive variance are predisposed to develop ulnar impaction syndrome. Positive ulnar variance is often idiopathic, but it can be caused by malunion of a distal radial fracture, premature physeal arrest of the distal radius, or an Essex–Lopresti injury (18). Ulnar impaction syndrome has been successfully treated by unloading the distal ulna. Treatment options have included debridement of the TFCC (18), the "wafer" procedure (19), hemiresection of the distal ulna (20), and ulnar-shortening osteotomy (21). All but the last of these procedures can be performed arthroscopically. The torn TFCC tear can be debrided arthroscopically, and a bur can be used to remove the distal 2 mm of the ulnar head (wafer procedure) through the enlarged perforation in the TFCC (22).

Carpal Instability

There are two main classes of carpal instability: carpal instability dissociated (CID) and carpal instability nondissocia-tive (CIND). In cases of CID, the interosseous ligaments of the proximal row are torn. Arthroscopy provides the best evaluation of the ligaments and joint surfaces and allows the surgeon to visualize these joints while they are being stressed by external manipulation or an arthroscopic probe (23).

Scapholunate Tears

Scapholunate tears may be as common as scaphoid fractures (24). Treatment, during the first 6 weeks when the soft tissues are healing, provides the best opportunity for ligamentous healing to prevent instability and the subsequent degeneration to scapholunate advanced collapse (SLAC wrist) (25). Unfortunately, early diagnosis can be difficult, and widening of the scapholunate gap may not appear until the secondary ligamentous restraints become lax (26). Arthrography cannot distinguish membranous perforations, which do not require treatment, from complete ligament tears.

A tear of the scapholunate or lunotriquetral ligament is seen as irregular, frayed tissue on radiocarpal arthroscopy. Instability associated with a tear is confirmed by midcarpal arthroscopy, because the joint surfaces are not obscured by the ligaments. Normally a probe will not be admitted into the scapholunate interval (Fig. 48.3). If a tear is present, there is loss of the normal alignment of the scaphoid and lunate, and an arthroscopic probe can be introduced into the interval (Fig. 48.4). Open interosseous ligament repair has been advocated, but it is difficult to perform because of the small size of the ligament. If scapholunate instability is confirmed, percutaneous fixation of this joint can be performed. Whipple et al. (27) reported 80% good results at 4 years for arthroscopic reduction and percutaneous fixation

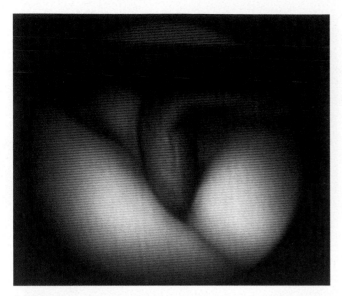

FIGURE 48.3 A normal midcarpal joint with a scapholunate interval that will not admit a probe.

of scapholunate and lunotriquetral tears. Results were superior for those patients who underwent repair less than 3 months after injury and had no static scapholunate diastasis on plain radiographs.

Lunotriquetral Tears

A lunotriquetral injury can occur after forced ulnar deviation of the wrist (24) or as part of a healed perilunate injury (28). Clinical assessment may identify localized tenderness, pain, and instability with ballotment (29). Plain radiographs

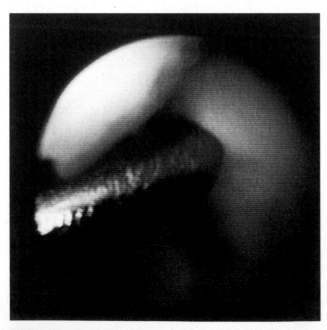

FIGURE 48.4 Disruption of the scapholunate interval, seen through the midcarpal radial portal, that will admit a probe.

are often normal, although there may be distal migration of the triquetrum on the anteroposterior radiograph. Clinical diagnosis can be difficult, and the differential diagnosis includes other causes of ulnar-side wrist pain. Assessment of lunotriquetral ligament tears with MRI is more difficult than for scapholunate ligament injuries because of the small size and oblique orientation of the ligament (13). These injuries can be assessed by arthroscopy and managed in the same manner as scapholunate tears.

Fractures of the Distal Radius

Arthroscopy is gaining popularity for the treatment of distal radial fractures (Fig. 48.5) for the following reasons: (a) It provides a thorough assessment of the articular surface of the distal radius; (b) It provides a thorough assessment of injuries to the carpus, intercarpal ligaments, and TFCC; (c) It aids in obtaining an anatomic reduction of the distal radius and carpus; and (d) Arthroscopy and percutaneous K-wire fixation minimize the soft tissue injury.

Knirk and Jupiter (30) established the causal relationship between intraarticular displacement and subsequent degenerative arthritis. The surgeon should aim for an anatomic reduction, because a 2-mm step leads to subsequent degenerative arthritis. Open reduction of comminuted unstable fractures is often difficult, requiring extensive soft tissue stripping, which produces a slower rehabilitation and a higher complication rate. The magnification provided by arthroscopy enables a more accurate reduction to be obtained. External manipulation, percutaneous K-wire "joysticks," and the arthroscopic hook probe can be used to manipulate intraarticular fragments. Percutaneous K-wires can be used to stabilize the fracture without the need to strip the soft tissues from the radius (31–34) (Fig. 48.6). The arthroscopic hook probe can be used to test the stability of frag-

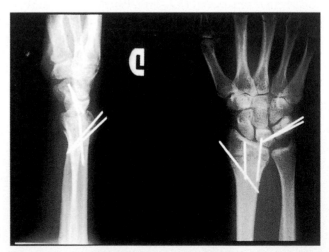

FIGURE 48.5 This patient had a distal radial fracture that was treated with Kapandji intrafocal pin fixation. Wrist arthroscopy revealed a triangular fibrocartilage complex tear, which was debrided, and a lunotriquetral tear, which was reduced with arthroscopic assistance and fixed with percutaneous K-wires.

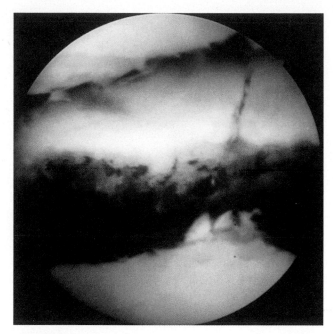

FIGURE 48.6 An intraarticular fracture of the distal radius seen through the 3-4 portal.

ments after fixation. With these new techniques, intraarticular steps can usually be reduced to less than 1 mm in all but the most comminuted fractures (Figs. 48.6 and 48.7).

In distal radius fractures, it is common to find associated tears of the interosseous ligaments and TFCC, which can be assessed and managed with the aid of arthroscopy. The incidence of TFCC disruption in distal radius fractures has ranged from 53% to 78% (35,36), and clinical symptoms have been reported in 5% to 15% of fractures (37).

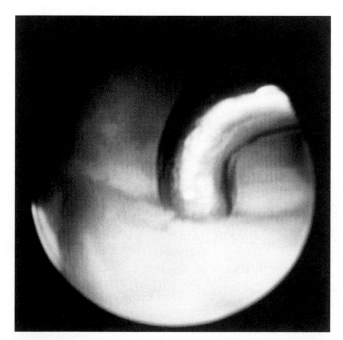

FIGURE 48.7 After arthroscopic reduction and fixation of the articular surface, the arthroscopic probe is used to assess the reduction and to test the stability of the fracture fragments.

Scapholunate ligament injuries have been reported in 22% to 54% of intraarticular distal radial fractures. Lunotriquetral ligament injuries have been reported in 7% to 15% of intraarticular distal radial fractures (35,38).

Scaphoid Fractures

Open reduction with internal fixation has been recommended for displaced acute fractures of the scaphoid. However, the volar approach breaches the important volar ligament, and the dorsal approach may compromise the blood supply to the scaphoid. Arthroscopic-assisted reduction of scaphoid fractures avoids these problems (39,40). The details of this technique are presented in Chapter 52.

Septic Arthritis

Septic arthritis is a condition that has been managed successfully with arthroscopy in the knee (41). Arthroscopy provides a thorough lavage of the joint and enables a biopsy of the synovium to be obtained. The surgeon can visualize the articular surface and the reactive synovitis.

Synovectomy

Synovectomy has historically been the first-line surgical treatment of joints affected by rheumatoid arthritis that have failed medical management (42,43). The concern with open synovectomy is the prolonged rehabilitation and the possibility of loss of motion. Arthroscopy provides a magnified view of the pathologic synovium, which typically accumulates on the volar ligaments of the radiocarpal joint (44,45) (Fig. 48.8). Adolfsson and Nylander (44) reported good results of arthroscopic synovectomy of the wrist in pa-

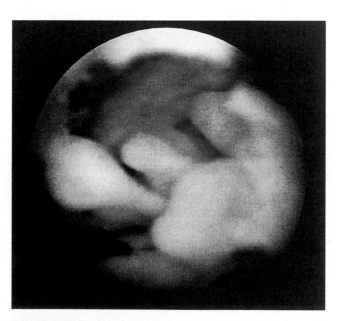

FIGURE 48.8 Extensive synovitis on the ulnar side of the radiocarpal joint, which can be arthroscopically resected.

tients with rheumatoid arthritis. All patients experienced a reduction in pain, and no patient experienced a decrease in the range of motion. There were no complications in their series.

Arthroscopic wrist synovectomy can be performed after open extensor tendon synovectomy.

Loose Bodies

Arthroscopy is a valuable technique to remove loose bodies, which usually occur after chondral defects or degenerative osteoarthritis and result in symptoms of pain and locking (46). Diagnosis can be confirmed with computed tomographic arthrography, and the loose body can be removed arthroscopically.

Ganglion

Ganglions of the wrist often originate from the dorsal aspect of the scapholunate ligament. The stroma of the ganglion and the reactive synovitis can be visualized and resected arthroscopically (39,47,48).

Chondral Defects

Chondral defects are common (49,50), but diagnosis remains difficult, even with imaging modalities such as MRI (11). If wrist pain persists despite conservative measures, wrist arthroscopy offers diagnosis and treatment. At arthroscopy, the size and stability of the chondral defects can be assessed. Chondral lesions can be smoothed to reduce mechanical symptoms and to minimize the production of intraarticular debris. Abrasion arthroplasty and joint lavage have been reported to be of value in some patients (50).

Roth and Poehling (50) reported a multicenter study of chondral defects in the wrist diagnosed with arthroscopy. Cartilage lesions were classified as primary if the source of symptoms was judged to be from the articular cartilage and secondary if it was from another cause (e.g., ligament instability, fracture). Eighty-three percent of patients with primary lesions improved, whereas only 55% of those with secondary lesions improved (50).

Degenerative Arthritis

Arthroscopic debridement of degenerative arthritis of the knee has been reported to produce good results (51–53,55–57), and similar results can be expected in the non–weight-bearing wrist joint. Arthroscopic debridement is most likely to be successful in patients with mechanical symptoms and minimal radiographic changes. Lavage and debridement of chondral flaps, osteophytes, and synovitis can be rewarding in some patients (54–57).

The scapho-trapezium-trapezoid (STT) joint is a common site of degenerative osteoarthritis. Arthroscopic de-

bridement can be performed via the STT or the radial midcarpal portal.

Resection Arthroplasty

Many procedures that were previously performed through an arthrotomy can now be performed arthroscopically. Proximal row carpectomy has been performed arthroscopically (54). Arthroscopy also allows the surgeon to accurately assess the articular surfaces of the capitate and the lunate fossa before proceeding with the proximal row carpectomy.

Hemiresection of the distal ulna has also been performed arthroscopically (53). Other arthroscopic procedures that have been reported include radial styloidectomy and excision of the proximal pole of the scaphoid (55). Open excision of the lunate for Kienböck's disease has been reported, but could be treated arthroscopically. Arthroscopic arthrodesis of the ankle has been reported (55), and similar techniques could be developed for the wrist fusion.

Chronic Wrist Pain

Chronic wrist pain can be considered as mechanical or dystrophic (57). Patients with mechanical symptoms such as catching, clicking, locking, and pain that increases with activity and decreases with rest are more likely to have a good result after wrist arthroscopy. In contrast, patients with dystrophic symptoms, such as burning pain that is often worse at night, exacerbated by minimal activity, or associated with cold insensitivity, dysesthesia, paresthesia, or vasomotor changes, are less likely to obtain symptomatic relief after arthroscopy (57).

Conventional studies including MRI often fail to delineate the problem (60). In patients with chronic wrist pain, ligamentous and cartilage injuries are often seen at arthroscopy (58,59) and result in a change in the diagnosis in up to 40% of patients (61). However, correlation of the arthroscopic findings with the clinical symptoms is important. Extraarticular causes of chronic wrist pain, such as neuromas and tendinitis, need to be excluded before arthroscopy.

Complications

The benefits of wrist arthroscopy must be compared with the possible complications. Complications after arthroscopy are rare, and the wrist is no exception. Major national surveys in France and the United States have revealed an overall complication rate of 0.56% (62,63). In the wrist, the major potential complications are infections, neuromas, tendon injuries, reflex sympathetic dystrophy, dorsal skin slough, tourniquet neuropraxia, compartment syndromes, and finger joint injury or skin slough from the finger traps. Adequate precautions during arthroscopy will prevent the majority of these complications. With the exception of the occasional case of reflex sympathetic dystrophy, none of these complications has occurred in our patients.

SUMMARY

Arthroscopy provides the surgeon with a magnified view of all intraarticular structures, including those areas that are difficult to access via arthrotomy. Advances in arthroscopic techniques and instrumentation have enabled the surgeon to extend the therapeutic possibilities of wrist arthroscopy. New instrumentation has enabled intraarticular surgery to be performed more efficiently. The wrist arthroscopist can now effectively manage scaphoid and distal radial fractures, TFCC tears, interosseous ligament tears, septic arthritis, chondral defects, and degenerative arthritis. The surgeon can use the anatomic principles that have been developed for open procedures and adapt them for use with the arthroscope. Arthroscopic surgery is minimally invasive; hence, patients rehabilitate quickly and with fewer complications. Arthroscopic surgery requires a high level of skill from the surgeon, but, when mastered, it provides considerable benefit to the patient.

REFERENCES

1. Takagi K. The classic arthroscope. *Clin Orthop* 1982;167:6–8.
2. Yung-Cheng C. Arthroscopy of the wrist and finger joints. *Orthop Clin North Am* 1979;10:723–733.
3. Roth JH. Hand instrumentation for small joint arthroscopy. *Arthroscopy* 1988;4:126–128.
4. Whipple TL. Powered Instruments for wrist arthroscopy. *Arthroscopy* 1988;4:290–294.
5. Cooney WP. Evaluation of chronic wrist pain by arthrography, arthroscopy and arthrotomy. *J Hand Surg Am* 1993;18:815–822.
6. Herbert TJ, Faithfull RG, McCann DJ, et al. Bilateral arthrography of the wrist. *J Hand Surg Br* 1990;15:233–235.
7. Dalinka MK. Is there a role for wrist arthrography now that MR imaging is readily available. *AJR Am J Roentgenol* 1994;162: 1494–1495.
8. Pretorius ES, Epstein RE, Dalinka MK. MR imaging of the wrist. *Radiol Clin North Am* 1997;35:145–161.
9. Gundry CR, Kursunoglu-Brahme S, Schwaighofer B, et al. Is MRI better than arthrography for evaluating the ligaments of the wrist? In vitro study. *AJR Am J Roentgenol* 1990;154:337–341.
10. Golimbu CN, Firooznia H, Melone C, et al. Tears of the triangular fibrocartilage of the wrist: MRI imaging. *Radiology* 1989;173:731–733.
11. Cerofolini E, Luchetti R, Pederzini L, et al. MRI evaluation of triangular fibrocartilage complex tears in the wrist: comparison with arthrography and arthroscopy. *J Comput Assist Tomogr* 1990;14:963–967.
12. Kang HS, Kindynis P, Brahme SK, et al. Triangular fibrocartilage and intercarpal ligaments of the wrist: MRI imaging. Cadaveric study with gross pathologic and histologic correlation. *Radiology* 1991;181:401–404.
13. Schweitzer ME, Brahme SK, Hodler J, et al. Chronic wrist pain: spin-echo and short tau inversion recovery MRI imaging and conventional and MRI arthrography. *Radiology* 1992;182: 205–211.
14. Mikic Z. The blood supply of the human distal radioulnar joint and the microvasculature of its articular disk. *Clin Orthop* 1984;187:26–35.
15. Osterman AL. Arthroscopic debridement of the triangular fibrocartilage complex tears. *Arthroscopy* 1990;6:120–124.
16. Darrow JC, Linscheid RL, Dobyns JH, et al. Distal ulnar recession for disorders of the distal radioulnar joint. *J Hand Surg Am* 1985;10:482–491.
17. Friedman SL, Palmer AK. Ulnar impaction syndrome. *Hand Clin* 1991;7:295–310.
18. Menon J, Wood VE, Schoene HR, et al. Isolated tears of the triangular fibrocartilage of the wrist: results of partial excision. *J Hand Surg Am* 1984; 9:527–530.
19. Feldon P, Terrono AL, Belsky MR. The "Wafer" procedure; partial distal ulnar resection. *Clin Orthop* 1992;275:124–129.
20. Bowers WH. Distal radioulnar joint arthroplasty: the hemiresection-interposition technique. *J Hand Surg Am* 1985;10:169–178.
21. Milch H. Cuff resection of the ulna for malunited Colles' fracture. *J Bone Joint Surg* 1941;23:311–313.
22. Feldon P, Terrono AL, Belsky MR. Wafer distal ulna resection for triangular fibrocartilage tears and/or ulna impaction syndrome. *J Hand Surg Am* 1992;17:731–737.
23. Cooney WP, Dobyns JH, Linscheid RL. Arthroscopy of the wrist: anatomy and classification of carpal instability. *Arthroscopy* 1990;6:133–140.
24. Jones WA. Beware of the sprained wrist: the incidence and diagnosis of scapholunate instability. *J Bone Joint Surg Br* 1988;70: 293–297.
25. Watson HK, Ballet FL. The SLAC wrist: scapholunate advanced collapse pattern of degenerative arthritis. *J Hand Surg Am* 1984;9:358–365.
26. Meade TD, Schneider LH, Cherry K. Radiographic analysis of selective sectioning at the carpal scaphoid: a cadaveric study. *J Hand Surg Am* 1990;15:855–862.
27. Whipple TL, Schengel D, Caffrey D, et al. Treatment of scapholunate dissociation by arthroscopic reduction and internal fixation. Presented at the International Wrist Investigators Workshop, Long Beach, CA, May 1990.
28. Mayfield JK, Johnson RP, Kilcoyne RK. Carpal dislocations: pathomechanics and progressive perilunar instability. *J Hand Surg* 1980;5:226–241.
29. Reagan DS, Linscheid RL, Dobyns DH. Lunotriquetral sprains. *J Hand Surg* 1984;9:502–513.
30. Knirk JL, Jupiter JB. Intra-articular fractures of the distal end of the radius in young adults. *J Bone Joint Surg Am* 1986;63: 647–659.
31. Mah E, Atkinson R. Percutaneous Kirschner wire stabilization following closed reduction of Colles' fractures. *J Hand Surg Br* 1992;17:55.
32. Greatting MD, Bishop AT. Intrafocal (Kapandji) pinning of unstable fractures of the distal radius. *Orthop Clin North Am* 1993;24:301–307.
33. DePalma A. Comminuted fractures of the distal end of the radius treated by ulnar pinning. *J Bone Joint Surg Am* 1952;34:651–662.
34. Rayhack J, Langworthy J, Belsole R. Transulnar percutaneous pinning of displaced distal radial fractures: a preliminary report. *J Orthop Trauma* 1989;3:107.
35. Richards RS, Bennett J, Roth JH, et al. Arthroscopic diagnosis of intraarticular soft tissue injuries associated with distal radial fractures. *J Hand Surg Am* 1997;22:772–776.
36. Lindau T, Arner M, Hagberg L. Intraarticular lesions in distal fractures of the radius in young adults: a descriptive arthroscopic study in 50 patients. *J Hand Surg Br* 1997;22:638–643.
37. Cooney WP, Dobyns JH, Linscheid RL. Complications of Colles' fractures. *J Bone Joint Surg Am* 1980;62:613–619.
38. Geissler WB, Freeland AE, Savoie FH, et al. Intracarpal soft-

tissue lesions associated with an intraarticular fracture of the distal end of the radius. *J Bone Joint Surg Am* 1996;78:357–365.

39. Whipple TL. The role of arthroscopy in the treatment of wrist injuries in the athlete. *Clin Sports Med* 1992;11:227–238.

40. Gan BS, Richards RS. Arthroscopically assisted internal fixation of scaphoid fractures. *Operative Techniques in Plastic Surgery* 1997;4:1–7.

41. Thiery JA. Arthroscopic drainage in septic arthritides of the knee: a multicentre study. *Arthroscopy* 1989;5:65–69.

42. Smiley P, Wasilewski SA. Arthroscopic synovectomy. *Arthroscopy* 1990;6:18–23.

43. Taylor AR. Synovectomy of the knee in rheumatoid arthritis patients. *J Bone Joint Surg Br* 1979;61:121.

44. Adolfsson L, Nylander G. Arthroscopic synovectomy of the rheumatoid wrist. *J Hand Surg Br* 1993;18:92–96.

45. Richards RS, Roth JH. Wrist arthroscopy: advances in diagnosis and treatment. *Adv Oper Orthop* 1991;1:203–225.

46. Whipple TL. Articular surface defects and loose bodies. In: Whipple TL. *Arthroscopic surgery of the wrist*. Philadelphia: JB Lippincott, 1992:93–102.

47. Whipple TL. *Arthroscopic surgery of the wrist*. Philadelphia: JB Lippincott; 1992:84.

48. Viegas SF. Intraarticular ganglion of the dorsal interosseous scapholunate ligament: a case for arthroscopy. *Arthroscopy* 1986; 2:93–95.

49. Whipple TL. Articular surface defects and loose bodies. In: Whipple TL. *Arthroscopic surgery of the wrist*. Philadelphia: JB Lippincott, 1992:93–102.

50. Poehling GG, Roth JH: Articular cartilage lesions of the wrist. In: McGinty JB, ed. *Operative arthroscopy*. New York: Raven Press, 1991:635–639.

51. Bert JM, Maschka K. The arthroscopic treatment of unicompartmental gonarthrosis: a five year follow-up study of abrasion arthroplasty plus arthroscopic debridement and arthroscopic debridement alone. *Arthroscopy* 1989;5:25–32.

52. Dandy DJ. Arthroscopic debridement of the knee [Editorial]. *J Bone Joint Surg Br* 1991;73:877–878.

53. McLaren AC, Blokker CP, Fowler PJ et al. Arthroscopic debridement of the knee for osteoarthritis. *Can J Surg* 1991;34:595–598.

54. Roth JH, Poehling GG. Arthroscopic "ectomy" surgery of the wrist. *Arthroscopy* 1990;6:141–147.

55. Whipple TL. Clinical applications of wrist arthroscopy. In: Lichtman DM, ed. *The wrist and its disorders*. Philadelphia: WB Saunders, 1988:118–128.

56. Ogilvie-Harris DJ, Lieberman I, Fitsialos D. Arthroscopically assisted arthrodesis for osteoarthritic ankles. *J Bone Joint Surg Am* 1993;75:1167–1174.

57. Poehling GP, Chabon SJ, Siegel DB. Diagnostic and operative arthroscopy. In: Gelberman RH, ed. *The wrist: master techniques in orthopedic surgery*. New York: Raven Press, 1994:21–48.

58. Koman LA, Poehling GG, Toby EB, et al. Chronic wrist pain: indications for wrist arthroscopy. *Arthroscopy* 1990;6:116–119.

59. North ER, Meyer S. Wrist injuries: correlation of clinical and arthroscopic findings. *J Hand Surg Am* 1990;15:915–920.

60. Levy HJ, Gardner RD, Lemak LJ. Bilateral osteochondral flaps of the wrists. *Arthroscopy* 1991;7:118–119.

61. Kelly EP, Stanley JK. Arthroscopy of the wrist. *J Hand Surg Br* 1990;15:236–242.

62. Kieser CH. A review of complications of knee arthroscopy. *Arthroscopy* 1992;8:79–83.

63. Small NC. Complications in arthroscopy: the knee and other joints. *Arthroscopy* 1986;2:253–258.

ARTHROSCOPY OF THE WRIST: OPERATING ROOM SETUP AND TECHNIQUE

ETHAN R. WIESLER
GARY G. POEHLING

Wrist arthroscopy has made significant progress over the last decade and is now a standard practice for many hand surgeons. Knowledge of anatomy and techniques is crucial for proper and safe evaluation and management of wrist disorders.

EQUIPMENT

There are now many sizes of arthroscopes available for arthroscopy for different joints. We are currently using a 2.7-mm, 30-degree arthroscope for virtually all procedures at the level of the radiocarpal and midcarpal joints of the wrist.

Similarly, there are many additional instruments available for the increasing indications and procedures possible in the wrist. Basket forceps, measuring 2 to 3 mm in diameter and at least 6 cm long, are ideal. There are options of suction, angled tips, square versus round ends, locking mechanisms, and spring-loaded devices readily available on the market. A motorized shaver is often useful for many of the procedures, and this shaver device also is available is a variety of sizes and shapes. An angled probe, measuring approximately 40 mm in length and 1.5–2.0 mm in diameter, is useful for palpation and evaluation of the intra-articular structures. Finally, grasping forceps, both curved and straight, are instruments we use commonly during wrist arthroscopy (Fig. 49.1).

OPERATING ROOM SETUP

Once the initial equipment is obtained, performing successful arthroscopic surgery of the wrist requires thorough understanding of the anatomy of the dorsal wrist, because the

E. R. Wiesler and G. G. Poehling: Wake Forest University Baptist Medical Center, Comprehab Plaza, Orthopaedic Surgery, Wake Forest University Baptist Medical Center, Winston-Salem, North Carolina.

major portal sites for wrist arthroscopy are from the dorsal approach. This chapter first describes the equipment and setup we use, followed by a description of the most common portals and relevant anatomy.

POSITION

We position the patient in the supine position, and use a distracting wrist tower (Dyonics) with disposable finger trap holders attached to it (Fig. 49.2). This device allows manual adjustment of traction, and we typically use 10 lb of traction.

3-4 Portal

The initial working portal for the radiocarpal joint is through the third and fourth dorsal compartments. An 18-gauge needle is inserted 0.5 cm distal to Lister's tubercle and angled approximately 20 degrees palmarly, replicating the palmar tilt of the distal radius. Sterile Ringer's lactate is injected into the joint space, and fluid (5 to 10 mL) is used to provide distention and allow the instruments to be more easily placed into the joint (Fig. 49.3). The skin is incised only to the depth of the dermis and in a longitudinal direction. This prevents transection of an extensor tendon. Furthermore, a small incision allows for a good soft tissue seal around the blunt cannula and prevents excessive fluid extravasation during the procedure as the instruments are exchanged. A blunt trocar is then introduced into the joint, again matching the palmar tilt of the distal radius articular surface to minimize iatrogenic injury to the radiocarpal joint surfaces. The borders of the portal are the extensor pollicis longus (EPL) radially, the extensor digitorum comminus (EDC) ulnarly, the radius proximally and the scapholunate (SL) ligament distally (Fig. 49.4). Initial visualization and inspection of the joint is most easily performed from this portal and, depending on the suspected pathology or

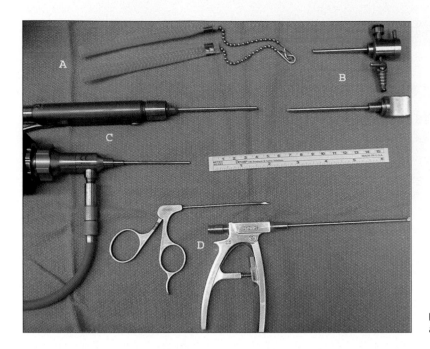

FIGURE 49.1 Instruments commonly used for wrist arthroscopy.

pathology appreciated at the time, further portals are then established for instrumentation.

6-R Portal

The 6-R portal is a commonly used portal for placement of instruments in the radiocarpal joint. It can be used for a variety of wrist pathology, including debridement of the SL ligament, debridement/repair of the triangular fibrocartilage complex (TFCC), evaluation of the lunotriquetral (LT) ligament, and arthroscopic-assisted distal radius fracture reduction. Its anatomic borders are the extensor digiti minimi (EDM) radially, the extensor carpi ulnaris (ECU) ulnarly, the TFCC and ulnar head proximally, and the lunate and triquetrum distally (Fig. 49.5). An 18-gauge needle is inserted just radial to the easily palpable ECU tendon and is visualized from the inside of the joint (Fig. 49.6). Once outflow is established through the needle and appropriate adjustments are made to center on the joint, the skin is incised as described previously, and the trocar is introduced in the joint.

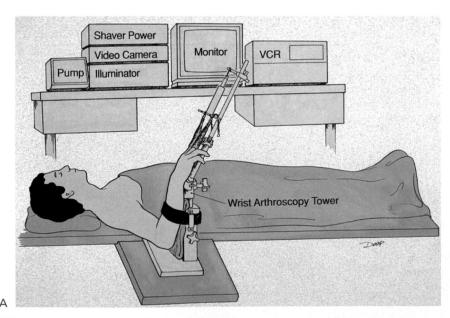

FIGURE 49.2   A–C: Operating room setup with arthroscopy tower and finger-distracting devices.

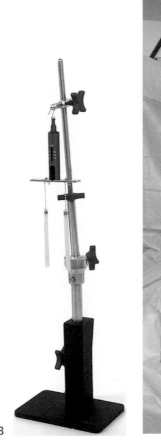

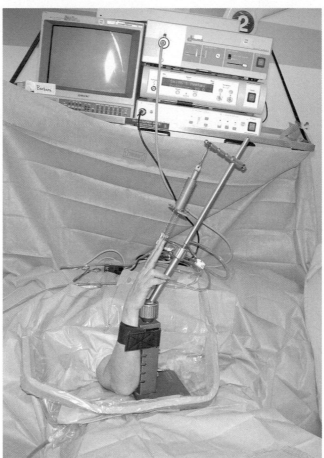

B   C

FIGURE 49.2 *(continued)*

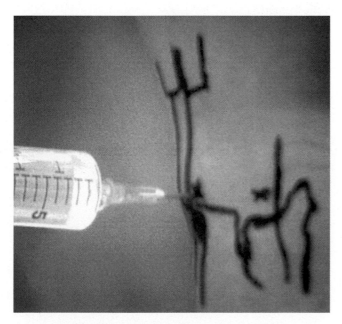

FIGURE 49.3 Joint distention in the 3-4 portal.

4-5 Portal

An additional portal, located between the fourth and fifth dorsal compartments, has been described and is useful for visualization and instrumentation around the LT interval. The radial border is the EDC, and the ulnar border is the EDM tendon. The same proximal and distal borders apply as for the 3-4 portal (Fig. 49.7).

ARTHROSCOPIC ANATOMY

The SL ligament is a thin proximal ligament that is easily defined by palpation with a probe. It has three anatomic regions: palmar, midsubstance, and dorsal. The stronger regions are the dorsal and palmar regions; they are made of strong, thick collagen fibers. The SL can easily be visualized

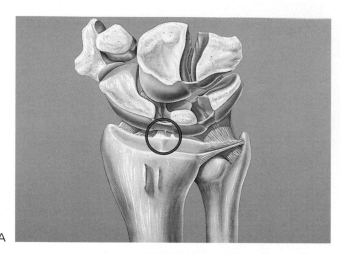

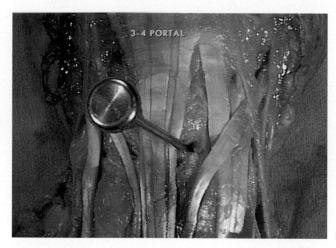

FIGURE 49.4 A: The 3-4 portal location anatomy. **B:** Anatomy of the 3-4 portal.

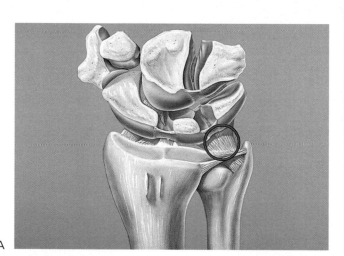

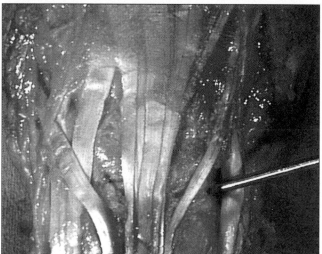

FIGURE 49.5 A and **B:** The 6-R portal.

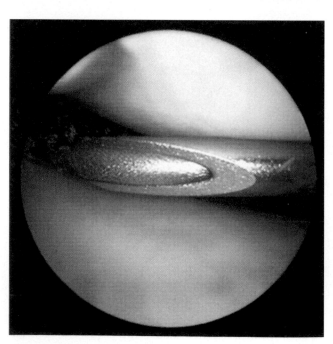

FIGURE 49.6 An 18-gauge needle in the 6-R portal, as seen from the inside of the radiocarpal joint.

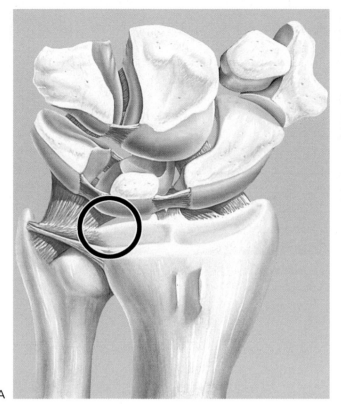

A

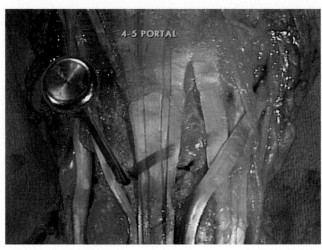

B

FIGURE 49.7 The 4-5 portal location **(A)** and anatomy **(B)**.

through the 3-4 and 6-R portals. It consistently has a fat pad at the palmar aspect that extends and covers the radioscapholunate (RSC) ligament, which helps identify the proper SL interval (Fig. 49.8). This small, Y-shaped ligament is often hidden by this fat pad, and the sagittal ridge at the base of this ligament divides the scaphoid and lunate fossae of the distal radius.

Radial Styloid and Radioscaphocapitate Ligament

The radial styloid and RSC ligaments are the most radial structures seen from the 3-4 portal. Just ulnar to the RSC ligament, one can often see the radiolunate (RL) ligament (Fig. 49.9).

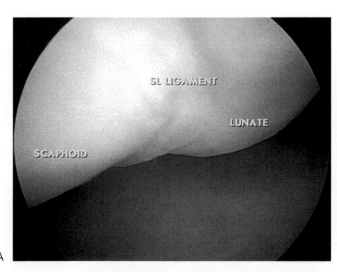

A

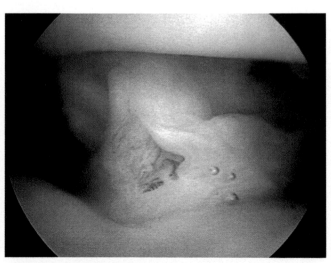

B

FIGURE 49.8   A: Scapholunate ligament (SL) seen from the 3-4 portal. **B:** Fat pad over the radioscapholunate (RSL) ligament seen through the 4-5 portal.

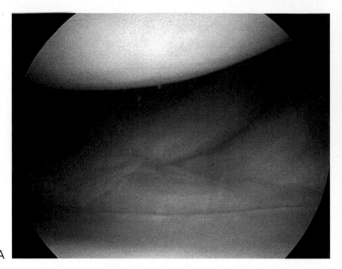

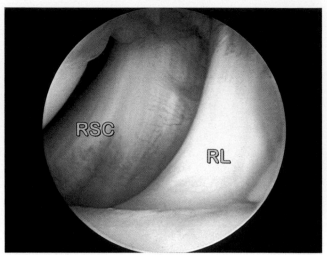

FIGURE 49.9   A: Radial styloid and radiocarpal ligaments. **B:** Radioscapholunate (RSC) and radi-olunate (RL) ligaments.

Ulnocarpal Ligaments

The ulnocarpal ligaments comprise the ulnolunate ligament and the ulnotriquetral ligament. They function as a strong palmar sling to the ulnar side of the wrist and insert onto the palmar margins of the lunate and triquetrum (Fig. 49.10).

TRIANGULAR FIBROCARTILAGE COMPLEX

The TFCC has a broad attachment on the ulnar border of the radius and the base of the ulnar styloid. Extraarticular attachments are also to the subsheath of the ECU tendon. The palmar side blends with the ulnocarpal ligaments, and

dorsally it integrates with the sheath of the ECU (Fig. 49.11).

MIDCARPAL JOINT

The midcarpal joint has two major portals, on the radial and ulnar sides of the capitate. The borders of the midcarpal radial (MCR) portal are the extensor carpi radialis brevis (ECRB) tendon radially, the ECU ulnarly, the capitate distally, and the lunate proximally (Fig. 49.12). The MCR portal is established by a technique similar to that mentioned previously for the radiocarpal 3-4 portal. An 18-gauge needle is inserted into the MCR portal, approxi-

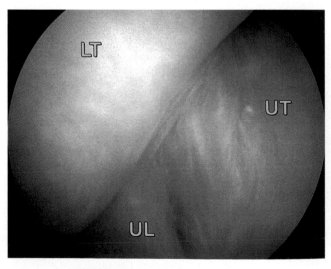

FIGURE 49.10 Ulnocarpal ligaments.

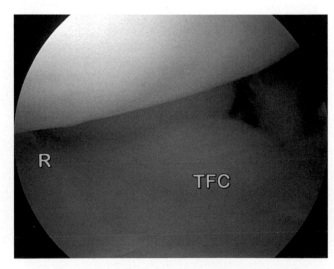

FIGURE 49.11 Triangular fibrocartilage complex (TFCC).

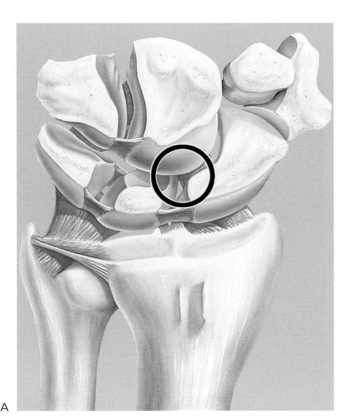

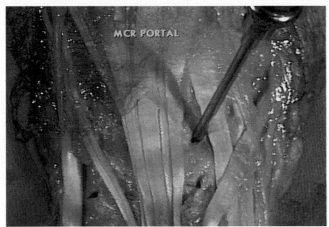

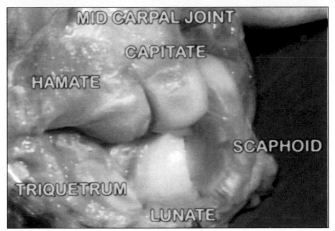

FIGURE 49.12 A: Midcarporadial (MCR) location. **B:** MCR portal. **C:** MCR anatomy.

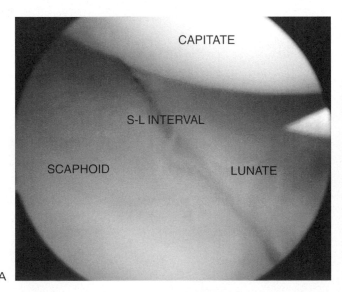

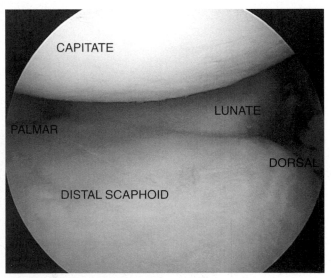

FIGURE 49.13 A and **B:** Views seen through the MCR portal.

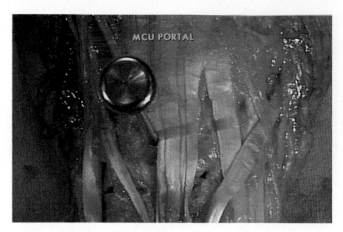

FIGURE 49.14 Midcarpoulnar (MCU) portal.

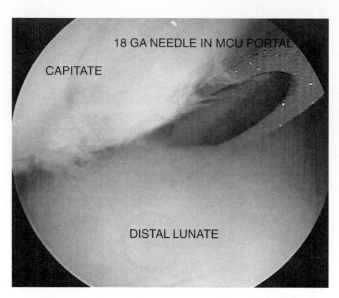

FIGURE 49.15 View seen through the MCU portal.

mately 2 cm distal to the 3-4 portal. The joint is distended with 5-7 mL of fluid, the skin is incised, and a blunt trocar is inserted. This allows visualization of the distal aspect of the scaphoid, lunate, and SL ligament. Additionally, the articular surfaces of the capitate and midcarpal alignment can be seen (Fig. 49.13).

The midcarpoulnar (MCU) portal is just on the ulnar border of the EDC tendon compartment in line with the center of the fourth metacarpal, 2 cm ulnar to the MCR portal (Fig. 49.14). A needle is introduced into the MCU space, and fine positioning is done through direct visualization from the MCR portal. The skin is incised in a longitudinal direction, and the trocar is introduced into the joint (Fig. 49.15).

Operative Arthroscopy, third edition. Edited by John B. McGinty, Stephen S. Burkhart, Robert W. Jackson, Donald H. Johnson, and John C. Richmond.
Lippincott Williams & Wilkins © 2003.

PALMER MIDCARPAL INSTABILITY

DAVID M. LICHTMAN
RANDALL W. CULP
ATUL JOSHI

Instability of the midcarpal joint was first described in 1934 by Mouchet and Belot (1). However, it was not until 1980 that midcarpal instability (MCI) was recognized to be a source of clinical symptoms (2). In 1981, Lichtman et al. described a small series of patients who had a palmar sag at the midcarpal joint and who complained of a spontaneous "clunk" at the triquetrohamate joint with ulnar deviation of the wrist (3). Anatomic studies at that time revealed that the ulnar arm of the arcuate ligament, also called the volar capitotriquetral ligament, was a significant stabilizer of the midcarpal joint. This ligament inserts proximally on the volar triquetrum, triquetrolunate ligament, and ulnar corner of the lunate. It then runs horizontally to the proximal hamate, to which it sends some fibers, and then inserts distally into the neck of the capitate. Sectioning of this sturdy ligament created midcarpal laxity that resembled the clinical picture of MCI. A more recent study (4) showed that, in addition to the horizontal fibers of the arcuate ligament, vertical fibers course from the volar triquetrum to the hook of the hamate and the pisohamate ligament. These fibers blend with the fascial insertion of the hypothenar muscles, as well as with the insertion of the tendon of the flexor carpi ulnaris around the pisiform. This confluence of structures is called the ulnar arcuate ligament complex (Fig. 50.1).

In 1990, Viegas et al. demonstrated that the dorsal radiolunotriquetral ligament (DRTL) also plays a major role in stabilizing the proximal row (5) (Fig. 50.2). After division of this ligament, a volar intercalary segmental instability (VISI) deformity occurs, reflecting hypermobility and excessive flexion of the entire proximal row (Fig. 50.3).

The pathomechanics of palmar MCI (PMCI) can be explained as follows: Laxity of the dorsal and palmar support ligaments permits the head of the capitate (and proximal ha-

mate) to sag volarly in the midcarpal joint. This volar translocation induces a passive VISI pattern or volar flexion deformity across the entire proximal row (Fig. 50.4). From this position, the normal articular interactions of the midcarpal joint cannot occur; that is, with radial to ulnar deviation, the normal smooth transition from proximal row flexion to proximal row extension is not seen. Instead, the VISI pattern (proximal row flexion) persists until ulnar deviation is complete, at which time a rapid "catch-up clunk" occurs as the proximal row jumps from excessive flexion into physiologic extension, and the head of the capitate and the hamate suddenly reseat themselves. Hypermobility of the proximal row is a hallmark of this condition.

What I have presented thus far is PMCI, which is, by far, the most common clinical type of MCI. A few cases of dorsal MCI have also been seen, but this condition is very rare. Combined dorsal and palmar MCI may also exist. Other authors have referred to instabilities at the midcarpal joint as capitolunate instability pattern (CLIP wrist) (6) and carpal instability nondissociative (7), but I believe that these terms are less descriptive names for essentially the same clinical condition described earlier (PMCI).

DIAGNOSIS

The diagnosis of PMCI can be made easily by history and physical examination once the examiner has had previous experience with this condition. The volar wrist sag can be seen by carefully looking at the wrist's configuration (Fig. 50.5). The clunk with ulnar deviation is obvious as the midpalmar sag reduces itself spontaneously. This reduction can be reproduced passively by the examiner by gentle axial compression, ulnar deviation, and intercarpal supination *(the midcarpal shift test)*. The patient will tell the examiner that this maneuver exactly duplicates the symptoms.

Radiographic and arthroscopic studies are essential to confirm the diagnosis. Aside from the characteristic VISI deformity and volar sag at the midcarpal joint (Fig. 50.2), the standard x-ray films are essentially normal. Because the

D. M. **Lichtman:** Department of Orthopaedic Surgery, John Peter Smith Hospital, Fort Worth, Texas.
R. W. **Culp:** The Philadelphia Hand Center, King of Prussia, Pennsylvania.
A. **Joshi:** Department of Orthopaedic Surgery, John Peter Smith Hospital, Fort Worth, Texas.

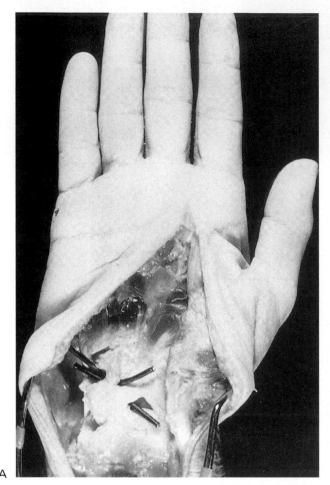
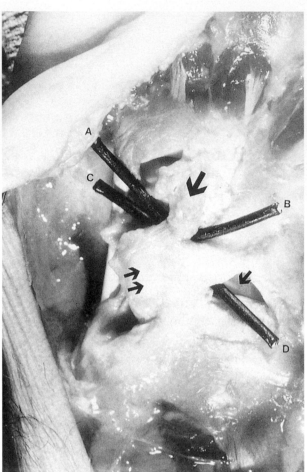

A   B

FIGURE 50.1   A: Overview of a dissected right cadaver hand and wrist. The contents of the carpal canal, the pisiform bone, and the pisohamate ligament have been removed. The radiolunate and radioscapholunate ligaments have also been removed to help visualization of the ulnar arcuate ligament complex. **B:** Close-up view of the same wrist. The *large arrow* points to the hook of the hamate. The *small arrow* points to the head of the capitate in the space of Poirier. The *double arrow* points to the triquetral facet of the pisotriquetral joint. Stick A-B runs beneath the vertical fibers of the ulnar arcuate ligament. Stick C-D runs under the vertical fibers distally and the broader horizontal fibers of arcuate ligament proximally.

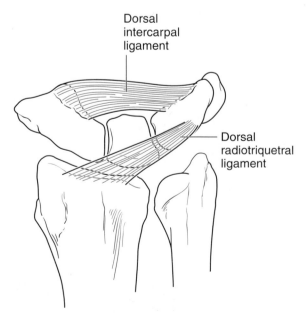

FIGURE 50.2 Doral capsular ligaments of the wrist: dorsal intercarpal ligament (DIL) and dorsal radiotriquetral ligament (DRTL).

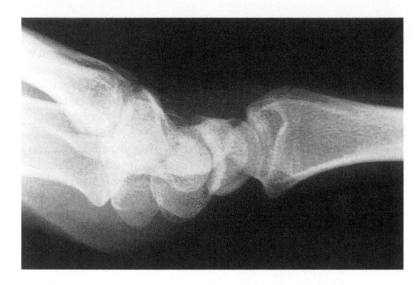

FIGURE 50.3 Lateral radiograph with the wrist in neutral deviation demonstrates the volar intercalary segmental instability deformity of the entire proximal row with volar positioning of the head of the capitate.

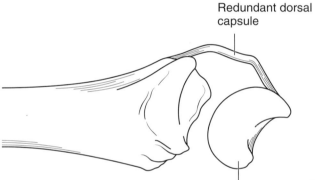

Redundant dorsal capsule

Lunate in volar tilt

FIGURE 50.4 Proximal volar intercalary segmental instability occurs after division or laxity of specific support structures (see text), which includes the dorsal radiotriquetral ligament.

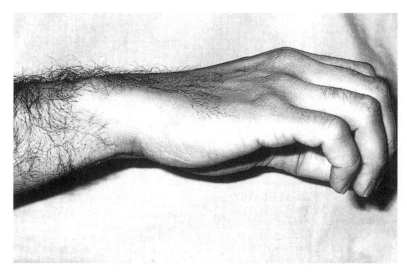

FIGURE 50.5 Volar wrist sag seen best from the ulnar side during clinical examination.

subluxation is easily reducible, plain films may not show the defect. In a few of my patients, a dissociative lesion of the proximal row has coexisted with the PMCI. In these cases, the x-ray picture can confuse the diagnosis because the signs and symptoms of PMCI almost always overshadow those of dissociative lesions, yet the latter are more striking on the x-ray films.

Video fluoroscopy always confirms the diagnosis of PMCI if the examiner knows what to look for. The sudden transition of the proximal row from VISI to DISI as the wrist goes into ulnar deviation coincides with the clunk. The entire proximal row rotates as a unit, and this feature distinguishes PMCI from triquetrolunate and scapholunate instability. When these dissociative lesions coexist with PMCI, the individual components can be identified, but it takes practice and patience to sort them out while viewing the videos.

Wrist arthroscopy is an important diagnostic adjunct to video fluoroscopy (9). It is essential to rule out dissociative lesions before surgical treatment of MCI. Gross triquetrolunate or scapholunate instability will compromise the surgical results of MCI repairs. Even mild dissociative lesions can be aggravated by procedures that stabilize the midcarpal joint. Although arthrography can demonstrate dissociative wrist lesions, this procedure is not as sensitive as arthroscopy. Bone scans do not add specific diagnostic information, and the indications for magnetic resonance imaging have not been fully defined for MCI.

NONSURGICAL TREATMENT

Conservative treatment of PMCI is always recommended initially. I start with splinting, avoidance of aggravating activities, and nonsteroidal antiinflammatory drugs. Most patients respond to simple conservative measures once the definitive diagnosis is made.

Clinical and laboratory investigations have shown that external dorsally directed pressure on the pisiform bone can eliminate the clunk of PMCI by reducing the proximal row VISI deformity and distal row sag. Upward pressure on the pisiform causes a downward rotation of the lunate and triquetrum out of the rotated VISI position. The proximal row becomes stabilized and colinear with the radius and distal row. Based on this finding, dynamic splints have been devised that support the proximal row in neutral while permitting active motion of the carpus and forearm.

Direct observation has also shown that active contraction of the extensor carpi ulnaris, flexor carpi ulnaris, and hypothenar muscles can also reduce the sagging (VISI) midcarpal joint. Some patients with MCI can eliminate the clunk by contracting these muscles before ulnar deviation of the wrist. More investigation needs to be done to determine the role of passive splinting as well as muscle rehabilitation in treating milder cases of PMCI.

SURGICAL TREATMENT

Surgery is indicated for patients in whom conservative management fails. Symptoms must be severe enough to interfere with activities of daily living. The patient must be also willing to sacrifice some loss of motion to relieve clunking and pain.

Initially, my surgical treatment of PMCI consisted of ligament reconstruction using a slip of extensor carpi ulnaris to stabilize the triquetrohamate joint. It then evolved to direct advancement and tightening of the ulnar arcuate ligament complex. Alternatively, arthrodesis of the midcarpal joint (triquetrum-hamate-lunate-capitate fusion) was performed for definitive stabilization.

More recently, I discontinued volar (ulnar arcuate ligament complex) reconstruction in favor of dorsal (DRTL) reefing. This procedure is based on the aforementioned findings that the DRTL is a major stabilizer of the midcarpal joint. I have confirmed this directly during surgical procedures on patients with MCI by temporarily reefing (clamping) the DRTL and noticing a significant improvement in the midcarpal shift test.

Dorsal reefing is a straightforward procedure. Begin with a dorsal longitudinal incision of 8 cm. centered over Lister's tubercle. Reflect full-thickness flaps of skin and subcutaneous tissue from the dorsal retinaculum. Remove the extensor pollicis longus from the third compartment. Divide the fourth compartment retinaculum for about 1 cm from its distal edge. Mobilize the dorsal extensor tendons from the wrist capsule. Reflect the extensor pollicis longus and dorsal wrist extensors radially and the common finger extensors ulnarly. The dorsal capsule is now exposed. Identify the DRTL coursing obliquely from the ulnar one-third of the distal radius to the dorsum of the triquetrum. Divide the ligament transversely by making a 3-cm incision in the dorsal wrist capsule, about 1 cm distal to the end of the radius with the patient's wrist distracted (Fig. 50.6A and B). Now, pull the distal capsular flap proximally to correct the volar rotation (VISI) of the lunate and proximal row (Fig. 50.6C). Check the lateral view on the C-arm to confirm neutral alignment of the proximal row and colinearity of the radius, lunate, and capitate. Now, place a 0.048-inch Kirschner wire (K-wire) subcutaneously from the triquetrum to the capitate to maintain midcarpal alignment. Next, place two rows of sutures (pants-over-vest) to shorten the dorsal capsule and maintain the tension on the proximal row (Fig. 50.6D). Place the extremity in a short-arm cast with the wrist in the neutral position. Remove the pin at 8 weeks, and begin gentle active range of motion at 12 weeks postoperatively.

In a published review of our first 16 operative cases (8), it was clear that midcarpal arthrodesis was the most reliable operative procedure, because 100% of patients treated with fusion obtained a satisfactory result. Nevertheless, when given a choice, many patients choose a soft tissue recon-

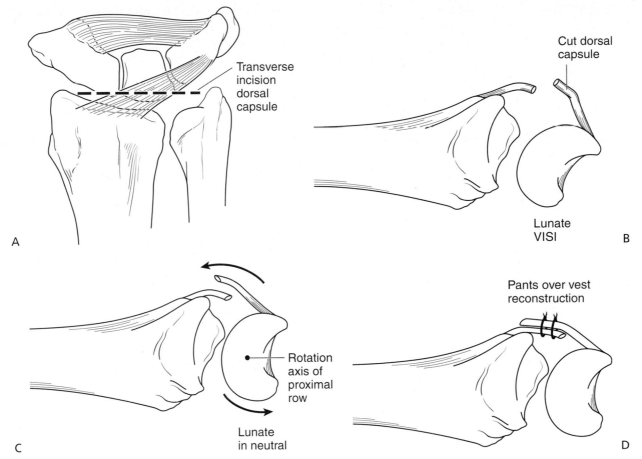

FIGURE 50.6 A and **B:** Location of the incision in the dorsal capsule and dorsal radiotriquetral ligament (DRTL). **C:** Volar intercalary segmental instability deformity can be corrected by pulling proximal distal flap of capsule and DRTL. This rotates the proximal row around its axis. **D:** Two rows of sutures (pants-over-vest) are placed to maintain capsular tightening.

struction, in the knowledge that if the clunk recurs, a fusion can be done at a later date. Future research in the area of wrist kinematics and anatomy should lead to more reliable methods of soft tissue stabilization.

ARTHROSCOPIC CAPSULAR SHRINKAGE

Electrothermal shrinkage techniques have gained popularity in the treatment of shoulder instability (10). Biologically, the efficacy of this method is based on the electrothermal disruption of the collagen bonds in capsular and ligamentous structures with subsequent healing in a shortened or tightened position (11). This understanding has led to the use of these techniques as a newer treatment option for MCI.

Technique

Place the patient supine on the operating table. Using a tower, provide 10 lb of traction through the index and long fingers. Inflate the wrist joint 1 cm distal to Lister's tubercle at the 3-4 portal and introduce the 2.7-mm arthroscope.

Evaluate the radiocarpal joint for any concomitant ligament or cartilage injuries. Advance the arthroscope between the radioscaphocapitate and long radiolunate ligaments palmarly. Remove the arthroscope, and place a switching stick into the arthroscopic cannula. The switching stick exits palmarly under the flexor carpi radialis tendon just proximal to the wrist crease. Make a small palmar incision to protect the flexor carpi radialis and neurovascular structures, and introduce the arthroscope over the switching stick to create a palmar portal. Identify the DRTL from this viewpoint (2). Now, replace the arthroscope into the 3-4 portal and identify the DRTL again by looking dorsoulnarly. Introduce a 1.5-mm electrothermal probe (Arthrocare, Sunnyvale, CA; or Oratec, Menlo Park, CA) into the palmar portal, and shrink the DRTL electrothermally with controlled temperatures. Adjust the tension by correcting any VISI deformity with a K-wire in the lunate under fluoroscopic control.

Develop a midcarpal radial portal by inflating the dorsal wrist joint on the radial side of the long metacarpal proximal to the capitate. Evaluate the midcarpal joint for other ligament or cartilage injuries. Identify the ulnar arm of the arcuate ligament complex, particularly the triquetrocapitate ligament, which runs obliquely from the triquetrum, across the proximal corner of the hamate, to the palmar neck of the capitate (2,4). Develop an ulnar midcarpal portal by entering the midcarpal joint at the center of the ring metacarpal proximal to the capitate and hamate. Introduce the electrothermal probe and thermally shrink the triquetrohamate ligament. Again, adjust the tension with correction of any VISI deformity.

Pin the midcarpal joint with 0.045 K-wires for 4 weeks to correct any VISI deformity. Have the patient begin a home program of early progressive range-of-motion and strengthening exercises using a removable splint between sessions.

Results

To date, five patients have undergone the procedure. The average age was 29 (range, 22 to 45) years. Follow-up has averaged 8 (range, 4 to 16) months. The midcarpal clunk resolved in four of the five patients with pain resolution. Range of motion decreased by an average of 20 degrees in the flexion-extension plane, whereas grip strengths increased by an average of 15%. Further follow-up will be needed to assess the efficacy of this newer procedure.

CONCLUSIONS

In summary, PMCI is an uncommon but not rare clinical condition. Improved understanding of the anatomy and physiology of the midcarpal joint has led to the development of promising new rehabilitative as well as operative techniques. Arthroscopic examination of the wrist is helpful in ruling out dissociative lesions of the proximal row, which,

if they exist, must be addressed before or concomitant with the surgical treatment of PMCI. Arthroscopic capsular shrinkage for PMCI is currently under investigation and has shown promising results in a limited number of cases.

REFERENCES

1. Mouchet A, Belot J. Poignet à résault (subluxation médiocarpienne en avant). *Bull Mem Soc Natl Chir* 1934;60:1243–1244.
2. Lichtman DM, Schnedier JR, Swafford AR. Midcarpal instability. Presented at the 35th annual meeting of the American Society for Surgery of the Hand, Atanta, GA, 1980.
3. Lichtman DM, Schnedier JR, Swafford AR, et al. Ulnar midcarpal instability: clinical and laboratory analysis. J Hand Surg 1981;6:515–523.
4. Lichtman DM, Niccolai TA, et al. The ulnar arcuate ligament complex: its anatomy and functional significance. Presented at the 43rd annual meeting of the American Society for Surgery of the Hand, Baltimore, MD, 1988.
5. Viegas SF, Patterson RM, Peterson PD, et al. Ulnar-sided perilunate instability: an anatomic and biomechanic study. *J Hand Surg Am* 1990;15:268–277.
6. Johnson RP, CarreraGF. Chronic capitolunate instability. *J Bone Joint Surg Am* 1980;68:1164–1176.
7. Dobyns JH, Linchied RL, Wadih SM, et al. Carpal instability, nondissociative (CIND). Presented at the annual meeting of the American Academy of Orthopedic Surgeons, San Francisco, CA, 1987.
8. Lichtman DM, Bruckner JD, Culp RW, et al. Palmer midcarpal instability: results of surgical reconstruction. *J Hand Surg [Am]* 1993;18:307–315.
9. Berger RA. Arthroscopic anatomy of the wrist and distal radioulnar joint. *Hand Clin* 1999;15:393–413.
10. Anderson K, McCarty EC, Warren RF. Thermal capsulorrhaphy: where are we today? *Sports Med Arthrosc Rev* 1999;7:117–127.
11. Naseef GS, Foster TE, Traunerk, et al. The thermal properties of bovine joint capsule. the basic science of laser and radio frequency-induced capsular shrinkage. *Am J Sports Med* 1997;25:670–674.

INTRAARTICULAR FRACTURES OF THE DISTAL RADIUS

GREGORY J. HANKER

Fractures of the distal radius remain extremely common injuries and represent the most frequent type of fracture in the upper extremity (1–4). The distal radius fracture occurs in all age groups, from children to the elderly. These injuries are more frequent in preadolescents and adolescents than in adults (5). In the adult population, distal radius fractures usually result from high-energy injuries, such as motor vehicle accidents, falls from moderate heights, or sports activities (6,7). After age 50 years, the injury rate in women is four times that found in men (5).

Although distal radius fracture is a common injury, there is no universal agreement about treatment regimens or classification systems. Older modalities of treatment that were not concerned with restoration of anatomic alignment, or intraarticular joint congruity, are no longer acceptable. It is now clear that postfracture deformity will lead to a significant functional hand impairment (8,9). Over the past decade, many orthopaedists have clearly focused our attention on the complexity of the distal radius fracture and on the critical importance of providing appropriate surgical treatment (1–4,10–16). We are beginning to appreciate the presence of associated injuries to the wrist cartilage and intraarticular soft tissue restraints, such as the intercarpal ligaments and the triangular fibrocartilage complex (TFCC) (17,18).

Our treatment goal in either the conservative treatment or the surgical management of displaced, intraarticular distal radius fractures is to restore the overall anatomy of the distal radius to within acceptable anatomic parameters. Knirk and Jupiter were the first to bring our attention to the importance of restoring articular congruity in the treatment of the distal radius fracture. Specifically, articular displacement in excess of 1 mm should not be accepted. Otherwise, the fracture is virtually guaranteed to develop posttraumatic osteoarthritis (19). Since the 1990s, multiple authors have found a high prevalence of intraarticular soft tissue lesions

associated with a distal radius fracture (17,18,20–25). The benefit of arthroscopic management of the intraarticular distal radius fracture has also been increasingly appreciated. Arthroscopic evaluation of the fractured wrist joint provides a new dimension of care for the treating surgeon and provides a direct tool to evaluate the complexity of the bony and soft tissue injuries thoroughly, to manage these injuries definitively, and to assist with the critical fracture reduction of the intraarticular segments (18,20–30).

ANATOMY

The wrist is an extremely complex joint. The multiple bony articulations gain additional support through a complex interconnecting array of extrinsic and intrinsic ligaments. The wrist is a system of multiple joints and articulations, which together permit the complex range of motion in six different directions, around three variable axes. All told, there are 15 bones that provide 45 articular surfaces within the wrist joint. The kinematics of this complex wrist system remains difficult to comprehend fully.

Distal radius fractures should initially be assessed with standard plain radiographs, including posteroanterior and lateral views, at the very minimum. Additional views, such as an oblique view, can be obtained as needed. From these plain radiographs, a determination can be made about the complexity of the fracture, and, possibly, information can be obtained about associated carpal or distal radioulnar joint (DRUJ) injuries. The posteroanterior and lateral radiographs of the injured wrist should be obtained using standard positioning of the extremity. By careful analysis of the radiographs, the degree of displacement from normal anatomic parameters can usually be ascertained with a significant degree of accuracy. In some complex cases of distal radius fractures, especially when there is significant impaction of the joint surfaces, computed tomographic scans and magnetic resonance imaging can help to shed additional light on the positioning of the fracture fragments and their degree of displacement.

G. J. Hanker: Hand and Upper Extremity Surgery, Southern California Orthopaedic Institute, Van Nuys, California.

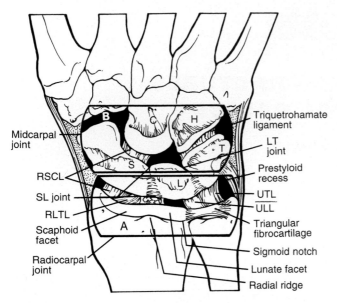

FIGURE 51.1 A: Arthroscopic appearance of the radiocarpal joint. The cartilaginous inferior surfaces of the proximal carpal row and the scaphoid and lunate facets of the distal radius can be clearly seen. The fracture pattern, displacement of the fracture fragments, injuries to the extrinsic and intrinsic ligaments, and the triangular fibrocartilage complex (TFCC) can be diagnosed by viewing through the dorsoradial and dorsoulnar portals. **B:** Arthroscopic appearance of the midcarpal joint. During the arthroscopic treatment of a distal radius fracture, the midcarpal joint is usually not entered unless it is necessary to treat an intrinsic ligament injury of the scapholunate ligament (SLL) or lunotriquetral ligament (LTL). Notice that the scapholunate joint (SLJ) and lunotriquetral joint (LTJ) are devoid of ligamentous attachments in this space, and thus a clear view of the anatomic relationship between the scaphoid and lunate or lunate and triquetrum can be obtained.

Because wrist arthroscopy is an important adjunct tool to assist with the evaluation of the bony and soft tissue intraarticular injuries, it is essential that the treating physician be familiar with normal arthroscopic anatomy (Fig. 51.1). Arthroscopic reduction and internal fixation (ARIF) of distal radius fractures has the distinct advantage of producing minimal surgical trauma and providing excellent visualization of the injured joint surface. This then allows for an accurate reassembly of the articular fracture fragments under direct visualization and definitive management of injuries to the cartilage, intrinsic ligaments, TFCC, and capsular tissues.

CLASSIFICATION

Multiple classification systems attempt to define the varying patterns of articular fracture at the distal end of the radius (1–4,31). The purpose of these fracture classification systems is to serve as a means of communication between treating physicians so common patterns of injury are described. The ideal classification system, one hopes, not only would serve as a basis for determining appropriate treatment of the

injury, but also would suggest outcomes after treatment. The classification system could also suggest the possibility or probability of associated internal injuries of the wrist, such as intrinsic ligamentous injuries with associated carpal instabilities, or TFCC injuries that could lead to DRUJ problems.

Many of these classification systems combine both intraarticular and extraarticular fracture patterns. The Frykman, Melone, Mayo, and AO/ASIF (Arbeitsgemeinschaft für osteosynthesefragen/Association for the Study of Internal Fixation) classification schemes help us to stratify the various patterns of bony injury: extraarticular versus intraarticular, and the relationship of intraarticular bony fragments with regard to displacement and comminution (Table 51.1). The Frykman classification focuses on the intraarticular extension of the fracture and involvement of the ulna styloid. It indirectly implies that the involvement of these structures contributes to the complexity of the fracture and the difficulty of treatment. In the Frykman system, displaced and nondisplaced fractures are considered equally important. Unfortunately, for this reason, the Frykman system cannot be used to predict outcome of treatment. The Mayo classification is similar to that of Frykman, that is, extraarticular versus intraarticular, but it introduces an additional variable that attempts to distinguish the extension of the distal radius fracture into the radioscaphoid or radiolunate joint. In the Mayo classification system, injury to the distal ulna is excluded.

The Melone classification was probably the first system to provide an accurate description of the pattern of the intraarticular fracture of the distal radius. This classification is relevant to intraarticular fractures only, because extraarticular fractures are not included in the scheme. The Melone classification system places importance on the medial portion of the articular fracture. The AO/ASIF classification system is the most comprehensive, but also the most detailed, thus making it somewhat difficult to remember the multiple fracture categories. In the AO/ASIF system, distal radius fractures are classified into three main types and are then further subdivided into subgroups. The classification is arranged in an ascending order of severity, according to the anatomic complexity of the fracture. Other classification systems exist, such as the Gartland and Werley, Sarmiento, Fernandez, McMurtry and Jupiter, and Cooney. Each of these classification systems is based on an analysis of the injury radiographs. The classification systems attempt to direct our attention to the pattern and degree of joint disruption. Unfortunately, several reports have indicated that these classification systems are of no predictive value for clinical outcome. The AO/ASIF classification scheme, because of its complexity, possesses the further problem of being highly unreliable because of high interobserver and intraobserver nonreliability. All the systems, unfortunately, possess poor reliability for the basic classification process itself. They are not easily reproducible. The treating physician

TABLE 51.1 CLASSIFICATION SCHEMES TO DESCRIBE FRACTURES OF THE DISTAL RADIUS

Frykman classification	
Type I	Extraarticular pattern
Type II	Extraarticular with distal ulna fracture
Type III	Intraarticular pattern involving only the radiocarpal joint
Type IV	Intraarticular into the radiocarpal joint with a distal ulna fracture
Type V	Intraarticular pattern involving only the distal radioulnar joint
Type VI	Intraarticular into the distal radioulnar joint with a distal ulna fracture
Type VII	Intraarticular into both radiocarpal and distal radioulnar joints
Type VIII	Intraarticular into radiocarpal and distal radioulnar joints with distal ulna fracture
Mayo classification	
Type I	Extraarticular
Type II	Intraarticular involving the radioscaphoid joint
Type III	Intraarticular involving the radiolunate joint
Type IV	Intraarticular involving the radioscapholunate joint
Melone classification	
Type I	Undisplaced or displaced four-part fracture but stable after reduction
Type II	Comminution and instability with displacement of the medial complex as a unit
Type III	Volar spike fragment present
Type IV	Profound displacement of the four-part fracture, with wide separation or rotation
Type V	Burst injury pattern
AO/ASIF classification	
Group A	Extraarticular, metaphyseal fracture
Group B	Intraarticular rim fracture
B1	Radial styloid fracture
B2	Dorsal rim fracture
B3	Volar rim fracture
Group C	Complex, intraarticular fracture disrupting the continuity of the epiphysis and metaphysis
C1	Radiocarpal joint congruity preserved, metaphysis fractured
C2	Articular displacement
C3	Diaphyseal-metaphyseal involvement

AO/ASIF, Arbeitsgemeinschaft für osteosynthesefragen/Association for the Study of Internal Fixation.

should be cognizant of the main issues involved when attempting to classify the nature of the distal radius injury. It is probably best to think in terms of fracture displacement, especially articular displacement. It is also important to consider angulation, shortening, the degree of fracture comminution, and the quality of bone stock represented on the injury radiographs. This simple assessment will more than

likely serve as a basis for the evaluating physician to determine the appropriate choice of treatment.

Unfortunately, none of these classification systems is helpful in ascertaining the likelihood of an associated complicating injury to the wrist joint soft tissue restraints. In my personal experience in treating distal radius fractures over the past 15 years, I have found that carpal or DRUJ instability is not specifically associated with any of the various fracture classification systems. This means that the occurrence of a wrist instability can happen randomly in any type of distal radius fracture. Thus, our current methods of classification are not very useful in determining which patients will have wrist instability. Conversely, there is no statistically significant relationship between any arthroscopic findings (i.e., ligament tear, TFCC tear, or cartilage injury) and the fracture classification systems discussed earlier. Therefore, the occurrence of a serious intrinsic or extrinsic ligamentous injury, TFCC injury, or cartilage injury can happen randomly in any type of distal radius fracture. Other authors have shown that ligamentous and TFCC injuries are easily overlooked and are frequently not considered when one interprets the initial injury radiographs. Arthrography of the fractured distal radius may be of some benefit, but it is certainly difficult to perform on an injured patient with substantial amount of wrist pain (32). It has come to the attention of several traumatologists that operative wrist arthroscopy is probably the most effective way to diagnose definitively a suspected ligamentous injury of the wrist, as well as associated soft tissue and cartilage injuries.

ASSOCIATED INJURIES

Arthroscopic evaluation of the fractured wrist joint provides the treating physician with the unique capability to examine the full extent of the internal pathologic process directly. A thorough visual examination of the radiocarpal joint and, if necessary, the midcarpal and distal radioulnar joints, will directly define the nature and extent of the bony, cartilaginous, and soft tissue ligamentous injuries. Significant associated injuries are the rule, not the exception. These ligamentous, cartilage, and fibrocartilaginous injuries were previously ignored (17). For that reason, appropriate treatment has been lacking regarding intrinsic ligamentous, cartilage, capsular, or TFCC injuries. It is now unacceptable simply to treat the bony injury of the distal radius and to ignore the associated internal soft tissue and cartilage injuries.

Over the past several years, especially since this chapter was initially written in the second edition of *Operative Arthroscopy* in 1996 (18), many investigative studies have been done describing in detail the importance of arthroscopic management of intraarticular distal radius fractures. Furthermore, the intercarpal soft tissue lesions associated with these intraarticular distal radius fractures have been

TABLE 51.2 FREQUENCY OF ASSOCIATED ARTHROSCOPIC FINDINGS WITH INTRAARTICULAR DISTAL RADIUS FRACTURES

Parameter	Frequency %
Triangular fibrocartilage complex tear, acute	64
Type 1A	4
Type 1B	3
Type 1C	6
Type 1D	51
Combination	8
Degenerative	13
Carpal instability	26
Scapholunate joint	9
Lunatotriquetral joint	12
Perilunate	5
Distal radioulnar joint instability	8
Osteochondral fracture	20
Intraarticular loose bodies	16
Dorsal capsular tears	70

identified, and their frequency has been fairly well determined.

I treated 205 cases of intraarticular fractures of the distal radius with the technique of ARIF (Table 51.2). An analysis of Table 51.2 reveals several obvious findings. There is an extremely high incidence of TFCC tears in association with intraarticular distal radius fractures (64%). Most of these TFCC tears are type 1D, because they result from an avulsion of the central disc off its attachment to the sigmoid notch of the distal radius (Fig. 51.2). The type 1D pattern is seen almost exclusively with the distal radius fracture. This

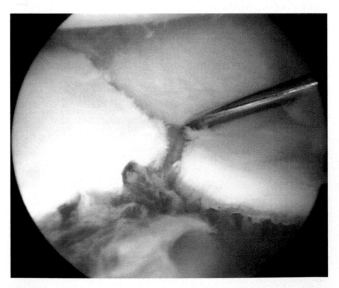

FIGURE 51.2 Arthroscopic appearance of an acute type 1D triangular fibrocartilage complex (TFCC) tear resulting from a Melone type IV intraarticular fracture. The probe is at the intersection of the torn TFCC *(to the right)* and the sigmoid notch *(to the left).*

injury can be arthroscopically repaired, as suggested by several authors. However, there is no justifiable reason to spend extra time and effort to repair the central disc avulsion from the sigmoid notch, because this portion is avascular, and it always runs the risk of improper healing. In addition, repair adds additional time and significant complexity to the overall fracture reduction process. I favor simple arthroscopic excision of the torn central portion of the disc. This uniformly results in a satisfactory result, and it is very easy to accomplish with standard arthroscopic instrumentation during the course of the ARIF.

The most common pattern of TFCC tear associated with a "sprained" wrist is the central type 1A, which is rarely seen with a distal radius fracture. Also noteworthy is that 8% of my patients had a complex tear of the TFCC, with an additional dorsal peripheral detachment from the capsule. Only 3% of patients had an ulnar detachment, despite a high incidence of ulna styloid fractures.

In 26% of the intraarticular distal radius fractures, carpal instability was present: 9% involving scapholunate joint (SLJ) instability primarily resulting from a complete tear of the scapholunate ligament (SLL) (Fig. 51.3A and B) and 12% involving lunotriquetral joint (LTJ) instability resulting from a full-substance lunotriquetral ligament (LTL) tear (Fig. 51.4). Perilunate injury patterns were noticed in 5% of patients and resulted from complete tears of both the SLL and LTL. DRUJ instability was present in a surprisingly high 8% of patients. The instability appeared to be primarily associated with the bony component of the fracture and, to a lesser degree, with the TFCC component. The dorsomedial fracture fragment is usually displaced, and it is often still attached to the dorsal portion of the torn TFCC. This leads to a widening and separation of the sigmoid notch and subsequent increased translation of the distal ulna at its articulation with the sigmoid notch of the distal radius. This significant disruption of the dorsomedial fracture component explains the presence of the DRUJ instability.

The dorsal capsule was torn in 70% of patients. Associated with disruption of the capsule is the possibility of tearing of the extrinsic dorsal capsular ligaments, and this could also lead to some degree of added instability. This may explain why the closed treatment of displaced and comminuted distal radius fractures using the technique of capsuloligamentodesis could fail to maintain the fracture reduction because of the loss of the extrinsic dorsal ligaments. Osteochondral fractures were seen in 20% of the cases and often involved the dorsal, inferior surface of the lunate. Intraarticular loose bodies were found in 16% of cases.

Since my initial presentation in 1993 to the American Society for Surgery of the Hand at the annual meeting in Orlando, Florida (17), there have been many other reports regarding the associated ligamentous and chondral injuries discovered during the arthroscopic evaluation of an intraarticular distal radius fracture. In 1995, Seibert et al. presented their work indicating that ARIF was a very helpful tech-

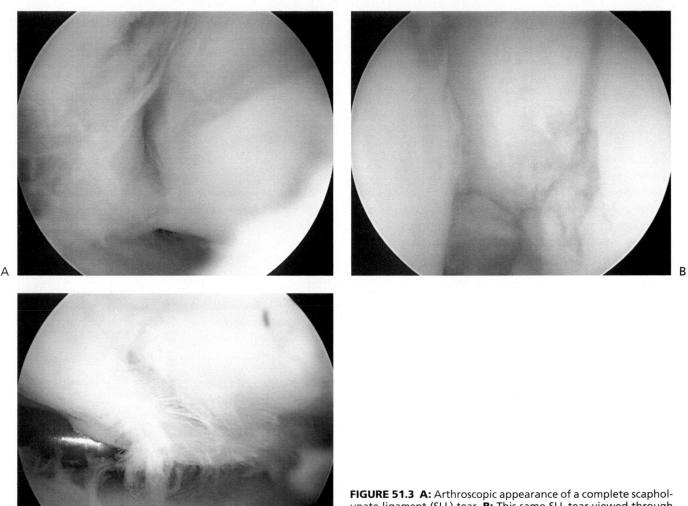

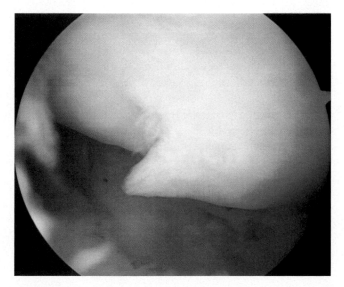

FIGURE 51.3 A: Arthroscopic appearance of a complete scapholunate ligament (SLL) tear. **B:** This same SLL tear viewed through the gross diastasis of the scapholunate joint (SLJ). This would be considered a grade IV intercarpal ligamentous tear, with SLJ instability. **C:** Incomplete tear through the membranous portion of the SLL. No instability is present.

FIGURE 51.4 Complete tear of the lunotriquetral joint (LTL) from its attachment to the inferior pole of the triquetrum. Dynamic instability is present.

nique. In their 18 patients who were treated with this technique, these surgeons found five TFCC tears, ten SLL tears, and five chondral fractures involving the proximal pole of the scaphoid (20). In 1996, Geissler et al. reported on 60 cases of intraarticular distal radius fractures, and these surgeons found 26 TFCC tears, 19 SLL tears, and nine LTL tears; in 13 of the 60 patients, there were at least two associated injuries. These investigators also proposed a classification system that allowed for arthroscopic evaluation of ligament tears (21). In 1997, Richards et al. presented their arthroscopic findings in the evaluation of 118 patients. These surgeons found a 35% incidence of TFCC tears, 22% SLL tears, 7% LTL tears, and 6% perilunate injuries. They also performed arthroscopy on a significant number of patients with extraarticular distal radius fractures. Surprisingly, there was a very high percentage of associated intraarticular injuries even with these extraarticular fractures. These investigators found the following in patients with the extraarticular fractures: 53% TFCC tears, 7% SLL tears, and 13% LTL tears. In their review of the preoperative radiographs, these surgeons found that shortening and dorsal angulation of the intraarticular fracture components correlated with the presence of a TFCC tear, but not with interosseous ligamentous tears (22). That same year, Lindau et al. found in their 50 patients a 78% incidence of TFCC tears, which they thought correlated to the presence of an ulna styloid fracture. These surgeons also found a 54% incidence of SLL tears and a 32% incidence of chondral lesions. In their 50 patients, no major instability was discovered. There were, however, significant numbers of combined injuries involving the TFCC, intrinsic ligaments, or combinations thereof (23).

More recently, in 1999, Geissler and Freeland reviewed their experience with associated injuries and found a 50% incidence of TFCC tears and described their arthroscopic technique to help classify tears of the intercarpal ligaments (24). In 2000, Mehta et al. found an incidence of 58% TFCC tears, 85% SLJ instability, 61% LTJ instability, and 19% osteochondral lesions (25).

From these data, it can be seen that the incidence of associated injuries is quite high. Triangular fibrocartilage complex injuries are the most common, and, as previously mentioned, they usually consist of an acute type 1D injury pattern. However, complex injuries can occur in which the TFCC is torn in several locations. The TFCC is arthroscopically evaluated from the dorsoradial, dorsoulnar, and ulnar wrist portals during the course of ARIF. The treatment of these TFCC tears follows standard recommendations for the arthroscopic management of acute TFCC injuries (33–35). Basically, central tears are arthroscopically debrided, leaving behind a healthy peripheral and stable rim of fibrocartilage; peripheral tears, usually dorsal from the wrist capsule or ulnarly from the styloid, can also be arthroscopically repaired, with the placement of appropriate sutures.

Ligamentous injuries should be evaluated during the course of the ARIF and then addressed after reduction of the distal radius fracture. Many possible injuries to the intrinsic ligaments can be seen arthroscopically. These include a severe grade II injury of the ligament in which the ligamentous fibers are attenuated, but the ligament itself is basically intact. There can be complete tearing of the membranous portion of the ligament, in which case debridement of the membranous tear is accomplished arthroscopically. If there is a complete tear of the intercarpal ligament with obvious instability, this will need to be managed with reduction of the unstable joint, and with either percutaneous pin fixation techniques or open ligamentous repairs (36–39).

Carpal bone chondral injuries are best managed with chondroplasty. This is usually performed with the full-radius shaver debriding injured and unstable cartilage fragments, while burring down to a cancellous bone base. This is done in an attempt to incite a fibrocartilaginous healing response. Loose bodies are harvested with the use of grasping instruments. Tears of the dorsal capsule are debrided with a full-radius shaver.

TREATMENT OF ACUTE DISTAL RADIUS FRACTURES IN ADULTS

In an adult patient with an intraarticular distal radius fracture, the physical examination should take into account the patient's age, gender, occupation, activity level, handedness, and overall physical condition. Any complicating injuries, such as nerve or tendon dysfunction, should be identified on the preoperative evaluation and appropriately treated. In the rare event that the fracture is open, immediate surgical treatment is necessary. In a closed injury, the first step is to obtain good-quality posteroanterior and lateral radiographs of the fractured wrist. In most cases, these plain radiographs are usually sufficient to determine a management plan, because the degree of comminution, angulation, shortening, and the quality of bone stock can be ascertained. The radiographic hallmarks of an unstable distal radius fracture are metaphyseal comminution and excessive articular fragmentation. When these features are present, some form of stabilization of the fracture fragments will be necessary. If there is any doubt about the complexity of the fracture and the displacement of the fracture fragments, it is best to obtain a computed tomography scan of the distal radius before deciding on a management program. However, this is rarely necessary because ARIF provides a more accurate assessment

Many excellent treatment algorithms can be used in the decision-making process to select the appropriate management of these displaced intraarticular distal radius fracture. Distal radius fractures that are undisplaced, or are displaced and stable, can usually be reduced with manipulation and then managed with cast immobilization and an early therapy program. The displaced, unstable fractures of the distal radius are best treated with closed reduction with the patient under anesthesia and with some form of percutaneous Kirschner wire (K-wire) fixation. This is usually the least invasive technique with the greatest potential for a successful outcome. Various alternative management techniques have been described in the literature. The surgical management of shearing fractures and articular compression fractures is well described by Jupiter, Fernandez, and Trumbull et al. (1,2,15). The choice of technique depends on the experience of the treating surgeon. Good to excellent results have been reported with a variety of surgical techniques, such as open reduction and internal fixation using AO/ASIF distal radius fracture plates, percutaneous Kapandji pinning or Py pinning, application of various external fixation frames (40–43), and supplemental bone grafting with either autogenous graft or injectable calcium phosphate compounds (44,45).

The surgical goal for all these management systems is to restore the distal radius anatomy, that is, radial height, radial inclination, palmar tilt. The articular component of the distal radius fracture requires an exact anatomic reduction, because even a minimal step-off in excess of 1 mm is often associated with the development of posttraumatic osteoarthritis. The intraarticular fractures obviously present the greatest challenge to the treating physician. As we have seen, even nondisplaced, stable intraarticular fractures can be associated with serious ligamentous or TFCC injuries. We are also now beginning to realize that nondisplaced, extraarticular fractures of the distal radius may also have a high association of significant intraarticular injuries. Certainly, the displaced and unstable intraarticular fracture of the dis-

tal radius will require some modality of surgical treatment. The intraarticular fracture pattern, as classified by Melone, is quite helpful in understanding the nature of the fracture and the possibility for associated injuries, as well as to anticipate problems of fracture fragment reduction (Fig. 51.5) (31).

The treatment of distal radius fractures in the athlete deserves special mention. The conservative medical or surgical management of an athlete's distal radius fracture, and any associated injuries, follows already well-established treatment principles of orthopaedic care discussed earlier. What is different in the management of the athlete's fractured wrist is the great pressure placed on the treating physician to minimize lost time from athletic competition. Specific orthopaedic treatment must be custom tailored to the following: the location of the injured tissues; the severity and extent of the tissue trauma; the athlete's age, in terms of preadolescent versus skeletally mature versus elderly; level of competition; and the sport-specific demands, especially if a unique performance task is required of a particular position in that sport. Sound orthopaedic principles should not be compromised in an attempt to return the athlete to early sports participation (6,7).

An arthroscopic examination of the intraarticular distal radius fracture complements fracture care (Fig. 51.6); it does not substitute for well-established surgical techniques to reduce and stabilize the fracture. Because the primary goal in the management of these fractures is to restore the articular congruity, the arthroscope affords a direct visual tool to monitor the success of the reduction. Several authors have discovered that arthroscopic visualization of the fractured

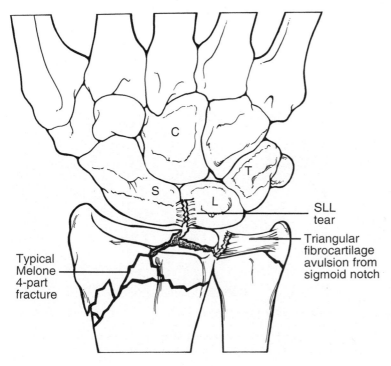

FIGURE 51.5 Typical four-part intraarticular distal radius fracture as described by Melone. In my experience, the sagittal fracture line is typically adjacent to the ridge separating the scaphoid from lunate facets. The force of the fracture extends into the radioscapholunate ligament and causes it to tear. Additional force leads to tearing of the scapholunate ligament (SLL) and possible carpal instability. The coronal fracture line extends ulnarly from the ridge and usually displaces two or more medial fracture fragments. The dorsomedial or volar medial fracture fragments may be impacted and difficult to reduce. If sufficient energy is available along the coronal fracture line, the force will cause tearing of the triangular fibrocartilage complex (TFCC). The central disc will be avulsed from its attachment to the sigmoid notch of the radius. In some cases, the coronal fracture line will be obliquely oriented and can lead to a dorsal peripheral tear of the TFCC or a volar tear of the ulnolunate ligament.

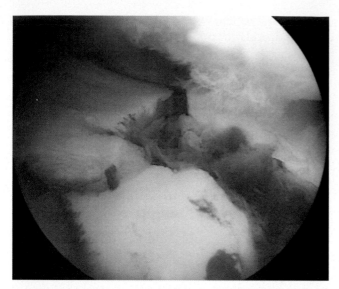

FIGURE 51.6 Arthroscopic appearance of a typical four-part intraarticular distal radius fracture.

cartilaginous surfaces of the distal radius is far superior to either fluoroscopic control or open arthrotomy. Since this chapter was last prepared in 1996, more than eight reports in the orthopaedic literature have recommended the technique of ARIF. These authors have found that the technique is helpful for obtaining an accurate and anatomic reduction of the displaced distal radius fracture fragments, is a useful adjunct to other surgical management options, is beneficial in reducing and fixing the dorsomedial fracture fragment, appears to provide a better result than standard open reduction and internal fixation (ORIF), and is basically effective and safe. The arthroscope provides an illuminated and magnified viewing field within the injured wrist joint. This presents the ideal situation in which the treating surgeon can then reconstruct the fractured distal radius joint surface and search for associated intercarpal injuries. The technique of ARIF also assists with placement of fixation devices to stabilize the distal radius fracture. The hope is that with the use of these improved adjunctive arthroscopic techniques, displacement of depressed distal radius fracture fragments can be avoided, thus minimizing any major postoperative problems such as malunion and subsequent posttraumatic degenerative joint disease (46). Distal radius malunion with resultant dorsal tilt of approximately 20 degrees can have significant alterations in the interosseous membrane tightness, which would then subsequently limit pronation and supination of the forearm, as well as general flexibility of the wrist (47). It is also responsible for the development of midcarpal instability.

Surgical outcome is improved with the use of assisted arthroscopy because of the added degree of accuracy in reducing the intraarticular components of the fracture, thus providing superior healing of the joint surface with less chance of posttraumatic wrist arthrosis. Thorough visualization of the injured wrist joint also provides the ability to de-

tect and treat the serious associated ligamentous, fibrocartilaginous, or cartilage injuries now known to occur in a high percentage of these cases. Such associated wrist problems—carpal instability, TFCC tears, or osteochondral injuries—would otherwise remain undetected and untreated and could lead to further chronic wrist disorders.

TECHNIQUE OF ARTHROSCOPIC-ASSISTED REDUCTION AND INTERNAL FIXATION

The fundamental principles of operating room setup, a well-trained surgical team, proper fracture instrumentation, and arthroscopic equipment are all necessary to carry out a successful procedure. Much equipment is needed to perform the arthroscopic surgical treatment of the displaced, intraarticular distal radius fracture. A large operating room is quite helpful (Fig. 51.7). The patient with the intraarticular distal radius fracture can be brought to the operating room at virtually any time after the injury. I have not noticed any difference in the technique if the operation is performed on the same day of the injury or is delayed for 7 to 10 days. There will usually be some degree of intraarticular bleeding through the fracture site, and this is easily managed with through-and-through irrigation and an upper arm pneumatic tourniquet. Usually, regional anesthesia such as an axillary block is performed. A small, portable fluoroscopic x-ray unit allows for easy manipulation about the surgical field without the bulk and awkwardness of the larger units.

After a pneumatic tourniquet is wrapped on the patient's upper arm and the limb is prepared and draped, the index, middle, and ring fingers are placed in finger traps and suspended in overhead traction through a standard shoulder boom affixed to the operating table. Seven to 12 lb of traction weight is exerted across the wrist, depending on the size of the patient's arm. If available, a traction tower can be used, but is not essential to carry out a successful procedure.

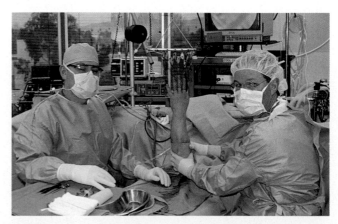

FIGURE 51.7 Operating room setup for arthroscopic reduction and internal fixation. A vast amount of arthroscopic, fluoroscopic, and fracture fixation equipment is necessary, and it must be properly positioned for ease of access.

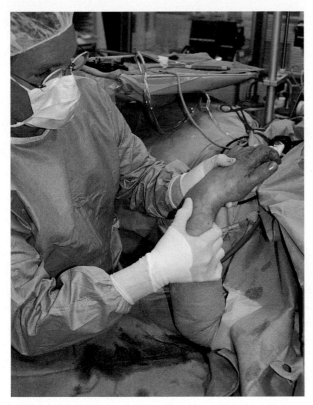

FIGURE 51.8 A closed reduction of the distal radius fracture can be performed either directly, as shown here; or with the limb in traction, as shown in Fig. 51.7.

The surgeon performs a closed reduction of the distal radius fracture by direct manual manipulation (Fig. 51.8). The portable fluoroscope is helpful at this point because the surgeon can use it to determine whether radial height, inclination, and palmar tilt have been restored. In addition, some preliminary information about the articular congruity can also be obtained. However, I caution that a significant step-off in the articular fracture fragments can exist, even when the fluoroscopic image looks as though an anatomic reduction has been achieved. On occasion, an intercarpal ligamentous injury that could lead to carpal instability may become apparent on the fluoroscopic image when traction is exerted across the wrist joint. A step-off or separation at the SLJ or LTJ could possibly represent a complete tear of the SLL or LTL, respectively.

The radiocarpal joint is infused with saline. The 3-4 dorsoradial portal is prepared, and the arthroscopic sheath with blunt trocar is introduced atraumatically into the wrist joint. Inflow is established through this cannula. I have not found it helpful to use a separate portal for inflow. I have also not experienced any significant extravasation of the arthroscopic fluid into the adjacent soft tissues about the dorsum of the hand or the forearm. If a computerized fluid management pump is being used, the pressure should be kept low, at approximately 20 torr. Outflow is usually done through the shaver or suction punch apparatus, which is in-

serted in a separate portal. At the beginning of the procedure, a 19-gauge hypodermic needle can be inserted in the vicinity of the 6R dorsoulnar portal. Lavage of the radiocarpal joint with saline can assist with the removal of intraarticular fracture debris, hematoma, and fibrin clot (Fig. 51.9).

The 2.7-mm, 30-degree small joint arthroscope is inserted into the 3-4 dorsoradial portal, and the injured wrist joint is examined systematically. Diagnostic arthroscopy is facilitated by placing a motorized full-radius shaver into the dorsoulnar portal to suction the remaining fracture debris from the joint. Full visualization of the fracture is not possible until all debris is removed (Fig. 51.10). The articular congruity of the distal radius intraarticular fracture fragments now can be assessed thoroughly. Visualization from both the dorsoradial and dorsoulnar portals is absolutely necessary to determine the position and alignment of the fracture fragments fully (Fig. 51.11). When all the fracture lines can be seen, the success of the initial reduction can be observed. Equally important is full evaluation of the integrity of all intrinsic wrist ligaments, volar extrinsic ligaments, TFCC, capsule, cartilaginous surfaces of the distal radius and carpal bones, and if at all possible, extrinsic dorsal wrist ligaments.

If the articular fracture fragments are still displaced more than 1 mm, an attempt must be made to disimpact the fragments and restore as smooth an articular surface as possible.

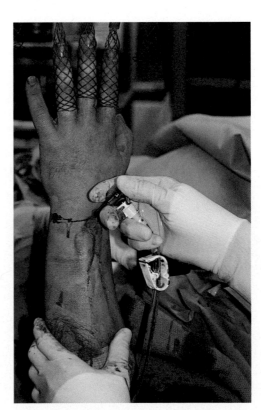

FIGURE 51.9 The fracture debris is lavaged from the radiocarpal joint.

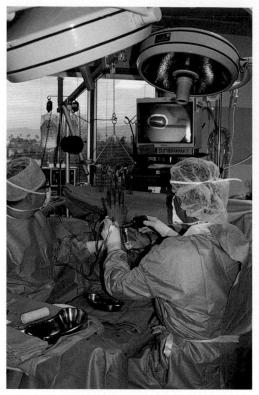

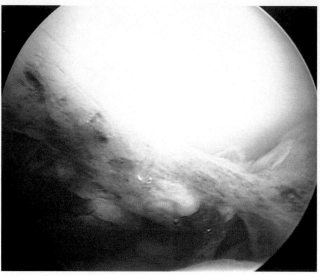

A   B

FIGURE 51.10 A: A motorized full-radius shaver is introduced through a second portal to assist with removal of fracture debris, thus providing a clear view of the injured joint. **B:** Arthroscopic appearance of the intraarticular fracture debris consisting of hematoma and fibrin clot.

A dissecting probe instrument can be introduced into the radiocarpal joint to assist with movement of the fracture fragments and to disimpact any die-punch fragments (Fig. 51.12). Alternatively, 0.045 or 0.062 K-wires can be passed percutaneously into the respective fracture fragments to act as "joysticks." The K-wires are passed into the subchondral areas of the fracture fragments and can be manipulated under direct arthroscopic visualization and fluoroscopic con-

trol (Fig. 51.13). When a satisfactory reduction of the fracture fragments has been confirmed both arthroscopically and fluoroscopically, the K-wires can be drilled into the radius bone to secure fixation of the fracture fragments (Fig. 51.14).

Once an acceptable reduction of the intraarticular fracture is confirmed, visually through the arthroscope and radiographically through the fluoroscope, secure fixation is ac-

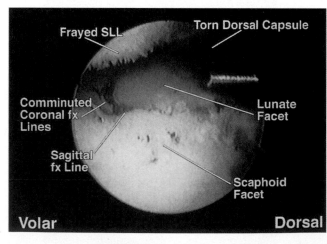

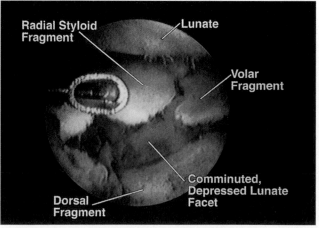

A   B

FIGURE 51.11 A: Arthroscopic view of the intraarticular fracture pattern as seen from the dorsoradial (3-4) portal. **B:** Arthroscopic view of the intraarticular fracture pattern as seen from the dorsomedial (6R) portal.

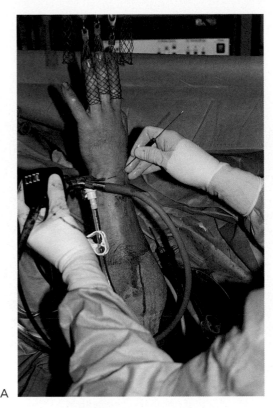

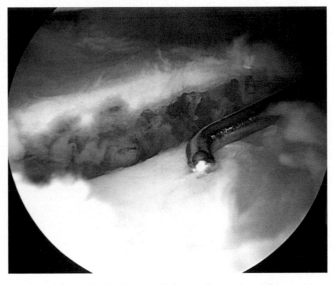

A

B

FIGURE 51.12 A: A spatula instrument is introduced through the dorsoradial portal to assist with fracture fragment manipulation. **B:** A probe is placed inside the joint to assist with elevation and reduction of the dorsomedial displaced fracture fragment.

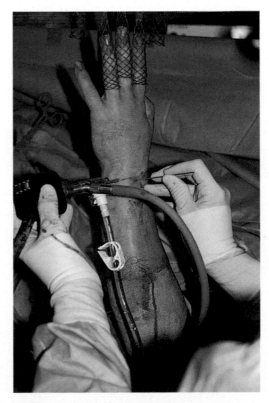

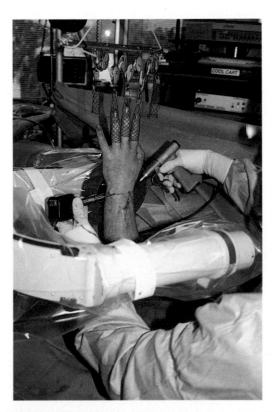

FIGURE 51.13 A 0.062 K-wire is placed into a depressed die-punch fracture fragment to assist with elevation.

FIGURE 51.14 The small, portable fluoroscope is essential to aid additional K-wire placement.

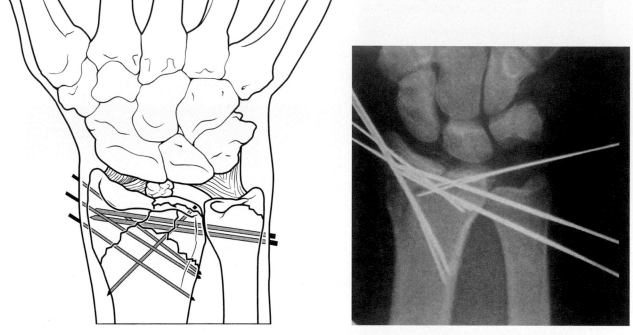

A

B

FIGURE 51.15 A: Schematic view of percutaneous K-wire fracture fixation. Open reduction of the intraarticular fracture components has been confirmed arthroscopically and fluoroscopically; fixation is obtained with two or three 0.045 K-wires through the radial styloid. If the dorsomedial fragment is difficult to maintain, an additional K-wire should be placed through the fragment. In many patients, I use Rayhack's technique of placing two 0.062 K-wires through the distal ulna and into the distal radius to act as an additional buttress to the unstable distal radius fracture fragments. **B:** Radiograph of the distal radius fracture. Percutaneous pins provide stable fixation.

complished using additional K-wires (Fig. 51.15). It is possible that an ORIF may be needed if reduction by manipulation and arthroscopic assistance does not lead to anatomic reduction of the fragments. If a significant bone defect is present during the course of the fracture reduction, then autogenous cancellous bone graft or possibly injectable calcium phosphate graft substitute can be installed to supplement fixation. In some extremely unstable fractures, external fixation may also be needed.

The surgeon should carefully assess the stability of the DRUJ and the carpus. Any instabilities should be treated accordingly (48–51). A spectrum of interosseous ligament injuries can be found, including attenuation of the ligament, partial full-substance tears of the membranous component of the ligament, and complete tears with gross instability leading to diastasis between the carpal bones. It is imperative to evaluate the SLL and LTL thoroughly through a variety of arthroscopic portals. In the case of a ligamentous injury, it is also necessary to use a midcarpal portal for evaluation of the SLJ and LTJ from the midcarpal space. Only in the midcarpal space are these respective joints clearly seen and their appropriate alignment discovered arthroscopically (Fig. 51.16). Attenuation of the intercarpal ligaments is usually observed with some hemorrhage in the substance of the ligament, but there is no evidence of instability. Attenuation and tearing of the interosseous ligament may lead to either dynamic or static instability. These in-

juries are difficult to treat, because the outcome is not known when a moderate grade II–type sprain of the ligament exists. It is probably best simply to debride any frayed portion of the ligament and then to immobilize the carpal bones in conjunction with postoperative immobilization of the distal radius fracture. When there is a complete liga-

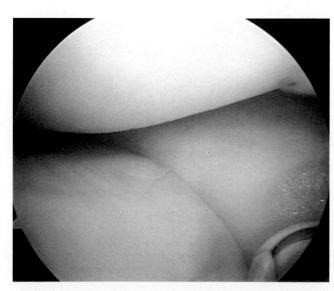

FIGURE 51.16 Arthroscopic view of the lunotriquetral joint (LTJ) from the midcarpal portal.

mentous tear, that is, a grade III injury, and gross instability, the carpal instability is best managed with possible arthroscopic reduction and percutaneous K-wire fixation of the injured joint. In my personal experience, this is easier to perform with the LTJ injuries than with SLJ injuries. The anatomy of the SLJ makes placement of percutaneous K-wires very difficult. There may also be a perilunate instability with tearing of both the SLL and LTL, and this is extremely difficult to manage arthroscopically. Usually, these more significant grade IV injuries, as classified by Geissler, require open surgical repair.

As previously mentioned, tears of the TFCC are usually managed with excision of the torn central disc. The most common acute type 1D tear is best managed with simple arthroscopic debridement of the central portion of the complex, by using standard arthroscopic technique and instrumentation. If there is an acute modified type 1C tear involving the dorsal peripheral portion of the TFCC, it can be surgically repaired. Suture techniques for accomplishing this have been well described in the literature.

RECOMMENDATIONS FOR TREATMENT OF DIFFERENT FRACTURE CLASSES

Compression Fractures

Melone's intraarticular fracture classification scheme helps us to understand the injury mechanism, and especially the importance of the medial fracture complex. In my experience, Melone type II and IV injuries are the most commonly encountered fracture patterns. Both involve comminution of the joint surface and displacement of the medial fracture complex. The type II injury does not contain a separate displaced volar medial fracture fragment, as is normally seen in the type IV injury. With this classification system, the lunate facet becomes the focus of a direct compression injury leading to dorsal displacement of the dorsomedial fracture fragment. Preinjury radiographs of this type of distal radius fracture often do not clearly show the significance of the displaced dorsomedial fracture fragment. Any time the posteroanterior radiograph, or more often the oblique radiograph, hints at the possible suggestion of a dorsomedial fracture fragment, it is usually found to be displaced by over 1 to 2 mm. In addition, very commonly associated with this dorsomedial fracture fragment is an acute type 1D tear of the TFCC. With the compression mechanism of injury to the lunate facet of the distal radius causing displacement of the dorsomedial fracture fragment, the energy propagates into the sigmoid notch and leads to tearing of the TFCC directly off the notch itself. This mechanism is clearly substantiated by the high proportion of type 1D TFCC tears seen with virtually all distal radius fractures.

Wrist arthroscopy is extremely helpful in identifying this displaced dorsomedial fracture fragment and in assisting with an anatomic reduction. Often, this fracture fragment is seen to be displaced 2 to 3 mm, and this displacement is not at all evident on fluoroscopic imaging. The arthroscope must be placed in both the dorsoradial and dorsoulnar portals to assess the position of the dorsomedial fracture fragment. Usually, one or two 0.045 K-wires are necessary to secure this fracture fragment anatomically. The reduction of this fracture fragment may assist with stabilization of the DRUJ.

The Melone type IV intraarticular fracture typically has four parts to the fracture that require accurate assessment and anatomic reduction. The radial styloid fracture fragment is usually contained in one piece, and this can be reduced initially with fluoroscopy and percutaneous pinning with two to three 0.045 K-wires. On occasion, the radial styloid fracture may itself be comminuted, and this adds to the complexity of the repair. In these situations, arthroscopic examination of the radial styloid fracture fragment is extremely helpful to ascertain the degree of comminution and the extent of the anatomic reduction. The dorsomedial and volar medial fracture fragments, primarily involving the entire lunate facet, are next anatomically reduced. Usually, these two fracture fragments can be teased back into position using an intraarticular probe or K-wires placed into the fragments themselves to assist with manipulation and elevation. In a die-punch fracture involving either the lunate or scaphoid facet, percutaneous manipulation with a 0.062 K-wire assists in elevating the fracture fragment back into position. Once again, anatomic reduction is confirmed with both fluoroscopy and arthroscopy to ensure that the fracture fragments are aligned within 1 mm. Even with die-punch injuries of 4 to 5 mm, I have not found it necessary to proceed with supplemental bone grafting. Certainly, if there is additional comminution or more significant impaction of the fracture fragments, bone grafting may then be necessary. As mentioned previously, cancellous graft or an injectable calcium phosphate material may be used to fill in the void.

In some situations, the volar medial fracture fragment may not be reducible, despite all attempts at manipulating the fragment. In this case, ORIF using the volar approach may be essential. When the fracture fragments are extremely unstable because of significant comminution of the metaphyseal area of the bone, that is, a Melone type V injury or an AO/ASIF C3 type injury, the use of an external fixator is recommended.

Shearing Fractures

Shearing fractures usually result in the development of marginal fracture fragments that displace palmarly, dorsally, or even radially. The three most common types are the volarly displaced Smith's fracture, the dorsally displaced Barton's fracture, or Chauffeur's fracture with displacement of the radial styloid. In my experience, the volar displaced fracture, that is, Smith's fracture, is virtually impossible to treat arthroscopically. This fracture fragment is extremely difficult to reduce arthroscopically and to pin percutaneously. My approach is to proceed with ORIF of the volarly displaced fracture fragment and to apply a buttress plate. I then proceed with wrist arthroscopy to assess the extent of the reduction. Often, it is found that the articular reduction of the Smith's fracture is not as anatomic as the treating surgeon would think. Even though the fracture fragments may be anatomically aligned along the volar cortex of the bone just beneath the buttress plate, there is no guarantee that the articular components of the fracture meet up within 1 mm of each other. The fluoroscope is also notoriously poor at assessing the congruency of the articular reduction. Wrist arthroscopy is invaluable in ensuring that the fracture has been anatomically reduced (Fig. 51.17). Furthermore, as previously mentioned, there is a high association of intraarticular soft tissue injuries with this type of fracture. I first apply the buttress plate to the palmar aspect of the bone after anatomic reduction of the fracture fragments is done. I place only one or two proximal screws in the plate. The distal screws are not attached until after the wrist arthroscopy is completed, to ensure that the reduction is anatomic. I usually place the distal three to four screws under direct arthroscopic evaluation. In this way, the fracture fragment is not displaced with the installation of the screws, and the anatomic reduction is arthroscopically visualized to be maintained. Because an open incision is made volarly, immediate access to the volar wrist capsule is obtainable. In many of these approaches, I use a volar arthroscopic wrist portal to assist with additional observation of the wrist joint (Fig. 51.18).

The dorsal Barton's-type fractures are more accessible to arthroscopic reduction and percutaneous pin fixation. In my experience, even significant comminution of the displaced dorsal marginal fracture is amenable to manipulation

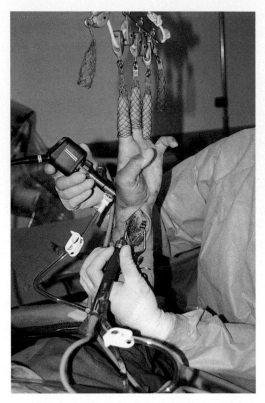

FIGURE 51.18 During the open reduction and internal fixation of a volar shear fracture, there is easy access to the volar wrist capsule allowing for safe establishment of a volar wrist portal.

through the use of longitudinal traction and direct compression on the fracture fragments, followed by percutaneous pin fixation. In some instances, this is stabilized with the application of an external fixator.

Displaced radial styloid fractures, that is, Chauffeur's fractures, are also amenable to arthroscopic reduction. If the

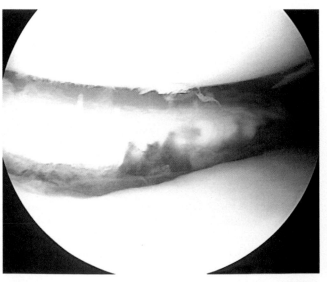

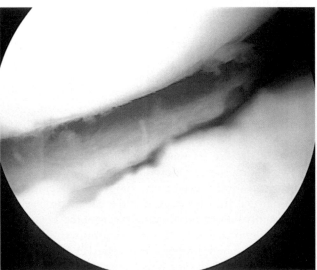

A   B

FIGURE 51.17 A: Shearing fracture line still displaced. **B:** Shear fracture now clearly visualized to be anatomically reduced.

radial styloid fracture fragment consists of one large piece, it can often be fixed with a cannulated screw or K-wires. With a radial styloid fracture, there is a higher incidence of associated scapholunate ligamentous injuries and instability. This is quite understandable, because the shear component of the fracture, propagating through the radial styloid, usually enters the wrist joint through the radial ridge, just below the SLJ. With sufficient energy, the force then leads to disruption of the SLL and the development of an instability. Wrist arthroscopy is extremely helpful not only in reducing the fracture fragment anatomically, but also in ascertaining the nature of the injury to the SLL. Standard treatment for an acute scapholunate ligamentous injury is then accomplished.

Ulna Styloid Injuries

In my experience, fractures of the ulna styloid are rarely associated with ulnar-sided tears of the TFCC or disruption of the DRUJ. I have only a few acute type 1B tears of the TFCC from its attachment to the ulna styloid in my patients with intraarticular distal radius fractures. On occasion, the ulna styloid fracture fragment is reducible and may be percutaneously pinned to help maintain reduction. Even if the ulna styloid fracture is left untreated, either a fibrous union or a bony union will ensue, and rarely is it ever a problem later in the management of the wrist fracture. It is, however, imperative to evaluate the entire TFCC arthroscopically. It is not unusual to find a dorsal peripheral tear and even, on a rare occasion, a volar peripheral tear, that will require further treatment. The dorsal peripheral tear of the TFCC can be repaired arthroscopically using a variety of techniques, either outside-in or inside-out. On occasion, the TFCC is torn from its attachment to the fovea of the base of the ulna styloid, and it must be reattached. This can also be done arthroscopically in a fashion similar to that of the dorsal peripheral tear, but in this case, the repair must be back to the bone.

In injuries to the TFCC or in the presence of Melone type IV fractures, assessment of stability of the DRUJ must always be made. If the dorsomedial and volar medial fracture fragments are significantly displaced, this will cause incongruity of the distal ulna with the sigmoid notch of the distal radius and can actually lead to gross instability of the DRUJ. This form of instability is usually treated with reduction of the fracture. In these cases, I favor placing two to three 0.062 K-wires percutaneously through the distal ulna and into the fractured epiphyseal area of the distal radius. This is done with the patient's wrist in a slight position of supination. The placement of these additional ulnar-sided pins accomplishes two goals: first, it reduces the DRUJ anatomically and stabilizes it, thus allowing for both bony and ligamentous healing; and second, the 0.062 K-wires add an additional buttressing effect to stabilize the distal radius fracture.

REHABILITATION

The percutaneously placed K-wires that were installed during the ARIF of the distal radius fracture may be left external to the skin or clipped below the level of the skin, depending on the preference of the surgeon. Both techniques appear to have good results, but a study done in our office indicates that when the pins are left external to the skin, there are fewer complications in the management of the patient. If ulnar-sided 0.062 K-wires are used to stabilize the DRUJ or to buttress the distal radius fracture, they are left external to the skin and are removed in approximately 3 to 4 weeks. In my experience, the placement of three or four of these ulnar-sided 0.062 K-wires usually leads to a significant buttressing effect, which then eliminates the necessity for the use of an external fixation frame. The short-arm splint or modified long-arm sugar-tong splint (Fig. 51.19) that is applied in the operating room is left in position until the patient returns for the first postoperative visit, 7 to 10 days later. The 0.045 K-wires that have been installed, usually about the radial and dorsomedial aspects of the distal radius, are removed in 6 to 8 weeks, depending on the rate of fracture healing. Once all K-wires have been removed, a comprehensive occupational hand therapy program is initiated. At each office visit for the first 4 weeks, posteroanterior and lateral radiographs of the wrist are obtained to ensure con-

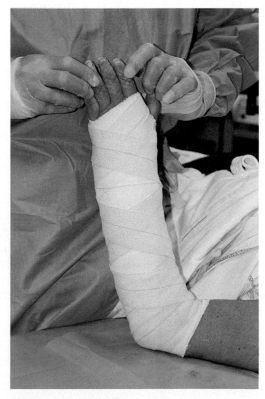

FIGURE 51.19 Modified long-arm sugar-tong splint.

tinued anatomic fracture healing and to assess for any possible migration of the K-wires. Immediately after the surgical procedure, the patient is thoroughly encouraged and educated in digital flexibility exercises.

Once an occupational therapy program is initiated, the patient can concentrate on stretching exercises to work out the wrist stiffness that always accompanies these distal radius fractures and then to begin to develop strength and endurance. In most patients, wrist stiffness persists for a minimum of 4 to 6 months. Many patients take 6 to 12 months to regain maximum strength.

Virtually every patient with a wrist fracture is treated as an outpatient. Regional anesthesia is often used. Wrist arthrotomy is avoided, unless absolutely necessary. The arthroscopic removal of intraarticular fracture debris appears to reduce postinjury adhesions and subsequent wrist joint stiffness significantly. The arthroscopically treated patients appear to have much less postoperative pain.

Complications associated with ARIF are rare. There have been no infections or sinus tracts developing at the arthroscopic portals. Complications associated with the percutaneous placement of K-wires are fairly common. Many patients complain of pain at the site of the wire, even if it is left external to the skin. Many times, the placement of these wires induces temporary sensory neuritis in either the radial sensory nerve or the dorsal sensory branch of the ulnar nerve. Several months after the K-wires are removed, this nerve irritability resolves. Ulceration of skin at the penetration site of K-wires can occur, usually in older patients. This is treated with removal of the K-wires and local wound management. Healing by secondary intention occurs within 2 to 3 weeks.

SUMMARY

Wrist arthroscopy allows for an increased measure of an accurate evaluation of the intraarticular bony and soft tissue components of complex intraarticular distal radius fractures. Residual fracture displacement can be visually corrected to within 1 mm, thus obtaining an accurate anatomic reduction. This added degree of accuracy in the intraarticular component of the fracture reduction provides for superior healing of the joint surface with less chance of posttraumatic wrist arthrosis. In fact, this finding has been substantiated in many reports in which wrist arthroscopy was used to treat intraarticular fractures of the distal radius. The studies clearly indicate that ARIF is both effective and safe, and outcome is improved. The authors of these studies highly favor ARIF over ORIF. They also reiterate that fluoroscopy alone is inadequate for the treatment of an intraarticular distal radius fracture, because it does not uniformly lead to accurate reduction of the fracture fragments. It is highly recommended that operative wrist arthroscopy be employed to verify and assist with the reduction of the intraarticular component of the fracture. In all instances, the use of ARIF is an excellent adjunct management tool. In my experience, the technique of ARIF is quite safe and poses no additional risk to the patient than the normal risks associated with surgical treatment of the distal radius fracture. On the contrary, the ability of the surgeon to reduce the complex, displaced fracture fragments accurately and to identify and treat commonly associated soft tissue and cartilage injuries is a major advance in the management of these challenging fractures.

REFERENCES

1. Jupiter JB. Complex articular fractures of the distal radius: classification and management. *J Am Acad Orthop Surg* 1997;5:119–129.
2. Fernandez D, Jupiter J. *Fractures of the distal radius: a practical approach to management.* New York: Springer, 1996.
3. Fernandez D, Palmer A. Fractures of the distal radius. In: Green DP, et al., eds. *Operative hand surgery,* 4th ed. New York: Churchill Livingstone, 1999:929–985.
4. Saffar P, Cooney W III. *Fractures of the distal radius.* Philadelphia: JB Lippincott, 1995.
5. Oskam J, Kingma J, Klasen H. Fracture of the distal forearm: epidemiological developments in the period 1971–1995. *Injury* 1998;29:353–355.
6. Whipple T. The role of arthroscopy in the treatment of wrist injuries in the athlete. *Clin Sports Med* 1998;17:623–634.
7. Hanker G. Radius fractures in the athlete. *Clin Sports Med* 2001; 20:189–201.
8. Bacorn RW, Kurtzke JF. Colles' fracture: a study of two thousand cases from the New York State Workmen's Compensation Board. *J Bone Joint Surg Am* 1953;35:643–658.
9. McQueen M, Caspers J. Colles' fractures: does the anatomical result affect the final function? *J Bone Joint Surg Br* 1988;70:649–651.
10. Cooney W III. Fractures of the distal radius. In: Cooney W III, et al., eds. *The wrist: diagnosis and operative treatment,* vol 1. St. Louis, MO: CV Mosby; 1998:310–355.
11. Cooney WP III, Berger RA. Treatment of complex fractures of the distal radius: combined use of internal and external fixation and arthroscopic reduction. *Hand Clin* 1993;9:603–612.
12. Leibovic S. Fixation for distal radius fractures. *Hand Clin* 1997; 13:665–680.
13. Rodriguez-Merchan E. Management of comminuted fractures of the distal radius in the adult: conservative or surgical? *Clin Orthop* 1998;353:53–62.
14. Hove L, Nilsen P, Fuanes O, et al. Open reduction and internal fixation of displaced intraarticular fractures of the distal radius. *Acta Orthop Scand* 1997;68:59–63.
15. Trumble T, Culp R, Hanel D, et al. Intraarticular fractures of the distal aspect of the radius. *Instr Course Lect* 1999;48:465–480.
16. Ring D, Jupiter J. Percutaneous and limited open fixation of fractures of the distal radius. *Clin Orthop* 2000;375:105–115.
17. Hanker GJ. Arthroscopic evaluation of intraarticular distal radius fractures. Presented at the 46th annual meeting of the American Society for Surgery of the Hand, Orlando, FL, 1991.
18. Hanker G. Intraarticular fractures of the distal radius. In: McGinty J, ed. *Operative arthroscopy,* 2nd ed. New York: Lippincott–Raven, 1996:987–998.
19. Knirk JL, Jupiter JB. Intraarticular fractures of the distal end of the radius in young adults. *J Bone Joint Surg Am* 1986;68:647–659.

20. Seibert F, Fellinger M, Grenhenig W, et al. Distal radius fractures "loco typico": arthroscopic diagnosis and minimally invasive treatment of additional lesions. *Arthroskopie* 1995;8:273–280.
21. Geissler W, Freeland A, Savoie F, et al. Intracarpal soft tissue lesions associated with an intraarticular fracture of the distal end of the radius. *J Bone Joint Surg Am* 1996;78:357–365.
22. Richards R, Bennett J, Roth J, et al. Arthroscopic diagnosis of intraarticular soft tissue injuries associated with distal radius fractures. *J Hand Surg Am* 1997;22:772–776.
23. Lindau T, Arner M, Hagberg L. Intraarticular lesions in distal fractures of the radius in young adults: a descriptive arthroscopic study of 50 patients. *J Hand Surg Br* 1997;22:638–643.
24. Geissler W, Freeland A. Arthroscopic management of intraarticular distal radius fractures. *Hand Clin* 1999;15:455–465.
25. Mehta J, Bain G, Heptenstall R. Anatomical reduction of intraarticular fractures of the distal radius: an arthroscopically assisted approach. *J Bone Joint Surg Br* 2000;82:79–86.
26. Abe Y, Doi K, Kuwata N, et al. Surgical options for distal radius fractures: indications and limitations. *Arch Orthop Trauma Surg* 1998;117:188–192.
27. Doi K, Hattari Y, Otsuka K, et al. Intraarticular fractures of the distal aspect of the radius: arthroscopically assisted reduction compared with open reduction and internal fixation. *J Bone Joint Surg Am* 1999;81:1093–1100.
28. Augë W, Velãzquez M. The application of indirect reduction techniques in the distal radius: the role of adjuvant arthroscopy. *Arthroskopie* 2000;16:830–835.
29. Adolfsson L, Jörgsholm P. Arthroscopically assisted reduction of intraarticular fractures of the distal radius. *J Hand Surg Br* 1998;23:391–395.
30. Geissler W, Freeland A. Arthroscopically assisted reduction of intraarticular distal radius fractures. *Clin Orthop* 1996;327:125–134.
31. Melone CP. Unstable fractures of the distal radius. In: Lichtman DM, ed. *The wrist and its disorders.* Philadelphia: WB Saunders, 1988:160–177.
32. Schweitzer ME, Brahme SK, Hodler J, et al. Chronic wrist pain: spin-echo and short tau inversion recovery MR imaging and conventional and MR arthrography. *Radiology* 1992;182:205–211.
33. Hanker G, Hanker K. Role of arthroscopy in the management of triangular fibrocartilage complex injuries and wrist fractures. In: Parisien JS, ed. *Current techniques in arthroscopy.* Philadelphia: Thieme, 1998:137–147.
34. Trumble T, Gilbert M, Vedder N. Arthroscopic repair of the triangular fibrocartilage complex. *Arthroscopy* 1996;12:588–597.
35. Whipple T. *Arthroscopic surgery: the wrist.* Philadelphia: WB Saunders, 1992.
36. Lenoble E, Dumontier C, Goutallier D, et al. Fractures of the distal radius: a prospective comparison between trans-styloid and Kapandji fixations. *J Bone Joint Surg Br* 1995;77:562–567.
37. Ruch D, Bowling J. Arthroscopic assessment of carpal instability. *Arthroscopy* 1998;14:675–681.
38. Stoffelan D, DeMulder K, Bross P, et al. The clinical importance of carpal instabilities following distal radius fractures. *J Hand Surg Br* 1998;23:512–516.
39. Peicha G, Seibert F, Fellinger M, et al. Mid-term results of arthroscopic treatment of scapholunate ligament lesions associated with intraarticular distal radius fractures. *Knee Surg Sports Traumatol Arthrosc* 1999;7:327–333.
40. Dunning C, Lindsay C, Bichnell R, et al. Supplemental pinning improves the stability of external fixation in distal radius fractures during simulated finger and forearm motion. *J Hand Surg Am* 1999;24:992–1000.
41. Krishnan J, Chipchase L, Slavotinek J. Intraarticular fractures of the distal radius treated with metaphyseal external fixation. *J Hand Surg Br* 1998;23:396–399.
42. Fihry T, Fadili M, Harfaoui A, et al. Distal radius fractures: Kapandji's or Py's pinning. *Ann Chir Main* 1998;17:31–40.
43. Zanolli R, Louis D. Intraarticular fractures of the distal end of the radius treated with an adjustable fixator system. *J Hand Surg [Am]* 1997;22:428–440.
44. Jupiter J, Winter S, Sigmar S, et al. Repair of five distal radius fractures with an investigational cancellous bone cement: a preliminary report. *J Orthop Trauma* 1997;11:110–116.
45. Ladd A, Pliam N. Use of bone graft substitutes in distal radius fractures. *J Am Acad Orthop Surg* 1999;7:279–290.
46. Wagner W, Tencer A, Kiser P, et al. Effects of intraarticular distal radius depression on wrist joint contact characteristics. *J Hand Surg Am* 1996;21:554–560.
47. Kihara H, Palmer A, Werner F, et al. The effect of dorsally angulated distal radius fractures on distal radioulnar joint congruency and forearm rotation. *J Hand Surg Am* 1996;21:40–47.
48. Geissler W, Fernandez D, Lamey D. Distal radioulnar joint injuries associated with fractures of the distal radius. *Clin Orthop* 1996;327:135–146.
49. Sennwald G, Zdaakovic V. Wrist arthroscopy: a prospective analysis of 53 post-traumatic carpal injuries. *Scand J Plast Reconstr Hand Surg* 1997;31:261–266.
50. Lindau T, Hagberg L, Adlercreutz C, et al. Distal radioulnar joint instability is an independent worsening factor in distal radius fractures. *Clin Orthop* 2000;376:229–235.
51. Lindau T, Adlercreutz C, Aspenberg P. Peripheral tears of the triangular fibrocartilage complex cause distal radioulnar joint instability after distal radius fractures. *J Hand Surg Am* 2000;25:464–468.

SCAPHOID FRACTURES

TERRY L. WHIPPLE

The incidence of carpal scaphoid fractures in the United States is uncertain but has been estimated to be between 30,000 and 200,000 new fractures annually, with approximately 5% to 10% of these fractures progressing to nonunion (1,2). The scaphoid represents an important mechanical link between the proximal and distal carpal rows. With wrist flexion, the scaphoid positions the proximal row to transfer axial load between the hand and the distal radius. Disruption of the linkage between the proximal and distal carpal rows changes the kinematics of the wrist and renders the carpus unstable for axial load transfer as the proximal row shifts in a volar direction and the distal row shifts in a dorsal direction. The proximal carpal row collapses into extension under loaded conditions (3), and the result is shear and concentrated compression between the scaphoid and the radial styloid and between the head of the capitate and the dorsal aspect of the lunate (4). Force overload eventually causes degenerative changes on the articular surface of the distal radius, the proximal pole of the scaphoid, and between the lunate and capitate.

Typical physiologic bending moments on the scaphoid produce compression of its volar cortex and tension dorsally. This finding explains the usual flexion displacement of the distal pole of the scaphoid after transverse fractures through its waist and the development of the characteristic humpback deformity.

Blood supply to the proximal pole of the scaphoid is provided principally through intraosseous channels and is usually disrupted by fractures through the waist of the bone. Deprivation of circulation to the proximal pole compromises fracture healing and causes the high incidence of delayed union and nonunion.

The natural history of carpal scaphoid fractures is well documented (1–3,5–10). Fracture treatment with cast immobilization may require up to 6 months, or even more, to achieve healing. Nonunion leads to progressive displacement of the fracture fragments in 50% of cases and radiographic evidence of degenerative arthritis in up to 97% of cases within 5 years (11,12). Timely and effective treatment of acute scaphoid fractures therefore becomes a crucial concern if catastrophic mechanical and degenerative consequences are to be avoided.

Plaster immobilization of scaphoid fractures has long been regarded as conservative treatment (13,14). Because cast immobilization may require many weeks to months, conservatism in terms of patient function and ultimate lost opportunity cost is questionable. Moreover, the appropriate method of cast immobilization remains unresolved. Various recommendations have included short-arm and long-arm casting, with and without inclusion of the thumb or even the index and long fingers. Positions of flexion and radial deviation to compress the fracture have been recommended, but there is equal enthusiasm for positions of wrist extension and ulnar deviation to prevent fracture collapse.

Operative treatment for scaphoid fractures has generally been considered a more aggressive approach. Recommended procedures include primary bone grafting and internal fixation of the fracture fragments with Kirschner wires, screws, and even small contoured plates (14–19). Operative treatment involves a greater initial cost and carries associated risks of infection, further fracture displacement, complications related to implanted hardware, and further disruption of osseous circulation, especially circulation to small proximal fragments.

Rational decisions regarding primary treatment for scaphoid fractures remain subjective. Certainly, it is generally agreed that motion at the fracture site is undesirable; motion increases the risk of nonunion with instability and ultimate fracture displacement (9,11,12). There is consensus in the literature that optimum treatment of scaphoid fractures must include effective immobilization of the fragments and that the best long-term results are seen when the normal geometry of the scaphoid is preserved. More rigid fracture immobilization can be accomplished with internal fixation than with casting, but the technical difficulties and risks of surgical treatment are undeniable. For these reasons,

T. L. Whipple: Department of Orthopaedic Surgery, Bowman Gray School of Medicine, Wake Forest University; Department of Orthopaedics and Rehabilitation, University of Virginia School of Medicine, Charlottesville, Virginia; Department of Orthopaedic Surgery, Medical College of Virginia, Richmond, Virginia.

I have sought ways to reconcile the generally recognized treatment goals, including maximum fracture stabilization, with the associated risks of operative treatment. In recent years, minimally invasive surgical procedures have been developed to accomplish proven objectives with reduced surgical morbidity. Among these have been accurate reduction and internal fixation of tibial plateau fractures and articular fractures of the distal radius under arthroscopic control. These procedures have permitted more accurate reduction of articular fracture fragments than can be achieved by closed ligamentotaxis, and they eliminate the need for arthrotomy or extensive surgical exposure for the application of internal fixation devices.

With techniques that are similar in principle and by employing newly designed instrumentation, a means has been devised for internally stabilizing fractures of the scaphoid through a limited incision using arthroscopic assistance. This technique offers the advantage of preserving soft tissue attachments to the scaphoid as well as its tenuous blood supply. It allows more rigid fracture stabilization than can be accomplished by casting alone and therefore reduces the required period of external wrist immobilization.

Fractures of the waist of the scaphoid can be seen and reduced during arthroscopic examination of the midcarpal space. Nondisplaced or minimally displaced fractures are apparent as a transverse line on the capitate articular facet (Fig. 52.1). The distraction necessary for manipulation of arthroscopic instruments in the midcarpal space assists in correcting acute flexion deformities. Other patterns of displacement may be more difficult to reduce, especially if one of the fragments is rotated. If, however, acute fractures require no reduction or can be reduced adequately with manipulation, minimally invasive internal fixation becomes an option.

FIXATION DEVICE

The device developed for this procedure can be used with certain advantages also in fractures treated by conventional surgical exposure. The Herbert-Whipple screw is a headless titanium screw with variably pitched threads at either end. It is similar to the Herbert screw. The newer device, however, has an increased diameter in the nonthreaded segment

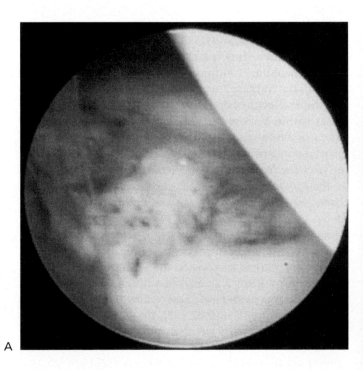

A

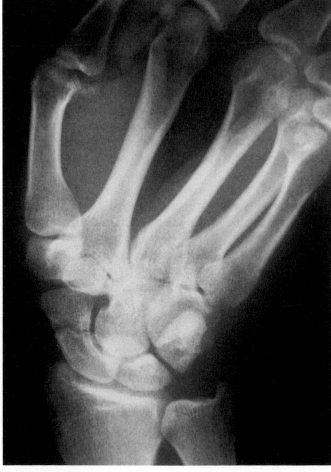

B

FIGURE 52.1 A: Arthroscopic view of an acute transverse waist fracture of the carpal scaphoid, right wrist, seen through the radial midcarpal (RMC) portal. **B:** Radiograph of the corresponding fracture of the right carpal scaphoid.

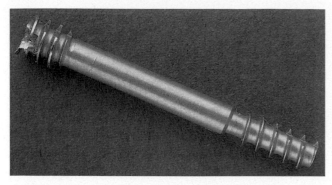

FIGURE 52.2 Herbert-Whipple screw: a cannulated device with self-tapping variably pitched threads and a wide nonthreaded portion to increase bending strength. (Courtesy of Zimmer, Inc., Warsaw, IN.)

to increase its bending strength and to resist fracture fragment rotation. It is also cannulated to allow installation over a preliminary guide pin (Fig. 52.2). Guide pin position can be confirmed radiographically and adjusted if necessary before the bone is drilled. The threads are self-tapping for more secure fixation in cancellous bone.

Engineering bench tests on this implant demonstrate equivalent pullout strength two and a half times the bending strength and one and a half times the torque strength compared with the Herbert screw. The variably pitched threads provide exactly 1 mm of fracture compression when the last trailing thread becomes buried in subchondral bone. The cannulated screw is decidedly easier to install than an uncannulated version and offers greater protection of the bone spicules that interdigitate between the threads of the screw compared with cases in which the bone is initially tapped, the tap is removed, and the screw is then installed during a third pass through the bone threads.

SURGICAL TECHNIQUE

The arthroscopically assisted procedure for scaphoid fracture fixation requires intraoperative fluoroscopy to confirm proper placement of the initial guide pin. A radially curved, longitudinal volar incision approximately 12 to 15 mm long is made radial to the flexor carpi radialis tendon, centered over the scaphotrapezial joint, which can be readily palpated. Blunt dissection is used to protect the palmar cutaneous nerve. With the wrist extended, the scaphotrapezial joint is exposed and is opened with a T-incision, thus peeling periosteum away from the volar surface of the trapezium. It is not necessary to open the radiocarpal space or to release any portion of the volar radioscaphocapitate ligament. This represents a distinct advantage over the conventional volar approach of the scaphoid used for Russe grafts and for scaphoid fracture fixation with the original Herbert screw. The volar tubercle of the trapezium is excised with a

5-mm osteotome to expose the articular surface of the distal pole of the scaphoid.

The patient's hand is placed in traction using finger traps applied to the index and long fingers. One may need 10 to 15 lb of distraction force for reduction of the displaced fragments, and a force of 8 to 10 lb is recommended for nondisplaced fractures. A 2.7-mm arthroscope can be inserted in the radial midcarpal portal, with irrigation inflow provided through the arthroscope sheath. Clearing the fracture hemarthrosis may require an evacuation needle or even a small shaver placed in the ulnar midcarpal portal. When the hemarthrosis has been cleared, the fracture is visualized and is reduced by manipulation of the distal pole. If necessary, a temporary Kirschner wire can be drilled percutaneously into the proximal pole of the scaphoid to aid fracture reduction.

The arthroscope then is transferred to the radiocarpal space in the 4-5 portal. A 1-2 portal is also established in the dorsal aspect of the anatomic snuffbox. The target hook of the Whipple compression jig is introduced through the 1-2 portal and is advanced to the dorsal aspect of the proximal pole of the scaphoid 1 to 2 mm radial to the scapholunate ligament. Here, the target hook is seated into the articular cartilage.

The guide barrel of the jig is slid down to the articular surface of the distal scaphoid, approximately 40% of the distance from the radial margin to the ulnar margin of the distal pole. Holding the thumb in hyperextension facilitates this distal exposure. The Whipple jig is then compressed firmly to secure the fracture. This completes the arthroscopic portion of the procedure unless repositioning of the guide pin becomes necessary.

A primary guide pin is measured to an appropriate length as gauged from the scale on the compression jig. The primary guide pin is drilled across the fracture site through the guide barrel, and pin placement is confirmed fluoroscopically. A secondary guide pin is drilled through the jig parallel to the primary guide pin to prevent rotation of the fracture fragments (Fig. 52.3). The scaphoid is drilled from distal to proximal with a cannulated step drill placed over the primary guide pin. The step drill is properly sized for the leading and trailing screw threads and contains built-in stops to control its depth of penetration. The broaching and drilling steps are done with a power drill because the guide pin ensures precise control.

The appropriate length Herbert-Whipple screw is inserted until it walks off the end of the screwdriver at the proper depth. Progression of the screwdriver is limited by a stop built into the compression jig, thus allowing the screw to advance while the screwdriver does not. After the jig is removed, the volar incision can be closed with subcutaneous and subcuticular sutures. In most cases, the jig compression and the additional screw compression completely stabilize the fracture. If the fracture pattern is very oblique, however, additional rotational control of the fragments can be obtained by leaving the secondary guide pin in place for 2 to 3

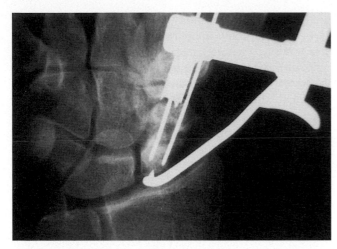

FIGURE 52.3 Whipple compression drill guide has directed the placement of a primary *(left)* and an accessory *(right)* guide pin across the scaphoid fracture from distal to proximal.

weeks postoperatively. This pin can be removed transcutaneously with ease.

A plaster splint, a short-arm cast, or an adjustable motion wrist splint should be applied for a short period to allow the incision to heal and for initial consolidation of the fracture. I have not found it necessary to immobilize the wrist for longer than 4 weeks, and most patients are permitted to move the wrist 2 weeks postoperatively.

Impact loading, torque, and extreme wrist positions are forbidden. To enforce this restriction, the VersaWrist splint (Smith & Nephew DonJoy, Inc., Carlsbad, CA) is useful (Fig. 52.4). It is a functional splint that can be locked in position for the initial immobilization period and then adjusted periodically to allow selected safe ranges of motion in the coronal and sagittal planes. Early motion is considered beneficial for articular cartilage nutrition and to prevent ligament fibrosis about the wrist. Early mobilization also min-

imizes demineralization from prolonged immobilization and enhances the patient's sense of functionality and well-being.

INDICATIONS

Arthroscopically assisted internal fixation of the scaphoid is not necessarily indicated for routine fracture management (Fig. 52.5). Comminuted fractures and those that cannot be anatomically reduced should be opened for accurate reduction and stabilization. For those fractures that must be opened, however, the same jig and fixation device are still appropriate, except in extremely comminuted fractures.

For reducible fractures, the minimally invasive procedure offers two distinct advantages: more rigid fracture immobilization than can be achieved with casting and the opportunity to reduce the period of cast immobilization to only 2 or 3 weeks, in most cases without major surgical exposure that compromises blood supply to the bone or disruption of additional ligamentous support. Absolute indications include nondisplaced or minimally displaced fractures in patients who can ill afford the possibility of casting for 10 to 26 weeks. This may include patients who would experience major loss of income from the inability to work or perform and those whose functional demands preclude prolonged casting.

Relative indications include nondisplaced or displaced reducible fractures in patients who would simply prefer surgical treatment to the possibility of prolonged casting and in patients with systemic disorders that could delay fracture healing or would contraindicate prolonged immobilization, such as peripheral vascular disease, rheumatoid arthritis, or contralateral hand dysfunction.

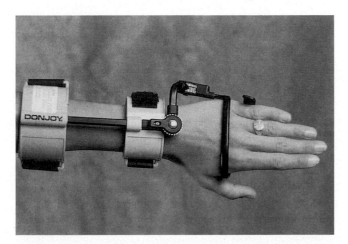

FIGURE 52.4 VersaWrist splint permits selection of safe ranges of motion in flexion, extension, and radial and ulnar deviation. (Courtesy of Smith & Nephew DonJoy, Inc., Carlsbad, CA.)

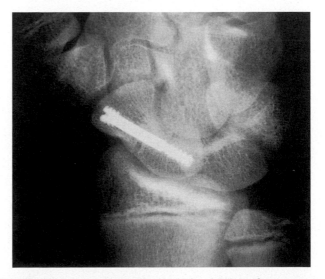

FIGURE 52.5 Arthroscopically assisted reduction of a transverse waist fracture of the scaphoid, internally stabilized and compressed with a Herbert-Whipple screw in a skeletally immature patient, right wrist.

All surgical procedures for the scaphoid are technically demanding. Nonunion, however, is associated with predictable adverse consequences, and union is predicated on effective fracture immobilization. This arthroscopically assisted approach to scaphoid fractures provides the combined advantage of internal fracture fixation and minimally invasive surgical technique. Patients are receptive to the approach, and the newer fixation devices have proven to be reliable and effective in comparison with other devices available for scaphoid fracture fixation.

REFERENCES

1. Eddeland A, Eiken O, Hellgren E, et al. Fractures of the scaphoid. *Scand J Plast Reconstr Surg* 1975;9:234–239.
2. Leslie IJ, Dickson RA. The fractured carpal scaphoid: natural history and factors influencing outcome. *J Bone Joint Surg Br* 1981; 63:225–230.
3. Fisk GR. Carpal instability and the fractured scaphoid. *Ann Coll Surg* 1970;46.63–76.
4. Weber ER. Biomechanical implications of scaphoid waist fractures. *Clin Orthop* 1980;149:83–89.
5. Barr JS, Elliston WA, Musnick H, et al. Fracture of the carpal navicular (scaphoid) bone: an end result study in military personnel. *J Bone Joint Surg Am* 1953;35:609–625.
6. Gilford WW, Bolton RH, Lambrinudi C. The mechanism of the wrist joint with special reference of fractures of the scaphoid. *Guys Hosp Rep* 1943;92:52–59.
7. Obletz BE, Haldstein BM. Non-union of fractures of the carpal navicular. *J Bone Joint Surg* 1938;20:424–428.
8. Stewart MJ. Fractures of the carpal navicular (scaphoid): a report of 436 cases. *J Bone Joint Surg Am* 1954;36:998–1006.
9. Verdan C, Narakas A. Fractures and pseudarthrosis of the scaphoid. *Surg Clin North Am* 1968;48:1083–1095.
10. Youm Y, McMurtry RY, Flatt AE, et al. Kinematics of the wrist: part I. An experimental study of radial-ulnar deviation and flexion-extension. *J Bone Joint Surg Am* 1978;60:423–431.
11. Mack GR, Bosse MJ, Gelberman RH. The natural history of scaphoid non-union. *J Bone Joint Surg Am* 1984;66:504–509.
12. Ruby LK, Stinson J, Belsky MR. The natural history of scaphoid non-union: a review of 55 cases. *J Bone Joint Surg Am* 1985;67: 428–432.
13. Mazet R Jr, Hohl M. Conservative treatment of old fractures of the carpal scaphoid. *J Trauma* 1961;1:115–127.
14. Soto-Hall R, Haldeman KO. The conservative and operative treatment of fractures of the carpal scaphoid (navicular). *J Bone Joint Surg* 1941;23:841–850.
15. Gasser H. Delayed union and pseudarthrosis of the carpal navicular: treatment by compression screw osteosynthesis—a preliminary report on 20 fractures. *J Bone Joint Surg Am* 1965;47:249– 266.
16. Herbert TJ. *The fractured scaphoid.* St. Louis, MO: Quality Medical Publishing, 1990.
17. Maudsley RH, Chen SC. Screw fixation in the management of the fractured carpal scaphoid. *J Bone Joint Surg Br* 1972;54:432– 441.
18. Russe O. Fracture of the carpal navicular: diagnosis, non-operative treatment, and operative treatment. *J Bone Joint Surg Am* 1960;42:759–768.
19. Unger HS, Stryker WC. Non-union of the carpal navicular: analysis of 42 cases treated by the Russe procedure. *South Med J* 1969; 62:620–622.

TRIANGULAR FIBROCARTILAGE LESIONS

LEE OSTERMAN

Injury of the triangular fibrocartilage (TFC) is frequently implicated as a cause of wrist pain. Wrist arthroscopy has become standard in the diagnosis and treatment of these injuries (1–6).

ANATOMY

The TFC is a cartilaginous disc interposed between the ulnar carpus and the distal ulna (7–9) (Fig. 53.1). It arises from the articular cartilage on the corner of the sigmoid notch of the radius and inserts into the base of the ulnar styloid and volarly in the ulnocarpal extrinsic ligaments, the ulnolunate and ulnotriquetral ligaments. This central disc portion of the TFC complex (TFCC) is the thinnest portion made up of interwoven obliquely oriented sheets of collagen fibers, oriented to withstand multidirectional and axial stress. This central disc portion is avascular and aneural. The TFCC includes the TFC articular disc as well as its merger with the ulnar extrinsic ligaments and the radioulnar ligaments (Fig. 53.2). The ulnar ligaments act as a sling to support the ulnar carpus. The dorsal and volar radioulnar ligaments are fibrous thickenings within the dorsal and volar edges of the TFC (Fig. 53.3). They function together to stabilize the distal radioulnar joint and thus limit rotational and axial migration. The peripheral portion of the triangular fibrocartilaginous disc is intimate with the floor of the fibrous sheath of the extensor carpi ulnaris (ECU) tendon.

The vascularity of the TFC has been carefully studied (7,10,11). The circulation of the TFCC arises from the ulnar artery through its radiocarpal branches and from the anterior interosseous artery through its dorsal and palmar branches. These vessels supply the TFC in a radial fashion. Histologic sections demonstrate that these vessels penetrate only the peripheral 10% to 40% of the discs (10). The central section and radial attachment of the disc are avascular (Fig. 53.4). *In vivo* studies in our laboratory, using a laser

Doppler probe, have confirmed the histologic studies. Thus, the vascular anatomy supports the concept that peripheral injuries of the TFC can heal, whereas tears of the avascular central portion cannot.

BIOMECHANICS

The TFCC has several important biomechanical functions. It transmits 20% of the axial applied load from the ulnar carpus to the distal ulna in an ulnar neutral individual. It is a major stabilizer of the distal radial ulnar joint and a stabilizer of the ulnar carpus (12,13). The amount of load transferred to the distal ulna is directly proportional to the ulnar variance. In neutral ulnar variance, approximately 20% of the load is transmitted. With positive ulnar variance, the load across the TFC is increased, and there is a corresponding decreased thickness to the central portion of the disc. There is also a dynamic load transmission resulting from rotation. In supination, the radius moves distally on the ulna to create a relative negative ulnar variance. In pronation, this is reversed. The ulna also moves within the sigmoid notch in a dorsal direction with pronation and volarly with supination. During this translation, the dorsal and volar radioulnar ligamentous portions of the TFCC become tense, as befits their stabilizing role (14).

MECHANISM OF INJURY

Traumatic injuries of the TFCC result from the application of an extension-pronation force to the axial loaded wrist such as in a fall on the outstretched hand. These can also occur from a dorsal rotation injury such as when a drill binds, thus rotating the wrist instead of the bit. Another mechanism of injury may occur from a distraction force applied to the volar forearm or wrist (15). Finally, tears of the TFC are commonly found in patients with fractures of the distal radius (16–21).

L. Osterman: Philadelphia Hand Center, Philadelphia, Pennsylvania.

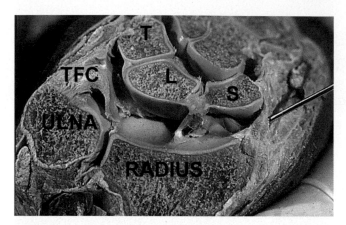

FIGURE 53.1 Frontal section, left wrist. The triangular fibrocartilage is seen separating the radiocarpal from the distal radial ulnar joint. It arises from the articular corner of the medial radius and inserts into the basifoveal area of the ulna. L, lunate; S, scaphoid; T, triquetrum; TFC, triangular fibrocartilage.

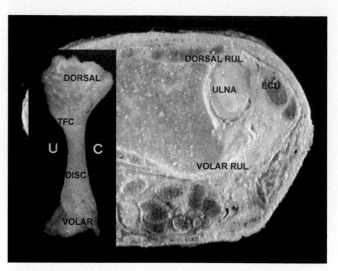

FIGURE 53.3 The radioulnar ligaments. The dorsal and volar radial ulnar ligaments merge with the central triangular fibrocartilage disc and serve as major stabilizers of the distal radial ulnar joint. In this picture, the majority of the triangular fibrocartilage disc has been removed to reveal the underlying distal ulna of this left wrist in pronation. The peripheral portion of the triangular fibrocartilage is intimate with the fibroosseous sheath of the extensor carpi ulnaris tendon (ECU).

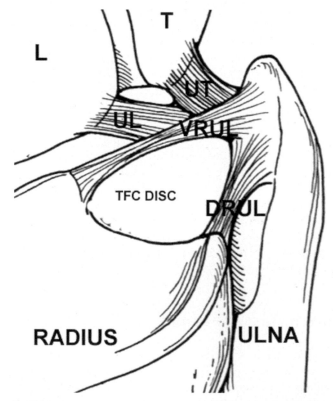

FIGURE 53.2 Diagram of the triangular fibrocartilage complex. It is composed of the following: the ulnar extrinsic ligaments ulnolunate (UL) and ulnotriquetral (UT); the volar and dorsal radial ulnar ligaments (VRUL and DRUL); and the triangular fibrocartilage disc itself.

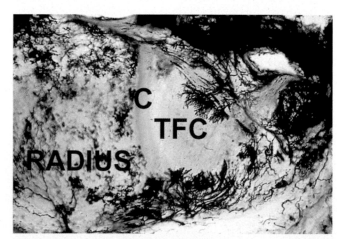

FIGURE 53.4 This axial view of the triangular fibrocartilage after vascular perfusion shows the rich vascular supply of the peripheral portions of the triangular fibrocartilage volarly, ulnarly, and radially. The central portion of the disc is avascular. The radial portion of the disc attaches to the articular surface of the medial radius, and when this cartilage is intact, there is poor vascularity to the radial attachment. TFC, triangular fibrocartilage; V, articular surface, radius. (From Bednar MS, Arnoczky, SP, Weiland AJ. The microvasculature of the triangular fibrocartilage complex: its clinical significance. *Gen Hand Surg Am* 1991;16:1101–1105, with permission.)

TABLE 53.1 TYPE 1: TRAUMATIC LESIONS

A. Central perforation	D. Radial avulsion
B. Ulnar avulsion	With sigmoid notch fracture
With distal ulnar fracture	Without sigmoid notch fracture
Without distal ulnar fracture	
C. Distal avulsion	

Not all perforations and defects in the TFC are traumatic. Several authors have shown an age-related correlation with lesions in the TFC (22,23). Many of these defects are asymptomatic. Patients with positive ulnar variance are more susceptible to such attritional lesions (24). In some instances, an acute injury is superposed on an otherwise asymptomatic tear.

CLASSIFICATION

Although several classification systems have been described (25–27), I have found the one by Palmer (28,29) to be the most useful. He divides the injuries into two basic categories, traumatic (type 1) and degenerative (type 2) (Table 53.1). Traumatic lesions are classified according to the location of the tear within the TFCC. Degenerative lesions are associated with positive ulnar variance and often have associated damage to surrounding structures such as the lunatotriquetral (or lunotriquetral) ligament and articular surfaces of the lunate triquetrum and the distal ulna.

A type 1A lesion represents an isolated tear in the central portion of the TFC disc (Fig. 53.5). The tear is several millimeters medial to the radial attachment, is usually oriented from volar to dorsal, and has the characteristics of an unstable flap. Type 1B (Fig. 53.6) lesions represent a peripheral tear of the TFC from its insertion on the distal ulna. This le-

sion can occur either with a fracture of the ulnar styloid or as a nonbony avulsion. The peripheral TFC is intimate with the floor of the ECU sheath. Thus, this type of injury can be associated with a concomitant disruption of the ECU sheath and clinical subluxation of ECU. This injury may also be associated with some mild clinical instability of the distal radioulnar joint.

Type 1C lesions (Fig. 53.7) represent a disruption of the TFCC from the volar ulnocarpal extrinsic ligaments. This lesion may result in a supination deformity of the carpus on the ulna.

Type 1D lesions (Fig. 53.8) represent avulsions of the TFC from its radial attachment. These are usually linear and are oriented in a volar dorsal direction. They occur within 1 to 2 mm of the medial corner of the radius and are often seen in distal radial fracture.

DIAGNOSIS

The mechanical symptoms of a TFC injury consist of ulnar-sided wrist pain, frequently with clicking (30). There may be a history of a fall on the pronated wrist, a traction injury, or a twisting injury. These symptoms should be mechanical, that is, improved by rest and worsened by load activity. The patient often has an associated tendinitis of the ECU tendon.

Generally, the symptoms should not be of a disabling intensity. The physical examination usually reveals tenderness over the ulnar side of the wrist. The TFC compression test is a provocative maneuver that is significant if it yields a painful response. The examiner axially loads the wrist (Fig. 53.9). Then with ulnar deviation or rotatory motion, a painful click that reproduces the symptoms can be elicited. As with all provocative maneuvers, it is important to compare the find-

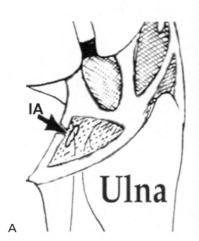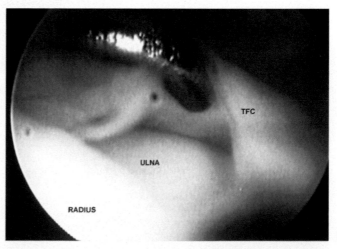

FIGURE 53.5 A: Schema of a traumatic type 1A central tear. **B:** Arthroscopic view from the 3-4 portal of a classic 1A tear. The probe shows the redundancy of the triangular fibrocartilage. The underlying ulna is noted to have a pristine articular surface and to be ulnar negative variant.

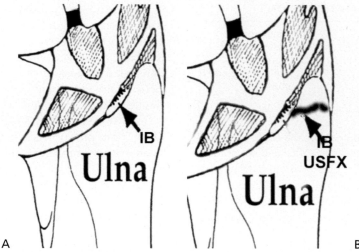

FIGURE 53.6 A: Schema of a type 1B peripheral avulsion of the triangular fibrocartilage disc from the dorsal ulnar aspect. **B:** Schema of a 1B peripheral TFC avulsion associated with fracture of the ulnar styloid.

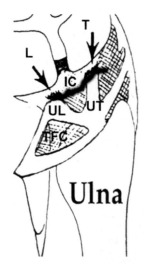

FIGURE 53.7 Schema of a type 1C distal avulsion from the ulnar extrinsic ligaments.

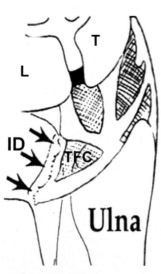

FIGURE 53.8 A type 1D lesion with avulsion of the triangular fibrocartilage from the radius.

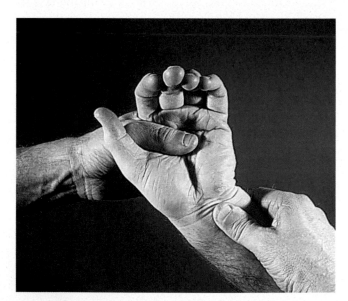

FIGURE 53.9 Triangular fibrocartilage axial load test.

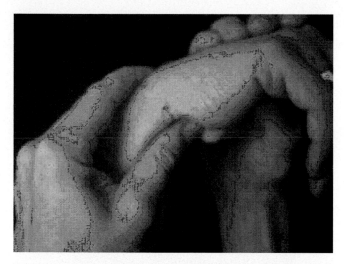

FIGURE 53.10 Ulnocarpal sag test. In the resting position, the ulnar carpus is seen to sag or lie in a supinated position relative to the ulna, which becomes more prominent. Upward pressure on the pisiform and downward pressure on the ulna can reduce the deformity. It generally represents either a type 1B or 1C triangular fibrocartilage lesion.

ings with those of the opposite wrist. The distal radioulnar joint should also be assessed for instability. Significant instability often presents as a positive "piano key" sign and a prominence of the distal ulna. Gross laxity represents a significant disruption of the TFCC. Repair of this lesion when necessary is often beyond the scope of arthroscope intervention. Arthroscopic repairs are most beneficial when any instability detected is mild. The ulnar carpus should be tested to see whether it supinates excessively on the distal ulna. When seen from the ulnar aspect, the carpus sags relative to the ulna (Fig. 53.10). This sign is suggestive of a type 1B or

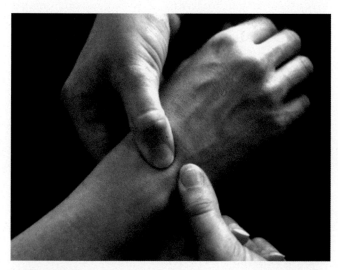

FIGURE 53.11 Lunatotriquetral ballottement test. The thumb and index finger on one hand stabilize the pisiform triquetral axis while the other hand stabilizes the lunate. A painful clicking in this area is often indicative of a lunatotriquetral ligament injury.

1C lesion. The lunatotriquetral joint should also be assessed to rule out concomitant lunatotriquetral ligament tear. Examination usually reveals point tenderness over the lunatotriquetral interval or the ulnar snuff box. A shuck test or lunatotriquetral ballottement test is often positive (Fig. 53.11). The ECU tendon should be checked for subluxation. Grip strength should be measured using a Jamar dynamometer; valid though weakened grip strength curves should be seen. (In some instances, differential anesthetic injection may be helpful in localizing the symptomatic source.) The differential diagnosis of ulnar-sided wrist pain consistent with TFCC injury includes ECU subluxation, lunatotriquetral ligament injury, pisotriquetral arthritis, chondral lesions of the ulnar lunate or midcarpal joint, ulnar artery thrombosis, and ulnar neuropathy at the wrist.

IMAGING STUDIES

Radiologic examination should include plain radiographs with neutral rotation posteroanterior and lateral views. These films allow assessment of carpal alignment, ulnar styloid morphology, and, most important, ulnar variance (31). Positive ulnar variance may be associated with an impaction-type cystic lesion in the ulnar half of the lunate. Configuration, alignment, and any arthritic change of the distal radioulnar joint should be noted. Clenched-fist radiographs in full ulnar deviation may show evidence of dynamic variance changes.

Advanced Imaging Studies

Advanced imaging techniques include arthrography, computed tomography, triple-phase bone scan, and magnetic resonance imaging (MRI). The role of each of these studies in the workup of a suspected TFC tear is debated. They should not replace a careful history, physical examination, plain radiography, or a reasoned correlation of signs and symptoms with the reported disorder.

Wrist arthrography can assess the integrity of the TFC and the intrinsic ligaments. Although it can be done as a static single radiocarpal injection, in my experience, the triple-injection arthrogram, as recommended by Levinsohn et al. (32), is best. The test involves initial injection of contrast material to the radiocarpal joint (Fig. 53.12). It is critical to observe the dye during the early flow phase as it is injected. If no dye leakage occurs in the midcarpal or distal radioulnar joints, then additional injections of the midcarpal and the distal radioulnar joint are administered after adequate time has passed to allow absorption of the contrast from the first injection. The midcarpal injection is most reliable for detecting tears of the lunatotriquetral ligament, and the distal radioulnar joint injection is reliable for detecting peripheral tears of the TFC. In both cases, one-way flaps may be missed on a single radiocarpal injection.

Several authors have questioned the significance of any arthrographic findings (31,33). A high incidence of symmetric findings has been reported in the opposite asymptomatic wrist. This finding led Metz and Reinus et al. (35,36) to conclude that, for an arthroscopic finding to be significant, it required bilateral triple-compartment arthrograms and a correlation of any asymmetric leakage with the patient's symptoms. Furthermore, arthrography cannot determine the size of the tear, its degree of instability, or whether there is associated synovitis or chondral change (35).

Computed tomography is best reserved when there is a question of instability or incongruency of the distal radial ulnar joint. Such a situation occurs very infrequently in the workup of TFC lesions.

A triple-phase bone scan has been helpful in identifying inflammation of the wrist. It can be considered a visual sedimentation rate of wrist inflammation and as a validity test in patients with poorly localized or excessive symptoms. A symptomatic TFC tear manifests a slight increased uptake ulnarly. In our study (38), there was a correlation with a positive bone scan ulnarly and a positive outcome after TFC debridement.

MRI has become the most widely used imaging study in the diagnosis of TFC tears (39–41). The advent of dedicated wrist coils has improved the resolution, but there is still poor sensitivity for detecting ulnar-sided TFC avulsions

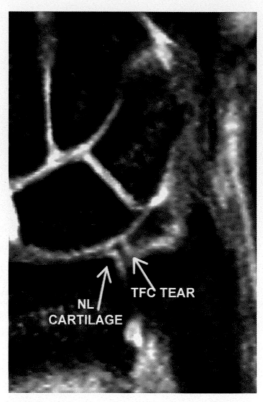

FIGURE 53.13 Magnetic resonance imaging of the wrist showing a tear of the triangular fibrocartilage. The clear area at the border of the radius is normal articular cartilage and does not represent a TFC tear.

and injury to the lunatotriquetral ligament. Our studies and those of others (42) have shown that the technique is 90% accurate for central and radial tears. The T2- or STIR-weighted images in the coronal plain are of the greatest diagnostic value (Fig. 53.13). The synovial fluid of the joint appears as a bright image with T2 weighting and outlines the tear of the TFC, similar to an arthrogram. Unlike arthrography, MRI can detect marrow changes, thus making it ideal to detect early avascular necrosis. Many patients with ulnar impaction have marrow changes on the ulnar side of the lunate, and this finding should not be confused with Kienböck's disease (Fig. 53.14).

Compared with these imaging studies, arthroscopy is more accurate in diagnosing lesions of the TFC (37,42,43). Arthroscopy can assess the size of the tear and can detect whether it has an unstable flap or associated synovitis or chondral or ligament lesions. The findings of active synovitis ulnarly associated with a tear usually correlate with this clinical significance (Fig. 53.15).

INDICATIONS FOR ARTHROSCOPIC TREATMENT

Initial treatment of most acute TFC injuries is by immobilization. Care should be taken to rule out any significant in-

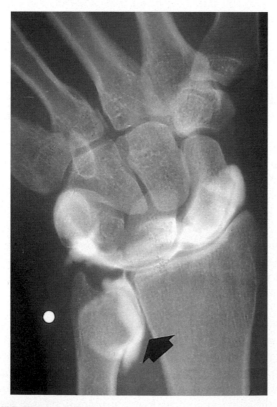

FIGURE 53.12 Radiocarpal arthrogram showing a classic communication with the distal radial ulnar joint through a triangular fibrocartilage tear. The *white dot* represents a pain marker.

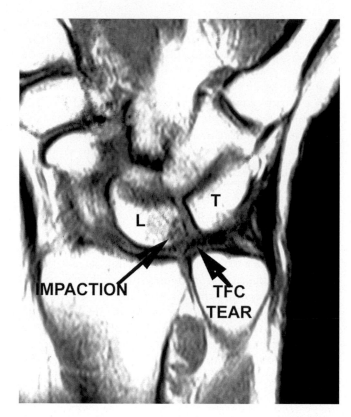

FIGURE 53.14 Ulnar impaction syndrome. This magnetic resonance imaging scan of the wrist shows the 1-mm positive ulnar variance with TFC disruption (better seen on the T2- or STIR-weighted image) and the impaction changes on the ulnar side of the lunate. These changes should not be confused with Kienböck's disease.

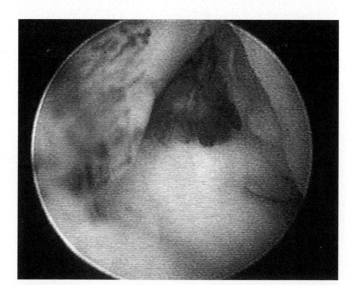

FIGURE 53.15 Arthroscopic view of active synovitis confirming the mechanical irritation caused by the adjacent triangular fibrocartilage tear.

stability of the distal radioulnar joint as well as associated injuries such as subluxation of the ECU tendon. If routine radiographs are negative and instability is not present, immobilization for 4 weeks is recommended (44,45). A peripheral tear would be expected to heal because of its good vascularity. In some patients, the judicious use of a steroid injection to calm local synovitis or ECU tendinitis, as well as a short course of wrist therapy, may also be helpful. Many central tears may also become asymptomatic even though they do not heal.

Studies by Mikic (22) have revealed age-related TFC perforations. In Mikic's studies, there were no TFC perforations in wrists of patients younger than 30 years. After the third decade, however, a linear progression of perforation with age was present such that all specimens from patients older than 50 years were found to have a TFC perforation. These anatomic findings support the concept that the defect in the central portion of the TFC can occur without symptoms. It is important to keep this fact in mind before attributing a patient's symptomatic pain fully to an observed perforation on an imaging study.

Indications for arthroscopic TFC surgery are a proven or suspected TFC injury with sufficient ulnar wrist symptoms that interfere with the patient's activities. The patient should have undergone a failed nonoperative treatment program of rest and immobilization and antiinflammatory drugs, as mentioned earlier. Generally, we wait a minimum of 3 to 4 months after the initial injury.

ARTHROSCOPIC TREATMENT

Type 1A Lesions

Type 1A lesions are isolated central tears of TFC without instability (Fig. 53.5). In patients with neutral or negative ulnar variance who have had no relief after nonoperative treatment, arthroscopic limited debrided of the unstable portion of the tear gives excellent relief of symptoms (26,30,46–48).

The biomechanical effect of excision of the central portion of the TFC has been examined (49,50). The excision of up to two-thirds of the central portion of the TFC with maintenance of the dorsal and volar and radial and ulnar ligaments and the ulnocarpal ligaments had no demonstrable effect on forearm axial load transmission or stability. Removal of greater than two-thirds of the disc or injury to the ligamentous portions will destabilize the distal radioulnar joint. Adams (49) emphasized that the peripheral 2 mm of the TFC must be maintained to avoid such stability problems.

A brief aside about the use of lasers and radiofrequency probes in wrist arthroscopy is appropriate (51). Currently, the holmium:yttrium-aluminum-garnet laser has been used to resect synovium and the TFC (52). The characteristics of this laser are its infrared spectrum, its fiberoptic capability, and its effectiveness in a liquid medium. Small 70-degree probes are now available that allow variable concentration of its energy to resect tissues efficiently ranging from synovium to bone. Concerns about damage to normal articular cartilage have been raised, but the major limitation to the widespread use of this technique continues to be its expense.

Small joint radiofrequency probes of both the monopolar and bipolar energy are now available. Such probes can be used for tissue resection and shrinkage. Although this method is cheaper than laser technology, similar concerns about long-term efficacy and effects been raised (53). Currently, standard arthroscopic instrumentation can successfully accomplish all therapeutic interventions relative to treating TFC lesions.

Regional anesthesia is generally used, and a well-padded tourniquet is placed on the patient's upper arm. The tourniquet is inflated approximately 50% of the time. After the induction of anesthesia, a careful clinical reexamination of the wrist is performed, including provocative maneuvers to identify the presence of any distal radial ulnar joint instability, abnormal clicks, or ECU subluxation. The wrist is then placed under traction, usually in a wrist traction tower. Initial placement of the arthroscope is through the 3-4 portal. After the systematic examination of the radial side of the wrist, the arthroscope is directed ulnarly. For the symptomatic lesion, synovitis is usually observed, particularly in the area of the prestyloid recess. Using an ulnar portal, most commonly the 6R portal, a 2.0- to 3.0-mm full-radius motorized suction shaver is inserted. As an alternative, a 4-5 portal can be used. The use of an 18-gauge needle can then be beneficial in establishing the exact placement and optimal position for the working portal.

After debridement of the synovitis, a small probe is inserted to palpate the instability of any flap tear as well as the tension in the TFC. Integrity of the ulnar extrinsic ligaments and of the intrinsic lunatotriquetral ligament should also be assessed visually and palpably.

For resection of the unstable flap, schutt punches and a small joint suction punch are used to excise the bulk of the lesion. A small joint banana blade is useful to transect the most ulnar portion of the unstable flap. If this technique is used, care should be taken not to use the underlying distal ulna as a cutting board and to use only the tip of the blade in cutting. The unstable portion is excised as an isolated fragment, very similar to a bucket-handle tear of the knee meniscus. The small-radius resector is then used to trim the edges. Occasionally, it is useful to switch the viewing portal to an ulnar portal and to bring the suction punch or shaver in from the radial side to smooth the ulnar remnant. Only the unstable portion is excised, with care taken to leave the peripheral attachments undisturbed (Fig. 53.16).

Patients with a traumatic central tear associated with positive ulnar variance may demonstrate chondromalacia and other impaction wear. These cases are best treated with limited debridement and ulnar recession by an arthroscopic wafer resection or osteotomy. This procedure is discussed in detail under the treatment of type 2 degenerative lesions.

After the completion of the radiocarpal portion of the arthroscopy through both radial and ulnar portals, the midcarpal joint should also be inspected. After completion of the procedure, the wrist is again reexamined while the patient is under anesthesia. Clicks that were generated by the TFC abnormality generally disappear after debridement. Portal sites are closed with either a Steri-strip or one nylon suture. A splint is used for the first week to support the wrist and extensor tendons. A splint is then worn intermittently for comfort for 3 weeks with restrictions on forceful grasping and repetitive rotatory activities. In some patients, a supervised therapy program may help to achieve a maximally improved outcome.

The outcomes of type 1A debridement have been rewarding, with between 80% and 85% of patients requiring

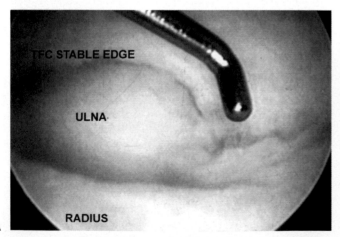

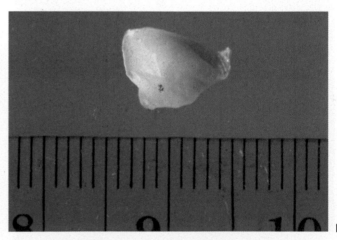

FIGURE 53.16 A: Arthroscopic view of a debrided type 1A triangular fibrocartilage (TFC) tear. Note the stable rim and *intact* ulnar cartilage. **B:** Excision of an unstable portion of a traumatic 1C TFC disc.

no further surgery and having an excellent to good result (38,46–48,54).

Type 1B Lesions

The diagnosis of a chronic type 1B peripheral tear (Fig. 53.6) can be difficult to make. Clinically, aside from ulnar wrist pain and a possible TFC stress test, there is often the suggestion of mild distal radial ulnar joint instability. In the isolated lesion without ulnar styloid fracture, plain radiographs are normal. Distal radial ulnar joint arthrography has been the most accurate modality, by identifying 60% of such tears compared with only 10% by radiocarpal arthrography and 40% by MRI (32).

Arthroscopy, however, is ideal in defining the peripheral lesion. From a viewing radial portal, the examiner may note synovitis peripherally and after debridement of this lesion, the peripheral tear may become obvious. The pathognomic finding is a loss of the normal tension of the TFC. With a probe brought through an ulnar portal, the tension in the TFC is palpated. As Hermansdorfer and Kleinman described (55), the tension in the TFC should be taut, like that of a drumhead or a trampoline. If the probe sinks into the TFC, as if into a feather bed, then a peripheral tear should be suspected (Fig. 53.17A and B).

One caveat in treating type 2B peripheral tears is that more than 50% of such lesions are associated with subluxation of the ECU tendon. The floor of the fibrous sheath of the ECU is intimate with the peripheral TFC. With hypersupination, both the floor of the ECU sheath and the peripheral TFC can be torn. In fact, Melone and Nathan (15) postulated a continuum of injury on the ulnar side of the wrist beginning with ECU sheath through the peripheral portion of the TFC continuing on through the ulnar extrinsic ligaments and lunatotriquetral ligaments. Thus, ECU subluxation accompanying a peripheral tear represents an early stage of this sequential injury pattern. Treatment requires not only arthroscopic repair of the peripheral TFC tear but also open reconstruction of the ECU sheath.

Several authors (55,56) reported the successful result of open repairs of this peripheral lesion of the TFC. In multiple studies (57–59), it is now clear that arthroscopic repair compares favorably with the open technique. There are two main techniques of arthroscopic repair. They both share an outside-to-inside approach but differ in the direction of that approach.

De Araujo et al. (57) popularized the Tuohy needle technique, by directing the sutures from the radial side of the wrist across the tear. The sutures are retrieved ulnarly and are tied. A concern of this repair technique is that the position of the counterincision and the exit point are somewhat difficult to control. Complications relative to irritation of the dorsal ulnar sensory nerve have been reported.

Currently, I favor an out-in technique from the ulnar side as originated by Whipple (6,59,60) (Fig. 53.17C). A standard arthroscopic setup is used, and the scope is directed from the 3-4 portal. After synovectomy, the edges of the tear are debrided with a full-radius resection to encourage healing and the stimulation of vascular ingrowth. A small, 1-cm incision is made just radial to the ECU tendon. The radial aspect of the sheath is opened for approximately 1 cm, with care taken not to disrupt the medial sheath or stability or stability of the ECU. Retracting the ECU ulnarly, two needles are passed through the capsule and across the tear under arthroscopic visualization (Fig. 53.17D and 17) Currently, I find the use of either the meniscus mender (6) or the TFC repair device most useful for this purpose. A wire loop is then passed through one needle to retrieve a 2-0 polydioxanone suture that has been passed through the other needle. This allows passage of a loop-type suture across the tear that, when drawn tight, will approximate the tear. Between two and four sutures may be required. The sutures are tied over the dorsal wrist capsule, rather than exteriorized over a button. The patient is immobilized in a Muenster cast for 4 weeks, and then a therapy program is started. Because this is a reparative procedure, outcome results have been excellent, with 85% to 90% achieving good to excellent results on long-term follow-up (6,58).

When a peripheral tear is associated with an ununited ulnar styloid fragment and instability, I have, in most cases, made the diagnosis arthroscopically. However, I have done an open procedure to address the ulnar styloid fragment with bony reattachment or excision of the fragment and reattachment of the TFC to the remaining distal ulna.

Type 1C Lesions

Type 1C lesions (Fig. 53.7) involve disruption of the TFC from the ulnar extrinsic ligament complex. Clinically, the patient may show a carpal supination deformity. Imaging techniques are not useful. For example, wrist arthrography often shows a communication to the pisotriquetral joint, but this exists as a normal variant of arthroscopy.

Arthroscopically, the diagnosis is made by a loss of tension or tear in the ulnar extrinsic ligaments (Fig. 53.18), as well as by the easy and direct visualization of the pisotriquetral joint. If the pisiform can be seen on radiocarpal arthroscopy, this usually represents a defect of these ulnar ligaments.

My Preferred Method

If the defect in the ulnar extrinsic ligaments is reparable, I make a small, 1-cm incision volar to the ECU tendon in the area of the triquetral snuff-box. Care is taken to avoid injury to the dorsal ulnar sensory nerve or volar ulnar neurovascular structures. The technique similar to the out-in repair of the peripheral TFC lesion. Needles are passed through the capsule through the defect in the ulnar extrinsic ligaments. The looped to sutures of 2-0 polydioxanone are then

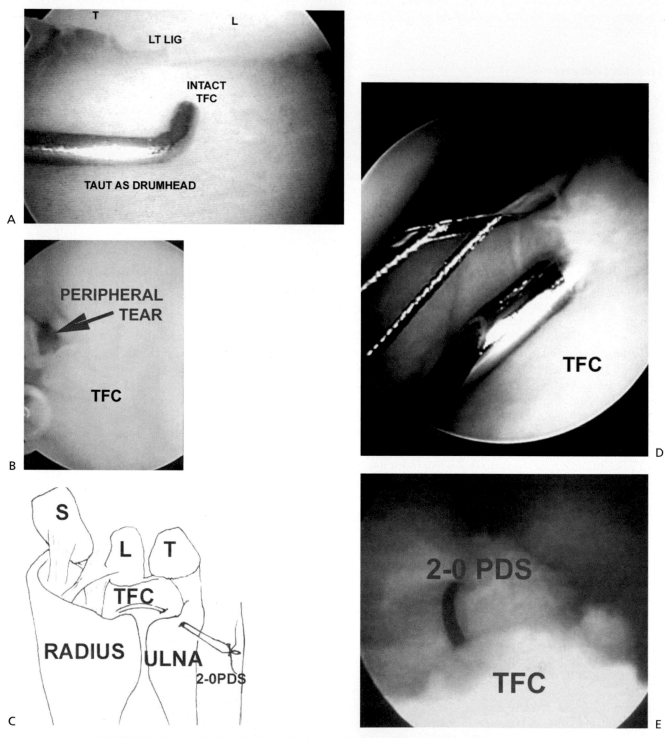

FIGURE 53.17 A: Arthroscopic view of an intact triangular fibrocartilage with normal drumhead compliance. If the triangular fibrocartilage were torn peripherally, the probe would sink into the triangular fibrocartilage as if it were a feather bed. **B:** Arthroscopic view of the peripheral tear, which is generally seen by viewing from the 3-4 portal toward the dorsal and ulnar aspect of the triangular fibrocartilage. This area must be debrided before the arthroscopic peripheral repair. **C:** Diagram of typical 1B arthroscopic peripheral repair. **D:** Using a meniscus mender, two needles are passed through the sheath of the extensor carpi ulnaris and across the tear. A loop is then passed through one needle. It is placed over the other needle, and a 2-0 polydioxanone suture is passed. **E:** Arthroscopic view of the suture repairing the peripheral tear. In general, one to three sutures are used.

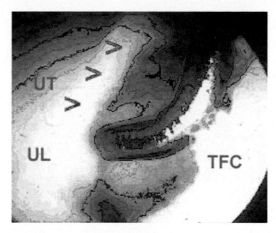

FIGURE 53.18 Arthroscopic picture of a type 1C lesion separating the triangular fibrocartilage from the ulnar extrinsic ligaments.

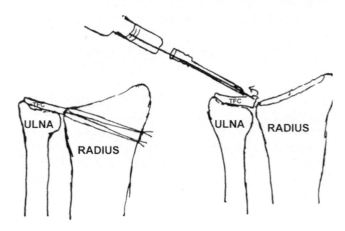

FIGURE 53.20 Diagram of a type 1D repair using an in-to-out technique with sutures tied over the lateral side of the radius in the area of the first extensor compartment.

brought out and are tied at the capsule level. When this lesion is present and repaired arthroscopically, it is often common to reef the dorsal ulnar portion of the TFC ligament as described for the type 1B lesion.

Type 1D Lesions

Type 1D lesions involve radial detachment of the TFC from the sigmoid notch to the distal radius (Fig. 53.8). Although not in Dr. Palmer's classification, this lesion could rightly be categorized with those that occur in isolation and those associated with a distal radial fracture (Fig. 53.19). Normally, the articular cartilage of the radius continues around the medial corner and into the sigmoid notch. The TFC originates from this articular location. Given this cartilage barrier, vascular studies suggest a poor potential for healing of such a radial tear. However, if this

cartilage is disrupted by fracture or mechanically, and the attachment site occurs on vascularized bone, then healing can occur. Arthroscopic repair techniques have been described by Sagerman and Short (61), by Jantea et al. (62), and by Jones and Trumble (63).

TFC tears within the 2-mm sigmoid rim that are oriented vertically from volar to dorsal are amenable to this technique. Standard arthroscopic traction setup is used. Once the tear has been identified and determined reparable, a small bur is introduced through the 4-5 portal, and the attachment site of the radius is abraded to bleeding bone (Fig. 53.20). In the interval between the flexor carpi ulnaris and ECU tendons, a 0.045 Kirschner wire (K-wire) is passed through the capsule to fix the detached TFC to the prepared radius. The jig, which is essentially a wire guide, is then placed over this K-wire to provide alignment of the entry point on the radial side of the wrist.

A

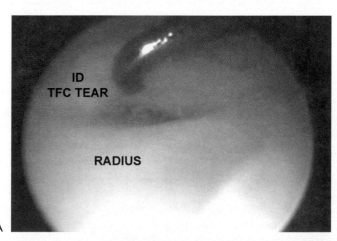

B

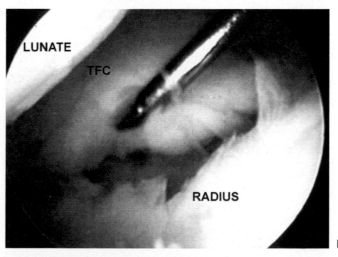

FIGURE 53.19 A: Classic type 1D tear not associated with a distal radius fracture. **B:** A type 1D tear associated with a fracture of the radius. This is a common lesion and is often triggered by pinning the triangular fibrocartilage back to its medial origin with a 4-5 K-wire.

A small longitudinal skin incision is then made between the first and second extensor compartments. Care is taken to avoid injury to the dorsal radial sensory nerve, radial artery, and extensor tendons. The jig and wire are adjusted to make sure these structures are avoided. An 18-gauge spinal needle is then placed in the jig and is drilled through the distal radius exiting at the prepared bone interface and then is passed through the TFC. In a similar fashion, a second 18-gauge spinal needle is introduced parallel to this. The trocars are removed from the 18-gauge needles, and a 2-0 polydioxanone suture is inserted through one needle and is retrieved through the opposite needle using a wire loop catcher. The suture is tied down over the radius, with the tension of the TFC confirmed under arthroscopic visualization. If necessary, a second suture is used. If the alignment jig is not available, then an alternative technique described by Trumble using a cannula and preloaded meniscal repair suture is equally effective.

When a radial TFC tear is identified during the arthroscopic treatment of a distal radial fracture, the radial portion of the TFC is pinned back to the radius using 0.035 K-wires. The TFC fixation pin is left percutaneously and is usually removed at 4 weeks. Arthroscopic and/or arthrographic evaluation in several of these patients has confirmed healing of the radial attachment.

TYPE 2 DEGENERATIVE TRIANGULAR FIBROCARTILAGE LESIONS

Degenerative tears are related to chronic overloading of the ulnar side of the wrist. The primary pathologic process is not in the TFC, but rather is the result of chronic ulnar abutment or impaction. Once symptomatic, the problem is progressive, and deterioration occurs over time (Table 53.2). For this reason, I recommend surgical correction in sufficiently symptomatic patients. The ulnar impaction may be primary or secondary. Wrists with neutral or positive ulnar

TABLE 53.2 DEGENERATIVE (ULNOCARPAL ABUTMENT SYNDROME STAGE) LESIONS

A. TFCC wear	E. TFCC perforation Lunate and/or ulnar chondromalacia Lunatotriquetral ligament perforation Ulnocarpal arthritis
B. TFCC wear Lunate and/or ulnar chondromalacia	
C. TFCC perforation Lunate and/or ulnar chondromalacia	
D. TFCC perforation Lunate and/or ulnar chondromalacia Lunatotriquetral ligament perforation	

TFCC, Triangular fibrocartilage complex.

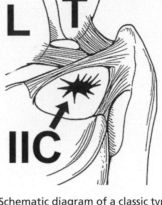

FIGURE 53.21 Schematic diagram of a classic type 2C degenerative tear. Note the stellate and fragmented appearance of the tear.

variance demonstrate tears or perforations in 73% compared with only 17% in specimens with negative ulnar variance (23). Secondary causes are generally traumatic and include distal radial fractures that heal with dorsal tilt and radial shortening. Short et al. (64) correlated increases in the dorsal tilt of the distal radius with forces transmitted to the distal ulna during axial loading. Other causes include distal radial growth arrest after physeal fractures in children and proximal migration of the radius after radial head resection. The ulnar impaction may also be dynamic, present only on load activities such as grip or forceful rotation. Thus, a patient with static neutral or even negative ulnar variance could dynamically have ulnar abutment. Arthroscopy plays a definite role in the treatment of primary ulnar impaction, whereas in secondary abutment, open surgery is often required.

In Palmer's schema, the progressive degenerative changes of ulnar abutment are subdivided into five categories: 2A, wear of the TFC without perforation of chondromalacia; 2B, wear of the TFC with chondromalacia of the lunate or ulna; 2C, true perforation of the TFC with lunate and/or chondromalacia (Fig. 53.21); 2D, TFC perforation plus lunate and/or ulnar chondromalacia and lunatotriquetral ligament perforation. No carpal instability patterns such as volar intercalary segmental instability is present (see Fig. 53.25); 2E, TFC perforation with generalized arthritic changes ulnarly involving the lunate and ulna. There is perforation of the lunatotriquetral ligament and ulnocarpal arthritis.

Diagnosis of a degenerative tear should be suspected in an older patient who complains of nontraumatic ulnar-sided wrist pain. Physical examination reveals tenderness over the distal ulna that increases with rotatory motion and loading of the wrist. The TFC compression test is often positive. Other provocative maneuvers, such as the shuck test, should be performed to assess the lunatotriquetral ligament stability. Distal radioulnar joint compression test may be positive if arthritis is present in this joint. Measurement of grip strength in pronation and supination may also be helpful.

As mentioned previously, ulnar variance radiographs are critical. Reservations relative to any cystic changes present on the ulnar aspect of the lunate or in the ulnar head should be recorded as well as the presence of any incongruency or arthritis of the distal radial ulnar joint. Arthrography is seldom used now, but radiocarpal injection can demonstrate the central TFC tear and midcarpal arthrography can detect the lunatotriquetral perforation.

MRI has been applied to the diagnosis of ulnar impaction. These symptomatic patients have focal signal intensity changes in the ulnar part of the lunate. Signal abnormality should not be confused with Kienböck's disease (Fig. 53.14). Imaeda et al. (40) noted focal abnormal signal intensity on the ulnar aspect of the lunate in 87% of patients with ulnar impaction; 43% showed similar changes on the triquetrum and 10% on the radial aspect of the ulnar head. After surgical correction, the signal intensity often returns to normal. MRI can also reveal tears in the TFC with a high degree of accuracy, but it is not sensitive to alterations in the lunatotriquetral ligament.

Diagnostic arthroscopy is the best way of staging the ulnar impaction lesion. Arthroscopy can directly evaluate the chondral surfaces for evidence of fibrillation or more severe chondral changes not visible on current imaging techniques. The TFC lesion is generally central and ragged as compared with the more linear traumatic tear. The lunatotriquetral ligament and stability of the lunatotriquetral joint should be assessed not only from the radiocarpal portal but also from the midcarpal portal.

Treatment

The primary goal in the treatment of ulnar impaction is to unload or decompress the ulnar carpus and ulnar head. This decompression can be accomplished by ulnar shortening osteotomy, partial ulnar head resection, or ulnar salvage procedures. Ulnar shortening osteotomy has been improved by the use of rigid fixation (65–67). Partial ulnar head resection, the so-called *wafer procedure,* removes the positive very distal portions of the ulna while leaving the distal radial ulnar joint intact. Feldon et al. (68) devised the open wafer technique, and it is now often performed arthroscopically (69). Distal radial ulnar joint salvage procedures such as a modified Darrach procedure and hemiresection interposition procedures are best reserved when there is arthritis of the distal radial ulnar joint.

Types 2A and 2B Lesions

A standard arthroscopic evaluation confirms the presence of any chondromalacia lesions and the continuity of the TFC and lunatotriquetral ligament. Any synovial inflammation is debrided. After the arthroscopy, an open ulnar shortening osteotomy is performed.

Type 2C Lesions

The ragged central tear is debrided with a suction punch to reveal the radial aspect of the ulna through the margins of the trimmed tear (Figs. 53.21 and 53.22). With a 3-4 viewing portal, a 4-mm bur is brought in through an ulnar portal, and the arthroscopic wafer procedure is begun. With the

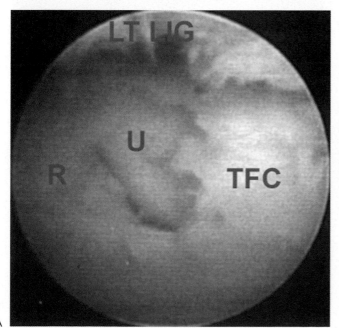

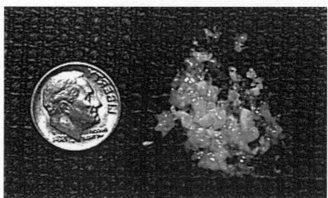

FIGURE 53.22 A: Arthroscopic view of a degenerative triangular fibrocartilage tear. Note the chondromalacia of the underlying distal ulna and the fraying of the lunate triquetrum and lunatotriquetral ligament. **B:** Typical excision remnants from a degenerative triangular fibrocartilage tear. Note the multiple fragments as compared with the traumatic type 1A tear in Fig. 53.16B.

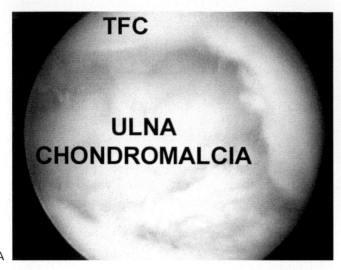
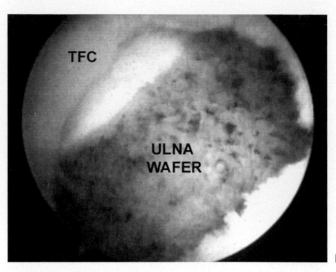

FIGURE 53.23 A: After debriding the triangular fibrocartilage, the arthroscopic view reveals significant ulnar impaction chondromalacia. This requires decompression with either arthroscopic resection or formal ulnar shortening osteotomy. **B:** Arthroscopic view after completion of the arthroscopic wafer.

bur, it is important to pronate and supinate the patient's wrist, to level the margins of the distal ulna evenly (Fig. 53.23). The medial corner of the radius serves as an anatomic landmark to assess the level of the resection. The limits of a resection that can be accomplished arthroscopically are between 3 and 4 mm.

Once the radial third of the ulna is resected through the tear, an 18-gauge needle is placed in the distal radial ulnar joint beneath the tear. The dislocation is confirmed from the 3-4 viewing portal. Using this needle as a marker, an operative portal to the distal radioulnar joint is established. Through this portal site, a bur or a small ⅛-inch osteotome is

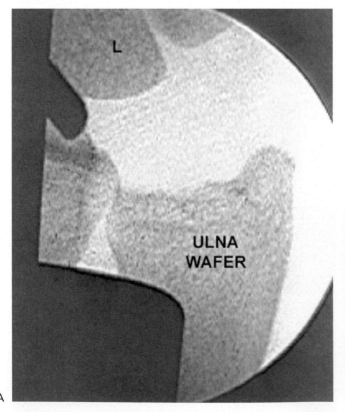
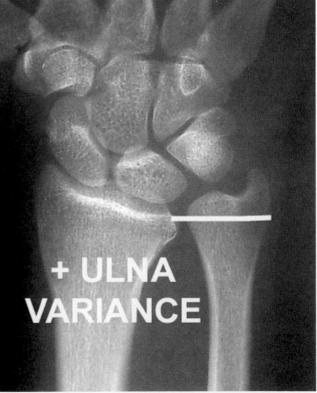

FIGURE 53.24 A: Arthroscopic view showing positive ulnar variance and an ulnar impaction lesion. **B:** Interoperative view after 3-mm wafer resection of distal ulna.

inserted. This allows clearance of the ulnar portion of the distal ulna beneath the remaining intact portion of the TFC. The leveling of the distal ulna is carried over to the basal styloid area. Frequent fluoroscopic evaluation is used to confirm the level of resection (Fig. 53.24). The final level of resection is assessed not only by the relationship to the medial corner of the radius but also under fluoroscopic control and in various rotatory positions. With adequate resection, the remaining portion of the TFC should be under no tension. The exact amount of cartilage and subchondylar ulnar bone to be resected is not precisely known. Wnorowski et al. showed that the excision of 3 mm of subchondylar bone decreased the force transmitted across the ulnar head by 50%. Further bone resection did little to decrease this poor transfer. In general, the arthroscopic resection seems to produce a negative ulnar variance of 2 mm. Postoperative treatment involves an intermittent short-arm splint for 4 weeks with active range-of-wrist motion exercises, followed by a graduated strengthening program at 4 weeks.

Types 2D and DE Lesions

These are the end stages of the ulnar impaction syndrome and represent disruption of the lunatotriquetral ligament with varying degrees of lunatotriquetral instability (Fig. 53.25). After arthroscopic debridement of the TFC as described in the type 2C lesion, a careful evaluation of a lunatotriquetral interval is done from both the radiocarpal and midcarpal joints.

If the ligament is frayed but the midcarpal joint shows no significant step-off at the lunatotriquetral interface and there are no chondromalacic changes on the hamate, then an arthroscopic wafer procedure is performed similar to that in type 2C lesions. This is particularly true in older patients.

If evidence of lunatotriquetral instability is noted such as fraying of the ulnar extrinsic ligaments, significant translation of the lunatotriquetral interface in the midcarpal joint, and chondromalacic changes on the hamate interface, then an ulnar shortening osteotomy is preferred. The frayed portions of the lunatotriquetral ligament are debrided, synovitic changes in the radiocarpal and midcarpal joint are debrided, and in some cases chondroplasty of the hamate is performed. After the ulnar shortening osteotomy, the lunatotriquetral interval is reassessed arthroscopically. Often there is improved stability of the lunatotriquetral interval secondary to tightening of the ulnar extrinsic ligaments, and no further treatment is indicated. If there is still significant instability, then percutaneous K-wire fixation of the lunatotriquetral interval is performed using two or three 0.045 K-wires. These wires are buried subcutaneously. If there are significant arthritic changes at the distal radioulnar joint, then salvage procedures are indicated.

A short-arm cast is worn between 4 and 8 weeks, and the percutaneous pins are removed in the office at between 6 and 8 weeks. A graduated therapy program is then begun, with maximum improvement reached by 4 months. The outcome of arthroscopic surgery for degenerative type 2 lesions requires long-term follow-up. Results at 3 to 5 years have yielded excellent to good clinical results in 75% of cases (38,52,70).

REFERENCES

1. Cooney WP. Tears of the triangular fibrocartilage of the wrist. In: Cooney WP, Linscheid RL, Dobyns JH, eds. *The wrist: diagnosis and operative treatment.* St. Louis, MO: CV Mosby, 1998:710–742.
2. Osterman AL. Wrist arthroscopy: operative procedures. In: Green DP, Hotchkiss RN, Pederson WC, eds. *Green's operative hand surgery,* 4th ed. Philadelphia: Churchill Livingstone, 1999: 207–222.
3. Palmer AK, Harris PG. Classification and arthroscopic treatment of triangular fibrocartilage complex lesions. In: McGinty JB, Caspari RB, Jackson RW, et al., eds. *Operative arthroscopy,* 2nd ed. Philadelphia: Lippincott–Raven, 1996:1015–1022.
4. Stanley J, Saffar P. *Wrist arthroscopy.* Philadelphia: WB Saunders, 1994.
5. Sagerman SD, Palmer AK, Short WH. Triangular fibrocartilage complex injury and repair. In: Watson HK, Weinzeig J, eds. *The wrist.* Philadelphia: JB Lippincott, 2001:607–614.
6. Bednar JM, Osterman AL. The role of arthroscopy in the treatment of traumatic triangular fibrocartilage injuries. *Hand Clin* 1994;10:605–614.
7. Chidgey LK, Dell PC, Bittar E, et al. Histologic anatomy of the triangular fibrocartilage. *J Hand Surg Am* 1991;16:1084–1100.
8. Chidgey LK. The distal radioulnar joint: problems and solutions. *J Am Acad Orthop Surg* 1995;3:95–109.
9. Kauer JMG. The articular disc of the hand. *Acta Anat* 1975;93: 590–605.
10. Bednar MS, Arnoczky SP, Weiland AJ. The microvasculature of the triangular fibrocartilage complex: its clinical significance. *J Hand Surg Am* 1991;16:1101–1105.
11. Thiru-Pathi RG, Ferlic DC, Clayton ML, et al. Arterial anatomy of the triangular fibrocartilage of the wrist and its surgical significance. *J Hand Surg Am* 1986;11:258–263.
12. Palmer AK, Werner FW. The triangular fibrocartilage complex of the wrist: anatomy and function. *J Hand Surg Am* 1981;6:153–162.

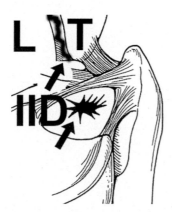

FIGURE 53.25 Schematic drawing of a classic type 2D triangular fibrocartilage lesion. Note the associated lunatotriquetral tear.

13. Palmer AK, Glisson RR, Werner FW. Relationship between ulnar variance and TFCC thickness. *J Hand Surg Am* 1984;9:681–683.

14. Kink GJ. Computerized tomography of the distal radioulnar joint: correlation with ligamentous pathology in a cadaveric model. *J Hand Surg Am* 1986;11:711–717.

15. Melone CP, Nathan R. Traumatic disruption of the triangular fibrocartilage complex. *Clin Orthop* 1992;275:65–73.

16. Culp RW, Osterman AL. Arthroscopic reduction and internal fixation of distal radius fractures. *Orthop Clin North Am* 1995;26:739–748.

17. Fischer M, Denzler C, Senwald G. Carpal ligament lesions associated with fresh distal radius fractures: arthroscopic study of 54 cases. *Swiss Surg* 1996;2:269–273.

18. Geissler WB, Freeland AE, Savoie FH, et al. Intra-articular soft tissue lesions associated with an intraarticular fracture of the distal end of the radius. *J Bone Joint Surg Am* 1996;78:357–365.

19. Lindau T. The role of wrist arthroscopy in distal radius fractures. *Atlas Hand Clin* 2001;6:285–305.

20. Richards RS, Bennett JD, Roth JH. Arthroscopic diagnoses of intraarticular soft tissue injuries associated with distal radius fractures *J Hand Surg Am* 1997;22:772–776.

21. Wolfe SW, Easterling KJ, Yoo AH. Arthroscopic assisted reduction of distal radius fracture. *Arthroscopy* 1995;11:706–714.

22. Mikic ZD. Age changes in the triangular fibrocartilage of the wrist joint. *J Anat* 1978;126:367–384.

23. Viegas SF, Ballantyne G. Attritional lesions of the wrist joint. *J Hand Surg Am* 1987;12:1025–1029.

24. Gan BS, Richards RS, Roth JH. Arthroscopic treatment of triangular fibro-cartilage tears. *Orthop Clin North Am* 1995;26:721–729.

25. Blair WF, Berger RA, El-Khoury GY. Arthrotomography of the wrist: an experimental and preliminary clinical study. *J Hand Surg Am* 1985;10:350–359.

26. Cooney WP, Linscheid RL, Dobyns JH. Triangular fibrocartilage tears. *J Hand Surg Am* 1994;19:143–154.

27. Whipple TL. Arthroscopic surgery. In: *The wrist*. Philadelphia: JB Lippincott, 1992.

28. Palmer AK. Triangular fibrocartilage complex lesions: a classification. *J Hand Surg Am* 1989;14:594–606.

29. Palmer AK. Triangular fibrocartilage disorders: injury patterns and treatment. *Arthroscopy* 1990;6:125–132.

30. Osterman AL, Terrill RG. Arthroscopic treatment of TFCC lesions. *Hand Clin* 1991;7:277–281.

31. Palmer AK, Glisson RR, Werner FW. Ulnar variance determination. *J Hand Surg Am* 1982;7:376.

32. Levinsohn EM, Rosen ID, Palmer AK. Wrist arthrography: value of the three compartment injection method. *Radiology* 1991;179:231–239.

33. Canter RM, Stern PJ, Wyrick JD, et al. The relevance of ligament tear or perforations on the diagnosis of wrist pain: an arthrographic study. *J Hand Surg Am* 1994;19:945–953.

34. Cooney WP. Evaluation of chronic wrist pain by arthrography, arthroscopy, and arthrotomy. *J Hand Surg Am* 1993;18:815–822.

35. Metz VM, Mann FA, Gilula LA. Lack of correlation between file of wrist pain and location of noncommunicating defects shown by three-compartment wrist arthrography. *AJR Am J Roentgenol* 1993;160:1239–1243.

36. Reinus WR, Hardy DC, Totty WG, et al. Arthrographic evaluation of the carpal triangular fibrocartilage complex. *J Hand Surg Am* 1987;12:495–503.

37. Roth JH, Haddad RG. Radiocarpal arthroscopy and arthrography in the diagnosis of ulnar wrist pain. *Arthroscopy* 1986;2:234–243.

38. Osterman AL. Arthroscopic debridement of triangular fibrocartilage complex tears. *Arthroscopy* 1990;6:120–124.

39. Golimbu CN, Firooznia H, Melone CP Jr, et al. Tears of the triangular fibrocartilage of the wrist: MR imaging. *Radiology* 1989;173:731–733.

40. Imaeda T, Nakamara R, Shionoya K, et al. Ulnar impaction syndrome: MR imaging findings. *Radiology* 1996;201:495–500.

41. Skahen JR, Palmer AK, Levinsohn EM, et al. Magnetic resonance imaging of the triangular fibrocartilage complex. *J Hand Surg Am* 1990;15:552–557.

42. Zlatkin MB, Chao PC, Osterman AL, et al. Chronic wrist pain: evaluation with high-resolution MR Imaging. *Radiology* 1989;173:723–729.

43. Pederzini L, Luchetti R, Soragni O, et al. Evaluation of the triangular fibrocartilage complex tears by arthroscopy, arthrography, and magnetic resonance imaging. *Arthroscopy* 1992;8:191–197.

44. Mikic Z, Ercegan GM. Healing of the articular disc of the wrist in dogs. *Int Orthop* 1993;17:282–285.

45. Mikic ZD. Treatment of acute injuries of the triangular fibrocartilage complex associated with distal radioulnar joint instability. *J Hand Surg Am* 1995;20:319–323.

46. DeSmet L, DeFerm A, Steenwerckx A, et al. Arthroscopic treatment of triangular fibrocartilage complex lesions of the wrist. *Acta Orthop Belg* 1996;62:8–13.

47. Gan BS, Richards RS, Roth JH. Arthroscopic treatment of triangular fibrocartilage tears. *Orthop Clin North Am* 1995;26:721–729.

48. Menon J, Wood VE, Schoene HR, et al. Isolated tears of the triangular fibrocartilage of the wrist: results of partial excision. *J Hand Surg Am* 1984;9:527–530.

49. Adams BD. Partial excision of the triangular fibrocartilage complex articular disc: a biomechanical study. *J Hand Surg* 1993;18:334–340.

50. Palmer AK, Werner FW, Glisson RR, et al. Partial excision of the triangular fibrocartilage complex. *J Hand Surg Am* 1988;13:391–394.

51. Nagle DJ, Geissler WB. Laser-assisted wrist arthroscopy. *Atlas Hand Clin* 2001;6:189–201.

52. Nagle DJ. Arthroscopic treatment of degenerative tears of the triangular fibrocartilage. *Hand Clin* 1994;10:615–624.

53. Sweet S, Weiss LE. Applications of electrothermal shrinkage in wrist arthroscopy. *Atlas Hand Clin* 2001;6:203–210.

54. Minami A, Ishikawa J, Suenaga N, et al. Clinical results of treatment of triangular fibrocartilage complex tears by arthroscopic debridement. *J Hand Surg Am* 1996;21:406–411.

55. Hermansdorfer JD, Kleinman WB. Management of chronic peripheral tears of the triangular fibrocartilage complex. *J Hand Surg Am* 1991;16:340–346.

56. Mooney JF, Poehling GG. Disruption of the ulnolunate ligament as a cause of chronic ulnar wrist pain. *J Hand Surg Am* 1991;16:347–349.

57. De Araujo W, Poehling GG, Kuzma GR, et al. New Tuohy needle technique for triangular fibrocartilage complex repair: preliminary studies. *Arthroscopy* 1996;12:699–703.

58. Zachee B, De Smet L, Fabry G. Arthroscopic suturing of TFCC lesions. *Arthroscopy* 1993;9:242–243.

59. Ruch DS, Ritter MR. Repair of peripheral triangular fibrocartilage complex tears. *Atlas Hand Clin* 2001;6:211–220.

60. Whipple TL, Geissler WB. Arthroscopic management of wrist triangular fibrocartilage complex injuries in the athlete. *Orthopedics* 1993;16:1061–1067.

61. Sagerman SD, Short W. Arthroscopic repair of radial-sided triangular fibrocartilage complex tears. *Arthroscopy* 1996;12:339–342.

62. Jantea CL, Baltzer A, Ruther W. Arthroscopic repair of radial-sided lesions of the triangular fibrocartilage complex. *Hand Clin* 1995;11:31–36.

63. Jones MD, Trumble TE. Arthroscopic repair of radial-sided triangular fibrocartilage complex tears. *Atlas Hand Clin* 2001;6: 221–239.
64. Short WH, Palmer AK, Werner FW. A biomechanical study of distal radial fractures. *J Hand Surg Am* 1987;12:529–534.
65. Bilos ZJ, Chamberland D. Distal ulnar head shortening for treatment of triangular fibrocartilage complex tears with ulnar positive variance. *J Hand Surg Am* 1991;16:1115–1119.
66. Boulas HJ, Milek MA. Ulnar shortening for tears of the triangular fibro-cartilaginous complex. *J Hand Surg Am* 1990;15:415–420.
67. Chun S, Palmer AK. The ulnar impaction syndrome: follow-up of ulnar shortening osteotomy. *J Hand Surg Am* 1993;18:46–53.
68. Feldon P, Terrono AL, Belsky MR. Wafer distal ulna resection for triangular fibrocartilage tears and/or ulna impaction syndrome. *J Hand Surg Am* 1992;17:731–737.
69. Wnorowski DC, Palmer AK, Werner FW. Anatomic and biomechanical analysis of the arthroscopic wafer procedure. *Arthroscopy* 1992;8:204–212.
70. Verheyden JR, Short WH. Arthroscopic wafer procedure. *Atlas Hand Clin* 2001;6:241–251.

Operative Arthroscopy, third edition. Edited by John B. McGinty, Stephen S. Burkhart, Robert W. Jackson, Donald H. Johnson, and John C. Richmond. Lippincott Williams & Wilkins © 2003.

INTEROSSEOUS LIGAMENTOUS INJURIES OF THE WRIST

WILLIAM P. COONEY III
RICHARD A. BERGER

Ligament injuries of the wrist constitute a significant problem second only to scaphoid fracture as a cause of pain and weakness in the wrist. Classic studies on the wrist (1–5) demonstrated the importance of interosseous ligaments in stability of the wrist. Failure of wrist ligaments as a result of trauma leads to a loss of carpal alignment, strength, and stability, now well known as *carpal instability* (3). Early diagnosis and treatment of interosseous ligament injuries are prerequisites if the orthopaedic or trauma surgeon who first encounters these patients is to expect satisfactory treatment results. Casual treatment of "sprains of the wrist" typically leads to chronic instability of the wrist, which is difficult to treat by ligament repair. To provide better outcomes from the treatment of ligament injuries of the wrist, early diagnosis is essential. In this chapter, we explore the role of arthroscopy in the diagnosis of instability of the wrist and its role in the treatment of both acute and chronic interosseous ligament injuries.

ANATOMY

Radiocarpal Joint

Intraarticular anatomy of the wrist consists of joint cartilage surfaces, intraosseous ligament connections referred to as *intraosseous ligaments,* and dorsal and palmar intracapsular ligaments (Figs. 54.1 and 54.2). The wrist consists of three joints—the radiocarpal, intercarpal and distal radioulnar—all of which can be involved in carpal instability. The proximal articular surface of the wrist consists of the scaphoid and lunate fossa of the distal radius, the intraarticular sulcus, and the triangular fibrocartilage (TFC) (Fig. 54.3). The proximal carpal row consists of the corresponding scaphoid, lunate, and triquetrum, which articulate with the distal radius and the TFC. Clear division between these structures is

enhanced during arthroscopy of the wrist by palpation with a triangulation probe (6–9). Palpation can demonstrate the differential consistencies among cartilage, bone, and ligaments and can allow the examiner a three-dimensional assessment of their integrity and consistency. Ligament tautness, cartilage firmness, and the trampoline resistance of the TFC can all be distinguished. Triangulation probing from the radial to ulnar and dorsal to palmar provides a contouring of the joint articular surfaces and interconnection ligaments (10,11), in effect a visual and tactile appreciation of the wrist. Differences in tactile feel assist in identifying pathologic conditions related to these intraarticular structures. For example, studies demonstrate that both the scapholunate (SL) and lunotriquetral (LT) ligaments have three components. Each ligament has (a) dorsal, (b) central, and (c) palmar components, which differ in their mechanical strength and function (Fig. 54.4) (12). Clinical studies and mechanical analysis further suggest that these structures can be injured individually as well as collectively. Arthroscopy of the wrist should always begin with inspection and palpation of the joint surfaces, intraosseous ligaments, and TFC (13–16).

Supporting the proximal carpal row of the wrist to the distal radius are several intracapsular ligaments. These should be examined next. These ligaments may be thought of as suspension cables that link the proximal carpal row to the distal radius (17–19) (Fig. 54.5). They are best viewed when the wrist is under traction (1,8–10,20). Although these ligaments resist tensile loads, more complex mechanical functions are present, and the exact role of both dorsal and palmar ligaments in maintaining carpal stability is under study. From a practical standpoint, it is extremely important to know that clear definition of these structures is possible only during wrist arthroscopy because they are intracapsular ligaments (19,20). In other words, they are not well delineated from an extracapsular view, and their function can be assessed only by wrist arthroscopy and not by gross anatomic or surgical observation of the wrist (Fig. 54.6).

W. P. Cooney III and R. A. Berger: Department of Orthopaedic Surgery, Mayo Clinic and Mayo Graduate School of Medicine, Rochester, Minnesota.

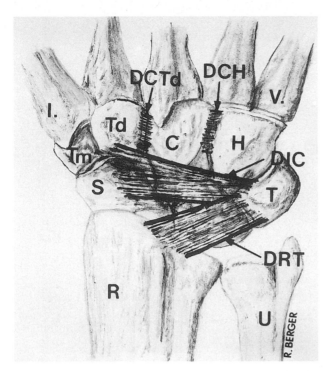

FIGURE 54.1 Dorsal carpal ligaments span between the distal radius (R) and triquetrum (T) and between the scaphoid (S), capitate (C), proximal hamate (H), and triquetrum (T). DIC, dorsal intercarpal ligament; DRT, dorsal radiotriquetral ligament; Td, trapezoid; Tm, trapezium. (From Cooney WP, Linscheid RL, Dobyns JH. Fractures and dislocations of the wrist. In: Rockwood CA Jr, Green DP, eds. *Fractures in adults,* 3rd ed. Philadelphia: JB Lippincott, 1991, with permission.)

During arthroscopy of the wrist, one examines the intracapsular ligaments by first looking palmarly and then sweeping the arthroscope in a radial to ulnar direction. One first can visualize the lateral radiocarpal ligament, often considered incorrectly as a collateral ligament, that extends from the radial styloid region to the distal scaphoid. Just palmar and ulnar to the radiocarpal ligament is the radioscaphocapitate ligament. This is a strong, thick ligamentous band of tissues that extends from the distal radius across the waist of the scaphoid to insert palmarly on the body of the capitate. The long radiolunate ligament and the short radiolunate ligament are observed and can be palpated next as one proceeds in a radial to ulnar direction along the palmar aspect of the wrist. These ligaments should be quite taut on palpation, especially under traction. One should, in fact, lessen the longitudinal traction to determine the functional continuity of these ligaments when assessing carpal instability. A third ligament, the radioscapholunate ligament, also referred to as the ligament of Testut (1–5) (Fig. 54.5), crosses over the short radiolunate ligament from a ulnar to radial direction. Originally believed to represent an important ligament constraint at the palmar aspect of the intraosseous SL ligament, it was subsequently shown to be a neurovascular, relatively weak, connection from the distal radius to the car-

pus, primarily serving proprioceptive and vascular functions.

Wrist arthroscopic observations moving from a radial to ulnar direction palmarly next demonstrate the palmar ulnotriquetral and ulnolunate ligaments, which originate from the palmar aspect of the TFC and only indirectly are attached to the fovea region at the base of the ulnar styloid. Once again, with traction applied and then released, the dynamic relationship of stress applied to the ulnar carpal ligaments and the TFC to the wrist during loading can be examined (5). These capsular ligaments and the intraosseous ligaments are best observed and tested by triangulation with a small intraarticular probe (21,22). We have been able to recognize differences in ligament appearance, tension, or response to stress loading (12,13), and pathologic changes or tears of the interosseous ligament can be determined with respect to length, width, and degree of potential carpal instability.

Midcarpal Joint

The midcarpal joint consists of the distal scaphoid, trapezium and trapezoid, lunate, capitate, triquetrum, and ha-

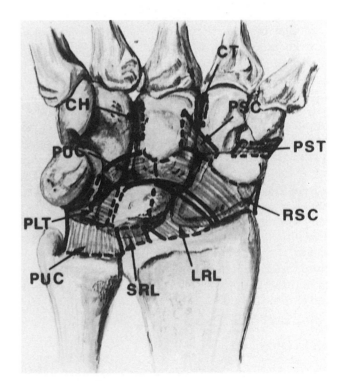

FIGURE 54.2 Palmar carpal ligaments (extracapsular view). CH, capitate hamate ligament; CT, capitate trapezoid ligament; LRL, long radiolunate ligament; PLT, palmar lunotriquetral ligament; PSC, palmar scaphocapitate ligament; PST, palmar scaphotrapezial ligament; PUC, palmar ulnocarpal ligament; PUC, palmar ulnocapitate ligament; RSC, radioscaphocapitate ligament; SRL, short radiolunate ligament. (From Cooney WP, Linscheid RL, Dobyns JH. Fractures and dislocations of the wrist. In: Rockwood CA Jr, Green DP, eds. *Fractures in adults,* 3rd ed. Philadelphia: JB Lippincott, 1991, with permission.)

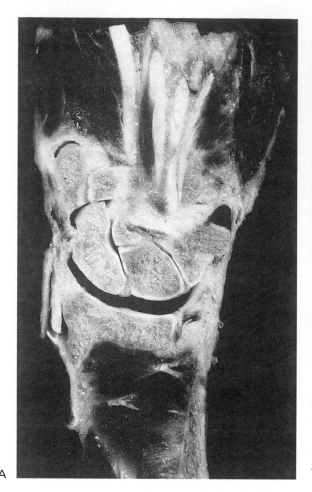

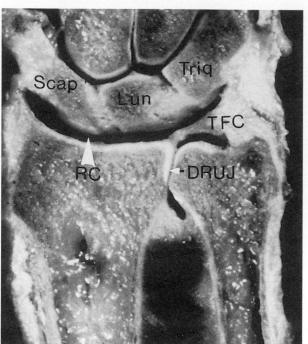

FIGURE 54.3 Cross-sectional anatomy of the right wrist. Articular cartilage covers the distal radius and triangular fibrocartilage (TFC) of the proximal aspect of the radiocarpal joint (RC) and the entire distal radioulnar joint (DRUJ). The articular surface of the scaphoid (Scap), lunate (Lun), and triquetrum (Triq) covers the distal surface of the radiocarpal joint and proximal surface of the midcarpal joint. (With permission of the Mayo Foundation.)

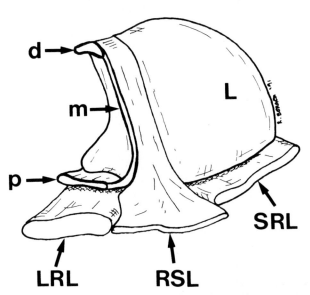

FIGURE 54.4 Components of the scapholunate ligament (A) dorsal third, (M) middle third, and (P) palmar third. LRL, long radiolunate ligament; RSL, radioscapholunate ligament; SRL, short radiolunate ligament. (With permission of the Mayo Foundation.)

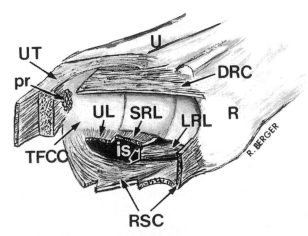

FIGURE 54.5 Suspensory nature of palmar intracapsular ligaments: scaphoid, lunate, and triquetrum removed. Axial view of the distal radius and support ligaments. DRC, dorsal radiocarpal (triquetral) ligament; IS, isthmus between radioscaphocapitate ligament and long radiolunate ligament; LRL, long radiolunate ligament; PR, prestyloid recess; RSC, radioscaphocapitate ligament; SRL, short radiolunate ligament; TFCC, triangular fibrocartilage complex; UL, ulnolunate ligament; UT, ulnotriquetral ligament. (With permission of the Mayo Foundation.)

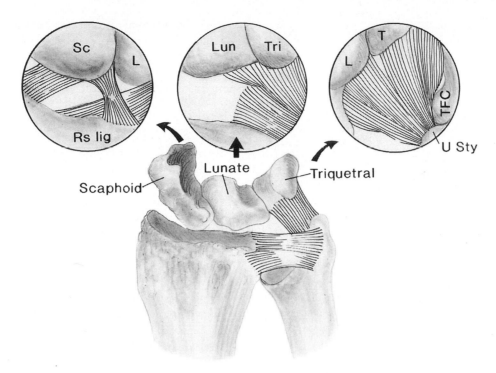

FIGURE 54.6 Arthroscopic view of the radiocarpal joint. *Left, top:* Arthroscopic portal view of the scaphoid (SC), lunate (L), and radioscapholunate ligament (RS Lig). *Center:* Arthroscopic view of central wrist, showing the lunate (Lun), triquetrum (Tri), and palmar ulnolunate and ulnotriquetral ligaments. **Right, top:** Arthroscopic view of the ulnar wrist, showing the lunate (L), triquetrum (T), ulnar styloid (USty), and triangular fibrocartilage (TFC). (With permission of the Mayo Foundation.)

mate. The joint articular surfaces, intraarticular spaces, and palmar wrist ligaments can be examined arthroscopically (22–24) (Fig. 54.3). Congruity of the joint articular surfaces of the proximal carpal row can be better appreciated from the midcarpal joint than from the radiocarpal joint (25). With a probe, one starts distally and palpates the scaphoid, trapezium, trapezoid joint surfaces, scaphocapitate joint, capitolunate joint, and hamate-triquetral joint, as well as the articulation between the hamate and the capitate. Some patients also have a hamate-lunate articulation, so-called *double-facet lunate.* One can closely examine the SL and LT joints with the triangulation probe, because there are no intervening interosseous ligaments. As mentioned later, one can determine degrees of carpal instability (Geissler stages I to IV) by probing the SL and LT joint with and without wrist traction (26,27). With a dynamic load applied and released, instability at both the SL and LT articulations can be appreciated. The palmar ligaments between the proximal and distal carpal rows can also be observed and palpated in the loose wrist when traction is applied. Synovitis between carpal bones or among the palmar ligaments, increased space between the SL or LT joints, and loss of cartilage between any of the midcarpal joint articulations are all readily appreciated with wrist midcarpal arthroscopy.

HISTORY AND EXAMINATION

Arthroscopic examination is an important aspect of the evaluation of the painful wrist. It is an essential component of a complete examination in the differential diagnosis of chronic carpal instability. Based on appropriate history and supportive clinical examination, the diagnosis of intraosseous ligament injuries and associated intracapsular ligament failure can clearly be made. Arthroscopy of the wrist has become the standard, with its better accuracy and definition than previously used wrist arthrography (13, 28–31).

With respect to the diagnosis of carpal instability, it is essential to have a history of a forceful hyperextension or flexion injury to the wrist. An inconsequential injury (sprain) rarely produces ligament disruption. A history of a significant fall, motor vehicle accident, or sports contact injury is required to make the diagnosis of an interosseous or intracapsular wrist ligament tear (3). The patient without this type of history is most unlikely to have posttraumatic carpal instability. The most typical presentation for wrist instability is a history of hyperextension force combined with forearm pronation or supination stress. A direct axial load may produce a fracture of the radius or carpometacarpal dislocation, but it does not usually result in carpal instability. The

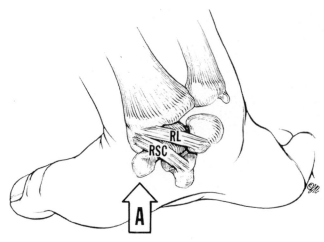

FIGURE 54.7 Mechanism of injury of most carpal instability problems. Hyperextension of the wrist combined with an axial force (A) applied as a ground reaction force to the outstretched hand. (From Fractures of the scaphoid. In: Taleisnik J. *The wrist.* New York: Churchill Livingstone, 1985, with permission.)

patient should be questioned carefully for information with respect to the mechanism of injury.

With hyperextension injury (Fig. 54.7), the capitate and hamate wedge themselves into the acetabular-shaped midcarpal articulation between the scaphoid and lunate, in effect driving the joint surfaces apart (2,14). Both intrinsic and extrinsic ligaments tighten under the stress of the loaded wrist (17,18). The extrinsic ligaments, which are weaker, appear to give way and attenuate first, followed by various portions of the interosseous ligaments. By nature of the anatomy of these intraarticular extrinsic ligaments, only the intrinsic SL and LT ligaments can be easily tested clinically with specific types of stress testing. Thus, it is essential that the reported injury mechanism should be assessed with respect to the clinical findings of tenderness, contusion, or ecchymosis or the location of positive stress testing. The mechanism of injury and clinical findings should be consistent with each other.

Physical Examination

The physical examination findings should support the diagnosis of carpal instability. After an acute injury, there should be swelling and tenderness, often diffuse. Patients note a loss of wrist motion and painful extremes of motion. Later, the tenderness should be more localized or specific to one side or area of the wrist. Combined dorsal radial or palmar ulnar tenderness is not unusual. Palmar tenderness is more typical of hyperextension injuries that cause tuberosity fractures (scaphoid, trapezium, hamate) or palmar capsular ligament injuries (Fig. 54.8). Dorsal tenderness is more typical of intraosseous ligament injuries or avulsion injuries such as the dorsal carpal ligaments from the triquetrum. Painful radial or ulnar deviation is associated with both capsular and in-

terosseous ligament tears. Rotational stress on the carpus should be performed but should be independent of forearm rotation. Stress testing of individual joints is also important, because it recreates the abnormal load between the scaphoid and lunate or the lunate and triquetrum (or perhaps the pisiform and triquetrum) and thereby produces pain or instability symptoms or both (Fig. 54.9). With a complete ligament dissociation on the radial side of the wrist (SL dissociation), palmar flexed rotatory subluxation of the scaphoid results, with loss of the palmar support ligaments. One can block flexion of the scaphoid by distal palmar pressure *(the Watson test)*. When the intrinsic SL and extrinsic palmar radiocarpal ligaments are competent, then the examination is negative. If the SL ligaments are torn, dorsal subluxation of the proximal scaphoid out of the scaphoid fossa of the distal radius can result, reproducing the patient's pain. One can also "rock" or ballotte or shift dorsally and palmarly the scaphoid on the lunate and determine whether this reproduces the patient's pain *(the Dobyns test)*. *Dynamic testing (stress loading)* of injured LT joints may also provoke pain. Ballottement and shearing the LT joint surfaces together can reproduce pain. A catch or click may be appreciated and may reproduce the patient's symptoms. *Strength testing* is another important diagnostic test for carpal instability. With repetitive grip in the normal wrist, the grip strength should remain the same. With carpal instability, however, the patient has a decrease in strength because pain fibers prevent repetitive forceful grip. Stress loading the wrist in flexion and extension or a combined scaphoid-lunate stress test should also reproduce pain if a significant ligament injury has occurred. Diagnostic blocks can be helpful, because pain should be reduced or absent in the affected joint or area of wrist injury after such an anesthetic block.

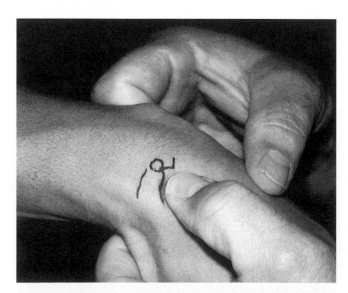

FIGURE 54.8 Dorsal tenderness between the scaphoid and lunate just distal to Lister's tubercle is present with scapholunate dissociation. (With permission of the Mayo Foundation.)

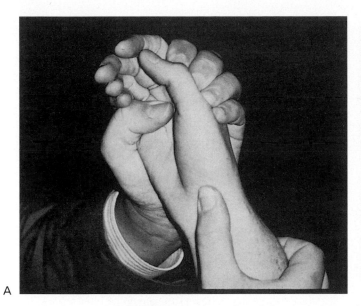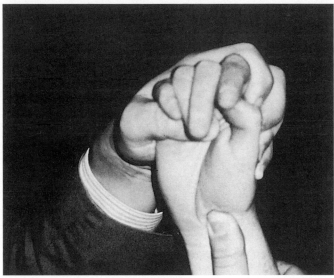

A   B

FIGURE 54.9 Stress testing of the scapholunate joint. **A:** Ulnar deviation of the wrist. The examiner's right thumb is placed on the distal scaphoid. **B:** Radial deviation of the wrist. The examiner's right thumb blocks scaphoid flexion and will force the proximal scaphoid dorsally over the dorsal rim of the distal radius. (With permission of the Mayo Foundation.)

Radiographic Examination

Radiographs of the wrist help to establish specific wrist injuries and separate skeletal from ligament disorders. Routine radiographs should include wrist posteroanterior, anteroposterior, and lateral views, as well as radial deviation and ulnar deviation. We also recommend the anteroposterior grip view (Figs. 54.10 to 54.12). The anteroposterior grip view demonstrates a gap between the scaphoid and lunate with SL dissociation that can be accentuated with firm grip

(Fig. 54.12). With SL dissociation, on the lateral wrist views, the scaphoid flexes palmarly, thus producing a clear deformity of a palmar flexed scaphoid and an extended lunate (the dorsal intercalary segmental instability deformity) (Fig. 54.11). Measurement of the SL gap and SL and lunocapitate angles with line drawings helps to identify increases in the bone angles that are pathologic signs of ligament injury.

Radiographic findings of LT dissociation are less common. With this injury, the scaphoid and lunate remain

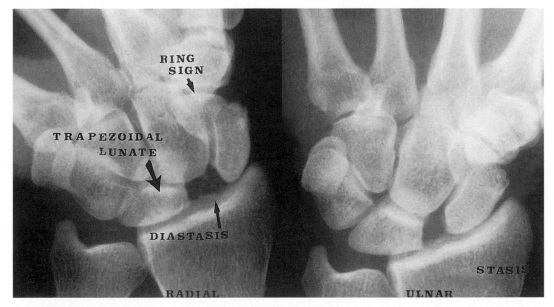

FIGURE 54.10 Scapholunate dissociation (anteroposterior view). Note the scapholunate gap (diastasis), flexion of scaphoid (ring sign), and hyperextension of lunate (trapezoidal shape of lunate).

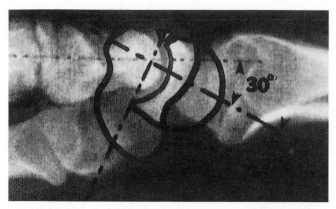

FIGURE 54.11 Scapholunate dissociation (lateral view). Note the dorsal flexed or extended position of lunate and palmar flexion of the scaphoid, producing more than a 90-degree scapholunate angle and a 30-degree capitate-lunate angle. (From Cooney WP, Linscheid RL, Dobyns JH. Fractures and dislocations of the wrist. In: Rockwood CA Jr, Green DP, eds. *Fractures in adults,* 3rd ed. Philadelphia: JB Lippincott, 1991, with permission.)

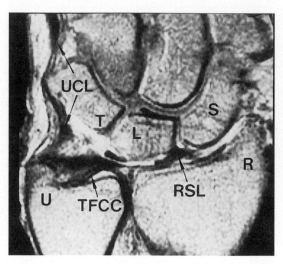

FIGURE 54.13 Magnetic resonance imaging of the wrist can show scapholunate and lunotriquetral ligament tears. L, lunate; R, radius; RSL, radioscapholunate ligament; S, scaphoid; T, triquetrum; TFCC, triangular fibrocartilage complex; UCL, ulnocarpal ligament complex.

linked together and fall into flexion, whereas the detached triquetrum extends and supinates. In some wrists, this injury can produce a break in the normally smooth carpal arcs (radiocarpal and midcarpal) and can lead to a palmar flexed lunate, which can be observed on the lateral radiograph (the volar intercalary segmental instability deformity). A positive ulnar variance increases the SL palmar tilt. Special views, such as a carpal tunnel view, are specific for palmar avulsion injuries. Supination oblique views help to show scaphoid fractures. Careful positioning of the wrist may assist in de-

tecting an SL gap, a scaphoid ring sign, or a break in the carpal row alignment not observed on routine films.

Special image testing can be useful. These tests include tomograms of the wrist (axial or computed tomography) and magnetic resonance imaging (Fig. 54.13) (32). We also recommend cineradiography of the wrist with stress (Fig. 54.12), and we now routinely perform stress test in the office with the newer small fluoroscopic imaging equipment. A bone scan is a useful screening tool to confirm suspected wrist instability, but it is not diagnostic. The ancillary test of greatest value for ligament injury is the wrist arthrogram. Triple injection studies provide important information about ligament continuity or damage. Correlation with clinical findings, however, is essential, because degenerative tears can be present that do not signify pathologic conditions. In patients who are more than 40 years old, bilateral studies of arthrography of the wrist commonly demonstrate symmetric lesions even in asymptomatic wrists, a finding bringing into question the diagnostic value of wrist arthrography. We recommend recording the arthrogram and performing stress testing during the arthrogram to provide a thorough examination that we can review with the patient later. Studying the results of the cine recording carefully adds to the diagnostic value of this test. Overinterpretation of the arthrogram, however, must be avoided, and findings should be confirmed by wrist arthroscopy before definitive treatments are determined.

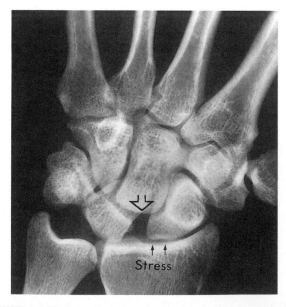

FIGURE 54.12 Grip view (posteroanterior) demonstrating increased scapholunate diastasis (gap) as the capitate *(arrow)* is forced between the scaphoid and lunate. (From Cooney WP, Linscheid RL, Dobyns JH. Fractures and dislocations of the wrist. In: Rockwood CA Jr, Green DP, eds. *Fractures in adults,* 3rd ed. Philadelphia: JB Lippincott, 1991, with permission.)

INDICATIONS FOR DIAGNOSTIC ARTHROSCOPY

One may consider wrist arthroscopy as a technique used only for the specific diagnosis of wrist instability or cartilage injury, but in reality it is an important extension of the physical and imaging examination of the wrist (4,6,8–11,13,33). Today, most hand surgeons believe that arthroscopy provides information that is unique and that cannot be obtained easily from any other source or technique of examination, including actual arthrotomy of the wrist (10,14–16). When one is planning surgical treatment of carpal instability or is in the process of diagnosis, wrist arthroscopy has the potential benefit of augmenting the clinical examination and, ultimately, assisting in making the correct diagnosis of pathologic features in almost every patient (8,33). Our indications for diagnostic wrist arthroscopy in carpal instability are generally twofold: (a) to confirm the suspected clinical diagnosis and to determine the extent (or degree) of specific carpal pathology and (b) to plan and carry out surgical treatment (including the choice of incision) based on the arthroscopic findings.

In our experience, arthroscopy is more accurate and sensitive than arthrography of the wrist when more than one wrist lesion is present (28,34). Internal derangements of the wrist can be better assessed by an arthroscopic examination, and the diagnosis can be made more accurately than by wrist arthrography (28). The location of certain ligament tears, for example, dorsal and central, versus palmar tears of the SL ligament can be better assessed, and treatment can planned based on these arthroscopic observations and careful triangulation probe assessment (Fig. 54.14) (6,13,35). In isolated SL dissociation, for example, the arthroscopic examination can direct us toward a dorsal versus palmar incision or can help to decide whether to consider SL ligament re-

pair, capsulodesis or tenodesis, or intercarpal fusion. We can examine the tension (redundancy) in palmar carpal ligaments (Fig. 54.15). The arthroscopic procedure also allows examination of the adjacent joint articular surfaces. Cartilage damage or advanced arthritis may change the operative treatment plan (10). If, for example, a scaphoid trapezial trapezoid (STT) fusion is planned for gross carpal instability and one observes articular cartilage loss from the proximal pole of the scaphoid, a procedure of ligament reconstruction and capsulodesis or even excision of the scaphoid with intercarpal fusion could be elected, rather than STT fusion. On the ulnar side of the wrist, if an LT tear is diagnosed, arthroscopy can assist in treatment planning. Should the LT ligament be repaired or reconstructed, or should an LT fusion with ulnar recession be performed based on the degree of LT tear and associated ulnocarpal abutment?

Midcarpal arthroscopy is essential in any evaluation of suspected carpal instability (Fig. 54.16) (9,13,23). With dynamic instability, midcarpal arthroscopy provides the best view of SL and LT joint articulation. The joint surfaces can be examined under stress loading, and loss of alignment or gap formation can be observed. The degree of gap or spacing between the SL and LT ligaments can be tested as described by Geissler (Table 54.1) (Fig. 54.16) (26). With minor instability (incomplete ligament tear), a triangulation probe does not usually enter the SL or LT interval. With a more significant instability (complete tear but without rotatory subluxation of the scaphoid), the probe enters the SL or LT joint and can be twisted in place. With a major tear and gross instability, both the probe and often the arthroscope

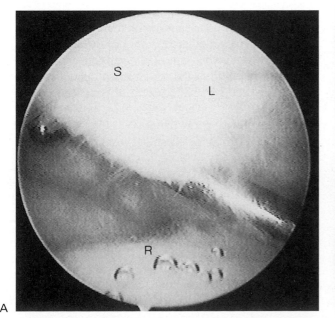
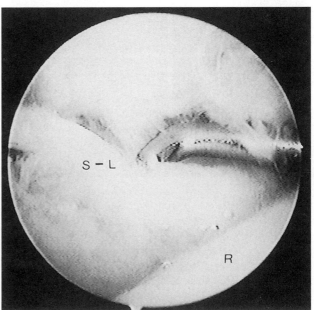

FIGURE 54.14 A: Arthroscopy of the radiocarpal joint with a triangulation probe lifting under a palmar scapholunate ligament tear. **B:** Probe between the scaphoid and lunate at the scapholunate (SL) ligament. L, lunate; R, radius; S, scaphoid.

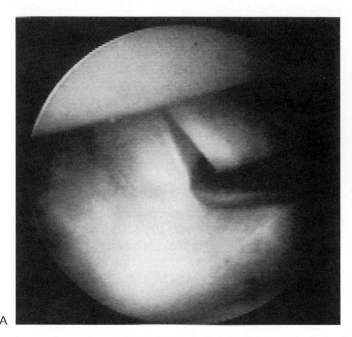
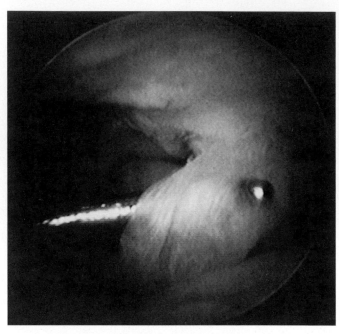

A   B

FIGURE 54.15 Radiocarpal arthroscopy of palmar carpal ligaments. **A:** Probe lifting an intact (taut) radioscaphocapitate ligament. **B:** Probe lifting a torn (redundant) long radiolunate (LRL) ligament.

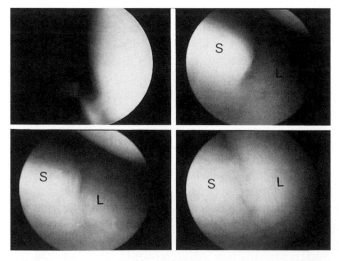

FIGURE 54.16 Midcarpal arthroscopy. Laxity of the scaphoid (S) and lunate (L) is demonstrated on stress loading the scaphoid and lunate under traction.

TABLE 54.1 ARTHROSCOPIC CLASSIFICATION OF WRIST INTEROSSEOUS LIGAMENT INSTABILITY

Grade	Description
I.	Attenuation or hemorrhage of interosseous ligament as seen from the radiocarpal joint; no incongruency of carpal alignment in midcarpal space
II.	Attenuation or hemorrhage of interosseous ligament as seen from the radiocarpal joint; incongruency or step-off midcarpal space; slight gap (less than the width of a probe) between carpal bones possibly present
III.	Incongruency or step-off of carpal alignment both the radiocarpal and midcarpal spaces; probe passable through the gap between bones
IV.	Incongruency or step-off of carpal alignment both the radiocarpal and midcarpal spaces; gross instability with manipulation noted; 2.7-mm arthroscope passable through the gap between carpal bones

can be inserted through the SL gap. Similarly, a break in the normal smooth contour of the proximal carpal row viewed from the midcarpal joint also suggests carpal instability. For advanced, static carpal instability, midcarpal arthroscopy provides a view of not only joint surface displacement but also the palmar carpal ligaments, which may be attenuated, torn, or hypervascular (Fig. 54.14). Secondary arthritic changes between the scaphoid and capitate or capitate and lunate SL advanced collapse (SLAC type II) may be present. With excessive rotational carpal instability, the STT joint can be inspected for secondary arthritic changes.

Diagnostic arthroscopy of both the radiocarpal and midcarpal joints is, in our opinion, an essential tool for assessing carpal instability (4,11,15), and a study demonstrated the added value of arthroscopy of both the midcarpal and radiocarpal joints. We recommend arthroscopy as a preliminary but essential procedure in the evaluation of nearly all primary repairs as well as surgical reconstructions for carpal instability. We plan a 10- to 15-minute arthroscopic evaluation to confirm suspected diagnoses and to assist in determining the optimum surgical exposure for the perceived pathologic process. We have changed surgical approaches based on arthroscopic findings.

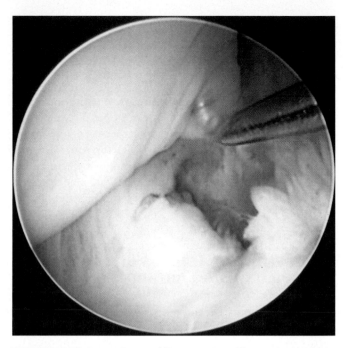

FIGURE 54.17 Lunotriquetral ligament tear. The probe is within a volar third lunotriquetral ligament tear; the triangular fibrocartilage and 60 portal are noted below the probe.

THERAPEUTIC ARTHROSCOPY

Indications for treatment of carpal instability by arthroscopy of the wrist are not well defined but are certainly in development (36–38). In patients with well-defined carpal instability, such as SL or LT ligament tears, we prefer open treatment techniques. Other surgeons suggest that arthroscopic reduction and pinning of the SL or LT joint may be of value when the patient presents early (less than 8 weeks from injury) with carpal instability (14). Arthroscopic examination has been considered appropriate for closed reduction and arthroscopically guided percutaneous pin fixation (Fig. 54.17). Observation of the reduction from the midcarpal joint of the scaphoid or lunate displacement can be combined with fluoroscopy and can result in a rewarding outcome for the patient. We have also had good preliminary results in dynamic carpal instability in which the ligaments are grossly intact but either stretched or attenuated. Multiple pin fixations across either the SL or LT interval appear to produce a chondrodesis sufficient for relief of symptoms and long-term wrist stability (Fig. 54.18). Series by several authors suggest a positive benefit from such treatment (12,14). There is no arthroscopic operative repair technique at this time described for the actual repair of SL or LT ligament injuries similar to repair of TFC or the glenoid labrum. Indirect methods of creating a fibrosis or chondrodesis across these joints may be beneficial, especially in the patient with an acute or subacute presentation.

With evidence suggesting that the central portions of the SL ligament and LT ligament are cartilaginous and

that they do not support tensile loads, arthroscopic debridement of a central deficit (tear) in the interosseous ligament may prove to have therapeutic benefit (19). The rationale is reasonable, but the benefits are not tested. It is not clear whether a cartilaginous tear of the SL or LT ligament or the central portion of the TFC has innervation sufficient to preclude wrist pain. Similarly, debridement of capsular adhesions within the radiocarpal joint or, occasionally, the midcarpal joint may have therapeutic benefit in selected patients. We have, for example, successfully treated a tennis professional by TFC debridement and radiocarpal synovectomy. Recreational and professional golfers have improved wrist motion and relief of symptoms (pain and weakness) after arthroscopic synovectomy (39,40). The reasons for these improvements must be considered, and the long-lasting benefits must still be demonstrated. Newer techniques including the use of lasers and capsular shrinkage procedures with thermal-couple probes may also prove beneficial (37,38).

For chronic carpal instability, which presents as radiocarpal arthritis (SLAC wrist), arthroscopic synovectomy combined with radial styloid excision has been successfully performed. The indication is usually chronic SL instability with arthritis limited to the scaphoid radial styloid articulation, but a similar approach may be reasonable for the established proximal pole scaphoid nonunion that cannot be treated by bone grafting. Arthroscopic excision of the proximal scaphoid and radial styloid can be effective in selected patients. For advanced arthritis associated with SL dissociation or scaphoid nonunion (now called SNAC wrist), complete proximal to middle-third scaphoid excision alone could be considered in the older patient who would not need a midcarpal wrist stabilization procedure. It would be theoretically possible to perform a complete proximal row carpectomy by arthroscopic techniques, but the advantage over an open carpectomy is not clear. Some degree of capsular contracture after proximal row carpectomy appears desirable to maintain wrist stability. One can anticipate the day when chronic carpal instability may be treated by arthroscopic techniques combining STT debridement of cartilage with injection of bone morphogenic protein and growth factor for fusion of the STT joint.

DIFFERENTIAL DIAGNOSIS OF CARPAL INSTABILITY USING ARTHROSCOPY

Carpal instability occasionally can be a subtle clinical finding and may not always be easy to confirm as the cause of persistent wrist pain. Patients may have symptoms suggesting carpal instability, but the diagnosis is elusive. Patients usually have a positive clinical history, local tenderness, provocative stress test, and loss of grip strength. On repeated examination, findings are consistent, but radiographs are completely normal. At this stage, we look to the bone scan

to help confirm a diagnosis of wrist instability (scan positive or negative). If the bone scan is positive and supporting clinical findings are present, two- or three-compartment wrist arthrography can be considered, combined with fluoroscopic recording of the arthrography. Stress testing after the arthrogram can demonstrate small ligament tears. More commonly today we proceed directly to diagnostic arthroscopy of the wrist (radiocarpal and midcarpal) to confirm and define the anticipated pathologic process (Figs. 54.19 and 54.20). If the bone scan is suggestive but not strongly positive and if wrist arthrography is not conclusive, wrist arthroscopy may be essential in evaluating functional wrist pain and in assessing Workers' Compensation cases. At a minimum, it can assist in separating intraarticular causes of wrist pain from extrinsic causes of pain, such as tendinitis or neuritis. Carpal instability can be excluded in the differential diagnosis.

Pathologic conditions of many types within the wrist such as intraosseous ganglia, occult fractures, and loose bodies can cause symptoms similar to those of carpal instability. These diagnoses can be either made or excluded with the assistance of wrist arthroscopy. Other examples include early rheumatoid arthritis, crystal deposit synovitis, occult sepsis (especially fungal or atypical mycobacterial infection), cartilage injuries (ulnar carpal abutment), and such rare conditions as pigmented villonodular synovitis and hemochromatosis.

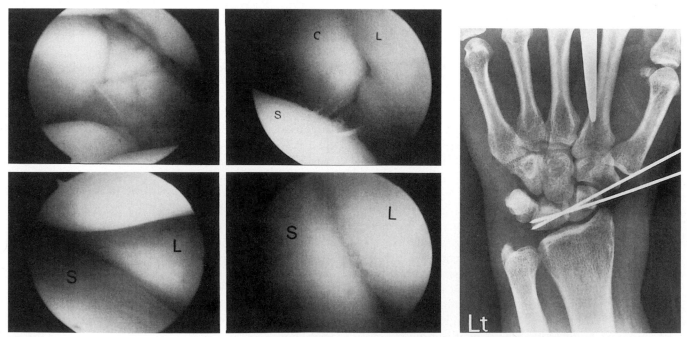

FIGURE 54.18 Midcarpal arthroscopy. **A:** Enlarged space between the scaphoid (S) and lunate (L), with compression of the capitate (L) onto the lunate *(top right)*. Wide scapholunate gap *(bottom left)* and closed (tight) scapholunate interval after percutaneous pinning. **B:** Percutaneous pin fixation of the scapholunate gap, reducing the scapholunate diastasis.

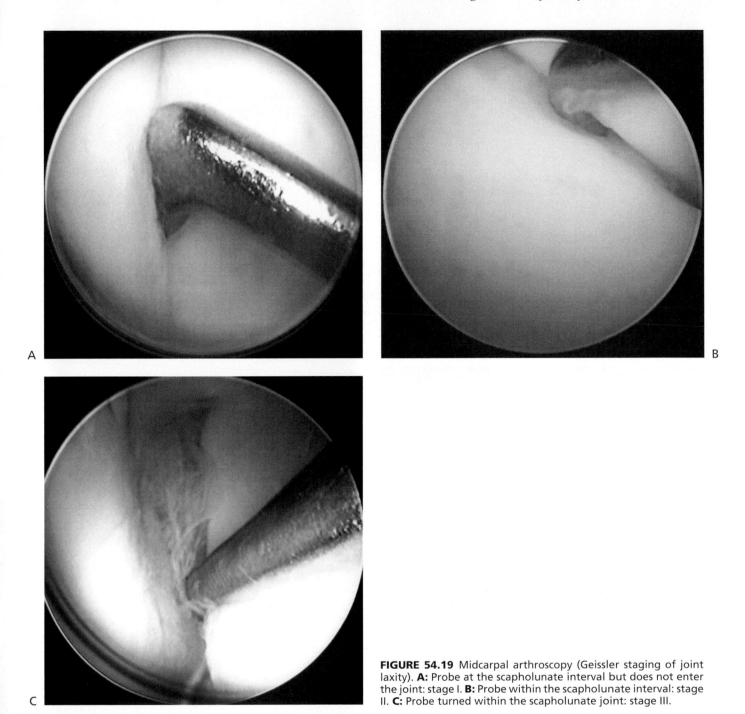

FIGURE 54.19 Midcarpal arthroscopy (Geissler staging of joint laxity). **A:** Probe at the scapholunate interval but does not enter the joint: stage I. **B:** Probe within the scapholunate interval: stage II. **C:** Probe turned within the scapholunate joint: stage III.

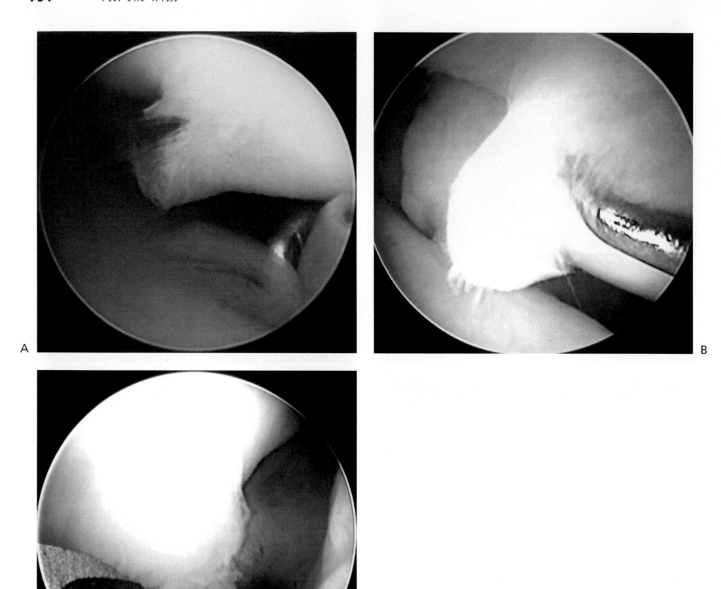

A

B

C

FIGURE 54.20 Therapeutic arthroscopy. **A:** Scapholunate ligament tear (scaphoid to left and lunate to right). **B:** Probing the scapholunate ligament demonstrates a middle to volar third tear; the dorsal ligament is intact. **C:** Arthroscopic debridement of the scapholunate ligament flap.

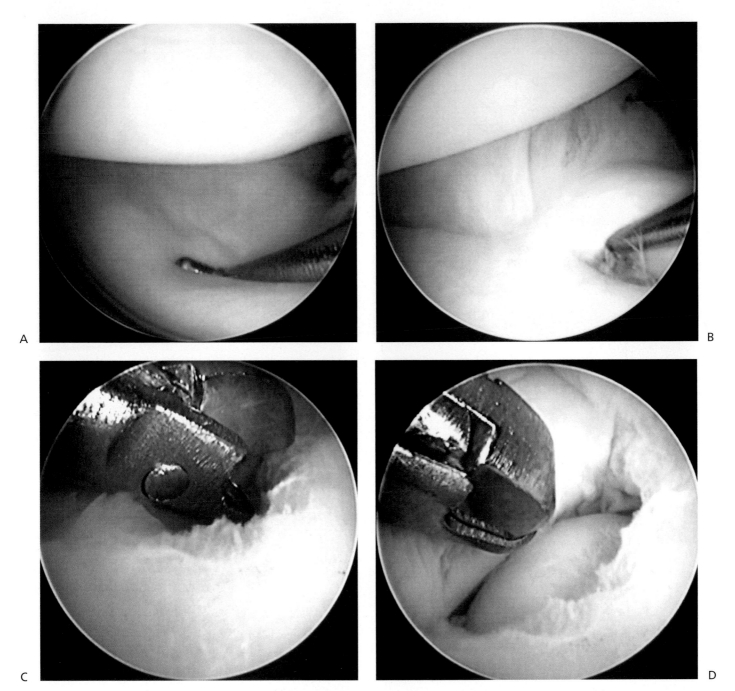

FIGURE 54.21 Triangular fibrocartilage tear. **A:** Palpation of the triangular fibrocartilage with loss of the trampoline effect. **B:** Probe under a torn triangular fibrocartilage; the lunate is above, and the ulnovolar carpal ligaments are noted. **C:** Debridement of the triangular fibrocartilage leading edge with suction punch. **D:** Appearance after debridement of the triangular fibrocartilage. Radius to left; ulnar head below; carpal instability with synovitis.

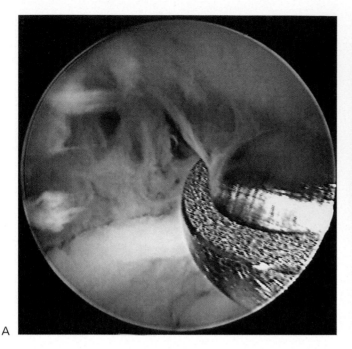
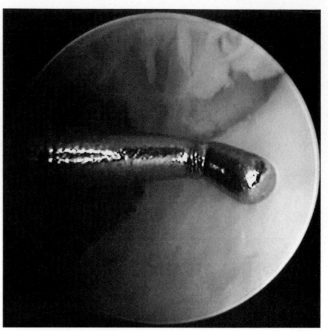

A   B

FIGURE 54.22 Radial shaver synovectomy of the radiocarpal joint: before **(A)** and after **(B)**.

SUMMARY

Arthroscopy of the wrist is an important diagnostic and potential therapeutic tool in the treatment of carpal instability. The subtle aspects of interosseous ligament injuries often require the direct inspection of these intracarpal ligaments that wrist arthroscopy provides. With a clear understanding of wrist anatomy, mechanics, and potential pathologic lesions, wrist arthroscopy becomes an essential tool in the evaluation and potential treatment of patients with wrist pain, both acute and chronic (Figs. 54.21 and 54.22). Earlier application of wrist arthroscopy in the patient who presents with a diagnosis of "wrist sprain" will bring about correct diagnoses and more effective treatments, both limited open and arthroscopically directed, to improve patient outcomes.

REFERENCES

1. Cooney WP, Dobyns JH, Linscheid RL. Arthroscopy of the wrist: anatomy and classification of carpal instability. *Arthroscopy* 1990;6:133–140.
2. Linscheid RL, Dobyns JH. The unified concept of carpal injuries. *Ann Chir Main* 1984;3:35.
3. Linscheid RL, Dobyns JH, Beabout JW, et al. Traumatic instability of the wrist: diagnosis, classification, pathomechanics. *J Bone Joint Surg Am* 1972;54:1612–1632.
4. Stanley J, Saffar P. *Wrist arthroscopy.* Philadelphia: WB Saunders, 1994.
5. Taleisnik J. *The wrist.* New York: Churchill Livingstone, 1985.
6. Botte M, Cooney WP, Linscheid RL. Arthroscopy of the wrist: anatomy and technique. *J Hand Surg Am* 1989;14:313–316.
7. Osterman AL. Arthroscopic debridement of triangular fibrocartilage tears. *Arthroscopy* 1990;6:120–124.
8. Ruch DS, Bowling J. Arthroscopic assessment of carpal instability. *Arthroscopy* 1998;14:675–681.
9. Roth JH, Poehling GG, Whipple TL. Arthroscopic surgery of the wrist. *Instr Course Lect* 1988;37:183–194.
10. Poehling GG, Roth JH. Articular cartilage lesions of the wrist. In: McGinty JB, Caspari RB, Jackson RB, et al., eds. *Operative arthroscopy.* New York: Raven Press, 1991:635–639.
11. Koman LA, Poehling GG, Toby EB, et al. Chronic wrist pain: indications for wrist arthroscopy. *Arthroscopy* 1990;6:116–119.
12. Peicha G, Seibert FJ, Fellinger M, et al. Lesions of the scapholunate ligaments in acute wrist trauma: arthroscopic diagnosis and minimally invasive treatment. *Knee Surg Sports Traumatol Arthrosc* 1997;5:176–183.
13. Poehling GG, Siegel DB, Koman LA, et al. Arthroscopy of the wrist. In: Green DP, eds. *Operative hand surgery.* New York: Churchill Livingstone, 1993.
14. Whipple TL. *The wrist.* Philadelphia: JB Lippincott, 1992.
15. Roth JH. Wrist arthroscopy. In: Lichtman DM, ed. *The wrist and its disorders.* Philadelphia: WB Saunders, 1988.
16. Whipple TL, Cooney WP, Poehling GG. Intraarticular fractures. In: McGinty JB, Caspari RB, Jackson RB, et al., eds. *Operative arthroscopy.* New York: Raven Press, 1991:651–654.
17. Logan SE, Nowak MD. Intrinsic and extrinsic wrist ligaments: biomechanical and functional differences. *Biomed Sci Instrum* 1987;23:9.
18. Berger RA. The anatomy of the ligaments of the wrist and distal radioulnar joint. *Clin Orthop* 2001;383:32.
19. Berger RA, Berglund LJ, An KN. Constraint and natural properties of the subregions of the scapholunate interosseous ligaments. *J Hand Surg [Am]* 1999;24:953.
20. North ER, Thomas S. An anatomic guide for arthroscopic visualization of the wrist capsular ligaments. *J Hand Surg Am* 1988; 13:815–822.
21. Westkaemper JG, Mitsionis G, Giannakopoulos PN, et al. Wrist

arthroscopy for the treatment of ligament and triangular fibrocartilage complex injuries. *Arthroscopy* 1998;14:479–483.
22. Kozin SH. The role of arthroscopy in scapholunate instability. *Hand Clin* 1999;15:435–444.
23. Hofmeister EP, Dao KD, Glowacki KA, et al. The role of midcarpal arthroscopy in the diagnosis of disorders of the wrist. *J Hand Surg* 2001;26:407–414.
24. Sennwald GR, Zdravkovic V. Wrist arthroscopy: a prospective analysis of 53 post-traumatic carpal injuries. *Scand J Plast Reconstr Surg Hand Surg* 1997;31:261–266.
25. Dautel G, Merle M. Chondral lesions of the midcarpal joint. *Arthroscopy* 1997;13:97–102.
26. Geissler WB, Freeland AE, Weiss AP, et al. Techniques of wrist arthroscopy. *Instr Course Lect* 2000;49:225–237.
27. Geissler WB, Freeland AE. Arthroscopic management of intraarticular distal radius fractures. *Hand Clin* 1999;15:455–465.
28. Cooney WP, Linscheid RL, Dobyns JH. Arthroscopy vs arthrography of the wrist *J Hand Surg Am* 1993;18:815–822.
29. North ER, Meyer S. Wrist injuries: correlation of clinical arthroscopic findings. *J Hand Surg Am* 1990;15:915–920.
30. Whipple TL. The role of arthroscopy in the treatment of wrist injuries in the athlete. *Clin Sports Med* 1998;17:623–634.
31. Huracek J, Troeger H. Wrist arthroscopy without distraction: a technique to visualize instability of the wrist after a ligamentous tear. *J Bone Joint Surg* 2000;82:1011–1012.

32. Schadel-Hopfner M, Iwinska-Zelder J, Braus T, et al. MRI versus arthroscopy in the diagnosis of scapholunate ligament injury. *J Hand Surg* 2001;26:17–21.
33. DeSmet L, Dauwe D, Fortems Y, et al. The value of wrist arthroscopy: an evaluation of 129 cases. *J Hand Surg* 1996;21:210–212.
34. Roth JH, Haddad RG. Radiocarpal arthroscopy and arthrography in the diagnosis of ulnar wrist pain. *Arthroscopy* 1986;2:234–243.
35. Tham S, Coleman S, Gilpin D. An anterior portal for wrist arthroscopy: anatomical study and case reports. *J Hand Surg Br* 1999;24:445–457.
36. Blackwell RE, Jemison DM, Foy BD. The holmium:yttrium-aluminum-garnet laser in wrist arthroscopy: a five-year experience in the treatment of central triangular fibrocartilage complex tears by partial excision. *J Hand Surg* 2001;26:77–84.
37. Tomaino MM, Shah M. Treatment of ulnar impaction syndrome with the wafer procedure. *Am J Orthop* 2001;30:129–133.
38. Nagle DJ. Laser-assisted wrist arthroscopy. *Hand Clin* 1999;15:495–499.
39. Dailey SW, Palmer AK. The role of arthroscopy in the evaluation and treatment of triangular fibrocartilage complex injuries in athletes. *Hand Clin* 2000;16:461–476.
40. Ekman EF, Poehling GG. Arthroscopy of the wrist in athletes. *Clin Sports Med* 1996;15:753–768.

CARPAL TUNNEL RELEASE

JAMES C.Y. CHOW

HISTORY OF CARPAL TUNNEL SYNDROME

The first carpal tunnel syndrome was described by Sir James Paget (1,2) in 1854 as median nerve compression after a fracture of the distal radius. In 1880, James Putman (3), a neurologist from Boston, described the symptoms suffered by a group of his patients. Although the term *carpal tunnel syndrome* was not used then, the symptoms he described would be considered classic for carpal tunnel syndrome today. In 1913, Marie and Foix (4) performed an autopsy on a patient and described advanced atrophy of the thenar muscle with no history of trauma or injury to the wrist region. There was enlargement of the median nerve, described as neuromata, proximal to the transverse carpal ligament. It was their opinion that the release of the transverse carpal ligament probably would have prevented the paralysis of the thenar muscles. The first surgical release of the transverse carpal ligament was described by Sir James Learmonth in 1933 (5). In 1946, Cannon and Love (6) reported 38 cases of tardy median nerve palsy. In 1947, W. Russell Brain, along with his colleague Marcia Wilkinson and the surgeon Dickson Wright (7), published the first article that described the details of the clinical signs, diagnosis, and pathophysiology of spontaneous compression of the median nerve in the carpal canal. Based on their findings, these investigators recommended early release of the transverse carpal ligament to prevent muscle or nerve deficits (7).

Beginning in the 1950s, George Phalen and colleagues (8–15) made the decompression of the median nerve of the wrist a well-known procedure to the surgeons in North America through a series of articles. He also described Tinel's and Phalen's signs to help in diagnosing this disease. Today, it is a better-known pathophysiology of the distal nerve compression with peripheral nerve involvement.

J. C. Y. Chow: Department of Surgery, Southern Illinois University School of Medicine, Springfield, Illinois.

ANATOMY OF THE CARPAL LIGAMENT

The transverse carpal ligament, a continuation of the deep fascia of the forearm, is made of compact, collagen fibers. In cross section, it has an appearance of an airplane's wing with a thicker, rounded edge distally and a thinner edge proximally. The thicker portion (distal portion) usually measures about 4 to 5 mm, whereas the thinner edge (proximal portion) measures from 1 to 2 mm. In cadaveric dissection, it has been noted that some carpal ligaments may be as thick as 8 mm, especially in a large hand or if there is some disease of the carpal ligament. The transverse carpal ligament extends across the opening on the palmar side of the wrist joint. This forms a roof over the transverse arch of the carpal bones and creates the canal called the *carpal tunnel.* This tunnel contains nine flexor tendons and the median nerve. The flexor tendons are usually covered by the synovial sheath, which allows their movement during the flexion of the wrist. Two bursae, ulnar and radial, can also be identified in the canal, with a thin bursal membrane on the top of the tendon sheath. The median nerve has numerous variances (16–25), including those of the motor branch as described in the excellent work of Lanz (20) in 1977. In this article, he described how the motor branch exits the carpal canal. For example, in 46% of the patients, it branches past the carpal canal and curves back to the thenar muscle. In 31% of the people, the motor branch exits under the carpal ligament after passing through the distal edge of the carpal ligament and then curves back to the thenar muscles. In 23% of the patients, the motor branches are actually transligamental, passes through the carpal ligament, and then enters the thenar muscles. Of course, there are other rare circumstances. For example, the presence of a high division of the median nerve or more than one motor branch that exits from the median nerve to the thenar muscle is present in less than 1% of the patients.

During the cadaveric dissections of the carpal ligament, it is possible to find two distinct layers: a superficial layer attached to the tubercle of the trapezium and a deep layer attached to the median lips of the groove of the trapezium (26). Guyon's canal is formed on the ulnar side of the hook of hamate between the two layers of fiber that form a triangular cross section. The ulnar nerve, ulnar artery, and ulnar veins are contained in this canal. The transverse carpal ligament extends 3.5 to 4 cm beyond the distal crease of the wrist. The principal source of the blood supply to the transverse carpal ligament can be divided into superficial and deep networks. The superficial network is formed by branches of the ulnar artery; the deep network is formed by branches of the superficial palmar arch (27).

PATHOPHYSIOLOGY OF CARPAL TUNNEL SYNDROME

The term carpal tunnel syndrome is now applied to all conditions that produce irritations or compression of the median nerve within the carpal canal. Basically, the condition occurs when either the space is too small for the contents or the contents are too large for the space; therefore, pressure is applied to the median nerve itself. Lundborg and Dahlin (28) described how they believe that the small capillary flow of the median nerve is shut down when pressure is applied, thus causing an ischemic factor. Most of the patients we have seen exhibited idiopathic, or spontaneous, carpal tunnel syndrome. I believe that some people may inherit a genetically narrow space at birth and develop this problem later. Any other conditions that reduce the capacity of the carpal canal produce symptoms, such as a deformed Colles' fracture, edema or swelling of the tendon sheath, soft tissue tumors in the canal, and increased thickness of the carpal ligament itself from repetitive trauma. In recent years, repetitive motion in the workplace has also been recognized as a factor in this problem. Many other systemic conditions may be related to the symptoms, including obesity, diabetes, thyroid dysfunction, Raynaud's dysfunction and disease, scleroderma, rheumatoid disease, systemic lupus erythematosus, or any other collagen disease. The last trimester of pregnancy is also known to produce symptoms in this area. Of course, many rare and unusual conditions cited in the literature could also be related to or produce carpal tunnel syndrome (29–102).

DIAGNOSIS OF CARPAL TUNNEL SYNDROME

The patient's history is most important in the diagnosis of carpal tunnel syndrome because it is a subjective condition. The patient usually complains of paresthesia, tingling, and numbness involving the long fingers, and symptoms are characteristically nocturnal. Sometimes, the patient may have pain referred to the forearm, upper arm, and even the shoulder and neck. The patient usually complains of decreasing grip strength, dropping things, and an inability to feel fine objects. Most predominant are the nocturnal symptoms. The patient reports problems sleeping at night because of waking up with numbness in the hand and having to rub the fingers to obtain some relief. Sometimes, a patient may wake up several times in a single night, and the result is very little sleep (8–15).

Carpal tunnel syndrome can be divided into three stages: early, progressive, and late. In the early stage, the symptoms appear only when provoked and are related to specific daytime activities. Most of the symptoms are sensory, without motor involvement. In the progressive stage, the symptoms are noticeable regardless of the daytime activities. The sensory findings are more pronounced, and the motor weakness begins to affect the hand. This is the stage when the patient usually seeks medical assistance because the symptoms suddenly worsen and begin to disturb sleep and daily activities. In the late stage, usually after the patient has had the symptoms for years, muscle atrophy becomes noticeable with weakness. Sometimes, the patient believes that the symptoms are improving because the pain and tingling sensation appear to have decreased; however, in reality, the condition has not really improved because permanent nerve injury has resulted. The patient usually demonstrates classical thenar muscle atrophy and loss of pinch-and-grip strength, an inability to oppose the thumb, and persistent numbness in the long fingers. In this stage, a nerve conductive velocity test may show a marked delay in the distal latency and, at times, may even be nonresponsive in either or both of the motor and sensory distal latency of the median nerve; this finding may suggest permanent nerve damage (27).

Physical examination assists in evaluating these patients. In classic carpal tunnel syndrome, the small finger is the only finger not involved. In acute cases, there is tenderness along the carpal canal area. Light percussion over the median nerve, at the wrist region, produces *Tinel's sign,* which is a tingling sensation that radiates to the long fingers and follows the median nerve distribution. *Phalen's sign,* or the wrist flexion test, is observed by having the patient hold the forearm vertically and drop both hands into complete flexion of the wrist. In this position, the median nerve is squeezed between the proximal edge of the carpal ligament, the adjacent flexor tendon, and the radius. If this maneuver duplicates the symptoms of tingling in the fingers within 60 seconds, then the findings are considered positive. Other examinations should include the monofilament test, two-point discriminations, reverse Phalen's test, and tourniquet test. Some clinicians even suggest a direct measurement of the pressure in the carpal canal. In the late stages of the symptoms, with thenar muscle atrophy, one can observe muscle wasting in the thenar area (8–15,103). Electromyography and nerve conductive velocity testing also help to detect this condition. However, the indications for surgery should not be decided or altered by the results of nerve conductive studies, especially when the results are normal but the patient persists with classical carpal tunnel syndrome clinically (104–108). A delay of the distal latency of the median nerve of 7.0 milliseconds or over represents significant compression of the median nerve. If this is present, surgical treatment should be considered without further delay.

A careful examination should be performed by the physician to exclude the possibility of cervical disc or thoracic outlet syndrome, pronator compression syndrome in the forearm, or other central nervous system diseases (109–112). Wrist radiography should be done routinely, including anteroposterior, lateral, and carpal tunnel views, to rule out any possibility of any bone or joint deformity, abnormality, or pathologic process. If a more extensive study is indicated, magnetic resonance imaging, computer tomography, ultrasonography, bone scanning, and arthrography of the wrist may be necessary (27,113–119).

CONSERVATIVE TREATMENT

Patients in the early stages of carpal tunnel syndrome normally respond to conservative treatment quite well. This conservative treatment should include the use of night splints, nonsteroidal antiinflammatory oral medication, rest for the afflicted hand, alteration of the daily activities or occupations, antivibration or protective work gloves, avoidance of repetitive movement or persistent pressure to the palm region, physical therapy, or even steroid injections in the carpal canal (120–124). In the advanced or progressive stage of the condition, patients usually do not respond to conservative treatment very well. Most of these patients have suffered for some time, and surgical treatment is under consideration. Patients in the late stage have had tingling and numbness of the hands for years with a marked delay, or no response, of the distal latency on the nerve conductive velocity test and thenar muscle atrophy. Some patients in this stage have lost the ability to button a shirt and cannot determine between one and two points during the two-point discrimination test. When a patient has reached this stage, surgical decompression of the carpal ligament is indicated without further delay. Of course, for late-stage patients with signs of permanent nerve injury, the prognosis after surgical treatment is guarded.

SURGICAL TREATMENT PRINCIPLES

The standard open surgical procedure has numerous different approaches by different surgeons (125–137). In general, it is a longitudinal curved incision over the palm region, ulnar and parallel to the thenar crest. Some surgeons prefer to extend the incision proximal to the flexor crease of the wrist joint, to form the shape of a lazy S. The reason for having the incision form a curve, or angle, to the flexor crease is that an incision straight across the crest would form a painful scar postoperatively. Some surgeons prefer to use magnification loupes, to preserve the small branches of the cutaneous nerve fibers as much as possible. The deep structures are exposed, and the median nerve is traced to the carpal ligament, which is then released under direct visualization (138). After the surgical procedure, a compression dressing, volar splint, or both should be applied to avoid bowstringing of the tendons or nerve.

Another surgical technique is to use a transverse incision over the distal wrist crease. The incision is approximately 5 cm in length, cut straight across the wrist area. Then, the surgeon uses scissors or a knife to cut the carpal ligament proximally to distally. This surgical technique involves a blind cut toward the distal carpal ligament. The danger in this technique is either cutting too far distally, thus increasing the chance of injury to the digital nerve or superficial palmar artery, or undercutting the ligament resulting in an incomplete release of the carpal ligament. Most surgeons have recommended abandoning this method (138).

In the past few years, endoscopic techniques have been developed in an attempt to decrease postoperative pain, pillar pain, and the painful scar of the open procedure. It has been proven that the patient has much less suffering and a faster recovery with the endoscopic technique than with the open procedure; however, it is a dangerous arthroscopic procedure if performed by inexperienced surgeons (139–142). Devastating complications have been reported throughout the United States by surgeons who have used the endoscopic carpal tunnel technique (143–146). This situation has raised a controversy regarding the value of endoscopic release of the carpal ligament. Many hand surgeons believe that the dangers of the procedure outweigh the benefits to the patient. Obviously, it would apply to all surgical procedures done by inexperienced surgeons. It has also been shown that endoscopic carpal ligament release can be performed safely by experienced surgeons and can give both the patient and the surgeon a great deal of satisfaction. I must say that the results are much better and the complication rates are a lot lower for the endoscopic release compared with my own open procedure for the carpal tunnel syndrome (147–151).

HISTORY OF THE ENDOSCOPIC RELEASE OF THE CARPAL LIGAMENT

When I began working on my technique in 1985, I did not know that Dr. Ichiro Okutsu, in Japan, or Dr. John Agee, in California, were working on similar goals at approximately the same time. Through trial and error of different approaches, the breakthrough of the idea of the slotted cannula came sometime around late 1986. The procedure was completed in May 1987, after 4 to 5 months of persistent practice on cadavers, before the procedure was performed on the first patient, in September 1987. Since that time, continued efforts have been made to improve of this procedure.

During the 1988 annual spring meeting of the Arthroscopy Association of North America (AANA), Dr. George Schonholtz, the president, presented a presidential address regarding the past, current, and future of arthroscopy. He presented a slide of Dr. Okutsu's that he had brought back from Japan of a view of the carpal ligament through a plastic tube. I believed that Dr. Schonholtz and I were probably the only two people present in that meeting who had ever seen the undersurface of the carpal ligament before. I also believe that this was the first presentation of an endoscopic view of the carpal ligament undersurface at an official meeting. At that time, Dr. Schonholtz predicted that endoscopic release of the carpal ligament would be developed in the near future. The first two articles regarding the endoscopic carpal tunnel release, Dr. Okutsu et al. and by me, were published in the March issue of *Arthroscopy Journal* in 1989 (147,152).

The first paper on endoscopic carpal tunnel release, based on my clinical results for the first 149 cases, was presented at the AANA's 1990 annual meeting in Orlando, Florida (148). In the fall of that same year, at the annual meeting of the American Society for Surgery of the Hand in Toronto, Dr. John Agee (153) presented his paper on the clinical results of his multicenter study. Therefore, three different studies, using three separate techniques of endoscopic carpal ligament release, were begun in different corners of the globe and were aimed at the same idea of minimizing the incision for releasing the carpal ligament for carpal tunnel syndrome by getting away from the traditional curved longitudinal incision in the palm region.

The three original techniques could be summarized as follows. The Chow procedure used a slotted cannula through dual portals, which allows the scope to be introduced at one end and the instrumentation at the other end, thus allowing for release of the carpal ligament with direct visualization (147–151). Dr. Okutsu (152), in Japan, used a clear plastic tube to introduce the scope so the carpal ligament could be visualized. A hook knife was then brought alongside the plastic tube to release the ligament. Dr. John Agee and colleagues (153,154) used a transverse incision to introduce a specially designed device. Under arthroscopic visualization, these investigators pulled a trigger that elevated the blade to cut the ligament. The common denominator of these three procedures is that we all used the current advancement of arthroscopic technology, enabling us to bring visualization of the surgical procedure to a television monitor with the use of a camera. Although our methods varied, the ideas were similar in that we were attempting to treat the patient with carpal tunnel syndrome and to preserve the normal hand structures.

Since the publication of the three original endoscopic carpal ligament release techniques, there has been considerable interest among surgeons. Many modifications and variations have been made to the three original ideas since their introduction to the public. For example, the Acufex Uni-portal (155) and Linvatec Endoscopic Releasing Kit (156) have been developed using the single portal, as described by Dr. John Agee, and the original slotted cannula idea from my technique. The Acufex Uniportal set uses a hook knife to cut distally to proximally, and the Linvatec Endoscopic Releasing Kit uses a push knife to cut proximally to distally. Mirza et al. (157) use a single palmar portal, as described for the alternative dual-portal Chow technique, and a sleeve-knife device attached to the endoscope. They use my basic concept of the slotted cannula to see and protect the important structures while creating a work space in the carpal canal to release the carpal ligament. However, by eliminating one additional portal, they sacrifice the visualization, flexibility, surgical ability, and mobility of the procedure and put the patient's safety in jeopardy. There are other modifications of the dual-portal technique as well. For example, Dr. Roman Lewicky (158) developed a plastic tube technique in which he uses a curved dissector to pass all the way from the proximal portal to the exit portal. He then passes the plastic tube from the distal portal to the proximal portal. He uses this plastic tube to guide the slotted cannula into the proper position and place. By doing so, he tries to increase the safety of placement of the slotted cannula.

SURGICAL TECHNIQUES

Chow's Dual-Portal Endoscopic Release For Carpal Tunnel Syndrome

Thanks to the effort of the Seven University Study Group (159,160), the original technique has been modified in an attempt to decrease the complications and the learning curve. The following is a description of the current dual-portal technique.

Setup

The patient is placed in a supine position, and a hand table is used. Two video monitors are preferred, but, of course, some surgeons can manage the procedure with only one. One of the two monitors should face the surgeon, and one should face the assistant (Fig. 55.1). The surgeon sits on the ulnar side of the patient, and the assistant faces the surgeon. Standard preparations and draping are performed as usual.

Anesthesia

Local anesthesia and intravenous medication are recommended for the procedure. The use of local anesthesia allows the patient and surgeon to communicate. An alert patient can inform the surgeon of any variance of nerve structure during the procedure (15–25). Usually, when the patient first comes into the room, 1 to 2 mg of midazolam hydrochloride (Versed) (Roche, Nutley, NJ) is given intravenously to help the patient relax and be more comfortable

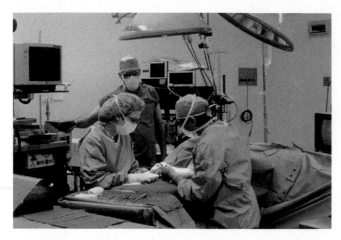

FIGURE 55.1 Setup for the Chow dual-portal technique. One of the two monitors should face the surgeon and one should face the assistant.

during the preparations and draping. Alfentanil hydrochloride (Alfenta) (Janssen Pharmaceutica, Inc., Piscataway, NJ), 200 μg, is given intravenously when the surgeon begins to mark the patient's hand. This is a short-acting analgesia with a peak action of 5 to 10 minutes. Normally, the surgical time for this procedure is less than 10 minutes. An injection of 1% lidocaine hydrochloride (Xylocaine) (Astra, Westboro, MA) without epinephrine is used at the entry and exit portals, but only to the skin, to avoid penetrating too deeply to affect the nerve.

Entry Portal

The proximal end of the pisiform is palpated and marked with a small circle. A 1- to 1.5-cm line is drawn radially from the proximal pole of the pisiform. A second line is drawn approximately 0.5 cm proximally to the end of the first line. A small, dotted line, approximately 1 cm in length, is drawn from the end of the second line to create the entry portal. If the palmaris longus is present, the center of the entry portal should be located at the ulnar border of the palmaris longus (Fig. 55.2).

Exit Portal

With the patient's thumb in full abduction, a line is drawn from the distal border, perpendicular to the long axis of the forearm. The second line is drawn from the third web space, parallel to the long axis of the forearm. These two lines should meet at a right angle. A bisecting line is drawn from the junction of these two lines, proximally 1 cm, to locate the distal portal. The surgeon should be able to palpate the hook of hamate. The exit portal should fall into the soft spot in the center of the palm and should line up with the ring finger, just slightly radial to the hook of hamate (Fig. 55.3).

Procedure

The 1% lidocaine hydrochloride is injected at both the entry and exit portal, approximately 1 mL at each portal. A small, transverse 1-cm incision is made at the entry portal mark. A hemostat is used for blunt dissection. Small digital nerves and vessels are pushed away (25,133,161–164). A tourniquet is normally not required if this dissection is handled properly. The fascia, with its distinguished fibers, should be able to be seen. A knife is used to make a small, longitudinal opening. This cut is extended with small, Stevens' curve, tenotomy scissors. If the palmaris longus is present, the longitudinal cut should be along the ulnar border of the palmaris longus. Care should be taken because, sometimes, there are two layers of fascia. Both these layers must be cut, and the ulnar bursa should be seen from underneath. With the small retractors, the distal border of the skin is lifted to create a vacuum that will separate the carpal ligament and the ulnar bursa. A curved dissector–slotted cannula assembly unit (Fig. 55.4) is slipped under the carpal ligament. When this unit is maneuvered back and forth, the rough undersurface of the carpal ligament, described as a "washboard" or "railroad track" effect, can be felt. With the tip of the unit touching the hook of hamate bone, the surgeon picks up the patient's fingers and hand and, maintaining this position, gently hyperextends the fingers and wrist. The assistant moves the hand rest down so the patient's hand rests comfortably on the frame. The slotted cannula assembly is gently advanced distally, pointing toward the

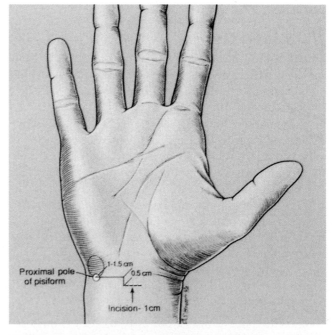

FIGURE 55.2 The entry portal is located by drawing a line 1 to 1.5 cm radially from the proximal pole of the pisiform, then drawing a second line approximately 0.5 cm for the end of the first line. A small dotted line, approximately 1 cm in length, is drawn from the end of the second line to create the entry portal.

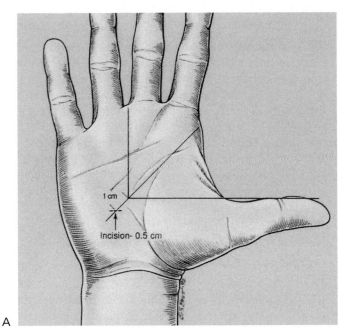

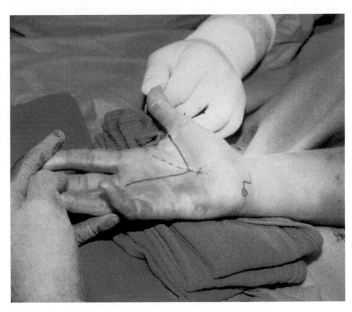

A B

FIGURE 55.3 A and **B:** The exit portal is located by drawing a line from the distal border of the fully abducted thumb, perpendicular to the long axis of the forearm. A second line is drawn from the third web space, parallel to the long axis of the forearm, and meeting at the first line in a right angle. A bisecting line is drawn from the junction of these two lines, proximal 1 cm, to locate the distal portal.

exit portal. A small, transverse or oblique incision is be made on the skin only. Arch suppressors are used to press down the structures, and the assembled unit exits through the distal portal (Fig. 55.5). The trocar is then removed so the slotted cannula remains in position under the carpal ligament. The patient's hand is then stabilized in the hand holder (Fig. 55.6).

Endoscopic Examination

The specially designed endoscope is inserted from the proximal opening of the slotted cannula. This is a short, 30-

degree scope with a light post that points up in the same direction of the 30-degree angle to ensure that the light post does not hit the patient's forearm. The camera and scope should rest comfortably in the first web space of the surgeon's hand. Usually, the surgeon braces the middle and ring fingers on the patient's forearm, or any firm object, to avoid shaking or moving the endoscope and to allow full control of the camera. A cotton swab can be inserted into the tube to clean the lens, and then the focus is adjusted to the best visualization (Fig. 55.7).

A blunt hook probe is inserted to palpate the undersurface of the carpal ligament proximally to distally (Fig.

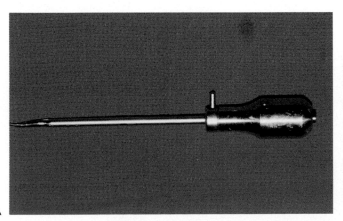

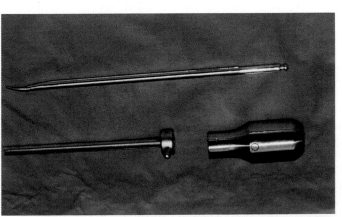

A B

FIGURE 55.4 A and **B:** Curved ECTRA SYSTEM dissector/slotted cannula assembly from Smith-Nephew Dyonics. (Courtesy of Smith-Nephew Dyonics.)

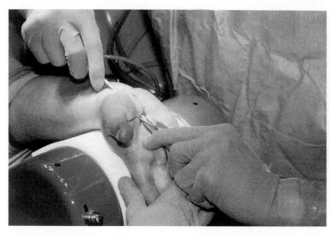

FIGURE 55.5 Arched suppressors are used to press down on the anatomic structures, to allow the unit to exit through the distal portal.

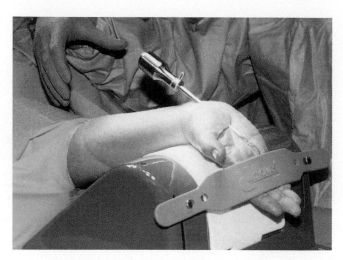

FIGURE 55.6 The hand is stabilized in the hand holder.

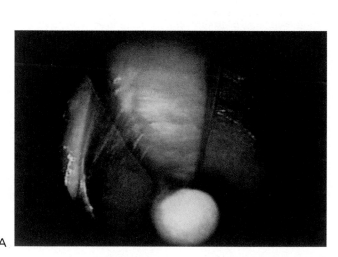

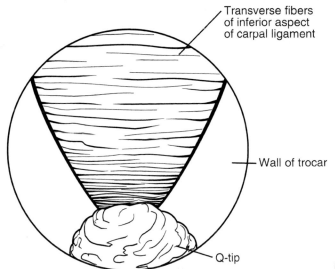

A

B

FIGURE 55.7 A cotton swab is inserted into the distal opening of the slotted cannula to clean the endoscope lens for better visualization.

Transverse fibers of inferior aspect of carpal ligament

Wall of trocar

Q-tip

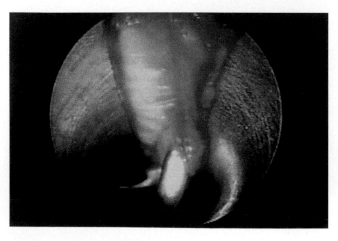

FIGURE 55.8 A blunt hook probe is inserted to palpate the under-surface of the carpal ligament carefully.

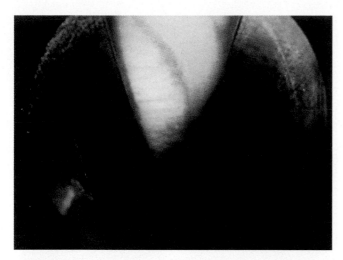

FIGURE 55.9 Median nerve seen through the slotted cannula.

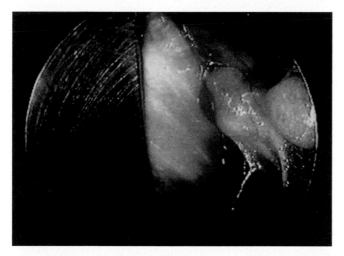

FIGURE 55.10 Tendon caught between the slotted cannula and the undersurface of the carpal ligament.

55.8). If any soft tissue appears in the opening of the slotted cannula, the blunt probe is used to palpate this tissue carefully. If the median nerve is present (Fig. 55.9), the patient will feel sharp or shooting pain to the fingers when the nerve is probed and will be able to inform the surgeon. Otherwise, it could either be synovial tissue or a portion of the ulnar bursa. If abundant soft tissue is noted in the opening of the slotted cannula, the surgical procedure should not be performed. The slotted cannula may need to be reinserted for better visualization; however, to avoid irreversible damage, surgery should not be carried out if tendons (Fig. 55.10), or other important structures, are caught between the slotted cannula and the undersurface of the carpal ligament.

If there is only a minimal amount of synovium obstructing the view, the trocar can be reinserted into the slotted cannula. The slotted cannula unit can then be rotated radially about 355 to 360 degrees to push the synovial tissue out of the way. I always emphasize to the physicians who attend the Endoscopic Carpal Tunnel Release (ECTRA) workshop course that surgeons should not be afraid or hesitate to convert an endoscopic procedure to an open, standard procedure if they are not able to obtain adequate visualization.

Ligament Cutting Technique

With the scope in the proximal portal and the instrumentation in the distal portal, the distal border of the carpal ligament is identified with the probe. The probe knife is used to make the first cut, distally to proximally (Fig. 55.11). Anything beyond the distal border of the carpal ligament should not be excised. The scope is withdrawn proximally about 1 cm (10 mm), and the triangle knife is used to make a small opening in the midsection of the carpal ligament

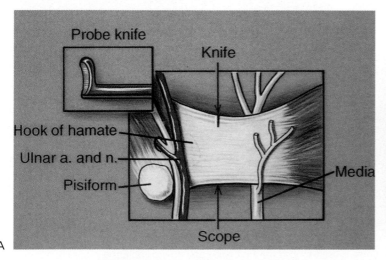

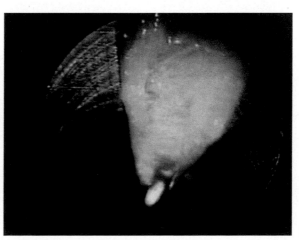

FIGURE 55.11 A and **B:** The probe knife is used to make the first cut, cutting distally to proximally.

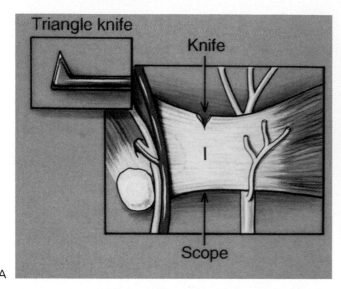

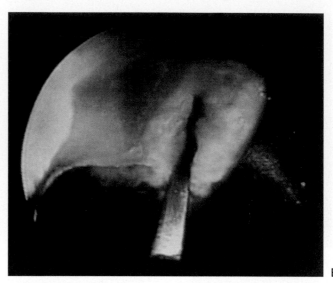

FIGURE 55.12 A and **B:** The triangle knife is used to make a small opening in the midsection of the carpal ligament.

(Fig. 55.12). The retrograde knife is brought in and placed in the second cut. Once the retrograde knife is well seated, it is pulled distally to join the first two cuts. Now, the distal portion of the carpal ligament is completely released (Fig. 55.13).

The scope is removed from the proximal opening of the slotted cannula and is inserted in the distal opening. The camera view on the screen now forms a mirror effect. The surgeon should realize that the previous ulnar side is now the radial side. By moving the scope proximally and distally, the previous distal cut is identified (Fig. 55.14). The probe knife is reinserted, and the carpal ligament is palpated to identify the proximal border. A small cut is then made with the probe knife proximally to distally (Fig. 55.15). The

probe knife is withdrawn, and the retrograde knife is inserted and seated in the proximal edge of the distal cut. It is then pulled proximally to join the proximal cut to excise the proximal carpal ligament completely (Fig. 55.16). If there are any additional fibers remaining, the triangle knife, or any other knife that feels appropriate, can be used to release these fibers until the surgeon is satisfied with a complete release.

Because of the position of the patient's hand, the cut edges of the carpal ligament should spring apart and disappear from the opening of the slotted cannula. If the edges can still be seen through the opening, the release is incomplete. While the assistant fully abducts the patient's thumb, the uncut portion of the ligament can be identified, and the

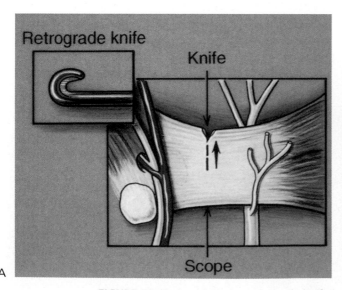

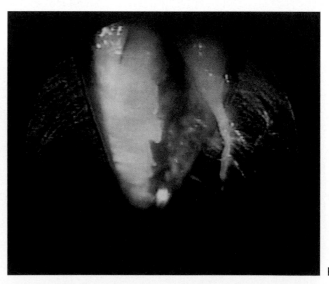

FIGURE 55.13 A and **B:** The retrograde knife is used to join the first two cuts, thus completing the release of the distal portion of the transverse carpal ligament.

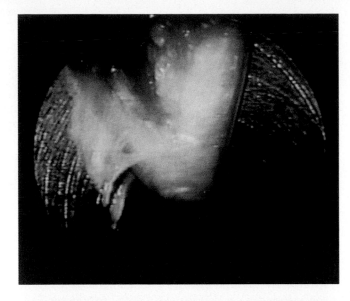

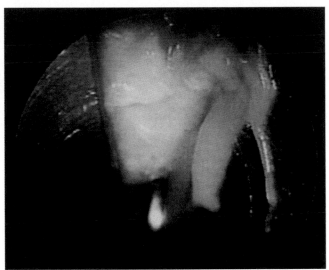

FIGURE 55.14 The endoscope is moved to the distal opening of the slotted cannula, and the previous cut is identified.

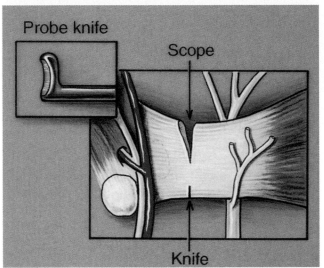

A

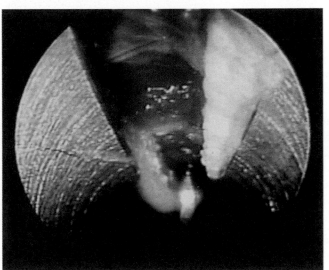

B

FIGURE 55.15 A and B: A small cut is made on the proximal border of the carpal ligament with the probe knife.

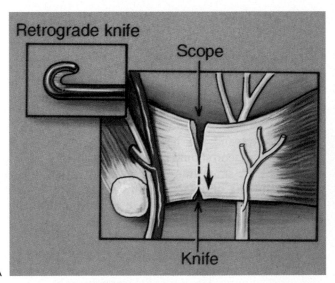

A

B

FIGURE 55.16 A and B: The retrograde knife is reinserted and seated in the proximal edge of the distal cut, then it is pulled proximally to the proximal cut, thus completing the dissection of the carpal ligament.

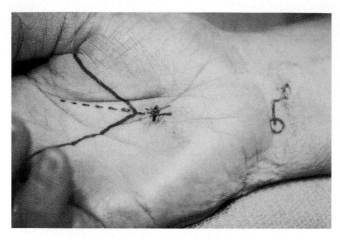

FIGURE 55.17 Only one suture is required to close each portal.

surgeon can complete the resection. By rotating the slotted cannula, the completely cut ligament can be seen endoscopically. There is a continuation fan volarly to the carpal ligament, and this should be preserved, as well as the palmaris brevis muscles, if present. This thin continuation fibrous fan from the thenar to the lesser thenar muscles prevents bowstringing of the flexor tendon and preserves muscle strength. There is seldom any bleeding, and only one suture is required for closing each portal (Fig. 55.17). Immediately after the procedure, the surgeon can examine the patient while still in a sterilized environment. If any intraoperative complications have occurred that may necessitate exposure of the hand, it can be preformed at the same time.

Postoperatively, active exercise begins immediately. The patient is advised to avoid heavy lifting or pushing down on the palm region until the discomfort disappears, usually 2 to 3 weeks. Active movement of the fingers decreases the formation of the scar tissue in the wrist region and therefore prevents adhesions on the tendons or nerve at the surgical site. Sutures are usually removed in 1 week. If the patient engages in heavy lifting too soon after the surgical procedure, there may be swelling and prolonged pain in the palm region. If these occur, fluidotherapy treatment for 20 minutes per day helps to decrease the condition within 1 week.

The carpal ligament does not have a rich blood supply or nerve fiber distribution; therefore, cutting only the carpal ligament definitely decreases postoperative pain, bleeding, and scarring. The palmaris longus tendon extension and muscle fibers are preserved by the endoscopic technique, which prevents bowstringing of the flexor tendon and the median nerve (165–170).

Alternative Dual-Portal Chow Technique: A Special Design for Hand Surgeons

Many hand surgeons are very uncomfortable with the blind insertion of the trocar exiting distally without seeing the distal superficial palmar arch and distal digital nerve; therefore, they may want to make the distal portal larger, to identify these structures before introducing the slotted cannula. This alternative technique is designed for those surgeons who are willing to take the time to explore the distal portal, especially for a hand surgeon who uses loupe magnification. So the important distal structures can be seen, the slotted cannula is placed in the same way but is inserted distally to proximally.

Procedure

The setup and marking of the portal setups are the same as described earlier. Whether a regional block or local anesthesia is used depends on the surgeon's preference; however, I strongly recommend the use of local anesthesia for the reason mentioned earlier. The entry portal for this alternative technique is made with a small, oblique incision (1 to 1.5 cm) over the distal palm region at the mark for the exit portal in the foregoing method. Magnified loupes are used while one carefully dissects down to identify the superficial palmar arch curving ulnarly to radially. Further careful dissection allows the identification of the median or digital nerve in the area.

The distal carpal ligament is identified, and the slotted cannula, curved side pointing upward, is inserted under the carpal ligament. The assembly should be touching the hook of hamate, gliding proximally. The "washboard" texture of the carpal ligament should be palpable with the curved dissector as the cannula is aimed toward the center of the wrist and the exit portal. The exit portal should be on the ulnar border of the palmaris longus, if it exists; otherwise, it should be aimed toward the center of the wrist marked as previously described, approximately 0.5 to 1.0 cm proximal to the flexor wrist crease. The fingers and the rest of the patient's hand are then hyperextended, and the hand is placed in the hand holder. The surgeon should be able to palpate the curved dissector tip. A small, transverse incision is then made, and the slotted cannula assembly is brought outside proximally. The rest of the procedure and cutting techniques can be carried out as previously described.

Agee's Technique

Dr. John Agee and colleagues (153,154) of California, in cooperation with the 3M Corporation, developed a surgical device that was shaped like a hand pistol (Fig. 55.18). This device is used to see and release the carpal ligament under direct visualization. This technique requires an incision that closely resembles the standard transverse incision on the wrist for carpal tunnel syndrome. However, instead of cutting blindly, this special pistol-shaped instrumentation allows the surgeon to visualize the undersurface of the carpal ligament while it is being cut. This instrument has a camera hookup located at the back of the handle and a disposable tip, which allow for viewing through an open window.

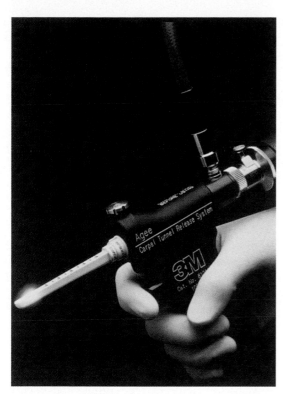

FIGURE 55.18 Pistol Grip Surgical Device developed by Dr. John Agee, in cooperation with the 3M Corporation. (Photos courtesy of 3M Corporation.)

Squeezing the trigger of the pistol-shaped instrument elevates a blade through the window, and withdrawing the entire instrument, distally to proximally, releases the carpal ligament.

Procedure

With the use of tourniquet control and regional block or general anesthesia, a 2-cm skin incision is placed in the wrist flexion crease between the flexor carpi radialis and the flexor carpi ulnaris tendons. A spreading subcutaneous dissection protects the underlying palmar cutaneous nerve. A probe inserted through a distally based U-shaped incision in the forearm fascia helps to define a proximal to distal path down the palmar-ulnar aspect of the carpal tunnel (Fig. 55.19). With the device aimed at the patient's ring finger and with the wrist in extension, the blade assembly of the device is inserted along the same path.

Through the window near the tip of the device's blade assembly, a strip of transverse carpal ligament that is free of all other structures is visualized. Once the distal edge of the ligament is clearly identified and the ulnar position and ring finger aim are checked, the trigger is pulled to elevate the blade in a triangular area defined by the ulnar half of the distal edge of the transverse carpal ligament, the ulnar border of the median nerve and/or its digital branches, and the proximal edge of the superficial palmar arch.

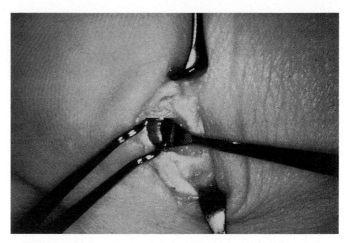

FIGURE 55.19 A 2-cm skin incision is placed in the flexion crease between the flexor carpi radialis and flexor carpi ulnaris tendons.

Application of upward pressure to hold the window against the deep side of the ligament as the device is gently withdrawn excludes flexor tendons and the median nerve during incision of the transverse carpal ligament. Additional passes may be necessary for complete release of the transverse carpal ligament, with endoscopic control permitting visualization of its cut edges (154).

Japanese Technique

Dr. Okutsu and his colleagues from Japan (152) developed a blunt, clear plastic tube, with an outer diameter of 6 mm, an inner diameter of 4 mm, and a barrel length of 175 mm. This tube is inserted into the carpal canal through a transverse incision made in the patient's forearm, ulnarly to the palmaris longus. The arthroscope is brought in through this clear plastic tube, and the carpal ligament is identified. A hook knife is passed along the ulnar side of the plastic tube to the distal border of the carpal ligament (Fig. 55.20). The

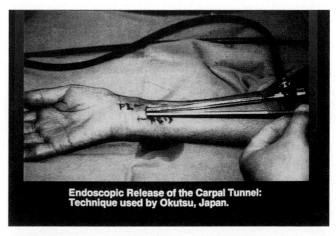

Endoscopic Release of the Carpal Tunnel: Technique used by Okutsu, Japan.

FIGURE 55.20 The arthroscope, in a clear plastic tube, is placed in the transverse incision made in the forearm, ulnar to the palmaris longus. A hook knife is passed along the ulnar side of the plastic tube to the distal border of the carpal ligament. (Photo courtesy of Dr. Okutsu.)

knife is hooked on the carpal ligament and is withdrawn to release the carpal ligament. The details of his procedure are described next.

Procedure

The operation is carried out using local anesthesia with 10 ml of 1% lidocaine solution that contains epinephrine in a concentration of 1:100,000, applied to the skin over the palmaris longus tendon, 3 cm proximal to the distal transverse carpal crease, and into the carpal tunnel. A pneumotourniquet is not used. A transverse incision of 5 to 10 mm is made at the anesthetized area, as well as at the fascia of the same region. The obturator is then gently inserted into the carpal tunnel from the radial side of the palmaris longus tendon, which helps to guide insertion of the scope to observe the median nerve. The clear plastic tube is introduced after the removal of the obturator. The scope slowly advances into the clear plastic tube. The median nerve, flexor tendons, and transverse carpal ligament are observed. With active or passive finger flexion and extension, the gliding motion of the tendon can be clearly observed under the scope. This maneuver is important to differentiate between the nerve and tendons. The transverse carpal ligament is examined through the universal subcutaneous endoscope placed in the carpal tunnel. The ligamentum fiber can be seen arranged in an arch form, running transversely.

To incise the transverse carpal ligament, the endoscope is removed from the carpal tunnel and is then inserted from the ulnar side of the palmaris longus tendon into the carpal tunnel through the same skin incision and is advanced to the palm. The location of the superficial palmar arch, which is located 10 to 15 mm distal from the distal end of the transverse carpal ligament, is checked. In some cases, arterial pulsation is observed under endoscopic vision. Then the arthroscope is drawn inside the sheath, which is located inside of the carpal tunnel in the proximal direction to check the transverse carpal ligament and visually to confirm the absence of the motor branch of the median nerve or any abnormalities at the site of the incision. Sometimes, the transverse carpal ligament is covered by the synovial membrane of the flexor tendons. In such cases, scraping the synovium with an L-shaped probe enables one to observe the transverse carpal ligament.

If the motor branch of the median nerve or any anatomic abnormality is evident at the site of the incision, the endoscopic procedure should be terminated, and open surgery should be performed. A retrograde hook knife is introduced along the ulnar side of the sheath from the previously made incision at the forearm. The transverse carpal ligament is caught by the knife under endoscopic vision and is then incised at the ulnar side. While one moves the arthroscope inside the sheath, which is located inside of the carpal tunnel, proximally, the knife is simultaneously drawn toward the operator. The transverse carpal ligament is released under complete endoscopic vision. When the ligament or forearm fascia is incised, subcutaneous fatty tissue of the wrist or forearm, respectively, should be visible through the endoscope. The entire length of the ligament can be completely divided with little bleeding. The skin incision at the forearm is closed with a single stitch, which completes the operation. On the day of the operation, patients elevate their hands to reduce the swelling and bleeding at the site of the operation. On the following day, patients are encouraged to perform gentle active range-of-motion exercises.

CLINICAL RESULTS

For 40 years, the standard open carpal ligament release and decompression for carpal tunnel syndrome claimed good to excellent results. It became the standard for treating carpal tunnel syndrome. After reviewing the literature carefully, however, it was actually found that the surgical failure rate varied from 7% to 20%, even when the safer longitudinal incision was used (171–184). The open procedure inherits obvious disadvantages with the palmar incision, including scar tenderness, pillar pain, hand weakness, carpal arch widening, bowstringing of the tendons and nerves, and many other reported complications (171–203). Of course, most of the complications of the open procedure are not reported in the literature. The idea for an endoscopic technique to release the carpal ligament came as an attempt to preserve normal tissue and anatomy of the hand and to decrease the problems that had been encountered with the open procedure. The smaller incision results in less skin damage and spares the palmar fascia, palmaris brevis muscles, and peripheral cutaneous nerves and vessels and, in turn, decreases scar tenderness, pillar pain, weakness, and bowstringing of tendons and nerves.

From September 1987 to September 1999, in Mt. Vernon, Illinois, 2,362 wrists in 1,674 patients with carpal tunnel syndrome underwent endoscopic release of the carpal ligament for carpal tunnel syndrome, using the dual-portal Chow technique. Of these patients, 1,082 were female and 592 were male, with ages ranging from 14 to 96 years. There were 790 right-hand procedures, 306 left-hand procedures, and 683 bilateral cases. All the patients in this series were carefully examined for other associated problems, including cervical disc or thoracic outlet syndrome, although some patients did have double-crush syndrome. All patients exhibited classic carpal tunnel syndrome symptoms including diminished sensation in the median nerve distribution, nocturnal pain, decreased pinch-and-grip strength, weakness of the hand, and persistent waking up during the night. The duration of the symptoms ranged from 1 week to 60 years, with 96% having a positive nerve conduction velocity test.

Among the 1,683 patients, there were 176 patients known to have thyroid disorders, 91 known to have rheumatoid disease, 201 with diabetes, 100 with a past history of trauma to the wrist, 148 with previously known wrist fractures, six known to have lupus erythematosus, and two who had scleroderma. One patient was known to have paraplegia, and 106 were known to have a ganglion cyst in the wrist region. Nine patients had a past history of stroke, 67 patients had a double-crush syndrome, and ten patients had recurrent carpal tunnel syndrome after having had an open procedure performed previously. The 14-year-old girl, the youngest of this series, was known to have a space-occupying lesion in the carpal canal preoperatively but refused to have the standard conventional surgical procedure to explore the carpal canal; therefore, endoscopic surgery was performed. All the patients had failed to respond to preoperative conservative treatment. Approximately 650 cases were performed using the original technique, whereas slightly more than 1,700 cases were performed using the modified technique described in this chapter.

Of the 2,362 cases, 268 (190 patients) were lost to follow-up; therefore, the results of this report are based on the remaining 2,094 cases (wrists) and 1,493 patients. The follow-up was 17 months to 11 years, 5 months. Most of the patient's symptoms were relieved, but there were 12 cases of recurrent symptoms for a recurrence rate of 0.57%, and 20 cases of continued problems after the endoscopic release of the carpal ligament, for a failure rate of 0.95%.

There were 642 of the original 2,362 cases, which were Workers' Compensation claims. Of these, 487 (76%) were engaged in heavy work, 146 (23%) were engaged in light work, and nine (1%) were no longer working. Of the remaining 1,720 non-Workers' Compensation cases, 432 (25%) were engaged in heavy work, 519 (30%) were engaged in light work, and 769 (41%) were retired or no longer working.

The clinical results of the 2,094 cases revealed that 651 (31%) returned to normal activity or work within 1 week, 1,305 (62%) returned to normal activity or work within 2 weeks, 1,601 (76%) returned to normal activity and work within 3 weeks, 1,800 (86%) returned to normal activity and work within 4 weeks, and 2,077 (99%) returned to work or normal activity after 4 weeks.

Of the 642 Workers' Compensation claim cases, 60 cases (12%) returned to work or normal activities within 1 week, 190 (36%) returned to work or normal activities within 2 weeks, 278 (53%) returned to work or normal activities within 3 weeks, 359 (69%) returned to work or normal activities within 4 weeks, and 517 (99%) returned to work or normal activities after 4 weeks.

Of the remaining 1,720 non-Workers' Compensation claim cases, 591 (38%) returned to work or normal activities within 1 week, 1,115 (71%) returned to work or normal activities within 2 weeks, 1,323 (84%) returned to work or normal activities within 3 weeks, 1,441 (91%) returned to work or normal activities within 4 weeks, and 1,560 (99%) returned to work or normal activities after 4 weeks.

Pinch-and-Grip Studies

A pinch-and-grip study was performed preoperatively and postoperatively. To avoid confusion, the number of patients and not the number of cases (number of wrists) was used in this pinch-and-grip study. Because of the geographic distance that some of the patients would have to travel, only 204 of 815 patients (25%) were able to return to complete the study. The preoperative strength was used in unilateral cases, and the better hand of two hands was used as a control in bilateral cases. The pinch-and-grip tests began 1 week postoperatively and were repeated each week until the patient regained normal, or better than normal, strength.

Of the 204 patients who returned for testing, 50 (25%) of the patients regained their pinch-and-grip strength within 1 week postoperatively, 120 (59%) regained normal strength within 2 weeks, 151 (74%) regained normal strength within 3 weeks, 164 (80%) regained normal strength in 4 weeks, 189 (93%) regained normal strength in 8 weeks, 199 (98%) regained normal strength in 12 weeks, and 203 (99.9%) regained their normal pinch-and-grip strength in 16 weeks.

COMPLICATIONS

Most of the complications of the standard open surgical release for carpal tunnel syndrome have not been reported; however, reviewing the available literature still reveals some existing complications. These include incomplete ligament release, nerve injuries, palmar hematomas, bowstringing of flexor tendons and median nerves, adhesions of nerves, reflex sympathetic dystrophy, deep wound infections, scar tenderness, pillar pain, persistent weakness of the hand, tendon lacerations, superficial palmar arch, and arterial injuries, even when the safer curved longitudinal incision was used (171–204). The nerve injuries include both median and ulnar nerve lacerations, motor branch and cutaneous branch of the median nerve injuries, and digital nerve injuries. Extensive reviews of the reported complications of conventional carpal ligament release surgery reveal a complication rate that varies from 1.4% in the report by Drs. Ariyan and Watson to 73% in the report by Drs. Clayburgh and Beckenbaugh (180,204).

The following discussion of complications involves the Chow technique and should not be confused with complications of the other endoscopic techniques. There was no permanent nerve or vessel damage, hematoma, or tendon laceration found in Chow's series. No permanent nerve or vessel damage, hematoma, or tendon laceration was reported among these 2,362 cases. One patient had superficial wound infections, two patients had transient ulnar nerve palsy, and two had incomplete release, for a complication rate 0.2% (5 of 2,362 cases). Since changing the direction of the retractor, there have not been any cases of neurapraxia.

One of the patients with an incomplete release was a 37-year-old woman who had a bilateral release. Both hands were completely asymptomatic after the surgical procedure, but 3 months after the patient returned to work, the left hand developed some minor symptoms. These symptoms, although not serious, continued to give her discomfort, especially as she increased her activities at work; therefore, the patient was offered a repeat endoscopic release of the carpal ligament or a standard decompression operation 8 months after the first surgical procedure. The patient chose to have the endoscopic release repeated, and the symptoms of the left hand were relieved after this second surgical procedure. The patient has had a follow-up period of more than 6 years with no more problems or complaints of carpal tunnel syndrome. She has returned to her normal duties; therefore, we conclude that the patient may have had an incomplete release of the carpal ligament during the first surgical procedure. The other patient who had an incomplete release had also undergone bilateral release; however, the patient continued to have problems with the left hand. The patient had a past medical history of keloid formation and a ridge of scar tissue at the portal sites; therefore, exploration and open decompression of the carpal canal were performed 3 months postoperatively. Large scar formation was found under the carpal ligament and attached to the median nerve. After the release of the carpal ligament, neurolysis was performed to free the median nerve. The patient was released back to work 5 weeks after the second surgical procedure, and after 3 years of follow-up, continues to do well. There were two patients who had transient ulnar nerve palsy. The first patient recovered spontaneously in 4 weeks. In this case, the patient was actually using her hand 10 days postoperatively with some inconvenience, along with slightly diminished sensation of the ulnar nerve distribution. Four weeks postoperatively, the ulnar nerve palsy had resolved completely, and the patient has had no further problems. The second patient had a bilateral carpal ligament release. The left hand had no problems, but the right hand developed a loss of interosseous muscle function immediately after the surgical procedure, although sensation appeared to be intact. It took almost 5 months before this patient fully recovered, and the patient now has full use of her hand with no residual problems.

Although my patients did not have any serious complications, several severe complications of this technique have been reported throughout the United States. In a multicenter prospective review of 640 endoscopic carpal tunnel releases using the Chow technique (159,160), a study performed by seven universities on a total of 640 cases of endoscopic carpal tunnel releases, the overall perioperative complication rate was 3.3%, or 21 complications of the 640 cases. Fourteen of these 21 complications involved neurapraxia, all of which resolved without sequelae, and no nerves were lacerated or transected. There was one laceration of the superficial flexor of the ring and small fingers,

four incomplete releases, and three late complications of the total 21 complications reported.

Merhdad Malek, D. Nagle, and I conducted a survey for complications using the dual-portal Chow technique among the ECTRA Workshop participants from 1993 to 1994 (144–146). A questionnaire was sent to the 844 surgeons who attended these workshop courses from December 1990 to September 1992, and 265 complete responses were received, for a total of 31.4% of the participants. The study was then based on the 265 surgeons, 73% of which were orthopaedic surgeons, with a total 10,246 cases and 9,562 patients. In this series, there was a total of 241 complications reported, or a complication rate of 2.3%. Of these, there were 154 nerve-related complications, for a total of 64% of all the complications. There were 104 of the 154 nerve-related complications that involved ulnar nerve; 89 were cases of ulnar nerve neurapraxia that resolved spontaneously, 12 were lacerations of the ulnar nerve, and three were complete transections of the nerve reported in this group. Median nerve neurapraxia with spontaneous recovery without permanent injury accounted for 21 of the 27 complications involving the median nerve; however, four lacerations and two transections of the median nerve were reported. There were 23 digital nerve complications; 20 of them were neurapraxias, and the remaining three were lacerations or transections of the digital nerve.

There were 38 complications related to blood vessels, 28 of which involved superficial palmar arch lacerations. There were 15 tendon injuries, eight complete and one partial laceration involving the fifth flexor tendon, three involving lacerations to both the fourth and fifth superficial flexor tendons, two lacerations of the fourth superficial flexor tendon only, and one partial laceration of the third superficial flexor tendon. There were 18 incomplete releases reported and six reflex sympathetic dystrophy complications. The remaining ten were listed as miscellaneous complications, including hematoma or superficial wound infection.

DISCUSSION AND HOW TO AVOID PITFALLS

Based on over 13 years of experience using the Chow technique for endoscopic release of the carpal ligament for carpal tunnel syndrome, I believe that it is a safe and reliable alternative for the treatment of carpal tunnel syndrome, but it does have its limitations. Surgeons who are interested in this technique should be aware of the steep learning curve and should realize that many details must be followed to avoid trouble (139–142). Damage to any of the important nerve and vessels in the carpal canal could result in irreversible damage to the patient; therefore, it is my suggestion that the surgeon who is seriously interested in the endoscopic release of the carpal ligament must become familiar with the anatomy, including the normal variances. The surgeon should also be familiar with the procedure itself, including using the proper instrumentation and endoscope. Obviously, the surgeon must be experienced in using a scope and must have proper motor skills.

Visualization is a critical portion of the procedure. If the surgeon's view of the undersurface of the carpal ligament is not adequate, or if it is blocked by anatomic structures, this procedure should not be performed. As I have indicated and strongly emphasized in the past, a blind surgeon is not a good surgeon. If, for any reason, the surgeon is not able to perform the endoscopic technique, the procedure should be abandoned without any feelings of guilt or shame to one's patient. The patient be informed of this possibility when informed consent is obtained before the surgical procedure.

From the experience in teaching cadaver laboratory courses, it has been found that ulnar placement of the entry portal is a very common mistake made by beginners. Therefore, checkpoints have been established to assist the surgeon who is interested in performing this procedure. The first checkpoint is to palpate the ulnar artery to ensure that the pulsations are not just below the incision line before marking the entry portal. Obviously, if the tourniquet is used, this important guideline is lost. The next checkpoint requires looking at the entire width of the wrist to ensure that the entry portal is centrally located. The third checkpoint is to be sure that the landmarks for the entry and exit portals are aligned along the long axis of the forearm. If there is any deviation, the portals should be rechecked before the incision is made. The fourth checkpoint is that the surgeon should palpate the hook of hamate and should mark it on the patient's hand, to ensure that both the entry and exit portals are located radially to the hook of hamate. The last checkpoint is that, during the entire procedure, instruments that are introduced into the wrist and hand should follow the long axis of the forearm.

Although the controversy regarding endoscopic release of the carpal ligament will persist, it took years for the standard carpal ligament release to become an established operative procedure with a decreasing complication rate. I believe that it will take time for the endoscopic release of the carpal ligament for carpal tunnel syndrome to establish its position; however, it does provide the surgeon with an alternative for decompressing the carpal canal.

CONTROVERSIES OF ENDOSCOPIC RELEASE OF THE CARPAL LIGAMENT

Blind Procedure

Obviously, this is the opinion of a surgeon who does not use a scope very often. For the arthroscopist, the scope is actually the eye; therefore, the surgeon is able to visualize the undersurface of the carpal ligament quite well. Actually, the endoscope enlarges the image 30 to 70 times, so the ligament and other anatomic structures can be seen more clearly than even with loupes, because of the higher magnification.

Inability to See the Entire Carpal Canal

In reply to this concern, first the question of whether the entire carpal canal needs to be seen must be answered. If so, endoscopic release of the carpal ligament would be the wrong choice for the patient. For example, if the surgeon believes that a tenosynovectomy needs to be performed for the patient with rheumatoid disease or if the surgeon believes that there may be a space-occupying lesion, the entire canal needs to be fully explored. If the surgeon believes that there is a high incidence of adhesion, some abnormality needs to be corrected, or if a neurolysis needs to be performed for any reason, an open procedure and exploration of the carpal canal are advised.

Increased Cost

Another controversy is the cost of the procedure. Recently, there has been more focus on the issue of cost. I do not believe that the cost of any other procedure has received as much scrutiny as endoscopic release of the carpal ligament in recent years. This cost includes the equipment cost for the high-technology instruments and the cost of the surgeon to learn this procedure, travel, and seminar expenses. However, several articles have indicated a weekly savings of approximately $443.00 per patient because of the shorter recovery period and economic savings in less production loss; therefore, the cost of this procedure is actually decreased and produces a savings in the long run (205–207). With regard to the learning expense for the surgeon, this would apply to all continuing education courses. The bottom line is: "Do you want to learn?"

Technically Demanding Procedure: Risks Outweigh Benefits

Obviously, this procedure is difficult, and it carries a steep learning curve. The procedure does require a certain skill, especially arthroscopic skill, before it can be performed, and, obviously, it is not for everyone. Some surgeons also suggest that it is a dangerous procedure and that the risks outweigh the benefits. I certainly agree that it is a dangerous procedure because of the important structures in the area of the carpal canal. Any injury to these important structures can cause irreversible damage to the patient. However, I believe that, when performed by experienced surgeons who fully understand anatomy, and when local anesthesia is used, it is a safer procedure compared with the open procedure. Because endoscopic release of the carpal ligament allows for visualization from the inside out as opposed to outside in, as in the standard procedure, the surgeon is actually able to see the nerve variance, if any, through the scope before the carpal ligament is released, rather than cutting the carpal ligament without seeing the important structures underneath it. It has been my experience, on several occasions, to have actually saved my patients from irreversible nerve injury because I was performing endoscopic release of the carpal ligament. For example, one of my patients had an ulnar, transligamental motor branch of the median nerve. The exit was so ulnar that, if I had been doing an open procedure, the motor branch could have been injured. Fortunately, I was performing the procedure through the scope; therefore, this extreme ulnar placement of the transligamental motor branch of the median nerve was seen and preserved. In more than 2,700 cases done in Mt. Vernon, Illinois over the past 14 years, similar extreme ulnar placement of the transligamental motor branch of the median nerve has been seen on ten occasions, for a ratio of 1:270 cases. Endoscopic release of the carpal ligament is a straightforward, simple procedure when performed by experienced surgeons. I believe the "risks," which concern some surgeons, involve only the beginner and the learning curve.

Gain of Immediate Benefits Postoperatively

Most surgeons believe that, in regard to the long-term results, the benefits are no different with the endoscopic release as compared with the open procedure. From the data we have so far, the success rate appears to be higher than that of the open procedure. I believe that preserving normal anatomic structure not only improves the results, but also decreases complications. Based on my long-term study (208), it appears that the endoscopic release gives immediate benefits postoperatively, and the long-term results show significant advantages.

CONCLUSION

According to the data gathered from the experience of the past 14 years, it is my belief that the results for the patient of endoscopic carpal ligament release are comparable to those of the standard open procedure for carpal tunnel syndrome. In fact, the data indicate a significant decrease in the incidence of reflex sympathetic dystrophy, bowstringing of the median nerve and flexor tendon, painful scars, pillar pain, and wrist stiffness compared with the standard open procedure. At this time, I believe that the endoscopic carpal tunnel release has already established its position. The obvious advantages are decreased postoperative pain, no loss of pinch-and-grip strength, faster recovery time, and a better success rate than can be achieved with the conventional open procedure for the treatment of carpal tunnel syndrome.

REFERENCES

1. Pfeffer GB, Gelberman RH, Boyes JH, et al. The history of carpal tunnel syndrome. *J Hand Surg Br* 1988;13:28.
2. Paget J. *Lectures on surgical pathology delivered at the Royal College of Surgeons of England,* 2nd US ed. Philadelphia: Lindsay & Blakiston, 1860.
3. Putman JJ. A series of paraesthesia, mainly of the hand, of periodical recurrence, and possibly of vasomotor origin. *Arch Med* 1880;4:147–162.
4. Marie P et Foix C. Atrophie isolée de l'eminence thénar d'origin nervitique: rôle du ligament annulaire antérieur du carpe dans la pathogénie de la lésion. *Rev Neurol* 1913;26:647–649.
5. Learmonth JR. The principle of decompression in the treatment of certain disorders of peripheral nerves. *Surg Clin North Am* 1933;13:905–913.
6. Cannon BW, Love JG. Tardy median palsy: median neuritis, median thenar neuritis amenable to surgery. *Surgery* 1946;20:210–216.
7. Brain WR, Wright AD, Wilkinson M. Spontaneous compression of both median nerves in the carpal tunnel: six cases treated surgically. *Lancet* 1947;5: 277–282.
8. Phalen GS, Gardner W, Lalonde A. Neuropathy of the median nerve due to compression beneath the transverse carpal ligament. *J Bone Joint Surg Am* 1950;32:109–112.
9. Phalen GS. Spontaneous compression of the median nerve at the wrist. *JAMA* 1951;145:1128–1133.
10. Phalen GS, Kendrick J. Compression neuropathy of the medial nerve in the carpal tunnel. *JAMA* 1957;164:524–530.
11. Phalen GS. The carpal tunnel syndrome: seventeen years experience in diagnosis and treatment of six hundred fifty-four hands. *J Bone Joint Surg Am* 1966;48:211–228.
12. Phalen GS. Reflection on 21 years' experience with carpal tunnel syndrome. *JAMA* 1970;212:1365–1367.
13. Phalen GS, Kendick J, Rodriguez J. Lipomas of the upper extremity. *Am J Surg* 1971;121:298–306.
14. Phalen GS. The carpal tunnel syndrome: clinical evaluation of 598 hands. *Clin Orthop* 1972;83:29–40.
15. Phalen GS. The birth of a syndrome, or carpal tunnel revisited. *J Hand Surg Am* 1981:109–110.
16. Mannerfelt L, Hybbinette CH. Important anomaly of the thenar motor branch of the median nerve. *Bull Hosp Jt Dis* 1972; 33:15.
17. Caffee HH. Anomalous thenar muscle and median nerve: a case report. *J Hand Surg* 1979;4:446.
18. Ogden J. An unusual branch of the median nerve. *J Bone Joint Surg Am* 1972;54:1779–1781.
19. Papathanassiou BT. A variant of the motor branch of the median nerve in the hand. *J Bone Joint Surg Br* 1968;50:156.
20. Lanz U. Anatomical variations of the median nerve in the carpal tunnel. *J Hand Surg Am* 1977;2:44.
21. Eiken O, Carsta N, Eddeland A. Anomalous distal branching of the median nerve. *Scand J Plast Reconstr Surg Hand Surg* 1971;5: 149.
22. Johnson RK, Shrewsbury MM. Anatomical course of the thenar branch of the median nerve, usually in a separate tunnel through the transverse carpal ligament. *J Bone Joint Surg Am* 1970;52: 269.
23. Seradge H, Seradge E. Median innervated hypothenar muscle: anomalous branch of median nerve in the carpal tunnel. *J Hand Surg Am* 1990;15:356–359.
24. Tountas CP, Birhle DM, MacDonald CJ, et al. Variations of the median nerve in the carpal canal. *J Hand Surg Am* 1987;12:708–712.
25. Carroll RE, Green DP. The significance of the palmar cutaneous nerve at the wrist. *Clin Orthop* 1972;83:24.
26. Cobb TK, Dalley BK, Posteraro RH, et al. Anatomy of the retinaculum. *J Hand Surg Am* 1977;2:44–53.
27. Chow JCY. Endoscopic carpal tunnel release. In: Whipple T, ed. *Arthroscopy of the wrist.* Philadelphia: JB Lippincott, 1993: 157–169.

28. Lundborg G, Dahlin LB. The pathophysiology of nerve compression. *Hand Clin* 1992;8:215–227.

29. Adamson JE, Srouji SJ, Horton CE, et al. The acute carpal tunnel syndrome. *Plast Reconstr Surg* 1971;47:332.

30. Aghasi MK, Rzetelny V, Axer A. The flexor digitorum superficialis as a cause of bilateral carpal tunnel syndrome and trigger wrist. *J Bone Joint Surg Am* 1980;62:134.

31. Amadio PC. Carpal tunnel syndrome, pyridoxine, and the work place. *J Hand Surg Am* 1987;12:875–880.

32. Badalamente MA, Sampson SP, Hurst LC, et al. Amyloid tenosynovial deposition in idiopathic carpal tunnel syndrome: a histological and ultrastructural study. Presented at the 48th annual meeting of the American Society for Surgery of the Hand, Kansas City, MO, 1993.

33. Barr WG, Blair SJ. Carpal tunnel syndrome as the initial manifestation of scleroderma. *J Hand Surg Am* 1988;13:366.

34. Barton NJ. Another cause of median nerve compression by a lumbrical muscle in the carpal tunnel. *J Hand Surg* 1979;4:189.

35. Bauman TD, Gelberman RH, Mubarak SJ, et al. The acute carpal tunnel syndrome. *Clin Orthop* 1981;156:151.

36. Bell GE Jr, Goldner JL. Compression neuropathy of the median nerve. *South Med J* 1956;49:966.

37. Bennet RM. The Fibrositis-fibromyalgia syndrome. In: Schumacher HR Jr, ed. *Primer on the rheumatic diseases,* 9th ed. Atlanta, GA: Arthritis Foundation, 1988:227–230.

38. Boyle JC, Smith NJ, Burke FD. Vibration white finger. *J Hand Surg Br* 1988;13:171–179.

39. Brown LP, Coulson DB. Triggering at the carpal tunnel with incipient carpal tunnel syndrome: report of an unusual case. *J Bone Joint Surg Am* 1974;56:623.

40. Brown EZ Jr, Snyder CC. Carpal tunnel syndrome caused by hand injuries. *Plast Reconstr Surg* 1975;56:41.

41. Brown FE, Tazer RC. Entrapment neuropathies of the upper extremity. In: Flynn JE, ed. *Hand surgery,* 3rd ed. Baltimore: Williams & Wilkins, 1982.

42. Burnham PJ. Acute carpal tunnel syndrome: median artery thrombosis as cause. *Arch Surg* 1963;87:645.

43. Butler B Jr, Bigley EC Jr. Aberrant index (first) lumbrical tendinous origin associated with carpal tunnel syndrome: a case report. *J Bone Joint Surg Am* 1971;53:160.

44. Heathfield KWG. Acroparaesthesiae and the carpal tunnel syndrome. *Lancet* 1957;2:226.

45. Chaudhuri KR, Davidson AR, Morris IM. Limited joint mobility and carpal tunnel syndrome in insulin-dependent diabetes. *Br J Rheumatol* 1989;28:191–194.

46. Chidgey L, Szabo R, Wiese D. Acute carpal tunnel syndrome caused by pigmented villondular synovitis of the wrist. *Clin Orthop* 1988;288:254–257.

47. Conklin JE, White WL. Stenosing tenosynovitis and its possible relation to carpal tunnel syndrome. *Surg Clin North Am* 1960;40:531.

48. Corradi M, Paganelli E, Pavesi G. Carpal tunnel syndrome in long-term hemodialyzed patients. *J Reconstr Microsurg* 1989;5:103–110.

49. De Abreau LB, Moreira RG. Median nerve compression at the wrist. *J Bone Joint Surg Am* 1958;40:1426.

50. Dellon AL. Clinical use of vibratory stimuli to evaluate peripheral nerve injury and compression neuropathy. *Plast Reconstr Surg* 1980;65:466.

51. DeLuca FN, Cowen NJ. Median nerve compression complicating a tendon graft prosthesis. *J Bone Joint Surg Am* 1975;57:533.

52. Entin MA. Carpal tunnel syndrome and its variants. *Surg Clin North Am* 1968;48:1097.

53. Evangelisti S, Reale V. Fibroma of tendon sheath as a cause of carpal tunnel syndrome. *J Hand Surg Am* 1992;17:1026–1027.

54. Eversmann WW Jr. Entrapment and compression neuropathies. In: Green DP, ed. *Operative hand surgery,* 3rd ed. New York: Churchill Livingstone, 1993:1346–1356.

55. Frymore JW, Bland J. Carpal tunnel syndrome in patients with myxedematous arthropathy. *J Bone Joint Surg Am* 1973;55:78.

56. Gama C, Franc CM. Nerve compression by pacinian corpuscles. *J Hand Surg* 1980;5:207.

57. Gellman H, Sie I, Waters RL. Late Complications of the weight bearing upper extremity in the paraplegic patient. *Clin Orthop* 1988;233:132–135.

58. Gilbert MS. Carpal tunnel syndrome in patients who are receiving long-term renal hemodialysis. *J Bone Joint Surg Am* 1988;70:1145–1153.

59. Golik A, Modai D, Pervin R, et al. Autosomal dominant carpal tunnel syndrome in a Karaite family. *Isr J Med Sci* 1988;24:295–297.

60. Hadler NM, Bunn WB. Work-related disorders of the upper extremity. *Occup Probl Med Pract* 1989;4:1–8.

61. Halperin JJ, Volkman DJ, Luft BJ, et al. Carpal tunnel syndrome in Lyme borreliosis. *Muscle Nerve* 1989;12:397–400.

62. Hecht O, Lipsker E. Median and ulnar nerve entrapment caused by ectopic calcification: report of two cases. *J Hand Surg* 1980;5:30.

63. Hunter JM. Recurrent carpal tunnel syndrome, epineural fibrous fixation, and traction neuropathy. *Hand Clin* 1991;7:491–504.

64. Jabaley ME. Personal observation on the role of the lumbrical muscles in carpal tunnel syndrome. *J Hand Surg* 1978;3:82.

65. Jackson IT, Campbell JC. An unusual cause of the carpal tunnel syndrome: a case of thrombosis of the median artery. *J Bone Joint Surg Br* 1970;52:330.

66. Kerr DC, Sybert DR, Albarracin NS. An analysis of the flexor synovium in idiopathic carpal tunnel syndrome: report of 625 cases. *J Hand Surg Am* 1992;17:1028–1030.

67. Kerrigan JJ, Bertoni JM, Jaeger SH. Ganglion cysts and carpal tunnel syndrome. *J Hand Surg Am* 1988;13:763.

68. Koris M, Gelberman RH, Duncan K, et al. Carpal tunnel syndrome: evaluation of a quantitative provocational diagnosis of dynamic carpal tunnel syndrome. *J Hand Surg Am* 1989;14:195–197.

69. Kremchek TE, Kremchek EJ. Carpal tunnel syndrome cause by flexor tendon sheath lipoma. *Orthop Rev* 1988;17:1083.

70. Kyle RA, Eilers SG, Linscheid RL, et al. Amyloid localized to tenosynovium at carpal tunnel release: natural history of 124 cases. *Am J Clin Pathol* 1989:393–397.

71. Linscheid RL. Carpal tunnel syndrome secondary to ulnar bursa distention from the intercarpal joint: report of a case. *J Hand Surg* 1979;4:191.

72. Lipscomb PR. Tenosynovitis of the hand and the wrist: carpal tunnel syndrome, de Quervain's disease, trigger digit. *Clin Orthop* 1959;13:164.

73. Loebe M, Heidrich H. The carpal tunnel syndrome: a disease underlying Raynaud's phenomenon? *Angiology* 1988;39:894–901.

74. Louis DS. Evaluation and treatment of median neuropathy associated with cumulative trauma. In: Gelberman RH, ed. *Operative nerve repair and reconstruction,* vol 2. Philadelphia: JB Lippincott, 1991:957–961.

75. Luchetti R, Mingione A, Monteleone M, et al. Carpal tunnel syndrome in Madelung's deformity. *J Hand Surg Br* 1988;13:19–22.

76. Lynch AC, Lipscomb PR. The Carpal Tunnel Syndrome and Colles's Fractures. *JAMA* 1963;185:363.

77. MacDougal B, Weeks PM, Wray RC Jr. Median Nerve Compression and Trigger Finger in the Mucopolysacchridoses and Related Diseases. *Plast Reconstr Surg* 1977;59:260.

78. Maeser VR, Hayes JM, Hyde AG An Industrial Case of Carpal Tunnel Syndrome. *J Hand Surg Am* 1986;11:222–227.

79. Mangini U. Some remarks on the etiology of the carpal tunnel compression of the median nerve. *Bull Hosp Jt Dis* 1961;63A:836.

80. Millender LH. Occupational disorders—the disease of the 1990's: a challange or a bane for hand surgeons [Editorial]. *J Hand Surg Am* 1992;17:193–194.

81. Millender LH. Occupational disorders in the upper extremity: orthopaedic psychosocial, and legal implications. In: Millender LH, Louis D, Simmons B, eds. *Occupational disorders of the upper extremity.* New York: Churchill Livingstone, 1992:1–4.

82. Oglivie C. Fulminating carpal tunnel syndrome due to gout. *J Hand Surg Br* 1988;13;42–43.

83. Omer GE. Median nerve compression at the wrist. *Hand Clin* 1992;8:317–324.

84. Orcutt SA, Kramer WG III, Howard MW, et al. Carpal tunnel syndrome secondary to wrist and finger flexor spasticity. *J Hand Surg Am* 1990;15:940.

85. Pecket P, Gloobe H, Nathan H. Variations in the arteries of the median nerve: with special considerations on the ischemic factor in the carpal tunnel syndrome (CTS). *Clin Orthop* 1973;97:144.

86. Prince H, Ispahani P, Baker MA. *Mycobacterium malmoense* infection of the hand presenting as carpal tunnel syndrome. *J Hand Surg* 1988;13:328–330.

87. Rubinstein MA. Carpal tunnel syndrome in lymphatic leukemia. *JAMA* 1970;213:1037.

88. Scelsi R, Zaniungo M, Tenti P. Carpal tunnel syndrome: anatomical and clinical correlations and morphological and ultrastrutural aspects of the tenosynovial sheath. *Ital J Orthop Trauma* 1989;15:75–81.

89. Schenck RR. Carpal tunnel syndrome: the new industrial epidemic. *Am Acad Occup Hlth Nurse J* 1989;37:226–231.

90. Schuind F, Ventura M, Pasteels JL. Idiopathic carpal tunnel syndrome: histologic study of flexor tendon synovium. *J Hand Surg Am* 1990;15:497.

91. Smith RJ. Anamolous muscle belly of the flexor digitorum superficialis causing carpal tunnel syndrome. *J Bone Joint Surg Am* 1971;53:1212.

92. Schultz RJ, Endler PM, Huddleston HD. Anomalous median nerve and an anomalous muscle belly of the first lumbrical associated with carpal tunnel syndrome: case report. *J Bone Joint Surg Am* 1973:55:1744.

93. Stein AH Jr. The relation of median nerve compresion to Sudeck's syndrome. *Surg Gynecol Obstet* 1962;115:713.

94. Suso S, Peidro L, Ramon R. Tuberculous synovitis with rice bodies presenting as carpal tunnel syndrome. *J Hand Surg Am* 1988;13:574–576.

95. Szabo DM, Steinberg DR. Nerve entrapment syndrome of the wrist. *J Am Acad Orthop Surg* 1994;2:115–123.

96. Tanzer RC. The carpal tunnel syndrome. *Clin Orthop* 1959;15:171–179.

97. Ullian ME, Hammond WS, Alfrey AC, et al. Beta-2-microglobulin–associated amyloidosis in chronic hemodialysis patients with carpal tunnel syndrome. *Medicine (Baltimore)* 1989;68:1, 7, 15.

98. Walton S, Cutler CR. Carpal tunnel syndrome: case report of unusual etiology. *Clin Orthop* 1971;74:138.

99. Weiss A, Steichen J. Synovial sarcoma causing carpal tunnel syndrome. *J Hand Surg Am* 1992;17:1024–1025.

100. Widder S, Shons AR. Carpal tunnel syndrome associated with extra tunnel vascular compression of the median nerve motor branch. *J Hand Surg Am* 1988;13:926–927.

101. Wieslander G, Norback D, Gothe CJ, et al. Carpal tunnel syndrome (CTS) and exposure to vibration, repetitive, wrist movements, and heavy manual work: a case-referent study. *Br J Ind Med* 1989;46:43–47.

102. Tompkins DG. Median neuropathy in the carpal tunnel caused by tumor-like conditions: report of the two cases. *J Bone Joint Surg Am* 1967;49:737.

103. Braun RM, Davidson K, Doehr S. Provocative testing in the diagnosis of dynamic carpal tunnel syndrome. *J Hand Surg Am* 1989:14:195–197.

104. Berman AT, Straub RR. Importance of preoperative and postoperative electrodiagnostic studies in the treatment of carpal tunnel syndrome. *Orthop Rev* 1974;3:57.

105. Grundberg AB. Carpal tunnel decompression in spite of normal electromyography. *J Hand Surg Am* 1983;8:348–349.

106. Shivde AG, Dreizin I, Fisher MA. The carpal tunnel syndrome: a clinical electrodiagnostic analysis. *Electromyogr Clin Neurophysiol* 1981;21:143.

107. Jackson DA, Clifford JC. Electrodiagnosis of mild carpal tunnel syndrome. *Arch Phys Med Rehabil* 1989;71:199–204.

108. Cioni R, Passero S, Paradiso C, et al. Diagnostic specificity of sensory and motor nerve conduction variables in early detection of carpal tunnel syndrome. *J Neurol* 1989:236:208–213.

109. Carroll RE, Hurst LC. The relationship of the thoracic outlet syndrome and carpal tunnel syndrome. *Clin Orthop* 1982;164:149.

110. Osterman AL. Double crush and multiple compression neuropathy. In: Gelberman RH, ed. *Operative nerve repair and reconstruction,* vol 2. Philadelphia: JB Lippincott, 1991:1211–1229.

111. Wood VE, Biondi J, Linda L. Double-crush nerve compression in thoracic-outlet syndrome. *J Bone Joint Surg Am* 1990;72:85–87.

112. Jones NF, Ming NL. Persistent median artery as a cause of pronator syndrome. *J Hand Surg Am* 1988;13:728–732.

113. Dellon AL, Fine IT. A noninvasive technique for diagnosis of chronic compartment syndrome in the first dorsal interosseous muscle. *J Hand Surg Am* 1990;15:1008.

114. Duran JA. A new diagnostic test for carpal tunnel syndrome. *J Bone Joint Surg Am* 1991;73:535.

115. Molitor PJ. A diagnostic test for carpal tunnel syndrome using ultrasound. *J Hand Surg Br* 1988;13:40–41.

116. Murphy RX, Chernofsky MA, Osborne MA, et al. Magnetic resonance imaging in the evaluation of persistent carpal tunnel syndrome. *J Hand Surg Am* 1993;18:113–120.

117. Mesgarzadeh M, Schneck CD, Bonakdarpour A, et al. Carpal tunnel—MRI: part II. Carpal tunnel syndrome. *Radiology* 1989;171:749–754.

118. Szabo RM, Gelberman RH, Dimick MP. Sensibility testing in patients with carpal tunnel syndrome. *J Bone Joint Surg Am* 1984;66:60–64.

119. Richman JG, Gelberman RH, Rydevik B, et al. Carpal tunnel volume determination by magnetic imaging 3-D reconstruction. *J Hand Surg Am* 1987;12:712.

120. Gelberman RH, Aronson D, Weisman MH. Carpal tunnel syndrome: results of a prospective trial of steroid injection and splinting. *J Hand Surg Am* 1992;17:1003–1008.

121. Gelberman RH, Rydevik BL, Pess GM, et al. Carpal tunnel syndrome: a scientific basis for clinical care. *Orthop Clin North Am* 1988;19:115–124.

122. Wood MR. Hydrocortisone injections for carpal tunnel syndrome. *Hand* 1980;12:62.

123. Stransky M, Rubin A, Lavaa NS, et al. Treatment of carpal tunnel syndrome with vitamin B$_6$: a double-blind study. *South Med J* 1989;82:841–842.

124. Weiss AC, Sachar K, Gendreau M. Conservative management of carpal tunnel syndrome: a re-examination of steroid injection and splinting. *J Hand Surg Am* 1994;19:410–415.

125. Heckler FR, Jabaley ME. Evolving concepts of median nerve decompression in the carpal tunnel. *Hand Clin* 1986;2:723–735.

126. Jakab E, Ganos D, Cook FW. Transverse carpal ligament reconstruction in surgery for carpal tunnel syndrome: a new technique. *J Hand Surg Am* 1991;16:202–206.

127. Lowery WE, Follender AB. Interfascicular neurolysis in severe carpal tunnel syndrome: a prospective, randomized, double-blind, controlled study. *Clin Orthop* 1988;227:251.

128. Mackinnon SE, McCabe S, Murray JF, et al. Internal neurolysis fails to improve the results of primary carpal tunnel decompression. *J Hand Surg Am* 1991;16:211–218.

129. Nissenbaum M, Kleinert HE. Treatment considerations in carpal tunnel syndrome with coexistent Dupuytren's disease. *J Hand Surg* 1980;5:544.

130. O'Malley MJ, Evanoff M, Terrono AK, et al. Factors that determine re-exploration treatment if carpal tunnel syndrome. *J Hand Surg Am* 1992;17:638–641.

131. Rowland SA. A palmar incision for release of the carpal tunnel. *Clin Orthop* 1974;103:89.

132. Freshwater MF, Arons MS. The effect of various adjuncts on the surgical treatment of carpal tunnel syndrome secondary to chronic synovitis. *Plast Reconstr Surg* 1978;61:93.

133. Taleisnik J. The palmar cutaneous branch of the median nerve and the approach to the carpal tunnel. *J Bone Joint Surg Am* 1973;55:1212–1217.

134. Gelberman RH, Pfeffer GB, Galbraith RT, et al. Results of treatment of severe carpal tunnel syndrome without internal neurolysis of the median nerve. *J Bone Joint Surg Am* 1987;69:896.

135. Garland H, Sumner D, Clark JMP. Carpal tunnel syndrome: with particular reference to surgical treatment. *BMJ* 1963;1:581.

136. Clayton M, Linscheid R. Carpal tunnel surgery: should the incision be above or below the wrist? *Orthopedics* 1988: 2:819–821.

137. Curtis RM, Eversmann WW Jr. Internal neurolysis as an adjunct to the treatment of the carpal tunnel syndrome. *J Bone Joint Surg Am* 1973;55:733.

138. Wright PE II, Milford LW. Carpal tunnel and ulnar tunnel syndromes and stenosing tenosynovitis. In: Crenshaw AH, ed. *Campbell's operative orthopaedics.* St Louis: CV Mosby, 1976: 3435–3438.

139. Levy HJ, Spofer TB, Kleinbart FA, et al. Endoscopic carpal tunnel release: an anatomic study. *Arthroscopy* 1993;9:1–4.

140. Rotman MB, Manske PR. Anatomical relationships of an endoscopic carpal tunnel device to surrounding structures: Joseph A. Boyes award paper. Presented at the 47th annual meeting of the American Society for Surgery of the Hand, Orlando, FL, 1991.

141. Seiler J III, Barnes K, Gelberman RH, et al. Endoscopic carpal tunnel release: an anatomic study of the two-incision method in human cadavers. *J Hand Surg Am* 1992;17:996–1002.

142. Schwartz TJ, Waters PM, Simmons BP. Endoscopic carpal tunnel release: a cadaveric study. *Arthroscopy* 1993;9:209–213.

143. Luallian SR, Toby EB. Incidental Guyon's canal release during attempted endoscopic carpal tunnel release: an anatomical study and report of two cases. *Arthroscopy* 1993;9:382–386.

144. Malek MM, Chow JCY. National study of the complications of over 10,000 cases of endoscopic carpal tunnel release. Presented at the 61st annual meeting of the American Academy of Orthopaedic Surgeons, New Orleans, LA, 1994.

145. Chow JCY, Malek MM. Complications of endoscopic release of the carpal ligament using the Chow technique. Presented at the AAOS 60th Annual Meeting of the American Academy of Orthopaedic Surgeons, San Francisco, CA, 1993.

146. Chow JCY, Malek M, Nagle D. Complications of endoscopic release of the carpal ligament using the Chow technique. Presented at the 4th annual meeting of the American Society for Surgery of the Hand, Phoenix, AZ, 1992.

147. Chow JCY. Endoscopic release of the carpal ligament: a new technique for carpal tunnel syndrome. *Arthroscopy* 1989;5:19–24.

148. Chow JCY. Endoscopic carpal tunnel release: clinical results of 149 cases. Presented at the 9th annual meeting of the Arthroscopy Association of North America, Orlando, FL, 1990.

149. Chow JCY. Endoscopic release of the carpal ligament: 22-month clinical results. *Arthroscopy* 1990;6:388–396.

150. Chow JCY. Endoscopic release of the carpal ligament: analysis of the 300 cases. Presented at the 58th annual meeting of the American Academy of Orthopaedic Surgeons, Anaheim, CA, 1991.

151. Chow JCY. The Chow technique of endoscopic release of the carpal ligament for carpal tunnel syndrome: 4 years of clinical results. *Arthroscopy* 1993;9:301–314.

152. Okutsu I, Nonomiya S, Takatori Y, et al. Endoscopic management of carpal tunnel syndrome. *Arthroscopy* 1989;5:11.

153. Agee JM, Tortsua RD, Palmer CA, et al. Endoscopic release of the carpal tunnel: a prospective randomized multicenter study. Presented at the 45th annual meeting of the American Society for Surgery of the Hand, Toronto, Canada, 1990.

154. Agee JM, McCarroll HR Jr, Tortosa RD, et al. Endoscopic release of the carpal tunnel: a ramdomized prospective multicenter study. *J Hand Surg Am* 1992;17:987–995.

155. Orr T. Endoscopic carpal tunnel release. Presented at the 22nd annual meeting of the American Society for Surgery of the Hand, Washington, DC, 1992.

156. Menon J. Endoscopic carpal tunnel release: a preliminary report. *Arthroscopy* 1994;10:31–38.

157. Mirza MA, King ET, Tanveer S. Palmar uniportal extrabursal endoscopic carpal tunnel release. *Arthroscopy* 1995;11:82–90.

158. Lewicky R. Endoscopic carpal tunnel release: the guide tube technique. *Arthroscopy* 1994;10:39–49.

159. Nagle DJ, Fischer T, Hastings H, et al. A multicenter prospective study of 641 endoscopic carpal tunnel releases using the Chow extrabursal technique. Presented at the 47th annual meeting of the American Society for Surgery of the Hand, Phoenix, AZ, November, 1992.

160. Nagle D, Fischer T, Harris G, et al. A multi-center prospective review of 640 endoscopic carpal tunnel releases using the Chow technique. *Arthroscopy* 1996;12:139–143.

161. Kessler I. Unusual distribution of the median nerve at the wrist. *Clin Orthop* 1969;67:124–126.

162. Kleinert J. The nerve of Henle. *J Hand Surg Am* 1990;15:784.

163. Shimizu K, Iwasaki R, Hoshikawa H, et al. Entrapment neuropathy of the palmer cutaneous branch of the median nerve by the fascia of flexor digitorum superficialis. *J Hand Surg Am* 1988;13:581–583.

164. Enger WD, Gmeiner JG. Palmar cutaneous branch of the ulnar nerve. *J Hand Surg* 1980;5:26.

165. Ritter MA. The anatomy and function of the palmar fascia. *Hand* 1973;5:263–267.

166. Shrewsbury MM, Johnson RK, Ousterhout DK. The palmaris brevis: a reconsideration of its anatomy and possible function. *J Bone Joint Surg Am* 1972;54:344–348.

167. Viegas S, Pollard A, Kaminksi K. Carpal arch alteration and related clinical status after endoscopic carpal tunnel release. *J Hand Surg Am* 1992;17:1012–1016.

168. Garcia-Elias M, Sanches-Freijo J, Salo J, et al. Dynamic changes of the transverse carpal arch during flexion-extension of the wrist: effects of sectioning the transverse carpal ligament. *J Hand Surg Am* 1992;17:1017–1019.

169. Richman JA, Gelberman RH, Rydevik BL, et al. Carpal tunnel syndrome: morphologic changes after release of transverse carpal ligament. *J Hand Surg Am* 1989;14:852–857.

170. Seradge H, Seradge E. Piso-triquetral pain syndrome after carpal tunnel release. *J Hand Surg Am* 1989;14:858–862.

171. Rhoades CE, Gelberman RH, Szabo RM, et al. The results of carpal tunnel release with and without internal neurolysis of the median nerve for severe and carpal tunnel release. *J Hand Surg* 1986;11:448.

172. Conolly WB. Ptifalls in carpal tunnel decompression. *Aust NZ J Surg* 1978;48:421–425.

173. Gellman H, Chandleer D, Petrasek J, et al. Carpal tunnel syndrome in paraplegic patients. *J Bone Joint Surg Am* 1988;70:517–519.

174. Hybbinette CH, Mannerfelt L. The carpal tunnel syndrome: a retrospective study of 400 operated patients. *Acta Orthop* 1975;46:610–205.

175. Gainer JV Jr, Nugent GR. Carpal tunnel syndrome: report of 430 operations. *South Med J* 1977;70:325–328.

176. Doyle JR, Carroll RE. the carpal tunnel syndrome: a review of 100 patients treated surgically. *Calif Med* 1968;108:263–267.

177. Harris CM, Tanner E, Goldstein MN, et al. The surgical treatment of carpal tunnel syndrome correletaed with preoperative nerve conduction studies. *J Bone Joint Surg Am* 1979;61:93–98.

178. Semple JC, Cargill AO. Carpal tunnel syndrome: results of surgical decompression. *Lancet* 1969;327:243–224.

179. Kulick MI, Gordillo G, Javidi T, et al. Long term analysis of patients having surgical treatment for carpal tunnel syndrome. *J Hand Surg Am* 1986;11:59–66.

180. Clayburgh RH, Beckenbaugh RD. Carpal tunnel release in patients with diffused peripheral neuropathy. *J Hand Surg Am* 1987;12:380–383.

181. Yu GX, Firrell JC, Tsai TM. Preopertive factors treatment outcome following carpal tunnel release. *J Hand Surg Br* 1992;17:646–650.

182. Nolan W III, Alkaitis D, Glickel S, et al. Results of treatment of severe carpal tunnel syndrome. *J Hand Surg Am* 1992;17:1020–1023.

183. Posch HL, Marcotte DR. Carpal tunnel syndrome: an analysis of 1201 cases. *Orthop Rev* 1976;5:25.

184. Gellman H, Kan D, Gee V, et al. Analysis of pinch and grip strength after carpal tunnel release. *J Hand Surg Am* 1989;14:863–864.

185. Duncan KH, Lewis RC, Foreman KA, et al. Treatment of carpal tunnel syndrome by members of the American Society for Surgery of the Hand: results of a questionnaire. *J Hand Surg Am* 1987;12:384–391.

186. Hansen AD, Amadio PC, DeSilva SP, et al. Deep postoperative wound infection after carpal tunnel release. *J Hand Surg Am* 1989;14:869–873.

187. Louis DS, Green TL, Noellert RC. Complications of carpal tunnel surgery. *J Neurol* 1985;62:352–335.

188. Langloh NC, Linscheid RL. Recurrent and unrelieved carpal tunnel syndrome. *Clin Orthop* 1972;83:41.

189. Lichtman DM, Rlorio R, Mack GR. Carpal tunnel release under local anesthesia: evaluation of the outpatient procedure. *J Hand Surg* 1979;4:544–546.

190. Das SK, Brown HG. In search of complications in carpal tunnel decompression. *Hand* 1976;8:243–249.

191. Fissette H, Onkelix A. Treatment of carpal tunnel syndrome: comparative study with and without epineurolysis. *Hand* 1979;11:206–210.

192. Gartsman GM, Kovach JC, Crouch CC, et al. Carpal arch alteration after carpal tunnel release. *J Hand Surg Am* 1986;11:372–374.

193. Downie AW. Misery in the hand: the carpal tunnel syndrome. *NC Med J* 1965;26:487–493.

194. Kessler FB. Complications of the management of carpal tunnel syndrome. *Hand Clin* 1986;2:401–406.

195. Cseuz KA, Thomas JE, Lambert EH, et al. Long term results of operation for carpal tunnel syndrome. *Mayo Clin Proc* 1966;41:232–241.

196. Lilly CJ, Magnell TD. Severance of the thenar branch of the median nerve as a complication of carpal tunnel release. *J Hand Surg Am* 1985;10:399–402.

197. MacDonald RI, Lictman DM, Hanlon JJ, et al. Complications of surgical release for carpal tunnel syndrome. *J Hand Surg* 1978;3:70–76.

198. Kuschner SH, Brien WW, Johnson D, et al. Complications associated with carpal tunnel release. *Orthop Rev* 1991;20:346–352.

199. Inglis AE. Two unusual operative complicatoins in the carpal tunnel syndrome. *J Bone Joint Surg Am* 1980;62:1208–1209.

200. Wood VE. Nerve compression following oppoensplasty as a result of wrist anomalies: report of a case. *J Hand Surg* 1980;5:279.

201. Terrino AL, Belskey MR, Feldon PG, et al. Injury to the deep motor branch of the ulnar nerve during carpal tunnel release. *J Hand Surg Am* 1993;18:1038–1040.

202. McCormack RM. Carpal tunnel syndrome. *Surg Clin North Am* 1960;40:517.

203. May JW, Rosen H. Division of the sensory ramus communicans between the ulnar median nerves: a complication following carpal tunnel release. *J Bone Joint Surg Am* 1981;63:836.

204. Ariyan S, Watson K. Palmar approach for the visualization and release of the carpal tunnel. An analysis of 429 cases. *Plast Reconstr Surg* 1977;60:539–547.

205. Brown RA, Gelberman RH, Seiler JG III, et al. Carpal tunnel release: a prospective, randomized assessment of open and endoscopic methods. *J Bone Joint Surg Am* 1993;75:1265–1275.

206. Palmar DH, Paulson JC, Lane-Larsen CL, et al. endoscopic carpal tunnel release: a comparison of two techniques with open release. *Arthroscopy* 1993;9:498–296.

207. Adams BD. Endoscopic carpal tunnel release. *J Am Acad Orthop Surg* 1994:2:179–184.

208. Chow JCY. Long term follow up of endoscopic release of the carpal ligament using the dual portal Chow technique. *Arthroscopy* 1999;15:417–421.

THE HIP

ARTHROSCOPY OF THE HIP— OVERVIEW: ASSESSMENT, IMAGING, INDICATIONS, CONTRAINDICATIONS, AND COMPLICATIONS

J. W. THOMAS BYRD

Arthroscopic surgery of the hip has followed a distinctly different evolutionary road than arthroscopic surgery of the knee. Knee arthroscopy evolved from traditional open methods to less invasive arthroscopic techniques. In contrast, many of the disorders that we currently address with arthroscopic surgery in the hip previously went unrecognized and untreated. Historically, arthrotomy of the hip was not a routine procedure, except for disorders of serious magnitude such as total hip arthroplasty for advanced degenerative disease, osteotomy for severe dysplasia, debridement for sepsis, and removal of bone fragments. Imaging methods could discern only the most obvious forms of disease. Current investigative studies have greater reliability in assessing intraarticular disorders of the hip. However, much of the impetus for discerning these lesions has been prompted by arthroscopic observation of both the type and the prevalence of their existence. Thus, our technical skills for performing hip arthroscopy continue to develop at the same time that we are trying to understand the normal arthroscopic anatomy, normal variants, and the morphology and etiology of intraarticular lesions.

In addition, the hip receives considerably less attention than other joints, especially in reference to sports injuries. Perhaps this joint is less vulnerable to injury. More likely, in the past we were less skilled at assessing these types of intraarticular problems and had few methods available to treat them. Arthroscopy has greatly expanded our knowledge of intraarticular disorders of the hip and now provides an effective means for addressing many of these problems.

Arthroscopy offers a less invasive alternative to arthrotomy for traditionally recognized forms of hip disease such as loose bodies or impinging osteophytes. Perhaps more important, arthroscopy offers a method of treatment for many conditions that previously went undiagnosed. In the past, these patients were simply resigned to living within the constraints of their symptoms.

ASSESSMENT

Clinical assessment, including the history and examination, focuses on whether the problem is intraarticular and thus potentially amenable to arthroscopic intervention (1). This discussion highlights the most salient features of the evaluation.

When one questions a patient regarding the onset of symptoms, it is important to determine whether there was a specific traumatic event. In general, problems resulting from significant trauma are more likely potentially to benefit from arthroscopy. When the onset of symptoms is insidious and gradual, or when it results from a seemingly minor precipitating episode, the response to arthroscopy is sometimes less predictable. This is because, in absence of a major injury, there is often some underlying predisposition or degenerative process that is less likely to be completely reversed by arthroscopy. These patients may still respond favorably, but this prospect should be kept in mind when one counsels patients on the potential benefits of arthroscopy.

Similarly, patients with mechanical symptoms such as catching, locking, or sharp stabbing are more likely to have a potentially correctable problem. Patients who simply have pain with activity or, worse yet, aching independent of activity are much less likely to respond favorably to arthroscopic intervention.

Daily activities that characteristically exacerbate hip joint disorders are outlined in Table 56.1. Twisting, such as when changing directions while bearing weight on the affected

J. W. T. Byrd: Nashville Sports Medicine & Orthopaedic Center, Department of Orthopaedics and Rehabilitation, Vanderbilt University School of Medicine, Nashville, Tennessee.

TABLE 56.1 CHARACTERISTIC HIP SYMPTOMS

Groin, anterior, and medial thigh pain	Pain when entering or exiting and automobile
Pain with ambulation	Difficulty with shoes, socks, or hose
Discomfort sitting with hip flexed	
Pain or catching on rising from the seated position	

leg, may cause pain, especially when turning toward the affected side, which effectively causes the hip to rotate internally. Sitting upright with the hip flexed may be uncomfortable, and patients often tend to slouch, listing away from the affected hip and keeping the leg slightly externally rotated. Rising from the seated position may often produce a painful catch. Ascending and descending stairs are usually more difficult than walking on level surfaces. Typically, when patients describe difficulty in getting their shoes and socks on and off, this suggests that they have developed restricted rotational motion.

The hip receives innervation from branches of L-2 to S-1 of the lumbosacral plexus, but its principal innervation is the L-3 nerve root. This explains why hip joint disease usually results in anterior groin pain and pain radiating to the medial thigh, which follows the L-3 dermatome distribution (Fig. 56.1). Posterior pain is rarely indicative of hip joint disease. Even posterior intraarticular lesions refer pain anteriorly or anterolaterally. Rarely, a joint problem causes posterior pain, and, if necessary, it can be substantiated if temporary relief is achieved by a fluoroscopically guided intraarticular injection of anesthetic.

The *C sign* is very characteristic of hip joint disease. The patient grips the hand above the greater trochanter with the thumb over the posterior aspect of the trochanter and cups the fingers into the groin (Fig. 56.2). The initial impression may be that these patients are describing lateral pain such as from the iliotibial band or trochanteric bursitis, but they are clearly demonstrating deep interior pain from the joint. One should remember this when assessing patients with hip disease.

Log rolling of the hip is the most specific test for intraarticular disease (Fig. 56.3). It rotates only the femoral head in relation to the acetabulum and capsule.

Other more sensitive maneuvers include forced flexion combined with internal rotation or abduction with external rotation (Fig. 56.4). These forceful maneuvers may normally cause some discomfort, so it is important to compare results with the uninvolved hip. In addition, with these maneuvers, a sense of catching or sharp pain may be elicited or perhaps even a click. This is somewhat analogous to McMurray's testing in the knee. Although a click may occasionally be found, mostly it is the reproduction of sharp pain that indicates disease.

Intraarticular lesions can usually be readily differentiated from external causes of "snapping hip." The iliopsoas tendon is the one most easily confused with a joint problem because the symptoms are situated deep within the anterior groin. It may produce a pronounced audible clunk that is characteristic and reproducible as the hip is brought from a flexed, abducted, externally rotated position into extension with internal rotation (Fig. 56.5). This occurs because the iliopsoas tendon transiently lodges against the anterior capsule or pectineal eminence. If necessary, snapping resulting from the iliopsoas tendon can be confirmed by iliopsoas bursography and then by fluoroscopically viewing the tendon flipping back and forth (Fig. 56.6).

Snapping of the iliotibial band is principally the result of the tensor fasciae latae flipping across the greater trochanter. The symptoms are located laterally, and the phenomenon is both visible and palpable. Patients can often stand and voluntarily demonstrate this snapping, which may have the visual appearance of subluxation of the hip, but this is rarely the case.

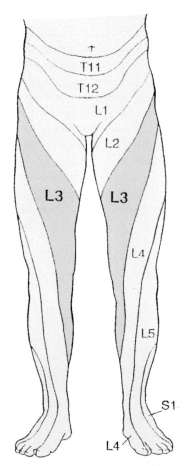

FIGURE 56.1 The L-3 dermatome crosses the anterior thigh and extends distally along the medial thigh to the level of the knee. (From Byrd JWT. Investigation of the symptomatic hip: physical examination. In: Byrd JWT, ed. *Operative hip arthroscopy.* New York: Thieme, 1998:25–41, with permission.)

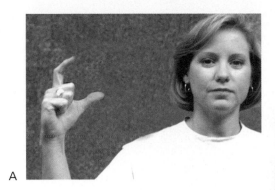

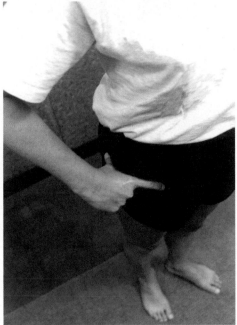

FIGURE 56.2 The C sign. **A:** Describing deep anterior hip pain, the patient cups the hand above the greater trochanter. **B:** The thumb rests over the posterior aspect of the trochanter while the fingers grip into the anterior groin.

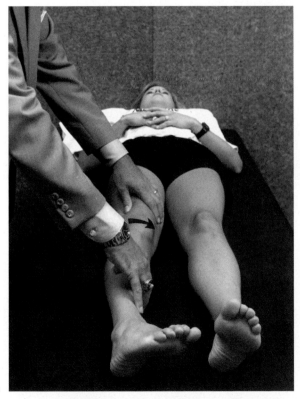

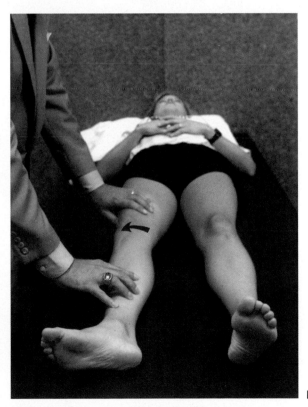

FIGURE 56.3 The log roll test is the most specific test for hip disease. Gently rolling the thigh internally **(A)** and externally **(B)** moves the articular surface of the femoral head in relation to the acetabulum but does not stress any of the surrounding extraarticular structures.

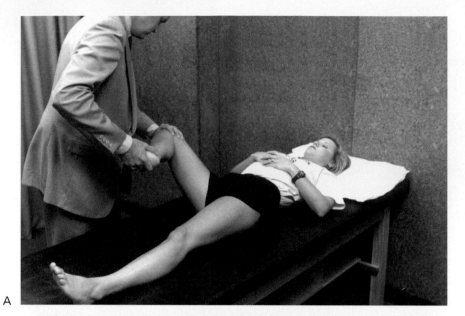

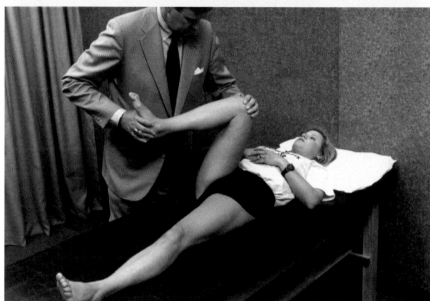

FIGURE 56.4 A: Forced flexion combined with internal rotation is often very uncomfortable and usually elicits symptoms associated with even subtle degrees of hip disease. **B:** Flexion combined with abduction and external rotation similarly is often uncomfortable and may reproduce catching-type sensations associated with labral or chondral lesions.

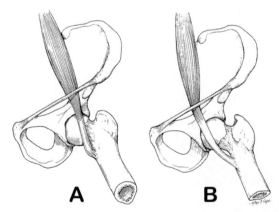

FIGURE 56.5 As the hip is brought from a flexed, abducted, externally rotated position **(A)** into extension with internal rotation **(B)**, the iliopsoas tendon transiently lodges against the anterior femoral head and capsule or pectineal eminence and creates the audible and palpable clunk. (From Allen WC, Cope R. Coxa saltans: the snapping hip revisited. *J Am Acad Orthop Surg* 1995:3;303–308, with permission.)

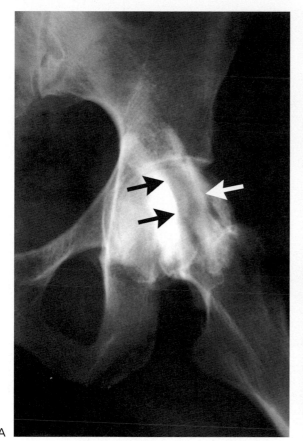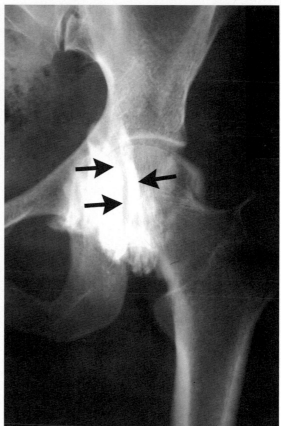

FIGURE 56.6 Iliopsoas bursography silhouettes the tendon *(arrows)* and allows visual confirmation of the snapping of the tendon as it is brought from flexion abduction and external rotation **(A)** into extension with internal rotation **(B)**.

IMAGING

Radiographs

Radiographs are an integral part of the assessment of a painful hip. Standard views consist of an anteroposterior pelvis view including both hips and a frog lateral view of the affected hip (Fig. 56.7). One should not embark on a treatment plan with an anteroposterior radiograph of only one hip. There are often subtle variations that can be interpreted only by comparing the image with that of the uninvolved side. Additionally, the view of the pelvis allows assessment of surrounding areas including the ilium, ischium, pubis, sacrum, and sacroiliac joint (Fig. 56.8). The frog lateral view is really a lateral view of the proximal femur and not a true lateral view of the joint, but it serves quite well as a useful screening radiograph. A cross-table lateral view may be important for some conditions, but it rarely provides additional information as a routine screening film. The false-profile view may be helpful in certain situations, to assess both narrowing of the anterior joint space and subtle subluxation, but again it is usually not necessary for routine radiographic assessment.

Magnetic Resonance Imaging

High-resolution magnetic resonance imaging (MRI) is increasingly reliable at discerning various forms of intraarticular disease. Adequate-quality imaging necessitates a 1.5-Tesla magnet and a dedicated hip surface coil. Lesser-quality studies, such as with small magnets or open scanners, are unreliable, except in detecting obvious disease such as avascular necrosis.

One useful finding may be the presence of an effusion. Even slight asymmetric fluid accumulation may be significant. The lack of capsular compliance around the hip typically does not allow for much effusion to develop. This must be carefully scrutinized because often slight variations may be superficially interpreted as normal. Conversely, the absence of an effusion does not preclude the existence of an intraarticular disorder because significant joint damage has been identified, even without an accompanying effusion.

Gadolinium Magnetic Resonance Imaging

MRI with an intraarticular injection of gadolinium (MRA) has greater sensitivity and specificity for intraarticular disor-

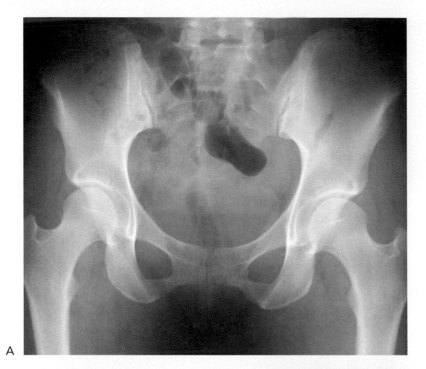

A

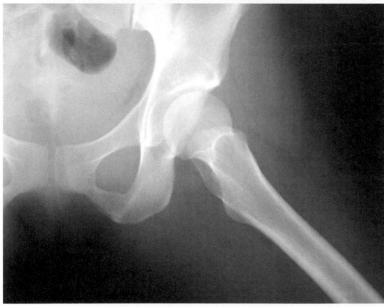

B

FIGURE 56.7 A: An anteroposterior radiograph of the pelvis is centered low to include the hips. Performed properly, this provides good radiographic assessment of the hip in the anteroposterior plane. Additionally, it allows radiographic visualization of the surrounding structures, including the lumbosacral junction, sacrum, coccyx, sacroiliac joint, ilium, ischium, and pubis. Of equal importance, it provides a comparison view of the contralateral hip, which is often helpful when trying to interpret subtle irregularities or variations present in the affected hip. **B:** The frog lateral view provides an excellent radiographic view of the proximal femur in a perpendicular plane to the anteroposterior film.

ders (2,3). It is especially helpful for radiolucent loose bodies, which are often overlooked by conventional MRI. Contrast medium may also extrude into tearing of the acetabular labrum or articular surface defects.

Historically, a fluoroscopically guided intraarticular injection of bupivacaine was the single most reliable test for discerning whether the source of symptoms was intraarticular and thus potentially amenable to arthroscopic intervention. With current gadolinium-enhanced arthrography techniques, it is especially helpful to inject an accompanying amount of bupivacaine; thus, information will be gained regarding localization of the patient's symptoms in addition to

the imaging information. It is important for the patient to be able to create the symptoms reliably before the injection, to tell whether there has been an element of relief after the injection.

Computed Tomography

Computed tomography (CT) is occasionally still superior to MRI for assessing bony architecture. Axial images may be greatly supplemented with reconstructed sagittal, coronal, and three-dimensional imagery. CT may clearly show intraarticular bony loose bodies and can be especially helpful

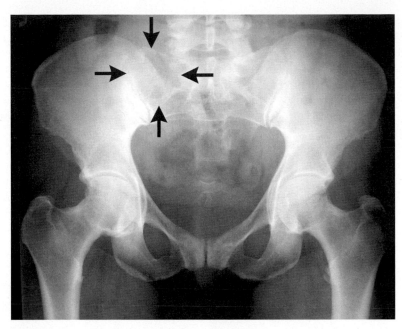

FIGURE 56.8 An anteroposterior pelvis radiograph of a 50-year-old woman with a chief complaint of right hip pain. Chronic bony changes are apparent around both hips, but an aggressive lytic lesion is identified in the right sacrum *(arrows)*.

in assessing peripheral osteophytes and avulsed fragments that may impinge on the joint or block motion.

Single- or double-contrast arthrography combined with CT has been very helpful in discerning radiolucent loose bodies. However, this method has been largely supplanted by MRA, which provides greater information regarding soft tissue details. Finally, under some circumstances, it may be easier to obtain a good-quality CT scan; a poor-quality MRI may be meaningless.

Radionuclide Scanning

Radionuclide scanning provides an image of the metabolic activity of bone. Traditional uses include investigation of arthritis, infection, stress fracture, tumor, and reflex sympathetic dystrophy. For most of these circumstances, MRI probably offers equal sensitivity and greater specificity. Bone scanning is still often helpful because it can provide a useful survey of surrounding areas. It is considerably less expensive than MRI, and, like CT, it may sometimes be easier to obtain a reliable-quality study.

INDICATIONS

The indications for hip arthroscopy continue to evolve. A summary of current applications is listed (Table 56.2). Although the indications are numerous, it is only the occasional patient who adequately fits these criteria. As mentioned in the section on assessment, one should be watchful of two specific parameters: the onset and the character of

symptoms. In general, patients with a specific episode of trauma are more likely to benefit. Absence of trauma or presence of a relatively minor precipitating event may be a harbinger of predisposition to injury or a degenerative process that may respond less successfully to arthroscopy (4). In addition, patients with mechanical symptoms such as catching, locking, or stabbing may potentially benefit more from debridement than those who simply ache or who have ill-defined pain during activities (5).

Loose Bodies

Removal of symptomatic loose bodies represents the clearest indication for hip arthroscopy (6–13). The diagnosis is usually readily apparent. Bony fragments can be defined by plain radiographs or CT scans. Radiolucent loose bodies are often evident with arthrography or arthrographic techniques combined with either CT or MRI. The importance

TABLE 56.2 INDICATIONS

Loose bodies	Instability
Labral tears	Joint sepsis
Degenerative disease	Status post total hip arthro-
Chondral injuries	plasty
Avascular necrosis	Unresolved hip pain
Synovial disease	Arthroscopy associated with
Ruptured ligamentum teres	open procedures
Impinging osteophytes	

From Byrd JWT. Indications and contraindications. In: Byrd JWT, ed. *Operative hip arthroscopy.* New York: Thieme, 1998: 7–24, with permission.

of loose body removal has been well documented, based on the work of Epstein (14). Arthroscopy offers the distinct advantage of lower morbidity, shortened recovery, and reduced cost compared with arthrotomy.

Most commonly, loose bodies are encountered as a result of previous trauma. The accompanying damage cannot be reversed, but removal of the fragments can result in marked symptomatic improvement and is known to slow the secondary damage caused by third-body wear (Fig. 56.9). Free fragments may sometimes develop simply as a consequence of degenerative joint disease (Fig. 56.10). It is important to distinguish this clinically because debridement has less predictable results and is possibly not necessary.

Numerous reports illustrate the successful role for removal of loose bodies resulting from synovial chondromatosis (Fig. 56.11) (9–11). Although there is always a potential concern of recurrent symptoms from residual disease, arthroscopy still offers a clear advantage over the morbidity associated with open synovectomy and debridement. In addition, synovial chondromatosis of the hip often presents a very occult clinical picture and may not be evident even with current imaging techniques. In one study, the diagnosis was evident preoperatively in only 44% of cases (11).

Loose bodies may also occur as a consequence of osteochondritis dissecans accompanying Perthes' disease and has been successfully treated by arthroscopic means (12,13).

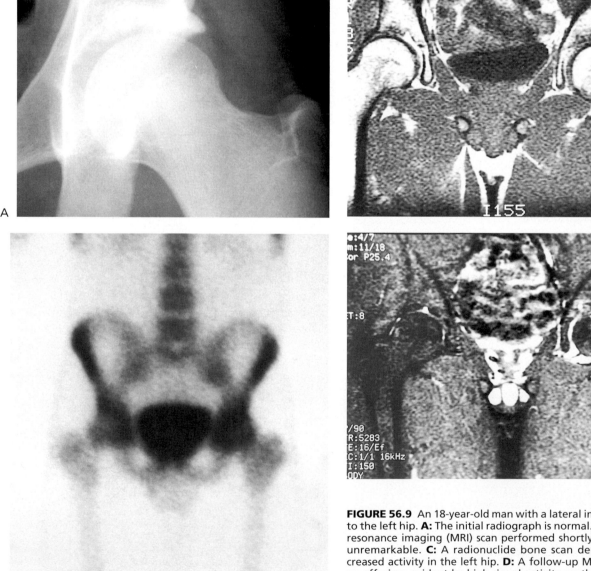

FIGURE 56.9 An 18-year-old man with a lateral impaction injury to the left hip. **A:** The initial radiograph is normal. **B:** A magnetic resonance imaging (MRI) scan performed shortly after injury is unremarkable. **C:** A radionuclide bone scan demonstrates increased activity in the left hip. **D:** A follow-up MRI scan reveals an effusion, evident by high signal activity on the T2-weighted image.

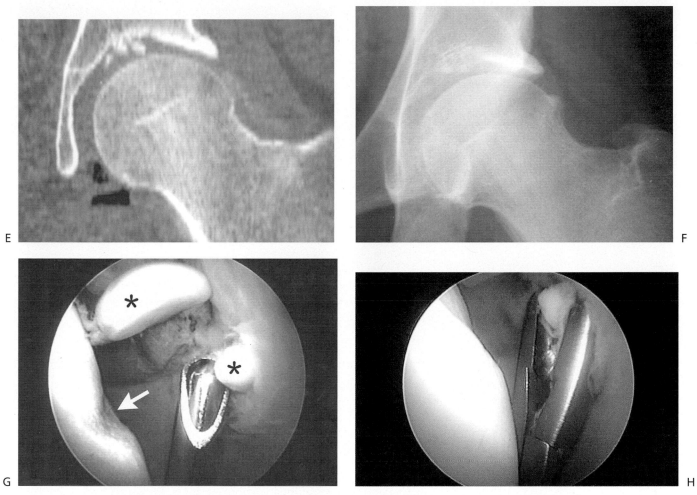

E

F

G

H

FIGURE 56.9 E: Computed tomography with coronal reconstruction demonstrates loose bodies. **F:** A follow-up radiograph, 13 months after the injury, reveals secondary changes including superolateral osteophyte formation on the femoral head. **G:** Two loose bodies are evident *(asterisks)* originating from the acetabulum. Scoring of the femoral head is evident *(arrow)* because of third-body wear. **H:** A pituitary rongeur has been introduced from the posterolateral position for retrieval of the loose bodies. (A to H, from Byrd JWT. Arthroscopy of select hip lesions. In: Byrd JWT, ed. *Operative hip arthroscopy.* New York: Thieme, 1998:153–170, with permission.)

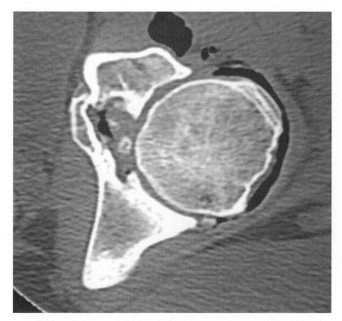

FIGURE 56.10 A 32-year-old man experiences worsening left hip pain 6 years after closed treatment of a posterior acetabular fracture. A computed tomography scan with double contrast arthrography reveals bone fragments within the fossa. However, symptoms are primarily the result of posttraumatic osteoarthritis characterized by joint space narrowing, subchondral sclerosis, and osteophyte formation. Arthroscopy revealed the fragments to be contained within the soft tissue of the fossa, not contributing to his symptoms.

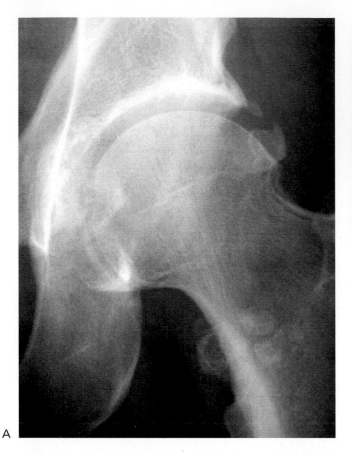

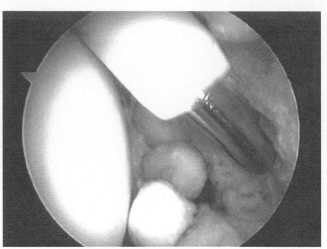

FIGURE 56.11 A 44-year-old man with a 1-year history of progressively worsening left hip pain. **A:** An anteroposterior radiograph demonstrates multiple densities characteristic of synovial chondromatosis with ossified lesions. **B:** An arthroscopic view reveals characteristic loose bodies, which were removed.

Additionally, foreign bodies such as bullets have been retrieved (15–17).

Labral Lesions

Historically, symptomatic labral tears have been elusive to conventional investigative studies. However, high-resolution MRI and gadolinium-enhanced MRA are increasingly reliable in discerning labral pathology (Fig. 56.12) (3). Debridement of labral tears can be very gratifying in terms of symptomatic improvement (7,18–23). However, the results may sometimes be less predictable and influenced by the origin of the tear, coexistent pathologic features, and an uncertain causal relationship of accompanying pain. Although acute tearing of a healthy labrum may occur, often there may be some underlying predisposition or degeneration

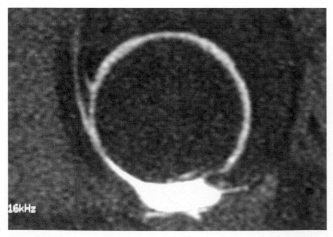

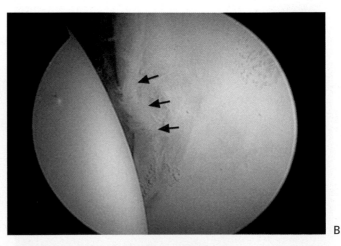

FIGURE 56.12 A 27-year-old woman with pain and catching of the left hip. **A:** A sagittal magnetic resonance imaging scan with gadolinium arthrography reveals a tear of the anterior labrum *(arrow)*. **B:** An arthroscopic view illustrates the tear of the anterior labrum at the articular labral junction *(arrows)*.

within the substance of the labrum that allows it to tear with relatively minor trauma. In these patients, it is unclear how effective simple debridement may be and even less certain whether this will influence further degeneration of this vulnerable hip. Second, labral tearing may accompany more generalized degenerative disease including articular surface erosion, and, in these cases, the results of treatment are dictated more by the extent of the global degenerative process (4,24). Finally, there is still much that we do not fully understand regarding the causal relationship of pain accompanying even large labral tears. Successful execution of the surgical procedure may simply not produce the expected result of marked symptomatic improvement. Santori and Villar found that only 67% of patients were pleased with the results of surgical treatment of labral disorders, regardless of whether articular damage was present (25).

Two unique areas warrant special mention. First is labral tearing in association with acetabular dysplasia (Fig. 56.13). It has been suggested that the presence of dysplasia may be a harbinger of poorer results (8). However, a more recent investigation of dysplastic hips found results of arthroscopy comparable to those in nondysplastic joints (26). The results were dictated more by the nature of the intraarticular disorder than by the presence or absence of dysplasia. Labral debridement must be selective, removing only the torn portion and preserving as much of the healthy tissue as possible. Overly aggressive debridement of the abnormally enlarged

labrum could accentuate instability of the joint. Moreover, arthroscopy is not a substitute "Band-Aid procedure" for patients who may be candidates for more definitive salvage procedures such as corrective osteotomy.

Second, a chronically inverted labrum (even without dysplasia) has been identified as a cause of subsequent osteoarthritis (27). As with other arthritic disorders, results of debridement of the torn inverted portion are often dictated more by the extent of accompanying articular damage (28). The characteristics of this entity are discussed in more detail in the next section.

Lage et al. described a classification system for labral tears (Fig. 56.14) (21). However, even the normal morphology of the acetabular labrum may be quite variable (19). A common variant is a cleft between the labrum and the acetabular articular surface (Fig. 56.15). This situation should not be misinterpreted as a traumatic detachment (29). The edges are smooth, and there are no signs of attempted healing or secondary associated trauma.

Degenerative Arthritis

Arthroscopic debridement for symptomatic degenerative disease of the hip is unpredictable. The most optimistic reports reflect a 60% likelihood of improvement, whereas other reports depict only 34% patient satisfaction (30,31). Even with careful patient selection, it is unlikely that the re-

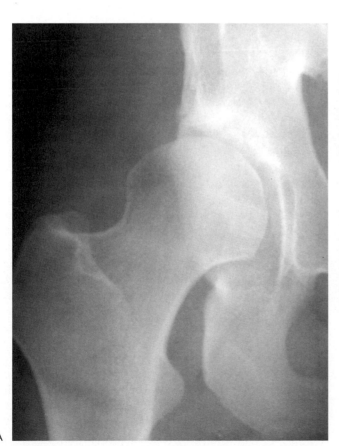

A

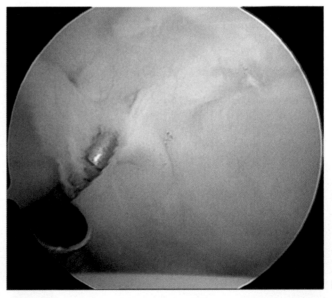

B

FIGURE 56.13 A 26-year-old woman developed spontaneous onset of pain and catching in her right hip. **A:** An anteroposterior radiograph reveals evidence of dysplasia. **B:** An arthroscopic view demonstrates an inverted lateral labrum with the torn edge reflected by the probe.

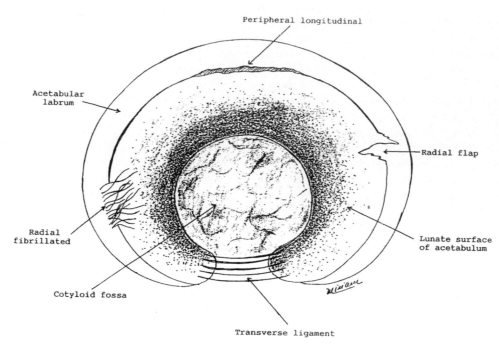

FIGURE 56.14 Diagrammatic representation of morphology of labral tears. (From Lage LA, Patel JV, Villar RN. The acetabular labral tear: an arthroscopic classification. *Arthroscopy* 1996;12:269–272, with permission.)

sults of simple debridement will approach those reported for other joints. Unlike the knee (a tricompartmental joint), in which patients can selectively unload portions by altering their gait pattern, the hip (a unicompartmental joint) cannot be as effectively unloaded, and this may partially explain the poorer results.

Moreover, it is not uncommon that plain radiographs may not reflect the extent of degenerative disease. Grade IV articular damage may accompany seeming joint space preservation. Even subtle asymmetry may indicate much

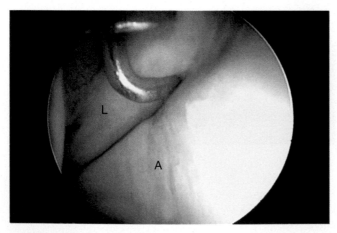

FIGURE 56.15 An arthroscopic view of the right hip from the anterior portal in a 25-year-old woman. Incidentally noted is the separation (probe) between the labrum (L) and the lateral aspect of the bony acetabulum (A).

more severe disease than would be initially suspected (Fig. 56.16). Santori and Villar found radiographs to be unreliable at detecting early stages of osteoarthritis, and, when disease was evident radiographically, there was usually significant degeneration on both sides of the joint when it was viewed arthroscopically (32).

Although arthroscopic debridement should not be considered an overly attractive alternative to arthroplasty, it is occasionally considered for younger patients with relatively well-preserved joint space and range of motion and relatively spontaneous onset of symptoms that could suggest a dislodged fragment. A final criterion is failure of response to conservative treatment, especially activity modification, but also physical therapy and antiinflammatory medications. In general, arthroscopy is considered only if symptoms are just about severe enough for the surgeon otherwise to be contemplating a joint replacement. This implies reasonable expectations on the part of the patient regarding the modest degree of improvement expected from the surgical procedure.

As mentioned earlier, a particular cause of osteoarthritis is the chronically inverted labrum, as described by Harris and Bourne (27). It has been reported that the diagnosis of this lesion can often be made radiographically, characterized by isolated superolateral joint space narrowing (Fig. 56.17A) (28). This condition may also give the appearance of dysplasia *(pseudodysplasia)* because the center edge (CE) angle is often normal. One must be especially careful of interpreting MRI scans in this setting that may clearly reveal labral tearing, but less clearly define the extent of articular

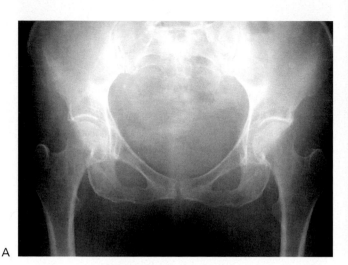

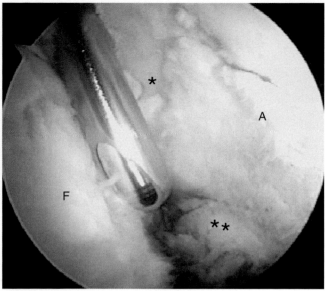

FIGURE 56.16 A: An anteroposterior pelvis radiograph of a 74-year-old woman with chronic rheumatoid arthritis who presented with recent onset of intractable mechanical left hip pain. Radiographs were reported as superficially normal, with only modest evidence of inflammatory degenerative changes, insufficient solely to explain the magnitude of her symptoms. However, there is subtle, but significant, joint space narrowing. **B:** An arthroscopic view of the left hip from the anterolateral portal reveals extensive articular surface erosion of both the femoral head (F) and the acetabulum (A) with areas of exposed bone *(asterisk)* and extensive synovial disease *(asterisks).* (From Byrd JWT. Investigation of the symptomatic hip: physical examination. In: Byrd JWT, ed. *Operative hip arthroscopy.* New York: Thieme, 1998:25–41, with permission.)

damage, which is ultimately the limiting factor in determining the response to treatment.

The results of arthroscopy in this population with an inverted labrum are no better than those reported for patients with other causes of degenerative arthritis (28). However, some patients have been found to have focal grade IV articular lesions of the lateral acetabulum, and, in the presence of healthy surrounding articular surface, these select patients may respond remarkably well to microfracture of the subchondral bone in addition to chondral and labral debridement (Fig. 56.17B to D). Typically, this treatment is followed by a strict protected weight-bearing status for 10 weeks, to neutralize the forces across the joint during maturation of the fibrocartilaginous healing response.

Chondral Injuries

Isolated chondral injuries are an excellent indication for hip arthroscopy. These may be especially evident in association with a dislocation or subluxation episode (7). Acute chondral injuries are also increasingly recognized in young, active adults (33,34). These injuries occur from a direct blow to the trochanter, such as from a fall. In thin patients without much subcutaneous padding, the force is transferred directly to the hip joint and results in acute chondral fragmentation on the medial femoral head or chondronecrosis of the medial acetabulum. This injury is seen in young

adults with high bone density, because older adults would more likely sustain a fracture and children would injure the growth plate. Investigative studies may not define the nature of the lesion, but it may reflect indirect evidence of injury such as effusion or subchondral edema on MRI or increased activity on a bone scan (Fig. 56.18). Removal of these unstable fragments can result in marked symptomatic improvement, but these fragments also provide an indicator of potential long-term problems.

Unstable articular fragments may also develop in association with Perthes' disease (13). An area of osteochondritis dissecans may not result in a true bony loose body, but it may dislodge an area of overlying articular cartilage. Excision of these unstable fragments can result in marked symptomatic improvement, even in the presence of a severely deformed radiographic appearance of the femoral head.

Avascular Necrosis

Arthroscopic debridement as a palliative procedure for end-stage avascular necrosis provides uniformly poor results (4,19). However, arthroscopy has found a role in earlier stages of the disease, especially in the assessment and management of potential candidates for free-vascularized fibular grafting (5,35,36). Arthroscopy allows inspection of the overlying articular surface of the femoral head to see whether there is adequate preservation for revascularization

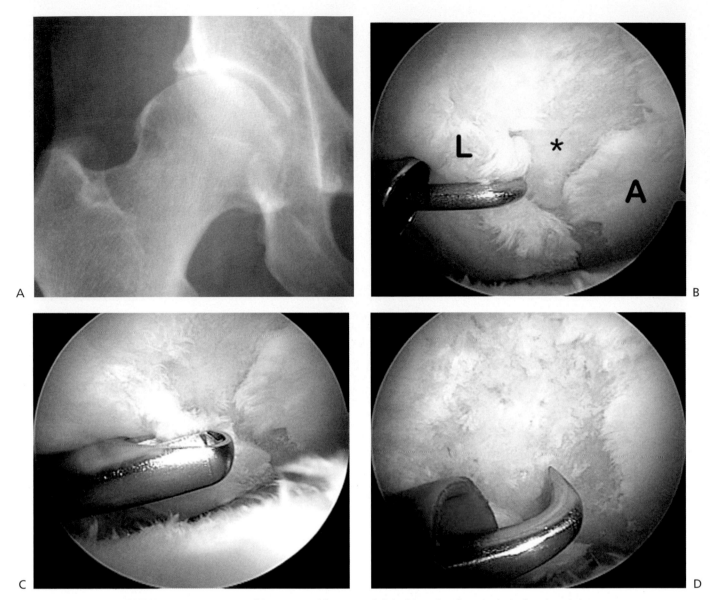

FIGURE 56.17 A 47-year-old woman with onset of right hip pain after a relatively minor injury. **A:** An anteroposterior radiograph reveals characteristic features of osteoarthritis associated with an inverted labrum: (1) joint space narrowing localized to the superolateral portion of the joint, (2) slight lateral uncovering of the femoral head suggesting mild acetabular dysplasia, and (3) radius of curvature of the acetabulum intersects the femoral head at the site of joint space narrowing. **B:** Degenerative tearing of the inverted portion of the labrum is evident (L) adjacent to the grade IV lesion of the acetabulum *(asterisk)* surrounded by relatively healthy acetabular articular surface (A). **C:** Debridement of the torn portion of the labrum and chondroplasty of unstable articular fragments is performed. **D:** The arthroscopic awl is used to create multiple perforations through the subchondral bone for vascular access. (B to D, from Byrd JWT. Arthroscopy of select hip lesions. In: Byrd JWT, ed. *Operative hip arthroscopy.* New York: Thieme, 1998:153–170, with permission.)

of the underlying bone to be effective. Other coexistent intraarticular diseases can also be addressed at the same time.

Synovial Disease

As with other joints, arthroscopic synovectomy has a recognized role in the hip, including various inflammatory arthritides and miscellaneous synovial conditions such as synovial

chondromatosis and pigmented villonodular synovitis (Figs. 56.11 and 56.19) (4,7,37–39). Although complete synovectomy cannot be performed, often adequate debridement is achieved for palliative or therapeutic purposes. Synovectomy for inflammatory disease such as rheumatoid arthritis should be carefully chosen but can result in improvement. As with other arthritic disorders, the response to treatment may be dictated by the degree of articular surface erosion.

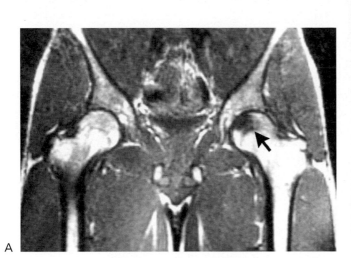
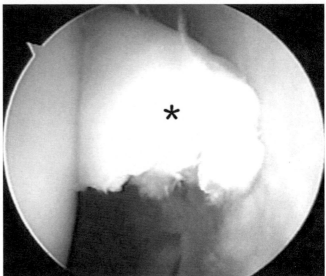

A   B

FIGURE 56.18 A 20-year-old male collegiate basketball player with painful catching of the left hip after a fall with lateral impaction of the joint. **A:** Magnetic resonance imaging revealed extensive signal changes in the medial aspect of the femoral head characterizing the subchondral injury associated with a fall. **B:** A full-thickness chondral flap lesion *(asterisk)* associated with the injury is identified. Excision resulted in complete alleviation of symptoms that allowed advancement to a professional career.

Synovial disorders of the hip tend to follow either a focal or a diffuse pattern. Focal patterns are limited to the area of the pulvinar within the acetabular fossa. Inflammatory processes contained in this region are sometimes quite painful and respond well to debridement, although the exact cause is not always well understood. Diffuse patterns involve the synovial lining of the capsule.

Arthroscopy can be quite effective in the management of synovial chondromatosis (9–11). Again, although complete debridement cannot be achieved, those fragments involving the weight-bearing portion of the joint, and thus causing symptoms, can be retrieved. As noted previously, the diagnosis of synovial chondromatosis in the hip can be much more elusive than in other joints. In many cases, the carti-

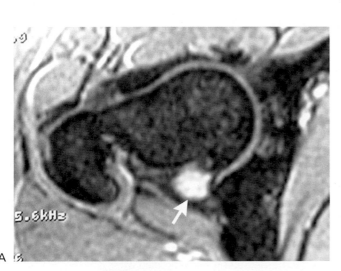
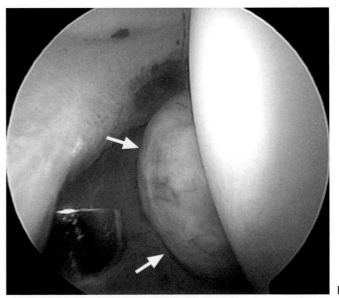

A   B

FIGURE 56.19 An 18-year-old woman presents with a 2-year history of ill-defined right hip pain. Magnetic resonance imaging suggested a posterior intraarticular cyst *(arrow)*. Arthroscopy reveals a nodular form of pigmented villonodular synovitis *(arrows)*. Excision resulted in resolution of symptoms.

laginous lesions may not ossify, and only a vague sense of synovial disease or intraarticular lesion may be present on investigative studies.

Ruptured Ligamentum Teres

Lesions of the ligamentum teres were classified by Gray and Villar (40). In general, these lesions may be traumatic or degenerative. Traumatic rupture invariably accompanies dislocation, but lesions can also occur in the absence of a dislocation episode (Fig. 56.20) (37,41–44). These lesions are often quite painful, with the disrupted fibers catching within the joint, and they respond well to arthroscopy. Indiscriminate debridement of the ligament should be avoided because of the ligament's potential contribution to the blood supply of the femoral head, but resection of the disrupted portion should not create a problem. Degenerative ruptures may also be symptomatic and respond to debridement, but most often these accompany more diffuse degenerative disease of the joint.

Impinging Osteophytes

Posttraumatic periacetabular osteophytes or malunited fragments can impinge on the joint and can cause pain and restrict motion. Excising a window in the capsule and dissecting peripheral to the joint, these types of osteophytes can be excised, thus eliminating the symptoms (Fig. 56.21) (7,13,37). This procedure requires good visualization and careful orientation to the surrounding extraarticular anatomic structures.

Rim osteophytes on the periphery of the femoral head may occasionally be sufficiently enlarged to block motion, impinge, and cause pain. Excision may similarly improve the symptoms, but otherwise, in general, debridement of de-

generative osteophytes is unproductive because the cause of pain is more closely associated with the accompanying articular erosion.

Instability

Thermal capsular shrinkage can be accomplished in the hip. More energy is necessary because of the thick capsule. The indication includes instability resulting from an incompetent capsule with normal joint geometry. Caution should be taken because of the many causes of the sensation of subluxation, in the absence of any true joint instability. Patient compliance is also imperative to a successful result. Currently, patients with hyperlaxity, usually from collagen disorder (i.e., Ehlers- Danlos syndrome) represent the population most likely to be candidates for this technique.

Sepsis

Numerous articles support the role of arthroscopic lavage and debridement in the treatment of joint sepsis of the hip (45–48). Arthroscopy offers an attractive alternative to the potential morbidity associated with an open procedure. Patient selection may be a factor because preferable outcomes are more likely in patients with an acute process with early intervention and a sensitive organism. These parameters especially apply for infection in the presence of total hip arthroplasty (48).

Status Post Total Hip Arthroplasty

Some case reports detailed the successful removal of entrapped material after total hip arthroplasty (49–51). Arthroscopy may also have a role in the management of disease accompanying polyethylene wear debris, but, in general,

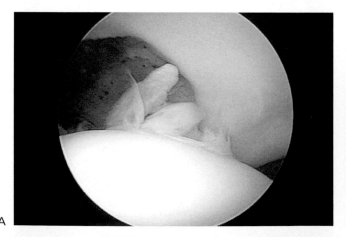
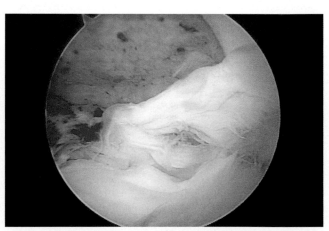

A   B

FIGURE 56.20 A 19-year-old woman experiences persistent mechanical right hip pain after a dashboard injury. **A:** Arthroscopy reveals a rupture of the ligamentum teres *(asterisks)* silhouetted by the pulvinar. **B:** A close-up view further defines the magnitude of the rupture *(asterisk)*. (From Byrd JWT. Arthroscopy of select hip lesions. In: Byrd JWT, ed. *Operative hip arthroscopy.* New York: Thieme, 1998:153–170, with permission.)

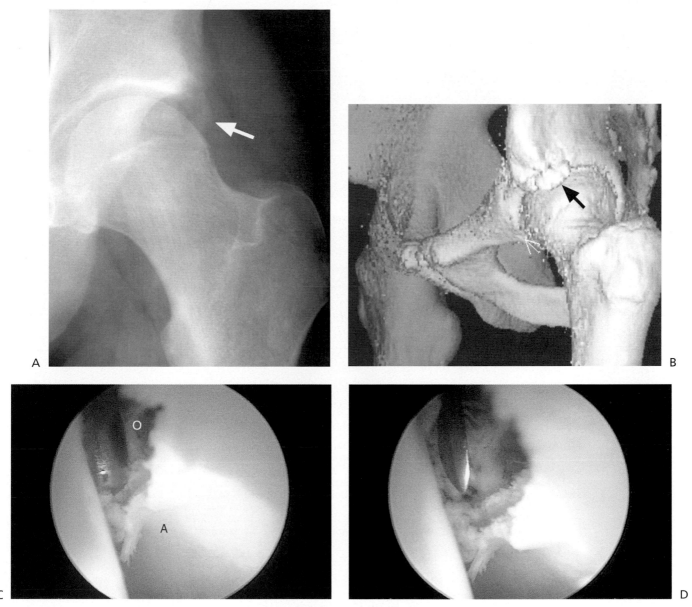

FIGURE 56.21 An 18-year-old high school football player experiences persistent pain and restricted motion after an avulsion fracture of the left anterior inferior iliac spine. **A:** An anteroposterior radiograph reveals ossification around the acetabulum *(arrow)*. **B:** Three-dimensional computed tomographic reconstruction defines the dimensions of the fragment creating a mechanical block to internal rotation *(arrow)*. **C:** A full-radius resector is used to develop the margins of the osteophyte (O), which lies anterior to the articular surface of the acetabulum (a).

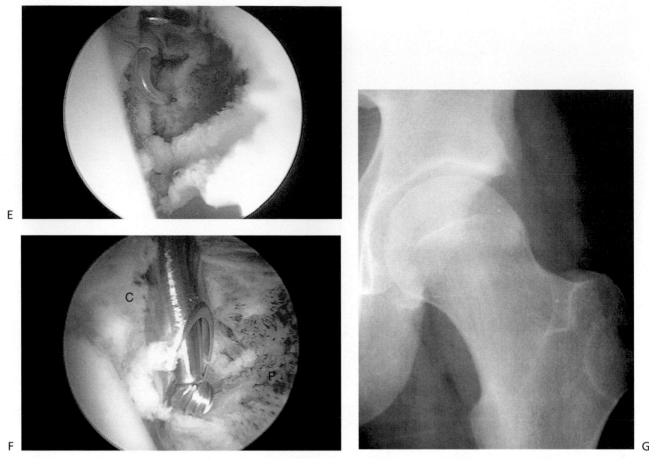

FIGURE 56.21 *(continued)* **D:** An arthroscopic knife is used to incise the capsule, partially contained within the fragment. **E:** Homeostasis, important for optimal visualization, is maintained with judicious use of the arthroscopic cautery. **F:** The anterior capsule (C) has been fully released, and a burr is used to excise the fragment, thus exposing the anterior column of the pelvis (P). The anterior margin of the acetabulum is at the bottom of the picture (A), and a portion of the femoral head is in view on the left (F). **G:** The postoperative radiograph reveals the extent of bony resection, and the patient regained full, pain-free range of motion. (C to F, from Byrd JWT. Arthroscopy of select hip lesions. In: Byrd JWT, ed. *Operative hip arthroscopy.* New York: Thieme, 1998:153–170, with permission.)

few causes of a symptomatic hip prosthesis are amenable to arthroscopic intervention (7,37). Hyman et al. reported successful arthroscopic management of eight consecutive patients with late acute infections of total hip arthroplasty (48).

Unresolved Hip Pain

Diagnostic arthroscopy is not a substitute for clinical diagnostic skills and appropriate evaluation ("looking is not a substitute for thinking"). However, arthroscopy has defined many elusive and often treatable causes of hip pain. This recognition has done much to potentiate the value and efficacy of other noninvasive investigative studies. As various imaging methods continue to improve, the role of diagnostic arthroscopy should diminish, but the literature still supports its role (52,53). There are numerous situations in which arthroscopy is contemplated without a clear diagno-

sis, but at least with a high degree of suspicion that the problem is intraarticular and potentially amenable to arthroscopic intervention.

Arthroscopy Associated with Open Procedures

Arthroscopy has been described either in conjunction with, or as a prelude to, select open procedures such as pinning for slipped capital femoral epiphysis, revascularization for avascular necrosis, osteotomy, or in association with miniarthrotomy (35,54–57).

CONTRAINDICATIONS

The clearest contraindication to hip arthroscopy is ankylosis of the joint. Lesser degrees of arthrofibrosis or capsular constriction may similarly preclude arthroscopy when the joint cannot be adequately distracted or distended for introduction of the instruments. Thus, the physical examination must include an assessment of reasonable rotational motion.

Significant alteration in the normal anatomy of the bone or surrounding soft tissues, whether from previous trauma or surgery, may contraindicate arthroscopy. Moreover, potential stress risers in the bone, which may occur from disease, trauma, or previous surgery, must be judiciously assessed in relation to the traction forces necessary to distract the joint for arthroscopy.

Severe obesity is a relative contraindication to hip arthroscopy. In patients with extremely dense soft tissues, even the extra-length instruments currently available may be inadequate for accessing the joint. Finally, advanced disease states with destruction of the hip joint are a contraindication to arthroscopy, but this contraindication reflects more on poor patient selection and emphasizes the importance of proper indications.

COMPLICATIONS

A review of 1,491 hip arthroscopy cases from seven leading centers around the world revealed the complications summarized in Table 56.3 (58). Twenty complications were defined, for an overall incidence of 1.34%. The most common feature of these complications was that they usually occurred early in the surgeons' experience. This finding reflects the learning curve associated with the developmental phase experienced by these pioneers in hip arthroscopy. This point is illustrated by two reports in the literature. Griffin and Villar reported their experience in 640 consecutive cases with a complication rate of 1.6%, none of which were major or long term (59). Conversely, Funke and Munzinger reported three complications among 19 procedures (60).

TABLE 56.3 COMPLICATIONS (NUMBER IN PARENTHESES) ASSOCIATED WITH 1,491 ARTHROSCOPIC HIP PROCEDURES

Transient pudendal nerve neuropraxia (5)	Partial lateral femoral cutaneous nerve neurapraxia (2)
Permanent pudendal nerve neuropraxia (1)	Laceration of the lateral femoral cutaneous nerve (1)
Transient sciatic nerve neuropraxia (4)	Scrotal skin necrosis (1)
	Femoral nerve palsy (1)
Intraabdominal fluid extravasation (3)	Instrument breakage (1)
	Heterotopic ossification (1)

From Byrd JWT. Complications associated with hip arthroscopy. In: Byrd JWT, ed. *Operative hip arthroscopy*. New York: Thieme, 1998: 171–176, with permission.

Complications are usually reported by those surgeons most experienced in arthroscopic techniques. Many serious problems, and the frequency with which they are encountered by inexperienced surgeons, may not be reported.

Neurovascular Traction Injury

Transient neuropraxia of the sciatic nerve resulting from traction was reported by Glick (61) in his early experiences, but not with his current technique. Hip flexion may partially relax the capsule, but it places the sciatic nerve under greater stretch during arthroscopy. I have not encountered any sciatic nerve disturbance but do not routinely employ flexion while distracting the joint.

The lateral femoral cutaneous nerve is divided into three or more branches at the level of the anterior portal (62). One of these small branches often lies close to the portal. Laceration is avoided by careful technique incising the skin. Neuropraxia of one of these branches can still occur when vigorous instrumentation is carried out from this portal, such as when removing loose bodies too large to be brought out through a cannula. I have experienced two such cases resulting in only a small area of decreased sensation in the lateral aspect of the thigh. One was transient. Nonetheless, the potential for neuropraxia of this structure should be mentioned in the preoperative discussion.

Direct Trauma to Neurovascular Structures

An anatomic study suggests that the major neurovascular structures are a safe distance from the portals when observing proper technique in portal placement (62). Clinical experiences have supported this finding as well. However, one case of femoral nerve palsy has been reported (Villar, *personal communication*), and I am aware of anecdotal information of femoral nerve laceration by an inexperienced surgeon.

Compression Injury to the Perineum

A case of soft tissue pressure necrosis of the perineum was reported by Eriksson et al. (63). I observed two cases of transient neuropraxia of the pudendal nerve before using a modified fracture table that incorporates a heavily padded, oversized perineal post. Similarly, Glick (61) reported this occurrence before implementing a custom distractor.

Common to all these cases was that they, too, occurred early in the surgeons' experience, a finding reflecting the learning curve associated with this technique. It also reflects the importance of a properly adapted fracture table or disrraction device. Additionally, it is prudent to use the minimal amount of traction force necessary to distract the hip and to keep the traction time to a minimum.

Fluid Extravasation

Three cases of fluid extravasation into the abdominal cavity have been reported (Glick, *personal communication*). All resolved without long-term sequelae. One did require paracentesis and ventilatory support overnight. One case occurred when arthroscopy was performed within a few days of an acetabular fracture, and it was speculated that extravasation occurred through the fracture into the pelvis. The other case occurred when arthroscopic release of the iliopsoas tendon was performed.

Bartlett et al. reported a case of cardiac arrest resulting from intraabdominal extravasation of fluid (64). The patient had an acute acetabular fracture that allowed flow from the joint into the abdominal cavity. The patient was successfully resuscitated, and the fluid was decompressed by laparotomy. Nonetheless, this complication highlights the potentially devastating consequences of inordinate extravasation.

Scope Trauma

The single most common complication, which is probably underreported, is "scope trauma." The dense soft tissue envelope and the tightly constrained joint limit the maneuverability of instruments. The convex articular surface of the femoral head is especially vulnerable to injury. This may occur during portal placement or subsequent instrumentation and requires a very thoughtful approach when carrying out operative arthroscopy of the hip.

The labrum is also susceptible to damage during portal placement. This is most likely to occur when one tries to use a more cephalad position for penetrating the capsule in an attempt to avoid the articular surface of the femoral head. The labrum may be inadvertently penetrated, potentially resulting in significant damage and uncertain, long-term consequences. During portal placement, it is best to approach low under the labrum but then direct upward to lift up to stay off the articular surface of the femoral head.

Instrument Breakage

The potential for instrument malfunction or breakage is increased by the dense soft tissue envelope, constrained architecture of the joint, and extra length of the instruments. Only sturdy instruments should be used, and extra-length instruments designed for other endoscopic uses should not be improperly applied to the hip joint. I am aware of two cases of instrument breakage by experienced surgeons. In both cases, the broken piece was retrieved arthroscopically,

but this problem reflects the importance of taking great technical care when instrumenting the joint.

Vascular Insult to the Femoral Head

Avascular necrosis of the femoral head as a consequence of hip arthroscopy has not been reported. Nonetheless, the effect of this procedure on the vascular flow to the femoral head remains unknown. I have observed one case of avascular necrosis that progressed after arthroscopy, and this was also observed by Villar (65). This condition may have been a consequence of the natural course of the disease, but it is uncertain whether this could have been precipitated by the arthroscopic intervention.

Heterotopic Ossification

I have observed a small focal area of heterotopic bone formation along a single portal tract. This was later excised uneventfully, but this demonstrates that arthroscopy is not entirely immune to complications more frequently attributed to open hip procedures.

Infection and Systemic Problems

Neither infection nor another systemic problem such as thromboembolic disease has been reported as a consequence of hip arthroscopy. However, these still remain potential complications. If patients have risk factors for thromboembolic disease, more aggressive anticoagulant prophylaxis would be appropriate. As a more local phenomenon, the occasional development of trochanteric bursitis in conjunction with the lateral portals has been observed and can be a stubborn problem.

REFERENCES

1. Byrd JWT. Investigation of the symptomatic hip: physical examination. In: Byrd JWT, ed. *Operative hip arthroscopy*. New York: Thieme, 1998:25–41.
2. Leunig M, Werlen S, Ungersbock A, et al. Evaluation of the acetabular labrum by MR arthrography. *J Bone Joint Surg Br* 1997; 79:230–234.
3. Czerny C, Hofmann S, Neuhold A, et al. Lesions of the acetabular labrum: accuracy of MR imaging and MR arthrography in detection and staging. *Radiology* 1996;200:225–230.
4. Byrd JWT, Jones KS. Prospective analysis of hip arthroscopy. *Arthroscopy* 2000;16:578–587.
5. O'Leary JA, Berend K, Vail TP. The relationship between diagnosis and outcome in arthroscopy of the hip. *Arthroscopy* 2001; 17:181–188.
6. Byrd JWT. Hip arthroscopy for post-traumatic loose fragments in the young active adult: three case reports. *Clin Sports Med* 1996;6:129–134.
7. Byrd JWT. Indications and contraindications. In: Byrd JWT, ed. *Operative hip arthroscopy*. New York: Thieme, 1998:7–24.

8. Sampson TG, Glick JM. Indications and surgical treatment of hip pathology. In: McGinty JB, ed. *Operative arthroscopy,* 2nd ed. New York: Lippincott–Raven, 1996:1067–1078.

9. Okada Y, Awaya G, Ikeda T, et al. Arthroscopic surgery for synovial chondromatosis of the hip. *J Bone Joint Surg Br* 1989;71:198–199.

10. Witwity T, Uhlmann RD, Fischer J. Arthroscopic management of chondromatosis of the hip joint. *Arthroscopy* 1988;4:55–56.

11. McCarthy JC, Bono JV, Wardell S. Is there a treatment for synovial chondromatosis of the hip joint. *Arthroscopy* 1997;13:409–410.

12. Bowen JR, Kumar VP, Joyce JJ, et al. Osteochondritis dissecans following Perthes' disease: arthroscopic-operative treatment. *Clin Orthop* 1986;209:49–56.

13. Medlock V, Rathjen KE, Montgomery JB. Hip arthroscopy for late sequelae of Perthes disease. *Arthroscopy* 1999;15:552–553.

14. Epstein H. Posterior fracture-dislocations of the hip: comparison of open and closed methods of treatment in certain types. *J Bone Joint Surg Am* 1961;43:1079–1098.

15. Goldman A, Minkoff J, Price A, et al. A posterior arthroscopic approach to bullet extraction from the hip. *J Trauma* 1987;27:1294–1300.

16. Glick JM. Hip arthroscopy. In: McGinty JB, ed. *Operative arthroscopy.* New York: Raven Press, 1991:663–676.

17. Cory JW, Ruch DS. Arthroscopic removal of a .44 caliber bullet from the hip. *Arthroscopy* 1998;14:624–626.

18. Altenberg AR. Acetabular labrum tears: a cause of hip pain and degenerative arthritis. *South Med J* 1977;70:174–175.

19. Byrd JWT. Labral lesions: an elusive source of hip pain: case reports and review of the literature. *Arthroscopy* 1996;12:603–612.

20. Ikeda T, Awaya G, Suzuki S, et al. Torn acetabular labrum in young patients. *J Bone Joint Surg Br* 1988;70:13–16.

21. Lage LA, Patel JV, Villar RN. The acetabular labral tear: an arthroscopic classification. *Arthroscopy* 1996;12:269–272.

22. Suzuki S, Awaya G, Okada Y, et al. Arthroscopic diagnosis of ruptured acetabular labrum. *Acta Orthop Scand* 1986;57:513–515.

23. Ueo T, Suzuki S, Iwasaki R, et al. Rupture of the labra acetabularis as a cause of hip pain detected arthroscopically, and partial limbectomy for successful pain relief. *Arthroscopy* 1990;6:48–51.

24. Farjo LA, Glick JM, Sampson TG. Hip arthroscopy for acetabular labrum tears. *Arthroscopy* 1999;15:132–137.

25. Santori N, Villar RN. Acetabular labral tears: result of arthroscopic partial limbectomy. *Arthroscopy* 2000;16:11–15.

26. Byrd JWT, Jones KS. Results of hip arthroscopy in the presence of dysplasia. Presented at the 20th annual meeting of the Arthroscopy Association of North America, Seattle, WA, 2001.

27. Harris WH, Bourne RB, Oh I. Intra-articular acetabular labrum: a possible etiological factor in certain cases of osteoarthritis of the hip. *J Bone Joint Surg Am* 1979;61:510–513.

28. Byrd JWT, Jones KS. Inverted acetabular labrum and secondary osteoarthritis: radiographic diagnosis and arthroscopic treatment. *Arthroscopy* 2000;16:417.

29. Nishina T, Saito S, Ohzono K, et al. Chiari pelvic osteotomy for osteoarthritis: the influence of the torn and detached acetabular labrum. *J Bone Joint Surg Br* 1990;72:765–769.

30. Farjo LA, Glick JM, Sampson TG. Hip arthroscopy for degenerative joint disease. *Arthroscopy* 1998;14:435.

31. Villar RN. Arthroscopic debridement of the hip: a minimally invasive approach to osteoarthritis. *J Bone Joint Surg Br* 1991;73:170–171.

32. Santori N, Villar RN. Arthroscopic findings in the initial stages of hip osteoarthritis. *Orthopedics* 1999;22:405–409.

33. Byrd JWT. Low velocity lateral impact injury to the hip: a source of occult hip pathology. *J South Orthop Assoc* 1997;6:151.

34. Byrd JWT. Lateral impact injury. A source of occult hip pathology. *Clin Sports Med* 2001;20:801–815.

35. Hunter DM, Ruch DS. Hip arthroscopy. *J South Orthop Assoc* 1996;5:243–250.

36. Sekiya JK, Ruch DS, Hunter DM, et al. Hip arthroscopy in staging avascular necrosis of the femoral head. *J South Orthop Assoc* 2000;9:254–261.

37. Byrd JWT. Arthroscopy of select hip lesions. In: Byrd JWT, ed. *Operative hip arthroscopy.* New York: Thieme, 1998:153–170.

38. Danzig LA, Gershuni DH, Resnick D. Diagnosis and treatment of diffuse pigmented villonodular synovitis of the hip. *Clin Orthop* 1982;168:42–77.

39. Gondolph-Zink B, Puhl W, Noack W. Semiarthroscopic synovectomy of the hip. *Int Orthop* 1988;12:31–35.

40. Gray AJR, Villar RN. The ligamentum teres of the hip: an arthroscopic classification of its pathology. *Arthroscopy* 1997;13:575–578.

41. Delcamp DD, Klarren HE, Van Meerdervoort HFP. Traumatic avulsion of the ligamentum teres without dislocation of the hip. *J Bone Joint Surg Am* 1988;70:933–935.

42. Barrett IR, Goldgert JA. Avulsion fracture of the ligamentum teres in a child: a case report. *J Bone Joint Surg Am* 1989;71:438–439.

43. Ebrahim NA, Salvolaine ER, Fenton PJ, et al. Calcified ligamentum teres mimicking entrapped intraarticular bony fragments in a patient with acetabular fracture. *J Orthop Trauma* 1991;5:376–378.

44. Kashiwagi N, Suzuki S, Seto Y. Arthroscopic treatment for traumatic hip dislocation with avulsion fracture of the ligamentum teres. *Arthroscopy* 2001;17:67–69.

45. Blitzer CM. Arthroscopic management of septic arthritis of the hip. *Arthroscopy* 1993;9:414–416.

46. Bould M, Edwards D, Villar RN. Arthroscopic diagnosis and treatment of septic arthritis of the hip joint. *Arthroscopy* 1993;9:707–708.

47. Chung WK, Slater GL, Bates EH. Treatment of septic arthritis of the hip by arthroscopic lavage. *J Pediatr Orthop* 1993;13:444–446.

48. Hyman JL, Salvati EA, Laurencin CT, et al. The arthroscopic drainage, irrigation, and debridement of late, acute total hip arthroplasty infections: average 6 year follow up. *J Arthroplasty* 1999;14:903–910.

49. Nordt W, Giangarra CE, Levy IM, et al. Arthroscopic removal of entrapped debris following dislocation of a total hip arthroplasty. *Arthroscopy* 1987;3:196–198.

50. Shifrin LZ, Reis ND. Arthroscopy of a dislocated hip replacement: a case report. *Clin Orthop* 1980;146:213–214.

51. Vakili F, Salvati EA, Warren RF. Entrapped foreign body within the acetabular cup in total hip replacement. *Clin Orthop* 1980;150:159–162.

52. Baber YF, Robinson AH, Villar RN. Is diagnostic arthroscopy of the hip worthwhile? A prospective review of 328 adults investigated for hip pain. *J Bone Joint Surg Br* 1999;81:600–603.

53. Dorfmann H, Boyer T. Arthroscopy of the hip: 12 years of experience. *Arthroscopy* 1999;15:67–72.

54. Futami T, Kasahara Y, Suzuki S, et al. Arthroscopy for slipped capital femoral epiphysis. *J Pediatr Orthop* 1992;12:592–597.

55. Hawkins RB. Arthroscopy of the hip. *Clin Orthop* 1989;249:44–47.

56. Ruch DS, Satterfield W. The use of arthroscopy to document accurate position of core decompression of the hip. *Arthroscopy* 1998;14:617–619.

57. Sekiya JK, Woytys EM, Loder RT, et al. Hip arthroscopy using a limited anterior exposure: an alternative approach for arthroscopic access. *Arthroscopy* 2000;16:16–20.

58. Byrd JWT. Complications associated with hip arthroscopy. In: Byrd JWT, ed. *Operative hip arthroscopy.* New York: Thieme, 1998:171–176.
59. Griffin DR, Villar RN. Complications of arthroscopy of the hip. *J Bone Joint Surg Br* 1999;81:604–606.
60. Funke EL, Munzinger U. Complications in hip arthroscopy. *Arthroscopy* 1996;12:156–159.
61. Glick JM. Complications of hip arthroscopy by the lateral approach. In: Sherman OH, Minkoff J, eds. *Current management of complications in orthopaedics: arthroscopic surgery.* Baltimore: Williams & Wilkins, 1990:193–201.
62. Byrd JWT, Pappas JN, Pedley MJ. Hip arthroscopy: an anatomic study of portal placement and relationship to the extra-articular structures. *Arthroscopy* 1995;11:418–423.
63. Eriksson E, Arvidsson I, Arvidsson H. Diagnostic and operative arthroscopy of the hip. *Orthopedics* 1986;9:169–176.
64. Bartlett CS, DiFelice GS, Buly RL, et al. Cardiac arrest as a result of intraabdominal extravasation of fluid during arthroscopic removal of a loose body from the hip joint of a patient with an acetabular fracture. *J Orthop Trauma* 1998;12:294–299.
65. Villar RN. *Hip arthroscopy.* Oxford, England: Butterworth-Heinemann, 1992.

Operative Arthroscopy, third edition. Edited by John B. McGinty, Stephen S. Burkhart, Robert W. Jackson, Donald H. Johnson, and John C. Richmond.
Lippincott Williams & Wilkins © 2003.

ARTHROSCOPY OF THE HIP: SUPINE POSITION

J. W. THOMAS BYRD

Hip arthroscopy can be performed with equal success whether the patient is placed supine or laterally. As with other joints, such as the shoulder and elbow, position selection is mostly dictated by the surgeon's preference.

The advantages of the supine position are as follows. Supine positioning is much easier than lateral positioning and can be accomplished in just a few minutes. It allows the use of a standard fracture table and avoids the necessity of highly specialized, infrequently used distraction devices. The layout of the operating room (OR) is user-friendly to the surgeon, assistants, and OR staff. Orientation to the joint is easy. Orthopaedic surgeons are accustomed to this position from their experiences in managing hip fractures. Establishing the anterior portal is perhaps a little easier supine, although access to the joint is readily achieved in either position.

Another potentially important advantage of the supine position regards the issue of fluid extravasation. As with any joint, some fluid will leak outside the capsule. However, there have been several reports of significant accumulation of fluid within the abdomen or retroperitoneum that resulted in transient vascular compromise of the lower extremities or even cardiac arrest (1,2). These reports were limited to the lateral position. This may be attributable to the effect of gravity as the abdominal and pelvic cavity create a sink into which the fluid collects. Although inordinate fluid extravasation is always a potential concern, these severe examples have not been encountered with the patient positioned supine.

DICTUMS ON HIP ARTHROSCOPY

There are several dictums about hip arthroscopy that need to be acknowledged. First, the key to a successful outcome lies in proper patient selection. A technically well executed procedure will fail if it is performed for the wrong reason. This may include failure of the procedure to meet the patient's expectations.

Second, regardless of whether the choice is supine or lateral, the patient must be properly positioned in order for the case to potentially go well. Poor positioning ensures a difficult procedure.

Third, simply gaining access to the hip joint is not an outstanding technical accomplishment. The paramount issue is accessing the joint in as atraumatic a fashion as possible. Because of the constrained architecture and dense soft tissue envelope of the hip joint, the potential for inadvertent iatrogenic arthroscope trauma is significant and, perhaps to some extent, unavoidable. Therefore, every reasonable step should be taken to keep this concern to a minimum. Perform the procedure as carefully as possible, and be certain that it is being performed for the right reason.

After accessing the joint, the techniques of operative arthroscopy for the hip mostly employ existing strategies established in other joints. However, because of the restraints imposed by the hip, technical deficiencies may be more apparent. With the technique described here and in previous literature (3–8), arthroscopy has been successfully performed in more than 300 consecutive cases. However, this may reflect more on successful patient selection rather than the superior merits of this particular technique. The surgeon must be cognizant of the contraindications to arthroscopy, including factors that may preclude access to the joint (see Chapter 54).

GENERAL SETUP

Anesthesia

The procedure is usually performed with the patient under general anesthesia. Epidural anesthesia is an appropriate alternative, but an adequate motor block is necessary to ensure muscle relaxation.

J. W. T. Byrd: Southern Sports Medicine & Orthopaedic Center, Department of Orthopaedics and Rehabilitation, Vanderbilt University School of Medicine, Nashville, Tennessee.

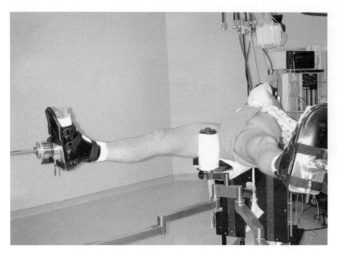

FIGURE 57.1 The patient is positioned on the fracture table so that the perineal post is placed as far laterally as possible toward the operative hip, resting against the medial thigh.

Patient Positioning

The patient is placed supine on the fracture table. A generously sized (12-cm diameter) perineal post made of well cushioned material is used. After the patient is placed against the post, the pelvis and trunk are then shifted away from the operative side of the table (Fig. 57.1). This lateralizes the post against the medial thigh of the operative leg, thus creating a slight lateral component to the direction of the traction vector (Fig. 57.2). This also distances the point of contact from the pudendal nerve, lessening the likelihood of transient neuropraxia.

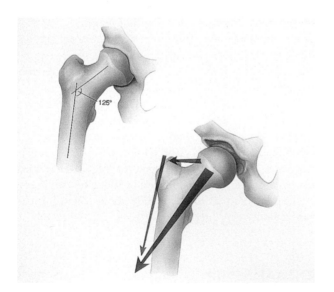

FIGURE 57.2 The optimal vector for distraction is oblique relative to the axis of the body and more closely coincides with the axis of the femoral neck than the femoral shaft. This oblique vector is partially created by abduction of the hip and partially accentuated by a small transverse component to the vector. (From Byrd JWT. The supine position. In: Byrd JWT, ed. *Operative hip arthroscopy.* New York: Thieme, 1998:123–138, with permission.)

The operative hip is positioned in extension and approximately 25 degrees of abduction. Slight flexion might help to relax the capsule, but it can make the sciatic nerve more vulnerable to stretch or unnecessarily draw it closer to the joint. Therefore, flexion is avoided during arthroscopy. Neutral rotation of the extremity during portal placement is essential, but freedom of rotation of the foot plate during arthroscopy facilitates visualization of the femoral head.

The contralateral extremity is abducted as necessary to accommodate positioning of the image intensifier between the legs. The contralateral foot is anchored with slight traction to provide a counterforce, which keeps the pelvis from shifting during distraction of the operative hip.

Traction is then applied to the operative extremity and distraction of the hip joint is confirmed by fluoroscopic examination. Adequate distraction typically requires 25 to 50 lb of traction. More force may be necessary for a tight hip but should be undertaken with some caution.

If adequate distraction is not readily achieved, allowing a few minutes for the capsule to accommodate to the tensile forces often results in relaxation of the capsule and adequate distraction without excessive force. Also, a vacuum phenomenon will be apparent fluoroscopically. This is created by the negative intracapsular pressure caused by distraction. This seal will be released when the joint is distended with fluid at the time of surgery and may further facilitate distraction. However, the effect is variable and should not be relied on to overcome inadequate traction (9).

Once the ability to distract the hip joint has been confirmed, the traction is released. The hip is then prepared and draped, and traction is reapplied when the team is ready to begin arthroscopy (Fig. 57.3). The surgeon, assistant, and scrub nurse are positioned on the operative side of the patient. The monitor and arthroscopy cart with an attached

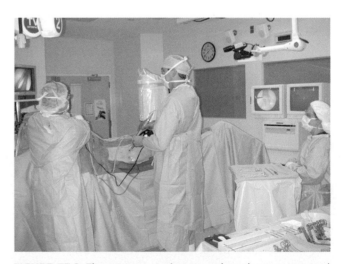

FIGURE 57.3 The surgeon, assistant, and scrub nurse are positioned on the operative side. The arthroscopy cart with monitor is on the nonoperative side. The C-arm, covered in a sterile drape, is positioned between the patient's legs with the fluoroscopic monitor at the foot.

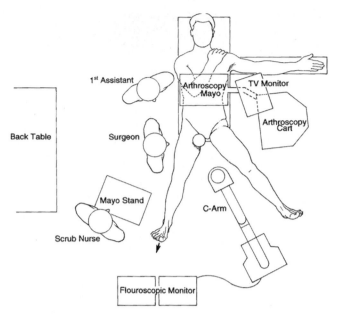

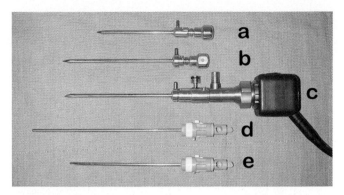

FIGURE 57.5 A standard arthroscopic cannula **(a)** is compared with the extra-length cannula **(b)**. A modified bridge **(c)** has been shortened to accommodate the extra-length cannula with a standard-length arthroscope. Extra-length blades **(d)** are also available and are compared with the standard-length blades **(e)**.

FIGURE 57.4 Schematic drawing of the operating room layout showing the position of the surgeon, assistant, scrub nurse, arthroscopy cart, monitor, Mayo stand, scrub nurse's Mayo stand, C-arm, and back table. (From Byrd JWT. The supine position. In: Byrd JWT, ed. *Operative hip arthroscopy.* New York: Thieme, 1998:123–138, with permission.)

sterile Mayo stand containing the video-articulated arthroscopes and power shaver are positioned on the contralateral side (Fig. 57.4).

Equipment

The image intensifier is routinely used for all cases. This is important for ensuring portal placement in the most accurate fashion.

Patient positioning for hip arthroscopy is simple and can be accommodated with any standard fracture table. An oversized, heavily padded perineal post more effectively distributes the pressure on the perineum and facilitates lateralization of the operative hip. The configuration of the post and positioning minimizes the risk of pressure neuropraxia of the pudendal nerve. A tensiometer is a valuable tool that can be incorporated into the foot plate of the fracture table. Because it must be zeroed after the patient is positioned and before longitudinal traction is applied, it provides a relative, not absolute, value of the traction force. However, the reading does provide an important intraoperative reference of how effectively traction is being maintained.

Both the 30-degree and the 70-degree video-articulated arthroscopes are routinely used to optimize visualization. Interchanging the two arthroscopes allows excellent visualization despite the limited maneuverability caused by the bony architecture of the hip and its dense soft tissue envelope. In general, the 30-degree arthroscope is best for viewing the central portion of the acetabulum and femoral head and the superior portion of the acetabular fossa. The 70-de-

gree arthroscope is best for visualizing the periphery of the joint, the acetabular labrum, and the inferior portion of the acetabular fossa.

A mechanical pump is advantageous for maintaining flow through the hip joint and aids in visualization. Use of a high-flow-rate fluid management system best allows for adequate flow without the use of excessive pressure, which could lead to inordinate extravasation of fluid.

Assorted 4.5-, 5.0-, and 5.5-mm extra-length cannulas are used to accommodate the dense soft tissue envelope that surrounds the hip. A shortened bridge allows use of these cannulas with a standard arthroscope (Fig. 57.5). Special 17-gauge 6-inch spinal needles allow passage of a guide wire into the joint. Special cannulated obturators then allow for passage of the cannula/obturator assembly over the guide wire (Fig. 57.6). The noncannulated obturators are sharper

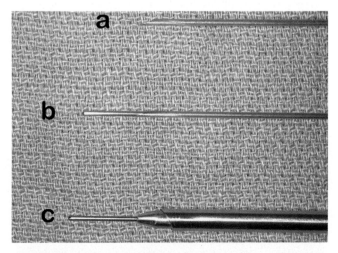

FIGURE 57.6 The cannulated obturator system allows for greater ease in reliably establishing the portals once proper positioning has been achieved with the spinal needle. The 6-inch 17-gauge spinal needle **(a,b)** accommodates passage of a Nitanol wire **(b,c)**. Specially treated, the wire is resistant to kinking. The cannulated obturator allows for passage of the obturator/cannula assembly over the guide wire **(c)**.

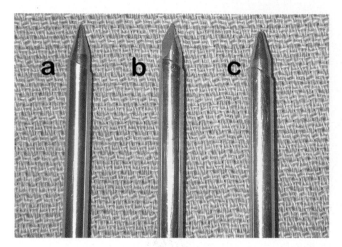

FIGURE 57.7 Close-up view comparing the standard obturator **(a)**, sharp trocar **(b)**, and custom sharp obturator **(c)**. The sharp obturator is better designed to penetrate the capsule while lessening the likelihood of inadvertent articular damage, occasionally attributed to the sharp trocar.

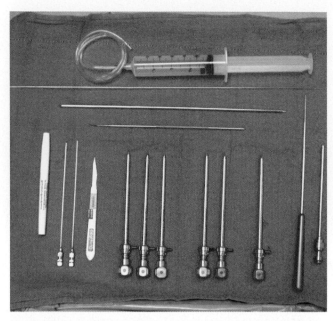

FIGURE 57.9 The nurse's Mayo stand contains basic instruments necessary for initiating the arthroscopic procedure, including a marking pen; no. 11 blade scalpel; 6-inch 17-gauge spinal needles; 60-mL syringe of saline with extension tubing; a Nitanol guide wire; three 4.5-, two 5.0-, and one 5.5-mm cannulas with cannulated and solid obturators; a switching stick; a separate inflow adapter; and a modified probe.

to facilitate penetration of the thick hip capsule, which is more difficult with a standard obturator. Its conical configuration is much more atraumatic than the triflanged tip of a trocar, which can create significant inadvertent articular damage (Fig. 57.7).

Extra-length curved shaver blades have been designed to allow for operative arthroscopy around the convex surface of the femoral head. Extra-length flexible cannulas allow for passage of these curved blades (Fig. 57.8).

Specially designed hand instruments must be sturdy as well as extra-long. The surgeon must avoid the temptation to use extra-length instruments designed for other endoscopic purposes, because they are often more fragile and more vulnerable to breakage when subjected to the manipulation necessary through the dense soft tissue envelope and around the bony contours of the hip joint.

Thermal energy, including the holmium yttrium–aluminum–garnet (YAG) laser and radiofrequency devices, may have particular advantage in the hip. Their maneuverability, despite the constraints imposed by the joint, optimizes access to various regions and often allows more effective tissue ablation than can be achieved with conventional shavers.

The scrub nurse's Mayo stand accommodates the instruments routinely needed for each case (Fig. 57.9). The 5.0-mm cannula is used for initial introduction of the arthroscope. The diameter allows adequate inflow from the fluid management system through the bridge. Once all three portals have been established, the inflow can be switched to one of the other cannulas, and the 5.0-mm cannula can be replaced with a 4.5-mm cannula. The routine use of three 4.5-mm cannulas allows complete interchangeability of the arthroscope, instruments, and inflow. The 5.5-mm cannula is also available for larger shaver blades.

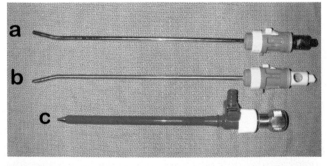

FIGURE 57.8 Extra-length curved blades with both a convex **(a)** and a concave **(b)** direction of the shaver face facilitate instrumentation around the femoral head. Extra-length disposable cannulas **(c)** accommodate these curved blades.

PORTALS

Three portals are used (Figs. 57.10 and 57.11): the anterior, the anterolateral and the posterolateral (10).

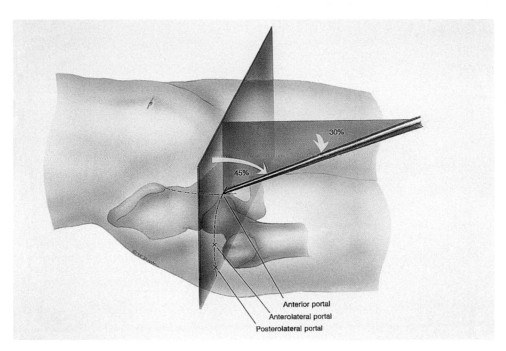

FIGURE 57.10 The site of the anterior portal coincides with the intersection of a sagittal line drawn distally from the anterior superior iliac spine and a transverse line across the superior margin of the greater trochanter. The direction of this portal courses approximately 45 degrees cephalad and 30 degrees towards the midline. The anterolateral and posterolateral portals are positioned directly over the superior aspect of the trochanter at its anterior and posterior borders. (From Byrd JWT. The supine position. In: Byrd JWT, ed. *Operative hip arthroscopy.* New York: Thieme, 1998:123–138, with permission.)

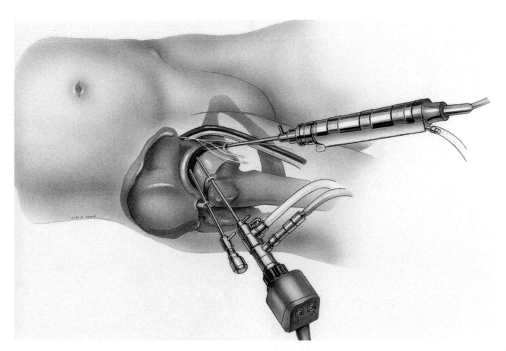

FIGURE 57.11 The relationship of the major neurovascular structures to the three standard portals is demonstrated. The femoral artery and nerve lie well medial to the anterior portal. The sciatic nerve lies posterior to the posterolateral portal. The lateral femoral cutaneous nerve lies close to the anterior portal. Injury to this structure is avoided by the use of proper technique in portal placement. The anterolateral portal is established first, because it lies most centrally in the safe zone for arthroscopy. (From Byrd JWT. The supine position. In: Byrd JWT, ed. *Operative hip arthroscopy.* New York: Thieme, 1998:123–138, with permission.)

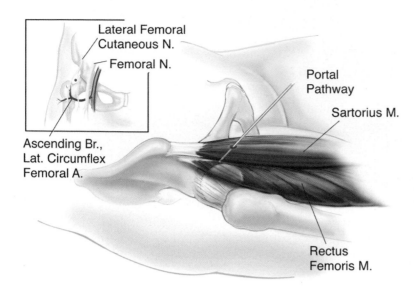

FIGURE 57.12 Anterior portal pathway and relationship to lateral femoral cutaneous nerve, femoral nerve, and lateral circumflex femoral artery. (Courtesy of Smith & Nephew Endoscopy, Andover, Massachusetts.)

Anterior Portal

The anterior portal (Fig. 57.12) lies an average of 6.3 cm distal to the anterior superior iliac spine. It penetrates the muscle belly of the sartorius and the rectus femoris before entering through the anterior capsule.

Typically, the lateral femoral cutaneous nerve is divided into three or more branches at the level of the anterior portal. The portal usually passes within several millimeters of one of these branches (Fig. 57.13). Because of the multiple branches, the nerve is not easily avoided by altering the portal position, but it is protected by the use of meticulous technique in portal placement. Specifically, it is most vulnerable to a skin incision that is placed too deeply, lacerating one of the branches.

Passing from the skin to the capsule, the anterior portal runs almost tangential to the axis of the femoral nerve and lies only slightly closer at the level of the capsule, with an average minimum distance of 3.2 cm (Fig. 57.14).

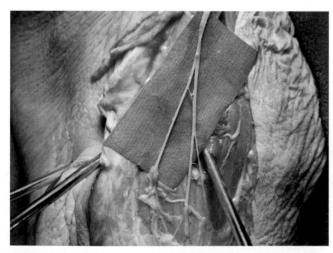

FIGURE 57.13 The relationship of the anterior portal to the multiple branches of the lateral femoral cutaneous nerve. Multiple branches at the level of the portal are characteristic, and the branches always extend lateral to the portal. (From Byrd JWT, Pappas JN, Pedley MJ. Hip arthroscopy: an anatomic study of portal placement and relationship to the extra-articular structures. *Arthroscopy* 1995;11:418–423.)

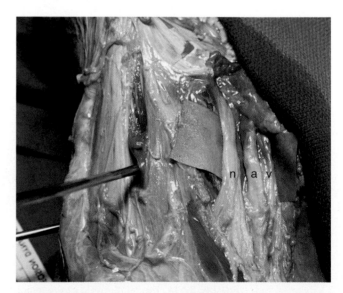

FIGURE 57.14 The femoral nerve **(n)** lies lateral to the femoral artery **(a)** and vein **(v)**. The relationship of the anterior portal as it pierces the sartorius is shown. (From Byrd JWT, Pappas JN, Pedley MJ. Hip arthroscopy: an anatomic study of portal placement and relationship to the extra-articular structures. *Arthroscopy* 1995;11:418–423.)

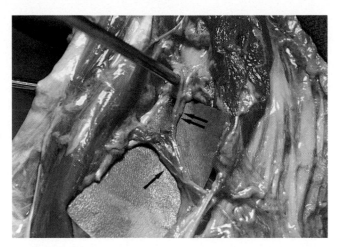

FIGURE 57.15 The ascending branch of the lateral circumflex femoral artery *(arrow)* has an oblique course distal to the anterior portal, seen here at the level of the capsule. This specimen demonstrates a terminal branch *(double arrow)* coursing vertically adjacent to the portal. (From Byrd JWT, Pappas JN, Pedley MJ. Hip arthroscopy: an anatomic study of portal placement and relationship to the extra-articular structures. *Arthroscopy* 1995;11:418–423.)

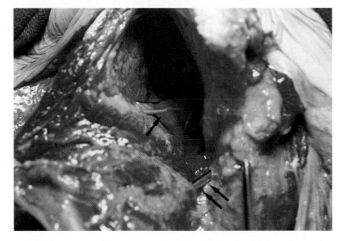

FIGURE 57.17 The superior gluteal nerve *(arrow)* is shown coursing transversely on the deep surface of the gluteus medius. It passes above the anterolateral portal *(double arrow)*, which is seen between the deep surface of the gluteus medius and the capsule. (From Byrd JWT, Pappas JN, Pedley MJ. Hip arthroscopy: an anatomic study of portal placement and relationship to the extra-articular structures. *Arthroscopy* 1995;11:418–423.)

Although variable in its relationship, the ascending branch of the lateral circumflex femoral artery is usually approximately 3.7 cm inferior to the anterior portal (Fig. 57.15). In some cadaver specimens, a small terminal branch of this vessel has been identified lying within millimeters of the portal at the level of the capsule. The clinical significance of this situation is uncertain, and there have been no reported cases of excessive bleeding from the anterior position.

Anterolateral Portal

The anterolateral portal (Fig. 57.16) penetrates the gluteus medius before entering the lateral aspect of the capsule at its anterior margin. The only structure of significance relative to the anterolateral portal is the superior gluteal nerve (Fig. 57.17). After exiting the sciatic notch, it courses transversely, posterior to anterior, across the deep surface of the

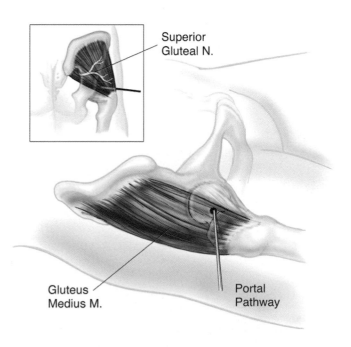

Superior Gluteal N.

Gluteus Medius M.

Portal Pathway

FIGURE 57.16 Anterolateral portal pathway and relationship to superior gluteal nerve. (Courtesy of Smith & Nephew Endoscopy, Andover, Massachusetts.)

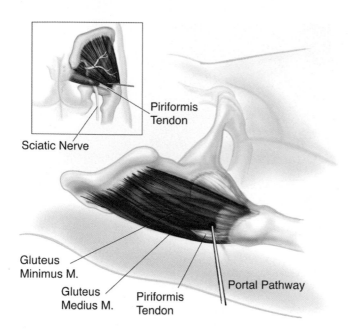

FIGURE 57.18 Posterolateral portal pathway and relationship to the sciatic nerve and superior gluteal nerve. (Courtesy of Smith & Nephew Endoscopy, Andover, Massachusetts.)

gluteus medius. Its relationship to both of the lateral portals is the same, with an average distance of 4.4 cm.

Posterolateral Portal

The posterolateral portal (Fig. 57.18) penetrates both the gluteus medius and the gluteus minimus before entering the lateral capsule at its posterior margin. Its course is superior and anterior to the piriformis tendon (Fig. 57.19). It lies closest to the sciatic nerve at the level of the capsule. The distance to the lateral edge of the nerve averages 2.9 cm.

SURGICAL PROCEDURE FOR NORMAL ARTHROSCOPIC EXAMINATION

The anterolateral portal is placed first because it lies most centrally in the "safe zone" for arthroscopy (10). Subsequent portal placements are aided by direct arthroscopic visualization. This initial portal is placed with the use of fluoroscopic inspection in the anteroposterior plane. However, orientation in the lateral plane is equally important. With the leg in neutral rotation, femoral anteversion leaves the center of the

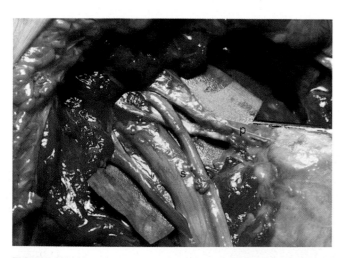

FIGURE 57.19 The relationship of the posterolateral portal to the piriformis tendon (p) and the sciatic nerve (s). Note the anomaly in which the sciatic nerve is formed from three divisions distal to the sciatic notch and the most lateral division passes through a split muscle belly of the piriformis. (From Byrd JWT, Pappas JN, Pedley MJ. Hip arthroscopy: an anatomic study of portal placement and relationship to the extra-articular structures. *Arthroscopy* 1995;11:418–423.)

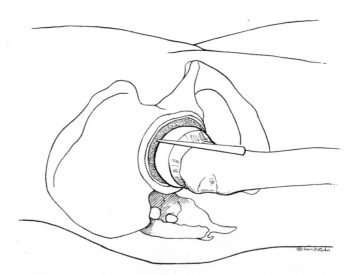

FIGURE 57.20 With the patient supine, the hip is in neutral rotation with the kneecap pointing toward the ceiling. A needle placed at the anterior margin of the greater trochanter (anterolateral position) is maintained in the coronal plane by keeping it parallel to the floor as it enters the joint. Because of femoral neck anteversion, the entry site will be just anterior to the joint's center. If the entry site is too anterior, it becomes crowded with the anterior portal. If it is too posterior, it becomes difficult to properly visualize the entry site for the anterior portal.

joint just anterior to the center of the greater trochanter. Therefore, the entry site for the anterolateral portal at the anterior margin of the greater trochanter corresponds to entry of the joint just anterior to its midportion. This correct entry site of the joint is achieved by keeping the instrumentation parallel to the floor during portal placement (Fig. 57.20).

When the hip is distracted, a vacuum phenomenon is often present (Fig. 57.21A). Prepositioning for the anterolateral portal is performed with a 6-inch 17-gauge spinal needle under fluoroscopic control (Fig. 57.21B). The joint is then distended with approximately 40 mL of fluid, and the intracapsular position of the needle is confirmed by back-

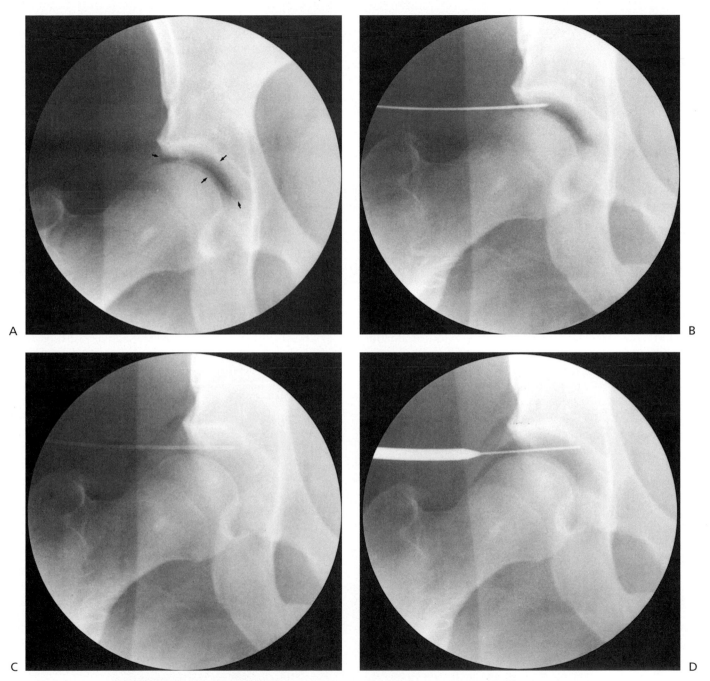

FIGURE 57.21 Anteroposterior fluoroscopic view of a right hip. **A:** A vacuum effect is apparent. It results from the negative intracapsular pressure created by distraction of the joint *(arrows).* **B:** A spinal needle is used in prepositioning for the anterolateral portal. The needle courses above the superior tip of the trochanter and then passes under the lateral lip of the acetabulum, entering the hip joint. **C:** Distention of the joint disrupts the vacuum and facilitates adequate distraction. **D:** The cannula/obturator assembly is passed over the Nitanol wire that was placed through the spinal needle. (From Byrd JWT. The supine position. In: Byrd JWT, ed. *Operative hip arthroscopy.* New York: Thieme, 1998:123–138, with permission.)

flow of fluid. Distention of the joint enhances distraction (Fig. 57.21C).

It is easy for the needle to inadvertently penetrate the lateral acetabular labrum during initial placement into the joint (11). This can be felt as pushing the needle through the labrum, in greater resistance than when just penetrating the capsule. If the needle pierces the labrum, once the joint has been distended, it is a simple process to back the needle up and reenter the capsule below the level of the labrum. Failure to recognize this situation can result in avoidable violation of the labrum by the cannula.

A stab wound is made through the skin at the entrance site of the needle. The guide wire is placed through the needle. The needle is then removed, leaving the wire in place. The cannulated obturator with the 5.0-mm arthroscopy cannula is passed over the wire into the joint (Fig. 57.21D).

While the portal is being established, the cannula/obturator assembly should pass close to the superior tip of the greater trochanter and then directly above the convex surface of the femoral head. It is important to keep the assembly off the femoral head to avoid inadvertent articular surface scuffing.

Initially, a variable amount of blood will be present within the joint owing to the distraction force necessary for separating the surfaces. This may be difficult to clear until a separate egress has been established. Simple venting with the spinal needle from anterior usually clears the field of view.

Once the arthroscope has been introduced, the anterior portal is placed; positioning is facilitated by visualization from the arthroscope as well as fluoroscopy. The 70-degree arthroscope works best for directly viewing where the instrumentation penetrates the capsule. Prepositioning is again performed with the 17-gauge spinal needle, entering the joint directly underneath the free edge of the anterior labrum. As the cannula/obturator assembly is introduced, it is lifted up to stay off the articular surface of the femoral head while passing underneath the acetabular labrum.

If proper attention has been given to the topographic anatomy in positioning the anterior portal, the femoral nerve will lie well medial to the approach (10). However, the lateral femoral cutaneous nerve lies quite close to this portal. It is best avoided by the use of proper technique in portal placement. The nerve is most vulnerable to laceration by a skin incision that is placed too deeply.

Rarely (less than 2% of cases in the series reviewed), access from the anterior portal is blocked by an overlying osteophyte or simply the architecture of the patient's acetabular bony anatomy. If necessary, arthroscopy can still be effectively performed by simply using the lateral two portals.

Lastly, the posterolateral portal is introduced. The fluoroscopic guidelines are similar to those for the anterolateral portal. Simply rotating the lens of the arthroscope posteriorly brings into view the site of entry underneath the posterior labrum. Placement under arthroscopic control is especially helpful to ensure that the instruments do not stray

posteriorly, potentially placing the sciatic nerve at risk. It is also important that the hip remain in neutral rotation during placement of the posterolateral portal. External rotation of the hip moves the greater trochanter more posteriorly. The trochanter is the main topographic landmark, and this mistake can place the sciatic nerve at greater risk for injury (Fig. 57.22).

Interchange of the instruments and arthroscope among the three established portals facilitates systematic examination and operative arthroscopy about the hip. Release of the capsule around the portal sites with an arthroscopic knife passed through the cannula improves maneuverability within the joint.

With the use of both the 30-degree and the 70-degree video-articulated arthroscopes, the structures that can dependably be visualized include the superior weight-bearing portion of the acetabulum; the fossa; the ligamentum teres; and the anterior, posterior and lateral aspects of the acetabular labrum. Most of the weight-bearing articular portion of the femoral head can be seen; visualization is facilitated by internal and external rotation of the hip intraoperatively.

The anterior wall and anterior labrum are best visualized through the anterolateral portal (Fig. 57.23). The posterior wall and posterior labrum are best visualized through the posterolateral portal (Fig. 57.24). The lateral labrum and its capsular reflection are best visualized through the anterior portal (Fig. 57.25). The fossa and ligamentum teres (Fig. 57.26) can usually be visualized through all three portals, with a different perspective from each.

To a lesser degree, the inferior aspect of the acetabulum and femoral head below the ligamentum teres, the inferior capsule, and the transverse acetabular ligament can be visualized (Fig. 57.27).

At the completion of the procedure, the traction is immediately released. The portals are reapproximated with nylon sutures, and a sterile dressing is applied.

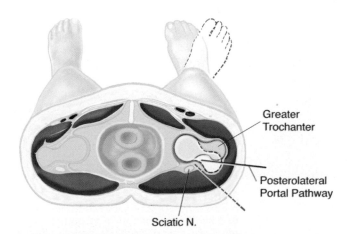

FIGURE 57.22 Neutral rotation of the operative hip is essential for protection of the sciatic nerve during placement of the posterolateral portal. (Courtesy of Smith & Nephew Endoscopy, Andover, Massachusetts.)

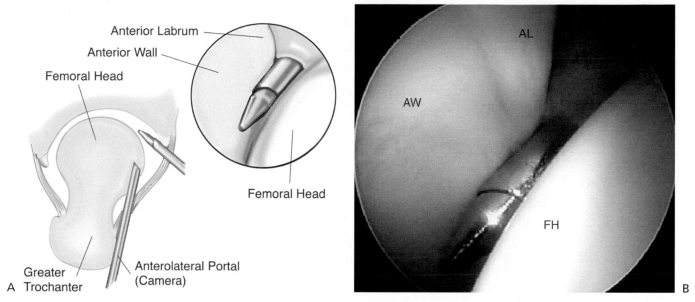

FIGURE 57.23 A: Arthroscopic view of a right hip from the anterolateral portal. (Courtesy of Smith & Nephew Endoscopy, Andover, Massachusetts.) **B:** Demonstrated are the anterior acetabular wall (AW) and the anterior labrum (AL). The anterior cannula is seen entering underneath the labrum, and the femoral head (FH) is on the right. (From Byrd JWT. The supine position. In: Byrd JWT, ed. *Operative hip arthroscopy*. New York: Thieme, 1998:123–138, with permission.)

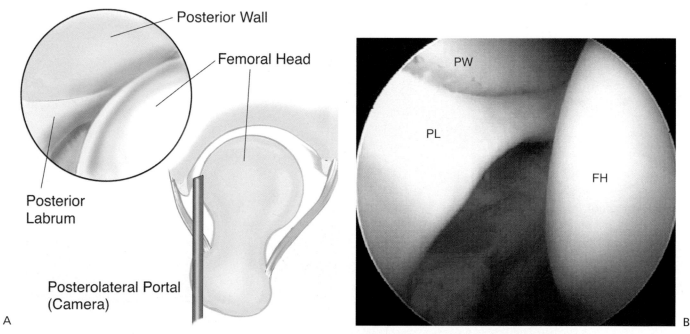

FIGURE 57.24 A: Arthroscopic view from the posterolateral portal. (Courtesy of Smith & Nephew Endoscopy, Andover, Massachusetts.) **B:** Demonstrated are the posterior acetabular wall (PW), posterior labrum (PL), and femoral head (FH). (Reprinted by permission.)

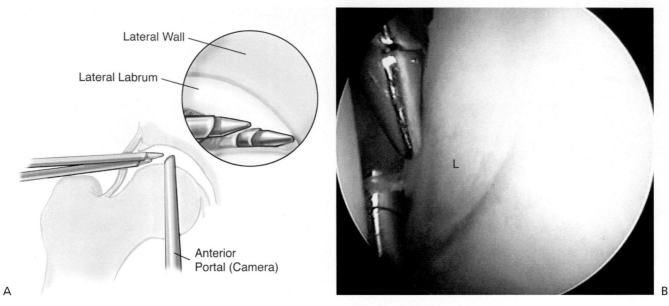

A

B

FIGURE 57.25 A: Arthroscopic view from the anterior portal. (Courtesy of Smith & Nephew Endoscopy, Andover, Massachusetts.) **B:** Demonstrated are the lateral aspect of the labrum (L) and its relationship to the lateral two portals. (From Byrd JWT. The supine position. In: Byrd JWT, ed. *Operative hip arthroscopy.* New York: Thieme, 1998:123–138, with permission.)

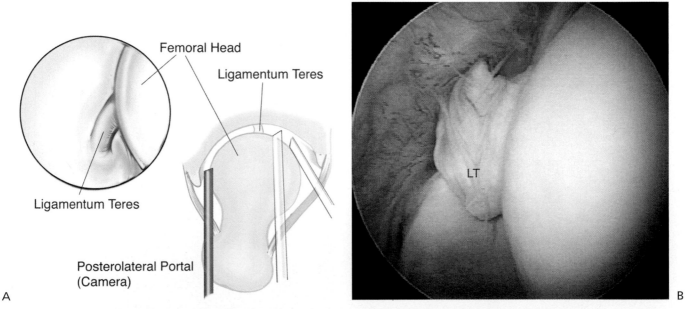

A

B

FIGURE 57.26 A: The acetabular fossa can be inspected from all three portals. (Courtesy of Smith & Nephew Endoscopy, Andover, Massachusetts.) **B:** The ligamentum teres (LT), with its accompanying vessels, has a serpentine course from its acetabular attachments. (From Byrd JWT. The supine position. In: Byrd JWT, ed. *Operative hip arthroscopy.* New York: Thieme, 1998:123–138, with permission.)

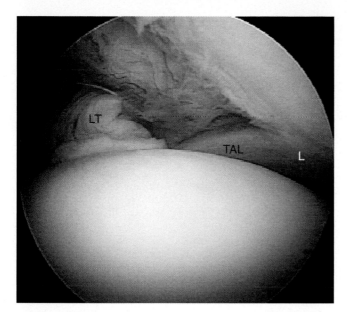

FIGURE 57.27 View from the anterior portal demonstrates where the inferior aspect of the anterior labrum (L) becomes contiguous with the transverse acetabular ligament (TAL) below the ligamentum teres (LT). (From Byrd JWT. The supine position. In: Byrd JWT, ed. *Operative hip arthroscopy.* New York: Thieme, 1998:123–138, with permission.)

POSTOPERATIVE CARE

Immediate ambulation is allowed. Crutches are typically used for 3 to 7 days until the gait pattern is normalized. For degenerative disease, protected weight bearing may be continued to tolerance for approximately 2 weeks. Only grade IV articular lesions addressed with abrasion arthroplasty or microfracture are kept on a strict protected weight-bearing status, which is maintained for 8 to 10 weeks.

The dressing is removed on the first postoperative day and replaced with Band-Aids. Portal sutures are removed within a few days. Supervised rehabilitation is implemented to facilitate and optimize recovery (12–14).

COMPLICATIONS

Among 265 consecutive procedures performed by this method, a total of 3 complications were encountered in 2 patients. One patient with numerous intraarticular loose bodies retrieved from the anterior portal developed a localized area of heterotopic ossification within the portal tract and neuropraxia of one branch of the lateral femoral cutaneous nerve. Another patient also developed a partial transient neuropraxia of the lateral femoral cutaneous nerve with complete resolution. Additionally, one patient simply felt that she was made worse as a consequence of the surgery; although not a complication, this is certainly a reason to give pause in the course of considering hip arthroscopy.

REFERENCES

1. Byrd JWT. Complications associated with hip arthroscopy. In: Byrd JWT, ed. *Operative hip arthroscopy.* New York: Thieme, 1998:171–176.
2. Bartlett CS, DiFelice GS, Buly RL, et al. Cardiac arrest as a result of intraabdominal extravasation of fluid during arthroscopic removal of a loose body from the hip joint of a patient with an acetabular fracture. *J Orthop Trauma* 1998;12:294–299.
3. Byrd JWT. Hip arthroscopy utilizing the supine position. *Arthroscopy* 1994;10:275–280.
4. Byrd JWT. The supine position. In: Byrd JWT, ed. *Operative hip arthroscopy.* New York: Thieme, 1998:123–138.
5. Byrd JWT. Diagnostic and operative arthroscopy of the hip. In: Andrews J, Timmerman L, eds. *Diagnostic and operative arthroscopy.* Philadelphia: WB Saunders, 1997:209–224.
6. Byrd JWT. *Hip arthroscopy: principles and application.* Andover, MA: Smith & Nephew Endoscopy, 1996.
7. Byrd JWT. Arthroscopy of the hip and applications: supine position. In: Chow JC, ed. *Advanced arthroscopy.* New York: Springer-Verlag, 2000:293–321.
8. Byrd JWT. *Operative hip arthroscopy* [Videotape]. New York: Thieme, 1998.
9. Byrd JWT, Chern KY. Traction vs. distension for distraction of the hip joint during arthroscopy. *Arthroscopy* 1997;13:346–349.
10. Byrd JWT, Pappas JN, Pedley MJ. Hip arthroscopy: an anatomic study of portal placement and relationship to the extra-articular structures. *Arthroscopy* 1995;11:418–423.
11. Byrd JWT. Avoiding the labrum in hip arthroscopy. *Arthroscopy* 2000;16:770–773.
12. Griffin KM, Henry CO, Byrd JWT. Rehabilitation after hip arthroscopy. *J Sport Rehabil* 2000;9:77–88.
13. Griffin KM, Henry CO, Byrd JWT. Rehabilitation. In: Byrd JWT, ed. *Operative hip arthroscopy.* New York: Thieme, 1998: 177–202.
14. Henry C, Middleton K, Byrd JWT. Hip rehabilitation following arthroscopy [Videotape]. Presented at the IOI Theater, American Academy of Orthopaedic Surgeons Annual Meeting, Orlando, FL, February 1995.

58

THE LATERAL APPROACH
TO THE HIP JOINT

JAMES M. GLICK
THOMAS G. SAMPSON

Since we first developed and reported on the arthroscopic lateral approach to the hip joint (1,2) we have been able to refine the technique so that the procedure is easier to perform. Initially, the arthroscopies were performed with the patient supine on a fracture table. We found it difficult to insert the arthroscope so that the hip could be completely visualized in two situations—in obese patients, and in those with spurs on the anterolateral aspect of the acetabulum. In fact, it was the inability to remove posterior inferior loose bodies in an obese patient that prompted us to develop the direct lateral approach. The fat drops away from the operative site when patients are placed on their sides, and the portals then provide a direct entry into the hip joint. The posterior portal in particular allows the surgeon to easily gain access to the joint when a large spur blocks the other portals of entrance. Our experience is based on more than 550 hip arthroscopies using the lateral approach.

OPERATIVE ROOM SETUP

The room setup is depicted in Fig. 58.1. The patient is on his or her side on an operating table. The foot is connected to the traction device. A padded post is placed in the perineum for countertraction. An image intensifier (fluoroscope) is positioned around the hip for anteroposterior views. After all the portals are completed, the image intensifier can be removed. The surgeon stands in front of the patient. The video monitor, image intensifier screen, and power and fluid pump equipment are to the rear of the patient so that the surgeon can view the television screen and the various LED readings comfortably. The nurse stands on the side and a little in back of the surgeon.

J. M. Glick: Department of Orthopaedic Surgery, University of California, San Francisco, California

T. G. Sampson: Department of Orthopaedic Surgery, University of California, San Francisco, and Healthsouth Surgery Center: Medical Direct, Total Joint Center, Saint Francis Memorial Hospital, San Francisco, California

Hip arthroscopy, whether performed in the lateral or in the supine position, requires extra-long and curved instruments. A longer arthroscope and longer instruments permit deeper penetration into the joint. Curved shavers and graspers should be available to reach underneath the circular femoral head and gain access to the corners and depths of the hip joint. Electrothermal or laser devices are also useful for reaching and cutting pathologic tissue that is obstructed by the curve of the acetabulum or is deep and in the corners of the joint. A slotted cannula helps in directing curved and malleable instruments into the joint (Fig. 58.2). Special traction devices are now available, but a fracture table can be used just as effectively (3) (Fig. 58.3). No matter what traction device is used, the safety factors to prevent neuropraxia of the sciatic and pudendal nerves must be adhered to.

TECHNIQUE

The patient, under general anesthesia or an epidural block, is placed in the lateral decubitus position with the hip to be treated on top. The foot is strapped into the distraction device, which places the hip in abduction (Fig. 58.4). The hip is then positioned in slight abduction, flexion, and external rotation to relax the capsule. If there is a hip flexion or adduction contracture, then the hip must be left in that position in order to distract the hip adequately with a safe amount of traction. The perineal post placed between the legs is pushed upward against the medial portion of the thigh on the involved leg. This produces slight upward distraction and keeps the post away from the branch of the pudendal nerve that crosses over the ischium. Two portals are made over the greater trochanter and one directly anterior (Fig. 58.5). Additional portals can be made, but instrument crowding may become a problem. Extra-long spinal needles are inserted into the skin at the planned portal sites to ensure accurate placement of the incisions. Important arteries and nerves are safely away from the insertion sites (Fig. 58.6). Branches of the lateral femoral

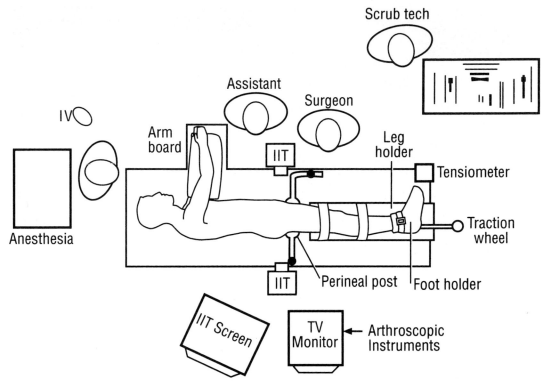

FIGURE 58.1 Room setup. Patient is in the left lateral decubitus position with the right hip upward. Note that the surgeon is working in front of the patient with the arthroscopic technician.

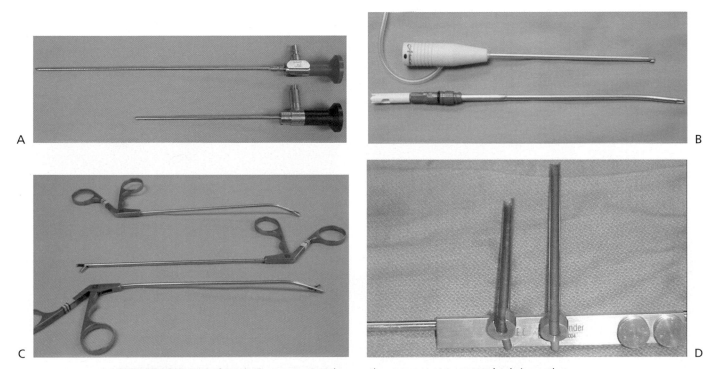

FIGURE 58.2 Extra-long instruments. **A:** A long arthroscope next to a standard-size arthroscope. **B:** A long curved shaver and an electrosurgical device. **C:** A long straight and curved graspers. **D:** Slotted cannulas.

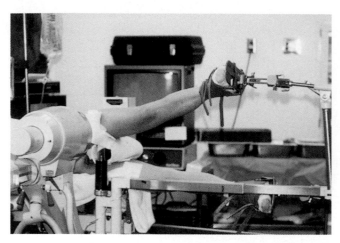

FIGURE 58.3 Patient in the lateral decubitus position on a fracture table. (From Glick JM. Hip arthroscopy: lateral approach. In: Parisien JS, ed. *Therapeutic arthroscopy.* New York: Raven Press; 1993:22.1–22.10, with permission.)

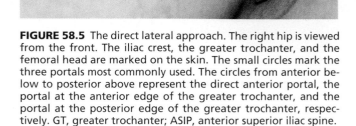

FIGURE 58.5 The direct lateral approach. The right hip is viewed from the front. The iliac crest, the greater trochanter, and the femoral head are marked on the skin. The small circles mark the three portals most commonly used. The circles from anterior below to posterior above represent the direct anterior portal, the portal at the anterior edge of the greater trochanter, and the portal at the posterior edge of the greater trochanter, respectively. GT, greater trochanter; ASIP, anterior superior iliac spine.

cutaneous nerve are near but not dangerously close to the direct anterior portal.

First, the hip is sterilely prepared and draped. The image intensifier should be draped out of the surgical field. Next, enough traction is applied to distract the hip at least 12 mm as noted on the image intensifier. The surgeon should not hesitate to apply more traction if necessary, but after all instruments have been inserted the traction should be reduced

back to 50 to 75 lb. After the traction is brought back to a safer level the distraction will remain, owing to muscle relaxation. Once the hip has been distracted sufficiently, an extra-long spinal needle is inserted over the anterior edge of the greater trochanter and advanced down the neck of the femur into the hip joint. A definite "give" is felt when the capsule is penetrated and the bony floor of the acetabulum then stops the needle. At this point, the position of the nee-

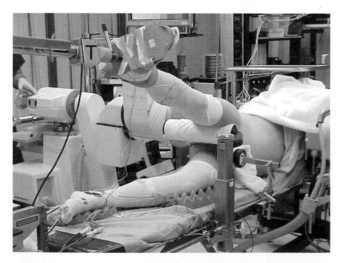

FIGURE 58.4 The right leg of a patient positioned in the foot piece of a traction device. The leg is positioned in slight flexion, abduction, and external rotation in order to relax the hip capsule. The perineal post is positioned upward against the medial side of the thigh so that it applies slight upward distraction and does not rest against the branch of the pudendal nerve that crosses over the ischium. (From Glick JM. Hip arthroscopy by the lateral approach. *Clin Sports Med* 2001;20:733–747, with permission.)

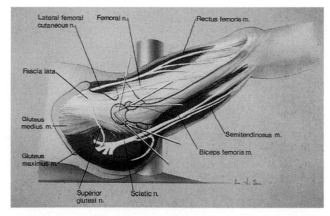

FIGURE 58.6 A diagram of the important nerves around the hip joint and their relations to the portals used for hip arthroscopy by the lateral approach. (From Glick JM. Complications of hip arthroscopy by the lateral approach. In: Sherman OH, Minkoff J, eds. *Arthroscopic surgery,* 1st ed. Baltimore: Williams & Wilkins; 1990:193–201, with permission.)

dle in the hip joint is verified with the image intensifier. If the joint has not been entered, the needle is manipulated into the joint under image intensification. Next, the stylet is removed and a syringe is used to inject 10 to 15 mL of room air into the joint to break the suction seal. Once the suction seal is broken, the hip will relax and more distraction will occur (Fig. 58.7). At this time, the hip is aspirated to deter-

mine whether fluid is present. Next, a Nitanol guide wire is inserted into the needle (Fig. 58.8) and the needle is removed, leaving the guide wire in the hip joint. With the guide wire in place, an incision is made around it with a no. 11 blade. Then, the arthroscopic sheath with its cannulated sharp stylet is introduced over the wire. In order to prevent damage to the articular cartilage, the advancement of the

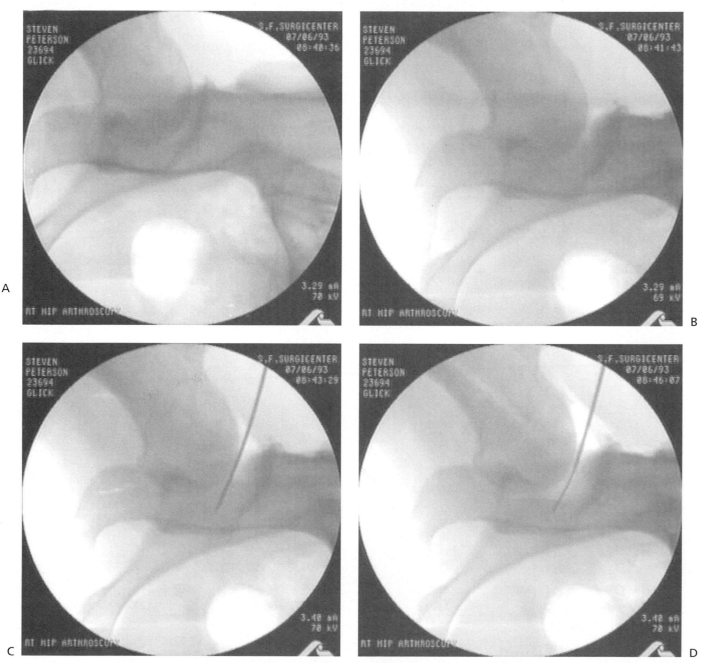

FIGURE 58.7 Fluoroscopic images of a right hip before and after the initial distraction. **A:** The hip without distraction. **B:** The hip distracted after the application of 50 to 75 lb of traction. **C:** The hip is distracted more after a needle is inserted and the suction seal is broken. **D:** The hip is distracted further after 10 mL of room air has been inserted with a syringe. (A and D from Glick JM. Hip arthroscopy by the lateral approach. *Clin Sports Med* 2001;20:733–747, with permission.)

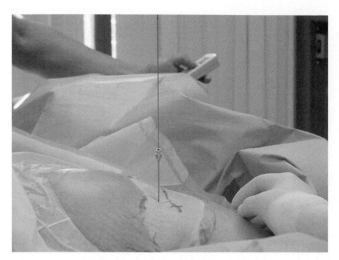

FIGURE 58.8 A Nitanol guide wire inserted into an extra-long spinal needle in the anterior paratrochanteric portal. (From Glick JM. Hip arthroscopy by the lateral approach. *Clin Sports Med* 2001;20:733–747, with permission.)

sheath and trocar is controlled by twisting the trocar and by watching its progress on the image intensifier (Fig. 58.9). Once the sheath is within the confines of the capsule, the trocar and wire are removed and the 30-degree fore-oblique arthroscope is coupled to it.

Most of the time, viewing the hip with its ambient air is all that is necessary to continue the next steps. If visualization is poor, fluid should be inserted through the stopcock on the arthroscope sheath to clean the joint. With the arthroscope in place, two more extra-long spinal needles are inserted in a similar manner, one over the posterior aspect of

the greater trochanter and the other directly anterior under direct vision. The surgeon must make sure that these two needles do not pierce the labrum. A 70-degree fore-oblique arthroscope is used if the edge of the acetabulum and the labrum are not well visualized with the 30-degree fore-oblique arthroscope. (4) When the other two needles are visualized within the joint, the image intensifier may be removed and the rest of the procedure performed under direct vision. Now, fluid is allowed to flow into the joint through the arthroscope sheath and outflow occurs through one of the remaining needles. We like to use the needle in the direct anterior portal for outflow and develop the posterior peritrochanteric portal as our first working portal. The process is then repeated for the posterior peritrochanteric portal. In most instances, the deep portions of the hip joint can be reached through the two peritrochanteric portals. If not, the anterior portal can be developed in the same manner as the two paratrochanteric portals (Fig. 58.10).

The last step is to widen the capsular portion of each portal, to increase instrument mobility and to improve access to all portions of the hip joint. To do so, an arthroscopic knife is inserted under direct vision and the capsule is cut in all directions as far as possible (Fig. 58.11). In addition, cutting the capsule permits easy passage of all instruments into the joint without maintaining the portal with a cannula. Usually, a curved shaver can easily be inserted into the joint once the capsule has been cut. However, a slotted cannula makes it easier to insert a curved instrument. Before the arthro-

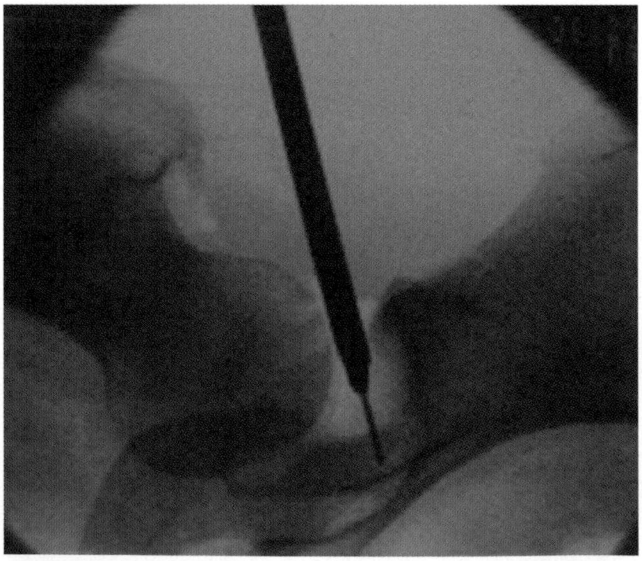

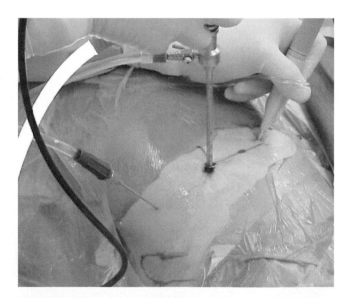

FIGURE 58.10 A view of a right hip from the head of the patient showing the three main portals for hip arthroscopy by the lateral approach. The arthroscope is in the anterior paratrochanteric portal, an electrothermal instrument is in the posterior peritrochanteric portal, and an extra-long spinal needle used for fluid outflow is in the direct anterior portal. GT, greater trochanter; ASIS, anterior superior iliac spine. (From Glick JM. Hip arthroscopy by the lateral approach. *Clin Sports Med* 2001;20: 733–747, with permission.)

FIGURE 58.9 Fluoroscopic view of the arthroscope sheath with its cannulated trocar over the guide wire in the hip joint (From Glick JM. Hip arthroscopy by the lateral approach. *Clin Sports Med* 2001;20:733–747, with permission.)

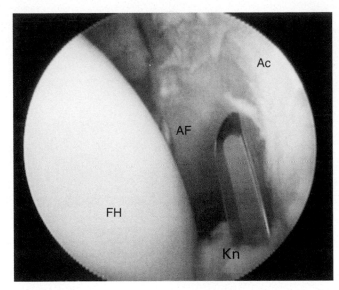

FIGURE 58.11 Cutting and elongating the right hip capsule with an arthroscopic knife. The knife is in the portal over the anterior edge of the greater trochanter, and the arthroscope is viewing from the posterior portal. FH, femoral head; Ac, acetabulum; AF, acetabular fossa; Kn, knife blade.

scopic knife is removed, a slotted cannula is inserted over it and the cannula is observed entering the joint. Then, the knife is removed and the curved instrument is directed along the slotted cannula (Fig. 58.12). Once the curved device is in the joint, the slotted cannula is removed so that the instrument can be moved freely around the joint. Before the curved instrument is removed, the slotted cannula is reinserted over it to maintain the portal.

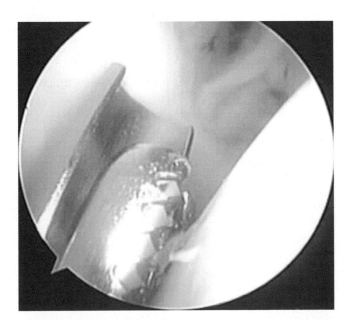

FIGURE 58.12 A view of a slotted cannula with a curved shaver entering the left hip through a direct anterior portal.

To visualize the periphery or capsular portion of the hip, the arthroscope is pulled back and the traction is reduced until the head retracts into the acetabulum. The contour of the femoral head is kept in sight. Then, a capsulotomy is performed with a motorized cutter and an electrothermal ablator. I have found that cuts made with the new high-radiofrequency ablators not only remove the synovium but also "marbleize" the tissue, so that the motorized cutters work more efficiently. The capsule is trimmed proximal and distally so that the junction of the head and the neck is easily visualized (Fig. 58.13). Debridement and synovectomy

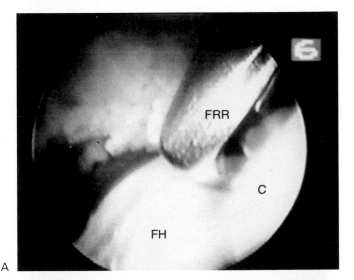

A

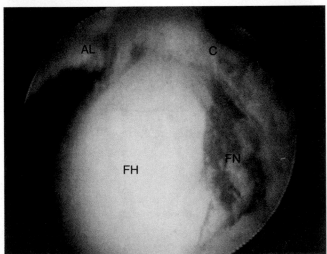

B

FIGURE 58.13 Views of the periphery of the hip joint. **A:** Trimming the capsule around the periphery of the left hip with a motorized full-radius resector inserted through the portal at the anterior edge of the greater trochanter. The arthroscope is viewing from the posterior portal. The traction has been reduced. **B:** View of the head–neck junction after resection of the capsule. FRR, full-radius resector; AL, acetabular labrum; FH, femoral head; FN, femoral neck; C, capsule. (From Glick JM. Arthroscopic surgery of the hip. In: Chapman MN, ed. *Operative orthopaedics*, 2nd ed. Philadelphia: JB Lippincott; 1993;2391–2401, with permission.)

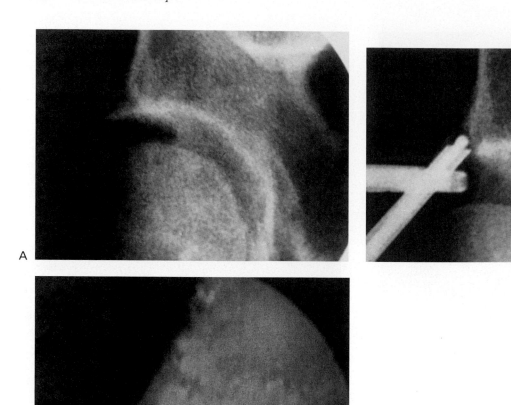

FIGURE 58.14 Resection of an anterior acetabular spur. **A:** Fluoroscopic view of the spur at surgery. **B:** Fluoroscopic view of the abrader cutting the spur. The abrader is in the portal at the anterior edge of the trochanter, and the arthroscope is viewing through the portal at the posterior edge of the trochanter. **C:** Arthroscopic view of the abrader removing the anterior spur. AR, acetabular rim; AB, abrader.

in this area are easily performed. Surgical instruments and the arthroscope can be interchanged among any of the portals. By rotating, adducting, abducting, flexing, and extending the leg and transferring the arthroscope to each portal, the surgeon can achieve a complete view of the hip.

When a large anterior spur is present, entrance into the hip joint is difficult and sometimes impossible. The spur may completely block the two anterior portals. The portal over the posterior aspect of the greater trochanter is not blocked and can be used effectively to enter the hip. We have found that the best way to develop the posterior portal is with the patient on his or her side. To start, the arthroscope is inserted into the posterior portal. The hip is distended with fluid inserted through the arthroscope sheath. Next, the anterior peritrochanteric portal is developed. The region of the spur is visualized through the arthroscope.

With the aid of the image intensifier, a motorized shaver is inserted blindly down to the spur and the soft tissue is debrided until the shaver tip comes into view. The electrothermal ablator can be used to speed up the debriding process once a space is made with the motorized shaver. Then a motorized abrader is inserted and under direct vision the spur is taken off (Fig. 58.14). Once the spur is removed, the third direct anterior portal may be developed.

ARTHROSCOPIC ANATOMY

The lateral approach provides a safe route for the arthroscope. The vital structures are away from the actual insertion sites and are in jeopardy if the bony landmarks are not recognized. The palpable bony landmarks are the greater

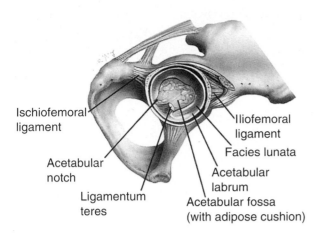

Ischiofemoral ligament

Iliofemoral ligament

Facies lunata

Acetabular notch

Acetabular labrum

Ligamentum teres

Acetabular fossa (with adipose cushion)

FIGURE 58.15 Diagram of the right acetabulum. Note the increased thickness of the anterior hip capsule caused by the iliofemoral ligament. (From Glick JM. Hip arthroscopy: lateral approach. In: Parisien JS, ed. *Therapeutic arthroscopy.* New York: Raven Press; 1993:22.1–22.10, with permission.)

trochanter and the anterior superior iliac spine. The deep bony landmarks are the neck and head of the femur and the acetabulum. These are palpated with the spinal needle and the trocar as the joint is approached. The instruments pass through the gluteus medius and minimus muscles as they are directed into the hip joint. A definite "give" on either side is felt as the capsule is pierced, and the bony floor of the acetabulum stops the instrument. If bone is struck before the capsule appears to be penetrated, the instrument has

been placed too superior, striking the outer wall of the acetabulum, or too inferior, hitting the head of the femur. The vital adjacent structures include the sciatic nerve posteriorly and the lateral femoral cutaneous nerve anteriorly. The femoral artery and nerve anteriorly and the superior gluteal nerve are far removed from the portals of entry (5), but their locations should be kept in mind.

With the surgeon in the anterior position, the video camera is oriented to provide the same image that the surgeon sees through the arthroscope. On the video screen, the head of the femur appears on the side opposite to that operated on. For example, in the right hip the femoral head is on the left, and in the left hip the femoral head is on the right; anterior is down and posterior is up in both the right and left hips. The entire acetabulum can be seen by the direct lateral approach. Figure 58.15 is a diagram of the acetabulum in relation to the arthroscope. The acetabular labrum is attached to the rim of the acetabulum and the transverse acetabular ligament at the site where the acetabular fossa opens inferiorly. The arthroscopic views displayed in Fig. 58.16 are what we see in a normal hip joint. Note the orientation and the position of the ligamentum teres. This structure is best seen with the arthroscope directed to the medial aspect of the joint. The capsular attachments define the joint and what can be seen with the arthroscope. Proximally, the capsule covers the labrum. Distally, it attaches to the intertrochanteric line on the anterior aspect of the neck and just proximal to the intertrochanteric crest on the posterior side of the neck. A

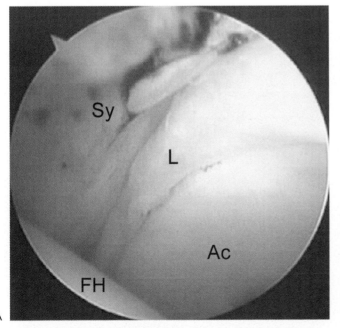

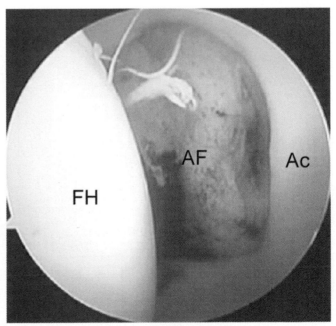

A · B

FIGURE 58.16 The right hip joint. **A:** The posterior aspect of the hip joint, which is the first part visualized after the arthroscope is inserted. **B:** The acetabular fossa.

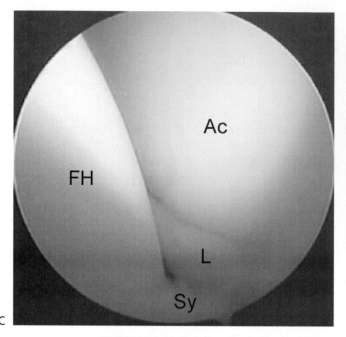

C

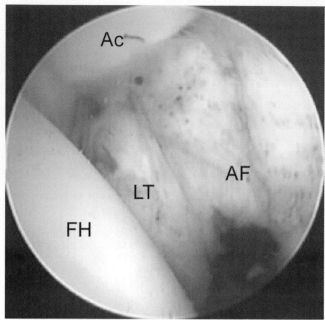

D

FIGURE 58.16 *(continued)* **C:** The anterior aspect of the hip joint. **D:** Deep in the acetabular fossa. AF, acetabular fossa; Ac, acetabulum; FH, femoral head; LT, ligamentum teres; L, labrum; Sy, synovium. (From Glick JM. Hip arthroscopy by the lateral approach. *Clin Sports Med* 2001;20:733–747, with permission.)

greater portion of the femoral neck is visible anteriorly than posteriorly because of the way the capsule attaches. The thick overlying ligaments of the hip form the folds in the capsule. The zona orbicularis is a ligament that forms a circular ring around the neck of the femur at the base of the head of the femur. Loose bodies frequently hide under this structure (Fig. 58.17).

DISCUSSION

The lateral approach provides an easy and safe access to the hip joint. The line from skin to the joint itself is a straight, downward drop (Fig. 58.18). The vital arteries and nerves are a safe distance from the portal sites. The potential problems that can arise from this procedure are from trac-

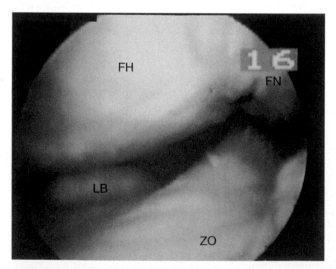

FIGURE 58.17 Arthroscopic view of the zona orbicularis at the head–neck junction of a left hip. A loose body is entrapped under the anterior aspect of the femoral head. FH, femoral head; FN, femoral neck; ZO, zona orbicularis; LB, loose body; A, anterior; P, posterior.

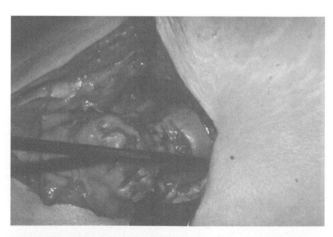

FIGURE 58.18 Cadaver specimen showing the direct lateral approach to the left hip joint. The large Steinmann pin is entering the hip joint over the greater trochanter. (From Glick JM: Hip arthroscopy by the lateral approach. *Therapeutic arthroscopy* 1993;22:1–22, with permission.)

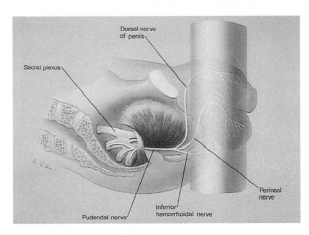

FIGURE 58.19 A diagram of the course of the pudendal nerve and its branches in relation to the pubic bone and the peroneal post placed between the legs of a patient. (From Glick JM. Complications of hip arthroscopy by the lateral approach. In: Sherman OH, Minkoff J, eds. *Arthroscopic surgery,* 1st ed. Baltimore: Williams & Wilkins; 1990:193–201, with permission.)

the chance of a significant sciatic nerve neuropraxia. To protect the pudendal nerve, Lyon et al. (7) suggested that the perineal post be at least 9 cm in diameter in order to distribute the forces in a wide area on the ischium, and that the surgeon make sure the pelvis is well supported so that the pressure of the post is not placed directly on the nerve. The perineal posts on most fracture tables are only 3 cm in diameter. They can be made larger by wrapping them with padding. In some fracture tables, the slats that support the lower leg can be removed and consequently the support on the pelvis is lost. For hip arthroscopy, the slats do not have to be removed.

The lateral approach provides a safe and simple way of performing hip arthroscopy. The instruments can easily be manipulated so that the entire confines of the joint can be visualized with the arthroscope and reached with operative instruments.

tion force that applies a compression force on the branches of the pudendal nerve as they cross the ischium (Fig. 58.19) and from traction force on the sciatic nerve (6). I have always maintained that traction should be treated like a tourniquet; that is, it should be applied for no longer then 2 hours. Furthermore, the amount of traction should not exceed 75 lb. I use a tensiometer, but it is not mandatory, because the major issue with the traction is the time of application. We have monitored the sciatic nerve using evoke potentials and, in some cases, motor potentials in more than 50 cases in the past year, and the poundage and time limits of the traction (75 lb and 2 hours) were verified. In addition, if the fracture table has a vertical post as well as a peroneal post, we set the vertical post in the back of the patient and not in the front. Flexing the hip around that post greatly increases the traction and at the same time places an extreme stretch on the sciatic nerve, setting up

REFERENCES

1. Glick JM, Sampson TG, Gordon RB, et al. Hip arthroscopy by the lateral approach. *Arthroscopy* 1987;3:4–12.
2. Glick JM, Sampson TG. Hip arthroscopy by the lateral approach. In: McGinty JB, Caspari RB, Jackson RW, et al., eds. *Operative arthroscopy,* 2nd ed. Philadelphia: Lippincott-Raven Publishers, 1996:1079–1089.
3. Glick JM. Hip arthroscopy using the lateral approach. *Instr Course Lect* 1988;19:223–231.
4. Byrd JWT. Avoiding the labrum in hip arthroscopy. *Arthroscopy* 2000;16:770–773.
5. Foster DE, Hunter JR. The direct lateral approach to the hip for arthroplasty. *Orthopedics* 1987;10:274–280.
6. Glick JM. Complications of hip arthroscopy by the lateral approach. In: Sherman OH, Minkoff J, eds. *Arthroscopic surgery,* 1st ed. Baltimore: Williams & Wilkins; 1990:193–201.
7. Lyon BS, Koval KJ, Kummer F, et al. Pudendal nerve palsy induced by the fracture table. *Orthopaedic Review* 1993;May:521–525.

PATHOLOGY AMENABLE TO ARTHROSCOPY OF THE HIP

JOSEPH C. MCCARTHY
LALIT PURI
JO-ANN LEE
WAEL BARSOUM

Arthroscopic surgery has enjoyed exponential growth in the current practice of orthopaedics as techniques and clinical applications have developed to allow minimally invasive diagnostic and therapeutic procedures, particularly for the knee and shoulder. Arthroscopic management of hip disorders has not received similar attention until recently. The concept of hip arthroscopy was first introduced in 1931 by Burman, but did not resurface in the North American literature until 1977, when Gross reported his experience with arthroscopy of congenitally dislocated hips (1,2). Sporadic reports of clinical application of arthroscopic techniques in the hip joint continued to appear in the literature through the early 1980s. In 1980 Vakilif and Warren (3) reported arthroscopic removal of entrapped cement after total hip arthroplasty, and in 1981 Holgersson et al. (4) reported the use of hip arthroscopy in the evaluation and treatment of juvenile chronic arthritis.

This relatively slow development of arthroscopy of the hip in North American centers is understandable. Anatomically the femoral head is deeply recessed in the bony acetabulum, and it is convex in shape, unlike the more planar surface of the knee. Volumetric distention of the hip joint is less than that of the knee, and the fibrocapsular and muscular envelope is thicker. Additionally, the relative proximity of the sciatic nerve, the lateral femoral cutaneous nerve, and the femoral neurovascular structures place them at potential risk (5,6).

Nevertheless, diagnostic and therapeutic applications of hip arthroscopy have developed over the last 10 years, and recent innovations in technique have allowed thoughtful advancement. Eriksson (7) recognized and quantitated the hip capsule distention and distraction forces necessary to allow adequate visualization of the femur and the acetabulum. Johnson (9) articulated techniques of needle positioning, anatomic landmarks, and cannula placement, and Glick (8) contributed his experience with lateral decubitus positioning and peritrochanteric portal placement. Adaptation of arthroscopy equipment and instruments specifically for the hip joint has led to safe visualization and instrumentation of the joint.

The advantages of hip arthroscopy include the ability to thoroughly inspect the joint and directly identify and address any previously undiagnosed or unmanageable pathology without an arthrotomy, and the ability to document and stage any pathology within the joint, thus potentially affecting future treatment—all with a minimally invasive procedure with short rehabilitation. The development of clinical and radiographic expertise in diagnosing intraarticular pathology has resulted in an increasing necessity for accessing the joint.

This chapter addresses the different pathologic processes amenable to diagnosis and treatment by hip arthroscopy. Current indications for this procedure include removal of loose bodies, synovial biopsy, subtotal synovectomy, management of labral tears, synovial chondromatosis, avascular necrosis with associated pathology, osteochondritis dissecans, chondral lesions, staging of chondral lesions, and the treatment of pyarthrosis (Table 59.1). In addition, those patients with long-standing, unresolved hip joint pain and positive physical findings may benefit from an arthroscopic evaluation for diagnostic as well as therapeutic reasons (10–19).

DIAGNOSIS

Hip pain, particularly in the young adult, is often functional in quality and may arise from a number of soft tissue structures in and around the hip joint. Most patients demonstrate improvement in function and a decrease in hip pain with conservative measures. If a patient's hip pain persists, is reproducible on physical examination, and does not re-

---

J. C. McCarthy, L. Puri, J-A Lee, and W. Barsoun: New England Baptist Hospital, Boston, Massachusetts.

TABLE 59.1 INDICATIONS FOR HIP ARTHROSCOPY

Loose bodies
Labral tears
Chondral lesions of the acetabular or femoral head
Osteonecrosis of the femoral head
Ruptured or impinging ligamentum teres
Dysplasia
Synovial abnormalities:
  Collagen disease (e.g., rheumatoid arthritis or systemic lupus
    erythematosus with impinging synovitis)
  Crystalline hip arthropathy (e.g., gout, pseudogout)
  Capsular shrinkage (e.g., Ehlers–Danlos syndrome)
  Synovial chondromatosis
  Hematologic disorders

Infection
After total hip arthroplasty (diagnosis of occult sepsis or removal
  of intraarticular wire or cement)
After trauma (dislocation, Pipkin fracture, removal of foreign
  body)
Osteoarthritis
Extraarticular conditions
Intractable pain (with positive physical findings)

spond to appropriate conservative measures including rest, ambulatory support, nonsteroidal antiinflammatory drugs, or physical therapy, hip arthroscopy may be of significant value (20).

The majority of conditions that cause pain in the region of the hip joint can be diagnosed from a comprehensive history, physical examination, and/or plain radiographs. These conditions include such clinical entities as iliotibial band tendonitis, greater trochanteric bursitis, inguinal or femoral hernia, hip fractures and/or dislocations, osteonecrosis, osteoarthritis, or calcified intraarticular loose bodies. For clinical entities such as iliopsoas tendonitis, inflammatory arthritis, early avascular necrosis, occult fractures, psoas abscess, tumor, upper lumbar radiculopathy, or vascular abnormalities, more sophisticated radiographic techniques, including computed tomography, magnetic resonance, and radioisotope studies, may facilitate diagnosis of persistent hip pain (10).

Despite vigorous investigation, a subset of patients have persistent symptoms but with negative or equivocal radiographic studies. Arthroscopy can lead to a definitive diagnosis in as many as 40% of these cases (21). Unexpected focal degenerative arthritis, chondromalacia, chondral flap tears, nonossified loose bodies, synovitis, labral lesions, and synovial chondromatosis have all been diagnosed in such circumstances.

Clinical Presentation

An intraarticular etiology causing intractable hip pain in the adult can manifest in a variety of ways. Patients can have referred pain to the anterior groin, anterior thigh, buttock, greater trochanter, and medial knee. Mechanical symptoms

of persistent clicking, catching, locking, giving way, and restricted range of motion can indicate an intraarticular etiology. Symptoms are usually preceded by a traumatic event, either a fall or a twisting injury, and can occur in any age group. In addition, symptoms are generally exacerbated with activity and improved with rest.

Patients who are candidates for hip arthroscopy should have reproducible symptoms and physical findings that are functionally limiting. Furthermore, an adequate trial of conservative treatment, including rest, use of nonsteroidal antiinflammatory drugs, ambulatory support, and physical therapy, must be pursued before surgical treatment is considered. In order to determine which patients would benefit from hip arthroscopy, McCarthy et al. (21) retrospectively reviewed 94 consecutive patients with intractable hip pain who underwent hip arthroscopy (21). They demonstrated statistically significant associations between preoperative clinical presentation and arthroscopic operative findings. The presence of loose bodies within the hip joint, whether ossified or not, correlated with locking episodes ($r = .845$, $p = .00$) and anterior inguinal pain ($r = 1$, $p = .00$). Acetabular labral tears detected arthroscopically correlated significantly with symptoms of anterior inguinal pain ($r = 1$, $p = .00$), painful clicking episodes ($r = .809$, $p = .00$), transient locking ($r = .370$, $p = .00$), or giving way ($r = .320$, $p = .0024$) and with the physical findings of a positive hip extension test ($r = .676$, $p = .00$). The findings of a chondral defect of the femoral head or acetabulum statistically correlated with anterior inguinal pain ($r = 1$, $p = .00$) but no other specific findings.

In addition, Fitzgerald (11), in a retrospective review of acetabular labral tears, found that 44 (80%) of 55 patients had a palpable or audible click, and 48 (87%) reported groin pain. However, only 48 patients were treated surgically and only 12 underwent arthroscopic confirmation.

Radiologic Evaluation

Radiologic workup of intractable pain referable to the hip can include plain radiographs, arthrography, bone scintigraphy, computed tomography (CT), and magnetic resonance imaging (MRI). Plain radiographs may demonstrate loose bodies or degenerative arthritis, but overall they have a very poor diagnostic yield for intraarticular pathology, including the early stages of degenerative joint disease. Arthrography may help with diagnosis, as was noted by Fitzgerald (11), who found that 44 of 50 patients with a suspected acetabular labral tear showed positive hip arthrography. However, only 12 of 55 patients underwent hip arthroscopy, without mention of arthrographic correlation to intraoperative findings. Bone scintigraphy has a low specificity for intraarticular abnormalities such as loose bodies, labral tears, and chondral defects. MRI also was found to have a poor diagnostic yield. Edwards et al. (10) prospectively studied 23 patients who had undergone MRI followed by hip arthroscopy

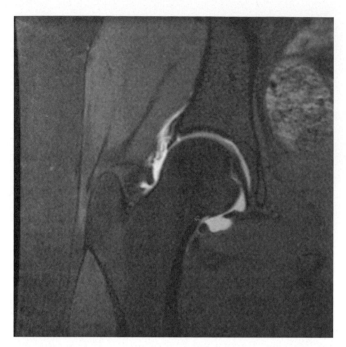

FIGURE 59.1 Gadolinium-enhanced magnetic resonance imaging view of right hip.

within a 3-week period. MRI was unable to detect pathology in patients with chondral softening, fibrillation, or partial-thickness defects less than 1 cm. In addition, MRI was unreliable for osteochondral loose bodies and labral tears found at the time of surgery.

Despite a normal radiologic workup, some patients continue to remain symptomatic. In the same study noted previously, McCarthy et al. (22) reported an 80% false-negative rate for all radiologic investigations (plain radiography, bone scintigraphy, CT, MRI, and arthrography) evaluating intractable hip pain (22). When diagnoses that were evident on plain films were excluded (e.g., loose bodies, stage III or IV degenerative joint disease), accurate diagnosis of unremitting hip pain by any radiologic modality was accomplished only 4% of the time. The most commonly overlooked cause of pain was acetabular labral lesions, for which there was no reliable radiologic means of diagnosis at that time. In their group of 94 patients with intractable hip pain, 52 (55%) had acetabular labral injuries, all of which were well visualized and debrided at arthroscopy.

Gadolinium-enhanced magnetic resonance (MR) arthrography of the hip is a relatively new technique devised to increase the sensitivity and specificity for detection of intraarticular hip pathology (23) (Fig. 59.1). Although MR arthrography represents an improvement over conventional MRI, it does have limitations when compared with direct visualization. The advantages of optical magnification, hip distraction, and direct probing at arthroscopy are considerable. Further improvements in MR resolution, image planning, and radiographic interpretive experience will increase detection of hip pathology.

CURRENT INDICATIONS

The current indications for hip arthroscopy are listed in Table 59.1.

LOOSE BODIES

The clinical presentation of locking or catching with activity can be associated with intraarticular loose bodies. Many conditions may lead to retained material which can become trapped in the acetabular fossa and cause pain. Arthroscopy is the least traumatic method of removing loose or foreign bodies from the joint.

Loose bodies may be ossified or not. If calcium is present, these bodies are readily identified by radiographic studies; if they are not evident on plain films, CT scanning, with or without contrast, is highly sensitive to visualize these structures. If symptoms are present, arthroscopy provides a minimally invasive technique for removal of those bodies.

If the loose bodies are not calcified, however, they can be extremely difficult to visualize. McCarthy and Busconi (18) showed that up to 67% of loose bodies may not be evident on conventional radiographic studies. If the bodies produce locking or catching symptoms, arthroscopy then becomes a means to establish the diagnosis and confirm the clinical suspicion, as well as to provide simultaneous treatment.

Loose bodies may occur as an isolated fragment, for example after a dislocation or as a result of osteochondritis dissecans. Alternatively, they may be multiples (2 to 300 bodies), as is seen in synovial chondromatosis. In this condition, some bodies may aggregate together in grape-like clusters 1 to 4 cm in diameter (Fig. 59.2). Often these bodies adhere

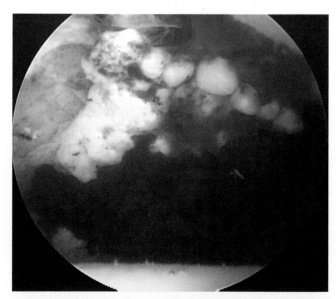

FIGURE 59.2 Intraoperative photograph of synovial chondromatosis.

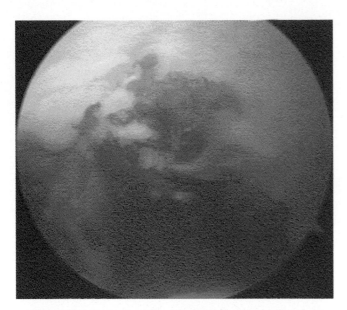

FIGURE 59.3 Intraoperative photograph of a foreign body.

to the synovium about the fovea and must be morcellized in order to be removed arthroscopically.

A number of authors have reported their experiences using the arthroscope to remove foreign material from the hip joint (3,24). As with arthroscopy in other joints, debris such as retained cement, wires, or projectiles may be visualized and removed (Fig. 59.3).

Labral Tears

Similar to loose bodies, a torn acetabular labrum may result in catching, locking, pain, or a click in the hip joint. Although labral tears have been recognized in the orthopaedic literature for some time, there has been increased attention to this clinical entity more recently (11,16,25–27). Altenburg (28) was the first to suggest that a torn acetabular labrum may predispose a patient to subsequent degenerative changes. Cartilage and Scott (29) and Ueo and Hamabuchi (30) independently implicated labral tears and degeneration in the subsequent development of coxarthrosis.

Labral tears may manifest without a prior history of trauma. Some tears are considered congenital and have been associated with acetabular dysplasia, slipped capital femoral epiphysis, and Legg–Calvé–Perthes disease (31). In these cases, radiographs may reveal a cystic indentation in the lateral roof of the acetabulum. Harris et al. (32) described an intraarticular labrum with degeneration in patients undergoing total hip arthroplasty for end-stage degenerative changes.

The acetabular labrum shares some similarity to the meniscus of the knee. Both contain avascular regions that preclude healing after injury. Minimal injury to the acetabular labrum, when subjected to repetitive motion and stress from the articulation of the femoral head, may progress. Re-

ciprocal injury to corresponding chondral surfaces of the femoral head can occur as well. Furthermore, the duration of symptoms and severity of labral injury found at arthroscopy have been statistically correlated (22).

Fitzgerald (11) showed that 45 (92%) of 49 labral injuries documented occurred at the anterior marginal attachment of the acetabulum. McCarthy et al. (22), in a series of 58 consecutive patients who were noted to have labral tears, also found that 96% occurred in the anterior quadrant (22). However, Ikeda et al. (16) looked at a younger patient population and noted an 86% incidence of posterosuperior labral injuries and tears.

Treatment of acetabular labral tears usually involves mechanical debridement of the unstable labral segment. Because of the excellent visualization provided by the arthroscope and the minimally invasive nature of the procedure, arthroscopic management of these lesions can be quite beneficial (Fig. 59.4).

Chondral Lesions of the Acetabulum and Femoral Head

Chondral lesions are one of the most elusive sources of hip joint pain. Because of the more constrained anatomy of the hip, compared with the shoulder, until recently these lesions were not believed to exist. The lack of a currently available radiographic test that can reliably diagnose the presence or extent of these lesions is frustrating for both patients and clinicians (18).

Gadolinium-enhanced MR arthrography has limitations in identifying chondral injuries. This lack of sensitivity may be explained in part by the examination's static nature and the lack of distraction during the study. Yet chondral lesions do occur with frequency. In a study of 457 hip arthroscopies

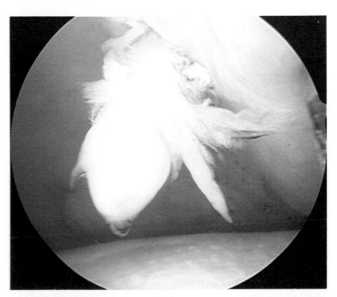

FIGURE 59.4 Intraoperative photograph of an anterior labral tear.

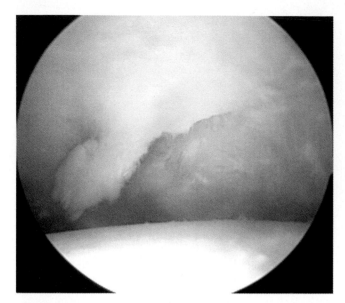

FIGURE 59.5 Intraoperative photograph of an acetabular chondral lesion.

during a 6-year period, chondral injuries occurred in the anterior acetabulum in 269 cases (59%), in the superior acetabulum in 110 cases (24%), and in the posterior acetabulum in 114 cases (25%). Although these lesions were seen most frequently in association with a labral tear, most disturbing was the unstable flap nature and extent of the full-thickness cartilage injury. The common initiating site for labral as well as chondral injuries has been termed the "watershed "zone (see Case Examples 1 and 2 at the end of this chapter). Seventy percent of the anterior, 27% of the superior, and 36% of the posterior chondral injuries were grade III or IV (Fig. 59.5). In addition, the senior author's classification of labral tears demonstrates a clear decrement in outcome once an associated chondral acetabular lesion of greater than 1 cm occurs (22).

Chondral injuries may occur in association with a multitude of hip conditions, including labral tears, loose bodies, posterior dislocation, osteonecrosis, slipped capital femoral epiphysis, dysplasia, and degenerative arthritis (Fig. 59.6). The difficulty in diagnosing these lesions as well as their effect on outcome provides a cogent rationale for arthroscopic hip surgery.

Osteonecrosis

The role of hip arthroscopy in avascular necrosis of the femoral head remains controversial. This theoretical debate centers on whether the increased pressure from joint distention further exacerbates the avascular status of the femoral head. Villar (20) reported possible progression after hip arthroscopy. Others have found arthroscopy to be helpful in staging the articular surface changes for possible osteotomy or bone grafting and have not observed progression attributable to the arthroscopic procedure (15).

The focus of most diagnostic as well as treatment efforts to date has been directed at the subchondral bone, to prevent its collapse. Revascularization, especially free-vascularized fibular grafting, has altered the natural history of this disease favorably.

However, because of the limitations of MRI and CT scanning to thoroughly evaluate the chondral joint surfaces, some unstable articular lesions have been missed. Arthroscopy allows a comprehensive mapping of the femoral head and acetabular joint surfaces, the labrum, and the synovium. In addition we have on several occasions viewed the intraosseous femoral head core track endoscopically and witnessed the clearcut demarcation of the avascular zone. Arthroscopy has no role in end-stage disease with a collapsed femoral head.

Therefore, the current rationale for arthroscopy in osteonecrosis is narrowly focused. It may facilitate staging of cases, especially before free fibular grafting (33–35).

We believe that arthroscopy should be reserved for those patients with evidence of mechanical symptoms such as locking, buckling, and catching that suggest a loose body, labral injury, or chondral flap lesion. In addition, it may have a role in the patient who fares poorly after revascularization, perhaps because of a chondral lesion. As noted previously, arthroscopy can be performed simultaneously with a core decompression.

Ruptured or Impinging Ligamentum Teres

This lesion, albeit infrequent, may occur as a result of trauma such as posterior dislocation or a Pipkin fracture. In addition, it may occur in association with degenerative arthritis. Isolated lesions of the ligamentum teres have occa-

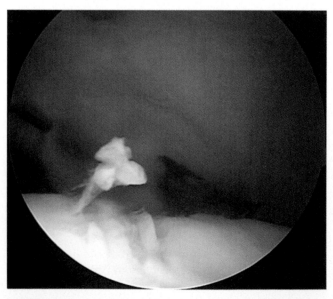

FIGURE 59.6 Intraoperative photograph of a femoral head chondral lesion.

sionally been reported (36–38). Gray and Villar (39) described this condition as a source of hip pain either alone or in conjunction with other articular pathology.

Dysplasia

Dysplasia can produce a hypertrophic labrum or ligamentum. As noted by Salter (40), the limbus is enlarged in dysplasia. By adult life, repetitive stretching of this structure may result in elongation, hypertrophic impingement, or both. In our experience, one such patient with Crowe I dysplasia presented with recurrent buckling, falling, and pain. After arthroscopic debridement of the ligament, these symptoms were alleviated. Six years later, identical symptoms in the opposite hip were eliminated by arthroscopic intervention.

Synovial Abnormalities

Deep-seated and unremitting hip joint pain can begin in the synovium, caused by a number of conditions with diverse etiologies, including inflammatory, hematologic, crystalline, collagenous, mechanical, viral, and tumoral disorders. Specific treatment is based on whether the condition is focal or diffuse, self-limited or unremitting in nature.

Arthroscopic synovectomy can be useful in the management of inflammatory conditions, but a total synovectomy is difficult if not impossible with current techniques (4,7,15,24,41). Traditional open synovectomy requires dislocation of the femoral head from the acetabulum, with the inherent risk of avascular necrosis and a prolonged rehabilitation period. Janssens et al. (17) described arthroscopic synovectomy as an adjunct to diagnosis and treatment of pigmented villondular synovitis. As the techniques for hip arthroscopy improve, the role of early arthroscopic intervention in inflammatory arthritis will expand.

Crystalline diseases such as gout or pseudogout can produce extreme hip joint pain. A joint effusion, best seen on T2-weighted MRI scanning, can be accompanied by an elevated or normal serum uric acid level. Joint fluid analysis with polarized light microscopic verification confirms the diagnosis. At arthroscopy, the senior author has witnessed high concentrations of crystals diffusely distributed throughout the synovium and embedded within the articular cartilage of the acetabulum. Arthroscopic treatment consists of copious lavage, mechanical removal of crystals, and, if necessary, synovial biopsy (Fig. 59.7). Crystalline diseases can often coexist with other pathology.

Collagen diseases such as juvenile rheumatoid arthritis, rheumatoid arthritis, lupus erythematosus, and Ehlers–Danlos syndrome occur in the hip, and it may be the presenting symptomatic joint. Patients with rheumatoid arthritis can present with an effusion, dense synovitis synechiae, and synovial cysts, as well as articular surface damage. Intense joint pain unresponsive to extensive conservative mea-

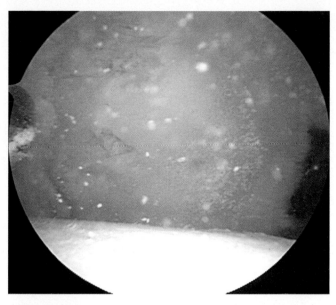

FIGURE 59.7 Intraoperative photograph of chondrocalcinosis.

sures is the rationale for arthroscopic intervention. The senior author has observed severe hypertrophic and hyperemic synovitis obscuring initial visualization of the femoral head and acetabulum. Arthroscopic treatment consists of synovial biopsy and/or synovectomy, evaluation and treatment of accompanying articular cartilage damage, and lavage. Procedural results are directly dependent on the stage of articular surface involvement.

As in the shoulder joint, Ehlers–Danlos syndrome can cause pain and instability in the hip. In combination with medical diagnosis, arthroscopic treatment has consisted of skin and synovial biopsy to further define disease classification. In addition, thermal capsular shrinkage has been performed judiciously (Fig. 59.8). The senior author's experience to date has been uniformly favorable. Longer-term follow-up is requisite to define this procedure's ultimate utility.

Synovial chondromatosis is a metaplastic synovial condition that results in the production of numerous loose bod-

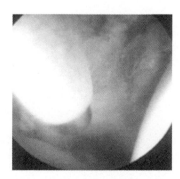

FIGURE 59.8 Intraoperative photograph of capsular shrinkage.

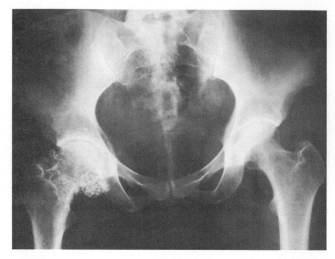

FIGURE 59.9 Plain radiograph of synovial chondromatosis.

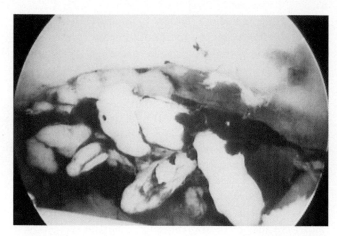

FIGURE 59.11 Intraoperative photograph of synovial chondromatosis.

ies. Although benign, this tumorous entity may be recurrent. The loose bodies, if nonossified, can make diagnosis of this disease extremely difficult. In a study of 10 cases, only 50% of patients were correctly diagnosed preoperatively by any radiographic means (Figs. 59.9 and 59.10). All of these hips had calcified bodies present, and none of the cases with nonossified bodies was evident before surgery, despite MRI scanning (23). Arthroscopic treatment in 20 cases to date has consisted of clarification of diagnosis, removal of between 5 to 300 loose bodies (especially those clustered within the fovea), treatment of articular damage, and synovectomy (Fig. 59.11). Although recurrence has been reported to occur in about 10% of cases despite intervention, a second arthroscopy may be performed without intercedent scarring. In addition, arthroscopy, in contrast to open arthrotomy, has been performed without the attendant risks of osteonecrosis, heterotopic bone, deep vein thrombophlebitis, neurovascular injury, or infection.

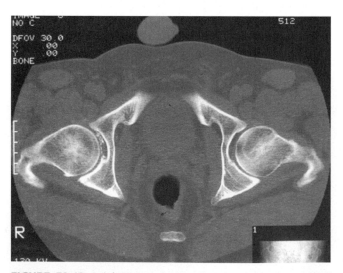

FIGURE 59.10 Axial CT scan image showing multiple calcified loose bodies in the fovea of the right hip.

Hematologic disorders such as sickle cell anemia, hemophilia, and pigmented villonodular synovitis can produce significant joint symptoms. Although medical management is usually effective when dysfunction becomes protracted, arthroscopic intervention may be warranted. This minimally invasive approach carries much less bleeding risk than open arthrotomy. Surgical treatment includes evacuation of hematoma, removal of synechiae, copious lavage, and synovectomy as necessary. There are no outcome data on this procedure, however symptomatically beneficial, to date.

Infection

Arthroscopy has a limited but important role in sepsis, particularly in pediatric patients (42). Acute bacterial joint involvement can be treated by decompression and lavage, with drains left in the joint, with minimal morbidity. In addition, for these cases in which joint aspiration is negative or equivocal, arthroscopy can provide definitive diagnosis through not only joint fluid analysis but also synovial biopsy. Simultaneously, joint irrigation and articular surface assessment and treatment can be performed.

Arthroscopy after Total Hip Replacement

Most patients with pain after total hip replacement do not require arthroscopic evaluation. The origins of symptoms after arthroplasty can usually be diagnosed by conventional means, including clinical examination (e.g., leg length discrepancy, abductor weakness), radiographic studies (e.g., component loosening, malposition, trochanteric nonunion), and special studies (e.g., bone scan, aspiration arthrogram for subtle loosening or sepsis).

If unexplained symptoms persist despite appropriate conservative treatment, arthroscopy can be beneficial. The senior author has performed arthroscopy in two patients with suspected sepsis but repeated negative joint aspirations. On both occasions, low-virulent organisms were recovered by fluid analysis as well as synovial biopsy. At the same time, debridement of exudates and impinging granulation tissue was performed, along with copious lavage and installation of a drainage catheter. On one occasion, the patient's advanced liver disease and coagulopathy precluded an open procedure; after successful arthroscopic intervention, he was ambulatory within 24 hours.

Another indication for a minimally invasive surgical approach is an intraarticular third body. The senior author has removed a broken trochanteric wire (16-gauge, 1.75 inches long) from a hip joint. The metallic fragment had migrated to within 5 mm of the prosthetic interface. In addition, two migrated porous beads have been arthroscopically. Recently, the senior author also removed an acetabular component screw that radiographs had shown to be progressively backing out (Fig. 59.12).

A potential use of arthroscopy may be to reverse symptomatically tight or impinging tendonous periarticular structures, such as the iliopsoas. Although attractive, arthroscopy to lavage the joint of wear-related enzymes does not address the primary implant-related cause of potential osteolysis. It should be noted that neither of these two applications has sufficient clinical data to warrant anything other than scrupulous judgment.

Trauma

Traumatic events about the hip joint are a frequent occurrence. Although most fractures of the femoral neck or acetabulum are successfully treated by reconstitution of the bony architecture, articular injuries can and do occur. Epstein et al. (43) reported that the high incidence of chondral damage present after a fracture-dislocation of the hip

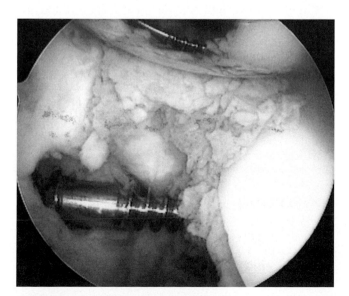

FIGURE 59.12 Intraoperative photograph of arthroscopic retrieval of a loose acetabular screw.

warranted an arthrotomy in every case. The high risks associated with open surgery in the early posttrauma period (infection, contracture, deep venous thrombosis, pulmonary embolism, heterotopic bone, neuromuscular dysfunction) have limited the enthusiasm for this approach. The minimally invasive nature of arthroscopy significantly reduces these risks. The senior author has treated a patient, who 5 days after a dislocation, experienced excruciating hip pain. At surgery, a large hematoma was evacuated, two chondral loose bodies were removed, and a torn posterior labrum was repaired. The patient was able to walk the next morning.

Dislocations and fracture-dislocations can produce, in addition to loose bodies and labral injuries, shear damage to the chondral surfaces of the femoral head or acetabulum. These are not often seen by MRI scanning. Pipkin fractures can result in displaced bone or cartilage from the femoral head or a ruptured ligamentum teres. Although it is difficult, we have successfully treated each of these conditions.

Intraarticular foreign bodies such as bullet fragments can affect the hip with or without an associated fracture. The senior author has removed a bullet that migrated into the joint 7 years after the patient's initial trauma. Most recently, a patient developed hip pain 2 years after attempted removal of a femoral intramedullary rod. A metallic fragment had migrated into the joint, embedding itself, like a piece of glass, into the superior lateral aspect of the acetabulum. At surgery the femoral head had already been scratched by this metallic shard. It was successfully removed endoscopically.

Osteoarthritis

The pain from osteoarthritic changes of the femoral head or acetabulum may far exceed the radiographic evidence of degenerative wear, usually characterized by joint space narrowing, osteophyte formation, subchondral sclerosis, and cystic changes. The absence of these finding on plain radiographs does not exclude osteoarthritis (21). Asymmetric, focal chondral degenerative changes, particularly in the anterior-superior aspect of the femoral head or acetabulum, may appear normal on anteroposterior pelvic radiographs. Arthroscopic examination can identify the exact extent and location of chondral degeneration and exclude other pathology (Fig. 59.13). However, if the is significant radiographic evidence of osteoarthritis, the condition usually is not amenable to arthroscopy. McCarthy and Glick have reported a direct correlation between the stage of cartilage loss, especially on the acetabular side, and poor outcome following arthroscopy (22).

Despite this cautionary note, arthroscopy can be beneficial in certain situations Arthroscopic lavage can give significant pain relief in patients with relatively advanced osteoarthritic changes, although this relief of symptoms is often temporary if other mechanical etiologic sources of pain are not identified and addressed (7,20). Debridement and chondral abrasion may have a role in the management

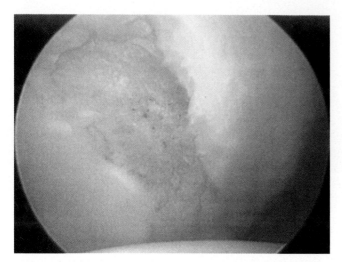

FIGURE 59.13 Intraoperative photograph of degenerative wear.

of osteoarthritis that is not advanced enough to justify more aggressive surgical options such as joint replacement (14). This is particularly applicable in young patients, in whom the surgeon may wish to avoid or delay total joint arthroplasty.

Extraarticular Conditions

The efficacy of arthroscopy in the treatment of pathologic conditions in encapsulated surgical environments (e.g., joints, bladder) has spawned interest in further applications. Advancements in general surgery and endoscopy of soft tissue cavities have allowed treatment of inguinal hernias and gallbladder disease. Similarly, orthopaedic arthroscopic procedures have begun to extend to nonarticular areas. As mentioned previously, a posttraumatic periarticular impinging ossification has been resected via the arthroscope. Glick also reported his experience with this technique for iliopsoas and iliotibial band release (44). It should be emphasized that the results are preliminary, and the recovery can be protracted, especially for the iliopsoas. Further study is necessary.

Intractable Hip Pain

Arthroscopy is not a substitute for clinical acumen. The myriad causes of inguinal and buttock pain include many extraarticular conditions. The vast majority of these cases are self-limited and will resolve with time and appropriate conservative management. Numerous psychologic, emotional, and legal as well as physical issues can contribute to pain intensity, extent, and protractedness. Occasionally an intraarticular joint injection with triamcinolone (Aristocort) and bupivacaine (Marcaine), done under fluoroscopic control, may help to clarify whether the source of pain is intracapsular.

Arthroscopic evaluation is considered when joint symptoms are unremitting, usually after more than 6 months, and radiographic studies are unable to provide a diagnosis. In such situations, Villar (45) reported that arthroscopy facilitated a diagnosis in 40% of cases.

The senior author has rarely operated for pain symptoms alone. Conversely, the patient with protracted mechanical symptoms (buckling, catching, locking) and positive physical findings (McCarthy hip extension sign, hip flexion adduction and external rotation painful impingement, and inguinal pain on resisted straight leg raising) represents an excellent candidate for surgery. Further evaluation of radiographic procedural sensitivity should diminish the number of hip diagnostic dilemmas.

CONTRAINDICATIONS

Arthroscopy is not a panacea for sound clinical judgment. Surgical intervention is proscribed for joint conditions that are amenable to medical management, such as the arthralgias associated with hepatitis or colitis. Similarly, hip pain referred from other sources (e.g., compression fracture of the first lumbar vertebra) precludes surgery.

Periarticular conditions such as stress fractures of the femoral neck, insufficiency fractures of the pubis ischium, and transient osteoporosis are best treated by nonendoscopic means.

Certain joint conditions, in the absence of mechanical symptoms, do not warrant arthroscopy. These include osteonecrosis and synovitis.

Acute skin lesions or ulceration, especially in the vicinity of anterior or lateral portals, would proscribe arthroscopy. In addition, sepsis with accompanying osteomyelitis or abscess formation requires open surgery.

Conditions that limit the potential for hip distraction may preclude arthroscopy. These include joint ankylosis, dense heterotopic bone formation, and significant protrusio.

Morbid obesity is a relative contraindication for arthroscopy, not only because of distraction limitations but also because of the requisite length of instruments necessary to access and maneuver within the deeply receded joint.

Finally, advanced osteoarthritis is in our opinion a contraindication for arthroscopy, as noted previously.

CONCLUSION

Hip arthroscopy is an exciting, evolving technique for the diagnosis and treatment of hip disease. Previously, the anatomic configuration of the hip joint, the paucity of equipment tailored to the procedure, and concerns about potential complications limited the number of cases performed. However, better understanding of appropriate por-

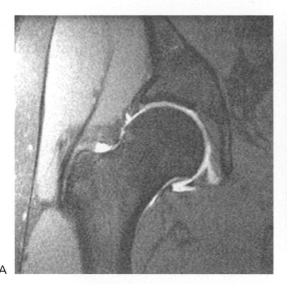

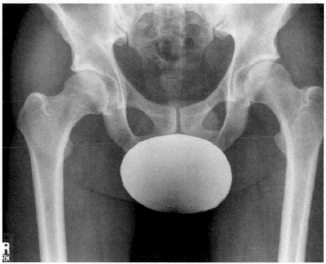

A   B

FIGURE 59.14 Gadolinium-enhanced MRI demonstrating a normal anterior acetabular labrum.

tal placement and experience with short periods of traction have made it possible to visualize the intraarticular structures of the hip joint in virtually every case.

Candidates for hip arthroscopy must have reproducible symptoms and physical findings that are functionally limiting and must have failed an adequate trial of conservative treatment. Improvements in arthroscopic technique and instrumentation have made it possible to arthroscopically diagnose and treat a variety of intraarticular causes of intractable hip pain that previously were misdiagnosed or required an open procedure. However, hip arthroscopy is extremely technique sensitive, requiring a thorough knowledge of anatomic relationships to prevent potentially catastrophic neurovascular complications. Anatomic cadaveric dissection and hip arthroscopic workshops are helpful in familiarizing the clinician with cross-sectional anatomy before performing hip arthroscopy.

Further advancements are necessary in optical equipment, manual and motorized instruments, and simple, reliable traction devices specific for this procedure. Refinements in patient selection and the increased availability of specific outcome data will help to define the role of hip arthroscopy in orthopaedic practice.

Case Example 1: A 35-year-old man presented with intractable anterior hip pain for at least 2 years which increased with daily activity. The pain onset was insidious and worsening over time. He demonstrated a positive hip extension test with an otherwise unremarkable examination. Gadolinium-enhanced MRI showed no definite intraarticular abnormality (Fig. 59.14A). The plain radiographs were within normal limits (Fig. 59.14B). Hip arthroscopy revealed a large flap at the watershed region with a torn anterior labrum (Fig. 59.15).

Case Example 2: A 27-year-old man with intractable anterior hip pain for 1 year complained of a popping sensation with occasional locking and buckling of his hip. The onset of symptoms was insidious. He was unable to run or participate in sports. The examination demonstrated a range of motion within normal limits but with a positive hip extension test. He walked with a slight limp. The gadolinium-enhanced MRI showed a torn anterior labrum with adjacent acetabular cartilage loss and subchondral cystic changes (Fig. 59.16). The plain radiographs were normal. Hip arthroscopy revealed a large flap at the watershed region with a torn anterior labrum (Fig. 59.17).

Case Example 3: A 34-year-old woman was referred to the senior author with synovial chondromatosis. The loose bodies

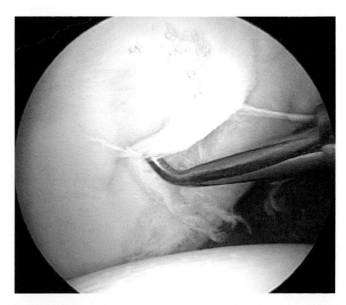

FIGURE 59.15 An arthroscopic probe demonstrating an unstable acetabular chondral flap in the watershed zone.

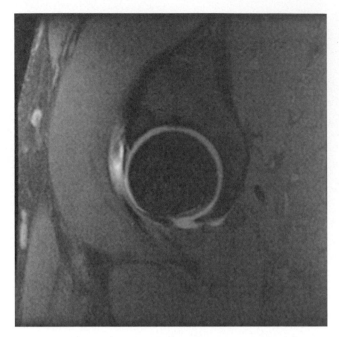

FIGURE 59.16 Arthroscopic MRI with a torn anterior labrum.

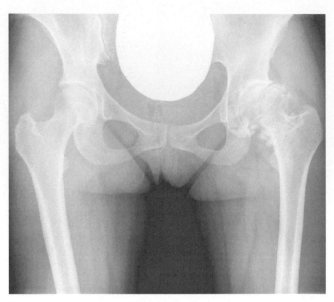

FIGURE 59.18 Multiple calcified loose bodies within the left hip joint.

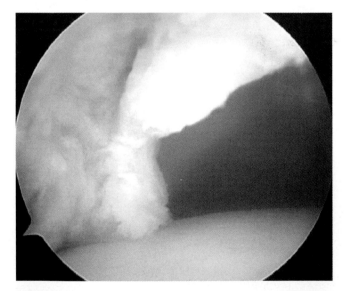

FIGURE 59.17 A torn, frayed anterior labrum with associated chondral flap.

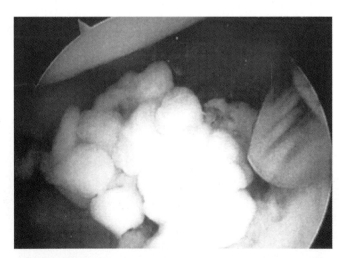

FIGURE 59.19 At surgery, grapelike clusters of loose bodies within the fovea.

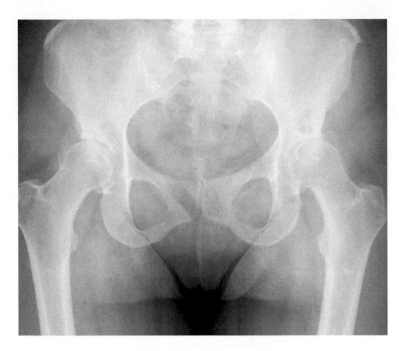

FIGURE 59.20 Radiograph showing dysplasia and joint space narrowing of the left hip joint.

were evident by MRI and plain radiographs (Fig. 59.18). She had constant anterior hip and groin pain that had increased over time. She was unable to exercise, and her walking was limited to 20 minutes. She walked with an obvious limp. On examination, external rotation was found to be limited by pain and locking. At hip arthroscopy, more than 75 loose bodies were removed (Fig. 59.19).

Case Example 4: A 49-year-old woman developed progressive and unremitting anterior hip and groin pain that had not responded to conservative therapy over the previous 3 years. She had occasional locking and buckling episodes with walking. She walked with an obvious limp. On examination, she had a positive hip extension test and resisted straight leg raising. Plain radiographs revealed acetabular dysplasia with mild

narrowing of the joint space superiorly (Fig. 59.20). An MRI revealed mild degenerative changes with some cyst formation in the acetabular roof. At arthroscopy, she was found to have an Outerbridge grade IV lesion in the anterior portion of the acetabulum adjacent to an enlarged and torn anterior labrum (Fig. 59.21). There were mild to moderate degenerative changes throughout the socket as well as the anterior femoral head.

REFERENCES

1. Burman M. Arthroscopy or the direct visualization of joints. *J Bone Joint Surg* 1931;4:669–695.
2. Gross R. Arthroscopy in hip disorders in children. *Orthop Rev* 1977;6:43–49.
3. Vakilif S, Warren R. Entrapped foreign body within the acetabular cup in THR. *Clin Orthop* 1980;150:159–162.
4. Holgersson S, Brattstrom H, Mogensen B, et al. Arthroscopy of the hip in juvenile chronic arthritis. *J Pediatr Orthop* 1981;1:273–278.
5. Dvorak M, Duncan CP, Day B. Arthroscopic anatomy of the hip. *Arthroscopy* 1990;6:264–00273.
6. Keene GS, Villar RN. Arthroscopic anatomy of the hip: an in vivo study. *Arthroscopy* 1994;10:392–399.
7. Eriksson E, Arvidsson I, Arvidsson H. Diagnostic and operative arthroscopy of the hip. *Orthopedics* 1986;9:169–176.
8. Johnson L. *Arthroscopic surgery principles and practice.* St Louis: CV Mosby, 1986.
9. Glick JM, Sampson TG, Gordon RB, et al. Hip arthroscopy by the lateral approach. *Arthroscopy* 1987;3:4–12.
10. Edwards DJ, Lomas D, Villar RN. Diagnosis of the painful hip by magnetic resonance imaging and arthroscopy. *J Bone Joint Surg Br* 1995;77:374–376.
11. Fitzgerald RH Jr. Acetabular labrum tears: diagnosis and treatment. *Clin Orthop* 1995:60–68.
12. Frich LH, Lauritzen J, Juhl M. Arthroscopy in diagnosis and treatment of hip disorders. *Orthopedics* 1989;12:389–392.

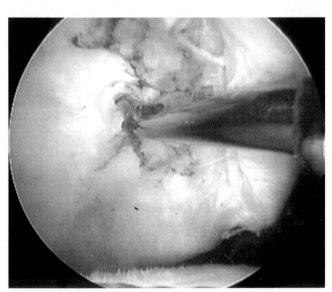

FIGURE 59.21 Outerbridge IV anterior acetabular lesion with exposed subchondral bone.

13. Gondolph-Zink B, Puhl P, Noack W. Semiarthroscopic synovectomy of the hip. *Int Orthop* 1988;12:31–35.
14. Hawkins RB. Arthroscopy of the hip. *Clin Orthop* 1989;(249):44–47.
15. Ide T, Akamatsu N, Nakajima I. Arthroscopic surgery of the hip joint. *Arthroscopy* 1991;7:204–211.
16. Ikeda T, Awaya G, Suzuki S, et al. Torn acetabular labrum in young patients: arthroscopic diagnosis and management. *J Bone Joint Surg Br* 1988;70:13–16.
17. Janssens X, Van Meirhaeghe J, Verdonk R, et al. Diagnostic arthroscopy of the hip joint in pigmented villonodular synovitis. *Arthroscopy* 1987;3:283–287.
18. McCarthy JC, Busconi B. The role of hip arthroscopy in the diagnosis and treatment of hip disease. *Orthopedics* 1995;18:753–756.
19. Okada Y, Awaya G, Ikeda T, et al. Arthroscopic surgery for synovial chondromatosis of the hip. *J Bone Joint Surg Br* 1989;71:198–199.
20. Villar R. Arthroscopic debridement of the hip: a minimally invasive approach to osteoarthritis. *J Bone Joint Surg Br* 1991;73:170–171.
21. McCarthy J, Day B, Busconi B. Hip arthroscopy: applications and echnique. *J Am Acad Orthop Surg* 1995;3:115–122.
22. McCarthy J, Wardell S, Mason J, et al. Injuries to the acetabular labrum: classification, outcome, and relationship to degenerative arthritis. Presented at the Annual Meeting of the American Academy of Orthopaedic Surgeons, San Francisco, CA, February 1997.
23. McCarthy J, Marchetti M, Newberg A, et al. *Improving diagnostic accuracy of chondral injuries: correlation of gadolinium MR imaging with arthroscopic surgery.* New Orleans: AAOS, 1997.
24. Goldman A, Minkoff J, Price A, et al. A posterior arthroscopic approach to bullet extraction from the hip. *J Trauma* 1987;27:1294–1300.
25. Collins DH, ed. *The pathology of articular and spinal diseases.* London: Edward Arnold & Co, 1949.
26. Dameron TB. Bucket handle tear of acetabular labrum accompanying posterior dislocation of the hip. *J Bone Joint Surg Am* 1959;41:131–134.
27. Nelson MC, Lauerman WC, Wells C. Avulsion of the acetabular labrum with intraarticular displacement. *Orthopaedics* 1990;13:889–891.
28. Altenberg AR. Acetabular labrum tears: a cause of hip pain and degenerative arthritis. *South Med J* 1977:70:174–175.
29. Cartilage IJ, Scott JHS. The inturned acetabular labrum in osteoarthrosis of the hip. *J R Coll Surg Edinburgh* 1982:6:339–344.
30. Ueo T, Hamabuchi M. Hip pain caused by cystic deformation of the labrum acetabulare. *Arthritis Rheum* 1984;27:947–950.
31. Harris WH. Etiology of osteoarthritis of the hip. *Clin Orthop* 1986;213:20–33.
32. Harris WH, Bourne RB, Oh I. Intraarticular acetabular labrum: a possible etiologic factor in certain cases of osteoarthritis of the hip. *J Bone Joint Surg Am* 1979;61:510–514
33. Lavernia CJ, Sierra RJ. Core decompression in atraumatic osteonecrosis of the hip. *J Arthroplasty* 2000;15:171–178.
34. Steinberg ME. Early diagnosis, evaluation, and staging of osteonecrosis. *Instr Course Lect* 1994;43:513–518.
35. Steinberg ME, Hayken GD, Steinberg DR. A quantitative system for staging avascular necrosis. *J Bone Joint Surg Br* 1995;77:34–41.
36. Delcamp DD, Klaaren HE, Pompe van Meerdervoort HF. Traumatic avulsion of the ligamentum teres without dislocation of the hip: two case reports. *J Bone Joint Surg Am* 1988;70:933–935.
37. Ebraheim NA, Savolaine ER, Fenton PJ, et al. A calcified ligamentum teres mimicking entrapped intraarticular bony fragments in a patient with acetabular fracture. *J Orthop Trauma* 1991;5:376–378.
38. Barrett IR, Goldberg JA. Avulsion fracture of the ligamentum teres in a child: a case report. *J Bone Joint Surg Am* 1989;71:438–439.
39. Gray AJ, Villar RN. The ligamentum teres of the hip: an arthroscopic classification of its pathology. *Arthroscopy* 1997;13:575–578.
40. Salter RB. Etiology, pathogenesis and possible prevention of congenital dislocation of the hip. *Can Med Assoc J* 1968;98:933–945.
41. Glick JM. Hip arthroscopy. In: McGinty JB, ed. *Operative arthroscopy.* New York: Raven Press, 1991:663–676.
42. Chung WK, Slater GL, Bates EH. Treatment of septic arthritis of the hip by arthroscopic lavage. *J Pediatr Orthop* 1993;13:444–446.
43. Epstein HC, Wiss DA, Cozen L. Posterior fracture dislocation of the hip with fractures of the femoral head. *Clin Orthop* 1985;(201):9–17.
44. Glick JM. Hip arthroscopy using the lateral approach. *Instr Course Lect* 1988;37:223–231.
45. Villar RN. Hip arthroscopy. *Br J Hosp Med* 1992;47:763–766.

ARTHROSCOPY OF THE HIP IN THE MANAGEMENT OF THE ATHLETE

MARC J. PHILIPPON

The hip joint appears to be the last frontier for the arthroscopic treatment of intraarticular injuries in athletes. The ability to visualize a joint arthroscopically that at times can be subjected to substantial forces of up to five times body weight during athletic activities such as running and jumping is exciting and certainly invaluable as a diagnostic tool (1). Injuries to the hip joint such as a torn labrum, loose bodies, torn ligamentum teres, chondral injuries, and capsular laxity with iliofemoral ligament deficiency can now be treated successfully arthroscopically (2–7). Athletes have a natural ability to recover from surgical intervention, and their discipline and focus make surgical intervention in these individuals a positive experience.

HIP PAIN IN ATHLETES

Injuries to the hip in athletes are mostly described as muscular strain as well as soft tissue contusion. It is important to be able to differentiate extraarticular from intraarticular pathology (Table 60.1). A complete history and hip/back examination is essential to arrive at the appropriate diagnosis. Pain is the most common complaint but is nonspecific. The athlete may complain of associated clicking, catching, snapping, and instability with guarding and decreased range of motion. The athlete will often describe his hip as being "tight" when suffering from a labral tear. The tightness may be explained by guarding of the iliopsoas and quadratus lumborum. It is important to apply the standard principles of physical examination when examining the athlete's hip (Table 60.2). It is essential when evaluating the athlete's hip to have good knowledge of the hip anatomy to be able to make good correlation with diagnostic imaging. Plain radiography, including a view of the anteroposterior (AP) pelvis, ultrasound, magnetic resonance imaging (MRI) with

arthrography, and computed tomography are invaluable tools to help in determining the cause of the hip pain in the athlete.

ANATOMIC FACTORS

The hip is an articulation between the head of the femur and the acetabulum. Its bony configuration is intrinsically stable except in situations where there is variation in the acetabular depth and femoral head geometry, which results in more reliance in the surrounding soft tissue. Craniomedial and craniolateral inclination of the weight-bearing surface has an effect on the joint capsule/ligaments of the hip and on the ligamentum teres as well as on the suction effect of the hip (8). The femoral head normally forms two thirds of a sphere and it is flattened in the area where the acetabulum applies its greatest load. When the body is in the anatomic position, the anterior part of the femoral head is not engaged in the acetabulum and the labrum augments the femoral head coverage by its extension from the bony acetabulum. The labrum runs circumferentially around the acetabulum perimeter to the base of the fovea and becomes attached to the transverse acetabular ligament posteriorly and anteriorly (9). The labrum has shown free nerve endings including proprioceptors and nociceptors, which may explain decreased proprioception and pain in an athlete with a torn acetabular labrum (5,10). The absence of significant vascularity in the labrum makes it difficult to heal. The vessels that penetrate the labrum are on the outermost layer on the capsular surface to a depth of approximately 0.5 mm, leaving most of the labrum avascular (11). The acetabular labrum is made of a triangular fibrocartilage and may act in enhancing stability by providing negative intraarticular pressure in the hip joint (12). It also may act as tension band to limit expansion during motion between the anterior and posterior columns during loading in the gait cycle (9). In analyzing the labral capsular complex, there is a theoretical concern about the potential rotational instability of a hip with a deficient labrum associated with redundant capsular tissue,

M. J. Philippon: Sports Medicine/Hip Disorders, University of Pittsburgh Medical Center, Center for Sports Medicine; Department of Orthopaedic Surgery, University of Pittsburgh School of Medicine, Pittsburgh, Pennsylvania.

TABLE 60.1 POTENTIAL CAUSES OF HIP PAIN

Extraarticular	Intraarticular
Adductor strains	Femoral neck stress fracture
Iliopsoas tendon strain	Osteonecrosis
Gluteus medius strain	Inflammatory arthritis
Hamstring strains	Osteoarthritis
Greater trochantic bursitis	Posttraumatic arthritis
Gracilis strain	Loose bodies
Iliopsoas bursitis	Acetabular labral tears
Ischial bursitis	Ruptured ligamentum teres
Rectus femoris tendonitis	Chondral injuries
External rotators tendonitis	Instability
Avulsion injuries	Capsular sprain
Stress fracture of the lesser	Developmental dysplastic hip
trochanter	Slipped capital femoral
Sacroiliac joint strain	epiphysis
Myositis ossifans	Legg-Calvé-Perthes disease
Hip pointer	Transient synovitis
Infection	

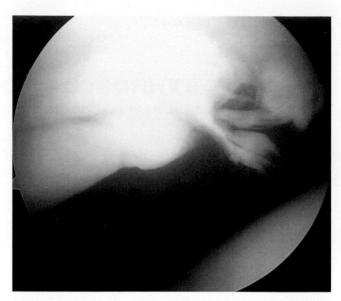

FIGURE 60.1 Anterior-superior labral tear in a professional athlete.

creating a potential abnormal load distribution due to a transient incongruous joint due to subtle subluxation (9).

The ligamentum teres is extracapsular and may have some stabilizing effect on the hip joint with a deficient labrum (13). The psoas tendon protects the anterior intermediate portion of the capsule, and by its anatomic location can be subjected to increased load in athletic activities especially in athletes with intraarticular pathology. The psoas bursa communicates with the hip joint in the adult in approximately 20% of the population.

GOLF

I have managed the hip injuries of 16 professional golfers (17 hips), including 13 players from the Professional Golfers' Association (PGA) Tour, one golfer from the Senior PGA Tour, one woman from the professional tour, and one professional golfer from the Asian tour. The athletes were treated for labral tear with associated capsular laxity (Fig. 60.1). Most of the tears were anterosuperior; however, in four golfers, posterior tears were present. Capsular laxity

with rotational instability was present in all of these athletes, including iliofemoral ligament deficiency in seven (Figs. 60.2 and 60.3). All of these athletes were treated in the supine position with hip arthroscopy with debridement of the torn portion of the labrum back to stable labral remnant. The capsule adjacent to the labral tear was assessed by probing, and focal thermal capsulorrhaphy was performed for capsular laxity. Hip rotation precaution was applied postoperatively for 18 days. All golfers were returned to their professional activities except for two patients. One athlete had concomitant shoulder surgery and is still rehabilitating his shoulder, and the other patient had surgery just 4 weeks ago. Overall, all patients had marked improvement in their symptoms and returned to competition without any pain.

TABLE 60.2 HIP EXAMINATION

Observation of gait and posture
Comparison from side to side
Palpation of hip bursae and surrounding soft tissue, including the anterior capsule
Analysis of active and passive range of motion
Assessment of overall generalized laxity
Dynamic fluoroscopic examination
Neurovascular examination
Provocative maneuvers

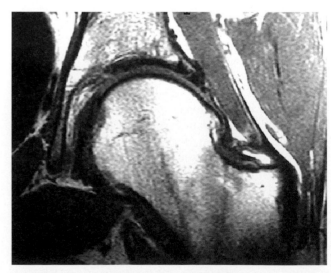

FIGURE 60.2 Iliofemoral ligament tear in a professional golfer with associated instability as detected by MRI.

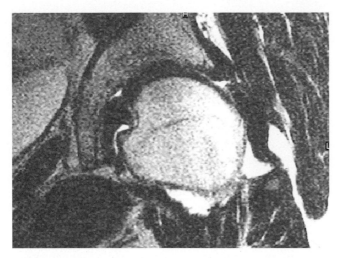

FIGURE 60.3 Same patient as in Fig. 60.2, 4 months after hip arthroscopy for labral tear debridement and thermal capsulorrhaphy adjacent to the torn iliofemoral ligament. Note the hypertrophied healed ligament.

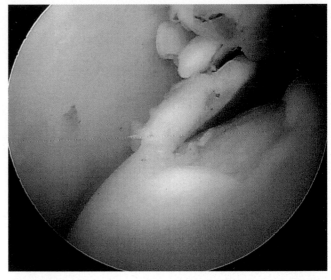

FIGURE 60.4 Chondral flap injury on the femoral head of a professional athlete.

An interesting outcome included improvement in the patient's driving distance and a greater sense of stability on the treated hip. Two patients went on to win PGA Tour tournaments. All patients had improvement in their modified Harris Hip Scale score.

We now have a better understanding of the mechanism of hip injury in golfers through our neuromuscular laboratory. Ten PGA professionals and six low-handicap amateur golfers diagnosed with acetabular labral tears and capsular redundancy of the hip of the hind limb have undergone laboratory testing for strength, proprioception, balance, flexibility, and swing-motion analysis conducted with electromyogram (EMG). This analysis demonstrated excessive hip abductor EMG activation, resulting in excessive anterior forces of the right hip during the golf swing in right-handed golfers. Negative uploading of the right hip at impact resulted in excessive anterior hip forces and painful position. It was also demonstrated that hip abductors/adductors EMG coactivation resulted in superior hip stabilization and less hip displacement forces. These findings are very important, and we are now working on injury prevention models and also are applying the analysis in our patient rehabilitation (10).

FOOTBALL

Football players are subjected to high-impact trauma as well as axial loading with rotational forces. I have treated five National Football League (NFL) players, three college football players, and two high school football players for athletic hip injuries. This group of patients also had labral tears, but the common finding was associated significant chondral injuries (Figs. 60.4 and 60.5). One patient had a fracture dislocation of the posterior wall of his acetabulum, which was treated with mini-arthrotomy, open reduction with internal fixation (ORIF), and arthroscopic debridement. This patient returned to activities, pain free. However, because of the nature of his dislocation, it was recommended that he not return to play for 1 year to minimize the risk of osteonecrosis. All athletes returned to football activities except one high school football player who had an intraarticular or loose body and is still in the rehabilitation phase. Positions played by these athletes include quarterback, wide receiver, tight end, and defensive back.

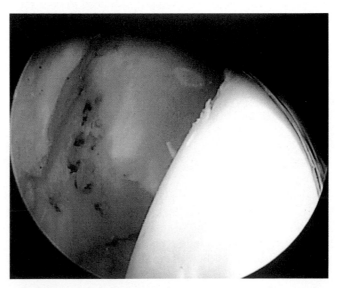

FIGURE 60.5 Chondral injury of the posterior acetabular wall of an NFL football player after microfracture treatment.

HOCKEY

Hockey players are subjected to significant, high-impact forces to their hip as well as significant abduction/external rotation movements. In these athletes the role of the iliofemoral ligament cannot be overemphasized. Strains are very common, as are hip flexors tendonitis. However, should these injuries show no improvement with time, consideration to diagnostic MRI-arthrogram should be given to exclude intraarticular pathology. I have treated two National Hockey League (NHL) hockey players arthroscopically for hip injuries. One patient had significant myositis ossification involving his hip abductor mass, and a anterior labral tear. He was treated with arthroscopic resection and debridement of the torn labrum. The patient improved significantly. He returned to skating pain free. The second patient had an anterior superior labral tear with associated chondral flap injury from the rim of the anterior wall and capsular laxity. He was treated with debridement and chondroplasty with focal thermal capsulorraphy. He had improvement in his symptoms, especially with hip rotation. He also subjectively felt improved strength in his hip. He also had associated iliopsoas tendonitis, which became a chronic problem that required extensive rest for recovery. It is important to note that the anterior capsule is reinforced laterally by the iliofemoral ligament. However, in the intermediate portion, there is capsular attenuation, and this area is being reinforced not by a ligament but by a tendon. Because there is significant load in this region, there is a bursa present between the joint and the actual tendon. In 20% of the adult population, this bursa communicates with the hip joint. It is certainly important to speculate that persistent flexor, strain, or tendonitis in hockey players, which is quite frequent, may have a relationship with intraarticular pathology such as a labral tear, chondral injury, or loose bodies, and persistent intraarticular synovitis can lead to fluid accumulation in the bursa, therefore compounding the problem and creating a vicious cycle if the intraarticular pathology is not addressed. It is also important to understand that in the rehabilitation phase of a hip treated arthroscopically for intraarticular pathology, a psoas tendonitis will resolve often approximately at the same rate as the intraarticular pathology is treated and healed.

BASEBALL

Baseball players are also subjected to significant axial loading at forces with rotational components. Baseball pitchers transfer weight at the end of the throw on their landing leg or have extra load on winding up during their early phase of throwing, and thus subject their hip joint. Baseball catchers are also subjected to extra load on their hip joint. I have treated two professional baseball pitchers and one baseball catcher. These patients had labral tear with adjacent capsular laxity, and one had significant chondral lesion on the femoral head adjacent to the labral tear. These patients were treated with debridement and chondroplasty. All three patients returned to their baseball activities without pain.

FIGURE SKATING

As in hockey players, the hip joint in figure skaters is subjected to strains from stroking. In addition, figure skaters are subjected to significant torsional force and centrifugal force from various components of their artistic routines. I have treated three Olympic-level figure skaters including one gold medallist. Labral injury with chondrosis was presented in all three patients as well as capsular laxity. Hip arthroscopy with torn labrum, focal thermal capsulorrhaphy, and chondroplasty was performed and all patients returned to their skating activities with marked improvement.

BALLET

Ballet dancers subject their hip to significant extreme of motion, especially rotation. This can lead to significant instability due to capsular stretching. Labral tear injunction with capsular and elongation can lead to rotational instability and to significant discomfort. This can be associated with flexor spasms and quadratus lumborum spasms and can lead to a false sense of hip tightness, which can result in unnecessary stretching of the above musculature and can create capsulitis and capsular elongation. Because of this, an MRI-arthrogram is important to detect intraarticular pathology in cases of persistent flexor tendinitis and/or "groin strain." I have treated five hips in four professional ballet dancers. These dancers all had capsular elongation with partial tear of their ligament teres and labrum tear at the time of surgery. Debridement and thermal capsulorrhaphy were performed. All patients had improvement in their symptoms and returned to their ballet activities with less pain. These patients require more progressive and extensive rehabilitation.

OTHER ATHLETES

I have also treated other professional athletes (Table 60.3).

Technique

All athletes in this series had surgery in the supine position except for one patient. They were placed over a fracture table to allow for distraction. The surgical hip was placed at 10 degrees of flexion, neutral abduction, and 5 degrees of internal rotation. This patient was treated in the lateral position because of a posterior acetabular fracture dislocation. The portals are established in the paratrochanteric region. The first portal is placed 1 cm proximal to the tip of the grater trochanter and 1 cm anterior. The second portal is

TABLE 60.3 HIPS TREATED BETWEEN MAY 1999 AND DECEMBER 2001:
***n* = 43**

Sport	No. of Treated Hips in Professional/Olympic Athletes	Returned to Active Competition	Improvement In Modified Harris Hip Scale Score
Golf	17	15	17
Football	5	4	5
Ice hockey	2	1	2
Baseball	3	3	3
Basketball	1	0	1
Tennis	1	1	1
Skateboarding	1	1	1
Gymnastics	2	2	2
Weightlifting	1	1	1
Ballet	5	3	5
Soccer	2	2	2
Tae-kwan-do	2	2	2
Olympic yachting	1	1	1
Figure skating	3	3	3

placed at the intersection of a line drawn in line with the anterior superior iliac spine. Fluoroscopic guidance is utilized for placement of the portals. Debridement of the labrum was performed with flexible radiofrequency instruments including a chisel and a monopolar heat probe that I developed. Chondroplasty was performed with a full radius motorized shaver as well as a thermal probe maintaining the temperature below 55°C. Good traction is essential, and the anesthesiologist maintains the patient completely relaxed and paralyzed during the procedure. Athletes who received thermal capsulorrhaphy had to respect rotation precaution for 18 to 21 days. The athletes were allowed only neutral rotation. If chondroplasty was performed, toe-touch weight bearing was recommended for 21 to 28 days.

DISCUSSION

Elite athletes are subjected to extreme forces and range of motion in their sport, which affects their hip joints and makes them prone to injuries. The mechanisms of injuries can be from repetitive motion or direct trauma. The surgeon should be aware of subtle radiographic evidence of hip dysplasia, which may be an underlying factor predisposing athletes to labral injury (2). Hip injuries in athletes that do not resolve or improve over a 4-week period should prompt the treating physician to look for intraarticular pathology.

Hip arthroscopy in the treatment of hip injuries in athletes appears to be very effective. This chapter discussed my experience with professional/Olympic athletes. These results are comparable in amateur, college, and high school athletes. Accelerated rehabilitation and prompt return to competition are strong benefits of the arthroscopic approach. Good technique and appropriate patient selection are essential for the success of this procedure.

REFERENCES

1. American Orthopaedic Society for Sports Medicine. Injuries to the pelvis, hip, and thigh. In: Griffin LY, ed. *Orthopaedic knowledge update. Sports medicine.* Rosemont, IL: American Academy of Orthopaedic Surgeons, 1994:239.
2. Byrd JW. Labral lesions: an elusive source of hip pain case reports and literature review. *Arthroscopy* 1996;12(5):603–612.
3. Dameron T Jr. Bucket-handle tear of acetabular labrum accompanying posterior dislocation of the hip. *J Bone Joint Surg* 1959; 41A:131–134.
4. Fitzgerald RH. Acetabular labral tears: diagnosis and treatment. *Clin Orthop* 1995;31:60–68.
5. Kim YT, Azusa H. The nerve endings of the acetabular labrum. *Clin Orthop* 1995;320:176–181.
6. Lieberman J, Altcheck D, Salvati E. Recurrent dislocation of a hip with a labral lesion: treatment with a modified Bankart-type repair. *J Bone Joint Surg* 1993;75A:1524–1527.
7. Santori N, Villar R. Acetabular labral tears: result of arthroscopic partial limbectomy. *Arthroscopy* 2000;16,1:11–15.
8. Bombelli R. *Structure and function in normal and abnormal hips*, 3rd ed. New York: Springer-Verlag, 1993.
9. Philippon MJ. The role of arthroscopic thermal capsulorrhaphy in the hip. *Clin Sports Med* 2001;20:817–828.
10. Lephart S, Philippon M, Draovitch P, et al. Golf injury prevention research models. Proceedings of the 2002 World Scientific Congress of Golf, St. Andrews, Scotland, July 26, 2002.
11. McCarthy JC, Noble PC, Wright J, et al. The role of labral lesions in the development of early degenerative hip disease. American Academy of Orthopedic Surgery, San Francisco, 2001.
12. Takechi H, Nagashima H, Ito S. Intra-articular pressure of the hip joint outside and inside the limbus. *J Jpn Orthop Assoc* 1982; 56:529–536.
13. Rao J, Zhou X, Villar RN. Injury to the ligamentum teres. *Clin Sports Med* 2001;20:791–799.

THE FOOT AND ANKLE

ANKLE ARTHROSCOPY

JAMES TASTO

Ankle arthroscopy was originally developed in Japan and was introduced into the United States in the early 1930s. Access to the joint was restricted, and the procedure never developed at that time. As the use of fiberoptic technology developed, access to smaller joints became more feasible. With the advent of smaller arthroscopes and instrumentation, as well as the development of wide-angle technology, all areas of the ankle joint became more readily accessible. Good to excellent results have been reported in the literature for the vast majority of cases (1–6).

INDICATIONS

The indications for ankle arthroscopy have developed over the past two decades. Originally it was used for diagnostic purposes and for removal of loose bodies. As techniques have improved, the indications have grown and promise to be even more comprehensive in the future (7–11).

As with most arthroscopic procedures, it may be valuable as a diagnostic tool when conventional methods do not allow a conclusive diagnosis. Other indications are removal of loose bodies or osteochondral fragments, chondroplasty, synovectomy, resection of soft tissue in the case of impingement syndrome, and removal of scar and adhesions (12,13) (Figs. 61.1, 61.2, and 61.3). In the case of osteochondritis dissecans, it can be used for removal or fixation of the fragment as well as abrasion or microfracture of the base. Arthroscopic ankle arthrodesis has developed as an alternative technique to the open procedure and affords a number of distinct advantages.

Repetitive trauma can give rise to tibial and talar osteophytes, which may be resected arthroscopically more precisely and less invasively than with conventional open procedures (Fig. 61.4). If an open stabilization is planned for ankle instability, it is a valuable adjunct to addressing any concomitant ankle pathology that may be present (14). There are some advocates of radiofrequency capsular shrink-

age for less severe cases of ankle instability, but no long-term data have been published. There are a variety of reports on the use of arthroscopy for debridement in the cases of degenerative arthritis of the ankle. In the more severe cases with some malalignment, the results are not that promising, but in less involved cases one can anticipate some short-term improvement.

Chronic syndesmosis injuries can be addressed through a debridement and partial synovectomy or debridement of the interosseous ligament and scar tissue with percutaneous screw fixation (15,16). It has also been advocated as a valuable adjunct in the diagnosis of chronic syndesmosis injuries if routine radiographs and stress films have not been definitive (17). Arthroscopic-assisted fracture fixation of ankle fractures has been described and has some distinct advantages in appropriate alignment of the chondral surfaces (18,19).

Tendoscopy is gaining acceptance as a technique to evaluate and treat disorders of the tendons around the ankle joint (Figs. 61.5, 61.6, and 61.7). In the future, we anticipate that many of the biologic resurfacing procedures will be done arthroscopically or with arthroscopic assistance.

CONTRAINDICATIONS

There are a few notable contraindications to performing an ankle arthroscopy. The presence of cellulitis or any active soft tissue infection in the lower extremity carries the risk of pyarthrosis. Severely restricted joint access is only a relative contraindication to ankle arthroscopy, because soft tissue distraction usually creates sufficient space to perform the procedure.

If an arthroscopic procedure is performed in the face of acute trauma, whether the injury is to soft tissue or a fracture, there may be a relative contraindication because of potential extravasation and the possibility of a compartment syndrome. It should be approached very cautiously in these cases, should be done with low pressure, and can be done as a "dry scope." Patients with poor vascular status and obesity have been shown to have much poorer results and may pre-

J. Tasto: Department of Orthopedic Surgery, University of California, San Diego; San Diego Medicine & Orthopedic Center, San Diego, California.

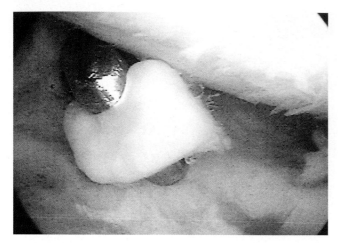

FIGURE 61.1 Arthroscopic removal of a loose body.

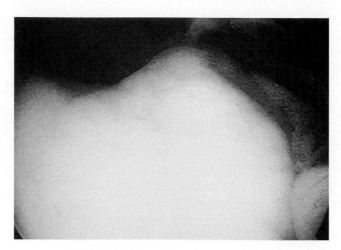

FIGURE 61.4 Anterior talar osteophytes.

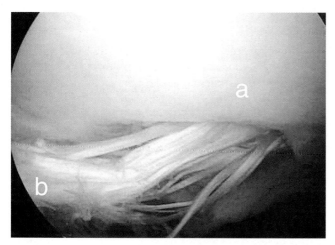

FIGURE 61.2 Partially torn posterior-inferior tibiofibular ligament. **A,** talus; **B,** posterior tibiofibular ligament.

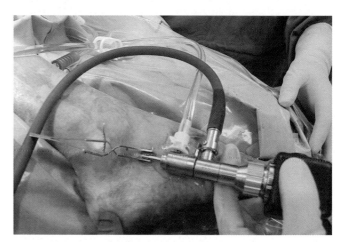

FIGURE 61.5 Peroneal tendoscopy.

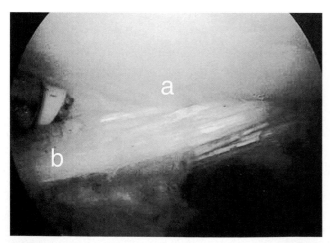

FIGURE 61.3 Radiofrequency modulation of partially torn posterior inferior tibiofibular ligament. **A,** talus; **B,** posterior tibiofibular ligament.

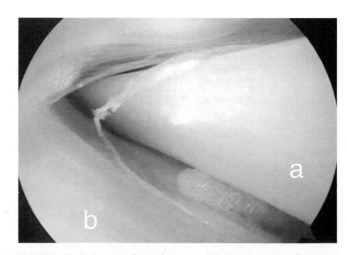

FIGURE 61.6 Peroneal tendons as visualized via tendoscopy. **A,** peroneus brevis; **B,** peroneus longus.

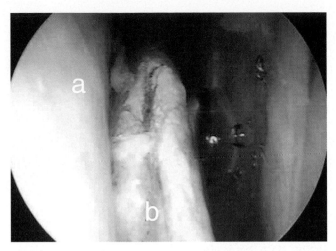

FIGURE 61.7 Ruptured peroneus brevis as visualized via tendoscopy. **A,** normal peroneus longus; **B,** ruptured peroneus brevis.

sent relative contraindications (20). Patients with suspect reflex sympathetic dystrophy or a sympathetic pain mediated syndrome may actually find their condition worsening if even a microinvasive procedure is performed.

IMAGING

Routine radiographs are essential before any surgical procedure. A variety of oblique views may be helpful to localize osteophytes and spurs responsible for osseous impingement syndrome. Stress films in the anteroposterior and lateral planes are a necessity if there is a question of instability. A Browden view will show any involvement of the posterior subtalar joint, which must also be taken into consideration for ankle and hind foot pain.

Magnetic resonance imaging scans are extremely helpful in identifying occult osteochondritis dissecans or defining the depth and perimeter of these lesions. Extraarticular causes of ankle and hind foot pain, such as tendon rupture or tenosynovitis, can be differentiated quite readily. Occasionally there is an indication for a computed tomographic scan when greater definition of the osseous components of ankle joint pathology is required. Bone scan can be helpful in some cases of occult syndesmotic injury and in the identification of early degenerative joint disease.

COMPLICATIONS

A thorough knowledge of the anatomy of the foot and ankle is critical in avoiding injuries to neurovascular structures and tendons (21–23). The majority of complications from ankle arthroscopy are neurologic in nature; although most resolve, permanent damage has been reported (24,25). Infections are probably no more prevalent than in similar arthroscopic procedures, but because of the increased incidence with open

foot and ankle procedures, meticulous surgical technique and attention to detail needs to be employed.

Fistula formation is somewhat unique to ankle arthroscopy, but the etiology is subject to debate. Current prevalent hypotheses include excessive debridement of soft tissue around portal sites, increased motion of the ankle postoperatively, proximity of skin portals to the ankle joint proper, and lack of suture closure. These fistulae can usually be effectively treated with a short period of immobilization.

Since the advent of soft tissue distraction, there have been few if any reports of complications secondary to skeletal distraction (26). It is recommended that traction not exceed 30 lbs or 1 hour, because traction in excess of these parameters has been shown to be responsible for ligament disruption and changes in nerve conduction velocity (27).

Compartment syndrome is a risk in ankle arthroscopy when dealing with fracture fixation, but it can be seen when inflow pressures get above safe levels and adequate outflow has not been established. Pseudoaneurysm has also been reported (28,29).

Other complications that can occur because of the restricted joint access are instrument breakage and chondral damage. Inadequate or excessive bone resection can occur if the surgeon incorrectly assesses the amount or location of bony lesions that need to be resected.

OPERATING ROOM SETUP

The patient is placed supine on the operating table, and either general or regional anesthesia is employed (30). Ankle arthroscopy generally requires distraction, and currently soft tissue distraction has completely replaced skeletal distraction (27). Commercially available outriggers can be attached to the operating room table and are attached to a soft tissue distraction strap. These ankle straps usually consist of a calcaneal component and dorsal containment strap (Fig. 61.8).

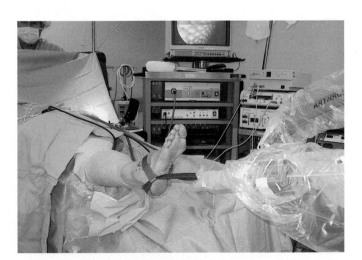

FIGURE 61.8 Soft tissue distraction strap and outrigger.

After the extremity has been thoroughly prepared and draped, the soft tissue distraction device is placed and traction is applied. Use of a tourniquet and leg holder is optional, but it does allow the surgeon to place the extremity in a neutral position for ready access to the variety of portals needed, and it provides countertraction for the ankle distraction. It is helpful to drop the foot of the table approximately 30 degrees, to aid in access to the ankle and to facilitate the creation of a posterolateral portal if necessary. This clearance also makes the manipulation of small instrumentation about the ankle easier to accomplish. The surgeon is positioned distal to the foot with arms straddling the traction device.

TECHNIQUE

Most ankle arthroscopy is carried out with a short, 2.7-mm wide-angle arthroscope (31). The choice of sheaths can determine the flow rate. A small shaver system is employed, usually with 3.5- or 2.0-mm blades. An 18-gauge needle is placed in the anteromedial portal and is critical in determining the appropriate angle to enter the joint. The ankle joint is distended with 8 to 10 mL of normal saline. If the portal is too high or too low, access will be very difficult. The needle guides the surgeon in portal placement and ensures that the appropriate location has been achieved.

Once the site is chosen, a nick and spread technique is employed with a no. 11 blade and a mosquito clamp. The anteromedial portal should be the primary portal that is established first (32–36). It is located just medial to the tibialis anterior tendon, and the angle of entrance is approximately 45 degrees to the long axis of the leg. The widest portion of the ankle joint is anteromedial through the notch of Harty and usually allows access to the posterior portion of the ankle joint. The anterolateral portal is established under direct vision with the needle, and again attention to the location as well as the angle is critical.

When using the nick and spread technique laterally, care is taken to avoid the dorsal intermediate branch of the superficial peroneal nerve. The safest location for the portal is just lateral to the peroneus tertius tendon. Once the outflow cannula is in place, a complete diagnostic arthroscopy is carried out. An accessory posterolateral portal may be used for outflow or as a working portal if necessary. This portal is created just lateral to the Achilles tendon and is placed about 0.5 cm distal to the posterior tibial plafond. It can also be placed under direct vision, with the entry site just inferior to the posterior-inferior tibiofibular ligament and again at about a 45-degree angle to the long axis of the joint (Fig. 61.9). Care is taken to avoid the sural nerve and the small saphenous vein.

Accessory portals can be established inferior to the standard portals and slightly peripheral. Placing needles in these portals can establish outflow when the routine working portal is being occupied by a curette or other instrument that does not allow outflow. Transmalleolar and transtalar portals are also used under special circumstances when approaching talar lesions. Posteromedial and anterior central portals are contraindicated because of the proximity of these portals to neurovascular structures.

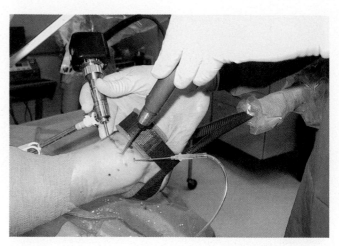

FIGURE 61.9 Portal placement with arthroscope in anteromedial portal, shaver in anterolateral portal, needle in accessory anterolateral portal, and outline of superficial branch of peroneal nerve.

If one moves the arthroscope and views from medial to lateral, the following anterior structures should be visualized (Figs. 61.10, 61.11, and 61.12):

- Deep deltoid ligament
- Medial gutter
- Anterior tibiotalar joint
- Anterior talar sulcus
- Anterior talofibular ligament
- Anterior tibiofibular ligament
- Trifurcation of the tibia, fibula and talus
- Lateral gutter

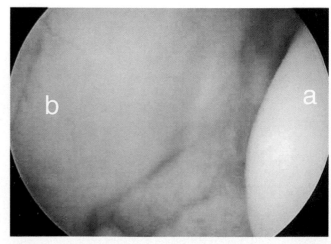

FIGURE 61.10 Anterior talar sulcus. **A,** talus; **B,** anterior capsule.

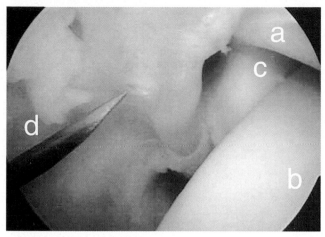

FIGURE 61.11 Anterior tibiofibular ligament. **A,** tibia; **B,** talus; **C,** fibula; **D,** needle pointing at anterior tibiofibular ligament.

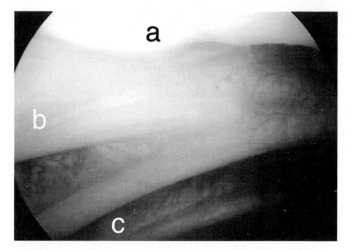

FIGURE 61.14 Posterior-inferior tibiofibular ligament. **A,** tibia; **B,** posterior-inferior tibiofibular ligament; **C,** transverse slip.

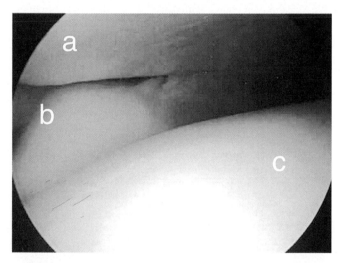

FIGURE 61.12 Trifiguration of tibia, fibula and talus. **A,** tibia; **B,** fibula; **C,** talus.

As the arthroscope is placed through the notch of Harty, moving from posterolateral to posteromedial, one visualizes the following (Figs. 61.13 and 61.14):

- Posterior-inferior tibiofibular ligament
- Transverse slip
- Posterior tibiotalar joint
- Reflection of the flexor hallucis longus
- Posteromedial gutter housing the neurovascular bundle

After carrying out a complete diagnostic examination from the anteromedial portal, the surgeon alternates portals and visualizes laterally, which provides a different perspective and allows the arthroscope to run deep into the fibular talar gutter and superior to the subtalar joint and capsule.

Most procedures can be done through two portals with occasional use of the posterolateral or accessory portals. Generous use of accessory portals using 18-gauge needles aids in fluid control and in delineating the succinct location of portal placement should any instrumentation be necessary.

Once the surgical procedure is carried out, Steri-Strips are applied to the wound and 10 mL of local anesthetic is instilled into the joint. A bulky, semirigid dressing is applied. Touch weight bearing and range of motion are limited for 5 to 7 days.

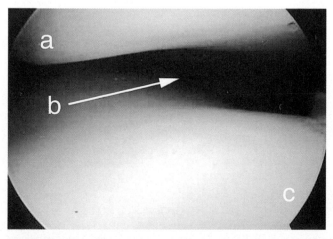

FIGURE 61.13 Notch of Harty. **A,** tibia; **B,** notch of Harty as visualized through the anteromedial portal; **C,** talus.

REFERENCES

1. Demaziere A, Ogilvie-Harris DJ. [Operative arthroscopy of the ankle: 107 cases.] *Rev Rhum Mal Osteoartic* 1991;58:93–97.
2. Martin DF, Baker CL, Curl WW, et al. Operative ankle arthroscopy: long-term follow-up. *Am J Sports Med* 1989;17:16–23.
3. Lundeen GW. Historical perspectives of ankle arthroscopy. *J Foot Surg* 1987;26:3–7.
4. Guhl JF. New techniques for arthroscopic surgery of the ankle. *Orthopedics* 1986;9:261–269.

5. Amendola A, Petrik J, Webster-Bogaert S. Ankle arthroscopy: outcome in 79 consecutive patients. *Arthroscopy* 1996;12:565–573.

6. Feder KS, Schonholtz GJ. Ankle arthroscopy: review and long-term results. *Foot Ankle* 1992;13:382–385.

7. Stetson W, Ferkel RD. Ankle arthroscopy: I. Technique and complications. *J Am Acad Orthop Surg* 1996;4:17–23.

8. Aroen A, Granlund OG. [Ankle arthroscopy: indications, findings and results.] *Tidsskr Nor Laegeforen* 1999;119:658–660.

9. Ogilvie-Harris DJ, Gilbart MK, Chorney K. Chronic pain following ankle sprains in athletes: the role of arthroscopic surgery. *Arthroscopy* 1997;13:564–574.

10. van Dijk CN, Scholte D. Arthroscopy of the ankle joint. *Arthroscopy* 1997;13:90–96.

11. Sandmeier RH, Renstrom PA. *Scand J Med Sci Sports* 1995;5:313.

12. DeBerardino TM, Arciero RA, Taylor DC. Arthroscopic treatment of soft-tissue impingement of the ankle in athletes. *Arthroscopy* 1997;13:492–498.

13. Branca A, Di Palma L, Bucca C, et al. Arthroscopic treatment of anterior ankle impingment. *Foot Ankle Int* 1997;18:418–423.

14. Kibler WB. Arthroscopic findings in ankle ligament reconstruction. *Clin Sports Med* 1996;15:799–804.

15. Ogilvie-Harris DJ, Gilbart MK, Chorney K. Chronic pain following ankle sprains in athletes: the role of arthroscopic surgery. *Arthroscopy* 1997;13:564–574.

16. Tasto JP, Laimins PD. Recent advances in ankle arthroscopic techniques. In: Parisien JS, ed. *Current Techniques in Arthroscopy.* New York: Thieme, 1998:181–194.

17. Takao M, Ochi M, Naito K, et al. Arthroscopic diagnosis of tibiofibular syndesmosis disruption. *Arthroscopy* 2001;17:836–843.

18. Thordarson DB, Bains R, Shepherd LE. The role of ankle arthroscopy on the surgical management of ankle fractures. *Foot Ankle Int* 2001;22:123–125.

19. van Dijk CN, Verhagen RA, Tol JL. Arthroscopy for problems after ankle fracture. *J Bone Joint Surg Br* 1997;27:280–284.

20. Japour C, Vohra P, Giorgini R, et al. Ankle arthroscopy: follow-up study of 33 ankles: effects of physical therapy and obesity. *J Foot Ankle Surg* 1996;35:199–209.

21. Takao M, Ochi M, Naito K, et al. Arthroscopic diagnosis of tibiofibular syndesmosis disruption. *Arthroscopy* 2001;17:836–843.

22. Lamy C, Stienstra JJ. Complications in ankle arthroscopy. *Clin Podiatr Med Surg* 1994;11:523–539.

23. Berger FA, Click J, Britt BT. Complications of ankle arthroscopy. *Foot Ankle* 1990;10:263–266.

24. Freedman DM, Barron OA. Iatrogenic posterior tibial nerve division during ankle arthroscopy. *Arthroscopy* 1998;14:769–772.

25. Ferkel RD, Heath D, Guhl JF. Neurological complications of ankle arthroscopy. *Arthroscopy* 1996;12:200–208.

26. Acevedo JI, Busch MT, Ganey TM, et al. Coaxial portals for posterior ankle arthroscopy: an anatomic study with clinical correlation on 29 patients. *Arthroscopy* 2000;16:836–842.

27. Dowdy PA, Watson VB, Amendola A, et al. Noninvasive ankle distraction: relationship between force, magnitude of distraction, and nerve conduction abnormalities. *Arthroscopy* 1996;12:64–69.

28. Thordarson DB, Bains R, Shepherd LE. The role of ankle arthroscopy on the surgical management of ankle fractures. *Foot Ankle Int* 2001;22:123–125.

29. O'Farrell D, Dudeny S, Manally S, et al. Pseudoaneurysm formation after ankle arthroscopy. *Foot Ankle Int* 1997;18:578–579.

30. Valentin A, Winge S, Stark A, et al. Late follow-up results of operative ankle arthroscopy in patients under local anesthesia. *Knee Surg Sports Traumatol Arthrosc* 1994;2:250–254.

31. Carson WG Jr, Andews JR. Arthroscopy of the ankle. *Clin Sports Med* 1987;6:503–512.

32. Takao M, Uchio Y, Shu N, et al. Anatomic bases of ankle arthroscopy: study of superficial and deep peroneal nerves around anterolateral and anterocentral approach. *Surg Radiol Anat* 1998;20:317–320.

33. Feiwell LA, Frey C. Anatomic study of arthroscopic portal sites of the ankle. *Foot Ankle* 1993;14:142–147.

34. Voto SJ, Ewing JW, Fleissner PR Jr, et al. Ankle arthroscopy: neurovascular and arthroscopic anatomy of standard and trans-Achilles tendon portal placement. *Arthroscopy* 1989;5:41–46.

35. Harty M: Ankle arthroscopy: anatomical features. *Orthopedics* 1985;8:1538–1540.

36. Andrews JR, Previte WJ, Carson WG. Arthroscopy of the ankle: technique and normal anatomy. *Foot Ankle* 1985;6:29–33.

Operative Arthroscopy, third edition. Edited by John B. McGinty, Stephen S. Burkhart, Robert W. Jackson, Donald H. Johnson, and John C. Richmond. Lippincott Williams & Wilkins © 2003.

SOFT TISSUE PATHOLOGY OF THE ANKLE

RICHARD D. FERKEL
TODD J. TUCKER

The prevalence of soft tissue pathology about the ankle historically has been underestimated. Patients often suffered from chronic painful conditions with few if any effective treatment options and rarely an accurate diagnosis. The advent of ankle arthroscopy has allowed a minimally invasive method for accurate diagnosis of ankle pathology. Disorders formerly thought to be untreatable and labeled as chronic sprains or nonspecific synovitis are often caused by recognized, discrete, and, most importantly, treatable lesions. Ankle arthroscopy has played a pivotal role in the growth of knowledge about ankle soft tissue pathology.

Several means of classification are possible for the soft tissue disorders of the ankle. The system shown in Table 62.1 is based on the cause of the synovial irritation.

PATIENT EVALUATION

A thorough history is critical to any patient evaluation. Many patients relate a discrete traumatic event as the onset of their symptoms; however, trauma may also exacerbate inflammation caused by a systemic process. Patients who complain of insidious onset, aching, or swelling, especially those with polyarthralgias, should be evaluated for possible systemic inflammatory causes. Likewise, a history of fevers, rubor, or possible joint inoculation should alert the physician to the possibility of an infectious cause.

After a thorough history and physical examination, routine three-view radiographs are appropriate diagnostic tools. Serum blood tests are indicated if a possible systemic or infectious cause for the patient's symptoms is suspected. Computed tomography is useful for accurate evaluation of osteochondral lesions (1). Magnetic resonance imaging (MRI) has been shown to be particularly useful in the diagnosis of soft tissue lesions about the ankle (2). The value of MRI studies depends on the experience of the radiologist and the surgeon as well as the use of appropriate imaging protocols. Three-phase bone scintigraphy is useful in differentiating soft tissue from bony inflammation (3). Tomography, arthrography, and tenograms are of limited usefulness in our opinion. Stress radiographs are very useful in differentiating primary soft tissue symptoms from those secondary to ankle instability.

SOFT TISSUE IMPINGEMENT

Anterior Soft Tissue Impingement

Chronic ankle pain after a sprain is frequently seen in an orthopaedic clinical setting. Pain is usually localized over the anterolateral ankle. An understanding of ankle anatomy is important in approaching this problem (Figs. 62.1, 62.2, and 62.3). The borders of the lateral gutter are the talus medially, the fibula laterally, and the tibia superiorly. The anteroinferior portion of the lateral gutter is bordered by the anterior talofibular ligament (ATFL) and the calcaneofibular (CF) ligament. The posteroinferior border consists of the posterior talofibular ligament (PTFL) and the CF ligament. Ankle inversion injuries commonly progress in the following sequence: torn ATFL, torn CF, torn PTFL. Symptoms of chronic ankle sprains are pain, loss of proprioception, and instability.

Wolin et al. (4), in 1950, were the first to describe "a pinching of a meniscoid mass" between the fibula and talus. They believed the tissue to be hyalinized connective tissue from the talofibular joint capsule. Their series included nine patients who all improved with open excision of the tissue. In 1982, Waller (5) described anterolateral corner compression syndrome and believed the symptoms to be caused by repetitive inversion injuries (Fig. 62.4). He found that these patients tended to have valgus heels and forefoot pronation. He believed the area of pathology to be a synovial or chondral compression at the lateral wall of the dome of the talus. He did not report patient results. Since then, several series of patients with soft tissue impingement or chronic pain after ankle sprains have been presented (6–11).

T. J. Tucker: Tucson Orthopedic Institute, Tucson, Arizona.
R. D. Ferkel: Southern California Orthopedic Institute, Van Nuys, California.

TABLE 62.1 CLASSIFICATION OF SOFT TISSUE DISORDERS

Soft tissue impingement
   Anterolateral
   Syndesmotic
   Posterior
   Medial

Posttraumatic arthrofibrosis
Synovial
   Rheumatic
      Rheumatoid arthritis
      Crystalline arthropathy
      Seronegative spondyloarthropathies
   Primary synovial disorders
      Synovial chondronatosis
      Pigmented villonodular synovitis

Hemophilia
Infectious
   Bacterial
   Fungal
Degenerative
Miscellaneous
   Ganglions
   Arthrofibrosis

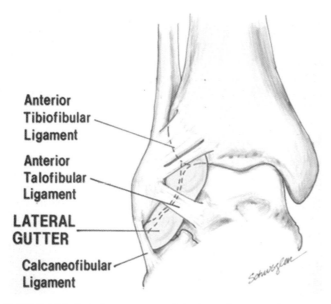

FIGURE 62.1 Anterior anatomy of the lateral gutter. The area is bordered by the tibia, fibula, and talus as well as the lateral ligamentous structures and joint capsule. Copyright R. Ferkel.

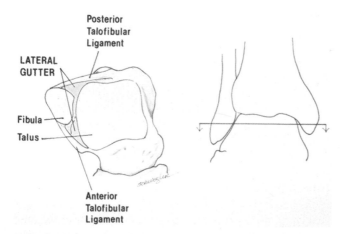

FIGURE 62.2 Axial anatomy of the anterior lateral gutter, syndesmotic area, and posterior gutter. The level of the cross section is demonstrated on the adjacent figure. Copyright R. Ferkel.

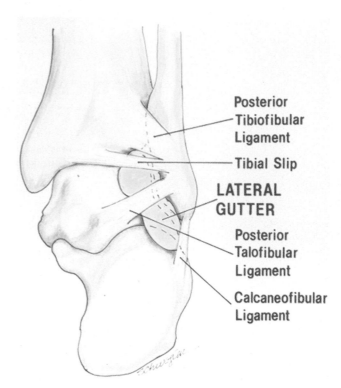

FIGURE 62.3 Posterior anatomy of the lateral gutter. Note that the transverse tibiofibular ligament courses from the fibula across toward the posteromedial tibia. Copyright R. Ferkel.

The differential diagnosis of anterolateral ankle impingement includes talar osteochondral lesions, symptomatic ossicles at the base of malleoli, peroneal subluxation or tears, tarsal coalition, degenerative joint disease, occult fracture of the talus or calcaneus, subtalar dysfunction, and reflex sympathetic dystrophy. Meyer et al. (12) demonstrated the value of computed tomography in the chronic ankle sprain. Their series included 13 patients with avulsed intraarticular

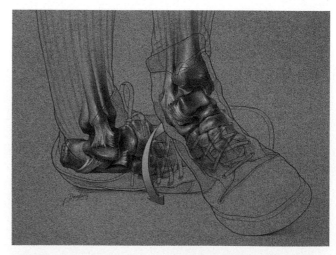

FIGURE 62.4 Mechanism for inversion injuries resulting in lateral ligament tears. Copyright R. Ferkel.

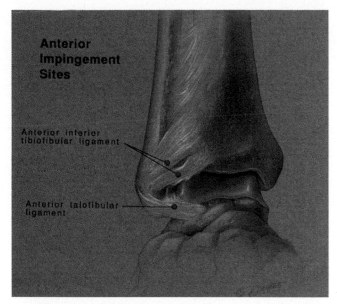

FIGURE 62.5. Anterior soft tissue impingement sites. Note the separate accessory fascicle of the anterior syndesmotic ligament that impinges across the lateral talar dome. Copyright R. Ferkel.

or juxtaarticular fragments not seen on plain films. In addition, MRI is useful in this circumstance.

There are three primary sites where anterior soft tissue impingement of the ankle occurs: the ATFL, the lateral gutter, and the anterior inferior tibiofibular ligament (AITFL) (Fig. 62.5). The clinical presentation is often a dull ache over the anterolateral ankle. Patients' symptoms are often exacerbated by activity, particularly sports (13). Because of the elusive nature of this diagnosis, patients tend to have seen several physicians without obtaining a correct diagnosis or adequate treatment.

On physical examination, tenderness may be elicited along the anterior syndesmosis, lateral gutter, or ATFL. It is sometimes difficult to differentiate the pain in the lateral gutter from subtalar pain (especially sinus tarsi pain). Radiographs may be helpful and can reveal calcification of ligaments, heterotopic bone, ossicles on the fibular base, or mild degenerative joint disease. However, radiographs are usually normal. Computed tomography, stress radiographs, and bone scan findings are usually normal. Previous studies have shown MRI to have a sensitivity of 39% to 42% and a specificity of 50% to 85% in detecting soft tissue impingement of the ankle (14,15). In our experience, MRI is 83% sensitive and 78% specific in diagnosing soft tissue impingement of the ankle (16) (Fig. 62.6). Differential injection may be useful if other diagnostic modalities fail. It is

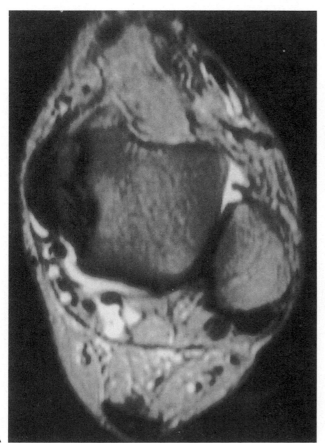

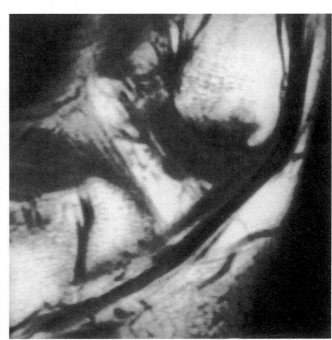

FIGURE 62.6 A: Axial T2-weighted image showing fluid in the lateral gutter and a torn remnant of the anterior inferior tibiofibular ligament. **B:** Sagittal T1-weighted image showing a soft tissue mass in the lateral gutter consistent with an impingement lesion. Copyright R. Ferkel.

important to note that some people have a communication between the ankle and subtalar joint that will confound injection results.

We treat this disorder arthroscopically at our institution. Arthroscopic examination of patients with soft tissue impingement usually shows a normal medial gutter and central ankle joint. Synovitis is typically present in the anterior syndesmosis and lateral gutter (Fig. 62.7). Fibrosis of the lateral gutter synovium with secondary chondromalacia of the lateral talar dome is often present. Rarely, a thick meniscoid lesion is present, extending from the anterolateral distal tibia to the distal lateral gutter. This lesion, as described by Chen (17), may contain tissue from capsule, torn ligament, and synovium. The term "meniscoid" came from the tissue's gross appearance, which resembles that of the meniscus of the knee joint.

The lateral gutter and syndesmosis are best visualized with a 2.7-mm, 30- or 70-degree arthroscope. The 70-degree lens is particularly useful when viewing from the anteromedial portal over the dome of the talus and into the lateral gutter (Fig. 62.8). This allows the anterolateral portal to serve as the working portal, giving more direct access to the tissues for debridement. It is important to reduce distraction during arthroscopy of the gutters, because increased traction narrows the gutters, making visualization and debridement more difficult. At surgery, the synovium, scar bands, chondromalacia, and loose bodies are removed with a combination of baskets, rongeurs, curettes, and motorized shavers. All of the abnormal tissue should be removed, with special care taken not to injure the remaining normal ATFL, capsule, and overlying subcutaneous nerves.

Postoperatively, wounds are closed with nylon sutures, and patients are placed in a short-leg, non–weight-bearing splint with crutches for 1 week. Sutures are then removed,

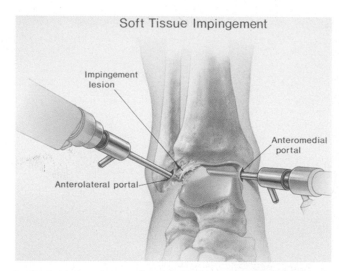

Soft Tissue Impingement

FIGURE 62.8 Technique for debridement of anterior soft tissue impingement lesions. Anterolateral impingement lesion is viewed through the anteromedial portal. The anterolateral portal is used for instrumentation. From Ferkel RD, Poehling GG, Andrews JR. *An illustrated guide to small joint arthroscopy.* Andover, Massachusetts: Smith & Nephew Dyonics, Inc., 1989 (Copyright R. Ferkel).

and patients are placed in a compressive stocking and short-leg walking boot and allowed to wean themselves over the next 2 to 4 weeks. Patients can usually resume sports 4 to 6 weeks postoperatively.

Histologic study of the impingement lesion demonstrates moderate synovial hyperplasia with subsynovial capillary proliferation. In addition, affected talar cartilage shows degenerative changes.

Between 1983 and 2000, we treated more than 250 patients arthroscopically for anterior soft tissue impingement. Previously, we reported on our initial treatment group of 31 patients with 84% good to excellent results (6). We have had similar results in an additional 220 cases. More recent stud-

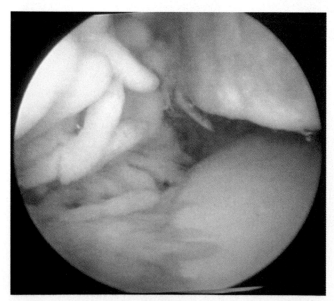

FIGURE 62.7 Chronically inflamed synovium due to anterolateral impingement. Note the papillary synovial projections in the lateral gutter. Copyright R. Ferkel.

TABLE 62.2 SEQUENCE OF LATERAL ANKLE IMPINGEMENT

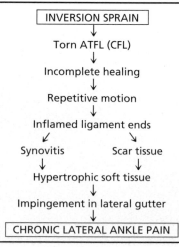

INVERSION SPRAIN
↓
Torn ATFL (CFL)
↓
Incomplete healing
↓
Repetitive motion
↓
Inflamed ligament ends
↙   ↘
Synovitis   Scar tissue
↓   ↓
Hypertrophic soft tissue
↓
Impingement in lateral gutter
↓
CHRONIC LATERAL ANKLE PAIN

ies have reported similar results in the treatment of this condition (10,18–20). It is important to rule out subtalar causes for lateral ankle pain, because patients with primary subtalar pathology will not benefit from ankle joint procedures.

The pathologic sequence of chronic lateral ankle pain is displayed in Table 62.2. In addition, the term "chronic ankle sprain" should be discarded in favor of the more appropriate term, "anterolateral ankle impingement."

Syndesmotic Soft Tissue Impingement

Injuries to the tibiofibular syndesmosis are among the most debilitating soft tissue injuries in the ankle (9,21). Unfortunately, the incidence of these injuries is very underestimated. Syndesmotic sprains are estimated to occur in approximately 10% of all ankle injuries, and they tend to be associated with collision sports. Syndesmotic sprain may include injury to any or all of the following structures: the ATFL, the PTFL, and the interosseous membrane (Fig. 62.9). On physical examination, patients have marked tenderness along the syndesmosis, as well as positive compression and external rotation tests (21,22). After injury, synovitis and scar formation can occur in the area of the AITFL, with subsequent soft tissue impingement in the area of the AITFL (Fig. 62.10). Arthroscopic evaluation reveals injected synovium surrounding the AITFL extending into the distal tibiofibular joint. Occasionally, the synovitis may ex-

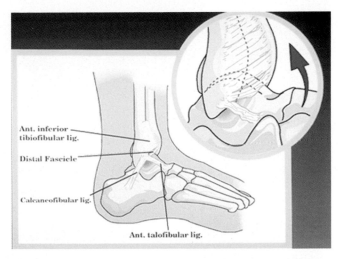

FIGURE 62.10 Impingement of a fascicle of the anterior inferior tibiofibular ligament across the lateral dome of the talus. With dorsiflexion, the distal fascicle of the anterior inferior tibiofibular ligament impinges on the lateral talar dome (*inset*). (Redrawn from Bassett FH, Gates HS, Billys JB, et al. Talar impingement by the anteroinferior tibiofibular ligament: a cause of chronic pain in the ankle after inversion sprain. *J Bone Joint Surg Sm* 1990;72: 55–59, with permission.) Copyright R. Ferkel.

tend along the joint line all the way to the posterior inferior tibiofibular ligament (PITFL). Bassett et al. (23) reported on syndesmotic impingement occurring with a separate distal fascicle of the AITFL (Fig. 62.11). A cadaveric study revealed the presence of this fascicle in 10 of 11 cadavers. The authors suggested that with anterior talofibular ligament laxity the talar dome may extrude anteriorly in dorsiflexion, leading to soft tissue impingement.

Treatment of syndesmotic impingement includes debridement of the AITFL and tibiofibular joint (Fig. 62.12). If a separate fascicle of the AITFL is present, it should be ex-

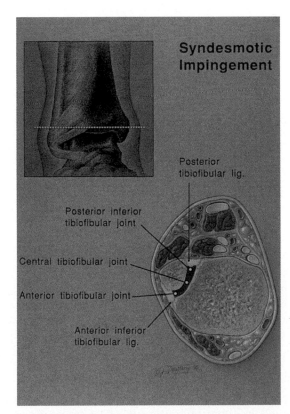

FIGURE 62.9 Cross-sectional view of possible syndesmotic soft tissue impingement sites. Note that impingement can occur anteriorly, centrally, or posteriorly. Copyright R. Ferkel.

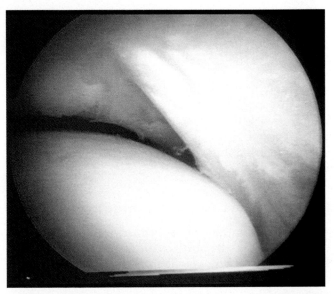

FIGURE 62.11 Separate fascicle of the anterior inferior syndesmosis impinging on the lateral talar dome. Copyright R. Ferkel.

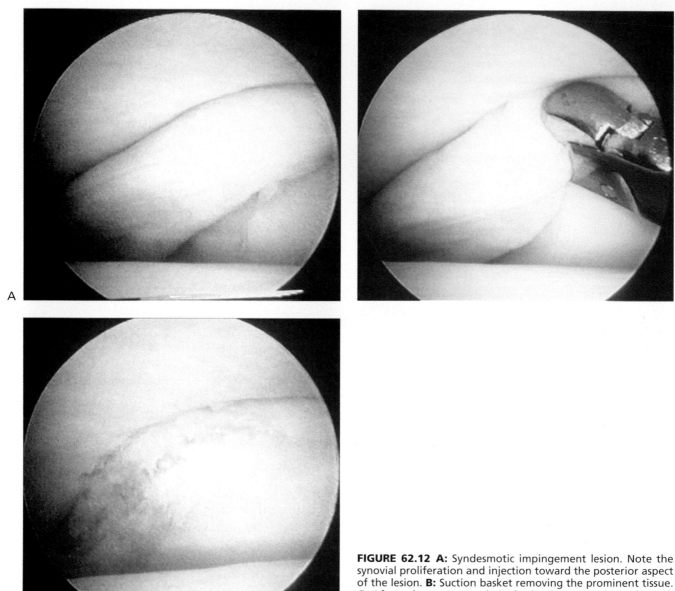

FIGURE 62.12 A: Syndesmotic impingement lesion. Note the synovial proliferation and injection toward the posterior aspect of the lesion. **B:** Suction basket removing the prominent tissue. **C:** After adequate resection, the impingement is eradicated. Copyright R. Ferkel.

cised. From anatomic studies at our institution, we have found that approximately 20% of the syndesmotic ligament is intraarticular. Therefore, complete removal of the intraarticular portion leaves approximately 80% of the ligament intact and does not predispose the patient to any iatrogenic instability.

Posterior Soft Tissue Impingement

Although it is less common, posterolateral impingement can occur. The areas of possible impingement include the PITFL, the transverse tibiofibular ligament, and occasionally a tibial slip (Fig. 62.13). A "posterior tibial slip," as described by Chen (17), is a band of tissue that originates from the PTFL and inserts on the posterior tibia and transverse ligament. This is distinct from the transverse tibiofibular lig-

ament, which courses obliquely from the distal fibula to the posterior tibia more proximally at its junction with the medial malleolus. Posterolateral impingement can occur as a solitary entity or along with anterior impingement. It usually is not detected by MRI or other radiographic studies and is easily missed if the arthroscopic examination does not include viewing from the posterolateral portal.

At surgery the PITFL, transverse tibiofibular ligament, and possibly a tibial slip can demonstrate hypertrophy or frank tearing with surrounding synovitis (Fig. 62.14). It has been postulated that patients with both a transverse tibiofibular ligament and a tibial slip are predisposed to posterior impingement. Excision of these hypertrophic tissues usually leads to significant improvement in symptoms. Anatomic variation in the size and shape of these structures is common, and care must be taken to excise only the pathologic tissue.

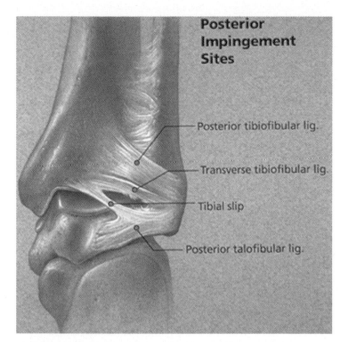

FIGURE 62.13 Potential posterior impingement sites. Note the "tibial slip" running obliquely from the posterior talofibular ligament to the transverse tibiofibular ligament. Copyright R. Ferkel.

Hamilton (24) described a "meniscus of the ankle" in ballet dancers. This posterior soft tissue rim could impinge in maximal plantar flexion. He also described tears in this meniscus that would displace, causing pain. An analogous structure exists in some marsupials. The clinical presentation is pain and posterior ankle tenderness anterior to the retrocalcaneal bursa. Pain may be aggravated by climbing up or down stairs. Occasionally, this lesion can be demon-strated on MRI. Treatment consists of excision of the torn or inflamed meniscoid tissue.

Medial Soft Tissue Impingement

Medial soft tissue impingement has recently been recognized as a cause for chronic ankle pain. van Dijk et al. (8) recently described a series of 30 patients with medial ankle pain after lateral ligament rupture. They described the method of medial chondral injury after inversion injury with lateral ligament rupture (Fig. 62.15). In their series, 20 patients were found to have an articular injury at the anterior distal medial malleolus with a kissing lesion on the medial talus. Six patients had a loose body. The authors found a statistical correlation between higher-energy injuries and the severity of chondral injury as well as a higher incidence of residual complaints at follow-up. Mosier-La-Clair et al. (7) implicated the anterior tibiotalar fascicle (ATTF) of the deltoid ligament as the source of pain in a series of 11 patients with medial posttraumatic ankle pain (Fig. 52.16). Six of the patients had suffered inversion injuries, four patients had previous ankle fractures, and one had a talus fracture. All patients showed synovitis around a thickened anterior tibiotalar fascicle. Treatment involved debridement of the synovitis, any associated chondral injury, and the ATTF of the deltoid ligament. Eight patients underwent concomitant removal of osteophytes. Overall, 9 of 11 patients had a good or excellent report. Of the two cases that were considered failures (one fair and one poor result), one patient had associated removal of osteophytes and the other did not. The authors did not comment as to what role they believe the removal of osteophytes played in patient outcome.

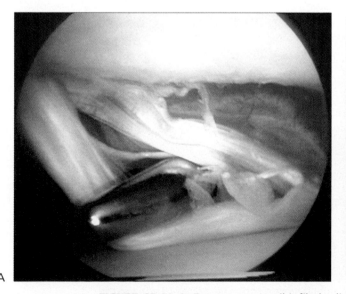

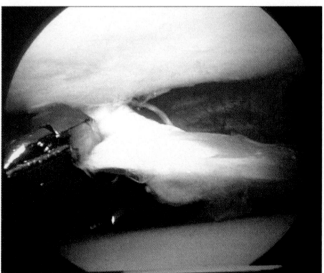

A   B

FIGURE 62.14 A: Torn transverse tibiofibular ligament causing posterior impingement. **B:** Removal of the torn tissue with a suction basket relieved the patient's symptoms. Copyright R. Ferkel.

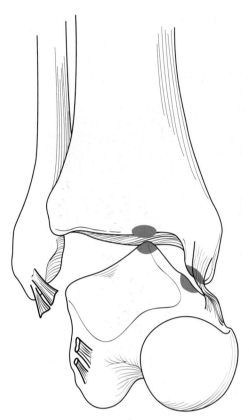

FIGURE 62.15 Mechanism for chondral injury associated with inversion injury with lateral ligament rupture. Note the potential areas for the development of chondral kissing lesions medially. (Redrawn from van Dijk CN, Verhagen RA, Tol JL. Arthroscopy for problems after ankle fracture. *J Bone Joint Surg Br* 1997;79: 280–284, with permission.) Copyright R. Ferkel.

POSTTRAUMATIC ARTHROFIBROSIS

Initially, joints respond to trauma with an inflammatory response. Often a localized or diffuse synovitis occurs. Fibrous bands and adhesions may form as the inflammatory tissue matures, causing further mechanical irritation. The patient with generalized nonspecific synovitis usually complains of swelling, aching, and pain. The onset of symptoms usually can be attributed to a specific event, but occasionally no specific event is remembered. If after adequate medical workup has failed to reveal a systemic cause and conservative treatment has failed, ankle arthroscopy is indicated. It is of paramount importance to rule out sympathetically mediated pain before considering arthroscopic evaluation. A patient with a history of minor trauma, who has pain out of proportion to the physical findings, color and temperature changes to the skin, or localized hair loss should undergo diagnostic workup for reflex sympathetic dystrophy. Surgical intervention in such patients often exacerbates the patient's symptoms.

At surgery, chronically inflamed synovium often is seen. Hemosiderin is rarely seen in the chronically inflamed ankle. Fibrous bands are often seen and tend to be located in the anterior joint (Fig. 62.17). The articular surfaces usually are minimally involved. Ankle sprains and fractures are the most common cause of nonspecific synovitis.

We have seen arthrofibrosis after ankle fractures undergoing open reduction and internal fixation. In a recent series of patients with continued pain after such treatment of an ankle fracture, van Dijk et al. (25) commonly noted arthrofibrosis,

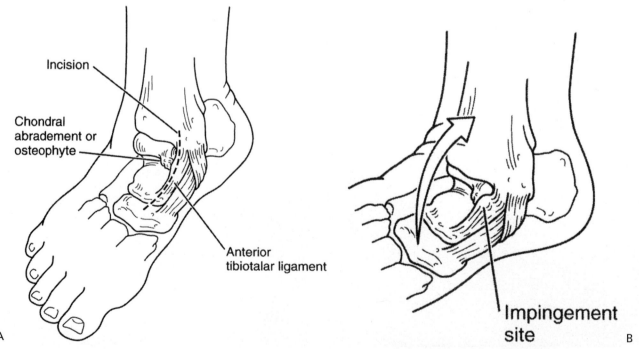

FIGURE 62.16 A: Site of author's skin incision for debridement and cheilectomy is shown on the medial side. **B:** Medial soft tissue impingement site at the anterior fascicle of the superficial deltoid ligament. (From Mosier-LaClair SM, Monroe MT, Manoli A. Medial impingement syndrome of the anterior tibiotalar fascicle of the deltoid ligament of the talus. *Foot Ankle Int* 2000;21: 385–391, with permission.)

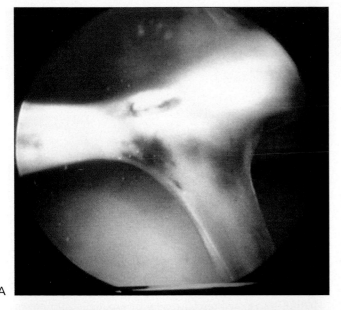

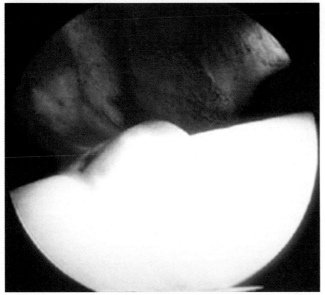

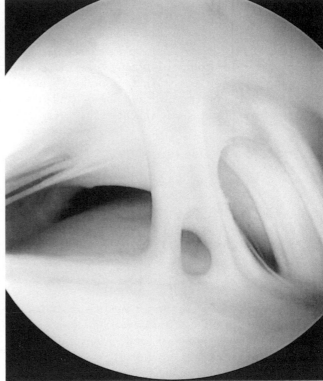

FIGURE 62.17 Posttraumatic fibrosis. **A:** Large anterolateral T-shaped scar formation. **B:** Note the thickened band of scar coursing over the talar dome. **C:** Advanced scar formation after fracture. Copyright R. Ferkel.

soft tissue impingement, and degenerative changes at the time of arthroscopy. Frequently, these patients have significant intraarticular scar formation at the time of arthroscopy. Adhesive bands, fibrosis, and synovitis are common findings that compromise arthroscopic visualization. On initial introduction of the arthroscope, it may be difficult to determine the intraarticular positioning of the instruments by direct arthroscopic visualization. The key to success in these cases is patience and good inflow. We use supine positioning with a thigh support and noninvasive distraction. A high inflow system using a posterolateral portal is invaluable in these situations.

The surgeon should begin in one quadrant of the ankle and slowly enlarge the field of view with a motorized shaver until the entire ankle joint is visualized. Both anterior portals and the posterolateral portal should be used for complete evaluation. Additional therapeutic measures (removal of loose

bodies, chondroplasty/microfracture) may proceed once adequate visualization has been obtained (26).

Postoperatively, the portals should be sutured. A posterior splint with stirrups is used until the first postoperative visit to facilitate wound healing. After the first postoperative visit, early joint mobilization is initiated to maintain range of motion (ROM). Most patients attain modest increases in ROM (6 to 8 degrees) but have more significant improvement in their symptoms.

SYNOVIAL DISORDERS

Nonspecific Localized Synovitis

Some patients develop pain and a localized synovitis in the medial or lateral talomalleolar region after an ankle sprain.

Examination shows localized tenderness, minimal swelling, and a normal ROM. Plain radiographs are normal; MRI occasionally shows a localized area of synovitis and some effusion but is often negative. If conservative treatment fails and other causes are ruled out, arthroscopy is indicated. On arthroscopic evaluation, patients have a localized synovial proliferation with papillary growth and fibrous band formation. Excision usually provides excellent results.

Rheumatologic Diseases

A discussion of rheumatic diseases is beyond the scope of this chapter, and the reader is referred to other texts (27). Rheumatic disease can affect any number of joints, including the ankle. The arthroscopist should be familiar with the diagnosis and treatment of rheumatic diseases.

Rheumatoid Arthritis

Rheumatoid arthritis is a chronic systemic inflammatory disorder that results in the destruction of multiple synovial joints. The etiology is unknown, and various causes have been postulated. Symptoms and findings in the rheumatoid ankle are similar to those in the hand, wrist, knee, and foot. Rheumatoid arthritis in the ankle manifests with joint destruction and limitation of motion of the tibiotalar and subtalar joints.

Surgery in the rheumatoid patient should be reserved for when chemotherapy fails to achieve adequate relief. It is critical to assess the patient's overall health as well as the local joint condition before considering surgery (28). The decision to proceed with surgery should be a joint decision that includes the surgeon, the patient, and the rheumatologist. Continued pain, effusions, and synovitis are the most common reasons for surgery.

At the time of surgery, distraction is especially important to achieve maximal room for visualization and instrumentation. Synovitis and chondromalacia are the most common findings in the rheumatoid ankle (Fig. 62.18). Chondromalacia is often advanced and often involves areas of necrotic cartilage on the talar dome and tibial plafond (29). Free flaps of cartilage and loose bodies are debrided with a small-diameter (2.9-mm) shaver. Occasionally, a smaller shaver is needed in especially tight ankles. A subtotal synovectomy should be performed to minimize future symptoms.

The histopathology of rheumatoid synovium shows synovial hyperplasia with papillary formation and necrosis. Due to areas of surface necrosis, many synovial villi have a creamy-yellow appearance. These are referred to as rice bodies. It is impossible to achieve a complete synovectomy (30), but attempts to remove as much as possible are warranted. The results of early synovectomy are better than for late synovectomy (31). Early synovectomy may provide the joint with several years of good function, but if advanced chondromalacia or bony changes are present, the results are gen-

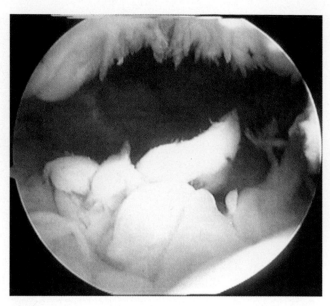

FIGURE 62.18 Arthroscopic view of a patient with advance rheumatoid arthritis of the ankle. Note the advanced fraying and chondral loss on the talar surface as well as generalized synovial proliferation. Copyright R. Ferkel.

erally poor. McEwen (32) questioned the benefit of ankle synovectomy for rheumatoid arthritis, but we believe it offers good patient relief if performed early in the disease progression. Even in the best situation, synovectomy slows joint destruction rather than preventing it.

If patients have advanced joint degeneration and continued pain, synovectomy should be avoided in favor of ankle arthrodesis. This can be performed arthroscopically or by traditional open means. Arthroscopic arthrodesis offers the benefit of a minimally invasive procedure in patients who are most likely taking multiple medications that impede wound healing. No results after subtalar synovectomy have been reported, but it may offer symptomatic relief in patients with refractory subtalar inflammation and minimal radiographic evidence of joint degeneration.

Pigmented Villonodular Synovitis

Pigmented villonodular synovitis (PVNS) is considered by some to be a benign neoplasm of the synovium (33). It occurs most frequently in the knee, but it can occur in the ankle. PVNS can exist in a localized (circumscribed) or a generalized form. Ankle lesions tend to be circumscribed lesions. The clinical presentation is a warm, swollen, tender joint with limited ROM. Aspiration of the joint produces a dark, serosanguineous fluid. Radiographs are occasionally helpful in making the diagnosis. Arthrography may show nodular filling defects, and MRI can demonstrate synovial proliferation and bone destruction (34) (Fig. 62.19). Diagnosis is confirmed at arthroscopy, which shows synovitis with papillary formation and hemosiderin deposition (Fig. 62.20).

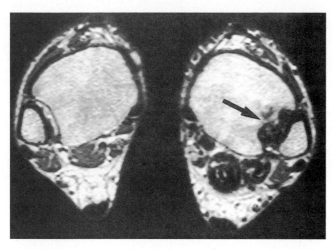

FIGURE 62.19 Magnetic resonance imaging scan of an ankle with pigmented villonodular synovitis. Note the synovial proliferation and bone erosion at the distal tibiofibular joint. Copyright R. Ferkel.

Treatment involves subtotal synovectomy. Again, the distracter is of paramount importance in facilitating visualization and instrumentation for the synovectomy.

Histologic examination of PVNS shows deep synovial cell proliferation, hypervascularity, fibrosis with lymphocytic infiltration, lipid-laden macrophages, and hemorrhage (35). Arthroscopic excision of the lesion is usually curative for the localized form of PVNS. Patients with the generalized form are prone to have recurrences after synovectomy.

Synovial Chondromatosis

Synovial chondromatosis is an uncommon disorder occasionally seen in the ankle (36). It is almost always monoarticular. The diagnosis is suggested by a limited ROM, mechanical symptoms, and swelling. Synovial chondromatosis is characterized by multiple foci of cartilage metaplasia within the synovium (37). As these masses grow, they can form nodules within the synovium and break free, becoming loose bodies with varying degrees of ossification. If these bodies ossify, they become radiopaque and the diagnosis is made with plain radiographs (Fig. 62.21). At other times, the lesions are radiolucent and are seen on arthrography or MRI.

The three phases of synovial chondromatosis as described by Milgram (38) are as follows:

1. *Active intrasynovial phase*—Synovial proliferation and nodule formation without formation of loose bodies occur.
2. *Transitional phase*—Active synovial disease and multiple intraarticular loose bodies characterize this stage. There is no osteoid formation in the early aspect of this phase, so plain films will be normal. Later in this stage, ossification occurs and the loose bodies are seen on plain radiographs.
3. *Burned-out phase*—This phase occurs when there is no more synovial hyperplasia or new nodule formation. There are multiple loose bodies, and degenerative changes occur in the joint as a result of third-body wear.

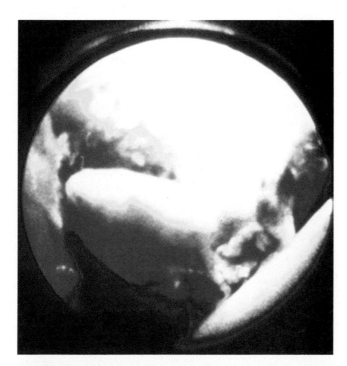

FIGURE 62.20 Arthroscopic view of pigmented villonodular synovitis showing characteristic reddened villous synovial proliferation. Copyright R. Ferkel.

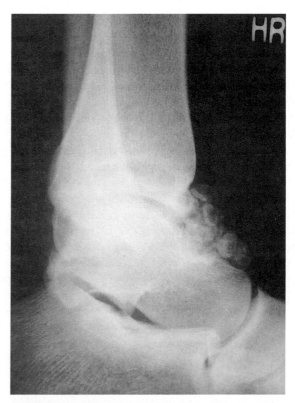

FIGURE 62.21 Lateral ankle radiograph showing multiple loose bodies caused by synovial chondromatosis. Copyright R. Ferkel.

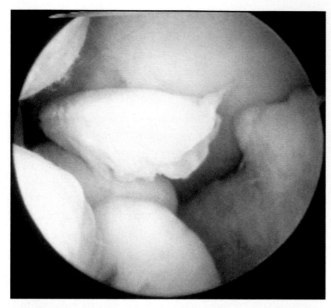

FIGURE 62.22 Arthroscopic view demonstrating multiple loose bodies caused by synovial chondromatosis. Copyright R. Ferkel.

Diagnosis is confirmed by arthroscopy and synovial biopsy. At arthroscopy, there is chronic synovitis with loose chondral or osteochondral bodies (Fig. 62.22). Degenerative changes are present in chronic cases. The presence of loose bodies in the joint does not confirm the diagnosis of synovial chondromatosis. Other disorders that can produce loose bodies are degenerative arthritis, osteochondral lesions of the talus, rheumatoid arthritis, trauma, Charcot arthropathy, and tuberculosis. The absence of chondroid metaplasia in the synovium helps exclude these other conditions in favor of synovial chondromatosis (39).

With the use of the distracter, loose bodies are removed arthroscopically. Some loose bodies are large and may need to be fragmented or removed through an extended portal incision. It is important to view the ankle from all portals, paying special attention to dependent regions of the ankle joint, to ensure that all loose bodies are removed. Once all loose bodies have been removed, synovectomy of the involved proliferative synovium is performed. The recurrence rate after open surgery is 5%. No series has been reported using arthroscopic technique, but one would expect to be able to remove all loose bodies and to perform a better synovectomy arthroscopically than is possible with an open technique.

An aggressive form of synovial chondromatosis has been described (40). It has a high recurrence rate with the potential for distant metastasis. If metastasis occurs, it should be treated as a synovial chondrosarcoma.

HEMOPHILIA

Classic hemophilia is a sex-linked recessive disease that manifests with decreased levels of factor VIII. Other variations include Christmas disease (factor IX) deficiency, and von Willebrand's disease (abnormal factor VIII and platelet dysfunction). From an orthopaedic standpoint, patients with hemophilia suffer from recurrent, painful hemarthroses that lead to rapid chondral breakdown and advanced secondary degenerative changes. Hemarthroses usually result from minor trauma, or they can be spontaneous in patients with very low factor levels. Patients with acute bleeds present with pain, warmth, and swelling of the affected joint. Treatment consists of factor replacement, immobilization, elevation, and ice.

Recurrent bleeds lead to chondral destruction and subsequent joint space narrowing and sclerosis. Arthroscopic synovectomy can be of benefit in preventing recurrent hemarthroses and joint degeneration. It is of paramount importance to have a multidisciplinary team caring for these patients if surgery is considered. Deficient factors should be replaced to 100% of normal levels preoperatively and maintained at 50% of normal for 10 days postoperatively.

Arthroscopy has been shown to be an effective tool for performing ankle synovectomy for the treatment of recurrent hemophilic ankle hemarthroses (41,42). Recently, synovectomy using two coaxial posterior portals to treat patients with hemophilia was described (41). This four-portal technique reportedly allows for a more complete synovectomy. The two posterior portals are located in the intermalleolar plane just posterior to each malleolus (Fig. 62.23). The posterolateral portal is created by an outside-in technique, and the posteromedial portal is made in an inside-out fashion using a blunt trocar. In the cadaveric aspect of this study, one cannula split the posterior tibial tendon, but there were no symptomatic tendon or neurovascular injuries in the clinical series of 29 ankles, with an average follow-up of 45 months. The authors attributed the cadaveric injury to possibly lower compliance and mobility in the cadaveric tissue.

We have no experience with this technique, but it may offer improved visual and mechanical access to the posterior recess of the ankle. The posterior and posteromedial ankle are often poorly visualized and instrumented in patients with proliferative synovitis, such as hemophiliacs. We agree with the authors of the study that only experienced ankle arthroscopists, who are very familiar with local anatomy, should consider this technique until it has a longer record of clinical follow-up.

INFECTION

Arthroscopy is also useful in the diagnosis and treatment of ankle infection. Biopsy allows for accurate diagnosis, and thorough lavage and debridement are therapeutic. This is especially helpful in fungal and more indolent infections, because tissue culture is more helpful than fluid culture in these settings.

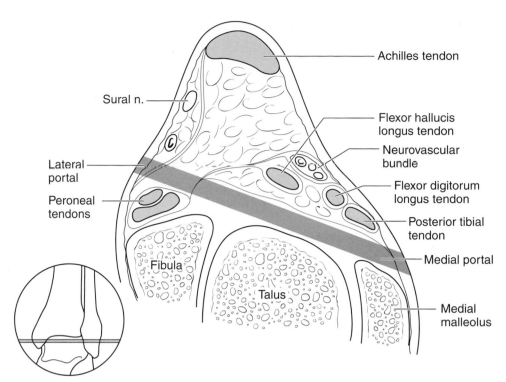

Achilles tendon

Sural n.

Flexor hallucis longus tendon

Neurovascular bundle

Lateral portal

Flexor digitorum longus tendon

Peroneal tendons

Posterior tibial tendon

Fibula

Medial portal

Talus

Medial malleolus

FIGURE 62.23 Diagram showing correct placement of coaxial posterior portals. Note the relationship of the portals to adjacent neurovascular structures. (Adapted from Acevedo JI, Busch MT, Ganey TM, et al. Coaxial portals for posterior ankle arthroscopy: an anatomic study with clinical correlation on 29 patients. *Arthroscopy* 2000;16:836–842.)

Coccidioidomycosis or "valley fever" is endemic in the southwestern United States. It is primarily a pulmonary infection, with 0.1% to 0.2% of patients developing systemic spread. Twenty percent of these patients develop bone or joint involvement. African American patients are more prone to develop systemic effects of coccidioidomycosis. Treatment is thorough lavage, debridement, and appropriate antimicrobial pharmacotherapy.

DEGENERATIVE PROCESSES

Degenerative changes affecting the ankle and subtalar joints are common causes of ankle pain. Arthroscopy with chondroplasty, partial synovectomy, and excision of fibrous bands can give some relief of symptoms in the early degenerative stages. If patients have bony impingement at the anterior tibiotalar articulation, arthroscopic osteophyte excision can provide excellent relief of symptoms from the impingement. This is accomplished by alternately viewing from the anterolateral and anteromedial portals, using a 3.5-mm full-radius shaver and burr in the complementary portal to remove the impinging soft tissue and bone. Bone recession continues until no impingement occurs with maximal dorsiflexion under direct arthroscopic visualization. When performing this procedure, it is critical to keep the tool blades facing the bone, away from the overlying neurovascular structures.

Patients with advanced degenerative changes respond poorly to arthroscopic debridement. Fusion, either open or arthroscopic, is a more appropriate treatment for these patients.

TECHNIQUE FOR ANKLE SYNOVECTOMY

In almost all the conditions discussed in this chapter, either a localized or subtotal synovectomy is part of the treatment. Basic details of ankle arthroscopy have been discussed, but several technical points are important to emphasize.

We prefer patients to be positioned supine with a thigh support and a bump underneath the ipsilateral buttock. The ankle is placed in a special strap to aid noninvasive distraction. We no longer routinely use invasive distraction for ankle arthroscopy. The noninvasive strap allows the foot to be secured while still allowing easy access to the anteromedial, anterolateral, and posterolateral portals. Distraction is an essential part of performing an excellent synovectomy.

We prefer to use 3.5- or 2.7-mm full-radius shavers for ankle synovectomy (Fig. 62.24). These are less aggressive than other shaver options, minimizing the risk of capsular or

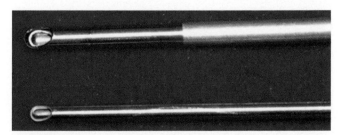

FIGURE 62.24 The 2.7- and 3.5-mm full-radius shavers used for ankle debridement. The small diameter of the instruments allows improved access to difficult-to-reach areas in the joint while minimizing the risk of iatrogenic chondral injury. Copyright R. Ferkel.

neurovascular injury from overexuberant shaving. In addition, it is important when shaving the anterior synovium to point the open face of the shaver away from the capsule to prevent injury to adjacent structures. We also use both 30- and 70-degree wide-angle lenses for maximal visualization.

The first key to a successful synovectomy is the use of a balanced, high-flow system. The use of a separate inflow cannula placed posterolaterally when working anteriorly, or in the third complementary portal when working or viewing posteriorly, is helpful in achieving this. The second key is to have an interchangeable cannula system that allows the arthroscope, baskets, shavers, and inflow to be quickly and easily switched. The third key is to perform a 21-point complete diagnostic arthroscopy before operative arthroscopy. Synovectomy and debridement should be performed sequentially and thoroughly, beginning with the arthroscope placed anteriorly and continuing with viewing from the posterolateral portal. Instruments are placed either anteriorly or posteriorly as needed until synovectomy is completed. The cannula system facilitates instrument switching. In addition, coaxial posterolateral and posteromedial portals (41), described earlier in this chapter, may provide improved visualization and more direct access to the posterior joint for debridement. We have no experience with these accessory portals, but their use may be beneficial in difficult cases.

As a caution, it should be remembered that patients with rheumatoid arthritis have a friable, thin synovium and joint capsule. When debriding anteriorly or posteromedially, extreme caution must be used not to injure the overlying neurovascular structures. In these patients, the whisker-blade shaver, rather than the full-radius shaver, should be used (Fig. 62.25).

After the synovectomy is complete, the tourniquet should be deflated. A drain should be placed if extensive bleeding is encountered. It is removed after 1 or 2 days. The portals are closed using one vertical mattress nylon suture for each portal. A compression dressing is applied, and the foot is splinted in plantigrade position for 10 days until the sutures are removed.

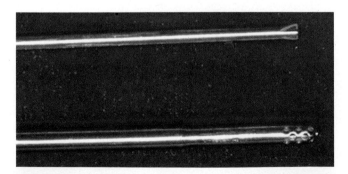

FIGURE 62.25 The 2.7- and 3.5-mm whisker blades should be used near the anterior capsule to prevent overly aggressive suction and subsequent injury to overlying neurovascular structures. Copyright R. Ferkel.

REFERENCES

1. Solomon MA, Gilula LA, Oloff LM, et al. CT scanning of the foot and ankle: I. Normal Anatomy. *AJR Am J Roentgenol* 1986; 146:1192–1203.
2. Ferkel RD, Flannigan B, Elkins B. MRI of the foot and ankle: correlation of normal anatomy with pathologic conditions. *Foot Ankle* 1991;11:290–305.
3. Freeman LM. *Freeman and Johnson's clinical radionuclide imaging,* 3rd ed. New York: Harcourt Brace Jovanovich, 1984.
4. Wolin I, Glassman F, Sideman F, et al. Internal derangement of the talofibular component of the ankle.
5. Waller JM. Hindfoot and midfoot problems of the runner. In: Mack RP, ed. *Symposium on the foot and leg in running sports.* St. Louis: Mosby, 1982.
6. Ferkel RD, Karzel RP, Del Pizzo W, et al. Arthroscopic treatment of anterolateral impingement of the ankle. *Am J Sports Med* 1991; 19:440–446.
7. Mosier-LaClair SM, Monroe MT, Manoli A. Medial impingement syndrome of the anterior tibiotalar fascicle of the deltoid ligament of the talus. *Foot Ankle Int* 2000;21:385–391.
8. van Dijk CN, Bossuyt PMM, Marti RK. Medial ankle pain after lateral ligament rupture. *J Bone Joint Surg Br* 1996;87:562–567.
9. Gerber JP, Williams GN, Scoville R, et al. Persistent disability associated with ankle sprains: a prospective examination of an athletic population. *Foot Ankle Int* 1998;19:653–660.
10. DeBerardino TM, Arciero RA, Taylor DC. Arthroscopic treatment of soft tissue impingement of the ankle in athletes. *Arthroscopy* 1997;13:492–498.
11. Martin DF, Curl WW, Baker CL. Arthroscopic treatment of chronic synovitis of the ankle. *Arthroscopy* 1989;5:110–114.
12. Meyer JM, Hoffmeyer P, Savoy X. High resolution computed tomography in chronically painful ankle sprain. *Foot Ankle* 1986; 8:291–296.
13. Ferkel RD. Arthroscopic treatment of osteochondral lesions, soft-tissue impingement, and loose bodies. AAOS Monograph Series: Chronic ankle pain in the athlete. San Francisco, American Academy of Orthopaedic Surgeons, 2000:43–70.
14. Liu SH, Nuccion SL, Finerman G. Diagnosis of anterolateral ankle impingement: comparison between magnetic resonance imaging and clinical examination. *Am J Sports Med* 1997;25:389–393.
15. Farooki S, Yao L, Seeger LL. Anterolateral impingement of the ankle: effectiveness of MR imaging. *Radiology* 1998;207:357–360.
16. Heinen GT, Applegate GR, Ferkel RD. *MRI evaluation of anterolateral ankle impingement.* San Francisco, American Academy of Orthopaedic Surgeons, 2001.
17. Chen Y. Arthroscopy of the ankle joint. In: Watanabe M, ed. *Arthroscopy of small joints.* New York: Igaku-Shoin, 1985.
18. Liu SH, Raskin BS, Osti L, et al. Arthroscopic treatment of anterolateral ankle impingement. *Arthroscopy* 1994;10:215–218.
19. Martin DF, Baker CL, Curl WW, et al. Operative ankle arthroscopy long-term follow-up. *Am J Sports Med* 1989;17:16–23.
20. Meislin RJ, Rose DJ, Parisien S, et al. Arthroscopic treatment of synovial impingement of the ankle. *Am J Sports Med* 1993;21:186–189.
21. Boytim MJ, Fischer DA, Neumann L. Syndesmotic ankle sprains. *Am J Sports Med* 1991;19:294.
22. Hopkinson WJ, St Pierre P, Ryan JB, et al. Syndesmosis sprains of the ankle. *Foot Ankle* 1990;11:325.

23. Bassett FH, Gates HS, Billys JB, et al. Talar impingement by the anteroinferior tibiofibular ligament: a cause of chronic pain in the ankle after inversion sprain. *J Bone Joint Surg Am* 1990;72:55–59.
24. Hamilton WG. Foot and ankle injuries in dancers. *Clin Sports Med* 1988;7:160–163.
25. van Dijk CN, Verhagen RA, Tol JL. Arthroscopy for problems after ankle fracture. *J Bone Joint Surg Br* 1997;79:280–284.
26. Ferkel RD. *Arthroscopic surgery: the ankle and foot.* Philadelphia: Lippincott-Raven, 1996.
27. Rodman GP, Schumacher R. *Primer on the rheumatic diseases,* 8th ed. Atlanta: Arthritis Foundation, 1983:187.
28. Goldie IF. A synopsis of surgery for rheumatoid arthritis (excluding the hand). *Clin Orthop* 1984;44:185–192.
29. Schoenholz GJ. *Arthroscopic surgery of the shoulder, elbow, and ankle.* Springfield, IL: Charles C Thomas, 1987:59–72.
30. Aschan W, Moberg E. A long-term study of the effect of early synovectomy in rheumatoid arthritis. *Bull Hosp Jt Dis* 1984;44: 106–121.
31. Goldie IF. Synovectomy in rheumatoid arthritis: theoretical aspects and a 14-year follow-up in the knee joint. *Reconstr Surg Traumatol* 1981;18:2–7.
32. McEwen C. Multicenter evaluation of synovectomy in the treatment of rheumatoid arthritis: report of results at the end of five years. *J Rheumatol* 1988;15:765–769.
33. Granowitz SP, D'Antonia J, Mankin HJ. The pathogenesis and long-term end results of pigmented villonodular synovitis. *Clin Orthop* 1976;114:335–351.
34. Beltran J, Noto AM, Mosure JC, et al. Ankle surface coil MR imaging at 1.5 tl. *Radiology* 1986;161:203–209.
35. Schumacher HR, Lotke P, Athreya B, et al. Pigmented villonodular synovitis: light and electron microscopic studies. *Semin Arthritis Rheum* 1982;12:32–43.
36. Holm CL. Primary synovial chondromatosis of the ankle. *J Bone Joint Surg Am* 1976;58:878–880.
37. Jeffreys TE. Synovial chondromatosis. *J Bone Joint Surg Br* 1967;49:530–534.
38. Milgram JW. Synovial osteochondromatosis. *J Bone Joint Surg Am* 1977;59:792–801.
39. Murphy FP, Dahlin DC, Sullivan CR. Articular synovial chondromatosis. *J Bone Joint Surg Am* 1962;44:77–86.
40. Goldman RL, Lichtenstein L. Synovial chondrosarcoma. *Cancer* 1964;17:1233–1246.
41. Acevedo JI, Busch MT, Ganey TM, et al. Coaxial portals for posterior ankle arthroscopy: an anatomic study with clinical correlation on 29 patients. *Arthroscopy* 2000;16:836–842.
42. Patti JE, Mayo WEB. Arthroscopic synovectomy for recurrent hemarthrosis of the ankle in hemophilia. *Arthroscopy* 1996; 12:652–656.

ARTHROSCOPIC-ASSISTED MANAGEMENT OF ANKLE FRACTURES

TODD J. TUCKER
RICHARD D. FERKEL

Ankle fractures are among the most common fractures treated by orthopaedic surgeons (1). The application of AO ASIF (Arbeitsgemeinschaft für Osteosynthesefragen/Association for the Study of Internal Fixation) technique, resulting in anatomic reduction and stable fixation, has led to excellent bony healing rates and improved outcomes compared with nonsurgical treatment for unstable fracture patterns (2–4). However, soft tissue injuries, associated either with the original injury or with surgical treatment, continue to pose difficult problems to the orthopaedist. Continued pain, residual stiffness, and posttraumatic degencrative changes are not uncommon sequelae after appropriate treatment of ankle fractures (5–7). Soft tissue damage, residual articular incongruity, or occult intraarticular chondral injury may be responsible for these continued symptoms (8–11).

Anatomic reduction of periarticular fractures is of paramount importance, because residual articular incongruity is associated with poor outcomes (3,12,13). Arthroscopic evaluation and reduction allows for precise restoration of normal joint architecture. In addition, chondral injuries, which would otherwise be unrecognized by traditional open surgical techniques, can be addressed at the time of arthroscopy.

INDICATIONS

Indications for arthroscopic treatment of fractures about the ankle include both intraarticular and extraarticular injuries that are likely to have significant concomitant articular injury. Chondral damage has been shown to be most commonly associated with injuries that involve the distal tibiofibular syndesmosis (14,15). Other fracture patterns are associated with chondral injuries to a lesser extent. Arthroscopic-assisted treatment is especially useful in posterior malleolar fractures, as well as medial malleolar and talar fractures. Simple fracture patterns involving the tibial plafond, such as Tillaux and triplane fractures, are amenable to arthroscopic treatment. Some authors are treating pilon fractures with arthroscopically assisted technique, but flow must be carefully monitored to prevent possible compartment syndromes. Complex pilon fractures are beyond the scope of treatment currently and pose a significant risk of extravasation-related complications.

Absolute contraindications are open fractures, severe edema, neurovascular injury, and infection. Advanced degenerative joint disease, chronic peripheral edema, vascular insufficiency, fracture-dislocations, and fractures with concomitant severe ligamentous disruption are relative contraindications. In addition, children with open physes should not undergo arthroscopic treatment with joint distraction because of the potential physeal injury associated with joint distraction. Children with triplane or Tillaux fractures who are nearing physeal closure are considered appropriate patients.

ARTICULAR INJURIES ASSOCIATED WITH FRACTURES

Damage to the articular surfaces of the ankle joint commonly occurs with ankle fractures. Feldman (16) reported on 15 extraarticular ankle fractures, 14 caused by supination with external rotation (SER) and one by pronation with external rotation (PER). Eleven (73%) of the ankles demonstrated associated articular injury. Seven patients had a talar chondral fracture, and four had a tibial osteochondral fracture. Hinterman et al. (15) prospectively studied 288 patients undergoing arthroscopy before prior to open reduction with internal fixation of ankle fracture. They found articular surface lesions in 79.2% of the patients. Talar lesions were more common than tibial lesions. In addition, the incidence and severity of articular lesions increased as fracture severity, using the Danis–Weber classification system, increased from B to C fracture pattern.

T. J. **Tucker:** Tucson Orthopedic Institute, Tucson, Arizona.

R. **Ferkel:** Southern California Orthopedic Institute, Van Nuys, California.

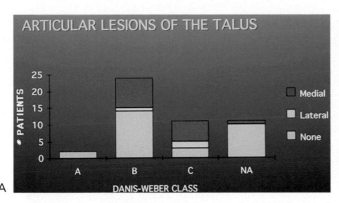

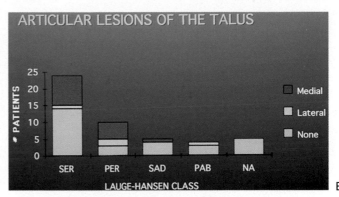

FIGURE 63.1 Distribution of traumatic articular surface lesions (TASLs) as they relate to type of ankle fracture. Incidence of TASLs as related to the Danis–Weber classification **(A)** and as related to the Lauge–Hansen classification **(B)**.

In the senior author's series (14), 48 acute ankle fractures were studied. The fractures were classified according to both to both the Lauge–Hansen and the Danis–Weber system (Fig. 63.1). The number of ankle fractures for each mechanism were as follows: SER, 24 (52%); PER, 10 (22%), pronation with abduction (PAB), 4 (9%), and supination with adduction, 5 (11%). Four patients had a Tillaux fracture, and one had a triplane fracture.

Using the Danis–Weber classification, 2 patients (4%) had Weber A fractures, 24 (52%) had a Weber B fracture pattern, and 11 patients (24%) had Weber C fractures. Again, one patient had a triplane fracture and four had Tillaux fractures. An additional six patients had isolated medial malleolus fractures and were not classified according to Danis–Weber.

None of the preoperative radiographs (anteroposterior, lateral, and mortise oblique views) showed an osteochondral lesion. On introduction of the arthroscope, almost all patients in this series were found to have fracture hematoma and fracture debris. Thirteen patients (28%) had free fragments requiring operative removal. Twenty-nine patients (62%) had traumatic articular surface injuries (TASL), including 19 talar and 10 tibial lesions (Fig. 63.2).

The incidence of TASLs was highest (8 [75%] of 12 fractures, 11 Weber C and 1 Weber B) among fractures that disrupted the syndesmosis (Fig. 63.3). This finding was statistically significant (*p* = .01). SER pattern Weber B fractures had a 42% (10/24) incidence of TASL, including 9 medial

FIGURE 63.2 Talar traumatic articular surface lesion associated with an ankle fracture. Note the full-thickness lesion and its extension between the bone and cartilage due to shear injury. Copyright R. Ferkel.

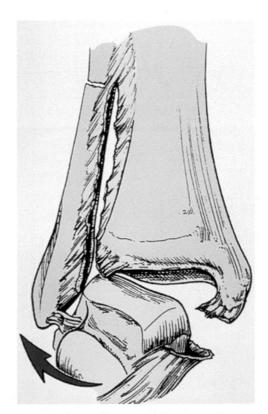

FIGURE 63.3 Mechanism for lateral talar chondral injury associated with Weber C, or Lauge–Hansen PER IV, fracture pattern. Copyright R. Ferkel.

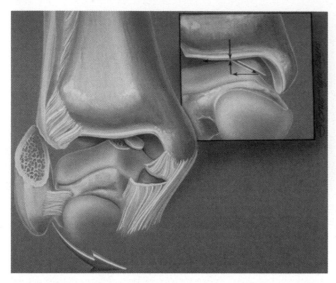

FIGURE 63.4 Mechanism for medial talar chondral injury from a Weber B ankle fracture. Copyright R. Ferkel.

and 1 lateral talar dome injury (Fig. 63.4). No talar TASLs were included among the two Weber A fractures, the two Tillaux fractures, and the single triplane fracture. Among the 34 ankles with a stable syndesmosis, only 10 (29%) had a talar TASL, and 9 of these were SER pattern fractures.

Talar lesions involved the medial dome in 15 patients and lateral wall in 4. All were devoid of subchondral bone, precluding internal fixation. Of the ten tibial lesions, five were at the posterior tibiofibular ligament origin, three at the anterior capsular insertion, and two at the central articular surface.

Of the ten tibial TASLs, two were central and eight were peripheral. Five of the peripheral lesions were avulsions of the posterior inferior tibiofibular ligament (5/8)(Fig. 63.5),

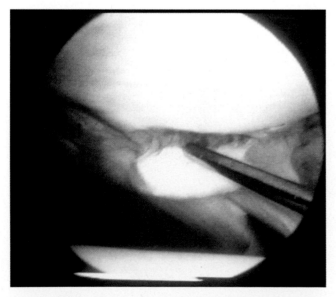

FIGURE 63.5 Avulsion of the posterior inferior tibiofibular ligament off the tibial surface. Copyright R. Ferkel.

and three were lesions of the anterior capsule. Seven of the eight peripheral tibial TASLs were associated with external rotation injury patterns.

It is clear that associated articular injury is common after ankle fracture (14–16). At this time, it is not clear what the long-term sequelae are from these injuries. The goal of arthroscopic-assisted fracture reduction and fixation is twofold: first, to ensure anatomic reduction, and second, to minimize the potential long-term morbidity from associated soft tissue and cartilaginous injuries suffered at the time of fracture. Arthroscopic evaluation allows for a precise evaluation of fracture reduction, and it is the only means to directly visualize articular surface injury in many ankle fractures.

PREOPERATIVE PLANNING

Ideally, arthroscopic evaluation and fracture treatment is done as soon as possible after injury. Within several hours after injury, edema precludes safe arthroscopic treatment. If significant edema is present, then placement in a bulky splint dressing and elevation of the ankle above heart level is indicated for 7 to 14 days, or until swelling resolves. An indication of edema resolution is the skin "wrinkle test." Preoperative radiographs should include the standard anteroposterior, lateral, and mortise views. Occasionally, with osteochondral fractures or triplane type injuries, computed tomographic scans may be of benefit in identifying fracture patterns. Once edema has resolved and the fracture type and treatment plan have been decided, then it is appropriate to proceed with treatment.

ARTICULAR INJURY TECHNIQUE

Fracture treatment can be done with the patient under general or regional anesthesia. He or she is positioned supine with a bolster under the ipsilateral hip (Fig. 63.6). The hip is flexed, and a thigh holder holds the limb in position. A thigh tourniquet is placed but is not inflated unless necessary. Manual or noninvasive distraction is used to avoid the potential for creation of an open fracture with invasive distraction. After sterile preparation, the surface anatomy is outlined and a standard anteromedial portal is established with care not to injure the saphenous neurovascular structures. Then a 2.7-mm, 30-degree arthroscope is introduced. Pressure is maintained with the use of gravity inflow. Adequate outflow is important to prevent extravasation of fluids. After joint lavage to clear any blood or debris, the anterolateral portal is made under direct visualization, with care to avoid injury to the intermediate dorsal cutaneous branch of the superficial peroneal nerve. After these two portals, the posterolateral portal is made under direct arthroscopic visualization with care to avoid the sural nerve.

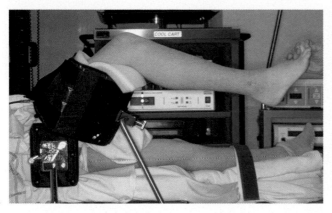
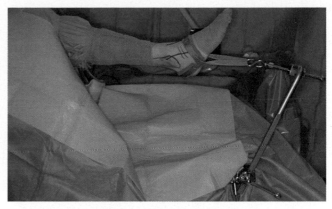

A   B

FIGURE 63.6 Proper positioning of a patient for ankle arthroscopy. **A:** Note that the hip is flexed approximately 45 degrees. **B:** Noninvasive distraction is applied with the use of the displayed outrigger device with an ankle strap. Copyright R. Ferkel.

To minimize the risk of neurovascular injury, all portal incisions should be through skin only, with the remainder of the portal penetration accomplished with blunt trocars. Motorized and manual tools are used as needed to clear any remaining clot and bony or chondral fragments. Once the entire joint is adequately clean, a routine evaluation is performed (17) using anterior and posterior visualization portals.

Before fracture reduction, fracture edges should be debrided and loose articular fragments devoid of bone should be removed with either motorized or manual tools. Full-thickness lesions should be debrided to the subchondral plate, and the edges should be debrided to leave a perpendicular cartilage edge. This allows for better clot retention after abrasion and microfracture.

Osteochondral loose fragments, if large enough, can be fixed with the use of absorbable pins or, less preferably,

Kirschner wires (Fig. 63.7). Large fragments may be amenable to fixation by countersunk screws.

Anterolateral talar lesions are either fixed or excised through the anterolateral portal. Inflow should be from the posterolateral portal for these lesions. Instruments through the anterolateral portal or the cannula itself can be used to manipulate the fragment for reduction. K-wires offer good temporary fixation once reduction is achieved. Polyglycolic acid pins allow good fixation coupled with bioabsorbability for these fractures.

Posterolateral talar lesions are best visualized through the posterolateral portal, with instruments passed from the anterolateral portal. Inflow is from the anteromedial portal. Occasionally, an accessory posterolateral portal is needed for visualization, and the primary posterolateral portal is used for instrumentation. Full-thickness cartilage injuries can be drilled, with the K-wire passed through the posterolateral

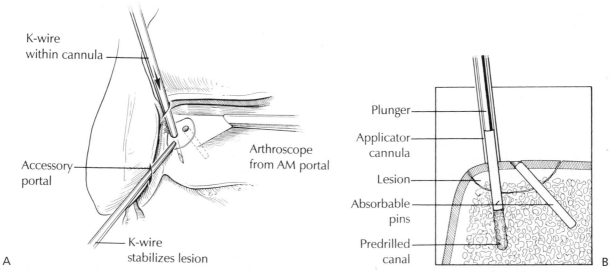

A   B

FIGURE 63.7 Technique for pinning a talar osteochondral fracture. **A:** After anatomic reduction, two K-wires are drilled across the fracture. **B:** Absorbable pins precut to the appropriate length are advanced across the fracture for fixation. (From Ferkel RD. *Arthroscopic surgery: the foot and ankle.* Philadelphia: Lippincott, 1996.)

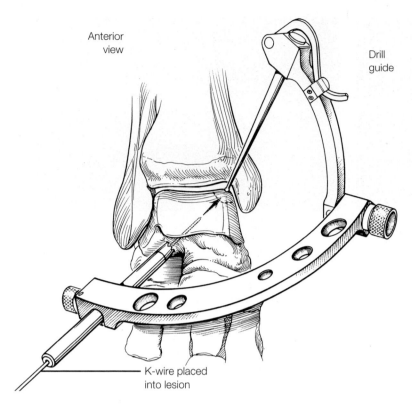

Anterior view

Drill guide

K-wire placed into lesion

FIGURE 63.8 Technique for retrograde drilling of an osteochondral defect of the posteromedial talus. Note the micro-Vector guide placed through the anteromedial portal for proper positioning of the drill holes and the drill entering inferolaterally through the sinus tarsi. The ankle of approach as well as the tip of the guide can be adjusted to attain multiple drill holes for revascularization. (From Ferkel RD. *Arthroscopic surgery: the foot and ankle.* Philadelphia: Lippincott, 1996.)

portal along with ankle dorsiflexion and plantar flexion to make multiple drill holes as needed.

Medial talar dome injuries tend to be posterior and are more difficult to address arthroscopically. Offset drill guides or ACL-type guides through a transmalleolar portal may be necessary. Another option is a retrograde approach through the sinus tarsi using a Micro-Vector or similar drill guide (Fig. 63.8). In rare cases, a medial malleolar osteotomy may be necessary. If a concomitant medial malleolar fracture is present, it may substitute for an osteotomy.

ARTHROSCOPIC-ASSISTED REDUCTION

After adequate arthroscopic examination and debridement, fracture reduction is addressed. Visualization from all three portals is recommended to facilitate proper understanding of fracture geometry. A probe or Freer elevator is used to disimpact depressed fragments. Reduction is achieved through a combination of extraarticular (manual manipulation or reduction forceps), and if necessary, intraarticular manipulation, while viewing the joint arthroscopically. Kirschner wires or guide wires may be useful for provisional fixation of articular fragments once reduction is achieved. Once temporary reduction and provisional fixation (if needed) are achieved, then standard internal fixation is performed (Fig. 63.9). It is convenient to use a cannulated screw system for this percutaneous technique. Once this is achieved, the arthroscope is used to confirm anatomic reduction, and the

joint is lavaged. Radiographic confirmation of the fracture reduction and fixation should be obtained before the patient leaves the operating room. Portals should be closed with skin sutures.

For uncomplicated fractures, a non–weight-bearing splint is worn for 2 weeks and the patient is instructed to elevate the leg. A removable splint is used for the next 2 weeks and is removed for range of motion (ROM) exercises. Partial weight bearing is begun in a boot or short leg cast starting at 4 weeks.

Complex or more unstable patterns may need as much as 3 months of non–weight-bearing treatment to allow for osseous union. If possible, non–weight-bearing ROM should be encouraged as soon as the fracture is mechanically stable to minimize the risk of postoperative stiffness.

Medial Malleolar Fractures

The first aspect of arthroscopic treatment for any fracture is adequate lavage and treatment of the associated articular pathology. After this is achieved, the fracture site is gently debrided with the use of small curettes from the anteromedial or anterolateral portals. At this time, a Freer or similar elevator is used to disimpact any depressed component of the fracture. If there is an associated fibular fracture, it should be reduced and fixed in order to attain and maintain fibular length before the medial malleolus is addressed. After fibular treatment (if needed), two guide wires from the AO 4.0-mm cannulated set are placed percutaneuosly

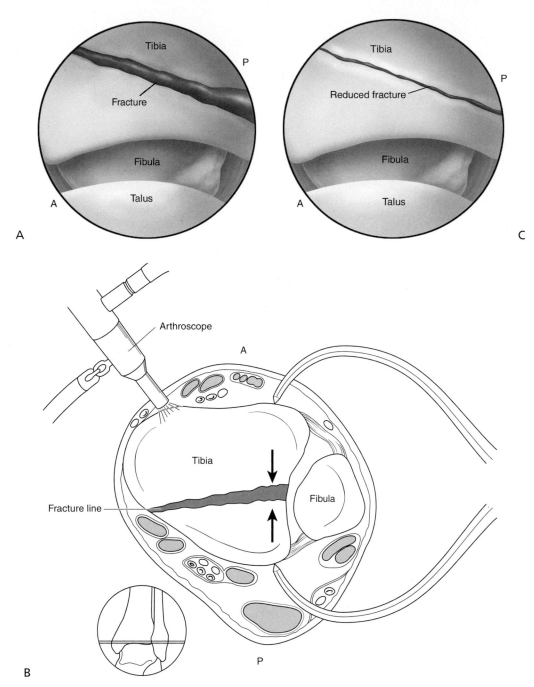

FIGURE 63.9 Technique for arthroscopic-assisted reduction and fixation of a posterior malleolus fracture in a left ankle. **A:** Arthroscopic view of fracture line with clot viewed from the antero-medial portal. **B:** Cross-sectional view through the left ankle joint, looking up at the distal tibial articular surface with the arthroscope, as reduction is achieved with the use of a percutaneous clamp between fracture fragments. Note the relation of the clamp placement to adjacent neurovascular structures. **C:** Arthroscopic view of reduction from anteromedial portal.

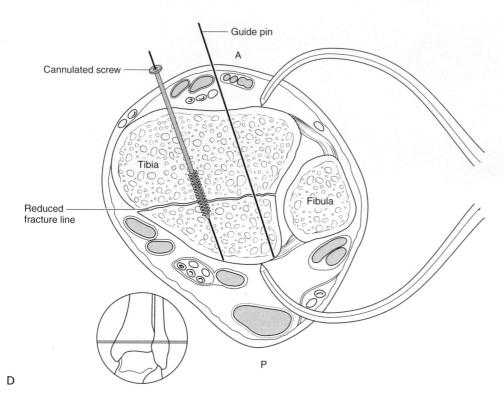

D

E

FIGURE 63.9 *(continued)* **D:** Cross-sectional view of the left ankle, looking up through the cancellous bone of the distal tibia, with temporary K-wire and definitive screw fixation. Note the placement of percutaneous screws to avoid overlying neurovascular structures. **E:** Final fixation after removal of external clamp and guide wires.

through the distal tip of the medial malleolus, stopping just distal to the fracture line. The guide wires can be used to skewer the fracture fragment and aid in manual manipulation as needed. With these techniques, the fracture is reduced anatomically under direct arthroscopic visualization. After reduction, the guide wires are advanced across the fracture site. Two 4.0-mm cannulated screws are advanced across the fracture for definitive fixation (Fig. 63.10). Radiographs should be taken in the operating room to confirm anatomic reduction. Arthroscopic portals and screw placement skin defects are closed with vertical mattress sutures.

Postoperatively, the patient is placed in a splint for 2 weeks, after which the splint and sutures are removed. The patient is placed in a removable boot for an additional 2 weeks of non–weight-bearing immobilization. During this time, the boot is periodically removed to allow for ROM exercises. At 4 weeks after surgery, the patient is allowed to begin progressive weight bearing in the boot.

Posterior Malleolar Fractures

Posterior malleolar fractures usually involve avulsion of the posterior inferior tibiofibular ligament. Less commonly, they are caused by talar rotation and impaction into the posterior lip of the tibia. Posterior malleolar fractures often reduce once the fibular fracture is reduced. For this reason, it is necessary to adequately treat the fibular fracture before assessment of the posterior malleolus. Indications for fixation are a tibial fragment that involves more than 25% of the articular surface or persistent displacement of the fracture of

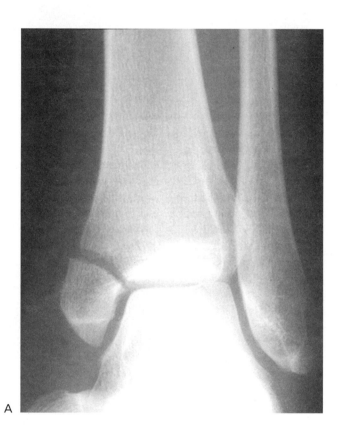

A

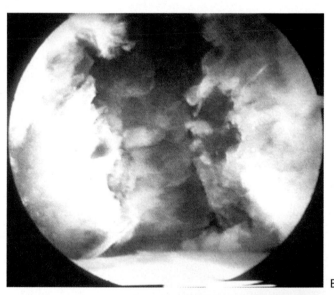

B

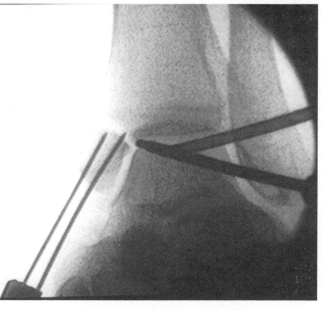

C

FIGURE 63.10 Arthroscopic-assisted technique for medial malleolus fracture. **A:** Radiograph of medial malleolus fracture. There is no accompanying proximal fibular fracture or syndesmotic injury. **B:** Arthroscopic view of fracture after debridement. **C:** Percutaneous guide wires advanced up to but not across fracture line.

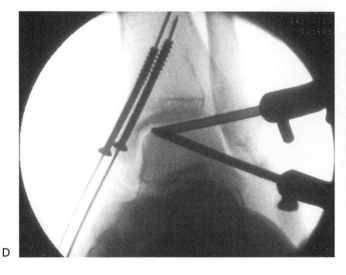

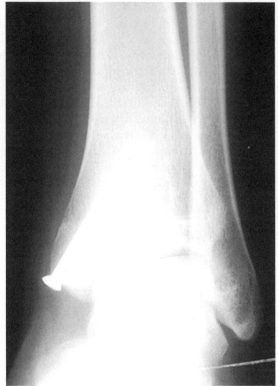

FIGURE 63.10 *(continued)* **D:** After arthroscopically verified anatomic reduction, the guide wires and screws are advanced across the fracture. **E:**Follow-up radiograph after removal of guide wires. Copyright R. Ferkel.

more than 2 to 3 mm (18). Nonconcentric reduction of the ankle joint in these situations puts the ankle at risk for post-traumatic degenerative joint disease (6).

Posterior malleolar fractures are ideal for arthroscopic-assisted reduction and fixation. It is often difficult to achieve anatomic reduction with a closed technique. If typical closed measures for reduction fail, a relatively large posterior approach is needed. In addition, the sural nerve is in close association with a traditional open approach. Arthroscopic-assisted reduction allows for anatomic reduction, which commonly involves disimpaction of tibial plafond fragments. This is difficult with traditional techniques.

After adequate debridement, the fracture is visualized from the anteromedial portal with inflow from the antero-lateral or posterior portal. With the use of a Freer elevator through the remaining posterior or anterolateral portal, the impacted aspect of the fracture can be elevated. Extension of the patient's great toe presses the flexor hallucis longus against the posterior malleolus and helps in reduction. Then, the pelvic reduction forceps is placed percutaneously (Fig. 63.11), and the anterior and posterior fragments are reduced and held in place. Direct arthroscopic visualization is used to confirm anatomic reduction. Lag screws are then placed percutaneously from anterior to posterior to fix the fracture. After fixation, the portals are closed and a sterile dressing is placed.

The leg is splinted with a posterior and U stirrup for 2 weeks of non–weight-bearing immobilization. At 2 weeks, the sutures are removed and a removable boot is used. Early ROM, avoiding plantar flexion, is begun after sutures are removed. Partial weight bearing in the boot is begun at 4 weeks and progressed to full weight bearing at 8 weeks. Once the ankle is clinically and radiographically healed, usually by 8 weeks, the boot is removed and unrestricted weight bearing is allowed.

Anterior Margin or Tillaux Fractures

Tillaux fractures involve an avulsion of the anterior inferior tibiofibular ligament (Fig. 63.12). After debridement and lavage, the fracture is reduced with the use of instruments from the anterolateral portal and internal rotation of the foot. Visualization is from the anteromedial portal (Fig. 63.13). The extraarticular portion of the Tillaux fragment is often an impediment to reduction. If so, the anterolateral portal incision can be extended proximally to allow for debridement of the interposed soft tissue. Reduction is confirmed by direct arthroscopic visualization from the anteromedial portal. Then, provisional guide wires are advanced percutaneously from anterior to posterior, with care to avoid neurovascular injury. Lag screws are placed by a standard AO technique. The wounds are closed with nylon vertical mattress sutures, and a splint is placed on the foot in neutral position.

The sutures are removed and the splint is replaced with a removable boot at 2 weeks after surgery. The boot is removed for ROM exercises. Non–weight bearing is continued until 4 weeks after surgery, at which time progressive weight bearing in the boot is begun.

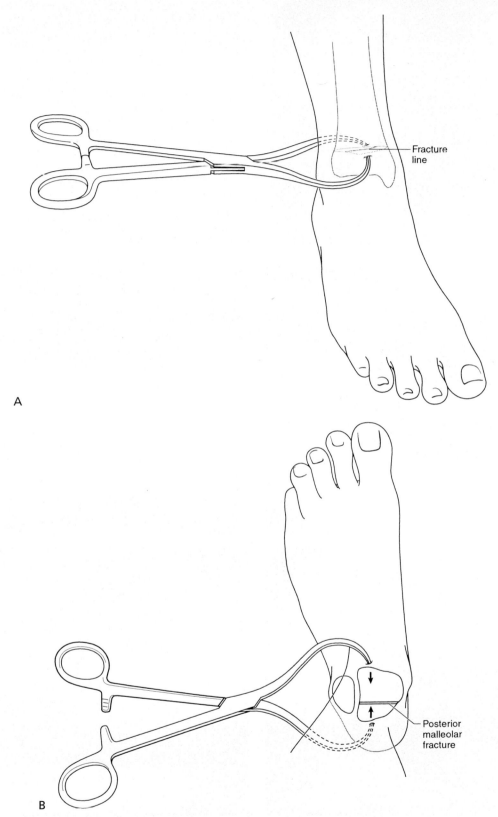

Fracture line

Posterior malleolar fracture

A

B

FIGURE 63.11 Fracture through distal tibia, including posterior malleolus. **A:** External view of percutaneous reduction of distal tibial fracture. **B:** Axial view looking down on fracture as reduction is achieved with the use of a pelvic reduction clamp.

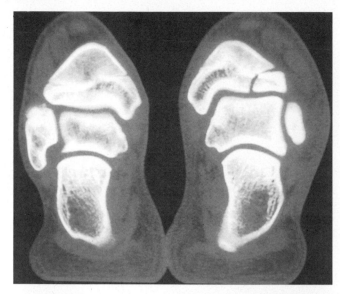

FIGURE 63.12 Computed tomographic scan showing minimally displaced Tillaux fracture fragment. Note the physis in the process of closing. Copyright R. Ferkel.

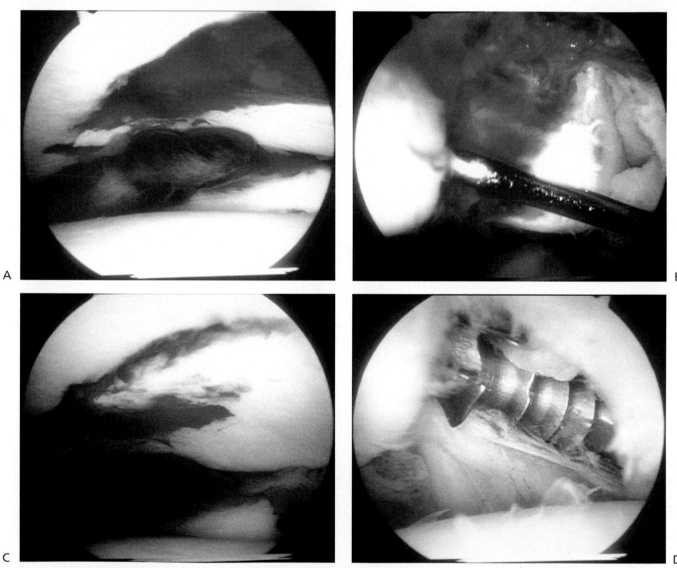

FIGURE 63.13 Reduction and fixation of displaced Tillaux fracture. **A:** Arthroscopic view of tibiotalar joint in a Tillaux fracture viewed from anteromedial portal. Note the fracture hematoma and fibula in the background. **B:** Additional view from anteromedial portal viewing the anterior edge of the Tillaux fragment. Note the probe coming from the anterolateral portal into the fracture. **C:** Reduction is achieved by a posteriorly directed force from the anterolateral aspect of the fracture fragment. **D:** Lag screw entering through the anterolateral portal into the anterolateral aspect of the Tillaux fragment.

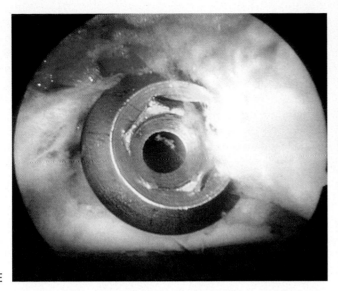

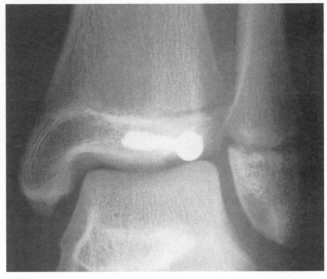

E   F

FIGURE 63.13 *(continued)* **E:** End-on view of the screw from the anterolateral portal after definitive fixation. **F:** Postoperative radiograph showing the fixed fracture. Copyright R. Ferkel.

Triplane Fractures

Triplane fractures are fractures of incomplete physeal closure. The peak age for this fracture is 12–14 years old. Their complex geometry is caused by the incomplete physeal closure of the distal tibia. The distal tibial physis closes from posteromedial to anterolateral. Triplane fractures are so named because the fracture lines propagate in three separate planes. There may be two to four fracture fragments; most commonly, there are three. The three primary fracture fragments are the distal tibial metaphysis, the posterior malleolus and medial epiphysis with a posterior metaphyseal spike, and the anterolateral epiphyseal fragment (Tillaux fragment) (Fig. 63.14).

The fracture lies in three different planes, necessitating cross-sectional as well as coronal and sagittal imaging. Computed tomographic scanning allows for precise diagnosis and treatment planning. The goal of treatment is anatomic reduction. As the physis is in the process of fusing, there is little risk of leg length discrepancy due to the physeal injury associated with triplane fractures.

Anatomic reduction of the articular aspect of the fracture is the primary goal in triplane fracture management. Patients with these fractures are by definition young, and any residual articular incongruity puts them at increased risk for long-term degenerative changes. Anatomic reduction and fixation of the Tillaux fragment facilitates anatomic reduction of the metaphyseal aspect of the fracture. The articular reduction and fixation takes precedence over the proximal fracture alignment.

A standard setup is used in the operating room, as are standard anteromedial, anterolateral, and posterolateral portals. The Tillaux fragment is reduced as described in the previous section. After reduction and fixation of the Tillaux fragment, percutaneous fixation of the metaphyseal fracture

component is performed by a standard AO technique. Occasionally, the metaphyseal aspect of the fracture has soft tissue interposed that prevents anatomic reduction. In this case, open reduction is necessary. Plastic deformation at the time of injury may also make proximal reduction more difficult. If this occurs, anatomic reduction of the joint line re-

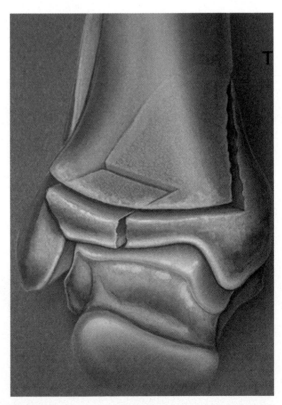

FIGURE 63.14 Three-part triplane fracture demonstrating complex nature of the fracture pattern. Note the coronal, sagittal, and axial components of the triplane fracture. Copyright R. Ferkel.

mains the primary goal and residual metaphyseal stepoff is acceptable.

Tibial Plafond Fractures

Fractures of the tibial plafond usually result from an axial load, often with a rotational component. Higher-energy fractures can result in marked comminution, soft tissue injury, and articular incongruity. These fractures require careful preoperative planning. Soft tissue compromise is the most common complication after operative treatment of these fractures (19–22). The trend has been toward minimally invasive reduction technique and limited internal fixation (23–26). Arthroscopic-assisted surgery has a role in Allgower 1 and 2 type fractures. Markedly comminuted or Ruedi–Allgower 3 fractures are beyond the scope of arthroscopic treatment. Extravasation of fluid poses a significant risk for development of compartment syndrome, and soft tissue must be monitored meticulously to minimize this risk. Operative arthroscopic time should be kept to a minimum, and gravity inflow, rather than pump systems, should be used.

The fractured extremity should be either treated immediately or splinted and elevated for several days to allow edema to reside. A standard setup is used, with the exception that a padded strap is used for traction. Alternatively, a spanning external fixator may be placed preoperatively to give adequate traction across the joint and to serve as postoperative immobilization (Fig. 63.15). This does make manipulation of arthroscopic tools more difficult intraoperatively. Traction should be adjusted to allow adequate visualization with the least possible tension across the fracture site. Standard arthroscopic portals are used. It is important to remember that landmarks are altered by the fracture and its associated swelling, so palpation of the talus may offer more reliable reference than tibial anatomy.

After successful portal placement, the ankle should be thoroughly lavaged and debrided of any loose fragments. Larger fragments may be amenable to fixation. A combination of closed reduction, intraarticular manipulation with a Freer elevator or similar tool and percutaneous manipulation with reduction forceps is used to achieve a reduction, starting at the articular surface and moving proximally. After reduction, limited internal fixation by an appropriate

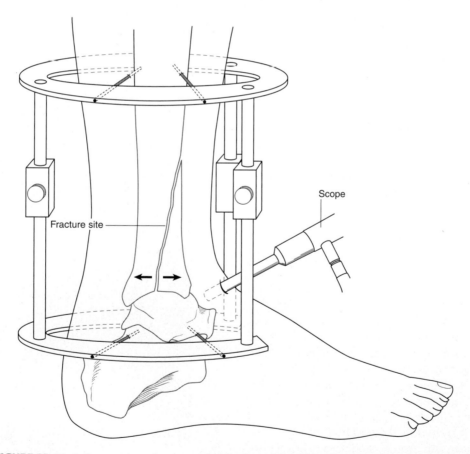

FIGURE 63.15 Arthroscopic evaluation and reduction of distal pilon fracture. Note the temporary external fixation that allows for maintenance of fracture length during reduction and fixation of the fracture. Note also the open aspect of the ring anteriorly to minimize interference with arthroscopic manipulation.

AO technique is employed. After fixation, fracture alignment is verified with timely arthroscopic visualization.

After surgery, the portals are closed with vertical mattress sutures. A carefully padded splint in neutral position is used for 2 weeks. The patient should return 1 week after surgery for a wound check. At the 2-week postoperative clinic visit, the sutures are removed and the splint is exchanged for a removable splint. An extended period of non–weight bearing may be necessary for adequate fracture healing. Plafond fractures each have their own personality, and immobilization and weight bearing schedules are adjusted accordingly. Up to 3 months of non–weight bearing is common after fixation of more complicated fractures.

COMPLICATIONS

Arthroscopic-assisted fracture care demands careful attention to fluid management, local anatomy, and the use of minimally traumatic technique. Compartment syndrome has not been reported in association with ankle arthroscopy, although the risk is present in the setting of an acute fracture. The surgeon must pay close attention to inflow and, more importantly, to outflow in the acutely fractured ankle. In our experience, extravasation can be kept to a minimum with adequate inflow and balanced outflow.

Normal surface anatomic relationships are altered in the setting of fracture. In addition, soft tissue swelling further confuses local anatomic landmarks. This increases the risk of superficial neurovascular injury from portal placement. Repetitive introduction and removal of instruments increases the risk of iatrogenic injury. This can be minimized by meticulous surgical technique and use of interchangeable small-joint cannulae for introduction of the arthroscope and instruments.

Infection risks can be minimized by the use of preoperative antistaphylococcal antibiotics, followed by 48 hours of a similar oral antibiotic. Wounds should be closed with nylon sutures. Postoperatively, the ankle should be elevated and immobilized at least until the portals are healed and the sutures removed.

CONCLUSION

Arthroscopic-assisted ankle fracture treatment allows for debridement of associated chondral and osteochondral injuries after ankle fracture. In addition, precise assessment of the fracture reduction is possible. Precise reduction of articular fractures is shown to decrease the long-term risk of post-traumatic arthritis.

The long-term sequelae of acute articular injury associated with fracture are unclear, but studies suggest that chondral injury may be a significant cause of late degenerative processes (11,27). Arthroscopy allows for treatment of associated chon-dral injury at the time of initial fracture treatment. It is not possible to determine whether acute intervention will decrease the incidence or severity of late functional deficits after ankle fracture; only a prospective, randomized trial could prove this. Lantz et al. (27) found a 49% incidence of talar chondral injury associated with ankle fracture. At follow-up, patients with talar chondral injury associated with malleolar fractures had decreased ankle ROM and function. Taga et al. (11), in a series of patients with chronic ankle instability who underwent arthroscopy and ligamentous repair, found that those with ligamentous injuries and more than 50% articular surface injury complained of persistent pain at follow-up. These series suggest that chondral injury does affect patient outcome. What remains unclear is the effect of surgical intervention on the outcome.

In a small, prospective study, Thordason et al. (28) demonstrated no difference in short-term outcomes after treatment for ankle fracture with and without arthroscopy. Nineteen patients were randomly assigned to one of two treatment groups; ten patients underwent standard open reduction with internal fixation, and nine underwent arthroscopic debridement before fixation. This study does address some interesting questions, but the average follow-up period was only 21 months (range, 6 to 39 months). We believe that the treatment of associated chondral injury would be a long-term benefit. Twenty-one months is too short a follow-up to determine the efficacy of this procedure. In addition, only nine patients underwent arthroscopy with a 4.5-mm arthroscope; eight had chondral injury, and one had a loose body. None of the patients needed significant debridement. A larger series of patients undergoing arthroscopy would probably show more varied chondral injuries. Also, the use of a 2.9-mm small-joint arthroscope, as we recommend, would allow better diagnostic accuracy. We believe that this study shows good preliminary data, but a larger series with longer-term follow-up is needed to determine the value of arthroscopic-assisted technique.

The senior author's series demonstrated that patients with injury to the syndesmosis are at highest risk for articular injury after ankle fracture. Arthroscopy allows accurate diagnosis and treatment of these potential lesions with minimal surgical trauma. Also, removal of loose fragments prevents future third-body articular wear. Judicious debridement of free ligament tears may also be beneficial in preventing late impingement.

Additionally, fracture patterns such as posterior malleolar fractures that do not reduce with closed techniques traditionally require relatively extensile open exposure. Arthroscopic-assisted reduction and intraarticular manipulation of depressed fragments is a valuable skill for the treating surgeon, obviating the need for patient repositioning and a posterior approach.

In summary, arthroscopic-assisted fracture treatment offers a less invasive treatment option for the surgeon. It allows accurate assessment of fracture patterns, treatment of associated soft tissue and chondral injuries at the index operation, and excellent evaluation of articular reduction. Although its benefit has not been proven, it is intuitively appealing. The trend of surgical technique is toward less invasive measures. Further study is needed to determine arthroscopy's place in the treatment of ankle fractures.

REFERENCES

1. Daly PJ, Fitzgerald RH, Melton LJ, ct al. Epidemiology of ankle fractures in Rochester, Minnesota. *Acta Orthop Scand* 1987; 58:539–544.
2. Ali MS, McLaren CA, Rouholamin E, et al. Ankle fractures in the elderly: nonoperative or operative treatment. *J Orthop. Trauma* 1987;1:275–280.
3. Hughes JL, Weber H, Willenegger H, et al. Evaluation of ankle fractures: non-operative and operative treatment. *Clin Orthop* 1979;138:111–119.
4. Yde J, Krisensen KD. Ankle fractures: supination-eversion fractures of stage IV. Primary and late results of operative and nonoperative treatment. *Acta Orthop Scand* 1980;51:981–990.
5. Bauer M, Bergstrom B, Hemborg A, et al. Malleolar fractures: nonoperative versus operative treatment. A controlled study. *Clin Orthop* 1985;198:110–117.
6. Bauer M, Jonsson K, Nilsson B. Thirty year follow-up of ankle fractures. *Acta Orthop Scand* 1985;56:103–106.
7. Cass JF, Morrey BF, Katoh Y, et al. Ankle instability: comparison of primary repair and late reconstruction after long-term follow-up study. *Clin Orthop* 1985;198:110–117.
8. Anderson IF, Crichton KJ, Grattan-Smith T, et al. Osteochondral fractures of the dome of the talus. *J Bone Joint Surg Am* 1989;71:1143–1152.
9. Renstrom, Per A. Persistently painful sprained ankle. *J Am Acad Orthop Surg* 1994;2:270–280.
10. Stone JW. Osteochondral lesions of the talar dome. *J Am Acad Orthop Surg* 1996;4:63–73.
11. Taga I, Shino K, Inoue M, et al. Articular cartilage lesions in ankles with lateral ligament injury: an arthroscopic study. *Am J Sports Med* 1993;21:120–126.
12. Pettrone FA, Gail M, Pee D, et al. A prospective randomized study of the management of severe ankle fractures. *J Bone Joint Surg Am* 1985;67:67–78.
13. Zenker H, Nerlich M. Prognostic aspects in operated ankle fractures. *Acta Orthop Trauma Surg* 1982;100:237–241.
14. Loren GJ, Ferkel RD. Arthroscopic assessment of occult intra-articular injury in acute ankle fractures. *Arthroscopy* 2002;18: 412–421.
15. Hinterman B, Regazzoni P, Lampert C, et al. Arthroscopic findings in acute fractures of the ankle. *J Bone Joint Surg Br* 2000;82: 345–351.
16. Feldman MD. Evaluation of intra-articular damage in displaced extra-articular ankle fractures. Eastern Orthopaedic Association, Annual Meeting. Scottsdale, AZ: EOA, 1997.
17. Ferkel RD. Diagnostic arthroscopic examination. In Ferkel RD. *Arthroscopic surgery: the foot and ankle.* Philadelphia: Lippincott-Raven, 1996:103–118.
18. Trafton PG, Bray TJ, Simpson LA. Fractures and soft tissue injuries of the ankle. In: Browner BD, Jupiter JB, Levine AM, et al. *Skeletal trauma,* 2nd ed. Philadelphia: WB Saunders, 1992: 1871–1957.
19. Dillin L, Slabaugh P. Delayed wound healing, infection, and nonunion following open reduction and internal fixation of tibial plafond fractures. *J Trauma* 1986;26:1116–1119.
20. Shelton ML, Anderson RL Jr. Complications of fractures and dislocations of the ankle. In: Epps CH Jr, ed. *Complications in orthopaedic surgery,* 2nd ed, vol 1. Philadelphia: Lippincott, 1986: 599–648.
21. Teeny SM, Wiss DA. Open reduction and internal fixation of tibial plafond fractures: variables contributing to poor results and complications. *Clin Orthop* 1993;292:108–117.
22. Teeny SM, Wiss DA, Hathaway R, et al. Tibial plafond fractures: errors, complications, and pitfalls in operative treatment. *Orthop Trans* 1990;14:265.
23. Babis GC, Vayanos ED, Papaioannou N, et al. Results of surgical treatment of tibial plafond fractures. *Clin Orthop* 1997;341: 99–105.
24. Marsh JL, Bonar S, Nepola JV, et al. Use of an articulated external fixator for fractures of the tibial plafond. *J Bone Joint Surg Am* 1995;77:1498–1509.
25. McDonald MG, Burgess RC, Bolano LE, et al. Ilizarov treatment of pilon fractures. *Clin Orthop* 1996;325:232–238.
26. Tornetta P III, Weiner L, Bergman M, et al. Pilon fractures: treatment with combined internal and external fixation. *J Orthop Trauma* 1993;7:489–496.
27. Lantz BA. McAndrew M. Scioli M, et al. The effect of concomitant chondral injuries accompanying operatively reduced malleolar fractures. *J Orthop Trauma* 1991;5:125–128.
28. Thordason DB, Bains R, Shepard LE. The role of ankle arthroscopy on the surgical management of ankle fractures. *Foot Ankle Int* 2001;22:123–125.

THE FOLLOWING REFERENCES ARE NOT CITED IN THE TEXT:

Berndt AL, Harty M. Transchondral fractures (osteochondritis dissecans) of the talus. *J Bone Joint Surg Am* 1959;41:988–1020.

Danis R. *Theorie et pratique de l'osto-synthse.* Paris, Masson & Cie, 1947.

DeBerardino TM, Arciero RA, Taylor DC. Arthroscopic treatment of soft-tissue impingement of the ankle in athletes. *Arthroscopy* 1997;13:492–498.

Ferkel RD, Karzel RP, Del Pizzo W, et al. Arthroscopic treatment of anterolateral impingement of the ankle. *Am J Sports Med* 1991;19: 440–446.

Ferkel RD, Orwin JF. Ankle arthroscopy: a new tool for treating acute and chronic ankle fractures. *Arthroscopy* 1993;9:352–353.

Ferkel RD, Orwin JF. Arthroscopic treatment of acute ankle fractures and postfracture defects. In: Ferkel RD. *Arthroscopic surgery: the foot and ankle.* Philadelphia: Lippincott-Raven, 1996:185–200.

Ferkel RD, Scranton PE Jr. Current concepts review: arthroscopy of the ankle and foot. *J Bone Joint Surg Am* 1993;75:1233–1242.

Holt ES. Arthroscopic visualization of the tibial plafond during posterior malleolar-fracture fixation. *Foot Ankle* 1994;15:206–208.

Lauge-Hansen N. "Ligamentous" ankle fractures: diagnosis and treatment. *Acta Chir Scand* 1949;97:544–550.

Lauge-Hansen N. Fractures of the ankle: II. Combined experimental-surgical and experimental-roentgenologic investigations. *Arch Surg* 1950;50:957–985.

Lauge-Hansen N. Fractures of the ankle: IV. Clinical use of genetic roentgen diagnosis and genetic roentgen reduction. *Arch Surg* 1952;64:488–500.

Lauge-Hansen N. Fractures of the ankle: V. Pronation-dorsiflexion fracture. *Arch Surg* 1953;67:813–820.

Lauge-Hansen N. Fractures of the ankle: III. Genetic roentgenologic diagnosis of fractures of the ankle. *AJR Am J Roentgenol* 1954;71:456–471.

Meislin RJ, Rose DJ, Parisien JS, et al. Arthroscopic treatment of synovial impingement of the ankle. *Am J Sports Med* 1993;21: 186–189.

Miller MD. Arthroscopically assisted reduction and fixation of an adult Tillaux fracture of the ankle. *Arthroscopy* 1997; 13:117–119.

Ogilvie-Harris DJ, Reed SC. Disruption of the ankle syndesmosis: diagnosis and treatment by arthroscopic surgery. *Arthroscopy* 1994; 10:561–568.

Outerbridge RE. The etiology of chondromalacia patellae. *J Bone Joint Surg Br* 1961;43:752–757.

Stauffer RN. Intraarticular ankle problems. In: Evarts CM. *Surgery of the musculoskeletal system,* vol 3. New York: Churchill-Livingstone, 1983.

Stetson WB, Ferkel RD. Ankle arthroscopy: I. Technique and complications. *J Am Acad Orthop Surg* 1996;4:17–23.

Stetson WB, Ferkel RD. Ankle arthroscopy: II. Indications and risks. *J Am Acad Orthop Surg* 1996;4:24–31.

Weber BG. *Die Verletzungen des oberen Sprunggelenkes: Aktuelle Probleme in der Chirugie,* 1st ed. Bern: Verlag Hans Huber, 1966.

Weber BG. *Die Verletzungen des oberen Sprunggelenkes: Aktuelle Probleme in der Chirugie,* 2nd ed. Bern: Verlag Hans Huber, 1972.

Whipple TL, Martin DR, McIntyre LF, et al. Arthroscopic treatment of triplane fractures of the ankle. *Arthroscopy* 1993;9:456–463.

Wolin I, Glassman F, Sideman S. Internal derangement of the talofibular component of the ankle. *Surg Gynecol Obstet* 1950;91: 193.

Yao I, Weis E. Osteochondritis dissecans. *Orthop Rev* 1985;14:190–194.

64

ARTHROSCOPIC TIBIOTALAR ARTHRODESIS

CRAIG D. MORGAN

Since 1900, more than 30 different surgical techniques through nine different open approaches have been described for fusion of the tibiotalar joint (1,2). A review of this literature shows that complication rates as high as 60% have been reported, with an average pseudoarthrosis rate of approximately 20% and infection rates ranging from 5% to 25% (3–8). In contrast, a simple open technique described by Morgan et al. (2) in 1985 showed successful fusion in 96%, with low morbidity in long-term (10-year average) follow-up of 101 cases. Salient features of this technique included maintenance of the normal bony contours of the ankle mortise and internal fusion fixation by two crossed transmalleolar screws (2). In general, the arthroscopic procedure described in this chapter recreates the open Morgan method of ankle arthrodesis using current arthroscopic technique (9,10).

OPERATIVE TECHNIQUE

As with the open method, this arthroscopic procedure includes three basic steps: (a) debridement of all hyaline cartilage and subchondral bone, (b) fusion reduction in a neutral position, and (c) internal fusion fixation in a neutral position with two transmalleolar crossed screws. Equipment necessary to perform this procedure includes an image intensifier and radiolucent operating table; a 30-degree, fore-oblique, 4-mm or 2.7-mm arthroscope with camera and television and video equipment; a high-speed motorized suction abrader and shaver; 15-degree angled arthroscopic rasps and ringed curettes, soft tissue noninvasive distraction straps, and a cannulated cancellous screw system for internal fixation.

The patient is placed in the supine position and usually is anesthetized on a standard operating table with a radiolucent foot and ankle extension that allows the ankle to be flu-

C. D. Morgan: The Morgan Kalman Clinic, Wilmington, Delaware; Department of Orthopaedic Surgery, Sports Medicine, University of Pennsylvania, Philadelphia, Pennsylvania.

oroscoped with an image intensifier during the procedure. A sandbag is placed under the buttock of the operative limb to avoid external rotation of the leg during the procedure. After routine preparation and draping from the proximal tibia to the toes, which allows adequate assessment of ankle alignment, a proximal thigh tourniquet is applied and inflated. The ankle and foot are suspended on a large sterile cloth bump placed behind the posterior aspect of the midcalf, which allows free access to the posterolateral aspect of the ankle (Fig. 64.1). Next, noninvasive distractive software straps are applied to the foot and ankle, which allow the surgeon to apply significant tibiotalar distractive forces when necessary to allow for adequate visualization, particularly in the middle and posterior joint spaces (Fig. 64.2).

Three standard arthroscopic portals are used: anterolateral, anteromedial, and posterolateral (Fig. 64.3). With the arthroscope placed anterolaterally, the amount of necessary distraction is assessed. Once good visualization is achieved, a posterolateral portal is established, and a large-bore cannula is placed through it; this can be used for fluid inflow and, later, for instrumentation to the posterior compartment (Fig. 64.3C). Next, a motorized arthroscopic abrader is used in a systematic fashion to debride the articular surfaces of the tibial plafond, talar dome, and medial and lateral talomalleolar surfaces of all remaining hyaline cartilage and subchondral bone, thus exposing viable cancellous bone (Fig. 64.4). During debridement, care is taken to maintain the normal bony contour of the talar dome and tibial plafond (i.e., talar convexity and concavity) while correcting any varus–valgus deformity that may exist. One should avoid squaring off the surfaces or resecting too much bone medially, because this creates a varus deformity, which should be avoided. A fusion in varus was shown by Morgan et al. (2) in long-term follow-up to lead to suboptimal clinical results caused by lateral forefoot metatarsalgia.

Debridement of the most posterior aspect of the talus and posterior malleolus may be done with the motorized abrader placed from posterolateral while viewing with the

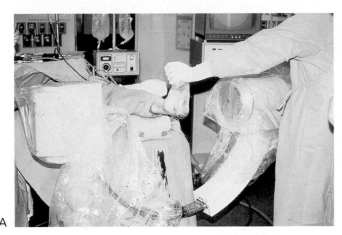

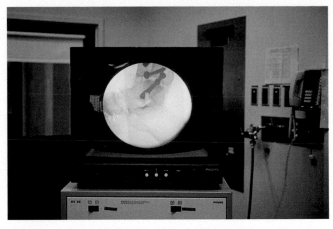

FIGURE 64.1 A: The left ankle is positioned on a large cloth bump, which allows circumferential access to the ankle and fluoroscopy with an image intensifier. **B:** Fluoroscopic monitor image of the case in progress in **(A)**—lateral view of completed closed left ankle fusion.

arthroscope from anterolateral or anteromedial (Fig. 64.3C). This may also be done using 15-degree curved handheld rasps and ring curettes from in front (Fig. 64.5). In general, the medial half of the debridement process is done with the arthroscope placed anterolaterally and the abrader placed anteromedially. Conversely, the lateral half of the debridement process is done with the arthroscope placed anteromedially and the abrader anterolaterally.

After debridement of the tibiotalar weight-bearing surfaces, a similar technique is used to debride the medial and lateral talomalleolar spaces. Because the talus anatomically is an apex superior wedge-shaped structure in both the sagittal and coronal planes that articulates with the plafond and both malleoli, failure to clean out both talomalleolar spaces

prevents apposition of the talar weight-bearing surface with the plafond during the reduction phase of the procedure (Fig. 64.6).

The final step in the debridement process involves removal of the usually large anterior tibial lip osteophyte, which otherwise would block adequate reduction of the talar dome convexity into the concavity of the tibial plafond and block dorsiflexion to the desired neutral position. The osteophyte may be removed with the use of the abrader and arthroscope placed anteriorly. Occasionally, if there is scarring of the anterior capsule to the osteophyte, the arthroscope may be placed posterolaterally to give better visualization and subsequent assessment of the amount of bone removal required.

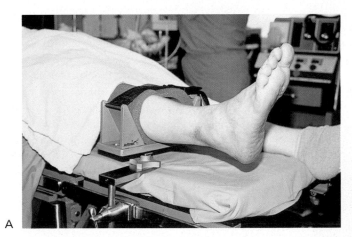

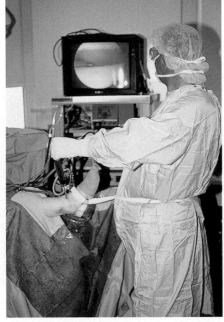

FIGURE 64.2 A: Right ankle with soft tissue noninvasive distraction system (Artrex, Naples, FL) applied. **B:** Note that the strap around the surgeon's back allows distraction to be adjusted by surgeon's leaning backward or forward.

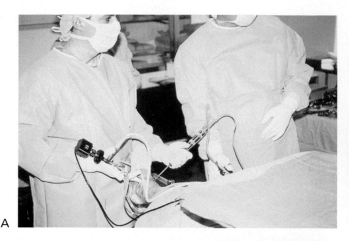

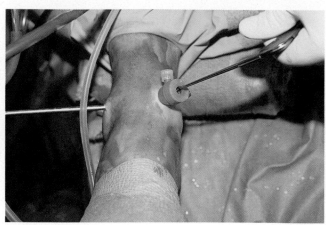

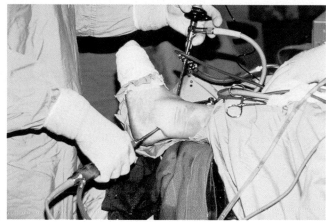

B

C

FIGURE 64.3 A and **B:** Standard anterolateral and anteromedial portals. **C:** Motorized instrumentation positioned from a posterolateral approach.

Once viable cancellous bone is visualized surrounding the fusion area, the distraction software is released and the fusion surfaces are reduced under image intensification by manual upward displacement of the hindfoot and dorsiflexion of the forefoot to a neutral position. With the talus held in this position, either manually or with the distraction straps removed, internal fixation is obtained by two cannu-

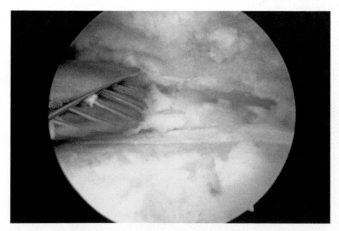

FIGURE 64.4 Arthroscopic view of motorized abrader debriding remnants of hyaline cartilage to subchondral bone.

lated 6.5- or 7.5-mm diameter cancellous screws placed percutaneously over guide pins, one from the medial distal tibial metaphysis and one from the distal fibular metaphysis into the body of the talus (2). These screws angle anteriorly approximately 40 degrees to gain maximum purchase into the talus without entering the subtalar joint (Fig. 64.7). Confirmation of the fusion reduction and screw placement is made using the image intensifier or permanent radiographic films. During this step, particular attention is directed to confirming that the subtalar joint has not been penetrated by the tip of either screw.

All portals are closed with a single 4-0 nylon stitch. The ankle is immobilized in a well-padded short-leg cast with the ankle and tarsus in a neutral position. The patient is kept from weight bearing for 6 weeks, followed by an additional 6 weeks in a short-leg walking cast.

INDICATIONS

The indications for ankle fusion are those previously reported by Morgan et al. (2) for the open procedure. Any condition that results in irreversible destruction of the hyaline cartilage surfaces of the ankle, leading to disabling pain and dysfunction unresponsive to conservative measures such

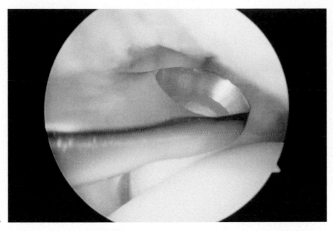
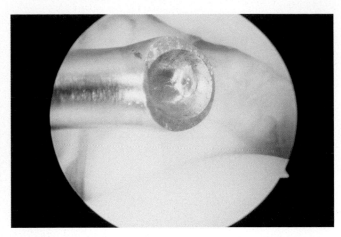

A   B

FIGURE 64.5 Fifteen-degree bent ringed **(A)** and standard **(B)** curettes used to debride existing hyaline cartilage to the subchondral plate.

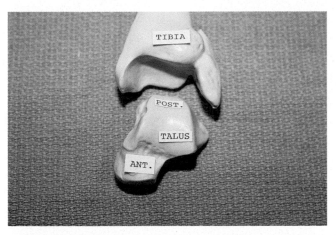

FIGURE 64.6 Note the anterior-to-posterior and inferior-to-superior wedge-shaped contour of the talar articular surfaces, which will block reduction of the talus to the tibial plafond during the reduction maneuver unless both talomalleolar spaces have been debrided of enough bone to prevent this effect.

An arthroscopic rather than an open approach to ankle fusion is believed to be most advantageous in patients with systemic problems associated with an increased risk of poor wound healing or infection. Such problems include hemophilia, rheumatoid arthritis, insulin-dependent diabetes mellitus, peripheral vascular disease, and long-term use of corticosteroids. In addition, an arthroscopic approach is favored in special situations such as posterior tibial artery occlusion or absence from prior trauma, and in the presence of prior anterior ankle skin grafts that preclude the use of an open anterior or anterolateral approach due to risk of vascular compromise from the exposure.

CONTRAINDICATIONS

An arthroscopic approach is contraindicated in patients with severe varus or valgus deformity of the tibiotalar articulation (greater than 15 degrees compared with the normal contralateral ankle). In such patients, only an open approach offers an adequate and accurate custom bone removal to allow for precise correction of severe deformity. Also, avascular necrosis of the talus is contraindicated for standard cross-screw ankle fusion by either an open or an arthroscopic procedure, because it usually results in a nonunion due to lack of blood supply on the talar side of the joint. In this situation, an open vascular anterior tibial sliding bone graft fusion (Blair type) is the procedure of choice.

Although arthroscopic ankle fusion is the only arthroscopic procedure I know of in which iatrogenic hyaline cartilage injury is not a problem, the procedure is quite tedious and requires great attention to detail. Before attempting it, the surgeon should be well versed in arthroscopic techniques and have substantial experience in arthroscopy of joints other than the knee, particularly the tibiotalar joint. Prior experience with open ankle fusion is also quite helpful.

as nonsteroidal antiinflammatory drugs, steroid injections, orthoses, and footwear modifications, produces a clinical arthropathy well suited for fusion of the joint. The most common indication is posttraumatic arthritis (Fig. 64.8). Other, less common indications include systemic diseases that may affect the ankle, such as rheumatoid arthritis, psoriatic arthritis, and various forms of hemophilia that produce hemophiliac arthropathy secondary to recurrent intraarticular bleeds. In addition, chronic longstanding talar osteochondritis dissecans, particularly posteromedial lesions, may destroy the joint and constitute an indication for fusion as a salvage procedure. Finally, neurologic motor deficits that lead to loss of foot and ankle position that is not well controlled or tolerated with braces or orthoses may become an indication for fusion of the tibiotalar joint. Postpolio residual, permanent foot drop secondary to peroneal nerve palsy, and postcompartment syndrome residual are examples of neurologic deficit indications.

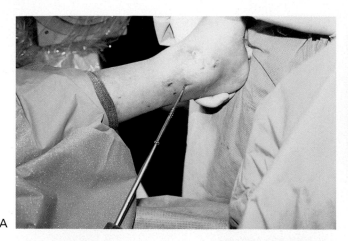

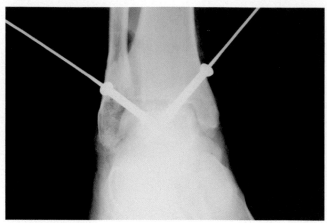

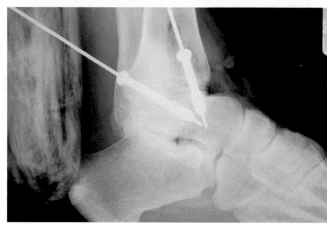

FIGURE 64.7 A: Left ankle, medial view of medial guide wire placement for medial screw. Note anterior angulation of guide pin and position of image intensifier to assist the surgeon with pin placement and fusion reduction. **B** and **C:** Radiographs of fusion reduction and cannulated screw placement over guide pins, anteroposterior **(B)** and lateral **(C)**.

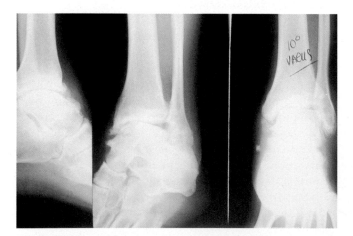

FIGURE 64.8 Radiographic appearance of a typical case of disabling posttraumatic tibiotalar arthritis in 10 degrees of varus malalignment.

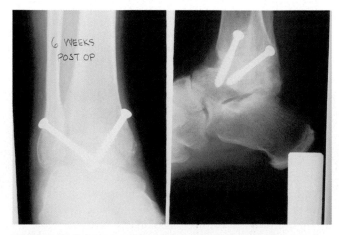

FIGURE 64.9 Postoperative radiographs at 6 weeks, showing solid arthrodesis in the recommended neutral position in the right ankle.

Should technical difficulties be encountered at any point during the arthroscopic procedure, the arthroscopic approach may be abandoned and the fusion completed with an open approach using either an anterolateral or a straight midline anterior exposure (2).

CLINICAL EXPERIENCE

Schneider (12; D. Schneider, *personal communication,* 1988) was the first to perform and report a successful arthroscopic ankle arthrodesis in 1983. Using the technique described in this chapter, I have fused 30 ankles with a minimum 8 years' follow-up (5 for hemophiliac arthropathy and 25 for posttraumatic arthritis). Radiographic bony union occurred in half of the patients by 6 weeks and in all by 12 weeks (Fig. 64.9). In this series, one complication occurred, consisting of a broken drill bit in the tibia, which happened during creation of the hole for a tibial distraction pin early in my experience, when I was using skeletal distraction with a modified Wagner device (Fig. 64.6B). In that case, the retained drill bit in an intramedullary location has caused no sequelae. In one additional case early in this series, I was unable to reduce the fusion adequately after the debridement step, and the fusion was completed by open arthrotomy. In that case, dense scarring in the medial and lateral talomalleolar spaces probably could have been removed arthroscopically.

In 1990, 39 cases were reported as a multicenter study (13), and one nonunion occurred that later fused with an open sliding bone graft procedure. Also, one complication, consisting of a dorsalis pedis arterial pseudoaneurysm, occurred secondary to the use of an anterocentral portal (13; J. Glick, *personal communication,* 1986). For this reason, the use of the anterocentral approach is not recommended. At this time, a continuation of the multicenter experience that began in 1983 (13) includes 75 cases with 1 to 11 years of follow-up (14). Results in this large series include a 96% rate of fusion, no infections, and 95% good-to-excellent functional clinical results (14). Others using similar techniques have achieved similar results (15).

In 1996, Glick et al. (16) reported long-term results of this arthroscopic procedure with favorable outcomes similar to those reported previously and equal to or better than those reported for the open procedure (16). In their series,

34 patients were evaluated at an average of 8 years after surgery and demonstrated a fusion rate of 97%, with 86% good-to-excellent functional clinical results.

In summary, long-term clinical experience with this arthroscopic technique has produced results that compare favorably with results of a similar procedure done by open arthrotomy, with the reduced morbidity inherent in an arthroscopic approach (2,16).

REFERENCES

1. White AA III. A precision posterior ankle fusion. *Clin Orthop* 1974;98:239–250.
2. Morgan CD, Henke JA, Bailey RW, et al. Long-term results of tibiotalar arthrodesis. *J Bone Joint Surg Am* 1985;67:546–550.
3. Ahlberg AKE, Henricson AS. Late results of ankle fusion. *Acta Orthop Scand* 1981;52:103–105.
4. Boobbyer GN. The long-term results of ankle arthrodesis. *Acta Orthop Scand* 1981;52:107–110.
5. Charnley J. Compression arthrodesis of the ankle and shoulder. *J Bone Joint Surg Br* 1951;33:180–191.
6. Johnson FW, Boseker EH. Arthrodesis of the ankle. *Arch Surg* 1968;97:766–773.
7. Morrey BF, Wiedeman GP. Complications and long-term results of ankle arthrodesis following trauma. *J Bone Joint Surg Am* 1980;62:777–784.
8. Said E, Hunka L, Siller TM. Where ankle fusion stands today. *J Bone Joint Surg Br* 1978;60:211–214.
9. Morgan CD. Arthroscopic tibiotalar arthrodesis. In: Guhl JF, ed. *Ankle arthroscopy, pathology and surgical techniques.* Thorofare, NJ: Slack, 1988:119–123.
10. Morgan CD. Arthroscopic tibiotalar arthrodesis. *Jefferson Orthop J* 1987;16:50–52.
11. Guhl JF. Portals and techniques: mechanical distraction. In: Guhl JF, ed. *Ankle arthroscopy, pathology and surgical techniques.* Thorofare, NJ: Slack, 1988:52–53.
12. Schneider D. Arthroscopic ankle fusion: a case report. Presented at the Annual Meeting of the Arthroscopy Association of North America, New Orleans, LA, 1983.
13. Glick JM, Myerson MS, Morgan CD, et al. Arthroscopic ankle arthrodesis. Presented at the 9th Annual Meeting of the Arthroscopy Association of North America, Orlando, FL, April 1990.
14. Morgan CD. Arthroscopic tibio-talar arthrodesis. *Jefferson Orthop J* 1987;16:50–52.
15. Ogilvie-Harris DJ, Lieberman I, Fitsialos D. Arthroscopically assisted arthrodesis of osteoarthritic ankles. *J Bone Joint Surg Am* 1993;75:1167–1174.
16. Glick JM, Morgan CD, Myerson MS, et al. Ankle arthrodesis method: long-term follow-up of 34 cases. *Arthroscopy* 1996;12:428–434.

OSTEOCHONDRAL AUTOGRAFT OF THE TALUS

F. ALLEGRA
A. AMELINA

HISTORICAL EVALUATION: ETIOLOGY AND EPIDEMIOLOGY

A chondral lesion was first described in 1856 by Aleksander Monro (1), who published in Berlin the discovery of loose bodies in the knee joint, caused by trauma. But it was not until 1870 that a further description of this lesion was given by Paget (2), and it was 1888 before the term *osteochondritis dissecans* (OCD), coined by König (3) was first used. König proposed the theory of a spontaneous osteonecrosis secondary to a vascular occlusion in the subchondral bone, describing loose bodies found in the joints of uninjured patients; he considered "phlogosis" of the bone and cartilage layers to be the cause of this typical lesion, defining osteochondritis as tissue inflammation and dissecans as fragmentation and separation of the chondral surface (from the Latin word *dissecare*, "to cut").

In 1898, Barth (4) came to the same conclusion, despite the fact that a traumatic etiology was not found in all cases. In 1922, Kappis (5) confirmed the presence of a common traumatic origin, referring for the first time to cases in which ankle joints were affected by osteochondral lesions. Although none of these authors had specific evidence, they suggested the hypothesis of an ischemic necrosis of the subchondral bone as the pathophysiologic basis of the lesions, with the typical presence of the separated fragment and its conversion into loose bodies.

Marks (6) in 1952 and Rödén and Tillegaard (7) in 1953 reported an analysis of 55 cases affected by OCD. Other similar lesions to the articular cartilage of the talar dome postulated a common traumatic origin.

In 1959, Berndt and Harty (8) gave a fundamental contribution to the epidemiology and to the nosologic classification, which had the benefit of dividing the evolution of the lesion into four radiologic stages. They examined 191 cases from 54 reports that had appeared in the literature between 1856 and 1956 in which transchondral fracture of the talar dome was described.

The AA added a personal group of 24 patients with the same pathology and also carried out experiments of a variety of imposed forces on 24 cadaveric ankles. They tried to demonstrate the theory that the so-called OCD lesions should be considered a transchondral fracture of the talar dome. This had been simulated on cadaveric specimens by forcing the foot into maximum dorsiflexion and inversion and compressing the lateral border of the talar dome against the chondral surface of the fibular malleolus, until the rupture of the lateral ligament and the beginning of avulsion of the osteochondral chip. They described a double evolution of the fragment as having to remain in site or having to displace the bony dome.

On the other hand, a combination of plantar flexion, rotation, and inversion of the foot produced the same progression in determining the medial chondral lesions with an application of the same forces. Furthermore, by histologic examination of the collected specimens, they demonstrated the presence of a deep layer of fibrous tissue, between deep bone with viable osteocytes and subchondral bone with a total lack of such cells. This tissue was overlain by an articular cartilage layer with chondral viable cells. O'Donoghue (9) in 1966 and Davidson et al. (10) in 1967 considered these kinds of lesions to be intraarticular fractures. During that same period (1966), Campbell and Ranawat (11) attempted to respond to the question about the etiology by matching the bony ischemia to the subsequent necrosis of the bone which evolves through a pathologic fracture to the osteochondral lesion.

As a result of these studies, many researchers have supported a traumatic etiology of the lesion. In 1980, Canale and Belding (12), in a group of 31 patients with an ankle affected by a chondral talar lesion, described in 29 of them the presence of an anamnestic trauma. This was demonstrated by the association of all lateral articular cartilage dome defects with a traumatic origin, but not on the medial side, because the association was demonstrated only in 64% of the ankles.

F. Allegra and A. Amelina: Department of Orthopaedic Surgery, Guarnieri Clinic, Rome, Italy.

Reviewing 25 patients with talar chondral lesions, Alexander and Lichtman (13) in 1980 supported the hypothesis of the former AA They demonstrated a correlation between lateral cartilage defects and an ankle trauma or sprain; however, this association was matched only in 18% of all the medial lesions.

In 1982, Guhl (14) first described an arthroscopic classification of the chondral lesions, agreeing with the traumatic etiology. Nevertheless, in a group of 22 patients, Flick and Gould (1985) described a history of ankle trauma in all patients presenting as a chondral lesion on the lateral side compared with those with a lesion on the tibial side, of whom only 82% had such a history (15). In a comprehensive survey, they compared the reports of 500 patients described in the literature who had a talar dome cartilage defect. On the peroneal side it was produced by trauma in 99% of patients, but on the medial side in only 70% of patients.

Further studies have shown trauma to be a unique cause of a chondral lesion, but this is not true for all patients. The hypothesis for a traumatic cause was supported in 1986 by Pritsch et al. (16), Parisien (17), and Baker et al. (18); in 1987 by Pettine and Morrey (19); and in 1989 by Van Buecken et al. (20) and Anderson et al. (21), with a variable percentage ranging from 75% in both sides lateral and medial (Pritsch et al.) to 85% in all examined patients (Anderson et al.).

ETIOLOGY

At present, there is no study that can confirm the exact etiology of OCD, in the talar dome or in any other articular cartilage surface: it remains controversial. According to Berndt and Harty's suggestions (8), fibular side chondral lesions found very often in a traumatic episode, such as a sprain, are the only cause and may produce a transchondral or osteochondral fracture of the talar dome. The theory of a traumatic origin is the most credited hypothesis for the lateral lesions: an acute traumatic episode or serial overuse "microtraumas" can lead to a chondral lesion.

However, the lesions on the medial side appear only in a variable percentage of cases in conjunction with a traumatic history; often the OCD is not attributable to a unique known factor. Other factors that may influence the appearance of the lesion include hormonal disorders, endocrine and hereditary situations, use of steroids, alcohol abuse, and "constitutional" abnormalities which are often present in these patients, although their role is still unknown. In these cases, members of the same family seldom present multiple joints affected by chondral lesions in addition to the ankle. In some described cases, the bilaterality of the lesions affects both of the ankles (22). Cited in several studies, these observations suggest lesions of a nontraumatic origin, such as an ischemic cause that can collapse the bone. As Ferkel (23) suggested, an ischemic event alone may determine the cartilage defect in the patient, affected by some constitutional

and/or acquired factors that can involve the microvessels in a reduction of blood supply and subsequent ischemia. An osteonecrotic process occurs in the compressed bone, until it is involved in a subchondral fracture and collapses. The progression of the lesion is noted by the presence of synovial joint fluid inside the trabecular broken bone, which marks the boundary of the lesion and prevents natural healing due to the lack of close soft tissue that could guarantee a sufficient blood supply.

TERMINOLOGY

In all studies and surveys referenced here, the authors have often used various terms and words to define the pathologic lack of the chondral or osteochondral surface of the talar dome: transchondral fracture, osteochondral fracture, talar dome fractures, flake fractures, OCD, and others, still reflecting the confusion regarding the mechanism. In other words, the term used typically represents the supposed etiology of the lesion, even though no theory or etiologic hypothesis is more accredited than another. To avoid any misunderstanding about the path of the lesion mechanism and origin, to define a collapse and a separation of the cartilage surface, with or without the underlying bone that caused by an inflammatory, traumatic, microtraumatic, congenital, family, or other origin, the AA agree with Ferkel (23) that *osteochondral lesion of the talus* (OLT) is the best term.

MECHANISM OF INJURY

To explain the injury mechanism of a traumatic cartilage talar dome defect, Berndt and Harty (8) reproduced the lesions in cadaveric specimens by forcing the foot into the pathologic position: inversion, dorsiflexion and tibial internal rotation can cause a lateral lesion, but inversion associated with plantar flexion and tibial external rotation can lead to a medial lesion.

This hypothesis was supported by Ferkel (23), who suggested the presence of shear stresses on the talar dome lateral margin and, respectively, on the posteromedial edge, which increases the effect of the impacting forces. The resulting impact crosses the border of the bone along the line determined by a component of shear forces; the subsequent fracture is displaced, depending on the resistance of its own bone–cartilage system.

However, in patients affected by chondral talar lesions not caused by a demonstrated single traumatic injury, the etiology can be explained by multiple factors, which lead to an "idiopathic osteonecrosis" through microtraumatic stresses. Microtraumas caused by repetitive articular cartilage surface loading or excessive stress can lead to cellular degeneration or death by disruption of the collagen fibril ultrastructure and by increased hydration, developing fissures on the chondral surface and thickening of the subchondral bone (24). These structural changes are not involved in deep chondral fractures caused by a single joint injury. The forces produce tension, shearing, and pressure by fluid over the chondral surface and can lead to articular damage such as chondral fissures or flaps and fractures. In this case, the bone has been respected, limiting the necrotic traumatic effects to the involved site in the chondrocyte layer, followed by spontaneous metabolic and mitochondrial activity by the cells in the border, tending to repair the defect (24,25). Because no bleeding and no inflammatory response occur, the injured chondral tissue is not repaired.

In the osteochondral fractures, the applied forces can extend the lesion through the chondral plate to the subchondral bone layer. The cellular activity increases; cellular proliferation and differentiation by chondroblast-like cells helps to remodel the defects, forming a new fibrocartilaginous area (24,26,27). Because of the local loss of blood from the bone and the inflammatory response activated by the injury, the formation of a fracture hematoma begins through the bony and chondral separated surfaces, the fibrin-cloth formation. Thanks to the activation of multiple growth factors, which stimulate the cellular vascular migration and the differentiation of the mesenchymal chondroblast-like cells, the production of a matrix with a high percentage of collagen type II and a lower percentage of type I, similar to the normal cartilage, should begin. This repaired tissue can often evolve into a remodeled one, or it can remain without any changes (28).

On the bony site, the new tissue is rich in osteoblast-like cells which mature and produce new definitive bone. The quality of the chondral tissue restoration seems to depend on the area of the defect: the wider the lesion, the higher the risk of repair failure (24,28). Nevertheless, the joint load can play an important role in determining the progression of the defect or the cartilage repair. An excess of loading, as occurs in overweight people, contributes to delay in the progression of the repair processes and accelerates the disruption of the chondral-defect surface (25). The immobilization and inability to bear weight can reduce the capability of the joint to repair spontaneously and can add the risk of chondral deterioration. On the other hand, passive motion, weight loss, controlled weight-bearing and partial joint loading can help to stimulate the biologic repair responses (28).

CLASSIFICATION OF OSTEOCHONDRAL LESIONS OF THE TALUS

Observing the bone of the talus immediately beneath the chondral surface, Berndt and Harty (8) in 1959 described findings found in plain ankle radiographic examinations and proposed their classification which is still widely valued (Table 65.1). They considered this system to be "arbitrary" because it was based only on radiographic observation, not

TABLE 65.1 BERNDT AND HARTY RADIOGRAPHS: CLASSIFICATION OF OSTEOCHONDRAL LESION OF THE TALUS

Classification	Description
Stage 1	Local and circumstricted compression of subchondral bone
Stage 2	Delimitation and partial detachment of a fragment from the chondral surface
Stage 3	Total detachment of the fragment, which remains in site of injury
Stage 4	The fragment is totally detached from the crater and floats in the joint space

From Berndt AL, Harty M. Transchondral fractures (osteochondritis dissceans) of the talus. *J Bone Joint Surg Am* 1959;41:988–1020, with permission.

on the comparison of radiographic findings with the results of surgical inspection.

In 1982, Guhl (14) developed the first arthroscopic classification by comparing arthroscopic findings with radiographic scans. In 1986, Pritsch et al. (16) compared the preoperative plain radiographs with the arthroscopic pathologic picture in 24 patients. In the surgical appearance, the lesions were graduated into three stages with, respectively, intact and shiny, soft but not fissured, and fragmented cartilage. Because the lack of a total correlation between the radiographic and arthroscopic findings, they suggested basing the treatment on the real condition of the chondral layer of the talus and foresaw the role of arthroscopy as fundamental in giving definitive information about the chosen treatment.

In 1989, Anderson et al. (21) examined 24 patients divided into two groups affected by ankle injury to compare magnetic resonance imaging (MRI) and computed tomographic (CT) scans with radiographic findings. They concluded that the two methods were comparable in final results: MRI offered the best subtle definition of a trabecular lesion, and CT offered the best imaging of bony fragment position. They also proposed an OLT classification based on the MRI pictures (Table 65.2), which we still prefer to follow.

TABLE 65.2 ANDERSON ET AL. MAGNETIC RESONANCE IMAGES: CLASSIFICATION OF OSTEOCHONDRAL LESION OF THE TALUS

Classification	Description
Stage 1	Subchondral trabecular bone compression respecting the chondral layer
Stage 2A	Appearance of local cystic lesion in the subchondral layer
Stage 2	Fragment in site of injury, but incompletely separated from chondral joint surface
Stage 3	The in site undisplaced fragment is separated by synovial fluid from the bony crater
Stage 4	The fragment is displaced in the joint space

From Anderson JF, Crichton KJ, Gattan–Smith T, et al. Osteochondral fractures of the dome of the talus. *J Bone Joint Surg Am* 1989;71:1143–1152, with permission.

TABLE 65.3 FERKEL AND SGAGLIONE COMPUTED TOMOGRAMS: CLASSIFICATION OF OSTEOCHONDRAL LESION OF THE TALUS

Classification	Description
Stage 1	Local cystic lesion inside the subchondral bone respecting the chondral layer
Stage 2A	Local cystic lesion in communication with chondral surface
Stage 2B	Open cystic lesion with a fragment in site of injury, but separated from chondral joint surface
Stage 3	The undisplaced fragment presents typical radiolucency
Stage 4	The detached fragment is displaced and can float in the joint space

From Ferkel RD, Sgaglione NA. Arthroscopic treatment of osteochondral lesions of the talus: long-term results. *Orthop Trans* 1993–1994;17:1011, with permission.

Nelson et al. (29), in 1990, comparing arthroscopic findings with MRI scans of knee and talar chondral defects, and Dipaola et al.(30), 1 year later, examining joint cartilage defects with MRI findings, classified the lesions into four stages. In 1993, Ferkel and Sgaglione (31) proposed a classification based on two planes of CT images correlated with arthroscopic pathologic findings (Table 65.3). The CT scans provided a big improvement in bone lesion delineation in the coronal and axial planes.

In 1995, Frank et al. (35) presented an arthroscopic classification based on surgical findings comparing preoperative radiographic, CT, and MRI scans with the intraoperative correlated lesions. They concluded that MRI is more reliable than CT, because of its ability to precisely show bone, cartilage, and soft tissues in their entirety, although CT is still the first choice in OLT diagnostic accuracy.

RADIOLOGIC AND MAGNETIC RESONANCE IMAGING EVALUATION

Therefore, despite its cost, MRI (Fig. 65.1) is considered to be more valuable than radiographs or CT scans because of its higher precision in the diagnosis of OLT. Frank et al. (32) in 1989, Bryant et al. (33) in 1993, and Stone (22) in 1996 recommended the CT scan as the most efficient means to show the borders of the bony crater but suggested applying MRI if associated soft tissue lesions are suspected.

Kelbérine et al. in 1999 (34), Chang and Lenczner (35), and Lahm et al.(36) in 2000 preferred to use preoperative MRI because it shows the osteochondral lesion peculiarities and the marrow bony edema, allowing for more precisely planned surgery. If an OLT is suspected, it is necessary to first obtain plain double-view radiographs of the ankle, both to detect the lesion on the affected side and to avoid the risk of missing a contralateral asymptomatic lesion, which is described in 8% to 25% of cases (18,22,23).

When the lesion is found, it is necessary to confirm the imaging with a CT scan to delineate the defect and to detect its borders, position, depth into the recipient bone, as well as the aspect and structure of the closer bony trabeculae. But only MRI offers the opportunity to define the type of osteochondral talar lesion and to detect the site and depth of the defect placement, to determine the quality of the surrounding chondral layer and the presence of a vascular bony reaction around the OLT, and to detect the extension of the trabecular alteration or damage under the chondral surface. In other words, MRI helps the surgeon to be more accurate in planning for surgery and in performing the right technique. For these reasons, our preference is plain radiographic scans and MRI, which all the operated patients undergo before surgery. On the other hand, MRI is conducive to follow the classification for an osteochondral talar defects preoperative evaluation, proposed by Anderson et al. (21). According to current opinion (37), MRI is performed using the T1-weighted, fat-suppressed, three-dimensional, spoiled gradient-echo technique and the T2-weighted, fast spin-echo technique. By comparing the results of both techniques in their dissimilarities, it is possible to visualize the cartilage layer and its areas of defect.

CLINICAL EVALUATION

If the OLT is caused by a trauma, the patient presents an acute inverted injured ankle with persistent edema, hematoma on the lesion side, and swelling and pain despite conservative treatment. But more often it is not trauma related, and the symptoms are defined by chronic pain on the side of the lesion, accompanied by episodes of walking pain, limited range of motion, occasional swelling, grinding and popping, never having healed despite medical and physical therapy, and an occasional limp that is much more frequent than expected.

All of the described symptoms can be intermittent and aggravated by weight bearing. Their persistence and the appearance of reflex sympathetic dystrophy appearance are symptomatic of chronic joint involvement. Joint instability, such as giving away and frequent inversion events, is more common than stiffness; nevertheless, stress radiologic examinations seldom confirm the presence of articular laxity and ligament lesions. For some patients, it is not possible to walk on low heels. They recover by replacing them with high heels. However, others have symptoms for the opposite reason. During the physical examination, palpation of the talar space anterior to the fibular malleolus, stressing the foot in plantar flexion, may show symptoms of an anterolateral defect, whereas symptomatic palpation of the articular surface posteriorly to the tibial malleolus, stressing the joint dorsally, may indicate a posteromedial defect. A definitive diagnosis often may be reached on direct arthroscopic visualiza-

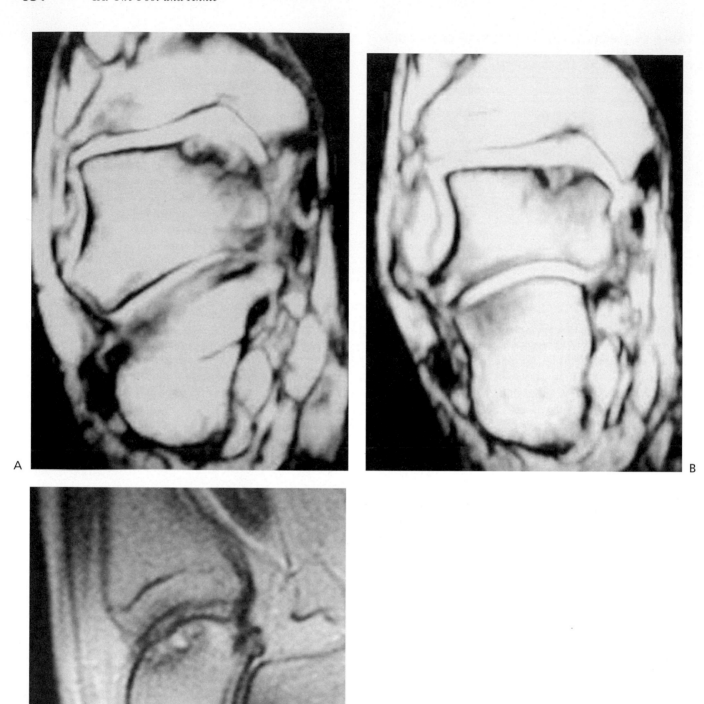

FIGURE 65.1 Magnetic resonance imaging views show a peripheral **(A)**, a central **(B)**, and a posterior **(C)** osteochondral lesion of the talus.

tion, because MRI has not reliably been able to identify chondral lesions of the talar dome.

After the surgery, patients have been clinically evaluated every 30 days until complete recovery and the return to former activities and sports. After a period of 6 to 12 months, all of our operated patients routinely and repeatedly undergo MRI examinations to check for whole graft ingrowth into the recipient healthy bone.

PRINCIPLES OF TREATMENT

The choice of treatment involves the success of a given therapeutic method to restore the articular defect and degenerated surface of the talus with new ingrown filling tissue into the chondral area, respecting as much as possible the mechanical properties of the original tissue in regard to the weight-bearing capability of the new surface.

The best cartilage repair should guarantee the complete restoration of the chondral tissue by cell proliferation, structure reorganization, and new collagen matrix composition—in other words, regeneration of a chondral-like original duplicated joint surface. However, the clinical results are not in direct relation with the capability of the surgeon to restore the defect. A perfect resurfaced refilling has been shown not to correlate with pain disappearance or range of motion recovery. The goal of any treatment is a cartilage restoration that guarantees long-term and lasting results in pain relief and joint motion. For these reasons, the choice of operative or conservative treatment it is still open to debate, as is its timing, partially because of the inadequacy of imaging results and studies on which the surgeon decides the choice of treatment, depending on the location of lesions, their intactness and size, the time of discovery, the presence of associated lesions, and the patient's age. All the studies before the MRI classification showed the difficulties of establishing the correlation between results and surgical treatment (8,12,15,19), which had been considered encouraging in medial stage 3 (12,15), always poor in lateral stage 3 (12), and comparable to the conservative therapy in medial undisplaced stage 3 (19). In all the studies, the results have been influenced by the delay in diagnosis and treatment.

CURRENT SURGICAL OPTIONS

Generally it is appropriate to treat chondral talar dome defects first by the least aggressive, cheapest, simplest, and lowest-risk treatment for the patient and the most experienced surgical technique that can guarantee a higher final result. For a talar dome articular defect, many surgical options have been described, including those that stimulate the formation of fibrin clot through a fibrochondral tissue growth stimulation and those that may substitute the defected area with a hyaline cartilage layer grafted or induced by a mesenchymal

cell growing mechanism. All the procedures may be performed arthroscopically or by open arthrotomy. If possible, it is still recommended to fix all the separated or intact fragments in their recipient defected areas using absorbable pins, K-wires, small metal screws, or absorbable arrows or darts, depending on the fragment size and the surgeon's skill.

For large and thick cartilage defects, all of the current surgical arthroscopic techniques (18,32,38) are based on ablation of the defect by the use of a burr shaver (chondroabrasion), by performing microfractures, as Steadman (41) described, or by drilling the defected chondral surface, following the technique reported by Ferkel (23,36,34). Surgical penetration of subchondral bone may disrupt intraosseous blood vessels, leading to fibrin-clot formation by release of growth factors, by the stimulation of local new blood vessels, and by new cells introduced into the cartilage defect: the final repair is a cloth of fibrocartilage. This represents, however, the limit of these techniques, never covering the defect by hyaline cartilage. For small and thin defects (stages 1 and 2), some authors propose articular cartilage sculpting by a thermal effect induced by radiofrequencies and arthroscopically performed (38), but the results still remain to be investigated.

To simply restore the chondral defected surface, periosteal and perichondral grafts widely diffused in the body have proven to be an attractive source. It seems they induce the growth of chondrocytes from mesenchymal cells, apparently influenced by motion and normal loading (41). Although few publications have referred to talar defects, these may also be refilled by implantation of mesenchymal stem cartilage-forming cells, expanded in culture, which produces a cartilaginous-like matrix more similar to the original cartilage layer than the mechanically induced one (42).

Some authors (42,43) have proposed an algorithm in the repair of articular cartilage defects but not specifically for the ankle joint, recommending a simple debridement for low-demand patients and small-size lesions, with subchondral perforations such as drilling or microfractures for high-demand patients and wider defects. If these procedures should fail, the surgeon may propose to the patient a treatment based on autologous chondrocyte transplantation or on osteochondral autologous transfer grafting (OATS or mosaicplasty).

PREFERRED APPROACH

It is suggested that plain radiographs and MRI scans may be very useful in ensuring a prompt and precise diagnosis of the patient's ankle joint problems, because they allow for defect classification and address the right surgical option and as well as determine the site, size, and depth of the chondral defect and associated articular lesions.

Secondly, if the lesion is acute, an arthroscopic procedure may be performed to palpate, to evaluate, to mobilize, to de-

TABLE 65.4 CHRONIC TREATMENT OF OSTEOCHONDRAL LESION OF THE TALUS

Classification	Description
Stage 1	Rest, physical therapy, casting, not weight-bearing
Stage 2	Arthroscopic debridement of the lesion, microfractures, subchondral drilling
Stage 3	Arthroscopic synoviectomy and debridement, drilling, microfractures, osteochondral grafting
Stage 4	Arthroscopic synoviectomy and debridement, autologous osteochondral grafting: open autologous chondrocyte transplantation, as autologous or allogeneic osteochondral grafting

bride, and to fix the displaced fragment with any means the surgeon is skilled to use, depending on fragment size and thickness.

Thirdly, if the lesion is chronic, larger than 1 square centimeter, and in an achievable position, the cartilage defect must be arthroscopically debrided to remove the scar tissue and to reach the bloody, bony subchondral layer. After that, it is appropriate to attempt an osteochondral autograft pressed into the recipient, preprepared socket. Autologous chondrocyte transplantation must be performed only with an open technique and requires a longer period of treatment and recovery.

Stage 1 lesions may respond to a conservative treatment and to rest (Table 65.4). It is possible for the patient to return to normal pain-free activity if the MRI shows a complete healing of the defect on the surface of the talus. Very seldom does it require a surgical repair.

Stage 2 lesions rarely respond to conservative therapy and will require a surgical option with an arthroscopic procedure, with the aim of performing debridement and a scar tissue removal from the defected area by stimulating the blood flow into the injured site. Subchondral drilling and microfractures are a surgical technique used to break through the thick subchondral bony layer and to stimulate the ingrowth of a new repair tissue.

Stage 3 and 4 lesions do not respond to conservative treatment and need a surgical therapy. Joint environment synovectomy and cartilage defect debridement may not be enough to repair the lesion (eg, perforation or disruption of an underlying sclerotic bony layer) and may not lead to a bone and cartilage restoration of the defected area. In our opinion, in these cases, the body of the talus may require an osteochondral grafting to ensure proper healing.

OSTEOCHONDRAL AUTOGRAFTING

Since 1998, we have applied the surgical technique for osteochondral autograft (OATS) proposed by Bobic (43) for repair of chondral lesions of the knee, to restore the cartilage surface of talar defects. The purpose is to replace the defected area of a chondral surface, previously prepared, with an autograft transferred from an intact chondral site of the ipsilateral knee on the external margin of the patellofemoral joint, using a dedicated instrumentation and disposable core system. The cartilage layer height of the donor site is sufficiently similar to the closer one around the recipient socket in the talar dome. Differences between the talar surface and the anteroexternal region of the external femoral condyle are less than expected.

This technique has been preferred to other, similar ones because it is possible to insert only one graft as large as necessary, precisely sized to the talar defect, instead of some smaller ones close to each other, assuming the aspect of the chondral dome surface. Only in some very selected cases, in the presence of an oval shaped OLT, are two big, close grafts required.

As initially supposed and now demonstrated by recent studies (44), longer and bigger grafts may be placed with a better press-fit compared with smaller ones, gaining better stability. To avoid problems in congruency limiting narrow spaces between the newly transplanted cartilage, which results in spaces' filling up with fibrocartilage, Hangody et al. (45) exchanged his previous technique for a new one which provides overlapping grafts with the aim of reducing the fibrous repair between the new chondral grafted surfaces. However, this technique still has some technical problems when performed arthroscopically and when restoring the typical double-curved talar dome surface.

Examining with an arthroscopic second-look biopsy a group of patients who had undergone autogenous osteochondral transfer graft or a mosaicplasty talar dome procedure, both Bobic (43) and Hangody et al. (45) showed donor sites filled with fibrocartilage around the grafts. The transplanted cartilage seems to maintain its own histologic features and its own chondral properties thanks to deep matrix integration.

Indications

The indications for the talar OATS treatment depend on the clinical and pathologic profile. We consider three different conditions. The first one is the stage of OLT: following the CT classification proposed by Ferkel and Sgaglione, we prefer to submit all the patients to a surgical arthroscopic treatment who are classified as type 2b, 3, or 4. The second factor is the patient's age: if the growing cartilage layer has not closed, the treatment is always to attempt to fix the detached chondral fragment, delaying any surgical repair which can be aggressive to the bone. The third factor is the site of the lesion, which strongly conditions the possibility of an arthroscopic repair. Following both classifications proposed by Ferkel and Anderson, we reserve OATS arthroscopic treatment for all the anterolateral and anteromedial

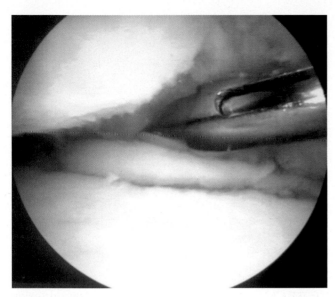

FIGURE 65.2 Lateral side defect area: the fragment is isolated from its bony bed (stage 3).

talar defects (Fig. 65.2) and for those posteromedial or posterolateral defects that are placed anteriorly to the middle transverse line of the talus (Fig. 65.3).

Surgical Technique

This surgical technique is performed arthroscopically using the three standard portals. The patient is assessed in the supine position, the knee in 30 to 40 degrees semiflexion is kept in a leg holder, and the ankle is positioned neutrally and is maintained in distraction with a traction of 5.5 to 6.5 lb. If necessary, the ankle should be allowed to move into maximum dorsal or plantar flexion. Beyond the arthro-

scope, shaver, and other basic instruments, the surgical instrumentation setup includes an inflation pump, a radiofrequency device, and the OATS instrumentation, which consists of various-sized single-use reamers for osteochondral autograft transfer.

The exploration of the ankle joint is performed starting with a complete 21-point examination, as proposed by Ferkel (23). All the articular surfaces must be accurately explored by checking the gliding surface and leaving no site unchecked. If the OLT is acute, as happens in younger patients, the lesion must be palpated with a probe and identified as to dimensions as well as size and width of the chondral layer. The same evaluation must also be performed on the subchondral bone, whose presence can guarantee a strong adhesion as big as the bony layer width. The fragment must be moved to explore the recipient socket and to clean it up from any free trabecular bony body with a shaver. Finally, it must be placed in its own correct position, pushed in, and stabilized. In this case, currently good options are bioabsorbable arrows or chondral darts, which must never be removed after the fragment integration. Nevertheless, it is possible to also use Kirschner wires, small metal screws, or other means available such as suture anchors (Fig. 65.4). The typical patient affected by a chronic OLT who is a candidate for this technique is an adult whose detached lesion has not been healed with conservative treatment or with a previous surgical techniques such as chondroabrasion, drilling, or microfractures and who presents an articular environment with a congruent uninjured chondral surface.

The arthroscopy is performed in the same way to explore the joint and to check the defected area. It is important to remove all of the synovia that might reduce joint visibility during the exploration of the articular space and gutters, limiting its removal from the anterior space, where its excess

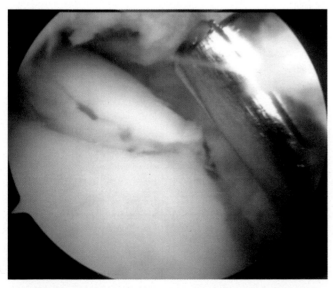

FIGURE 65.3 Medial side defect area: the fragment is totally detached and is loosening the talus surface (stage 4).

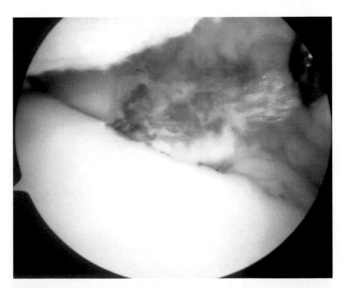

FIGURE 65.4 An acute detached fragment is put in place and fixed with a suture anchor (stage 4).

can be symptomatic due to the impingement between both tibial and talar chondral surfaces. However, synovia should be respected in its integrity as much as possible, because this membrane is the only one to produce the joint fluid necessary to feed the superficial chondral layers of the joint. If found, any loose body must be removed (Fig. 65.5). The anterior tibial osteophyte, when present, can reduce the ankle's range of motion and may be symptomatic. Osteophytes may be located in an intraarticular, intracapsular, or extraarticular position and should be carefully evaluated if placed more medially or laterally in respect to the median line of the joint. The angle seen in a lateral view between the talar neck and the anterior distal bony tibial surface must be 60 degrees or greater; if it is narrower, the osteophyte must be resected. Before sizing its width, the defected area must be cleaned up by removing the scar tissue from the lesion bed through abrasion by a small bur or through thermal effect radiofrequency-induced ablation (coblation).

When the defected area (Fig. 65.6) is spotted on the talar articular surface, its position should be accurately evaluated on both the frontal and the lateral planes. On the frontal plane, the lesion may be found in an almost central position (central lesions), on the talar median line or near the talus lateral borders but sufficiently separated from them, without the involvement of the lateral or medial vertical chondral surface. Otherwise, the lesion may be discovered in a more external position on the rounded angle of the talus, between the two changes of inclination of the talar articular surface (peripheral lesions).

In the first case, only the superior joint surface of the bone along the anteroposterior convexity of the talus is involved; in the second case, the site of the chondral lesion is extended through the 90-degree angled articular surface to create a sharp margin step, which may strongly conflict with

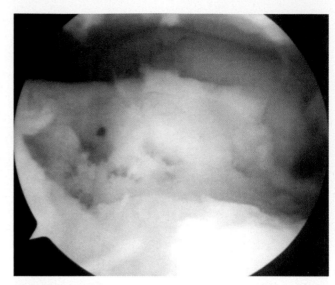

FIGURE 65.6 A big anterolateral osteochondral talar dome defected area.

the correspondent tibial or fibular malleolus internal side. This kind of OLT is more severe because of the involvement of both the anteroposterior and the lateromedial convexity of the talar profile. To repair the central lesion, the graft must have a wide-bending radius shaped in the anteroposterior diameter, but in restoring the peripheral lesion, the graft harvesting should have a wide-bending radius shaped in the sagittal plane and 90 degrees curved in the front plane. Considering the lateral view, the OLT may be placed anteriorly (anterior lesion) or posteriorly (posterior lesion) to the median line that divides in two halves the body of the talus. Those placed anteriorly can be easily treated arthroscopically; those placed posteriorly may be repaired only if closer to the median line, which can be shown with a gentle plantar rotation of the talus. More posterior chondral defects should be exposed from the anterior tibial coverage applying a plantar stress to the ankle; otherwise no arthroscopic grafting repair can be performed.

If the defected area still remains partially covered by tibial bone, it is possible to gain up to 10 to 15 degrees of foot plantar flexion and to expose more talar surface, by gently forcing the foot in plantar position after performing a tibial anterior arthroscopic capsulectomy by shaver (Fig. 65.7A). To permit the placement of the graft as far posterior and perpendicular as possible into a posterior lesion, it is possible to remove some bone with a bur from the reentrant bony margin, a sulcus located between the lateral or medial malleolus and the anterior distal tibial central tuberosity, which wraps the anterior talar central chondral surface (Figs. 65.7B and 65.8). A limited bone removal does not relax or stiffen the joint. To achieve a posterior OLT by putting the foot in plantar flexion as described, with the aim of maintaining the vertical position of the lesion while pushing the graft into the prepared socket, a new anterior portal is opened. It is lo-

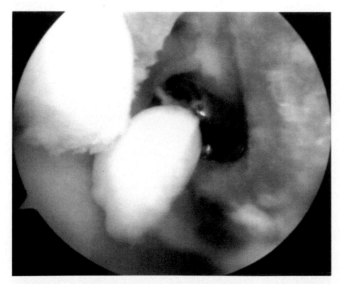

FIGURE 65.5 A cartilage loose body.

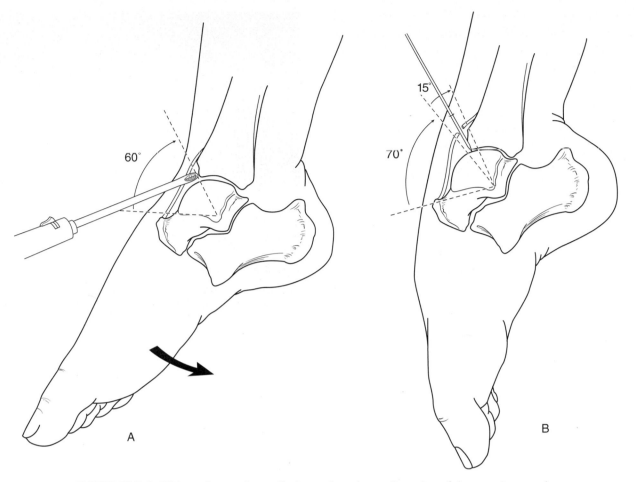

FIGURE 65.7 A: With maximum plantar flexion and maximum distention of the anterior capsule, the 50% articular surface of the talus is exposed off the tibia coverage, in the range between 0 and 60 degrees of the whole talar dome arch of 140 degrees. **B:** If an anterior capsular release is performed, the chondral exposition increases 55% to 60%, up to the 70-degree range. By removing some bone with a bur from that side of the tibia between the anterior tibial central distal tuberosity and the medial malleolus or between the same surface and the lateral malleolus, the local exposition of the talar articular surface should be increased 10 to 15 degrees, permitting the surgeon to reach some spotted area of defect, more posteriorly placed.

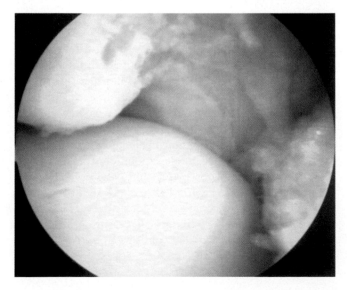

FIGURE 65.8 The reentrant margin as a sulcus between medial malleolus and the anterior distal tibial central tuberosity, which wraps up the anterior talar central chondral surface, partially deepened by bur.

cated as superior as possible, and as lateral or medial as necessary to allow a probing spinal needle, slipped along the anterior tibial surface, to keep the vertical position on the talar defected area. The location of this portal is particularly important for achieving the best graft placement and for achieving a satisfactory final result.

The defected area borders have been chopped off with a sharp-dimensioned reamer that is pushed in gently by a mallet. The A.A. consider that drilling-induced healing may burn up the new vascular bony connections in the recipient socket, although some surgeons prefer drilling (45) because the thickness of the talus may expose the patient to the risk of a vascular deficiency induced by mallet strokes. After the OLT disclosure and cleanup is finished, it is necessary to size its width to establish how many and how big the grafts should be that are harvested from the donor side. This generally depends on shape of the defected area; usually it is more roundish than oval, and it is often enough to cover it up with only one graft.

A graft length between 10 and 15 mm is generally considered standard because of the relatively reduced height of the talar bony body. The autograft is removed from the upper lateral patellofemoral ipsilateral knee joint, far from the patellar groove. This region is preferred to the femoral intercondylar notch because it has recently been demonstrated (46) to be significantly less pressured in the full range of joint motion.

On the knee joint, an anteroexternal portal is used for the arthroscope and a superoexternal one for the core-reamer, which is beaten into the donor site with a mallet up to the planned filling completion and turned away from the bone. The selection of the spotted area, where to remove the graft from, depends on the shape and the position of the defect on the talar convexity site and influences the final result. From the knee area it is possible to remove one or more autografts as necessary, being absolutely sure of the viability of the cartilage layer it is removed from (i.e., a healthy joint). If the OLT is a central lesion, it should be repaired with a graft from the superior-external femoropatellar joint on the anterior femoral articular surface, whose flat-shaped convexity in the anteroposterior diameter is the closest to that of the central talar dome. Going from a superior to an inferior direction, the rather flat bending radius increases to a more angled value, making the right angulation selection of the graft easier.

But if the lesion is peripheral, the donor site must be located on a more inferior and more lateral position of the external femoropatellar joint, directly over the lateral angle of the femoral chondral surface (Fig. 65.9). In this case, the graft must be harvested considering the double-bending profile of the talar defected area (Fig. 65.10). The selected articular surface of the lateral femoral condyle equally increases its bending radius both in the sagittal plane, going from the superior to inferior direction, and in the 90-degree

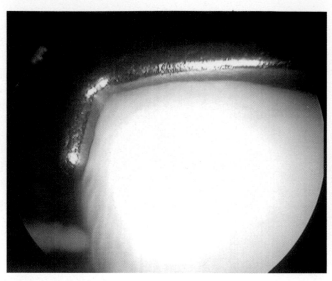

FIGURE 65.9 Evaluation with a probe of the convexity of the femoral lateral condyle articular surface, to select the donor area.

curved front plane, from a medial to a lateral position. All of the grafts are placed in their definitive site (Fig. 65.11) by pushing gently in with the mallet (Fig. 65.12) or by turning the sliding tip of the handle.

To reach the most anatomic position, the autograft must be placed into the talar dome defected area with the idea of restoring the chondral surface plane to as continuous a surface as possible. Therefore, the graft articular surface must be rotated or inclined as necessary to avoid the risk of interruption or step over the curved articular profile of the dome. In central lesions it must be placed vertically, and in the peripheral ones it must be considered an oblique placement into the talar bone, to respect the continuity of the articular chondral layer between the host bone and the grafted cartilage.

Postoperative Care

All patients are immobilized with a cast for 10 days, until stitches are removed, and medication is administered at the first clinical evaluation. Partial weight bearing is permitted with clutches for 2 weeks. Rehabilitation starts from the tenth day with exercise to restore ankle movements and proprioceptivity. Total weight bearing is allowed after 3 to 4 weeks, depending on the residual pain and the capability of the patient of complete gait restoration. All patients are evaluated after the surgery for 1 year; some patients have undergone a second MRI (Fig. 65.14) to check the ingrowth of the graft or an arthroscopic second-look surgery (Fig. 65.13) to check the resurfacing of the articular cartilage. The return to sports and former activities confirms a positive outcome and the reliability of the technique.

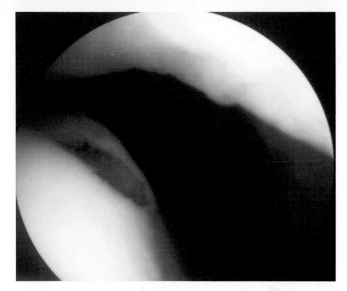

FIGURE 65.10. A femoral lateral condyle articular surface. The selected grafting area has been harvested.

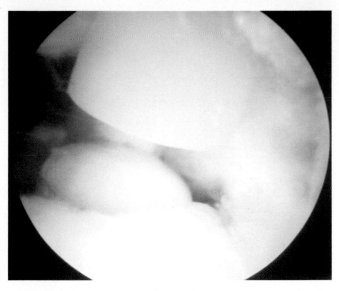

FIGURE 65.11 The autograft is definitely pulled into the defected area.

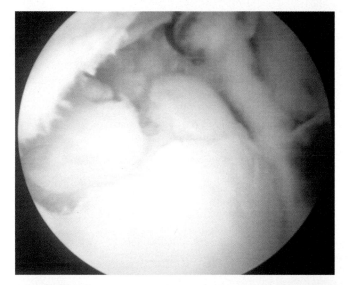

FIGURE 65.12 The final check of twin grafts placed to repair a big, oval-shaped osteochondral lesion of the talus. The space in between them will refill with fibrocartilage.

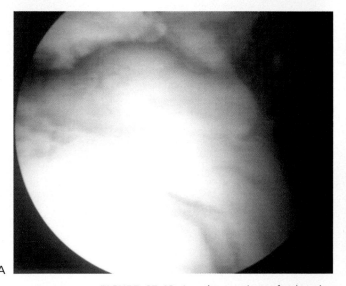

A

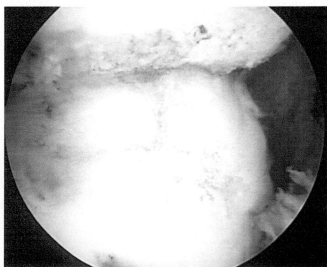

B

FIGURE 65.13 A arthroscopic graft placed at second look to refill posteromedial–peripheral **(A)** and lateral **(B)** lesions. Note the integration of the chondral layer and the restoration of the medial border articular surface.

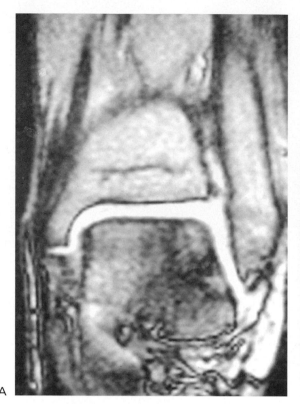
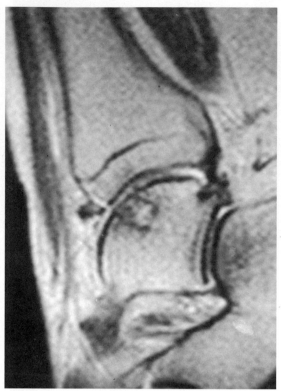

FIGURE 65.14 Postoperative magnetic resonance imaging views: a repaired peripheral osteochondral lesion of the talus **(A)** and a repair in a posterior-central osteochondral lesion of the talus **(B)**.

CONCLUSIONS

Despite the limited capability of a defected cartilage area to repair and to regenerate, injured synovialized joints may have some capacity to spontaneously repair chondral lesion defects, especially if the patient is undergoing a decrease in weight bearing, rest, and treatment of the subchondral bone with penetrating means to stimulate a new ingrowth of cell population to repair the defect.

The value of the proposed surgical arthroscopic treatment on an articular surface such as the talar dome in regard to thickness, shape, and range of motion must be correlated with the long-term clinical outcomes of articular function and symptom reduction, and never only to the possibility of resurfacing restoration of the chondral defect.

With this critical study based on our own personal experience, we simply want to offer a further therapeutic option in restoring chondral talar dome defects using a reproducible arthroscopic procedure. The more the progression of studies on cartilage repair, the more the effort of research appears to offer the best therapeutic choice to the surgeon. At the same time, the more the understanding of such complex restoration processes, the more questions that can be asked than answered.

Despite significant improvements in knowledge of the biologic changes during chondral surface degeneration, only a little additional information on spontaneous repair and

restoration of the defected cartilage is available. More advanced studies should be referred to those scientists who ask difficult questions and make an effort to answer them.

REFERENCES

1. Monro A. *Microgeologie.* Berlin: Th. Billroth, 1856:236.
2. Paget J. On the production of the loose bodies in joints. *St. Bartholomew's Hospital Rep* 1870;6:1.
3. König F. Uber freie Körper in den Gelenken. *Deutsch Zeit Chirurg* 1888:27:90–109.
4. Barth A. Die Enstehung und das Wachsthum der Frein Glenkkor per. *Arch Klin Chir* 1898;56:507.
5. Kappis M. Weitere Beiträge zur traumatisch-mechanischen Enstehung der "spontanen" Knorpelablösungen (sog. Osteochondritis dissecans). *Deutsch Zeit Chir* 1922;171:13–29.
6. Marks KL. Flake fractures of the talus progressing to osteochondritis dissecans. *J Bone Joint Surg Br* 1952;34:90–92.
7. Rödén S, Tillegaard P, Unander-Scharin L. Osteochondritis dissecans and similar lesions of the talus: report of 55 cases with special references to etiology and treatment. *Acta Orthop Scand* 1953;23:51–66.
8. Berndt AL, Harty M. Transchondral fractures (osteochondritis dissecans) of the talus. *J Bone Joint Surg Am* 1959;41:988–1020.
9. O'Donoghue DH. Chondral and osteochondral fractures. *J Trauma* 1966;6:469.
10. Davidson AM, Steele HD, McKenzie DA. A review of 21 cases of transchondral fractures of the talus. *J Trauma* 1967;7:378.
11. Campbell CJ, Ranawat CS. Osteochondritis dissecans: the question of etiology. *J Trauma* 1966;6:201.

12. Canale ST, Belding RH. Osteochondral lesions of the talus. *J Bone Joint Surg Am* 1980;62:97–102.

13. Alexander AH, Lichtman OM. Surgical treatment of transchondral talar dome fractures (osteochondritis dissecans). *J Bone Joint Surg Am* 1980;62:646.

14. Guhl JF. Arthroscopic treatment of osteochondritis dissecans. *Clin Orthop* 1982;167:65–74.

15. Flick AB, Gould N. Osteochondritis dissecans of the talus (transchondral fractures of the talus): review of the literature and new surgical approach for medial dome lesions. *Foot Ankle* 1985;5:165–185.

16. Pritsch M, Horoshowsky H, Farine I. Arthroscopic treatment of the chondral lesions of the talus. *J Bone Joint Surg Am* 1986;68: 862–865.

17. Parisien JS. Arthroscopic treatment of osteochondral lesions the talus. *Am J Sports Med* 1986;14:211–217.

18. Baker CJ, Andrews JR, Ryan JB. Arthroscopic treatment of transchondral talar dome fractures. *Arthroscopy* 1986;2:82–87.

19. Pettine KA, Morrey BF. Osteochondral fractures of the talus: a long term follow-up, 1987. *J Bone Joint Surg Br* 1987;69:89–92.

20. Van Buecken K, Barrack RL, Alexander AH, et al. Arthroscopic treatment of transchondral talar dome fractures. *Am J Sports Med* 1989;17:350–356.

21. Anderson JF. Crichton KJ, Gattan-Smith T, et al. Osteochondral fractures of the dome of the talus. *J Bone Joint Surg Am* 1989;71:1143–1152.

22. Stone JW. Osteochondral lesions of the talar dome. *J Am Acad Orthop Surg* 1996;4,2:63–73.

23. Ferkel RD. *Arthroscopic surgery: the foot and the ankle,* 1st ed. Philadelphia: Lippincott-Raven Press, 1996.

24. Frenkel SR, DiCesare PE. Degradation and repair of articular cartilage. *Front Biosci* 1999;4:671–685.

25. Bukwalter JA, Mow VC, Ratcliffe A. Restoration of injured and degenerated articular cartilage. *J Am Acad Orthop Surg* 1994;2: 192–201.

26. Shapiro F, Koide S, Glimcher M. Cell origin and differentiation in the repair of full-thickness defects of articular cartilage. *J Bone Joint Surg Am* 1993;75:532–553.

27. Mitchell N, Shepard N. The resurfacing of adult rabbit cartilage by multiple perforations through the subchondral bone. *J Bone Joint Surg Am* 1976;58:230–233.

28. Mankin HJ, Mow VC, Bulkwater JA, et al. Form and function of articular cartilage. In: Simon SR, ed. *Orthopedic basic science.* Rosemont, IL: American Academy of Orthopedic Surgeon, 1994:1–44.

29. Nelson DW, Dipaola J, Colville M, et al. Osteochondritis dissecans of the talus and knee: prospective comparison of MR and arthroscopic classifications. *J Comp Assist Tomogr* 1990;14:804–808.

30. Dipaola J, Nelson DW, Colville M. Characterizing osteochondral lesions by magnetic resonance imaging. *Arthroscopy* 1991;7:101–106.

31. Ferkel RD, Sgaglione NA. Arthroscopic treatment of osteochondral lesions of the talus: long term results. *Orthop Trans* 1993–1994;17:1011.

32. Frank A, Cohen P, Beaufils P, et al. Arthroscopic treatment of osteochondral lesions of the talar dome. *Arthroscopy* 1989;5:57–61.

33. Bryant DD, Siegel MG. Osteochondritis dissecans of the talus: a new technique for arthroscopic drilling. *Arthroscopy* 1993;9:238–241.

34. Kelbérine F, Frank A. Arthroscopic treatment of osteochondral lesions of the talar dome: a retrospective study of 48 cases. *Arthroscopy* 1999;15:89–95.

35. Chang E, Lenczner E. Osteochondritis dissecans of the talar dome treated with an osteochondral autograft. *Can J Surg* 2000; 43:217–221.

36. Lahm A, Erggelet C, Stainwachs M, et al. Arthroscopic management of osteochondral lesions of the talus: results of drilling and usefulness of magnetic resonance imaging before and after treatment. *Arthroscopy* 2000;16:299–304.

37. McClauley TR, Disler DG. Magnetic resonance imaging of the articular cartilage of the knee. *J Am Acad Orthop Surg* 2001;9: 2–8.

38. Kaplan L, Uribe JW, Saksen H, et al. The acute effects of radiofrequency energy in articular cartilage: an in vitro study. *Arthroscopy* 2000;16:2–5.

39. Steadman JR, Rodkey WG, Singleton SB, et al. Microfractures technique for full-thickness chondral defects: technique and clinical results. *Oper Tech* 1997;7:300–304.

40. O'Driscoll SW, Keeley FW, Salter RB. Durability of regenerated articular cartilage produced by free autogenous periosteal grafts in major full-thickness defects of joint surfaces under the influence of continuous passive motion: a follow-up report at one year. *J Bone Joint Surg Am* 1988;70:595–606.

41. Peterson L, Minas T, Brittberg M, et al. Two to nine year outcome after autologous chondrocyte transplantation of the knee. *Clin Orthop* 2000;374:212–234.

42. Minas T, Peterson L. Advanced technique in autologous chondrocyte transplantation. *Clin Sports Med* 1999;18:13–44.

43. Bobic V. Arthroscopic osteochondral autograft transplantation in anterior cruciate ligament reconstruction: a preliminary clinical study. *Knee Surg Sports Traumatol Arthrosc* 1996;3:262–264.

44. Duchow J, Hess T, Kohn D. Primary stability of press-fit-implanted osteochondral grafts. *Am J Sport Med* 2000;28:24–27.

45. Hangody I, Kish G, Kárpáti Z, et al. Treatment of osteochondritis dissecans of the talus: the use of mosaicplasty technique. Preliminary report. *Foot Ankle Int* 1997;18:628–635.

46. Simonian PT, Sussmann PS, Wieckiewicz TL, et al. Contact pressure at osteochondral donor site in the knee. *Am J Sports Med* 1998;26:491–494.

SUBTALAR ARTHROSCOPY

JAMES TASTO

Subtalar arthroscopy was first described by Parisien and Vangsness in 1985 (1). The subtalar joint is a very complex joint which functionally is responsible for inversion and eversion of the hindfoot (2–9). The majority of the arthroscopic procedures described are performed in the posterior compartment. The use of smaller instrumentation with improved optics has made this procedure more widely accepted.

ANATOMY AND BIOMECHANICS

The subtalar joint comprises three articulations: the posterior, middle, and anterior joints or facets (Figs. 66.1 and 66.2). There are numerous extraarticular ligaments that stabilize the subtalar joint. The major ligaments encountered during subtalar arthroscopy are the intraarticular components, which consist of the interosseous talocalcaneal ligament, the lateral talocalcaneal ligament, and the anterior talocalcaneal ligament (Fig. 66.3). These coalesce to form the division between the posterior and the middle facets of the subtalar joint. The interosseous ligament is a broad, stout structure measuring approximately 2.5 cm in breath from medial to lateral. It is an important landmark and marks the arthroscopic boundary for posterior subtalar arthroscopy. The subtalar joint is a single-axis joint that acts like a mitered hinge connecting the talus and calcaneus (10,11). The direction of the axis of movement about this joint is backward, downward, and lateral, running from the dorsal medial talus to the posterolateral calcaneus. It is a determinative joint which influences the biomechanics of the distal portion of the midfoot and forefoot. The more horizontal the hinge, the greater the influence of torque and rotation on the midfoot and forefoot. Various authors performing anatomic cadaver studies have reported the range of motion of the subtalar joint to be from 20 to 60 degrees of combined inversion and eversion (10–12).

The three articulations of the subtalar joint are able together to provide rotation between the talus and calcaneus about a common axis of rotation (10–12). At the end of its normal range of motion, the curves of the three articulations suddenly become incongruous, no longer providing motion about a common axis of rotation (10–12). Further motion disarticulates the subtalar joint. This force must be rotational and must exceed the compressive forces holding the talus and calcaneus together (10,11).

At the end of its normal range of motion, the subtalar joint stops and the ligaments continue to be relaxed. Only when the transverse rotational force is increased to the extent that it exceeds the compressive force do the ligaments tighten. The ligaments therefore become taut only at the beginning of an imminent dislocation or subluxation (10,11). The subtalar joint is separated into an anterior and a posterior compartment by the sinus tarsi and the tarsal canal. The tarsal canal contents include the cervical ligament, the talocalcaneal interosseous ligament, the medial root of the inferior extensor retinaculum, the fat pad, and a variety of blood vessels. The anterior portion of the subtalar joint includes both the anterior and the middle facets. It also contains the talonavicular articulation as well as the spring ligament. The posterior subtalar joint has a long axis that is located obliquely about 40 degrees to the midline of the foot, faces lateral, and consists of a convex posterior facet of the calcaneus and a concave facet of the talus. The capsule of the posterior subtalar joint is reinforced laterally by the cervical ligament and the calcaneofibular ligament.

INDICATIONS

As with most arthroscopic surgery, the procedure can be done for diagnostic purposes if there are clinical indications that point to the disorder's being isolated to this joint. Some of the more common indications include synovitis and partial disruptions of the interosseous ligament in the sinus tarsi. Other indications include arthrofibrosis, residual post-

J. Tasto: Department of Orthopedic Surgery, University of California, San Diego; San Diego Medicine & Orthopedic Center, San Diego, California.

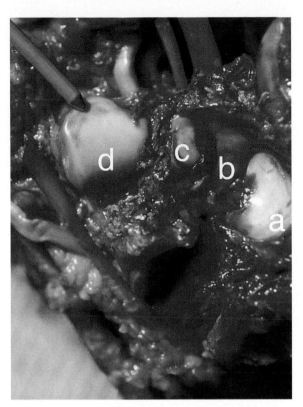

FIGURE 66.1 Topographic view of a prosected anatomic specimen, the posterior subtalar joint: **a**, undersurface of talus; **b**, middle facet of talus; **c**, anterior facet of talus; and **d**, superior surface of calcaneus.

traumatic scar formation, and unstable chondral or osteochondral lesions. It may also be useful in the treatment of fractures of the lateral process of the talus, loose bodies, subtalar impingement, and subtalar arthrodesis. It can be used in combination with an ankle arthroscopy in the evaluation and treatment of combined ankle and subtalar instability for diagnostic and possible therapeutic treatment (1,3,4,7).

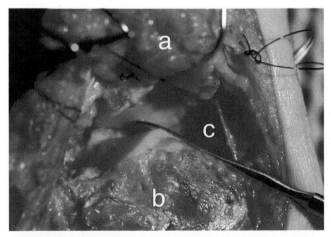

FIGURE 66.2 Anatomic dissection of lateral posterior subtalar joint: **a**, talus; **b**, calcaneus; and **c**, subtalar joint.

CONTRAINDICATIONS

The subtalar joint is a relatively tight joint and access is not always easy. In the case of previous fracture and restricted joint access with concomitant arthrofibrosis, there may be a relative contraindication to an arthroscopic procedure, particularly if the articular surfaces are malaligned. The presence of internal fixation devices may obscure either the anterior portals or the posterior portal and may make an arthroscopic procedure impossible to perform. The obvious presence of a cellulitic reaction around the hindfoot is certainly a contraindication to any elective arthroscopic procedure.

IMAGING

Conventional radiographs should include the routine anteroposterior, lateral, and mortise films of the ankle. A Browden view is quite valuable and is generally taken with the forefoot in plantar flexion and the ankle rotated approximately 40 degrees. This view is particularly helpful to isolate the posterior subtalar joint and appreciate subtle changes. A magnetic resonance imaging (MRI) scan is often useful to differentiate intraarticular pathology from the soft tissue causes of lateral hindfoot pain. If subtle arthritis is expected, a computed tomography (CT) scan may be helpful to define the osseous morphology more accurately.

Arthrography plays very little role currently in the diagnostic workup for ankle and subtalar pain. Differential injections, however, have proven to be an excellent adjunct in differentiating lateral ankle pain from subtalar pain.

SURGICAL TECHNIQUE

The arthroscopic technique for subtalar arthroscopy was previously described by Parisien and Frey (1,3,7). The patient is placed in the lateral decubitus position with the legs and hips appropriately padded. The operative procedure is generally done with the aid of an inflated thigh tourniquet. No traction is applied to the extremity as is done in ankle arthroscopy. The application of a soft tissue distraction device actually obliterates the portal. Only a slight amount of inversion is allowed on the ankle; if extreme inversion is applied, the surrounding soft tissues can obliterate the portals and make the arthroscopic procedure more difficult.

Should an ankle arthroscopy be contemplated at the same time, the subtalar arthroscopy should be done first. This is to avoid the normal extravasation that occurs with an ankle arthroscopy, which might hinder a subsequent subtalar arthroscopy. A marking pen is then used to delineate the outline of the fibula, the superficial peroneal nerve, and the sural nerve. All three portals are marked (Fig. 66.4).

The subtalar joint is preinjected with about 7 mL of saline. One must be very careful to make sure that the in-

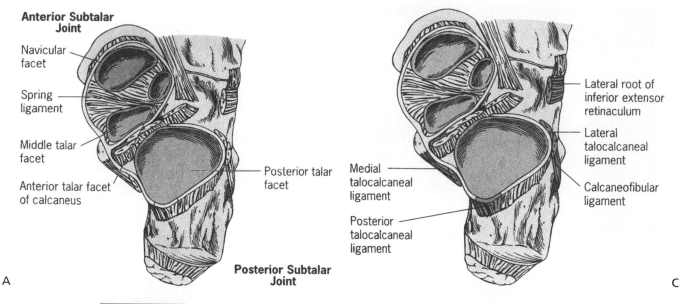

Anterior Subtalar Joint

- Navicular facet
- Spring ligament
- Middle talar facet
- Anterior talar facet of calcaneus
- Posterior talar facet
- **Posterior Subtalar Joint**

A

- Lateral root of inferior extensor retinaculum
- Lateral talocalcaneal ligament
- Medial talocalcaneal ligament
- Posterior talocalcaneal ligament
- Calcaneofibular ligament

C

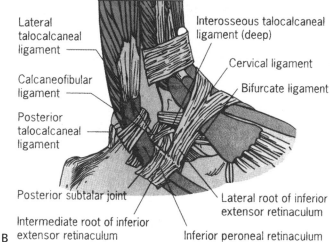

- Lateral talocalcaneal ligament
- Calcaneofibular ligament
- Posterior talocalcaneal ligament
- Posterior subtalar joint
- Intermediate root of inferior extensor retinaculum
- Interosseous talocalcaneal ligament (deep)
- Cervical ligament
- Bifurcate ligament
- Lateral root of inferior extensor retinaculum
- Inferior peroneal retinaculum

B

FIGURE 66.3 A: The subtalar joints. **B:** Lateral view of the right ankle showing the peripheral ligaments. **C:** Axial view of the ankle showing the peripheral ligaments. (From Parisien JS. Arthroscopy of the posterior subtalar joint. In: Parisien JS, ed. *Current techniques in arthroscopy.* New York: Theime, 1998:161–168; adapted from Ferkel RD. Subtalar arthroscopy. In: Ferkel R, ed. *Arthroscopy surgery: the foot and ankle.* Philadelphia: Lippincott-Raven; 1996:231–254, with permission.)

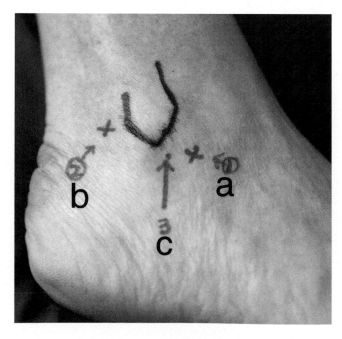

FIGURE 66.4 Portal sites for subtalar arthroscopy: **a,** anterolateral portal; **b,** posterolateral portal; **c,** accessory lateral portal.

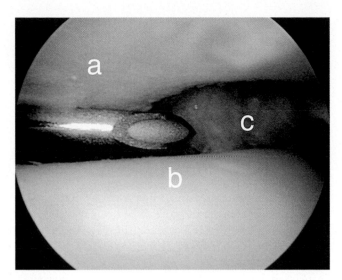

FIGURE 66.5 Arthroscopic view of a right posterior subtalar joint: **a,** talus; **b,** calcaneus; **c,** posteromedial corner.

jection is not placed in the subcutaneous tissue. This also gives reassurance to the surgeon, if a large-bore needle is used, that the joint has been entered, and it provides an appropriate angle for the initial placement of the arthroscopic sheath and trocar.

The anterolateral portal is established first by a nick and spread technique with a no. 11 blade. This is usually located in the region of the sinus tarsi and approximately 1.5 to 2 cm anterior and 1 cm distal to the tip of the lateral malleolus. The skin only is incised; further dilation and spreading is done with a small mosquito clamp. The 2.7-mm dull tro-

car and sheath are then placed in the anterior portal. The arthroscope should now be located posterior to the interosseous ligament. If better visualization is required initially, then an 18-gauge needle can be placed in juxtaposition to establish appropriate flow. The posterolateral portal is then established by palpating the soft tissues and establishing the entry site with an 18-gauge needle using an outside-in technique while visualizing through the anterior portal. This portal is usually located approximately 1 cm proximal and 1 cm posterior to the distal tip of the fibula. Care is taken to avoid the sural nerve and the small saphenous vein while making this portal. The nick and spread technique is used in a vertical fashion to avoid damaging these structures. If a large amount of synovium and scar is encountered in the anterior portal and visualization is impaired, then an accessory portal is established (Fig. 66.4) and a small shaver is placed in to debride this area.

Initially visualization is done from the anterolateral portal with outflow established in the posterior portal. Later, these portals may be reversed. A pump is employed to keep complete control over the pressure and avoid excessive extravasation and a potential compartment syndrome. The pressure is usually maintained at about 35 mm Hg pressure.

A complete diagnostic subtalar arthroscopy is now carried out. Distal to the anterolateral portal will be the interosseous talocalcaneal ligaments and proximal will be the talocalcaneal joint (Fig. 66.5). One can now visualize the lateral recess, the reflection of the calcaneofibular ligament, the lateral talocalcaneal ligament, the os trigonum, and the lateral process of the talus (Fig. 66.6). Through this portal

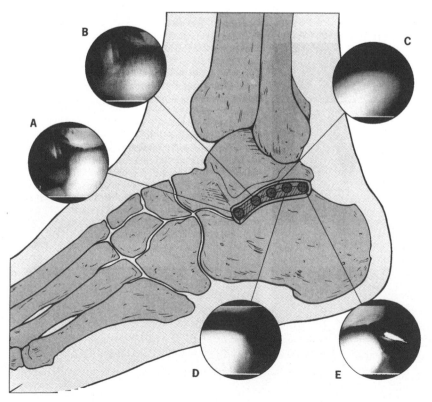

FIGURE 66.6 Arthroscopic visualization of various areas of the posterior subtalar joint in a patient with subtalar instability. Shown are the interosseous ligament area **(A)**, anterior aspect of the joint **(B)**, midaspect of the joint **(C)**, posterior aspect of the joint **(D)**, posterior pouch of the subtalar joint **(E)**. (From Parisien J. Arthroscopy of the posterior subtalar joint. In: Parisien JS, ed. *Current techniques in arthroscopy.* New York: Theime, 1998:161–168; adapted from Parisien JS. Arthroscopy of the posterior subtalar joint and great toe. In: Parisien JS, ed. *Techniques in therapeutic arthroscopy.* New York: Raven, 1993:20: 1–10, with permission.)

one can visualize the posterior compartment but does not see the anterior and middle facets or the anterior compartment of the subtalar joint. If there is a complete disruption of interosseous ligaments, however, it can be visualized. It is possible to enter these compartments with the arthroscope if a portal is extended through the interosseous ligament going distally.

Conventional 2.0- and 3.5-mm shavers can be used to perform a debridement and synovectomy early in the procedure to improve visualization. Small, loose-body forceps can be used to remove loose bodies, and occasionally radiofrequency can be used to perform ablation and modulation of the synovium and abnormal soft tissue. A full and detailed description of the technique for an arthroscopic subtalar arthrodesis (ASTA) follows.

RESULTS AND COMPLICATIONS

Favorable results have been reported with this technique if appropriate indications are defined and meticulous attention to detail is adhered to. In a series of 49 subtalar arthroscopies, Frey et al. reported 94% good-to-excellent results (4). The patients had injuries to the interosseous ligament, arthrofibrosis, degenerative joint disease, and fibrous coalitions of the calcaneonavicular joint.

Complications of subtalar arthroscopy have been reported by Williams and Ferkel (4,13–15). A wide variety of pathologic conditions were encountered, as previously discussed. The complications in these series included several cases of neurapraxia, of both the sural nerve and the superficial branch of the peroneal nerve, sinus tract infections, and wound infections. As in ankle arthroscopy, the most prevalent complication is neurapraxia of the superficial peroneal nerve and sural nerve. This can be avoided in most cases with careful attention to the anatomy as well as a careful nick and spread technique when establishing portals.

ARTHROSCOPIC SUBTALAR ARTHRODESIS

Operative procedures designed for subtalar fusion have been in existence for almost 90 years. Nieny performed the first subtalar arthrodesis in 1905. There have been numerous techniques reported in the literature, which have utilized both intra-articular as well as extra-articular methods (16–24). Results have generally been favorable, with a variety of complications reported (25–27). Data on rate of fusion, time until union, complications, and long-term follow up are noticeably missing in both the older and the more recent literature. A number of other procedures for subtalar pathology have been described, including arthroscopy, arthroplasty, triple arthrodesis, and sinus tarsi exploration. Surgical open reduction of calcaneal fractures has gained acceptance when attempting to restore the normal anatomic

alignment of the joint surfaces. This is an effort to avoid the sequelae of posttraumatic degenerative arthritis of the subtalar joint. Both operative and conservative care of calcaneal fractures continues, however, to be plagued with long-term symptomatic degenerative changes in the subtalar joint.

ASTA as a surgical procedure was developed in 1992 and first reported at the 1994 annual meeting of the Arthroscopy Association of North America (AANA) in a preliminary review. The procedure was designed to improve traditional methods by using a microinvasive technique. The decision to proceed with this surgical technique grew out of the success with arthroscopic ankle arthrodesis (28). Subtalar arthroscopy has been described by a number of authors, but few cases or attempts at arthroscopic subtalar fusion have been published (14). Recent work by Solis has paralleled some of my earlier work (29).

The development of an arthroscopic technique was intended to yield less morbidity if it could be performed with the use of the same techniques and principles as an arthroscopic ankle fusion. It was hypothesized that perioperative morbidity could be reduced, blood supply preserved, and proprioceptive and neurosensory input enhanced. A prospective study was initiated to document the effectiveness of the procedure and to determine the time until complete fusion, the incidence of delayed union and of nonunion, and the prevalence of complications.

Indications and Workup

The indication for ASTA is intractable subtalar pain secondary to rheumatoid arthritis, osteoarthritis, or posttraumatic arthritis. Other indications include neuropathic conditions, gross instability, paralytic conditions, and posterior tibial tendon rupture. Most of the earlier literature in subtalar surgery was centered on the stabilization of paralytic deformities secondary to poliomyelitis. The majority of patients encountered in today's medical environment that require this procedure have posttraumatic and arthritic disorders.

A small segment of the population present with posterior tibial tendon dysfunction or a talocalcaneal coalition.

Patients must have failed conservative management in order to qualify for arthroscopic subtalar fusion. Conservative treatment comprises a variety of modalities, including orthotics, nonsteroidal antiinflammatory drugs, activity modification, and occasional cortisone injections into the subtalar joint. Patients must also be apprised of the possibility that an open procedure might be required should this technique not be technically feasible.

The patient's history is usually one of lateral hindfoot pain that can be confused quite easily with ankle pathology. Increased symptoms with weight bearing on uneven ground is a classic complaint. History of a previous calcaneal fracture should immediately alert one to the possibility of subtalar pathology. The clinical findings consist of pain over the sinus tarsi and the posterolateral subtalar joint. Patients also report reproduction of the symptoms on inversion and eversion of the subtalar joint with the ankle locked in dorsiflexion.

The clinical work up for this patient profile is quite simple. Often a good history and physical examination, confirmed by plain radiographs, is sufficient to confirm the diagnosis (Fig. 66.9). On occasion, CT or MRI may be necessary (30). There is little need for a bone scan or arthrography (31). Differential injections continue to be a valuable diagnostic aid to confirm as well as separate out ankle pain from subtalar pain. Radiographs do not have to show profound degenerative changes, because only small alterations in the biomechanics of this joint can produce significant symptoms.

The contraindications to this procedure are previously failed subtalar fusions, gross malalignment requiring correction, infection, and significant bone loss. On occasion, a patient with moderate malalignment is a candidate for *in situ* stabilization. Although significant bone loss has not been encountered frequently, it did not present a serious problem in a series of arthroscopic ankle arthrodesis (28).

Each procedure was done in an ambulatory surgery center environment, with the patient discharged on the same day. The only exception was the occasional patient treated at the Veterans' Administration Medical Center affiliated with this teaching institution. Patients were given preoperative, intraoperative, and postoperative antibiotics for a total of three doses because of the use of internal fixation. General anesthesia was used in the majority of the cases.

Arthroscopy: Technique

Patients are placed in the lateral decubitus position with the patient lying on the unaffected side. Two pillows are placed between the legs while the affected ankle and subtalar joint are allowed to hang over a blanket roll in a natural position of plantar flexion and inversion. After thorough preparation and draping of the patient, anatomic landmarks and portal sites are identified and marked with a surgical pen. The tourniquet is then elevated. In general, the operative procedure is completed within one tourniquet time (1 hour 45 minutes).

Establishment of the portal sites is one of the more difficult portions of the procedure. The full description of this technique was outlined in the beginning of this chapter. It is critical to predetermine the angles of the subtalar joint, because its unique geometry and limited access leave little room for error. The surgeon should not hesitate to use fluoroscopy to confirm portal location if necessary.

The anterolateral and the posterolateral portals are the two conventional portals. If necessary, an accessory portal may be established approximately 1 cm posterior to the anterolateral portal. This portal can be used for debridement or for outflow enhancement. It can also be used for visual-

ization on occasion. Both the anterolateral and the posterolateral portal are used in an alternating fashion during the procedure for viewing and for instrumentation. Occasionally, significant arthrofibrosis is present and makes entry and visualization difficult. In such cases, the accessory anterolateral portal is quite useful.

The arthroscope used for this procedure should be a 2.7-mm, wide-angle, short, small-joint arthroscope. It should be equipped with a choice of sheaths to accommodate limited or increased flow. The blunt trocar and sheath is introduced through the anterolateral portal and the posterolateral portal can be established at this time. In the initial cases, a small laminar spreader was used in the anterolateral portal to increase access. This was later abandoned as a routine, but it may still be used if distraction is a significant problem. Arthroscopic resection of the interosseous ligament may also be used for additional distraction, but I have not used it.

It is important to be certain that the arthroscope is in the subtalar joint and that the ankle joint or the fibular talar recess has not been inadvertently entered. All debridement and decortication is done posterior to the interosseous ligament, because only the posterior facet is fused. The middle and anterior facets are not visualized under normal circumstances unless the interosseous ligament is absent. The majority of the procedure is done with the arthroscope in the anterolateral portal and the instruments in the posterolateral portal. The remaining and final debridement is accomplished by alternating these two portals.

A primary synovectomy and debridement is necessary for visualization, as with other joints. The articular surface is debrided, which makes the joint more capacious and instrumentation easier. Complete removal of the articular surface down to subchondral bone is the next phase of the procedure (Fig. 66.7). The talocalcaneal geometry is quite unique and requires a variety of instruments. In general, multiangular curettes and a complete set of burs suffice.

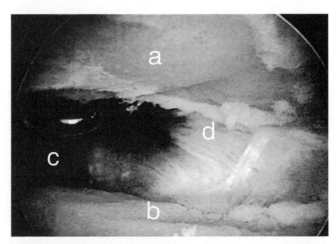

FIGURE 66.7 Posterior subtalar joint, viewing from posterolateral portal. **a,** talus; **b,** calcaneus; **c,** sinus tarsi; **d,** interosseous ligament.

Once the articular cartilage has been resected, approximately 1 to 2 mm of subchondral bone is removed to expose the highly vascular cancellous bone. Care must be taken not to alter the geometry and not to remove excessive bone. This would lead to poor coaptation of the joint surfaces. Once the subchondral plate is removed, small "spot-weld" holes measuring approximately 2 mm in depth are created on the surfaces of the calcaneus and talus to create vascular channels (Fig. 66.8). Careful assessment of the posteromedial corner must be made, because residual bone and cartilage could be left there which could interfere with coaptation. Often the curette safely breaks down this corner and also provides the surgeon with additional tactile feedback. The neurovascular bundle is directly posteromedially and must be taken into consideration at all times and protected.

After viewing from both portals to ensure complete debridement and decortication, the tourniquet is released and careful assessment of the vascularity of the calcaneus and talus is made. The joint is then thoroughly irrigated of bone fragments and debris. No autogenous bone graft or bone substitute is needed for this procedure.

The fixation of the fusion is done with a large cannulated 7.0-mm screw. The guide pin is started at the dorsal anteromedial talus and is angled posteriorly and inferiorly to the posterolateral calcaneus but does not violate the calcaneal cortical surface. Under fluoroscopy, the guide wire is placed with the ankle in maximum dorsiflexion to avoid any possible screwhead encroachment or impingement on the anterior lip of the tibia. Once the guide wire has been placed under these conditions, the ankle can then be relaxed, the screw inserted under fluoroscopic control, and the fusion site compressed. With this technique, the screw runs along the natural axis of rotation of the subtalar joint. Starting the

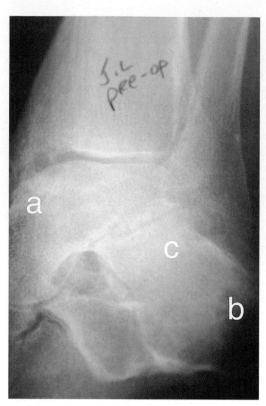

FIGURE 66.9 Browden view of an arthritic posterior subtalar joint: **a,** talus; **b,** calcaneus; **c,** subtalar joint.

screw from the dorsal and medial aspect of the talus avoids painful screwhead prominence over the calcaneus and the necessity of a second procedure for screw removal. To date, there have been no fractures or complications with this fixation technique (Fig. 66.10).

Steri-Strips are used instead of sutures to allow adequate drainage. A bulky dressing and a short-leg bivalve cast are applied. The patient is discharged home after appropriate circulatory checks in the recovery room. The first clinical evaluation takes place in the office within 48 hours. After approximately 1 week, the cast is removed and the patient is fitted immediately with an ankle–foot orthosis (AFO) if the swelling is minimal. Full weight bearing is allowed as tolerated at any time after surgery. In general, patients can tolerate full weight bearing without crutch support within 7 to 14 days after surgery. Although patients wear the AFO almost 24 hours a day, they are able to bathe as well as to take the ankle and foot through a range of motion without the brace. The AFO is removed after full union has been achieved. The standard three views of the ankle plus a Browden view are the radiographs of choice used in follow-up assessment.

Results and Complications

Since September of 1992, 25 patients have undergone arthroscopic subtalar fusion with sufficient follow-up time

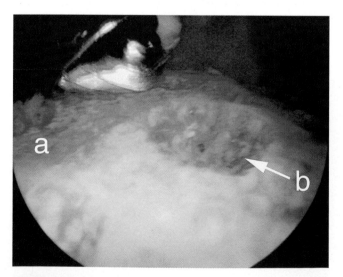

FIGURE 66.8 Superior surface of calcaneus after removal of articular surface, decortication, and "spot-welding": **a,** calcaneus; **b,** "spot-weld."

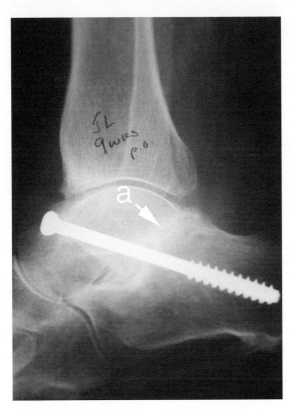

FIGURE 66.10 Lateral radiograph of a fused subtalar joint with a single cancellous screw across the posterior facet.

to determine the effectiveness of this procedure. The fusion rate, time until complete union, surgical technique, and complications were analyzed. One standard surgical procedure was used, and the method of internal fixation was not altered during this entire series. The posterior subtalar joint was the only joint fused during this procedure. Three of the 25 patients underwent a combined arthroscopic ankle and subtalar fusion. In this series, there were 8 patients with osteoarthritis, 10 with posttraumatic arthritis, 4 with posterior tibial tendon dysfunction, 2 with rheumatoid arthritis, and 1 with talocalcaneal coalition. Every patient had a radiographic evaluation at 2-week intervals to determine the rate and quality of fusion. For an arthrodesis to be considered completely fused, both clinical and radiographic evidence are required. The parameters required for a successful arthrodesis are the following: evidence of bone consolidation across the subtalar joint, no motion at the screw, clinical absence of pain with weight bearing, and pain-free forced inversion and eversion. The average mean follow-up time was 22 months (range, 6 to 92 months). All 25 patients have clinical and radiographic union; the average time until complete fusion was 8.9 weeks (range, 6 to 16 weeks).

There are considerable advantages to this technique compared with open procedures. It is a minimally invasive technique that theoretically preserves the blood supply of the calcaneus and talus. This is especially important considering that many of these patients had previously undergone open surgery. Conventional open procedures by definition interrupt the blood supply and compromise vascular ingrowth and eventual fusion. Avoidance of incisions coupled with early range of motion and weight bearing helps avoid stress deprivation and enhance proprioception, reducing the devastating effects of reflex sympathetic dystrophy.

There have been no reoperations in this series, with the exception of one screw removal. One patient had a painful screw at the calcaneus; the screw penetrated the cortex, and the possibility of a stress fracture was entertained. Symptoms resolved after screw removal. Two patients had some residual anterolateral pain with some radiographic and clinical evidence of minor degenerative joint disease in the ankle. These findings were noted on preoperative films. One patient responded with complete relief to a diagnostic and therapeutic steroid and lidocaine (Xylocaine) injection into the ankle joint. One patient eventually underwent arthroscopic ankle arthrodesis because of preexisting osteoarthritis of the ankle. Valgus tilting of the ankle joint after subtalar arthrodesis has been reported, but it is unclear whether this was secondary to the fusion or merely a natural progression of the disease (32). Two cases not included in this series could not be completed arthroscopically because of significant malformation of the calcaneus and arthrofibrosis of the subtalar joint. These patients underwent a modified miniopen posterior subtalar arthrodesis. An identical screw fixation and postoperative protocol was used in these two patients. Skin problems about the hindfoot can be catastrophic and are obviously avoided by this technique. There were no superficial or deep infections in this series. All arthroscopic procedures have had reported reductions in infection, and one would hope that this procedure would also fall into that same category. There have not been sufficient cases, however, to validate this hypothesis.

Most open series show a longer time until union, with some prevalence of nonunions. Although too early to validate, preliminary observations would indicate a more rapid time until union as well as an increased rate of union. There has been a paucity of literature on isolated open subtalar arthrodesis with adequate follow-up statistics over the last 25 years.

CONCLUSION

The obvious advantages are quite dramatic. Early weight bearing and AFO immobilization allow patients an early return to work. Outpatient surgery is a cost-effective benefit. Patient satisfaction and comfort are greatly enhanced, and only oral pain medication is required. All patients have tolerated their postoperative regimen and same-day discharge.

ASTA is a technically demanding procedure that requires some rather advanced arthroscopic skills to perform. Joint access is tight and restricted, requiring small instrumentation. Deformities cannot be corrected; therefore, at this stage, this must be considered a fusion *in situ*. The learning curve is steep because of the smaller patient population available for enhancement of surgical skills.

Overall, this procedure has stood the test of time and follow-up. The results appear to be excellent in terms of patient satisfaction, fusion rate, time until union, and postoperative morbidity. The recognition and enhancement of this technique as well as the development of more advanced technology will certainly allow this ASTA technique to mature even further over time.

REFERENCES

1. Parisien JS, Vangsness T. Arthroscopy of the subtalar joint: an experimental approach. *Arthroscopy* 1985;1:53–57.
2. Cahill DR. The anatomy and function of the contents of the human tarsal sinus and canal. *Anat Rec* 1965;153:1–17.
3. Frey C, Gasser S, Feder K. Arthroscopy of the subtalar joint. *Foot Ankle Int* 1994;15:424–428.
4. Frey C, Feder S, DiGiovanni D. Arthroscopic evaluation of the subtalar joint: does sinus tarsi syndrome exist? *Foot Ankle Int* 1999;20:185–191.
5. Kjaersgaard-Andersen P, Wethelund JO, Helmig P, et al. The stabilizing effect of the ligamentous structures in the sinus and canalis tarsi on movements of the hindfoot. *Am J Sports Med* 1988;41:19–27.
6. Lehman WB, Lehman M. The surgical anatomy of the interosseous ligament of the subtalar joint as it relates to clubfoot surgery. *Bull Hosp Jt Dis Orthop Inst* 1981;41:19–27.
7. Parisien JS, ed. *Arthroscopy surgery.* New York: McGraw-Hill, 1988.
8. Perry J. Anatomy and biomechanics of the hindfoot. *Clin Orthop* 1983;177:9–15.
9. Resnick D. Radiology of the talocalcaneal articulations: anatomic considerations and arthrography. *Radiology* 1974;3:581–586.
10. Inman VT, Mann RA, Duvries. *Surgery of the foot.* St. Louis: CV Mosby, 1973:27–19.
11. Root M, Orien WP, Weld J. Normal and abnormal functions of the foot. *Clin Biomech* 1977;2:79.
12. Hicks JH. *The mechanics of the foot. Vol 1: the joints.* J Anat 1953;87:345–357.
13. Williams MM, Ferkel RD: Subtalar arthroscopy; indications, technique, and results. *Arthroscopy* 1994;10:345.
14. Ferkel RD: Subtalar arthroscopy. In: Ferkel R, ed. *Arthroscopy surgery: the foot and ankle.* Philadelphia: Lippincott-Raven, 1996:231–254.
15. Tasto JP, Frey C, Laimans P, et al. Arthroscopic ankle arthrodesis. *Instr Course Lect* 2000;49:259–280.
16. Thomas FB. Arthrodesis of the subtalar joint. *J Bone Joint Surg* 1967;2:93–97.
17. Dick IL. Primary fusion of the posterior subtalar joint and the treatment of fractures of the calcaneus. *J Bone Joint Surg Br* 1953;35:375.
18. Gallie WE. Subastragalar arthrodesis and fractures of the os calcis. *J Bone Joint Surg* 1943;25:731.
19. Grice DS. An extra-articular arthrodesis of the subastragalar joint for correction of paralytic flat feet in children. *J Bone Joint Surg Am* 1952;35:927.
20. Grice DS. Further experience with extra-articular arthrodesis of the subtalar joint. *J Bone Joint Surg Am* 1955;37:246.
21. Hall MC, Pennal GF. Primary subtalar arthrodesis in the treatment of severe fractures of the calcaneus. *J Bone Joint Surg Br* 1960;42:336.
22. Geckler EO. Comminuted fractures of the os calcis. *Arch Surg* 1943;61:469.
23. Harris RI. Fractures of the os calcis. *Ann Surg* 1946;124:1082.
24. Wilson PD. Treatment of fractures of the os calcis by arthrodesis of the subtalar joint. *JAMA* 1927;89:1676.
25. Gross RH. A clinical study of bachelor subtalar arthrodesis. *J Bone Joint Surg* 1976;58:343–349.
26. Mallon WJ, Nunley JA. The Grice procedure: extra-articular subtalar arthrodesis. *Orthop Clin North Am* 1989;20:649–654.
27. Moreland JR, Westin GW. Further experience with Grice subtalar arthrodesis. *Clin Orthop* 1986;207:113–121.
28. Tasto JP. *Arthroscopic ankle arthrodesis: a seven year follow up.* Rosemont, IL: American Academy of Orthopaedic Surgeons, 1997.
29. Solis VH. *Personal communication,* 1996.
30. Seltzer SE, Weisman B. CT of the hindfoot with rheumatoid arthritis. *J Arthritis Rheum* 1985;28:12–42.
31. Goosens M, et al. Posterior subtalar joint arthrography. A useful tool in the diagnosis of hindfoot disorders. *Clin Orthop* 1989;(249):248–255.
32. Fitzgibbons, et al. *Valgus tilting of the ankle joint following subtalar arthrodesis.* Dublin: International Society of Foot and Ankle Surgery, 1995.

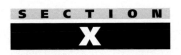

THE SPINE

MINIMALLY INVASIVE SURGERY OF THE SPINE

DONALD L. HILTON, Jr.

Endoscopic access through shoulder and knee arthroscopy brought minimally invasive surgery to the level of routine standard of care. Laparoscopy has made general and gynecologic surgery short-stay procedures. Spine surgery has lagged somewhat behind. Minimally invasive procedures such as the nucleotome, papain treatment and other percutaneous intradiscal procedures have not provided access to the epidural space for treatment of free disc pathology or foraminal stenosis (1–8).

Microendoscopic discectomy (MED) first provided endoscopic visualization of the epidural space combined with open port access to allow standard microdiscectomy instrumentation to be utilized (9). There have been several thousand cases of MED performed since its inception in the middle to late 1990s. MED has been compared to the gold standard of microdiscectomy (10). The main advantage of MED over microdiscectomy would appear to be the use of a small muscle splitting port as opposed to a muscle-stripping retractor. Disadvantages include a smaller working space (16-mm tube), further limited by the endoscope and two-dimensional visualization of the dura and associated anatomy.

The MED tube has previously been used as a retractor for microscopic access (11). We initially began using variable-length muscle splitting tubes in San Antonio in October 1998. This initial prototype was subsequently modified and expanded into the present MEDTRx-MD system (Medtronic Sofamor Danek), which continues to offer the endoscopic option.

The MEDTRx-MD system consists of a series of muscle-splitting tubes of varying diameters (14, 16, 18 mm) and lengths (3 to 8 cm in 1-cm increments). This allows tube selections to match the individual patient (Fig. 67.1) and provides access to a larger patient population than MED would

allow. The MED endoscope attachment is removed to eliminate unnecessary length.

These modifications provide versatility and allow even morbidly obese patients to be treated. The cervical spine can be accessed with posterior foraminotomy and discectomy also, and even recurrent discs can be safely treated. The visualization is obtained with a neurocapable operating microscope (Zeiss-Leica or comparable model), and bayonetted instruments (Fig. 67.2) are used to operate in much the same way that transsphenoidal pituitary surgery has been done for years in neurosurgery. The visualization is three-dimensional, and the procedure is in essence a microdiscectomy. The tube thus descriptively becomes a minimally invasive tubular retractor (MITR).

SURGICAL TECHNIQUE: LUMBAR, STANDARD APPROACH

The MEDTRx-MD system provides a series of MITRs and bayonetted instruments (Medtronic Sofamor Danek).

The patient is placed in the prone position on a Wilson-type frame or on shoulder rolls to allow adequate abdominal relaxation to adequately decompress the epidural veins. Intraoperative lateral fluoroscopy is used for localization (Figs. 67.3 and 67.4). A spinal needle is passed to the facet complex at the level of the disc approximately 1.5 cm lateral to the midline or approximately 1 cm to the palpable edge of the spinous process. This is done for the initial localization with fluoroscopy. When this placement is optimal, a localizing guide wire is passed to the same trajectory. This guide wire is passed down below the fascia in the same trajectory as the localizing spinal needle. Care is taken not to enter the canal (Fig. 67.5). A stab wound of approximately 1.5 cm is made that incorporates the guide wire, and the dilators are then placed over the guide wire to dilatate the muscles (Figs. 67.6 and 67.7). The appropriate tube is then selected to allow the tube to lie flush with the skin and provide a minimal working distance (Fig. 67.8).

D. L. Hilton, Jr.: Neurological Associates of San Antonio; Department of Neurosurgery, Southwest Texas Methodist Hospital, San Antonio, Texas.

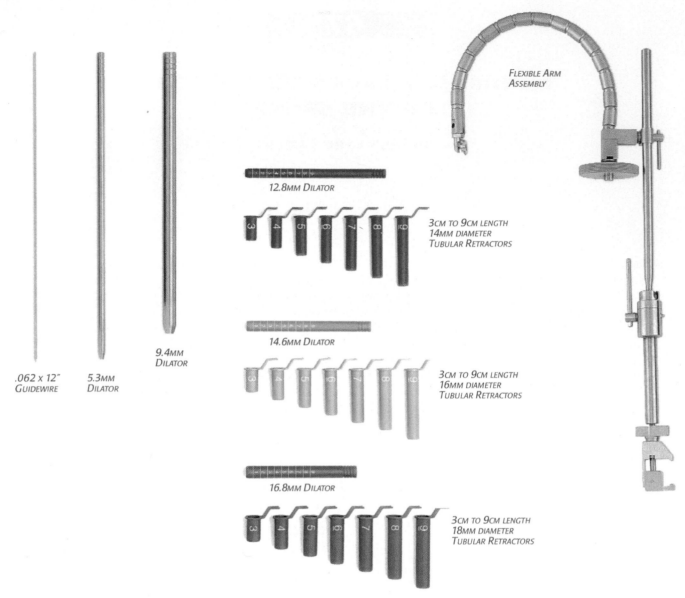

FIGURE 67.1 Dilator, tubes, and arms of the MEDTRx-MD system. (Courtesy of Medtronic Sofamor Danek.)

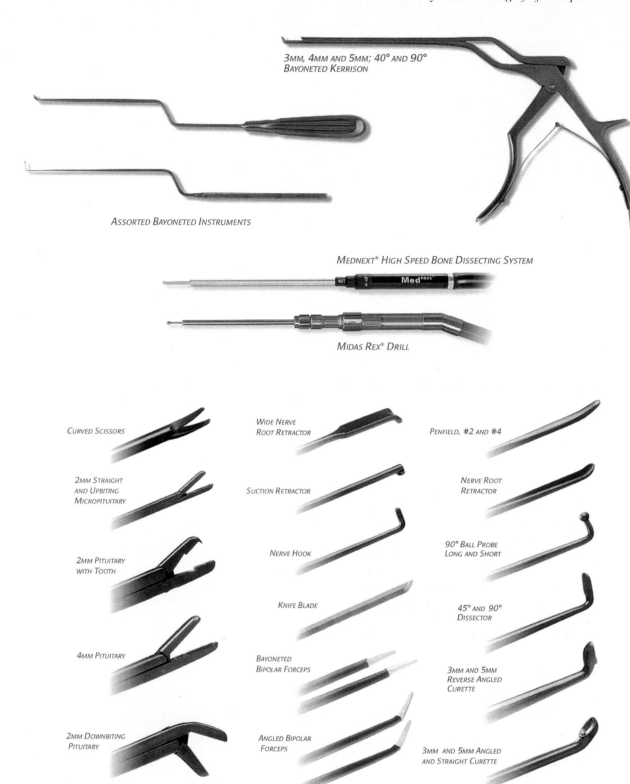

FIGURE 67.2 Bayonetted instruments of the MEDTRx-MD system. (Courtesy of Medtronic Sofamor Danek.)

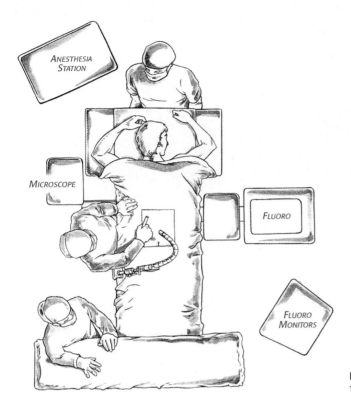

FIGURE 67.3 Operating room setup. (Courtesy of Medtronic Sofamor Danek.)

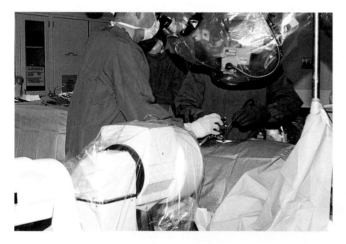

FIGURE 67.4 Surgeon and assistant with microscope and fluoroscope. (Courtesy of Donald L. Hilton, Jr., M.D., Southwest Texas Methodist Hospital.)

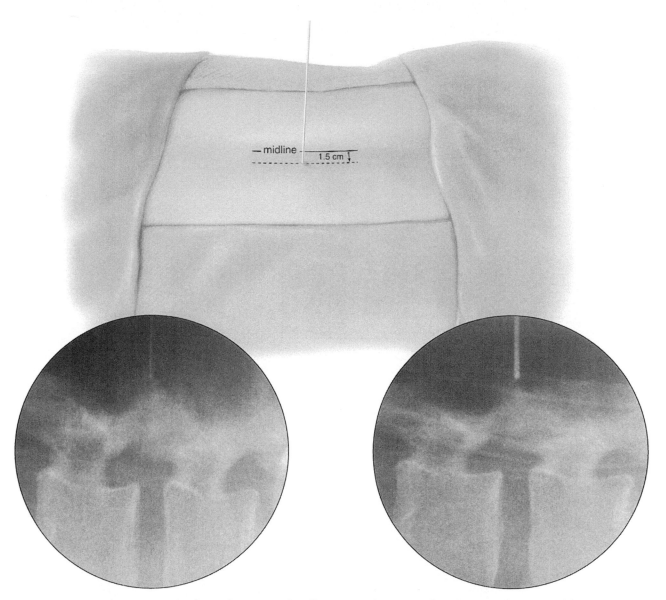

FIGURE 67.5 Guide wire and corresponding fluoroscopy. (Courtesy of Medtronic Sofamor Danek.)

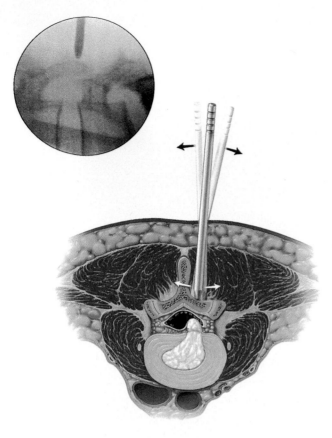

FIGURE 67.6 Initial dilator in position. (Courtesy of Medtronic Sofamor Danek.)

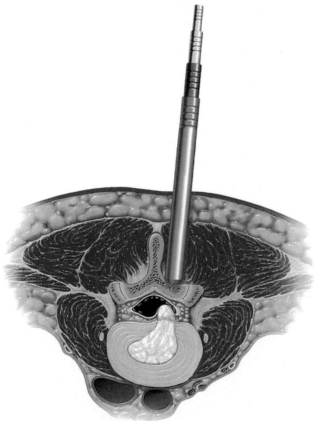

FIGURE 67.7 Successive dilation of operating port. (Courtesy of Medtronic Sofamor Danek.)

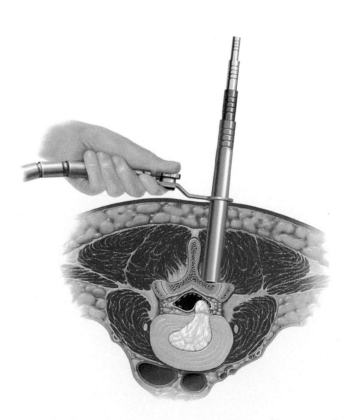

FIGURE 67.8 Tube in position over dilator. (Courtesy of Medtronic Sofamor Danek.)

Dilators are removed, and the microscope is brought into position (Fig. 67.9). High power is generally preferred, and the focus should be adjusted to allow adequate working space between the tube and the microscope (Fig. 67.10). An extended-length monopolar electrocautery is used to coagulate the thin layer of soft tissue over the facet and lamina (Fig. 67.11), and the inferior laminar edge is palpated and defined (Fig. 67.12). Kerrison rongeurs and/or power drills (Midas Rex, TDQ guide/TDQ 130D tool) are used to perform a laminotomy and medial facetectomy. The tube is advanced as the laminar edge is removed to allow the advancing edge of the bone to remain in visualization (Fig. 67.13). Initially this is a rostral march of the tube as it is wanded to allow progressive exposure of the ligamentum flavum until the free edge is seen. Bayoneted instruments are then used. A short ball hook is used to free the edge of the ligament from the dura, and right-angle Kerrison rongeurs are then used to carefully remove the ligament. This is possible to do safely with three-dimensional visualization to avoid a dural laceration even with a tight dura (Fig. 67.14).

The tube is then angled progressively caudally and laterally as the ligament is removed until the free edge and shoulder of the root are seen. Fluoroscopy may be used with probes placed in the canal to ascertain the exact location with regard to the pathology as seen in imaging studies. For axillary fragments well below the disc, dissection is continued in a caudal direction until the pathology is accessed; the converse is done for superiorly migrated fragments. A nerve root retractor may be used (Fig. 67.15). Up, straight and down binding pituitary-type rongeurs may be used in the interspace, as may ring curettes as desired. A modified knife may be used to incise the ligament as necessary. The wound is closed with subcuticular sutures, Steri-Strips, and a Band-Aid (Fig. 67.16).

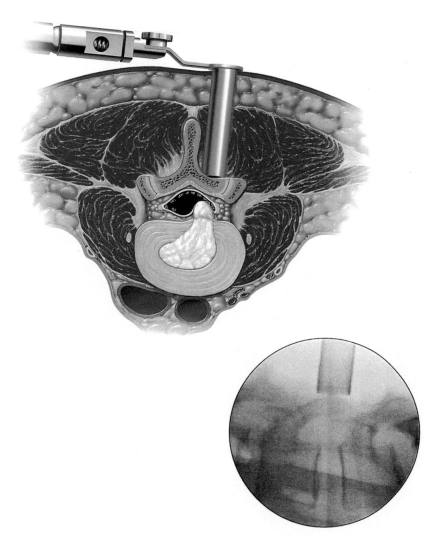

FIGURE 67.9 Tube in operating position. (Courtesy of Medtronic Sofamor Danek.)

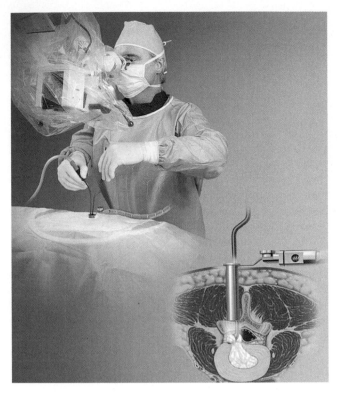

FIGURE 67.10 Relative position of microscope and tube allows sufficient working room with bayonetted instruments. (Courtesy of Medtronic Sofamor Danek.)

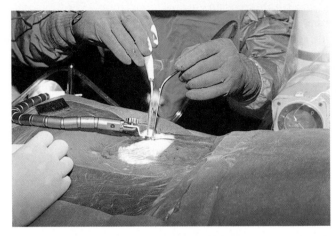

FIGURE 67.11 Monopolar cautery with suction removing soft tissue from lamina. (Courtesy of Donald L. Hilton, Jr., M.D., Southwest Texas Methodist Hospital.)

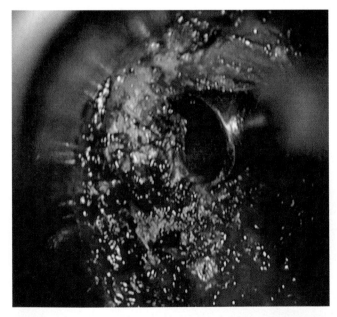

FIGURE 67.12 Curette defining laminar edge seen through 14-mm-diameter tube using Leica microscope. (Courtesy of Donald L. Hilton, Jr., M.D., Southwest Texas Methodist Hospital.)

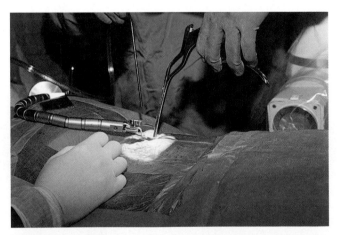

FIGURE 67.13 Kerrison rongeur removing laminar bone. (Courtesy of Donald L. Hilton, Jr., M.D., Southwest Texas Methodist Hospital.)

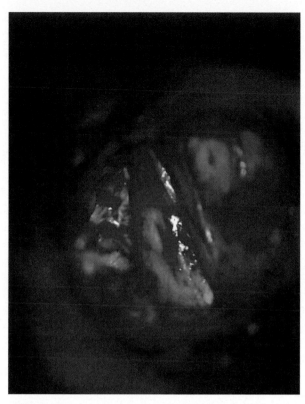

FIGURE 67.14 Dura seen with gel foam temporarily placed in epidural space for hemostasias. (Courtesy of Donald L. Hilton, Jr., M.D., Southwest Texas Methodist Hospital.)

SURGICAL TECHNIQUE: LUMBAR, LATERAL APPROACH

Foraminal or extraforaminal disc herniations may be approached laterally with a muscle-splitting technique. A point is marked approximately 5 to 6 cm lateral to the lateral edge of the spinous process. The point is chosen to be

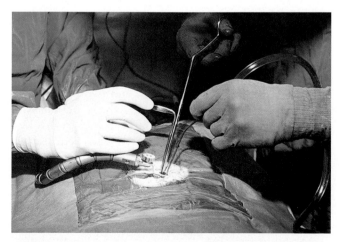

FIGURE 67.15 Pituitary rongeur removing disc material with concurrent suction; assistant holds nerve root retractor. (Courtesy of Donald L. Hilton, Jr., M.D., Southwest Texas Methodist Hospital.)

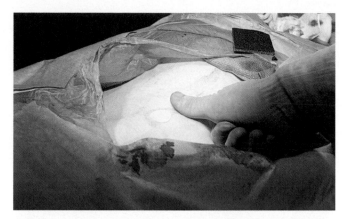

FIGURE 67.16 Round Band-Aid is placed after 14-mm diameter procedure. (Courtesy of Donald L. Hilton, Jr., M.D., Southwest Texas Methodist Hospital.)

essentially in line with the disc on fluoroscopy. The spinal needle is angled toward the facet, with intraoperative fluoroscopy used to guide the needle toward the facet at the level of the pedicle. Care is taken not to enter the foramen. The spinal needle is removed, and the guide wire is then passed below the fascia in this trajectory. It is not necessary to actually encounter the bone; simply penetrating the fascia usually suffices. A stab wound is made, as is done for the standard lumbar technique. The tubular dilator is then used to dilate the muscles, and the desired length and diameter MITR is chosen and placed over the dilators.

After the arm is locked in position, the microscope is brought in. The soft tissue over the lateral facet and the transverse process is removed. Usually only a small amount of bone is removed to obtain adequate exposure. A small amount of the caudal portion of the transverse process and the lateral portion of the facet is removed. Usually a few bites of the pars may be taken without destabilizing it; in this way the neural foramen is open. The intertransverse membrane is also divided. The nerve root is carefully identified as it passes around the pedicle. It may then be mobilized to find and remove the disc fragment and to completely open the neural foramen.

SURGICAL TECHNIQUE: POSTERIOR, CERVICAL APPROACH

This procedure is essentially a posterior cervical foraminotomy. It allows decompression of the foramen and/or removal of disc pathology. It has been described using MED with lateral fluoroscopy (12). The patient is anesthetized and generally placed in Mayfield pins for adequate control of the head and protection of the forehead and checks. The patient is then placed in the prone position. Intraoperative anteroposterior fluoroscopy is used (Fig. 67.17). After preparation and draping, the fluoroscope is used for the ini-

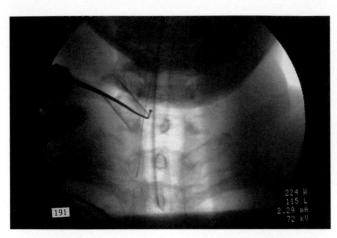

FIGURE 67.17 Anteroposterior fluoroscopic view showing ball probe. (Courtesy of Donald L. Hilton, Jr., M.D., Southwest Texas Methodist Hospital.)

tial portion of the procedure with localization. A point is selected approximately 2 to 2.5 cm lateral to the edge of the palpable spinous process. The entry point is usually estimated. The spinal needle is passed down under intraoperative fluoroscopic guidance until it safely encounters the lateral portion of the lateral mass. The fluoroscope is oriented in an anterior-posterior direction and angled slightly off vertical to be in line with the patient's spine. The spinal needle is passed down to the lateral mass under direct vision to make certain that the needle does not slide medially into the spinal canal. It is quite easy to visualize even C-7 through T-1 in this manner, which is difficult or impossible with lateral

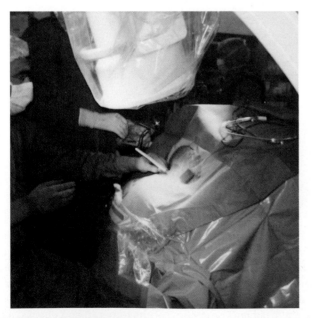

FIGURE 67.18 Cervical procedure with dilation, fluoroscope in position. (Courtesy of Donald L. Hilton, Jr., M.D., Southwest Texas Methodist Hospital.)

fluoroscopy. The tubular dilators are then used (Fig. 67.18). The cervical fascia is generally more resilient than the lumbar fascia. A firm twisting motion to dilators usually allow them to slide down over the wires and over successive dilators. The appropriate tubular retractor is selected and locked into position with the arm, with anteroposterior intraoperative fluoroscopy again being used to confirm the proper level. The fluoroscope is then moved away but it is kept sterile for possible subsequent localization as needed.

The microscope is brought in. The surgeon sits at the head of the patient and usually uses an armrest. The microscope is brought in over the surgeon's left shoulder, and the assistant may sit to the right. The microscope is generally used under high power, especially when 14-mm tubes are selected. This diameter has been found to be very satisfactory for cervical and lumbar surgery. The laminar–facet junction is identified, and a small Kerrison rongeur is used to remove first the superior edge of the inferior lamina at the desired level. The bony removal proceeds caudally, then laterally to the pedicle below, and then rostrally to the pedicle above, so that the foramen is completely open. The root is then carefully mobilized. The axilla is first explored. Usually fragments will be found in the axilla. The shoulder may also be explored as indicated. Excellent hemostasis is obtained, and the wound is closed in a fashion similar to that used for lumbar closures.

SURGICAL EXPERIENCE

In this series, the initial 60 to 70 MITR procedures were performed using three tubes of different lengths, each being 16 mm in diameter. One tube was shorter than the original MED tube at approximately 3.5 cm, and the longer tube was approximately 2 cm longer than the original tube. The endoscopic attachment portion was removed. These initial prototype variable-length MITR tubes were used in late 1998 and early 1999. The remainder of the cases were done using the MEDTRx-MD system.

There were a total of 228 patients in this series, including 139 men and 89 women; the average age was 43.6 years. Ten patients had either two levels of the same side or the same level on both sides operated, and two patients had three unilateral levels done through a single incision with 14-mm tubes used. The majority of the pathology involved disc herniation, although four synovial cysts were also addressed, as was foraminal stenosis in several cases. The largest patient was in the range of 390 lb, and for this patient an 18-mm-diameter tube, 12 cm long was used; it was specifically engineered to specification by Medtronic Sofamor Danek for this patient.

The initial posterior cervical procedure using a variable-length MITR was done on March 24, 1999. Twenty-two cervical MITR procedures have been performed to date.

RESULTS

There were 13 recurrent disc herniations in this series. Four occurred early (within 1 month), nine occurred in a more delayed fashion. The early recurrences were treated using the 14-mm-diameter tubular retractor, and the last four delayed recurrences using the 18-mm retractor. We did not encounter a cerebrospinal fluid leak in any of the recurrent procedures. Three-dimensional visualization allowed even the recurrent disc herniations to be done through the MITR tube with excellent visualization. These patients went home as outpatients. There have been no recurrent disc herniations in lateral procedures, of which 10 have been performed.

Overall we have encountered five cerebrospinal fluid leaks. None of these involved large rents in the dura. We chose to treat these with fibrin glue and gel foam placed over the dura and recumbency for 1 to 2 days. None of these patients had any immediate or delayed sequelae as the result of this complication.

Table 67.1 summarizes the overall clinical outcomes dating from September 1998 to the present. Ninety percent of the patients considered their discomfort to be less than before surgery, and 87% were very pleased and required no further treatment or follow-up. There were 13 recurrent disc herniations. Of those reoperated for recurrent disc herniation, all are now free of pain and require no further follow-up at this point.

In the posterior cervical series, 18 of the 22 patients consider their results to be excellent and describe no pain whatsoever. Two of these have some residual discomfort but are pleased with the result and require no further follow-up. One patient has continued pain but has also had multiple anterior procedures in the past and required a subsequent posterior procedure. This patient underwent MITR foraminotomies bilaterally. One of the foraminotomies completely relieved the pain, this being at the C5-6 level. The foraminotomy performed at C6-7 required a subsequent posterior fusion. There have been no infections in the cervical series. One patient developed a vertebral artery dissection 2 weeks after surgery with a hemianopsia resulting.

TABLE 67.1 CLINICAL OUTCOMES AFTER SPINAL MINIMALLY INVASIVE SPINAL SURGERY (AVERAGE FOLLOW-UP, APPROXIMATELY 8 MO)

Outcome	No. Patients
No sciatic pain	156
Minimal intermittent discomfort requiring no further treatment	42
Significant residual discomfort but better than preoperative pain	8
Preoperative pain unchanged	7
Pain worse than preoperative	2

This patient had experienced relief of her arm pain and no complication whatsoever with minimal bleeding at the time of the surgical procedure. Another patient experienced a recurrent disc herniation and subsequently underwent an anterior procedure approximately 4 months after the posterior procedure. He had experienced complete relief of his arm pain until this recurrence.

There have been two subsequent anterior procedures for patients having previous posterior procedures. One of these was in a patient with previous anterior surgery in whom a foraminotomy was performed. This patient still required a subsequent anterior procedure. The other patient required a subsequent anterior procedure after developing recurrence herniation.

The average surgical time for all procedures was 72 minutes. This surgical time has remained fairly standard. The average stay in the day surgery unit before discharge was 3 hours 28 minutes. Average blood loss was 56 mL. For the first 87 patients, the average return to work for those uninvolved with Workers' Compensation claims was 19.6 days, and for those with Workers' Compensation claims it was 63 days. If anything, we have seen these numbers decrease in the last hundred patients or so. Those involved with vocations not requiring bending, stooping, or lifting are generally returned to work quickly, usually within 3 to 7 days. For instance, four physicians in this series returned to work within 1 week, and two of these within 3 days. To date there have been no deep infections.

DISCUSSION

The MITR procedure is in essence a muscle-splitting microdiscectomy performed through an exceptionally small port that allows three-dimensional visualization. Although it is advantageous for all patients, the large or even morbidly obese patient receives a much less invasive procedure than would otherwise be possible with a standard microdiscectomy. Variable-length tubes allow access to patients that cannot be serviced with MED given the nonvariability of the tube length.

In San Antonio MED was initially used sparingly, because there was virtually universal concern about the adequacy of the visualization. In the last 3 years the MITR procedure has become widely used by both orthopaedic and neurologic surgeons. Approximately 500 MITR procedures have been performed in this 2.5- to 3-year period. I have performed approximately 250 procedures, and six other surgeons have performed approximately 250 among them, for a total of approximately 500 cases. A core of surgeons in San Antonio consider the MITR procedure the standard of care, particularly in the treatment of lumbar herniated discs. In several instances the issue of informed consent has been raised by patients who had standard discectomies by other surgeons who believed that they had not been fully informed about the MITR procedure.

Morbidly Obese Patients

Perhaps in no other subset of patients is the advantage of MITR seen more clearly than in the morbidly obese patients. Some surgeons may argue that they can do a very small standard microdiscectomy and send their patient home either as an outpatient or within 1 to 2 days. Few will claim, however that a 400-lb patient could be safely be treated with a 1.5- to 2-cm incision, as is allowed with the MITR tube. We have performed many procedures using the longest tubes in many patients who weighed well over 200 lb without any extra difficulty. The 14-mm tube has been used in the 8-cm length without difficulty numerous times, including in a 250-lb patient treated at three unilateral levels with a single incision. The extra length really does not hamper visualization given the optical capabilities of the operating microscope.

A specific case that deserves mention was that of a woman who weighted 380 to 400 lb. She had experienced severe sciatic pain secondary to a large free fragment. Even the longest tube in the MEDTRx-MD set would have been inadequate to access the spine in this patient. The length had been determined preoperatively, and I requested that Medtronic Sofamor Danek produce an 18-mm-diameter tube of 12-cm length. The versatility is illustrated in Fig. 67.19, with the 3-cm-long, 14-mm-diameter tube pictured next to this large tube. This tube was manufactured within 2 days, and this morbidly obese patient was operated on with an incision that was dressed with a Band-Aid. This patient has done well. She is a diabetic and certainly would have been at increased risk for wound infection if a large wound had been necessary.

This represents significant improvement in the ability to treat the morbidly obese. It is both the variable-length tube

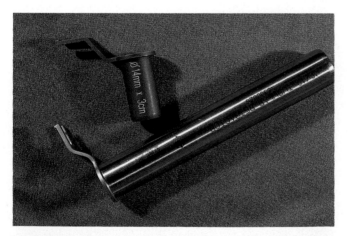

FIGURE 67.19 Custom-made, 18-mm-diameter, 12-cm long tube, shown with 14-mm-diameter, 3-cm long tube. (Courtesy of Medtronic Sofamor Danek.)

and the microscope which combine to provide this advantage.

Lateral Disc Herniation

The subset of patients with lateral disc herniation also illustrates the clear advantage of the muscle-splitting technique over the standard lumbar procedure. Most surgeons performing even a lateral muscle-splitting extraforaminal approach would require a larger incision to access the lateral foramen. This procedure truly provides superior visualization with a minimum of trauma to the tissues.

Cervical Minimally Invasive Tubular Retractor

The cervical patients have also done extremely well with this procedure. It has long been recognized that the posterior cervical foraminotomy is an excellent procedure that allows lateral and foraminal cervical disc disease to be addressed without fusion. The significant disadvantage was the frequently troubling cervical spasm and pain encountered with the muscle-stripping posterior approach. I have used the 14-mm-diameter tube in virtually all cases, both lumbar and cervical. These patients go home happily with a minimum of discomfort even on the day of surgery. One patient in this series was a retinal surgeon who was able to return work and to operate within 3 days.

A special caution is noted with the cervical procedure: I believe strongly that this procedure is safely done when anteroposterior fluoroscopy is used to avoid any chance of entering the spinal canal. It is also impossible to adequately visualize the lower cervical spine in most patients with only lateral fluoroscopy.

Recurrent Disc Herniation

The initial recurrent disc herniations in this series were opened in a standard fashion. The early recurrences were subsequently reoperated using the same 14-mm tube as was used for the initial procedure, and these patients have done well and have also gone home as outpatients.

Another distinct and important advantage of the MITR procedure over the MED is the ability to address recurrent disc herniation even when this is not in the immediate postoperative period and scarring is involved. Most surgeons would have been very uncomfortable addressing a delayed recurrent disc herniation with the original MED procedure, given the limitation in visualization. The microscope allows the scarred anatomy to be visualized adequately and even exceptionally. I have found that an 18-mm tube allows enough working distance to define the lateral bony edge, free the scar, and define the planes as is necessary in addressing recurrent disc pathology.

Multilevel Pathology

The MITR procedure lends itself well to performing at multiple levels. I initially used separate incisions when performing multilevel procedures unilaterally. Recently, however, several have been performed through the same incision. The entry point is placed halfway between the two discs, and the trajectory is adjusted to address each disc separately. When one disc level has been treated, the tube is removed; then the same incision is used to dilate and place the retractor at the other disc level. Several levels could be done in this manner, and one patient with three-level disease was treated through a single incision using 14-mm tubes. The MITR procedure allows different tubes to be selected to make this possible. For instance, in performing a three-level procedure, a 5-cm-long tube may be adequate at the L4-5 level, but when the trajectory is changed to angle superiorly or inferiorly to either the L3-4 or the L5-S1 level, a 6- or 7-cm tube may provide the extra length to allow the other level to be addressed. These patients, including one with a three-level procedure have also gone home as outpatients.

CONCLUSION

Minimally invasive surgery of the spine has received increased interest particularly in the last few years. The MITR procedure allows the surgeon to address the epidural space with instrumentation essentially identical to that considered to be the standard of care for microdiscectomy. This procedure is in essence simply a microdiscectomy done through the smallest possible working port.

The interest with which the MITR procedure has been received in San Antonio has been impressive. Surgeons who previously were skeptical about MED now consider the MITR procedure to be their standard of care. The MEDTRx-MD system has renewed interest in muscle-splitting tube surgery, particularly for many surgeons who were disappointed with the visualization of MED. I believe that this procedure will become the standard of care as more surgeons become familiar with it. It has been argued that the standard of care is the microdiscectomy, but the MITR procedure is actually a very small microdiscectomy,

particularly when a 14-mm-diameter tube is used. The versatility of this system will allow many patients to enjoy its decreased morbidity, as more surgeons become proficient with it.

ACKNOWLEDGMENT

The author gratefully acknowledges the assistance of Maria Biediger, RN who performed invaluable services with clinical followup.

REFERENCES

1. Choy DSJ, Case RB, Fielding W, et al. Percutaneous laser nucleolysis of lumbar discs. *N Engl J Med* 1987;317:771–772.
2. Grevitt MP, Shackleford IM, Mulholland RC. Automated percutaneous lumbar discectomy. *J Bone Joint Surg Br* 1992;77:949–956.
3. Hijakata S, Yamgishi M., Nakayama T, et al. Percutaneous discectomy: a new treatment method for lumbar disc herniation. *J Toden Hosp* 1975;5:5–13.
4. Onik G, Helms CA, Ginsberg L, et al. Percutaneous lumbar discectomy using a new aspiration probe. *AJR Am J Roentgenol* 1985; 144:1137–1140.
5. Onik G, Mooney V, Maroon JC, et al. Automated percutaneous discectomy: a prospective multi-institutional study. *Neurosurgery* 1990;26:228–233.
6. Schreiber A, Suezawa Y. Transdiscoscopic percutaneous nucleotomy in disc herniation. *Orthop Rev* 1986;15:35–38.
7. Schaffer JL, Kambin P. Percutaneous posterolateral discectomy and decompression with a 6.9-millimeter cannula: analysis of operative failures and complications. *J Bone Joint Surg Am* 1991;73:822–831.
8. Smith L. Enzyme dissolution of the nucleus pulposus in humans. *JAMA* 1964;265:137–140.
9. Foley KT, Smith MM. Microendoscopic discectomy. *Tech Neurosurg* 1997;3:301–307.
10. Dirksmeier PJ, Parsons IM, Kang JD. Microendoscopic and open laminectomy and discectomy in lumbar disc disease. *Semin Spine Surg* 1999;11:138–146.
11. Branch CL Jr. AANS/CNS joint section on spine, 14th Annual Meeting. Rancho Mirage, February 1998.
12. Adamson TE. Initial experience with endoscopic posterior cervical laminoforaminotomy for the treatment of cervical radiculopathy. Presented at the Meeting of the Cervical Spine Research Society, Atlanta, GA, 1998.

SUBJECT INDEX

Entries followed by *f* indicate figures; those followed by *t* indicate tables.